AN INVITATION
TO HEALTH

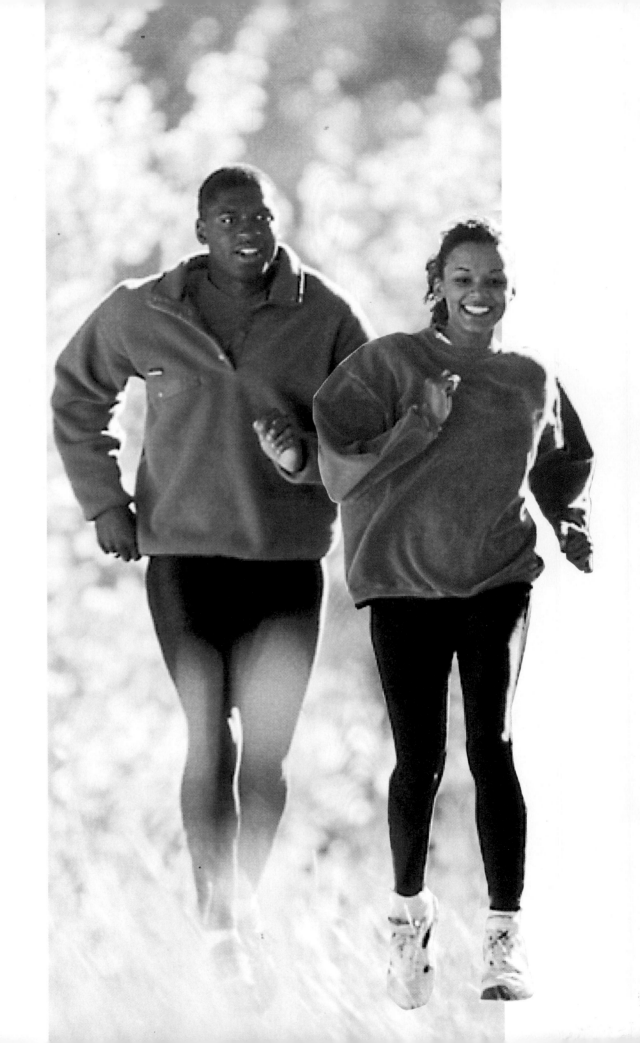

AN INVITATION TO HEALTH

Eighth Edition

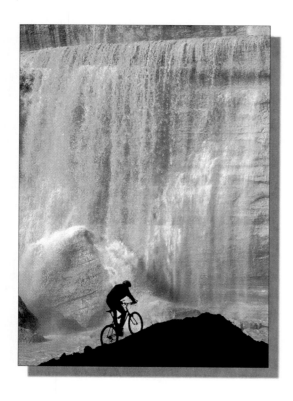

The Power of Prevention

DIANNE HALES

Brooks/Cole Publishing Company

ITP® *An International Thomson Publishing Company*

Pacific Grove • Albany • Belmont • Bonn • Boston • Cincinnati • Detroit • Johannesburg • London
Madrid • Melbourne • Mexico City • New York • Paris • Singapore • Tokyo • Toronto • Washington

Sponsoring Editors: *Denis Ralling and Vicki Knight*
Marketing Team: *Michael Campbell, Alicia Barelli, Deanne Brown, Jean Thompson, and Aaron Eden*
Editorial Assistant: *Stephanie Andersen*
Project Development Editors: *Megan Rundel and Jim Strandberg*
Production Service: *HRS Electronic Text Management; Lorraine Burke, Erica Smythe*
Production Coordinator: *Mary Anne Shahidi*
Permissions Editor: *Lillian Campobasso*

Interior Design: *HRS Electronic Text Management; Karen Mahakian*
Cover Design: *E. Kelly Shoemaker*
Cover Photo: *Bill Hatcher/Adventure Photo & Film*
Cover Photo Manipulation: *Bob Western*
Photo Research: *HRS Electronic Text Management*
Typesetting: *HRS Electronic Text Management*
Printing and Binding: *Von Hoffmann Press*

For more information, contact:

BROOKS/COLE PUBLISHING COMPANY
511 Forest Lodge Road
Pacific Grove, CA 93950
USA

International Thomson Editores
Seneca 53
Col. Polanco
11560 México, D. F., México

International Thomson Publishing Europe
Berkshire House 168–173
High Holborn
London WC1V 7AA
England

International Thomson Publishing GmbH
Königswinterer Strasse 418
53227 Bonn
Germany

Thomas Nelson Australia
102 Dodds Street
South Melbourne, 3205
Victoria, Australia

International Thomson Publishing Asia
60 Albert Street
#15–01 Albert Complex
Singapore 189969

Nelson Canada
1120 Birchmount Road
Scarborough, Ontario
Canada M1K 5G4

International Thomson Publishing Japan
Hirakawacho Kyowa Building, 3F
2-2-1 Hirakawacho
Chiyoda-ku, Tokyo 102
Japan

Printed in the United States of America.

10 9 8 7 6 5 4 3

Library of Congress Cataloging-in-Publication Data
Hales, Dianne
    An invitation to health: the power of prevention / Dianne Hales.—8th ed.
    p.   cm.
    Includes bibiographical references and index.
    IBSN 0-534-35733-4 (paperback)
    1. Health   2. Self-care, Health.   I. Title
    RA776,H148   1999
    613—dc21   98-22337
                                  CIP

To my husband, Bob, and my daughter, Julia, who make every day an invitation to joy.

To the Student

An Invitation to Health is an invitation to you. What you learn in this class will have a direct impact on how you'll look, feel, and act—now and for decades to come.

Perhaps you are in good health and think that you know all that you need to know about how to take care of yourself. If so, take a minute and ask yourself some questions:

- How well do you understand yourself? Are you able to cope with emotional upsets and crises? Do you often feel stressed out?

- How nutritiously do you eat? Are you always going on—and off—diets? Do you exercise regularly?

- How solid and supportive are your relationships with others? Are you conscientious about birth control and safer-sex practices?

- Are you caught up in any compulsive behaviors? Do you get drunk or high occasionally? Do you smoke?

- If you needed health care, do you know where you'd turn or how you'd pay? What do you know about your risk for infectious diseases, heart problems, cancer, or other serious illnesses?

- Have you taken steps to insure your personal safety at home, on campus, or on the streets?

- What are you doing today to prevent physical, psychological, social, and environmental problems in the future?

As you consider these questions, chances are that there are some aspects of health you've never considered before—and others that you feel you don't have to worry about for years. Yet the choices you make and the actions you make now will have a dramatic impact on your future.

Your health is your personal responsibility. Over time, your priorities and needs will inevitably change, but the connections between various dimensions of your well-being will remain the same: The state of your mind will affect the state of your body, and vice versa. The values that guide you through today can keep you mentally, physically, and spiritually healthy throughout your lifetime. Your ability to cope with stress will influence your decisions about alcohol and drug use. Your commitment to honest, respectful relationships will affect the nature of your sexual involvements. Your eating and exercise habits will determine whether you develop a host of medical problems.

An Invitation to Health, Eighth Edition, is packed with information, advice, recommendations, and research, and provides the first step in taking full charge of your own well-being. An important theme of this book is prevention. Ultimately, the power of prevention belongs to you—and it's a lot easier than you might think. You might simply add a walk or workout to your daily routine. You might snack on fruit instead of high-fat foods. You might cut back on alcohol. You might buckle your seat belt whenever you get in a car. These things may not seem like a big deal now, yet they may well make a crucial difference in determining how active and fulfilling the rest of your life will be.

The *Study Guide*, available through your bookstore, will also help you reach your goal of better health. You can use it to identify and review the main concepts in each chapter, practice your test-taking skills, and, through observation and self-assessments, incorporate concepts from the text into your life. But keep in mind that a personal health class is unlike any other course you'll take in college. You can't simply read the text, do your assignments, and pass the exams; you have to live what you learn. To help you on your way, the *Personal Health Interactive* CD-ROM, is also available through your bookstore. Besides providing study aids and chapter reviews, *Personal Health Interactive* features a Wellness Clinic, which provides you with the opportunity to set personal health goals and assess your progress toward achieving those goals.

This textbook is an invitation—an invitation to health in its broadest sense, to personal fulfillment, to life itself. Its pages provide the practical tools you need to work toward achieving your full potential. I hope that you keep this book and use it often as your personal health manual. I also hope that you accept this invitation in another sense—that you live what you learn and make the most of your life—now and through all the years and adventures the future may bring you.

May you live long and prosper.
Dianne Hales

To the Instructor

We have entered a new era in health care, and its hallmark is prevention. *An Invitation to Health*, Eighth Edition, introduces students to this new way of thinking about their health and their future. Subtitled *The Power of Prevention*, it outlines the keys to preventing the major killers of Americans—heart disease, cancer, and accidents—and to preparing for a life of health in the fullest sense of the word.

In this text, health is defined in the broadest possible way—not as an entity in itself, but as a process of discovering, using, and protecting all the resources within the individual, family, community, and environment. I emphasize how health is a subject that encompasses body, mind, and spirit, and the eighth edition brings this vision more fully to life by providing students with the information and inspiration they need to make healthful decisions and changes.

The Eighth Edition

This edition includes a wealth of new research, references, and pedagogical features. I have tried to "invite" students in new ways, to entice and excite them by making the content as relevant to their lives as possible. Yet my essential themes will be familiar to those who have used previous editions. I continue to place a strong emphasis on personal responsibility, a commitment to prevention, practical applications of knowledge, and a focus on behavioral change. These concepts are fundamental for any health course, and do not change from year to year.

Because the field of health science is so broad and it changes so rapidly, keeping up with the most recent developments provides an enormous challenge. In preparing the latest edition of *An Invitation to Health*, I have had the same goal in mind as aspired to in the past: creating the best health textbook on the market. The response from students and instructors to past editions has been enthusiastic and gratifying. But that positive feedback is due to the tradition of keeping this textbook *extraordinarily current*, and responding to input from reviewers who teach this course. For the eighth edition, I have continued that tradition.

The eighth edition of *An Invitation to Health* includes several hundred citations from 1996–1998 references. The majority are from primary sources, including professional books; medical, health, and mental health journals; health education periodicals; scientific meetings; federal agencies; publications from research laboratories and universities; and personal interviews with specialists in a number of fields. For those who have come to expect the very latest in the best available health information in *An Invitation to Health*, you won't be disappointed.

New information covered in this eighth edition includes the goals of Healthy People 2010, recent research findings on the effects of different types of fat in the diet, the phenomenon of sexual communication and fantasy in cyberspace, 1998 cancer incidence estimates, the health risks associated with cigar-smoking, the latest drug therapies for treating AIDS, and much, much more. Every chapter has been revised, and I encourage you to take a look at the following overview of this new edition.

Overview of the New Eighth Edition

The eighth edition of *An Invitation to Health* is organized into six sections, with a total of 21 chapters. Users of the seventh edition will find the chapter sequencing remains the same. Feedback from users of the previous edition and from reviewers indicated that the current organization worked very well and should be retained. The book's organization is flexible, however, so you can use the chapters in any order that suits your needs.

The chapters present key concepts in health in a comprehensive manner and cover the most current, as well as most controversial, issues in the field. The following is a chapter-by-chapter listing of some of the key topics I've added, expanded, or revised for this edition.

Chapter 1: An Invitation to Health for the Twenty-First Century

- The section on Health for the 21st Century has been fully revised, incorporating the latest statistics and research on longevity, causes of death, and other public health information.

- Healthy People 2000 is revisited with updated information on progress toward implementing its aims, and the new plans and goals for Healthy People 2010 are described.

- Expanded coverage of spiritual health, including the healthy effects of prayer, religion, and faith. New Figure 1-3 provides a graphic presentation of the practices of several different religions to promote physical health.

- Recent statistics on ethnic and racial groups facing different health risks have been added to the section on "Can Race Be Hazardous to Your Health?"

- The new *Campus Focus* feature makes its debut—a color, graphic illustration that will appear in over half of the chapters. Based on the 1995 National College Health Risk Behavior Survey of 4,600 students at 136 institutions, these figures represent a "snapshot" of the state of college students' health. In this first Campus Focus graphic, a series of pie charts showing a demographic breakdown of those who participated in this survey are shown.

- The first of the new *Health Online* feature boxes has been added (every chapter will have a Health Online box), which encourages the student to use the Internet and visit one particular website to investigate how it might serve to promote his or her health. The focus in this chapter is on "MedAccess Motivator", a website aimed at helping an individual establish personal wellness goals and assess progress towards these goals. As with all Health Online feature boxes, critical thinking questions are added to encourage the student to do more than simply visit the website.

Chapter 2: Managing Stress

- Revised and updated coverage on stress and college students, including new research findings on who is most at risk for high stress.

- Updated information on posttraumatic stress disorder.

- Results of a new study on the relation between stress and heart disease discussed in section on "The Cardiovascular System."

- Strategies for helping to avoid stress-related stomach aches are now described, with an emphasis on drinking plenty of water, eating fiber-rich foods, and neither skipping meals nor overeating.

- New Health Online feature box on "The Behavioral Institute of Boston's Stress Audit" website, which provides a comprehensive on line assessment of one's stress levels in many areas of life including job, family, social, financial, and emotional stress.

Chapter 3: Feeling Good

- A new Self Survey—"The Well-Being Scale"—replaces the survey in the previous edition, and freshens this chapter with a new self assessment appropriate for college students.

- New coverage added on emotional intelligence and its role as a factor in promoting overall health, and updated research on how happiness impacts brain functions.

- New Health Online feature box on "What's Your Emotional Intelligence Quotient?" This website, sponsored by the Utne Reader magazine, offers a ten-item quiz to help assess your level of emotional intelligence.

Chapter 4: Caring for the Mind

- Updated research presented on appropriate treatment for obsessive-compulsive disorder, and characteristic symptoms of those suffering manic depression (bipolar disorder).

- New and updated information on suicide incidence, with the new Campus Focus graphic depicting percentages of college students who had thought seriously and those who had actually attempted suicide.

- The section on Schizophrenia has been revised, offering an updated analysis of how antipsychotic drugs can and do make a positive difference.

- New information on psychiatric drugs has been added, including the prevalence of their use, and what their effects may be.

- New Health Online feature box highlights the "New York University Department of Psychiatry Online Screening," a website that provides screening tests for depression, anxiety, sexual disorders, attention deficit disorder, and personality disorders.

Chapter 5: The Joy of Fitness

- New section on "Making the Commitment," on how to get motivated to start a fitness program.

- New Campus Focus graphic on percentages of college students who participate in vigorous physical activity.

- New Health Online feature box looks at "Cool Tools," a website where you can calculate your target heart rate and your energy expenditure during exercise. The site also includes tips for those who would like to start a fitness program but don't know where to begin.

Chapter 6: Nutrition for Life

- The "Knowing What You Eat" section has now been moved to after the material on the Food Pyramid.

- Updated throughout with new information on the health benefits of healthy eating.

- New Campus Focus feature on eating habits of college students.

- Updated information on food irradiation, and updated statistics on the incidence and cost of food poisoning.

- New research cited on the health effects of fats, including the 1998 study showing a relationship between a diet high in monounsaturated fats and a lower risk of breast cancer. On the other side of the equation, recent research indicating the danger of trans fats is described.

- New information provided on olestra, the new fat replacement product.

- The Vegetarian Food Pyramid is now included.

- New Health Online feature box focuses on the "Cyber Diet" website, where an individualized "Nutritional Profile" can be put together and students can assess their current diet and learn more about fast foods.

Chapter 7: Eating Patterns and Problems

- New introductory material on the epidemic of obesity in America.

- Revised and updated coverage of unhealthy eating behaviors of college students.

- New Campus Focus feature graphic on college students and dieting.

- New material on the controversy about to what extent obesity leads to a shorter life.

- New coverage on the downfall of fen-phen.

- New Health Online feature box encourages students to visit the website for the "Healthy Body Calculator," to input their personal characteristics, determine a healthy weight range, and obtain additional information regarding nutrition, healthful waist-to-hip ratios, and more.

Chapter 8: Communicating and Relating

- New Self-Survey on "How Strong is the Communication and Affection in Your Relationship?"

- Updated information on the increased number of adults living with parents or living alone.

- Revised and updated coverage of the state of marriage in the United States, and new information on two-career couples.

- Updated statistics on divorce, and new Figure 8-7 on the rate of divorce in the U.S.

- New Health Online feature box on "The Marriage Toolbox," a website devoted to helping couples maintain, fix, or improve a relationship.

Chapter 9: Personal Sexuality

- New research on female sexual development cited, including the 1997 analysis showing a significant discrepancy in early-onset puberty between whites and African-Americans.

- Revised coverage of premenstrual syndrome.

- Revised and updated coverage of circumcision.

- Revised and updated information on adolescent sexuality.

- New Campus Focus feature graphic on the percentage of college students in different categories who have had sexual intercourse, and the percentage who have had six or more sex partners.

- Updated coverage of sex on campus, including the modified behavior of gay college men in light of the AIDS crisis.

- Significantly expanded and updated coverage of adult sexuality.

- Revised section on Homosexual Lifestyles.

- New sub-section added on "Sex in Cyberspace" in the Fantasy section.

- New Spotlight on Diversity feature box on "Cultural Variations in Sexual Arousal."

- New Table 9-2 on the Sexual Effects of Some Drugs.

- Revised and updated section on Erectile Disorders, noting Viagra and other medicines on the horizon to treat this condition, and new Figure 9-9 depicting The Incidence of Erectile Disorder and Age.

- New Health Online feature box spotlights an educational website from New York University that offers an "Online Sexual Disorders Screening" questionnaire for men and women who think they may have a sexual disorder.

Chapter 10: Reproductive Choices

- New Campus Focus feature graphic depicting the percentages of college students of different demographic groups who had used contraception during last sexual intercourse, and the percentages specifically using a condom.

- New Figure 10-3 depicts the percentages of women using contraception, by type of method used.

- Updated information on the IUD as a method of emergency contraception.

- Updated information on future contraceptives, including a male birth control pill.

- Updated coverage of abortion rates, methods of abortion, and public opinion on abortion. New Figure 10-17 on number of legal abortions in the United States from 1972-1995, and new Figure 10-18 on "A Cross-Cultural View of Abortion," showing the number of abortions per 1,000 women in selected countries.

- Revised section on Pregnancy and Age, including rates of teen pregnancy and parenthood after age 40.

- New information on the emotional impact of pregnancy loss.

- Updated information on infertility.

- New Health Online feature box on "Successful Con-

traception," a website sponsored by the Association of Reproductive Health Professionals. The interactive site includes an interactive program to help an individual choose the best birth control method, with individual preferences and behaviors taken into account.

Chapter 11: Defending Yourself from Infectious Diseases

- New Self-Survey—an STD Attitude Scale—replaces previous Self-Survey.

- Updated and expanded section on Allergies.

- Table 11-1 showing the Recommended Childhood Immunization Schedule, revised with the latest information.

- New information on popular new cold remedies, including zinc lozenges and echinacea.

- New section on the flu vaccine and treatments for influenza.

- Table 11-3 on Common Sexually Transmitted Diseases thoroughly updated.

- Thoroughly revised and updated coverage of HIV/AIDS, including the latest incidence rates in the U.S. and worldwide, and the new protease inhibitor drugs and "cocktail therapy" regimens.

- New Health Online feature box on "Cells Alive!", a website which provides interactive animations, illustrations, and descriptions to help explain how pathogens interact with the body's immune system.

Chapter 12: Keeping Your Heart Healthy

- New research noted on the effects of smoking and passive smoke in speeding up the process by which arteries become clogged, thus increasing the risk of heart attacks and strokes.

- Updated information about the controversy over the best medications for treating hypertension.

- New research cited on the association between oral contraceptive use and stroke, noting that the low-dose oral contraceptives have not shown evidence of an increased stroke risk.

- Updated coverage of levels of blood fat and the risk of stroke.

- The New Health Online feature box is on "Virtual Body: The Heart," a website which takes an animated, interactive tour of the human heart, and provides other valuable information on heart health.

Chapter 13: Lowering Your Risk of Cancer and Other Major Diseases

- Updated information on the declining overall cancer death rates in the United States, and how these can be attributed to changes in lifestyle and early detection.

- Figure 13-2 on Leading Sites for New Cancer Cases and Deaths completely updated with 1998 estimates from the American Cancer Society.

- New Table 13-1 on The Most Survivable Cancers.

- New research cited on so-called "breast cancer genes."

- Updated discussion of the debate over mammography for women under 50, as well as the latest computer technology to interpret mammograms with greater precision.

- Heavily revised and updated section on Prostate Cancer, including the latest screening procedures.

- New statistics on the incidence of diabetes in the United States, including estimates of undiagnosed cases.

- Heavily revised and updated section on Asthma, including new treatments recently introduced.

- New Health Online feature box for this chapter directs students to a website on "An Introduction to Skin Cancer"—its causes, how to determine personal risk, prevention, and treatment.

Chapter 14: Drug Use, Misuse, and Abuse

- New section, The Biology of Addiction, focusing on the influence of dopamine in addiction, with a new Figure 14-2 depicting the effect on a brain cell.

- Updated coverage of drug use in America, including the recent decline or leveling off (as of late 1997) in the overall use of drugs among teenagers, but the increased use of marijuana among older teens.

- New coverage of legal drugs now being used for purposes other than which they were intended, including Rohypnol, the so-called "date-rape drug," and ketamine, or "K," an anesthetic used by veterinarians.

- New Campus Focus feature graphic on College Students and Illegal Drug Usage.

- New Health Online feature box on "DAPA-PC," a website offering anonymous drug abuse screening.

Chapter 15: Alcohol Use, Misuse, and Abuse

- Updated information citing a 1997 study showing that one drink a day might have some health benefit in regard to heart disease.

- Thoroughly revised and updated coverage of Drinking on Campus, including the most recent problems with binge drinking.

- New Campus Focus feature graphic on College Students and Alcohol Use.

- Updated statistics regarding the effectiveness of tougher policies and educational campaigns on reducing the number of deaths caused by drunk drivers.

- New Health Online feature box directs students to the website "Drinking: A Student's Guide," where an online quiz can assess an individual's risk for developing an alcohol problem.

Chapter 16: Tobacco Use, Misuse, and Abuse

- Updated information on the effects of smoking on overall health.

- Updated statistics on the incidence of smoking among children, teens, and college students.

- New Campus Focus feature graphic on College Students and Smoking.

- New subsection on the link between smoking and depression.

- Revised and updated section on Cigars and the health risks associated with this new fad.

- Updated research cited on the effects of environmental tobacco smoke.

- The section on The Politics of Tobacco has been rewritten to reflect the tentative government settlement with the tobacco industry.

- Updated information on recent anti-smoking legislation around the country.

- New Health Online feature box highlights the website for "Quitnet," an organization dedicated to helping cigarette smokers to kick the habit. This website includes quizzes, strategies, and an online forum to discuss with others the experience of quitting smoking.

Chapter 17: Protecting Yourself

- New Campus Focus feature graphic on College Students and Road Safety.

- New section on Road Rage and steps one can take to avoid it.

- Updated statistics on the decline in overall crime rates in the United States during the 1990s.

- New Personal Voices feature box on survivors of domestic abuse.
- New section on Date Rape Drugs, including Rohypnol.
- New Health Online feature box on personal safety, directing the student to a website to "Rate Your Risk," an online questionnaire sponsored by the Nashville Police Department.

Chapter 18: Living Longer and Better

- Latest information on the biological bases of aging incorporated into the material, including new discoveries about the role of the enzyme telomerase.
- New Figure 18-3 on effects of aging on the body.
- Expanded and updated section on menopause and hormone replacement therapy, based on the very latest research.
- New coverage added on gender differences associated with aging of the brain.
- New information provided on tests that can detect low bone density, including DXA, DPA, SXA, QCT, and RA.
- New information on the somewhat greater risk to women of Alzheimer's, as well as research indicating postmenopausal women who have undergone estrogen replacement to be at a lower risk.
- New Health Online feature box on "Caregiver Alliance," an organization with a website providing good information and support to those who care for older family members or friends.

Chapter 19: When Life Ends

- New information on the needs of dying patients, including the need to hear what their lives have meant to their loved ones.
- New information on the multiple causes of mortality.
- New Health Online feature box on "Crisis, Grief, and Healing," a website for those who are suffering from grief.

Chapter 20: Taking Charge of Your Health

- New coverage on the medical self-help movement and the role of the Internet in providing not only the latest health information, but person-to-person communication and support. The limitations of the Internet in regard to obtaining reliable health information are also discussed.
- Updated information on Managed Care, including new Table 20-3 on The Growth of Managed Care.
- New Table 20-4 on the increase in the number of Americans without health insurance.
- Updated coverage of acupuncture, including recent research studies showing the effectiveness of acupuncture in treating certain conditions.
- New Health Online feature box highlights a website on "A Guide to Health Care Reform for Young Americans."

Chapter 21: Working Toward a Healthy Environment

- New Self-Survey: Are You Doing Your Part for the Planet?
- Updated information on the rate of world population growth.
- New Table 21-1 on deaths in various regions of the world resulting from either indoor or outdoor air pollution, and new coverage of the fires in Indonesia and Southeast Asia in 1997.
- New Health Online feature box focuses on the website for the "Sierra Club," offering a good source of information for those interested in helping to influence environmental policy.

Hales Health Almanac

- New Appendix to the 8th Edition: Health Information on the Internet. Part One of this appendix provides a description of how to navigate through the Internet in search of useful and accurate health information. The focus is on the positive nature of this new communication technology and how to make use of it in exploring health issues. But, due to the danger of obtaining misinformation about health on the web, this appendix also contains tips on sorting out reliable from less-than-reliable websites. Part Two of this appendix includes the web addresses for well over a hundred health-related sites, as well as the addresses for dozens of news groups online.
- Your Health Directory has been revised, with updated addresses, phone numbers, and web addresses provided.

Special Features and Pedagogy in the Eighth Edition

The response to the features and pedagogy in the seventh edition of *An Invitation to Health* was overwhelmingly positive, so the eighth edition retains nearly all of these popular enrichment elements and student study aids. Two new features have been added to the new edition: *Campus Focus*, and *Health Online.*

NEW! Campus Focus. How much vigorous exercise do college students get? How many have contemplated suicide? How many are eating nutritious meals? How many are using contraception if they engage in sexual intercourse? How many smoke, drink alcohol, and/or take drugs? These and other questions were the focus of a 1995 study, the National College Health Risk Behavior Survey. The results of this survey, published in a September 1997 article in the *Journal of American College Health*, are displayed in new pie charts and bar graphs prepared for this edition. Starting in Chapter 1 with a description of this study and a graph depicting the demographic breakdown of the 4,600 students who filled out the questionnaire, graphic illustrations of the results of this study appear in relevant chapters. For example, in Chapter 7, a Campus Focus graphic depicts

the numbers of students who had dieted, and the number of those who had vomited or took laxatives to lose or keep from gaining weight.

NEW! Health Online. With the use of the Internet soaring over the past few years, the potential for using the web to attain practical, up-to-date, and vital health information is phenomenal. Each chapter of the eighth edition includes a Health Online feature box, focusing on one informative website pertaining to material covered in that chapter, that the student is encouraged to visit. The websites chosen are dynamic ones—offering online assessments, interesting animations, or especially practical advice. For example, in Chapter 14, a commercial website offers an online quiz on How to Determine If You're At Risk for Alcoholism. In Chapter 17, the Nashville Police Department offers an online Rate Your Risk assessment of personal safety. Chapter 8's feature is The Marriage Toolbox, with a wealth of information pertinent to maintaining or fixing loving relationships. The value of good websites on the Internet is brought home, and practical health information is conveyed in yet another format to enhance each chapter. Moreover, this feature offers an additional resource: critical thinking questions appear at the end of Health Online, asking students to evaluate what they have seen at the website.

CAMPUS FOCUS: NUTRITION ON CAMPUS

Ate at least five servings of fruits and vegetables on the previous day

Ate two or fewer servings of high-fat food on the previous day

SOURCE: Douglas Kathy et al. "Results from the ... Survey", *Journal of American College Health*, ...

Health Online

Biobehavioral Institute of Boston's Stress Audit
http://www.bbinst.org/stressaudit/stress3.cgi
The Behavioral Institute of Boston's Stress Audit is a comprehensive assessment of your stress levels in many areas of life, including job, family, social, financial, and emotional stress. After you take the survey, the Stress Audit will tell you how you compare with the general population in each area of stress. It will also analyze your general susceptibility to stress, the sources of stress in your life, and the symptoms of stress you now show. You will also get some advice on how to lower your vulnerability to stress.

Think about it ...
- According to the Stress Audit, how does your stress level compare with that of the general population? What might you do to reduce your stress in areas where it is especially high?
- Why do you think the things in the Susceptibility to Stress inventory are especially important?
- If you were to design a new inventory for this site on School Stress, what might you include?

Wellness Inventory. The eighth edition begins with a *Wellness Inventory,* abridged from the *Wellness Workbook* by John W. Travis, M.D. This self-inventory provides students with a dynamic starting point for the course, and for relating the concept of wellness to all aspects of daily life.

Pulsepoints. This popular feature, appearing in every chapter, offers a snappy list of relevant, practical health tips. For example, in Chapter 6, the Pulsepoints lists and describes the "Top Ten Ways to Cut Fat," or, in Chapter 8, "Ten Characteristics of a Good Relationship."

Self-Survey. A popular feature, most of these assessments, which appear in every chapter, have been retained or only slightly modified. To freshen the book, however, some of the Self-Surveys have been replaced in the eighth edition, including those for Chapter 3, Chapter 8, Chapter 11, and Chapter 21.

Personal Voices. Another retained feature, Personal Voices boxes appears in a number of chapters, providing a focused look at one individual in relation to a topic covered in that chapter. For the eighth edition, a new Personal Voices has been added to Chapter 17 on surviving domestic abuse.

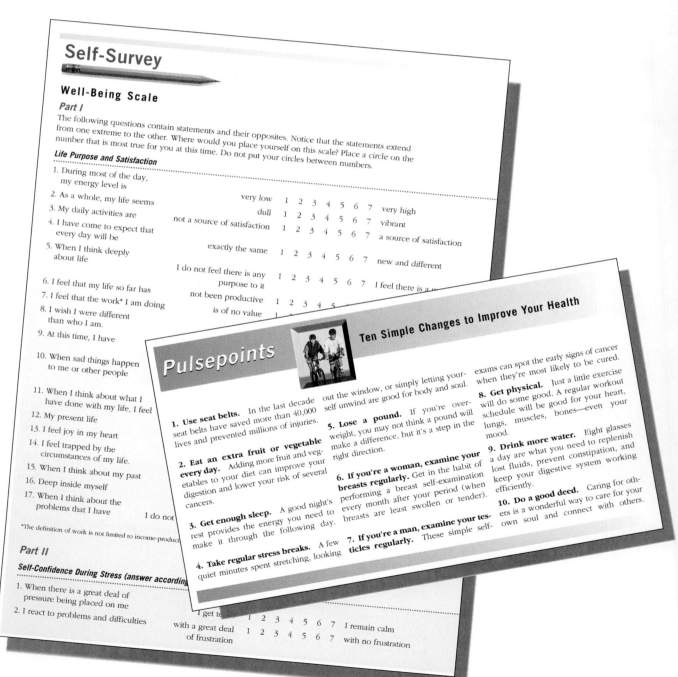

Strategies for Prevention. The Power of Prevention is the book's subtitle and is a major focus throughout the book. To help bring that theme home, checked lists of Strategies for Prevention appear in every chapter. These offer practical strategies for preventing health problems and reducing health risks.

Strategies for Change. To offer guidance for taking charge of every facet of healthful living, *An Invitation to Health* incorporates behavioral strategies within the text of every chapter, and emphasizes these strategies with

this special feature. Like Strategies for Prevention, these checked lists are meant to offer practical advice on how to make the changes needed to achieve better health.

Spotlight on Diversity. This feature highlights issues of cross-cultural or multicultural diversity pertinent to specific chapters. A new Spotlight on Diversity in Chapter 9 explores "Cultural Variation in Sexual Arousal."

Pedagogy. The eighth edition contains a wealth of pedagogical assistance to help students master the essential material.

Spotlight on Diversity
Closing the Minority Health Gap

How long can you expect to live? Are you at a higher-than-average risk for potentially deadly diseases? Do you have access to health services? If you are ill or injured, can you expect to receive the best possible care?

To some extent, your answer to these questions depends on your racial and ethnic background. As a growing number of studies indicates, many minority groups in the United States have shorter life expectancies, higher risks of illness, more limited access to services, and more negative expectations of and experiences with the health-care system than the population as a whole.

In the words of a National Institutes of Health (NIH) report, minorities have carried "an unequal burden with respect to disability, resulting in a lower life expectancy, minorities in the United States—African American, Asian Americans, Pacific Islanders, Native American other groups—experience as many as 75,000 than they would if they lived under the same tions as the white population.

But race itself isn't the primary reason for the lems faced by minorities in the United Stat Without adequate insurance or ability to pay make the lifestyle choices or afford the tests that could prevent illness or overcome it at the ble stages. According to public health expe may account for one-third of the racial diffe rates for middle-aged African-American adu pressure, high cholesterol, obesity, diabete are responsible for another third. The final blamed on "unexplained factors," which m poor access to health care and the stress of l in which skin color remains a major barrie the American Medical Association's Counc Judicial Affairs has reported, many minorit require health care but are less likely to r vices."

NIH has established an Office of Rese Health (ORMH) with the goal of "closing rently exists between the health of minoriti ity population." Since 1992, ORMH has p research and prevention efforts aimed at in health. Some focus on prenatal care to rates. Others are educating minority youth tion and AIDS.

80 SECTION I | A Lifetime of Wellness

Feeling in Control

Although no one has absolute control over destiny, there is a great deal that we can do to control how we think, feel, and behave. By assessing our life situations realistically, we can make plans and preparations that allow us to make the most of our circumstances. By doing so, we gain a sense of mastery. In nationwide surveys, Americans who feel in control of their lives report greater psychological well-being than those who do not, as well as "extraordinarily positive feelings of happiness."[36]

Developing Autonomy

One goal that many people strive for is **autonomy**, or independence. Both family and society influence our ability to grow toward independence. Autonomous individuals are true to themselves. As they weigh the pros and cons of any decision, whether it's using or refusing drugs or choosing a major or career, they base their judgment on their own values, not those of others. Their ability to draw on internal resources and cope with challenges has a positive impact on both their psychological well-being and their physical health, including recovery from illness.[37] Those who've achieved autonomy may seek the opinions of others, but they do not allow their decisions to be dictated by external influences. Because of this, it is said that their **locus of control**—that is, where they view control as originating—is *internal* (from within themselves) rather than *external* (from others).

Becoming Assertive

Being **assertive** means recognizing your feelings and making your needs and desires clear to others. Unlike aggression, a far less healthy means of expression, assertiveness usually works. You can change a situation you don't like by communicating your feelings and thoughts in nonprovocative words, by focusing on specifics, and by making sure you're talking with the person(s) who is directly responsible.

Becoming assertive isn't always easy. Many people have learned to cope by being passive and not communicating their feelings or opinions. Sooner or later they become so irritated, frustrated, or overwhelmed that

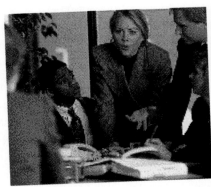

Practicing assertiveness allows you to express yourself actively and without aggression, to communicate and accomplish your goals.

they explode in an outburst—which they think of as being assertive. However, such behavior is so distasteful to them that they'd rather be passive. But assertiveness doesn't mean screaming or telling someone off. You can communicate your wishes calmly and clearly.

Even at its mildest, assertiveness can make you feel better about yourself and your life. The reason: When you speak up or take action, you're in the pilot seat. And that's always much less stressful than taking a back seat and trying to hang on for dear life.

Strategies for Change
Asserting Yourself

✔ Remind yourself that as an individual, you have certain rights—including the right to make mistakes, to change your mind, to say "I don't understand" or "I don't know."

✔ Don't expect an instant transformation. Assertiveness is a skill that takes time and practice to acquire.

✔ Decide what's really important and what's not before speaking up and setting limits.

✔ Don't think you have to be obnoxious in order to be assertive. It's most effective to state your needs and preferences without any sarcasm or hostility.

- *Learning Objectives.* Each chapter opens with a set of learning objectives, outlining the most essential information on which students should focus while reading the chapter.

- *Key Terms.* Key terms are boldfaced when they first appear in the chapter, are listed (with page references) at the back of each chapter, and are defined in the Glossary at the end of the book.

- *Making This Chapter Work for You.* Each chapter ends with a bulleted, detailed summary titled "Making This Chapter Work for You," which lists the key points covered in the chapter.

- *Review Questions.* A set of review questions appears at the back of each chapter, helping students to assess whether or not they have mastered the most important information.

- *Critical Thinking Questions.* Moving beyond just a review, a number of questions are also included at the end of the chapter which ask students to consider some applications of the chapter's coverage, or weigh in on some health-related controversy.

NEW! Connections to Personal Health Interactive. In-text icons at strategic places in the chapters of the eighth edition indicate topics for which a pertinent study aid is available on Brooks/Cole's health CD-ROM, *Personal Health Interactive.* Produced by Arthur and Wendy Kohn of Kwamba Multimedia Productions, this CD contains a Wellness Clinic—providing a variety of tools to help students assess their own health—and a study guide built around the chapter organization of *An Invitation to Health,* including key terms, study questions, and quizzes tied directly to the book. Each icon is numbered, and at the end of each chapter a legend is provided, matching the icon number with the relevant study aid on *Personal Health Interactive. Personal Health Interactive* is sold separately.

Ancillary Package

Instructors adopting the eighth edition of *An Invitation to Health* receive an extraordinary package of complimentary support materials to use with the textbook.

Instructor's Guide. The eighth edition features an updated Instructor's Guide prepared by Barbara Sayad. The IG includes chapter outlines and summaries, learning objectives, discussion questions, ideas for guest speakers, self-assessment exercises, references, readings, resources, and transparency masters.

Test Bank. Prepared by Dale Wagoner of Chabot College, an outstanding test bank of over 1,500 items is available, including multiple choice, short answer, and essay questions. Correct answers are referenced to the pages in the text, and multiple choice questions are categorized as factual, applied, or conceptual. In addition to the printed test bank, the questions are available on computer disks in Windows or Macintosh format, and Tele-Testing is also available.

75 Full-Color Transparency Acetates. Instructors adopting the eighth edition of *An Invitation to Health* may request a set of Transparency Acetates, containing 75 full-color acetates taken from main text figures. The set of transparencies will also be available on CD-ROM.

Health Study Center on Brooks/Cole's Website. Brooks/Cole's Health Study Center is located at http://healthstudy.brookscole.com, and features a variety of resources for the health instructor as well as the student. Adopters of the eighth edition of *An Invitation to Health* will be given the passwords to make full use of the site. Students will be able to visit the Health Study Center online and take practice tests for each chapter.

Brooks/Cole Video Library for Health. Adopting departments may select from the Brooks/Cole Video Library, an evolving list of documentary-style videos dealing with such subjects as weight control and fitness, AIDS and sex, sexual communication, peer pressure, compulsive and addictive behavior, and the relationship between alcohol and violence. Most of these videos, including several offered exclusively by Brooks/Cole, use interviews with students, professors, and experts to make the subject more real and personal. Contact your Brooks/Cole ITP representative for details and eligibility.

"Trigger" Video Series. These video complements—one on stress, the other on fitness—to the eighth edition of *An Invitation to Health* are designed to promote or "trigger" class discussion on a variety of important topics related to stress and fitness. These sixty-minute videos contain five 8-10 minute clips, followed by questions for discussion. Each segment is keyed to material in the text.

Dine Healthy Software (Windows and Macintosh). Dine Healthy teaches you how to eat sensibly, eliminating the need for crash diets. Clear, concise bar charts show how well you eat, with recommendations for food-choice changes. An exercise section enables you to track caloric expenditures and calculate ideal caloric intakes. A recipe analysis feature suggests how your favorite recipes can be improved nutritionally. An expandable database lets you add new food products as they come into the marketplace. Each adopting department is eligible to receive one copy of this powerful personal trainer for nutrition and fitness.

Diet Analysis Plus Software (Windows and Macintosh). This user-friendly software program helps simplify the process of diet analysis. It contains comprehensive information on nutrients in foods and energy expenditures from exercise. *Diet Analysis Plus* calculates the Recommended Dietary Allowances, analyzes daily intakes, identifies diet deficiencies and excesses, calculates comparisons and ratios, helps locate alternative foods, and helps plan an exercise program, as well as a weight-gain or -loss program. The database has been updated to include more foods common to college students as well as a comprehensive list of microwaveable foods.

The University of California at Berkeley Wellness Newsletter. Instructors who adopt the eighth edition of *An Invitation to Health* will receive a complementary one-year subscription to the *University of California at Berkeley Wellness Newsletter.* Adopters should contact Brooks/Cole's Marketing Department at 1-800-354-0092 to arrange for this subscription to be sent.

In addition, the following items are available for sale:

Study Guide. Written by Barbara Sayad, the Study Guide for the eighth edition includes learning objectives, study questions, and personal assessment and observation exercises.

Personal Health Interactive CD-ROM. Produced by Arthur J. Kohn and Wendy Kohn of Kwamba Multimedia Productions, this CD-ROM contains a Wellness Clinic and an interactive study guide for use with this text. In the Wellness Clinic, a variety of interactive tools are offered to help students assess their own health and monitor progress towards wellness goals. The interactive study guide is built around the chapter organization of *An Invitation to Health,* and includes a variety of innovative study aids. At the end of each chapter, it offers review sections comprised of key terms, study questions, and quizzes tied directly to the content of each chapter. New to the eighth edition, in-text icons appear in the text to highlight those topics in each chapter that have a relevant study aid on this CD-ROM. For instructors, an important benefit of *Personal Health Interactive* is its innovative LectureMaker program, which allows professors to prepare lectures quickly and easily and to export multimedia elements to popular presentation packages, such as PowerPoint, Persuasion, and Astound. The built-in "LecturePresenter" program enables instructors to present professional-quality multimedia lectures.

Dallas Telecourse Ancillaries

An Invitation to Health, Eighth Edition, has been adopted by the Dallas County Community College Telecourse, entitled "Living with Health." This award-winning course is distributed nationally to approximately 200 schools. Instructors offering the Telecourse receive the following complimentary special support materials:

- *Telecourse Study Guide for Living with Health.* The Study Guide for the Telecourse, *Living with Health,* contains a brief summary of each lesson, followed by learning objectives, study assignments for the text and video, key terms, a list of the experts interviewed with their affiliations, video focus points, individual health plan assignments, enrichment opportunities, and practice tests with page-referenced answers.

- *Telecourse Instructor's Manual.* This supplement helps instructors to implement the Telecourse at their school.

- *Test Bank.* Telecourse schools receive a customized test bank.

To Order

To adopt *An Invitation to Health,* Eighth Edition, contact your local ITP representative. To receive a review copy of this book, send your request on department letterhead to:

Brooks/Cole Publishing Company
Dept. Hales 001
511 Forest Lodge Road
Pacific Grove, CA 93950-5098
Or, visit the Brooks/Cole website at
http://www.brookscole.com/brookscole.html,
or e-mail us at info@brookscole.com.

Acknowledgments

I am deeply indebted to the many instructors and students, reviewers, editors, and others without whom this book would never have enjoyed so many years of success.

For the eighth edition, I was fortunate to work with a great team at Brooks/Cole. Marianne Taflinger, Denis Ralling, and Vicki Knight all provided their editorial expertise at different points along the way. In-house developmental editor Jim Strandberg and freelance developmental editor Megan Rundel provided invaluable input and assistance to improve the manuscript and keep the eighth edition on track. Mary Anne Shahidi oversaw the production process at Brooks/Cole, and deserve tremendous credit for coordinating the many pieces that go into a 4-color health textbook. I greatly appreciate the talents of Kelly Shoemaker and Bob Western in working up the wonderful cover, and thanks to Lillian Campobasso for her work on the permissions for this edition. Erica Smythe and Lorraine Burke of HRS Electronic Text Management have again worked their magic to design and produce a beautiful book on a demanding schedule. Jean Thompson has done a wonderful job preparing promotional materials for the eighth edition, and Michael Campbell and Alicia Barelli are directing an exceptional marketing effort. Thanks also to Faith Stoddard for her coordination of the outstanding supplements package, and to Stephanie Andersen, Deanne Brown, and Aaron Eden for their assistance in numerous aspects of this project.

Finally, let me express my thanks to the reviewers whose input has been so valuable through these many editions. For this eighth edition, I thank the following for their helpful assistance:

Rick Barnes, East Carolina University

Lois Beach, SUNY-Plattsburgh

James Brik, Willamette University

Stephen Haynie, College of William and Mary

Becky Kennedy-Koch, Ohio State University

Darlene Kluka, University of Central Oklahoma

Sabina White, University of California—Santa Barbara

Roy Wohl, Washburn University

For their help as reviewers or focus group participants for the seventh edition, I want to thank the following:

Marcia Ball	James Madison University	*Lorraine J. Jones*	Muncie, Indiana
David Black	Purdue University	*Mark J. Kittleson*	Southern Illinois University
Jill M. Black	Cleveland State University	*Debra A. Krummel*	West Virginia University
Cynthia Pike Blocksom	Cincinnati Health Department	*Roland Lamarine*	California State University, Chico
Mitchell Brodsky	York College		
Jodi Broodkins-Fisher	University of Utah	*Beth Lanning*	Baylor University
James G. Bryant, Jr.	Western Carolina University	*Loretta Liptak*	Youngstown State University
Marsha Campos	Modesto Junior College	*S. Jack Loughton*	Weber State University
James Lester Carter	Montana State University	*Michele P. Mannion*	Temple University
Lori Dewald	Shippensburg University	*Esther Moe*	Oregon Health Sciences University
Julie Dietz	Eastern Illinois University		
Gary English	Ithaca College	*Anne O'Donnell*	Santa Rosa Junior College
Michael Felts	East Carolina University	*Randy M. Page*	University of Idaho
Kathie C. Garbe	Kennesaw State College	*Carolyn P. Parks*	University of North Carolina
Gail Gates	Oklahoma State University	*Anthony V. Parrillo*	East Carolina University
Dawn Graff-Haight	Portland State University	*Janet Reis*	University of Illinois at Urbana-Champaign
Carolyn Gray	New Mexico State University		
Janet Grochowski	University of St. Thomas	*Steven Sansone*	Chemeketa Community College
Michael Hoadley	University of South Dakota		
Linda L. Howard	Idaho State University	*Larry Smith*	Scottsdale Community College
Jim Johnson	Northwest Missouri State University	*Carl A. Stockton*	Radford University
		Linda Stonecipher	Western Oregon State College
Chester S. Jones	University of Arkansas	*Emogene Johnson Vaughn*	Norfolk State University
Herb Jones	Ball State University	*David M. White*	East Carolina University
Jane Jones	University of Wisconsin, Stevens Point	*Robert Wilson*	University of Minnesota
		Martin L. Wood	Ball State University

Please R.S.V.P.

This book is an invitation to good health in its broadest sense—to personal fulfillment, to life itself. Its pages provide the practical tools students need to achieve their full potential. I also hope that your students accept this invitation in another sense: that they live what they learn and make the most of their health and of their lives.

I also have another invitation for you—a request to tell us what you think. *An Invitation to Health* was created for your students and for you. I would like to know what I'm doing right, what could be done better, and what I might include or drop in future editions. Your opinions and ideas matter a great deal to me, and I look forward to hearing from you.

Dianne Hales
c/o Brooks/Cole Publishing Company
511 Forest Lodge Road
Pacific Grove, California 93950-5098

About the Author

Dianne Hales, one of the most widely published free-lance writers in the country, is the author of numerous trade books and reference books in addition to *An Invitation to Health* and *Your Health*. A contributing editor of *Ladies Home Journal*, she has written more than 1000 articles for national consumer and health publications. She has won several national writing awards, including the prestigious National Media Award from the American Psychological Association and excellence-in-writing awards from the Council for the Advancement of Scientific Education. Her works have been translated into French, German, Spanish, Swedish, and Portuguese and have been published around the world.

BRIEF CONTENTS

CONTENTS

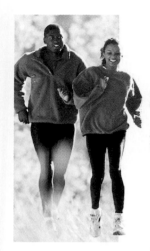

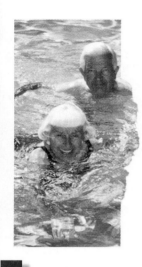

SECTION II
HEALTHY LIFESTYLES 117

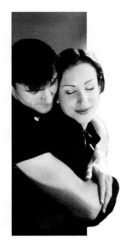

SECTION III
RESPONSIBLE SEXUALITY   211

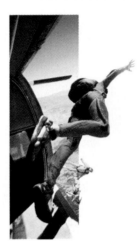

SECTION IV
PERSONAL HEALTH RISKS 329

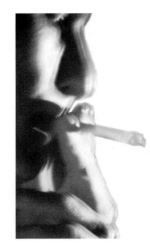

SECTION V
AVOIDING HARMFUL HABITS 437

17 Protecting Yourself 532

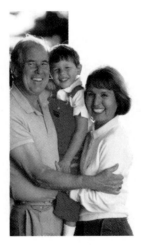

SECTION VI
THE CIRCLE OF LIFE 567

18 Living Longer and Better 568

FEATURES

Pulsepoints

Self-Survey

Spotlight on Diversity

Personal Voices

CAMPUS FOCUS

Strategies for Change

Strategies for Prevention

Health Online

What Is Wellness?

by John W. Travis, M.D.

Most of us think in terms of illness, and assume that the absence of illness indicates wellness. There are actually many degrees of wellness, just as there are many degrees of illness.

The Illness/Wellness Continuum (below) illustrates the relationship of the treatment model to the wellness model:

Moving from the center to the left shows a progressively worsening state of health. Moving to the right of center indicates increasing levels of health and well-being. The treatment model (drugs, herbs, surgery, psychotherapy, acupuncture, etc.) can bring you up to the neutral point where the symptoms of disease have been alleviated. The wellness model, which can be used at any point on the continuum, helps you move toward higher levels of wellness. The wellness model is not intended to replace the treatment model, but to work in harmony with it. If you are ill, treatment is important, but don't stop at the neutral point. Use the wellness model to move towards high-level wellness.

Remember, only you can implement the wellness model, calling on other people and resources as is appropriate. This questionnaire is designed to stir up your thinking about many areas of wellness.

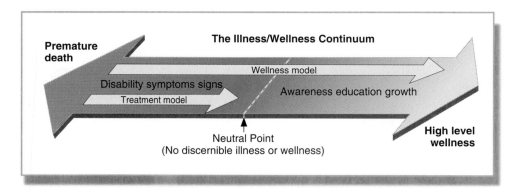

The Illness/Wellness Continuum

Premature death

Wellness model

Disability symptoms signs

Awareness education growth

Treatment model

Neutral Point
(No discernible illness or wellness)

High level wellness

While people often lack physical symptoms, they may still be bored, depressed, tense, anxious, or generally unhappy with their lives. Such emotional states often set the stage for physical and mental disease. Even cancer may be brought on through the subsequent lowering of the body's resistance from excessive stress. The same feelings can also lead to abuse of the body through smoking, overdrinking, and overeating. These behaviors are usually substitutes for other more basic human needs such as recognition from others, a more stimulating environment, caring and affection from friends, and greater self-acceptance.

Wellness is not a static state. High-level wellness involves giving good care to your physical self, using your mind constructively, expressing your emotions effectively, being creatively involved with those around you, and being concerned about your physical, psychological and spiritual environments.

The Wellness Energy System

Please refer to the illustration below. There you will see twelve arrows representing different kinds of energy. These correspond to the twelve sections of the Wellness Inventory.

Think of yourself as the person in the center. Notice the three sources from which you receive energy. You then channel this energy through your body, mind and being, converting it into nine other forms of energy before returning it to the environment around you.

Now think of your body as a pipeline or conduit of energy. Wellness results from the balanced flow of these energies through you. The presence of disease is a message that some form of energy is not flowing smoothly in your life. You are in some way blocking, overusing or ignoring one or another form of energy.

Energy Input

The three major ways by which you receive energy from the environment (see the inward arrows) are 1) Breathing oxygen (Section 2), 2) Sensing stimuli in your envi-

The Wellness Energy System

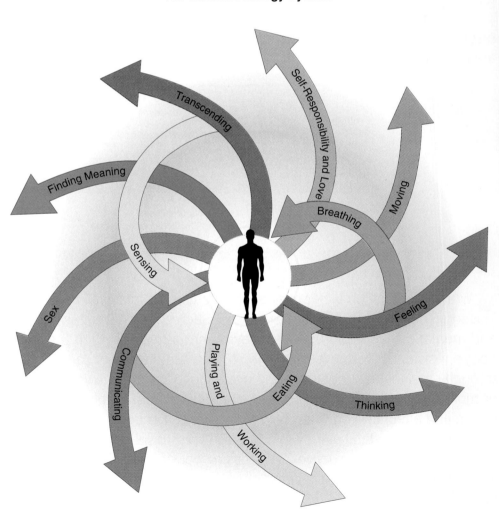

ronment (Section 3), and 3) Eating food which is oxidized by cells and is also used to build and repair body tissues (Section 4).

You convert some of the energy you take in to maintain the channel—your body—by generating heat and nerve impulses, replenishing and distributing blood, nutrients and hormones, and repairing tissues.

Energy Output

Now observe the remaining arrows which represent the outflow of energy to the environment. Begin with the arrow labeled Self-Responsibility and Love (Section 1). This is a form of energy which manifests as the attitude you choose toward your life. Wellness is enhanced by living your life with self-responsibility and love.

The next arrow is Moving (Section 5). Not only do you move your body through your external environment (exercise and fitness), but you move internal muscles to provide blood circulation, digestion, reproduction, etc. Continuing clockwise, energy is used for Feeling and expressing emotions (Section 6). The brain's activity of Thinking also includes intuition and dreaming (Section 7). Playing/Working are how you spend most of your waking hours (Section 8).

Communicating is a complex form of energy encompassing many of the preceding forms of energy (Section 9). Sex covers the whole spectrum of life-energy, not just genital feelings (Section 10).

Finding Meaning gives purpose and direction to the above forms of energy (Section 11). Transcending goes beyond the rational and connects us with all-that-is (Section 12).

The world will be changed by your transformation of energy. We will be changed by your communicating and touching, your work and play, your laughter and your tears. And your loving will change us all.

Instructions:

Set aside a half hour for yourself in a quiet place where you will not be disturbed while taking the Inventory. Record your responses to each statement in the columns to the right where:

2 = Yes, usually

1 = Sometimes, maybe

0 = No, rarely

Select the answer which best indicates how true the statement is for you presently.

After you have responded to all the appropriate statements in each section, compute your average score for that section and transfer it to the corresponding box provided around the Wellness Inventory Wheel at the end of the questionnaire.

Your completed Wheel will give you a clear presentation of the balance you have given to the many dimensions of your life. If your wheel is not well balanced, or small in size, we urge you to study the corresponding areas in the Wellness Workbook. Begin with those that interest you most and take your wellness journey at a gradual pace. We caution against undertaking massive and sweeping life changes. Gentle, steady progress is longer lasting.

You will find some of the statements are really two in one. We do this to show an important relationship between the two parts—usually an awareness of an issue, combined with an action based on that awareness. Mentally average your score for the two parts of the question.

Each statement describes what we believe to be a wellness attribute. Because much wellness information is subjective and "unprovable" by current scientific methods, you (and possibly other authorities as well), may not agree with our conclusions. Many of the statements have further explanation in a footnote (noted with an asterisk). If an idea sounds strange to you, read any footnotes or see the chapter reference in the Wellness Workbook. We ask only that you keep an open mind until you have studied available information, then decide.

This questionnaire was designed to educate more than to test. All statements are worded so that you can easily tell what we think are wellness attributes (which also makes it easy to "cheat" on your score). This means there can be no trick questions to test your honesty or consistency—the higher your score, the greater you believe your wellness to be. Full responsibility is placed on you to answer each statement as honestly as possible. It's not your score, but what you learn about yourself that is most important.

If you decide that a statement does not apply to you, or you don't want to answer it, you can skip it and not be penalized in your score.

The Wellness Inventory Wheel

Transfer your average score from each section to the corresponding box around the Wheel at right. Then graph your score by drawing a curved line between the "spokes" that define each segment. (Use the scale provided—beginning at the center with 0.0 and reaching 2.0 at the circumference.) Lastly, fill in the corresponding amount of each wedge shaped-segment, using different colors if possible.

Conclusions

When you have completed the Wellness Inventory, study your wheel's shape and balance. How smoothly would it roll? What does it tell you? Are there any surprises in it? How does it feel to you? What don't you like about it? What do you like about it?

We recommend that you use colored pens to go back over the questions, noting the ones on which your scores were low and choosing some areas on which you are interested in working. It is easy to overwhelm yourself by taking on too many areas at once. Ignore, for now, those of lower priority to you. Remember, if you don't enjoy at least some aspects of the changes you are making, they probably won't last.

Sample Questions

	Yes, usually	Sometimes, maybe	No, rarely
	2	**1**	**0**
1. I am an adventurous thinker.	✓		
2. I have no expectations, yet look to the future optimistically.		✓	
3. I am a nonsmoker.	✓		
4. I love long hot baths.			✓

Total points for this section = 5   4 + 1 + 0

Divided by __4__ (number of statements answered) = __1.3__ Average score for this section.

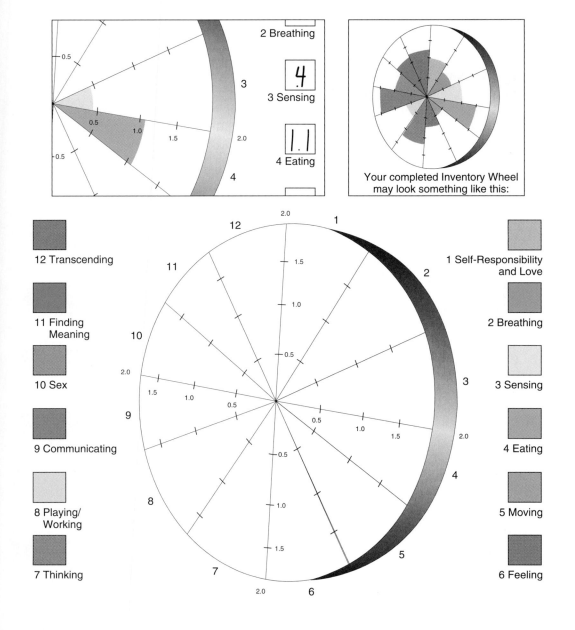

2 Breathing

3

3 Sensing

$\boxed{.4}$

4 Eating

$\boxed{1.1}$

4

Your completed Inventory Wheel
may look something like this:

12 Transcending

11 Finding Meaning

10 Sex

9 Communicating

8 Playing/ Working

7 Thinking

1 Self-Responsibility and Love

2 Breathing

3 Sensing

4 Eating

5 Moving

6 Feeling

Section 1 Wellness, Self-Responsibility and Love

	Yes, usually	Sometimes, maybe	No, rarely
	2	1	0

1. I believe how I live my life is an important factor in determining my state of health, and I live it in a manner consistent with that belief.
2. I vote regularly.[1]
3. I feel financially secure.
4. I conserve materials/energy at home and at work.[2]
5. I protect my living area from fire and safety hazards.
6. I use dental floss and a soft toothbrush daily.
7. I am a nonsmoker.
8. I am always sober when driving or operating dangerous machinery.
9. I wear a safety belt when I ride in a vehicle.
10. I understand the difference between blaming myself for a problem and simply taking responsibility (ability to respond) for that problem.

Total points for this section = _____ + _____ + _____

Divided by _____ **(number of statements answered)** = _____ **Average score for this section.**
(Transfer to the Wellness Inventory Wheel on p.5)

Section 2 Wellness and Breathing

	Yes, usually	Sometimes, maybe	No, rarely
	2	1	0

1. I stop during the day to become aware of the way I am breathing.
2. I meditate or relax myself for at least 15 (to 20) minutes each day.
3. I can easily touch my hands to my toes when standing with knees straight.[3]
4. In temperatures over 70° F (21° C), my fingers feel warm when I touch my lips.[4]
5. My nails are healthy and I do not bite or pick at them.
6. I enjoy my work and do not find it overly stressful.
7. My personal relationships are satisfying.
8. I take time out for deep breathing several times a day.
9. I have plenty of energy.
10. I am at peace with myself.

Total points for this section = _____ + _____ + _____

Divided by _____ **(number of statements answered)** = _____ **Average score for this section.**
(Transfer to the Wellness Inventory Wheel on p.5)

[1] Voting is a simple measure of your willingness to participate in the social system which ultimately impacts your state of health.
[2] Besides recycling glass, paper, aluminum, etc. if you purchase products which are reusable rather than disposable, and are packaged with a minimum of material, you will reduce the drain of resources and the toxic load on the environment caused by the disposal of wastes.
[3] A lack of spinal flexibility is usually a symptom of chronic muscle tension as well as indicative of a poor balance of physical activities.
[4] If your hand temperature is below 85°F (30° C) in a warm room, you're cutting off circulation to them via an overactive sympathetic nervous system. You can learn to warm your hands with biofeedback and to thereby better relax.
[5] Full-spectrum light, like sunlight, contains many different wavelengths. Most eyeglasses, and the glass windows in your home or car, block the "near" ultra violet light needed by your body. Special bulbs and lenses are available.
[6] Loud noises that leave your ears ringing cause irreversible and cumulative nerve damage over time. Ear plugs/muffs, obtained in sporting goods stores, should be worn around power saws, heavy equipment, and rock concerts!

Section 3   Wellness and Sensing

	Yes, usually	Sometimes, maybe	No, rarely
	2	**1**	**0**
1. My place of work has largely natural lighting or full spectrum fluorescent lighting.[5]	____	____	____
2. I avoid extremely noisy areas or wear protective ear covers.[6]	____	____	____
3. I take long walks, hikes or other outings to actively explore my surroundings.	____	____	____
4. I give myself presents, treats or nurture myself in other ways.	____	____	____
5. I enjoy getting, and can acknowledge, compliments and recognition from others.	____	____	____
6. It is easy for me to give sincere compliments and recognition to other people.	____	____	____
7. At times I like to be alone.	____	____	____
8. I enjoy touching or hugging other people.[7]	____	____	____
9. I enjoy being touched or hugged by others.[8]	____	____	____
10. I get and enjoy backrubs or massages	____	____	____

Total points for this section = [   ]   ____ + ____ + ____

Divided by ____ **(number of statements answered)** = ____ **Average score for this section.**
(Transfer to the Wellness Inventory Wheel on p.5)

Section 4   Wellness and Eating

	Yes, usually	Sometimes, maybe	No, rarely
	2	**1**	**0**
1. I am aware of the difference between refined carbohydrates and complex carbohydrates and eat a majority of the latter.[9]	____	____	____
2. I think my diet is well balanced and wholesome.	____	____	____
3. I drink fewer than five alcoholic drinks per week.	____	____	____
4. I drink fewer than two cups of coffee or black (non-herbal) tea per day.[10]	____	____	____
5. I drink fewer than five soft drinks per week.[11]	____	____	____
6. I add little or no salt to my food.[12]	____	____	____
7. I read the labels for the ingredients of all processed foods I buy and I inquire as to the level of toxic chemicals used in production of fresh foods—choosing the purest available to me.	____	____	____
8. I eat at least two raw fruits or vegetables each day.	____	____	____
9. I have a good appetite and am within 15% of my ideal weight.	____	____	____
10. I can tell the difference between "stomach hunger" and "mouth hunger," and I don't stuff myself when I am experiencing only "mouth hunger."[13]	____	____	____

Total points for this section = [   ]   ____ + ____ + ____

Divided by ____ **(number of statements answered)** = ____ **Average score for this section.**
(Transfer to the Wellness Inventory Wheel on p.5)

[7, 8]Long recognized by hospitals as therapeutic, touch can be a powerful preventative as well.

[9] Refined carbohydrates (white flour, sugar, white rice, alcohol, etc.) are burned up by the body very quickly and contain no minerals or vitamins. Complex carbohydrates (fruits and vegetables) burn evenly and provide the bulk of dietary nutrients.

[10] Coffee and non-herbal teas contain stimulants which, when over-used, abuse your body's adrenal glands.

[11] Besides caffeine, the empty calories in these chemical brews may cause a sugar "crash" shortly after drinking. Artificially sweetened ones may be worse. Consider the other nutrients you won't be getting, and the prices!

[12] In addition to a presumed connection with high blood pressure, salting of foods during cooking draws out minerals which are lost when the water is poured off.

[13] Stomach hunger is a signal that your body needs food. Mouth hunger is a signal that it needs something else (attention/acknowledgement), which you are not getting, so it asks for food, a readily available "substitute."

Section 5 — Wellness and Moving

	Yes, usually **2**	Sometimes, maybe **1**	No, rarely **0**
1. I climb stairs rather than ride elevators.[14]	____	____	____
2. My daily activities include moderate physical effort.[15]	____	____	____
3. My daily activities include vigorous physical effort.[16]	____	____	____
4. I run at least one mile 3 times a week (or equivalent aerobic exercise).[17]	____	____	____
5. I run at least three miles 3 times a week (or equivalent aerobic exercise)	____	____	____
6. I do some form of stretching/limbering exercise for 10 to 20 minutes at least three times per week.[18]	____	____	____
7. I do some form of stretching/limbering exercise for 10 to 20 minutes at least six times per week.	____	____	____
8. I enjoy exploring new and effective ways of caring for myself through the movement of my body.	____	____	____
9. I enjoy stretching, moving, and exerting my body.	____	____	____
10. I am aware of and respond to messages from my body about its needs for movement.	____	____	____

Total points for this section = ☐   ____ + ____ + ____

Divided by ____ **(number of statements answered)** = ____ **Average score for this section.**
(Transfer to the Wellness Inventory Wheel on p.5)

Section 6 — Wellness and Feeling

	Yes, usually **2**	Sometimes, maybe **1**	No, rarely **0**
1. I am able to feel and express my anger in ways that solve problems, rather than swallow anger or store it up.[19]	____	____	____
2. I allow myself to experience a full range of emotions and find constructive ways to express them.	____	____	____
3. I am able to say "no" to people without feeling guilty.	____	____	____
4. I laugh often and easily.	____	____	____
5. I feel OK about crying and allow myself to do so when appropriate.[20]	____	____	____
6. I listen to and consider other's criticisms of me rather than react defensively.	____	____	____
7. I have at least five close friends.	____	____	____
8. I like myself and look forward to the rest of my life.	____	____	____
9. I easily express concern, love and warmth to those I care about.	____	____	____
10. I can ask for help when needed.	____	____	____

Total points for this section = ☐   ____ + ____ + ____

Divided by ____ **(number of statements answered)** = ____ **Average score for this section.**
(Transfer to the Wellness Inventory Wheel on p.5)

---

[14] If a long elevator ride is necessary, try getting off five flights below your destination. Urge building managers to keep stair doors unlocked.
[15] Moderate = rearing young children, gardening, scrubbing floors, brisk walking, etc.
[16] Vigorous = heavy construction work, farming, moving heavy objects by hand, etc.
[17] An aerobic exercise (like running) should keep your heart rate at about 60% of its maximum, (120-150 bpm) for 12-20 minutes. Brisk walking for 20 minutes every day can produce effects similar to aerobic exercise.
[18] The stretching of muscles is important to maintaining maximum flexibility of joints and ligaments, etc. It feels good, too.
[19] Learning to take charge of your emotions and using them to solve problems can prevent disease, improve communications, and increase your self awareness. Suppressing emotions or using them to manipulate others is destructive to all.
[20] Crying over a loss relieves the body of pent-up feelings. In our culture males often have a difficult time allowing themselves to cry, while females may have learned to cry when angry, using tears as a means of manipulation.

Section 7 Wellness and Thinking

	Yes, usually **2**	Sometimes, maybe **1**	No, rarely **0**
1. I am in charge of the subject matter and the emotional content of my thoughts; and am satisfied with what I choose to think about.[21]	___	___	___
2. I am aware that I make judgements wherein I think I am "right" and others are "wrong."[22]	___	___	___
3. It is easy for me to concentrate.	___	___	___
4. I am conscious of changes (such as breathing pattern, muscle tension, skin moisture, etc.) in my body in response to certain thoughts.[23]	___	___	___
5. I notice my perceptions of the world are colored by my thoughts at the time.[24]	___	___	___
6. I am aware that my thoughts are influenced by my environment.	___	___	___
7. I use my thoughts and attitudes to make my reality more life-affirming.[25]	___	___	___
8. Rather than worry about a problem when I can do nothing about it, I temporarily shelve it and get on with the matters at hand.	___	___	___
9. I approach life with the attitude that no problem is too big to confront, and some mysteries aren't meant to be solved.	___	___	___
10. I use my creative powers in many aspects of my life.	___	___	___

Total points for this section = [ ]   ___ + ___ + ___

Divided by ___ **(number of statements answered) =** ___ **Average score for this section.**
(Transfer to the Wellness Inventory Wheel on p.5)

Section 8 Wellness and Playing/Working

	Yes, usually **2**	Sometimes, maybe **1**	No, rarely **0**
1. I enjoy expressing myself through art, dance, music, drama, sports, etc., and make time to do so.	___	___	___
2. I regularly exercise my creativity "muscles."	___	___	___
3. I enjoy spending time without planned or structured activities and make the effort to do so.	___	___	___
4. I can make much of my work into play.	___	___	___
5. At times I allow myself to do nothing.[26]	___	___	___
6. At times I can sleep late without feeling guilty.	___	___	___
7. The work I do is rewarding to me.	___	___	___
8. I am proud of my accomplishments.	___	___	___
9. I am playful and the people around me support my playfulness.	___	___	___
10. I have at least one activity (hobby, sport, etc.) that I enjoy regularly but do not feel compelled to do.	___	___	___

Total points for this section = [ ]   ___ + ___ + ___

Divided by ___ **(number of statements answered) =** ___ **Average score for this section.**
(Transfer to the Wellness Inventory Wheel on p.5)

[21] When you are unconscious of the content of your thoughts, they are more likely to control you. Observing them objectively develops self-awareness and strengthens your ability to take charge.
[22] Rather than trying to completely stop yourself from judging, you can observe your judgements as efforts by your ego to avoid getting on with life and hiding behind "right/wrong" game playing.
[23] Both biofeedback and the field of psycho-neuro-immunology have shown the connections between the mind, nervous system wend body. The more you become consciously aware of that connection, the greater responsibility you can take your health.

Section 9   Wellness and Communicating

	Yes, usually	Sometimes, maybe	No, rarely
	2	1	0

1. In conversation I can introduce a difficult topic and stay with it until I've gotten a satisfactory response from the other person.
2. I enjoy silence.
3. I am truthful and caring in my communications with others.
4. I assert myself (in a non-attacking manner) in an effort to be heard, rather than be passively resentful of others with whom I don't agree.[27]
5. I readily acknowledge my mistakes, apologizing for them if appropriate.
6. I am aware of my negative judgements of others and accept them as simply judgements—not necessarily truth.[28]
7. I am a good listener.
8. I am able to listen to people without interrupting them or finishing their sentences for them.
9. I can let go of my mental "labels" (ie., this is good, that is wrong) and judgemental attitudes about events in my life and see them in the light of what they offer me.
10. I am aware when I play psychological "games" with those around me and work to be truthful and direct in my communications.[29]

Total points for this section = [ ]   ____ + ____ + ____

Divided by ____ **(number of statements answered)** = ____ **Average score for this section.**
(Transfer to the Wellness Inventory Wheel on p.5)

Section 10   Wellness and Sex

	Yes, usually	Sometimes, maybe	No, rarely
	2	1	0

1. I feel comfortable touching and exploring my body.
2. I think it's OK to masturbate if one chooses to do so.
3. My sexual education is adequate.
4. I feel good about the degree of closeness I have with men.
5. I feel good about the degree of closeness I have with women
6. I am content with my level of sexual activity.[30]
7. I fully experience the many stages of lovemaking rather than focus only on orgasm.[31]
8. I desire to grow closer to some other people.
9. I am aware of the difference between needing someone and loving someone.
10. I am able to love others without dominating or being dominated by them.

Total points for this section = [ ]   ____ + ____ + ____

Divided by ____ **(number of statements answered)** = ____ **Average score for this section.**
(Transfer to the Wellness Inventory Wheel on p.5)

[24] Being aware of your internal distortion of perceptions can allow you to step back and re-assess a situation more objectively.

[25] Honesty, tempered with care and concern, clears out many negative thoughts which can clutter up your mind thus making your reality more fun. " Positive thinking" without honesty and truthfulness can backfire by suppressing valid concerns which must be addressed.

[26] Doing "nothing" can give us access to the more creative and non-verbal aspects of our being, so from another perspective, doing nothing becomes doing much more.

[27] Attacking others rarely accomplishes your goals in the long run. Persisting in your convictions without using force is more effective and usually solves the problem without creating new ones.

[28] It is important to recognize that our internal judgements of others are based on personal biases that often have little objective basis.

Section 11   Wellness and Finding Meaning

	Yes, usually	Sometimes, maybe	No, rarely
	2	**1**	**0**
1. I believe my life to have direction and meaning.	____	____	____
2. My life is exciting and challenging.	____	____	____
3. I have goals in my life.	____	____	____
4. I am achieving my goals.	____	____	____
5. I look forward to the future as an opportunity for further growth.	____	____	____
6. I am able to talk about the death of someone close to me.	____	____	____
7. I am able to talk about my own death with family and friends.	____	____	____
8. I am prepared for my death.	____	____	____
9. I see my death as a step in my evolution.[32]	____	____	____
10. My daily life is a source of pleasure to me.	____	____	____

Total points for this section = ☐   ____ + ____ + ____

Divided by ____ **(number of statements answered)** = ____ **Average score for this section.**
(Transfer to the Wellness Inventory Wheel on p.5)

This portion of the Inventory goes beyond the scope of most generally accepted "scientific" principles and expresses the values and beliefs of the authors. It is intended to stimulate interest in these areas. If you have beliefs strongly to the contrary, you can skip the questions or make up your own.

Section 12   Wellness and Transcending

	Yes, usually	Sometimes, maybe	No, rarely
	2	**1**	**0**
1. I perceive problems as opportunities for growth.	____	____	____
2. I experience synchronistic events in my life (frequent "coincidences" seeming to have no cause-effect relationship).[33]	____	____	____
3. I believe there are dimensions of reality beyond verbal description or human comprehension.	____	____	____
4. At times I experience confusion and paradox in my search for understanding of the dimensions referred to above.	____	____	____
5. The concept of god has personal definition and meaning to me.	____	____	____
6. I experience a sense of wonder when I contemplate the universe.	____	____	____
7. I have abundant expectancy rather than specific expectations.	____	____	____
8. I allow others their beliefs without pressuring them to accept mine.	____	____	____
9. I use the messages interpreted from my dreams.	____	____	____
10. I enjoy practicing a spiritual discipline or allowing time to sense the presence of a greater force in guiding my passage through life.	____	____	____

Total points for this section = ☐   ____ + ____ + ____

Divided by ____ **(number of statements answered)** = ____ **Average score for this section.**
(Transfer to the Wellness Inventory Wheel on p.5)

---

[29] Psychological games, defined by Eric Berne in Games People Play, are complex unconscious manipulations which result in their players getting negative attention and feeling bad about themselves.

[30] Including the choice to have no sexual activity.

[31] A common problem for many people is an overemphasis on performance and orgasm, rather than on enjoying a close sensual feeling with their partner, regardless of their having an orgasm.

[32] Seeing your death as a stage of growth and preparing yourself consciously is an important part of finding meaning in your life.

[33] Modern physics reveals that the idea of cause and effect may be as limited as Newton's theory of a mechanical universe. It suggests that we must expand our view to see that everything in the universe is connected to everything else. (Synchronicity describes that experience.)

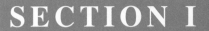

A LIFETIME OF WELLNESS

*H*ealth may be a science; living is an art. The principles that can help you understand the science and practice the art are simple and timeless and form the basic premise of this book: You have more control over your life and well-being than does anything or anyone else. Through the decisions you make and the habits you develop, you can influence how well—and perhaps how long—you will live. This section defines the dimensions of health and provides the information you need to take charge of your well-being now and in the years to come.

CHAPTER 1

AN INVITATION TO HEALTH FOR THE 21ST CENTURY

After studying the material in this chapter, you should be able to:

Identify and **explain** the dimensions of health and how they relate to total wellness.

Explain the principles and goals of prevention, and **differentiate** prevention from protection.

Explain the principles of health promotion.

Discuss the relationship between culture, economics, and health care.

Describe the factors that influence the development of health behavior.

Create a complete plan to change or develop a health behavior.

"How are you?" You may hear that question dozens of times each day. "Fine," you answer, without thinking. But how often do you ask yourself how you *really* are? How do you feel about yourself and your life? Are you under pressure to get good grades? Are you eating well and exercising regularly? Do you have close friends with whom to share your triumphs and traumas? If you choose to be sexually active, what do you do to prevent unwanted pregnancy or sexually transmitted illnesses? Do you smoke or use drugs? How much do you drink? Are you taking steps to prevent major illnesses? Do you get regular health checkups? Are you aware of safety and environmental threats to your health? How are you going to make the most of your life? What do you hope to accomplish before you die?

This book asks these questions and many more. It is a book about you: your mind and your body, your spirit and your social ties, your needs and your wants, your past and your potential. It's about exploring options; about discovering possibilities; about what makes you unique and what makes your life worthwhile.

This is also a book about living in a human body, thinking with a human mind, responding to a world of ideas and experiences with a human spirit. You are the owner of an incredible machine, the most complex and sophisticated on Earth. The human body is remarkably robust, resilient, and superbly equipped to deal with the challenges of daily living. Even processes we sometimes think of as malfunctions—a cough, a runny nose, diarrhea—can be indications of the body's capacity to heal itself.

While the body has its limits, there's no reason to tiptoe cautiously through life. We are designed to move, to think, to act—to stretch ourselves in every way. Muscles lose their tone if unexercised. Minds stagnate if we don't open them to new ideas and perspectives. If we don't make the most of what we are, we risk never discovering what we might become.

Health involves more than physical well-being. It is a state of body, mind, and spirit that must be viewed within the context of community, society, and environment. By providing the information and understanding you need to take care of your own health, *An Invitation to Health* can help you live more fully, more happily, and more healthfully. It also goes beyond the basics of health maintenance. Its primary themes—prevention of health problems, protection from health threats, and promotion of the health of others—can establish the basis for good health now and in the future.

The invitation to health that we extend to every reader is one offer you literally cannot afford to refuse: the quality of your life depends on it.

The Dimensions of Health

By simplest definition, **health** means being sound in body, mind, and spirit. The World Health Organization defines health as "not merely the absence of disease or infirmity," but "a state of complete physical, mental, and social well-being."[1] Health is the process of discovering, using, and protecting all the resources within our bodies, minds, spirits, families, communities, and environment. (See Figure 1-1.)

Health has many components: physical, psychological, spiritual, social, intellectual, and environmental. This book takes a *holistic* approach, one that looks at health and the individual as a whole, rather than part by part. Your own definition of health may include different elements, but chances are that you and your classmates would agree that it includes at least some of the following:

- A positive, optimistic outlook.

- A sense of control over stress and worries; time to relax.

- Energy and vitality; freedom from pain or serious illness.

- Supportive friends and family, and a nurturing intimate relationship with someone you love.

- A personally satisfying job.

- A clean environment.

Increasingly, Americans are striving to achieve the state of optimal health known as **wellness**. Wellness has been defined as purposeful, enjoyable living or, more specifically, a deliberate lifestyle choice characterized by personal responsibility and optimal enhancement of physical, mental, and spiritual health. Wellness means more than not being sick; it means taking steps to prevent illness and to lead a richer, more balanced, and

Figure 1-1 Wellness is the process of discovering, using, and protecting all the resources within our bodies, minds, spirits, families, communities, and environment.

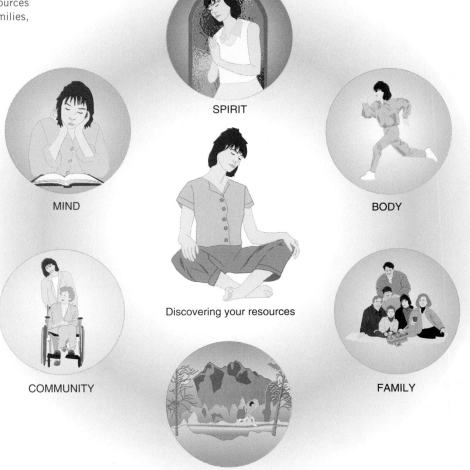

SPIRIT

MIND

Discovering your resources

BODY

COMMUNITY

ENVIRONMENT

FAMILY

Pulsepoints

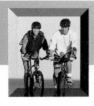

Ten Simple Changes to Improve Your Health

1. Use seat belts. In the last decade seat belts have saved more than 40,000 lives and prevented millions of injuries.

2. Eat an extra fruit or vegetable every day. Adding more fruit and vegetables to your diet can improve your digestion and lower your risk of several cancers.

3. Get enough sleep. A good night's rest provides the energy you need to make it through the following day.

4. Take regular stress breaks. A few quiet minutes spent stretching, looking out the window, or simply letting yourself unwind are good for body and soul.

5. Lose a pound. If you're overweight, you may not think a pound will make a difference, but it's a step in the right direction.

6. If you're a woman, examine your breasts regularly. Get in the habit of performing a breast self-examination every month after your period (when breasts are least swollen or tender).

7. If you're a man, examine your testicles regularly. These simple self-exams can spot the early signs of cancer when they're most likely to be cured.

8. Get physical. Just a little exercise will do some good. A regular workout schedule will be good for your heart, lungs, muscles, bones—even your mood.

9. Drink more water. Eight glasses a day are what you need to replenish lost fluids, prevent constipation, and keep your digestive system working efficiently.

10. Do a good deed. Caring for others is a wonderful way to care for your own soul and connect with others.

---

more satisfying life. (See Pulsepoints: "Ten Simple Changes to Improve Your Health".)

While physical well-being is essential to health, the term *wellness*, as used by health professionals, has a broader meaning. To understand how the concepts of wellness and health fit together, think of an automobile transmission: Having a disease (illness) is like being in reverse; absence of disease (health) puts you in neutral; but positive health changes (wellness) push you into drive—forward motion. When your entire lifestyle is based on health-enhancing behaviors, you're in high gear and going at top speed—and you've achieved total wellness.

In wellness, health, and sickness, there's considerable overlap in the functions of the mind, body, and spirit. As scientists have shown again and again in recent decades, psychological factors play a major role in enhancing physical well-being and preventing illness, but they can also trigger, worsen, or prolong physical symptoms. "The mind clearly can have a profound effect on every aspect of physiologic functioning," says James Gordon, M.D., Director of the Center for Mind-Body Studies in Washington, DC. "Individuals who are chronically pessimistic, angry, anxious or depressed are clearly more susceptible to stress and illness, including heart disease and cancer."[2] Similarly, almost every medical illness affects people psychologically as well as physically. For example, depression is common among individuals who suffer kidney failure or neurologic disorders, such as Parkinson's disease. (See Personal Voices: "Making the Most of the Mind-Body Connection.") Understanding the various dimensions of health can help you appreciate these complex interactions.

Physical Health

The various states of good and ill physical health can be viewed as points on a continuum (see Figure 1-2). At one end is early and needless death; at the other is optimal wellness, in which you feel and perform at your very best. In the middle, individuals are neither sick enough to need medical attention nor well enough to live each day with zest and vigor. For the sake of optimal physical health, we must take positive steps away from illness and toward well-being. We must feed our bodies nutritiously, exercise them regularly, avoid harmful behaviors and substances, watch out for early signs of sickness, and protect ourselves from accidents.

Psychological Health

Like physical well-being, psychological health is more than the absence of problems or illness. Psychological health refers to both our emotional and mental states—

Figure 1-2 The wellness-illness continuum.

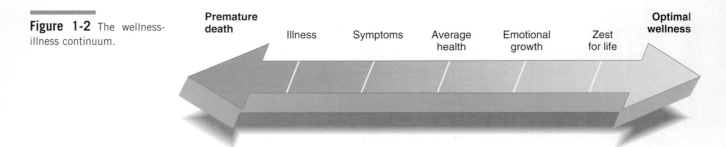

Premature death | Illness | Symptoms | Average health | Emotional growth | Zest for life | Optimal wellness

that is, to our feelings and our thoughts. It involves awareness and acceptance of a wide range of feelings in oneself and others, the ability to express emotions, to function independently, and to cope with the challenges of daily stressors. (Chapter 3 provides more information on psychological health.)

Spiritual Health

Being *spiritual* doesn't mean belonging to a formal religion. Its essential component is a belief in some meaning or order in the universe, a higher power that gives greater significance to individual life. Spiritually healthy individuals identify their own basic purpose in life; learn how to experience love, joy, peace, and fulfillment; and help themselves and others achieve their full potential. They concern themselves with "giving, forgiving, and attending to others' needs before one's own," says psychiatrist Roger Smith, M.D., of Michigan State University. Smith notes that spiritual development "produces a new meaning in one's life through a connectedness to something greater and mysterious."[3]

Americans tend to be both spiritual and religious. According to the most recent in a series of national Gallup polls conducted over the last 60-plus years, 90% of Americans believe in God—an all-time high. Most Americans also say that prayer is an important part of their lives, that they believe that miracles are performed by a divine power, and that they are sometimes conscious of the presence of God. Faced with physical or psychological difficulties, most Americans turn to prayer, reading the Bible, or meditation as a way of coping. Doctors share such beliefs: In a 1996 Yankelovich poll of family doctors, 99% said religion can aid healing. About one-third of America's medical schools now offer courses on spirituality and healing. And a growing number of doctors, while not endorsing any one approach to religion, are encouraging patients to cultivate a spiritual commitment—for the sake of their mortal bodies as well as their immortal souls.[4]

Increasingly, health professionals have recognized the power and potential of spirituality. For 30 years,

Herbert Benson, M.D., head of the Mind/Body Medical Institute at Harvard Medical School, has conducted rigorous experiments to document the influence of the spirit on health. His conclusion: The combination of relaxation and behavioral methods, such as prayer and meditation (described in Chapter x), with standard surgical and medical treatments can help relieve a host of medical problems, including chronic pain, arthritis, insomnia, and premenstrual symptoms.[5]

"Religion is very, very good for you," says psychiatrist David B. Larson, M.D., president of the National Institute for Healthcare Research. In an extensive review of the medical literature, he found not only that faith, belief, and religious commitment are positive influences on physical and mental health, but also that a lack of religious practice constitutes a clear and consistent health risk factor. In a study of medical students at Johns Hopkins University, an absence of religious belief was the single strongest predictor of the one in seven physicians who would develop an alcohol problem in the decades after graduation.[6]

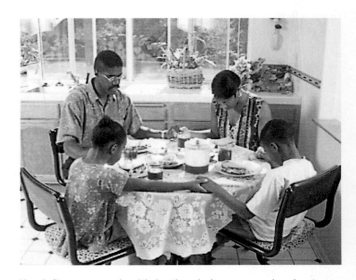

You influence your health by the choices you make about your body, your mind, and your place in the world. Take care of your health—your physical, psychological, spiritual, social, intellectual, and environmental well-being—because it can determine what you'll accomplish and become in your life.

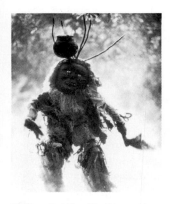

African Spirituality Dance is an essential ritual in many healing traditions of Africa. Constant rhythmic movements induce an ecstatic state that stimulates and ultimately relaxes the mind and body by shifting the focus from the self.

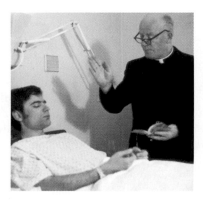

Catholicism During the sacrament of anointing of the sick, the seriously ill are anointed with oil that has been blessed by a bishop. As the oil is massaged into the forehead, the laying on of hands helps soothe and calm the patient.

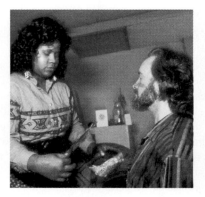

Native American Healing Each religion has its own rituals. Members of the Dakota/Lakota tribe, for example, conduct sweat ceremonies to heal the sick. Friends and family gather in a sweat lodge with the patient (or on her behalf) to sing and pray. It's believed that sweating heals the spirit and helps rid the body of illness.

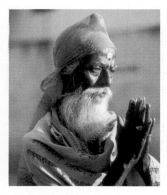

Hinduism Many followers fast regularly to cleanse their bodies of impurities. A person might also fast on behalf of a relative, hoping to please a god who can bestow health.

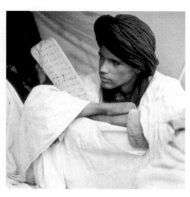

Islam When a Muslim becomes sick, loved ones read specific verses from the Koran to encourage her to be patient with her suffering.

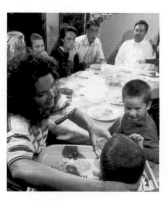

Mormonism The Mormon Word of Wisdom, a health code written in 1830, closely resembles today's nutrition guidelines, suggesting that meat be eaten sparingly and that fruits, vegetables, and grains be the foundation of the diet.

Figure 1-3 A sample of Religious Healing Rituals. The world's religions have developed practices to promote the physical health of their followers. **SOURCE**: Elizabeth Shaw, "Faith and Healing," *American Health*, November 1997.

"Deeply religious people of all faiths appear to benefit in five major areas," reports Dale Matthews of Georgetown School of Medicine, who reviewed more than 300 studies on healing and religion. These are: less substance abuse; lower rates of depression and anxiety, especially among women; enhanced quality of life; quicker recovery from injury or illness; and longer life expectancy. Four in five studies that looked at religion and survival found that people who went to church regularly, prayed frequently, or found religion important

Personal Voices Making the Most of the Mind-Body Connection

When Connie T. of San Francisco learned at age 44 that she had a very aggressive form of breast cancer, she was devastated. "I began gathering old letters and photos into a trunk so my three children would have something to remember me by. I was getting ready to die until I stopped myself and said, 'I'm going to concentrate on getting ready to live.' My goal was to live as long as I could to be here for my kids. I refused to listen to the statistics. I closed off negative thoughts. If I had a one-in-a-million shot, I decided I was going to be the one who makes it."

Connie received state-of-the-art medical treatment, including a mastectomy, chemotherapy, and a bone marrow transplant. But that was only part of her healing. "I'm an attorney, a highly rational person, but I tried everything. I shopped around for a support group until I found one made up of people who'd been given death sentences but were beating the odds. I meditated. I went to the beach and danced. I took joy in the smallest things. I relied on a strong, extensive network of friends, family, and coworkers who were pulling for me. And I never doubted that I was going to live."

Did Connie's positive emotional outlook help save her life? "Nobody knows for sure," she says, "But my doctors say my attitude made a big difference. At one point in my treatment, my heart stopped, and I had to be resuscitated. I saw the tunnel that people near death talk about. But I had told myself I was going to make it—and I did." More than five years later, Connie remains cancer-free.

Fifteen years ago Redford Williams was a heart attack waiting to happen. "I was a bear," says psychiatrist Williams of Duke University Medical Center, author, with his wife Virginia, of *Anger Kills*. He'd lose his temper often. He'd swear at drivers who dawdled. He'd find fault with everything Virginia did. "At the same time that my wife was complaining about the way I treated her, I was studying hostility and finding that guys like me—cynical, mistrustful, critical—were four to seven times more likely to die of heart disease and other causes by age 50. I realized that I had a health-damaging personality type, and if I didn't want to end up in a cardiac care unit at an early age, I'd have to change."

And so he did. Today, Williams, who is in excellent health, describes himself as a "recovering hostile guy" who's learned to replace potentially toxic attitudes and actions with positive ones. "Now, when Virginia isn't ready to go to church on time, instead of getting angrier and angrier, I reason with myself: I say, 'This is not that important. The worse that can happen is that we'll have to sit in back.' Then I pick up a book and read until she's ready."

Adrienne K., 69, of Holden, Massachusetts, lost her husband in March. Her diabetes and arthritis worsened; she underwent hip replacement surgery. Struggling with pain and disability, she worried about her deteriorating health. "I had been through a lot of changes, and I felt that my emotional processes were affecting my physical well-being," she says. And so she turned to the University of Massachusetts' Stress Reduction and Relaxation Program—the oldest and largest such center in the United States—to tune into her inner self through training in breathing exercises, relaxation, and meditation.

"I learned so much—that I'm valuable as a person, that it's okay to have all sorts of feelings, that it's important to focus on the present moment because it will never come again. I came to realize that there is beauty even in sorrow, that there is acceptance in living with pain." She's also seen dramatic improvements in her health. "I no longer need medication for my pain. I've been able to switch from insulin injections to oral medication for my diabetes. And my whole outlook is more positive and hopeful."

When Ann U., 43, of San Francisco learned that she had breast cancer, her large, loving family rallied around her and offered constant support through nine months of chemotherapy, a stem-cell transplant, and radiation treatment. But she found something different yet equally enriching in her support group: "In the group, you're able to talk about what's most frightening and challenging to you without feeling that you're burdening or scaring anyone. The other people don't get tired of the subject; they don't want to talk about something cheerier. And because you can share so openly, you're able to move through your fears and anxiety."

Looking back, Ann feels that the emotional aspects of her illness and recovery were the most important. "Cancer forces you to confront the reality that you're not going to live forever. It's the emotional work you do that lets you come to terms with that. Ultimately, you reach a point where you're changing, not because you want to keep the cancer from coming back, but because this is how you want to live for the rest of your life—whether that means one year, ten years, or fifty. D.H.

lived longer than those who didn't.[7] As Solomon noted centuries ago, good faith can indeed "add length of days to your life."

"In every culture, there's belief in higher powers or forces," notes mind-body pioneer Benson. "It's almost as if we're wired for God, as a survival instinct. Whether or not God exists, for many people believing in the Almighty is the most powerful belief a person can have. It gives us strength and solace, and that's healing in the truest sense of the word." [8]

Social Health

Social health refers to the ability to interact effectively with other people and the social environment, to develop satisfying interpersonal relationships, and to fulfill social roles. It involves participating in and contributing to your community, living in harmony with fellow human beings, developing positive interdependent relationships with others (discussed in Chapter 9), and practicing healthy sexual behaviors (discussed in Chapters 10 and 11).

As a growing number of research studies show, social isolation increases the risk of sickness and mortality. In a landmark study of 4725 men and women in Alameda County, California, death rates were twice as high for "loners" as for those with strong social ties. In other studies, social isolation greatly increased the risk of dying of a heart attack. In one study of 1368 patients undergoing cardiac catherization (a diagnostic test described in Chapter xx), those who were unmarried or did not have a close confidant were more than three times as likely to die as those with spouses or a close friend.[9] Heart attack patients have a better chance of long-term survival if they believe they have adequate help in performing daily tasks from family and friends.[10] Social contacts can even help ward off the common cold. In a study of 276 healthy volunteers, those with many diverse social connections (with spouses, friends, families, colleagues, and social group members) were less likely to develop colds when exposed to a virus than those who had the fewest such social ties.[11]

Health educators are placing greater emphasis on social health in its broadest sense as they expand the traditional individualistic concept of health to include the complex interrelationships between one person's health and the health of the community and environment. This change in perspective has given rise to a new emphasis on **health promotion**, which enhances health by building knowledge and skills among individuals and modifying their environment to foster healthier lifestyles.

Intellectual Health

The brain is the only organ capable of self-awareness. Every day you use your mind to gather, process, and act on information; to think through your values; to make decisions, set goals, and figure out how to handle a problem or challenge. Intellectual health refers to your ability to think and learn from life experience, your openness to new ideas, and your capacity to question and evaluate information. Throughout your life, you'll use your critical thinking skills, including your ability to evaluate health information to safeguard your well-being.

Another important component of intellectual well-being is "emotional intelligence," which is discussed in Chapter 2.

Environmental Health

You live in a physical and social setting that can affect every aspect of your health. Environmental health refers to the impact that your world has on your well-being. It means protecting yourself from dangers in the air, water, and soil, and in products you use—and also working to preserve the environment itself. (Chapter 21 offers a thorough discussion of environmental health.)

Health for the 21st Century

At the eve of the 20th century, the average American could expect to live for about 50 years. Infectious diseases, such as smallpox and tuberculosis, claimed tens of thousands of lives, particularly among the young and the poor. A high percentage of women died during childbirth or shortly afterward. By 1900, the average American woman could expect to live to an age of 50.9 years, compared with 47.9 years for a man. By 1950, women's projected lifespan had grown to 71.1 years and men's to 65.6.[12]

We have come a very long way. According to the National Center for Health Statistics, life expectancy in 1996 reached an all-time high: 76.1 years. The projected lifespans of both white and black males are longer than ever: 73.8 years and 66.1 years, respectively. The race differential has narrowed more than in the past, as has the gender gap. American women are expected to outlive men by six years, compared with a difference of 6.4 years in 1995.[13]

Infant mortality has reached another all-time low of 7.2 deaths per 1000 live births. The white infant mortality rate declined 5% in 1996 from the previous year (from 6.3 to 6), while the black rate dropped 6% (from 15.1 to 14.2). An estimated 15% decline in mortality rates stems from a decline in Sudden Infant Death Syndrome (SIDS).

TABLE 1-1   THE TOP 10 KILLERS

	Number of victims in the U.S.
Diseases of the heart	737,563
Cancer	538,455
Stroke	157,991
Chronic lung diseases	102,899
Accidents	93,320
Pneumonia and flu	82,923
Diabetes	59,254
HIV infection	43,115
Suicide	31,284
Chronic liver disease and cirrhosis	25,222

SOURCE: National Center for Health Statistics. Totals are for 1995, the latest year for which figures are available.

What Are Your Odds?

Diseases of the heart: Nearly two Americans in five—men and women—will eventually die of heart disease.

Cancer: One in two men and one in three women in this country will be diagnosed with cancer sometime during their lifetime. Three families in four will have to deal with cancer.

Stroke: One out of every 15 deaths in the United States is the result of a stroke. For those over 55, the incidence of stroke more than doubles in each successive decade. Among Americans aged 65 to 69, about 5% of the men and 2% of the women die from strokes. Nearly 10% of the men aged 80 to 84 die from strokes, as do 8% of the women 85 and older.

SOURCES: American Cancer Society and American Heart Association.

The top killers of Americans remain the same as the previous year (see Table 1-1), but there has been a dramatic decline in mortality related to Human Immunodeficiency Virus (HIV) infection and Acquired Immune Deficiency Syndrome (AIDS). In 1995, HIV/AIDS was the leading cause of death among 25- to 44-year-olds. In a single year, mortality declined 26% and slipped into second place behind accidents and injuries. HIV/AIDS mortality had increased an average of 16% per year between 1987 and 1994 before leveling off in 1995.

Homicide and suicide declined as causes of death in 1996 for the total population, but among young persons 15 to 24 years of age, they remain, respectively, the sec-

ond and third leading causes of death. Accidents are the number-one cause of death in this age group.

According to the Women's Research and Education Institute, gender is the single most important factor in predicting a person's life expectancy—more important than race, income, education, or lifestyle. Throughout the industrialized world, the gender that lives longer—by an average of 5 to 10%—is female. Insurance industry statistics indicate that every year, for every 100,000 Americans, 803 men and just 447 women die. The gender difference in mortality rates emerges before birth. From the moment of conception, baby girls are less likely to die in the womb or after delivery than baby boys. Once past age 30, women consistently outnumber and outlive men. By age 85, there are three women for every man. By the year 2020, according to current projections, the average woman's life may increase by ten years—and the average man's by just six.[14]

Not everyone sees women's longer lifespan as a bonus. "It's not that women live longer," says one observer. "They just take longer to die." Disease, in fact, spares no one. The sexes differ primarily in their susceptibility to specific illnesses.[15] Before age 50, men are prone to more lethal diseases, including heart attacks, cancer, and liver failure. But women are twice as likely as men to be disabled at any age, largely because of chronic problems such as arthritis, osteoporosis, and autoimmune disorders.

According to the U.S. National Center for Health Statistics, each year women spend 35% more days than men in bed because of nonfatal health conditions. These range from problems such as varicose veins, hemorrhoids, constipation, and eczema to complex conditions such as colitis (inflammation of the colon) and anemias. As women age, they're more prone to such problems. According to the Commonwealth Fund, more than 80% of American women aged 65 to 85 suffer at least one persistent illness.[16]

Healthy People 2000 and 2010

Ever since 1990, the U.S. Public Health Service, state health departments, and professional and voluntary organizations have been working to meet national health goals first outlined in a publication called *Healthy People 2000*. By 1995, this program had met 8% of its target goals and was showing movement in the direction of the accomplishment of 40% of the others. Progress has continued in many areas. According to a 1997 update, disparities in health services have declined for several minority groups. Infant mortality rates have dropped among Hispanic Americans, for instance, although they are still higher than for the U.S. population as a whole. The percentage of Hispanic women receiving prenatal care and undergoing regular Pap smears and mammograms (for women over 50) has increased. However, other health problems, including obesity and diabetes, remain more prevalent among Hispanic Americans than the population as a whole. Of all ethnic and racial groups in the United States, Hispanic Americans and Asian Americans and Pacific Islanders (AAPIs) are the least likely to have health insurance and are less likely to have regular sources of primary care than other Americans.

The campaign for better health for all Americans will not end with the 20th century. Plans have been proposed for a new Healthy People 2010. Its two overarching goals are increasing years of healthy life and eliminating health disparities. In addition, policy-makers have suggested four enabling goals: promoting healthy behaviors, protecting health, achieving access to quality health care, and strengthening community prevention. New areas of focus include the needs of the disabled, people with low incomes, and the chronically ill.[17]

How Healthy Are We?

Americans themselves are feeling good about their health. In a 1997 survey of a nationally representative sample of 1752 men and women, ages 18 and older, two-thirds said they are in "excellent" or "good" health. More than half said they have changed to healthier eating habits and are avoiding fats and eating more fruits and vegetables. But most Americans could be taking better care of themselves—and know it.[18]

According to the survey findings, half of Americans do not exercise—but 87% say that they should. Moreover, 57% describe themselves as overweight; 26% smoke; and 39% do not get annual checkups. "In terms of awareness and knowing about good health, I'd give Americans an A− or B+," comments Nancy Dickey, M.D., president of the American Medical Association. "But in terms of doing what we should, most of us only deserve a C or C−."

Compared with other nations, the United States ranks at neither the top nor the bottom. The citizens of many other industrialized nations—including Japan and many Western European countries—have longer life expectancies. In others, such as the former Soviet Union, life expectancy is actually falling. In developing countries, infectious diseases—old threats that have been vanquished in the Western world, as well as emerging infectious illnesses that spread rapidly and kill quickly (see Chapter 11)—continue to take an enormous toll in lives lost. In nations such as Uganda, Zambia, and the Central African Republic, life expectancy is under 50 years of age.

Worldwide, the top killers (see Table 1.1) are heart disease, respiratory infections such as pneumonia (which targets mainly children under age 5), stroke, diarrhea (in children under age 3), chronic obstructive pulmonary disease, tuberculosis, malaria, and measles. HIV continues to be a growing threat worldwide, particularly in Africa and Asia.

Without question, illness causes a great deal of suffering throughout the world—yet much of it can be prevented. According to the World Health Organization's 1995 survey of global health, at any one time more than 2 billion people—about 40% of the world's population—are ill, mostly with preventable diseases. The single most common underlying cause of their symptoms isn't a pathogen (disease-causing microorganism) but poverty. One-fifth of the world's 5.6 billion people live under conditions that provide little or no resources for preventing or treating illness. More than half cannot get essential medications; about a third of the world's children do not get enough to eat.[19]

Diversity and Health

We live in the most diverse nation on Earth. Look around your classroom or campus: Your fellow students come from dozens of different ethnic, racial, religious, and cultural groups. Minority students, who represented about 6% of undergraduates in 1960, now make up 25%.[20]

Your own family background may be woven of threads reaching back to several other countries and other cultures. For society, this variety can be both enriching and divisive. Tolerance and acceptance of others have always been part of the American creed. By working together, Americans have created a country that remains a symbol of opportunity around the world. Yet members of different ethnic groups still have to struggle against discrimination. Today, in this country's third century, all Americans still aren't equal in every way, includ-

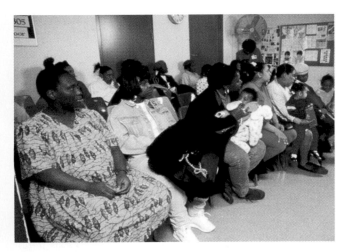

Neighborhood clinics can provide medical care that is sensitive to language differences and culturally diverse attitudes about health and medicine.

ing their health and health care. Poverty remains the single greatest barrier to better health for minorities in the United States. Without adequate insurance or ability to pay, many cannot afford the tests and treatments that could prevent illness or overcome it at the earliest possible stages. Some groups, particularly African Americans, also rate the health services in their communities as lower than those available to white Americans and have more negative opinions of the health care they receive.[21]

In the last two decades, America has become more culturally and racially diverse than ever before, with increases in Asian and Pacific Islander populations, Latinos, African Americans, Eskimos, and Native Americans. By the year 2050, the majority of people living in this country will belong to groups now called "minorities."[22] This is already the case in some states.

The growing influence of diverse racial and ethnic groups on our culture will affect national health priorities for many decades. As medical scientists are learning, there are clear differences with regard to disease and disability among different peoples. However, as public health experts explore the links between race, culture, and health, they are moving beyond any narrow definition of "minority" to the broader concept of "underserved," a group made up of many cultures that also includes the homeless, rural Americans, and women. Special problems also exist for illegal Americans, who often live in extreme poverty, perform difficult, hazardous jobs, and have little or no access to health ser-

vices. Even when they desperately need medical care, they may be so fearful of deportation that they do not seek help.

Diversity poses special challenges in health care. In some cultures, physicians are seen as less effective than other healers, who are believed to cure illness caused by bad karma or evil spirits. Language difficulties can create communication barriers. In addition, American physicians, trained to believe that high-tech medicine is best, may not understand or appreciate traditional healing practices. In many communities, innovative programs have begun to educate patients from other cultures about the American health-care system, as well as to educate American health-care providers about the beliefs and health practices of their diverse patients.

Can Race Be Hazardous to Health?

Different racial and ethnic groups often face different health risks. Consider the following statistics:

- The infant mortality rate for African-American babies remains higher than that of white babies.[23]

- Life expectancy for African Americans, though increasing, is 6.5 years lower than that for whites.[24]

- African Americans have higher rates of high blood pressure (hypertension), develop this problem earlier in life, suffer more severe hypertension, and have higher rates of hypertension-related deaths than whites.

- African Americans have higher rates of glaucoma, systemic lupus erythematosus, liver disease, and kidney failure than whites.[25]

- The death rate for heart disease among middle-aged black women is 150% higher than among white women the same age; among those with diabetes, their death rate is 134% higher than white female diabetics. Twice as many black as white women die of strokes and more than twice as many of diabetes.[26]

- Among young African-American women, breast cancer is a special threat. Of all black women diagnosed with breast cancer, 37% are younger than 50—compared with 22% of white women.[27]

- Native Americans have the highest rates of diabetes in the world. Among the Pima Indians, half of all adults have diabetes.[28]

- Southeast Asian men have a higher incidence of lung and liver cancer than the population as a whole.[29]

- Native Hawaiian women have a higher rate of breast cancer than women from other racial and ethnic groups.[30]

- Native Americans, including those indigenous to Alaska, are more likely to die young, primarily as the result of accidental injuries, cirrhosis of the liver, homicide, suicide, pneumonia, and the complications of diabetes than the population as a whole.[31]

Are these increased susceptibilities the result of racial or ethnic background, the stress of living with discrimination, an unhealthy lifestyle, lack of access to health services, or poverty? It is hard to say precisely. Certainly, poverty presents the greatest barrier to making healthy lifestyle choices, seeking preventive care, and getting timely and effective treatment.

Genetic and environmental factors also may play a role. Take, for example, the high rates of diabetes among the Pima Indians. Until 50 years ago, these Native Americans were not notably obese or prone to diabetes. However, after World War II, the tribe started trading handmade baskets for lard and flour. Their lifestyle became more sedentary, and their diet, higher in fats. In addition, as researchers have since discovered, many Pima Indians have an inherited resistance to insulin that increases their susceptibility to diabetes. The combination of a hereditary predisposition and environmental factors may explain why the Pimas now have epidemic levels of diabetes.

Other groups have other vulnerabilities. Caucasians, for instance, are prone to osteoporosis (progressive weakening of bone tissue); cystic fibrosis; skin cancer; and phenylketonuria (PKU), a metabolic disorder that can lead to mental retardation. Women with Chinese or Latino backgrounds face a significantly greater risk of developing diabetes during pregnancy than African Americans or whites. Asians and Asian Americans metabolize some medications faster than whites and thus require much smaller doses. Latinos have higher rates of death from diabetes and infectious and parasitic diseases than African Americans or whites.

Health-care providers often fail to recognize such factors, in part because the discussion of ethnicity in health is politically controversial. Some fear that it could lead to misconceptions about genetic superiority or inferiority. Yet recognition of different health needs and risks is the first step toward overcoming the health problems of many Americans. (See Spotlight on Diversity: "Closing the Minority Health Gap.")

The Health of College Students

As one of the nation's 12 million full- or part-time college students, you belong to one of the most diverse groups in America. A quarter of all 18- to 24-year-olds in the United States—some 7.1 million in all—are enrolled at one of the nation's 3600 colleges and universities. Some of you are reentry students, back on campus for the second time; half of all college dropouts return to school within 15 years. Within the next few years, older students—most working full-time—will make up the majority of college enrollments.

Although more than half of all young people ages 20 to 24 years have attended college, little is known about the health of college students nationwide. Some studies have focused on drinking, drug use, and sexual activity, but none assessed the health behaviors of students. To correct this information gap, in 1995 the National College Health Risk Behavior Survey surveyed the health behaviors of more than 4600 students at 136 institutions. The findings—featured throughout this edition of *Invitation to Health* in our new "Campus Focus" feature—represent a snapshot of the state of college students' health.

The primary finding from the mass of data collected was that many college students in the United States engage in behaviors that put them at risk for serious health problems. Here are some of the key findings:[32]

- One-third of those surveyed reported consuming five or more drinks on a single occasion in the last month, drinking and driving during this same period, or drinking while boating or swimming.

- Almost one in three (29%) college students smoke.

- Only one-fourth of the students (27.9%) who reported having sexual intercourse during the 30 days prior to the survey had consistently used condoms.

- One in five college students is overweight. About three-fourths (73.7%) do not meet the federal guidelines for daily fruit and vegetable consumption. One-fifth (21.8%) ate three or more high-fat foods the day preceding the survey.

- Somewhat more than a third of students (37.6%) had participated in vigorous exercise for at least 20 minutes on three or more of the seven days preceding the survey.

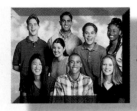

Spotlight on Diversity
Closing the Minority Health Gap

How long can you expect to live? Are you at a higher-than-average risk for potentially deadly diseases? Do you have access to health services? If you are ill or injured, can you expect to receive the best possible care?

To some extent, your answer to these questions depends on your racial and ethnic background. As a growing number of studies indicates, many minority groups in the United States have shorter life expectancies, higher risks of illness, more limited access to services, and more negative expectations of and experiences with the health-care system than the population as a whole.

In the words of a National Institutes of Health (NIH) report, minorities have carried "an unequal burden with respect to disease and disability, resulting in a lower life expectancy." Each year minorities in the United States—African Americans, Latinos, Asian Americans, Pacific Islanders, Native Americans, and other groups—experience as many as 75,000 more deaths than they would if they lived under the same health conditions as the white population.

But race itself isn't the primary reason for the health problems faced by minorities in the United States. Poverty is. Without adequate insurance or ability to pay, many cannot make the lifestyle choices or afford the tests and treatments that could prevent illness or overcome it at the earliest possible stages. According to public health experts, low income may account for one-third of the racial differences in death rates for middle-aged African-American adults. High blood pressure, high cholesterol, obesity, diabetes, and smoking are responsible for another third. The final third has been blamed on "unexplained factors," which may well include poor access to health care and the stress of living in a society in which skin color remains a major barrier to equality. As the American Medical Association's Council on Ethical and Judicial Affairs has reported, many minorities "are likely to require health care but are less likely to receive health services."

NIH has established an Office of Research on Minority Health (ORMH) with the goal of "closing the gap that currently exists between the health of minorities and the majority population." Since 1992, ORMH has provided funds for research and prevention efforts aimed at improving minority health. Some focus on prenatal care to improve survival rates. Others are educating minority youths about HIV infection and AIDS.

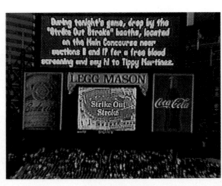

The "Strike Out Stroke" campaign in the southern United States features prevention messages and offers free blood pressure screenings in ballparks. Such community-based campaigns increase awareness of hypertension.

One of the most effective health promotion programs has taken aim at hypertension, a deadly threat to African Americans, who are at high risk for blood pressure problems. To increase awareness, the National Heart and Blood Institute has produced one-minute news and feature spots on hundreds of gospel and news talk stations. These public service announcements emphasize the importance of watching one's weight, being active, and getting regular checkups. In the South—known as the Stroke Belt because of its high incidence of cerebrovascular disease—a "Strike Out Stroke" campaign broadcasts preventive messages on scoreboards at local ballgames and offers free blood pressure readings at ballparks.

This community education effort seems to be paying off. In surveys completed in 1980, only 66% of African Americans knew they had high blood pressure, while fewer than 40% were getting treatment, and 13% had their blood pressure under control. A national survey, conducted a decade later and published in 1995, found that 73% of hypertensive African Americans are aware of their condition—the same as for the population as a whole. Of those with hypertension, 56% were being treated (compared with 55% for the population as a whole), and 28% had their blood pressure under control (compared with 31% for the population as a whole).

ORMH director John Rufin, M.D., expects such progress to continue: "The time is right for minority health in this country. We've seen progress in the last few years in terms of increased public awareness and heightened sensitivity toward this issue, but we have a long way to go before all Americans can look forward to a healthy future."

SOURCES: Blendon, Robert, et al., "How White and African Americans View Their Health and Social Problems," *Journal of the American Medical Association*, Vol. 273, No. 4, January 25, 1995. Goldsmith, Marsha. "Polished or Tarnished, the Golden Door," *Journal of the American Medical Association*, Vol. 273, No. 21, June 7, 1995. Sullivan, Mary. "Improved Health for Women and Minorities Is of Major Importance to NIH," *NIH News & Features*, Spring 1995. Voelker, Rebecca. "Speaking the Languages of Medicine and Culture," *Journal of the American Medical Association*, Vol. 273, No. 21, June 7, 1995. Murray-Garcia, J., "African-American Youth: Essential Prevention Strategies for Every Pediatrician," *Pediatrics*, Vol. 98, No. 2, July 10, 1995. Ford, Denyce, and Carolyn Goode, "African American College Students; Health Behaviors and Perceptions of Related Health Issues," *Journal of American College Health*, Vol. 42, No. 5, March 1994.

- Twice as many college men as women (12.3 versus 6.6%) rarely or never used safety belts when driving.

- White students were more likely than African American students to smoke, use smokeless tobacco, drink alcohol frequently, smoke marijuana or try cocaine, not use condoms consistently, and not participate in moderate physical activity. Black students were more likely than whites or Hispanics to report having had sexual intercourse, having six or more sexual partners, being overweight, and eating more high-fat foods.

The survey findings are important because they reveal a gap between what students know they should be doing to ensure good health and what they actually do. And college may be an ideal time to make permanent, life-enhancing changes.

Whether you're still in your teens or well into middle age, college can represent a turning point in your life. If you're a young adult, college offers the opportunity to shape your identity, define your goals, forge strong relationships, and prepare yourself for the future.

If you've returned to school or are starting college at midlife or later, you may already know what you need and want from school. If you're taking courses solely to enrich yourself, you can savor the opportunity to make your mind a more interesting place to live for the rest of your life. Whatever your age or stage of life, knowing how to prevent health problems can help you reach your goals.

Just by educating yourself, you're likely to improve your health—now and in the future. In a study of 2380 Californians, Stanford University researchers found that education may be a better road to health than either more income or a more prestigious job. Many risk factors for disease—including high blood pressure, elevated cholesterol, and cigarette smoking—decline steadily as education increases, regardless of how much money people make. Education may be good for the body as well as the mind by "influencing lifestyle behaviors, problem-solving abilities, and values," the researchers noted.[33] People who earn college degrees gain positive attitudes about the benefits of healthy living, learn how

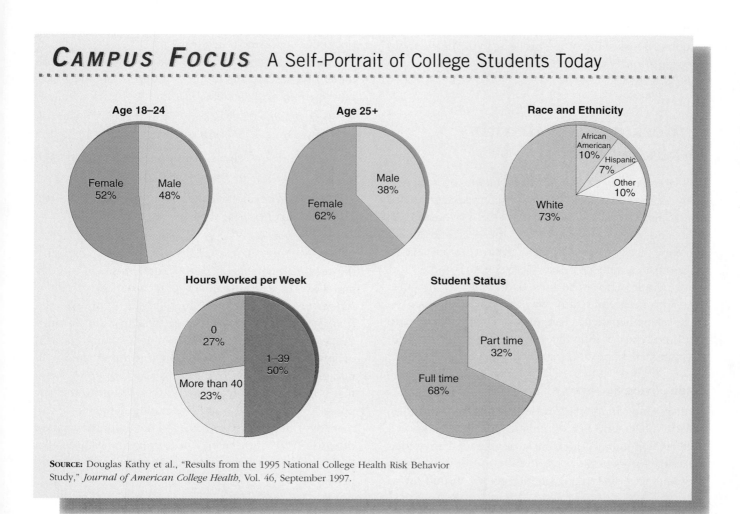

CAMPUS FOCUS A Self-Portrait of College Students Today

Age 18–24
Female 52%
Male 48%

Age 25+
Male 38%
Female 62%

Race and Ethnicity
African American 10%
Hispanic 7%
Other 10%
White 73%

Hours Worked per Week
0 27%
1–39 50%
More than 40 23%

Student Status
Part time 32%
Full time 68%

SOURCE: Douglas Kathy et al., "Results from the 1995 National College Health Risk Behavior Study," *Journal of American College Health,* Vol. 46, September 1997.

to gain access to preventive health services, join peer groups that promote healthy behavior, and develop higher self-esteem and greater control over their lives.[34]

Becoming All You Can Be

Many external factors can and often do affect us—from the weather, which can temporarily dampen or brighten our mood, to genetic predispositions that can result in certain health conditions. In addition, those who are poor, disabled, or discriminated against have fewer options for preventing illness or promoting health. But even if you can't control all your life circumstances, you are responsible for making the most of those circumstances. The first step is understanding that your own behaviors and choices can pose threats to your health.

By taking the Wellness Inventory, "What Is Wellness," that precedes this chapter, you can get a snapshot of the current state of your overall health and wellness. You also can get a sense of the aspects of your life that could use some attention and improvement. Use this course as an opportunity to zero in on at least one less-than-healthful behavior and improve it. The following sections discuss some of the processes you'll have to go through in order to make a successful change for the better.

Understanding Health Behavior

Behaviors that affect your health include exercising regularly, eating a balanced, nutritious diet, seeking care for symptoms, and taking necessary steps to overcome illness, and restore well-being. If there is one health behavior that you would like to improve, you have to realize that change isn't easy. Between 40% and 80% of those people who try to kick bad health habits lapse back into their unhealthy ways within six weeks. To make lasting beneficial changes, you have to understand the three types of influences that shape behavior: predisposing, enabling, and reinforcing factors (Figure 1-4).

Predisposing Factors

Predisposing factors include knowledge, attitudes, beliefs, values, and perceptions. Unfortunately, knowledge isn't enough to cause most people to change their behavior; for example, people fully aware of the grim consequences of smoking often continue to puff away.

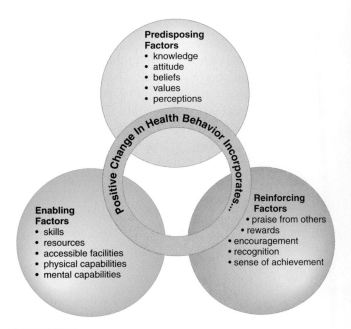

Figure 1-4 Factors that shape positive behavior.

Nor is attitude—one's likes and dislikes—sufficient; an individual may dislike the smell and taste of cigarettes but continue to smoke regardless.

Beliefs are more powerful than knowledge and attitudes, and researchers report that people are most likely to change health behavior if they hold three beliefs.

- *Susceptibility.* They acknowledge that they are at risk for the negative consequences of their behavior.

- *Severity.* They believe that they may pay a very high price if they don't make a change.

- *Benefits.* They believe that the proposed change will be advantageous to their health.

There can be a gap between stated and actual beliefs, however. Young adults may say they recognize the very real dangers of casual, careless sex in this day and age. Yet, rather than act in accordance with these statements, they may impulsively engage in unprotected sex with individuals whose health status and histories they do not know. The reason: Like young people everywhere and in every time, they feel they are invulnerable, that nothing bad can or will happen to them, that if there were a real danger, they would somehow know it. Often it's not until something happens—a former lover may admit to having a sexually transmitted disease (STD), or there may be a pregnancy scare—that their behaviors become consistent with their stated beliefs.

The value or importance we give to health also plays a major role in changing behavior. Many people aren't concerned about their health just for the sake of being healthy. Usually they want to look or feel better, be more productive or competitive, or behave more independently. They're more likely to change, and to stick with a change, if they can see that the health benefits also enhance other important aspects of their lives.

Perceptions are the way we see things from our unique perspective; they vary greatly with age. As a student, you may not think that living a few hours longer is a significant gain; as you grow older, however, you may prize every additional second.

Enabling Factors

Enabling factors include skills, resources, accessible facilities, and physical and mental capacities. Before you initiate a change, assess the means available to reach your goal. No matter how motivated you are, you'll become frustrated if you keep encountering obstacles. That's why breaking a task or goal down into step-by-step strategies is so important in behavioral change.

Reinforcing Factors

Reinforcing factors may be praise from family and friends, rewards from teachers or parents, or encouragement and recognition for meeting a goal. Although these help a great deal in the short run, lasting change depends not on external rewards, but on an internal commitment and sense of achievement. To make a difference, reinforcement must come from within.

A decision to change a health behavior should stem from a permanent, personal goal, not from a desire to please or impress someone else. If you lose weight for the homecoming dance, you're almost sure to regain pounds afterward. But if you shed extra pounds because you want to feel better about yourself or get into shape, you're far more likely to keep the weight off.

Strategies for Change

Setting Realistic Goals

Here's a framework for setting goals and objectives, the crucial preliminary step for making changes:

- ✔ Determine your goal or objective. Define it in words and on paper. Then test your definition against your own value system. Can you attain your goal and still be the person you want to be?
- ✔ Set small, manageable goals.
- ✔ Think in terms of evolution, not revolution. Revolutionary changes only inspire counterrevolutions. If you want to change the way you eat, start by changing just one meal a week.
- ✔ Identify your resources. Do you have the knowledge, skills, finances, time—whatever it takes? Find out from others who know. Be sure you're ready for the next step.
- ✔ Systematically analyze barriers. How can missing resources be acquired? Identify and select alternative plans. List solutions for any obstacles you foresee.
- ✔ Choose a plan. Think it through, step by step, trying to anticipate what might go wrong and why.

Making Decisions

Every day you make decisions that have immediate and long-term effects on your health. You decide what to eat, whether to drink or smoke, when to exercise, and how to cope with a sudden crisis. Beyond these daily matters, you decide when to see a doctor, what kind of doctor, and with what sense of urgency. You decide what to tell your doctor and whether to follow the advice given, whether to keep up your immunizations, whether to have a prescription filled and comply with the medication instructions, and whether to seek further help or a second opinion. The entire process of maintaining or restoring health depends on your decisions; it cannot start or continue without them.

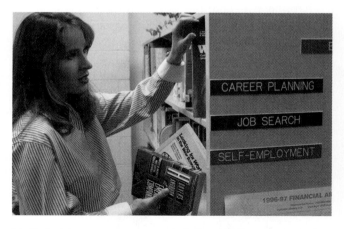

Large decisions may seem overwhelming, but they can be broken down into manageable steps to help you gather information and focus on what's best for you.

The small decisions of everyday life—what to eat, where to go, when to study—are straightforward choices. Larger decisions—which major to choose, what to do about a dead-end relationship, how to handle an awkward work situation—are more challenging. However, if you think of decision making as a process, you can break down even the most difficult choices into manageable steps:

- Set priorities. Rather than getting bogged down in details, step back and look at the big picture. What matters most to you? What would you like to accomplish in the next week, month, year? Look at the decision you're about to make in the context of your values and goals (both discussed in Chapter 3).

- *Inform yourself.* The more you know—about a person, a position, a place, a project—the better you'll be able to evaluate it. Gathering information may involve formal research, such as an on-line or library search for relevant data, or informal conversations with teachers, counselors, family members, or friends.

- *Consider all your options.* Most complex decisions don't involve simple either-or alternatives. List as many options as you can think of, along with the advantages and disadvantages of each.

- *Tune in to your gut feelings.* After you've gotten the facts and analyzed them, listen to your intuition. While it's not infallible, your "sixth sense" can provide valuable feedback. If something just doesn't feel right, try to figure out why. Are there any fears you haven't dealt with? Do you have doubts about taking a certain path?

- *Consider a "worst-case" scenario.* When you've pretty much come to a final decision, imagine what will happen if everything goes wrong—the workload becomes overwhelming, your partner betrays your trust, your expectations turn out to be unrealistic. If you can live with the worst consequences of a decision, you're probably making the right choice.

Changing Health Behavior

Change is never easy—even if it's done for the best possible reasons. When you decide to change a behavior, you have to give up something familiar and easy for something new and challenging. Change always involves risk—and the prospect of rewards.

Researchers have identified various approaches that people use in making beneficial changes. In the "moral" model, you take responsibility for a problem (such as smoking) and its solution; success depends on adequate motivation, while failure is seen as a sign of character weakness. In the "enlightenment" model, you submit to strict discipline in order to correct a problem; this is the approach used in Alcoholics Anonymous. The "behavioral" model involves rewarding yourself when you make positive changes. The "medical" model sees the behavior as caused by forces beyond your control (a genetic predisposition to being overweight, for example) and employs an expert to provide advice or treatment. For many people, the most effective approach is the "compensatory" model, which doesn't assign blame but puts responsibility on individuals to acquire whatever skills or power they need to overcome their problems.

Before they reach the stage where they can and do take action to change, most people go through a process comparable to religious conversion. First, they reach a level of accumulated unhappiness that makes them ready for change. Then they have a moment of truth that makes them want to change. One pregnant woman, for instance, felt her unborn baby quiver when she drank a beer and swore never to drink again. As people change their behavior, they change their lifestyles and identities as well. Ex-smokers, for instance, may start an aggressive exercise program, make new friends at the track or gym, and participate in new types of activities, like racquetball games or fun runs.

Social and cultural **norms**—behaviors that are expected, accepted, or supported by a group—can make change much harder if they're constantly working against a person's best intentions. You may resolve to eat less, for instance, yet your mother may keep offering you homemade fudge and brownies because your family's norm is to show love by making and offering delicious treats. Or you might decide to drink less, yet your friends' norm may be to equate drinking with having a good time.

If you're aware of the norms that influence your behavior, you can devise strategies either to change them (by encouraging your friends to dance more and drink less at parties, for example) or adapt to them (having just a bite of your mother's sweets). Another option is to develop relationships with people who share your goals and whose norms can reinforce your behavior.

The Keys to Successful Change

Awareness of a negative behavior is always the first step toward changing it. Once you identify what you'd like to change, keep a diary for one or two weeks, noting what you do, when, where, and what you're feeling at the time. If you'd like, enlist the help of friends or family to call attention to your behavior. Sometimes self-observation in itself proves therapeutic: just the act of keeping a diary can be enough to help you lose weight or kick the smoking habit.

Once you've identified the situations, moods, thoughts, or people that act as cues for a behavior, identify the most powerful ones and develop a plan to avoid them. For instance, if you snack continuously when studying in your room, try working in the library, where food is forbidden.

Planning ahead is a crucial part of successful change. If you can't avoid certain situations, anticipate how you might cope with the temptation to return to your old behavior. Develop alternatives. Visualize yourself walking past the desserts in the cafeteria or chewing gum instead of lighting a cigarette.

Some people find it helpful to sign a "contract," a written agreement in which they make a commitment to change, with their partner, parent, or health educator. Spelling out what they intend to do and why, underscores the seriousness of what they're trying to accomplish (see Figure 1-5).

Above all else, change depends on the belief that you can and will succeed. In his research on **self-efficacy**, psychologist Albert Bandura of Stanford University found that the individuals most likely to reach a goal are those who believe they can. The more strongly they feel that they can and will change their behavior, the more energy and persistence they put into making the change.[35] Other researchers have linked positive health change with optimism. Individuals who see themselves as optimists may underestimate their susceptibility to problems, such as hypertension, because they always expect things to turn out well. Individuals who perceive themselves as susceptible—that is, who anticipate potentially negative consequences—may be more cautious.[36]

Another crucial factor is **locus of control**. If you believe that your actions will make a difference in your health, your locus of control is internal. If you believe that external forces or factors play a greater role, your locus of control is external. Individuals with an external locus of control for health are less likely to seek preventive health care, are less optimistic about early treatment, rate their own health as poorer, and spend more time in bed because of illness than those with an internal locus of control.[37]

Reinforcements—either positive (a reward) or negative (a punishment)—also can play a role. If you decide to set up a regular exercise program, for instance, you might reward yourself with a new sweat suit if you stick to it for three months or you might punish yourself for skipping a day by doing ten minutes of exercises the following day.

Your **self-talk**—the messages you send yourself—also can play a role. In recent decades, mental health professionals have recognized the conscious use of positive self-talk as a powerful force for changing the way individuals think, feel, and behave. (Chapter 5 discusses self-talk as a principle of cognitive therapy.) "We have a choice about how we think," explains psychologist Martin Seligman, Ph.D., author of *Learned Optimism*. As he notes, by learning to challenge automatic negative thoughts that enter our brains and asserting our own statements of self-worth, we can transform ourselves into optimists who see what's right rather than pessimists forever focusing on what's wrong. "Optimism is a learned set of skills," Seligman contends. "Once learned, these skills persist because they feel so good to use. And reality is usually on our side.[38]

Strategies for Change
....
How to Make a Change

✔ Get support from friends, but don't expect them to supply all the reinforcement you need. You may join a group of overweight individuals and rely on their encouragement to stick to your diet. That's a great way to get going; but in the long run, your own commitment to losing weight has got to be strong enough to help you keep eating right and light.

✔ Focus on the immediate rewards of your new behavior. You may stop smoking so that you'll live longer, but take note of every other benefit it brings you—more stamina, less coughing, more spending money, no more stale tobacco taste in your mouth.

✔ To boost your self-confidence, remind yourself of past

My Contract For Change

Date: _____

Personal Goal: _____

_____

Motivating Factors: _____

_____

Change(s) I Promise to Make to Reach This Goal:

_____

Plan for Making This Change: _____

_____

Start Date: _____

Assessment Plan: _____

_____

_____

_____

If I Need Help: _____

_____

_____

Target Date for Reaching Goal: _____

Reward for Achieving Goal: _____

Penalty for Failing to Achieve Goal: _____

_____

Signed: _____

Witnessed By: _____

Figure 1-5 A sample health-change contract.

successes you've had in making changes. Give yourself pep talks, commending yourself on how well you've done so far and how well you'll continue to do.

✔ Reward yourself regularly. Plan a pleasant reward as an incentive for every week you stick to your new behavior—sleeping in on a Saturday morning, going out with some friends, or spending a sunny afternoon outdoors. Small, regular rewards are more effective in keeping up motivation than one big reward that won't come for many months.

✔ Expect and accept some relapses. The greatest rate of relapse occurs in the first few weeks after making a behavior change. During this critical time, get as much support as you can. In addition, work hard on self-motivation, reminding yourself daily of what you have to gain by sticking with your new health habit.

A New Era in Health Education

In the past, health education focused on individual change. Today many educators are using a new framework in which behavior change occurs within the context of the entire environment of a person's life. The primary themes that bring together personal health, social context, and a community focus are prevention, protection, and promotion.

The Power of Prevention

No medical treatment, however successful or sophisticated, can compare with the power of **prevention**. Two out of every three deaths and one in three hospitalizations in the United States could be prevented by changes in six main risk factors: tobacco use, alcohol abuse, accidents, high blood pressure, obesity, and gaps in screening and primary health care. Preventive efforts have already proved helpful in increasing physical activity, quitting smoking, reducing dietary fat, preventing STDs and unwanted pregnancy, reducing intolerance and violence, and avoiding alcohol and drug abuse.

Prevention can take many forms. Primary or "before-the-fact" prevention efforts might seek to reduce stressors and increase support in order to prevent problems in healthy people. Consumer education, for instance, provides guidance about how to change our lifestyle—the way we care for the basic needs of body

and mind—to prevent problems and enhance well-being. Other preventive programs identify people at risk and "empower" them with information and support so they can avoid potential problems. Prevention efforts may target an entire community and try to educate all of its members about the dangers of alcohol abuse, for instance, or environmental hazards, or they may zero in on a particular group (for instance, seminars on safer sex practice offered to teens) or an individual (one-on-one counseling about substance abuse).

In the past, physicians did not routinely incorporate prevention into their professional practices. Instead, consumers played the role of Humpty-Dumpty: as long as they sat quietly on the wall, they were ignored. When they fell, the medical equivalents of all the king's horses and all the king's men came running to put them back together again. Often, however, even the best these professionals could provide was still too little, too late.

But times have changed. Medical schools are providing more training in preventive care. The U.S. Public Health Service has issued a 400-page handbook that provides practical advice on how physicians can practice prevention.[39] In addition, researchers are demonstrating, in a growing number of studies, that prevention

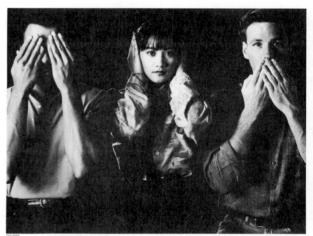

Prevention includes education and training that empowers us and enhances our well-being.

saves not only money, but also productivity, health, and lives. As many as 50% to 80% of the deaths caused by cardiovascular disease, strokes, and cancer could be avoided or delayed by preventive measures. Eliminating smoking could prevent more than 300,000 deaths each year, for instance, while changes in diet could prevent 35% of unnecessary deaths from heart disease.[40]

Strategies for Prevention

Working Toward Wellness

✔ Know what your real needs are and how to meet them.

✔ Act assertively to create the life you really want, rather than just reacting to what seems to happen to you.

✔ Nurture your body through good nutrition, regular exercise, and healthful sleep.

✔ Learn how to create and cultivate close relationships with others and how to communicate your emotions to others.

✔ Engage in projects that are meaningful to you and reflect your most important inner values.

✔ Respond to challenges in life as opportunities to grow in strength and maturity. Trust that your personal resources are your greatest strengths for living and growing.

The Potential of Protection

There is a great deal of overlap between prevention and **protection**. Some people might think of immunizations (discussed in Chapter 11) as a way of preventing illness; others see them as a form of protection against dangerous diseases. In many ways, protection picks up where prevention leaves off. You can prevent STDs or unwanted pregnancy by abstaining from sex. But if you decide to engage in potentially risky sexual activities, you can protect yourself by means of condoms and spermicides (discussed in Chapter 10). Similarly, you can prevent many automobile accidents by not driving when road conditions are hazardous. But if you do have to drive, you can protect yourself by wearing a seatbelt and using defensive driving techniques (discussed in Chapter 17).

The very concept of protection implies some degree of risk—immediate and direct (for instance, the risk of intentional injury from an assailant or unintentional harm from a fire) or long-term and indirect (such as the risk of heart disease and cancer as a result of smoking). In order to know how best to protect yourself, you have to be able to assess risks realistically.

Hereditary Risks

In all, more than 4000 diseases have been traced to flaws in the basic genetic blueprints for life. "With the exception of walking across the street and being hit by a car, all disease may be genetic," says geneticist Reed Pyeritz, M.D., of Johns Hopkins School of Medicine in Baltimore. "In addition to the classical genetic disorders, most of the common diseases that get us later in life—like atherosclerosis and cancer—involve a genetic predisposition.[41]

Each individual carries about twenty abnormal genes, including seven or eight deadly ones. Most are hidden, but in combination with other genes or in certain environmental conditions, they can become dangerous. According to the American Society of Human Genetics, about 5% of adults under age 25 have a genetically linked disease; among adults over 25, 60% develop a genetically influenced disorder.

In addition to rare genetic syndromes, hereditary diseases include common problems such as certain types of cataracts, glaucoma, gall bladder disease, hypertension, nearsightedness, ulcers, and dyslexia. "The general perception is that all hereditary diseases are unalterable and deadly, but that's not the case," observes Pyeritz. "The vast majority don't necessarily shorten life, although they can cause pain and suffering."

Most adult-onset illnesses, such as cancer, heart disease, and alcoholism, are caused by the interaction of multiple genes and environmental factors. Other disorders can be traced to a single gene. If the gene is stronger, or dominant (as is the case for Huntington's chorea, a progressive, incurable brain disorder), each child of a carrier faces a 50% risk of inheriting the disease. If the gene is weaker, or recessive (as in cystic fibrosis, a disorder of the mucous and sweat glands), each child faces a 25% chance of having the disease and a 50% chance of becoming a carrier. If the X gene contributed by the mother—which joins with a Y gene from the father to create a boy or an X gene from the father to create a girl—has the harmful trait (as in hemophilia), each son has a 50% risk of inheriting the disorder; each daughter has a 50% risk of being a carrier.

In the future, millions of Americans may be able to undergo tests to find out if they have genes that increase their risk of cancer, heart disease, alcoholism, and other common problems. But how many will want to know their possible fate? "That may depend on the type of problem," says geneticist Helga Toriello, M.D., of the American Society of Human Genetics, "Knowledge can be frightening when little, if anything, can be done to alter the course of a disease. But in most cases, forewarned is forearmed."[42]

Yet genetic testing may never be able to tell individuals all they want to know. "A test can tell you only whether you have a gene or a predisposition for a disorder," says geneticist Pyeritz, "It doesn't tell you when you might develop the disease, how it might affect you, whether your symptoms will be mild or severe or what the course of the illness will be." In addition, he notes, "testing is a double-edged sword. Consumers aren't the only ones eager to find out about inherited risks. Insurance companies and employers also want to know who may be vulnerable. Testing could lead to genetic discrimination."

Testing also may provide false reassurance. "If you discover that you don't have the gene that's been linked to alcoholism, does that give you permission to drink as much as you want?" asks Toriello, pointing out that among 70 people in a recent study, 28% of those *with-*

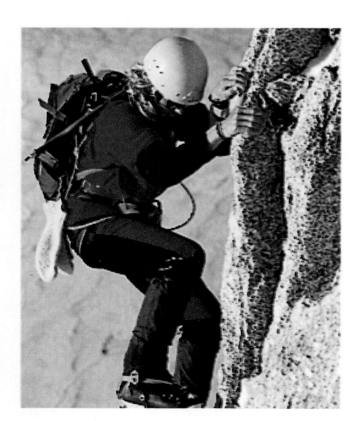

Wearing a helmet is a health choice that diminishes your risk of serious injury.

out the gene became alcohol-dependent and 23% of those *with* the gene did not.

Given the complexities and varied implications of learning about genetic risks, how much would you want to know? The answer is always profoundly personal. Knowledge can give you the power to prevent some problems or to seek early treatment for others. Yet it also can be a burden. As one woman at risk for a potentially fatal genetic disorder puts it, "You have to decide which is worse: the awful uncertainty of not knowing or the possibility of finding out that your worst fears will come true."

Assessing Risks

At this point in time, you cannot change your genes—or the risks they carry. This isn't true of all health risks. The risk of head injury is very real every single time you get on your mountain bike; however, it diminishes greatly when you put on a helmet. While the world can be a dangerous place, the greatest health threats stem from high-risk behaviors—smoking, excessive drinking, not getting enough exercise, eating too many high-fat foods, and not getting regular medical checkups, to name just a few. That's why changing unhealthy habits is the best way to reduce risks and prevent health problems.

Environmental health risks are the stuff newspaper headlines are made of (see Chapter 20 for a discussion of medical news). Every year brings calls of alarm about a new hazard to health: electromagnetic radiation, fluoride in drinking water, hair dyes, silicone implants, radon, lead. Often the public response is panic. Consumers picket and protest. Individuals arrange for elaborate testing. Yet how do we know whether or not alleged health risks are acceptable? Some key factors to consider:

- *Possible benefits.* Advantages or payoffs—such as the high salary paid for working with toxic chemicals or radioactive materials—may make some risks seem worthwhile.

- *Whether the risk is voluntary.* All of us tend to accept risks that we freely choose to take, such as playing a sport that could lead to injuries, as opposed to risks imposed on us, such as pollution from a nearby factory.

- *Is it fair?* The risk of skin cancer, which is increasing because of ozone depletion (see Chapter 21), affects us all. We may worry about it and take action to protect ourselves and our planet, but we don't resent it the way we resent living with the risk of violent

Education about health choices is a major aspect of health promotion.

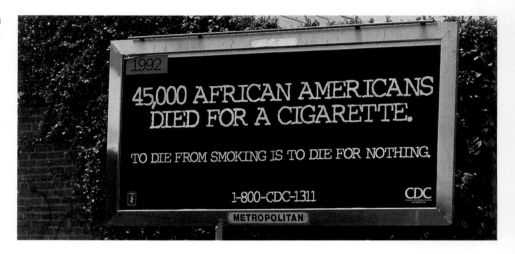

45,000 AFRICAN AMERICANS DIED FOR A CIGARETTE.

TO DIE FROM SMOKING IS TO DIE FOR NOTHING.

1-800-CDC-1311

CDC

METROPOLITAN

crime because the only housing we can afford is in a high-crime area.

- *Are there alternatives?* As consumers, we may become upset about cancer-causing pesticides or food additives when we learn about safer chemicals or methods of preservation.

- *"Framing."* Our thinking about risks often depends on how they're presented or framed—for instance, if we're told that a new drug may kill 1 out of every 100 people, instead of that it may save the lives of 99% of those who use it.

The Promise of Promotion

If the best defense is a good offense, health **promotion** represents the ultimate form of prevention and protection. The World Health Organization defines health promotion as the process of enabling people to improve and increase control over their health. Other health specialists define it as "a science and an art devoted to helping people achieve a state of optimal health."

Health promotion programs emphasize health-enhancing behaviors, such as exercising regularly; eating nutritious foods; managing stress well; avoiding tobacco, excess alcohol, and drugs; forming fulfilling relationships with friends; living in a community with clean air; and having purpose in life. They may focus on risk avoidance, such as staying out of the sun at midday, and risk reduction, such as using sunscreen.

One of the best examples of how effective health promotion can be is the dramatic reduction in smoking among young African Americans. In the past, black male teenagers started smoking earlier and in much greater numbers than white adolescents. But the African-Ameri-

can community began to send messages to its youth. Some people whitewashed billboards advertising cigarettes. Black musicians, athletes, and celebrities stopped using cigarettes in a public, glamorized way. Most powerful of all were the messages sent from teen to teen: that smoking was a bad, uncool habit that exploited the African-American community. African-American adolescents now smoke much less than white teens, with fewer than 5% of black teenagers describing themselves as regular smokers—compared with 22.9% of whites.[43]

Peer counseling—support offered by one student to another—has proven effective in many areas, from awareness of the dangers of casual, unprotected sex to education about what constitutes sexual harassment and coercion. However, often it's not enough to provide information and focus on an individual's responsibility to practice safer sex, eat less fat, exercise regularly, or stop a dangerous behavior. The reality is that all health decisions are made within the complex context of culture and community.

Increasingly, health educators are realizing that overemphasizing individual responsibility sets people up to fail and, with repeated failures, to blame themselves, even in circumstances beyond their control. A college student, for instance, may decide to eat more nutritiously. However, if the only available choices are high-fat foods in vending machines and campus cafeterias, all the good intentions and willpower in the world won't lead to success.

Many health promotion efforts look beyond the campus to make the same opportunities for nutritious food, leisure, exercise, and support open to others. To develop social responsibility in students, they encourage volunteering at community centers, homeless shelters, nursing homes, environmental agencies, and advocacy groups. Their goal is to help students define health, not

Personal Health 1.3 INTERACTIVE

Health Online

MedAccess Motivator   http://www2.medaccess.com/motivatorCF.login.cfm

The MedAccess Motivator is a site you can visit again and again to establish and achieve your personal wellness goals. This page first sets your baseline profile and helps you think through your own health goals based on a series of questions. It will then help you track your progress; give you advice, information, and behavior change contracts; and help you start or join a support group if you wish.

Think about it ...

- What health goals did you come up with using the MedAccess Motivator? Were they things that you had previously identified as goals, or did you come up with some new ones?

- What advantages, if any, would using an electronic system like MedAccess Motivator have over low-tech methods like using a paper and pencil to work out a behavior change plan?

- Try keeping track of your progress in meeting one health goal every day for one week. Does using a Web site help you stay motivated? What improvements could be made in this site?

only in terms of their own behaviors and well-being, but also in terms of what they can do to reach out and help others in the broader community make healthier choices and changes.

Making This Book Work for You
Taking Charge of Your Future

Through every chapter of this book, you'll recognize some familiar themes, messages that apply to every aspect of your health. Among the most important are the following:

- You're not simply a creature of mind, body, or spirit, but of all three. Physical, psychological, spiritual, social, intellectual, and environmental factors are interrelated in complex and crucial ways that affect your health.

- Prevention has the power to enhance the quality and duration of your life. Rather than waiting for bad health habits to take their toll, you can delay or eliminate many problems by adopting healthful behaviors now.

- Positive lifestyle changes—the basics of health promotion—enhance your health and enrich your well-being.

- You can take charge of your health and prevent illness by changing your health behaviors. The keys to success are motivation, accurate information, workable strategies, and a belief in your ability to change.

- You are not alone. Your ties to the people around you and to the environment in which you live give richness and meaning to your life.

- You face undeniable risks in life, but you can do a great deal to avoid or minimize their impact on your well-being.

To help safeguard your health, you need to understand basic theories about human health and life and to have up-to-date information about health practices. With the aid of your health instructors, *An Invitation to Health* can provide the basic knowledge and skills you need for a lifetime of well-being. But knowledge isn't enough; action is the key. The habits you form now, the decisions you make, and the ways in which you live day by day will all shape your health and your future.

This book can give you the understanding you'll need to make good decisions and establish a healthy lifestyle, but you can't simply read and study health the way you study French or chemistry—you must decide to live it.

This is our invitation to you.

Key Terms

The terms listed here are used within the chapter. Page numbers are included for each term.
A definition of each term is given in the green Glossary pages at the end of this book.

health *16*

locus of control *31*

norms *30*

prevention *33*

promotion *36*

protection *34*

reinforcements *31*

self-efficacy *31*

self-talk *31*

wellness *16*

Review Questions

1. What are the dimensions of health? How do they relate to total wellness?

2. How does lifestyle affect health prevention?

3. What strategies can promote wellness? What are some possible benefits of practicing these strategies?

4. What kinds of factors shape the development of health behavior? How so?

5. What should health-care providers know about cultural and gender differences? Why?

6. What are some overall strengths and weaknesses of the health of college students?

7. What could you do to change or develop a health behavior on your own? What kinds of strategies might you use? What could be the benefits?

Critical Thinking Questions

1. What is the definition of health according to the textbook? Does your personal definition differ from this, and if so, in what ways? How would you have defined health before reading this chapter?

2. Where do you lie on the wellness-illness continuum? What variables might affect your place on the scale? What do you consider your optimum state of health to be?

3. In what ways would you like to change your present lifestyle? What steps could you take to make those changes?

Connections to Personal Health Interactive

To enhance your understanding of the material covered in this chapter, check out the following study aids on the Personal Health Interactive CD-ROM. Each numbered icon within the chapter corresponds to an appropriate activity listed here.

1.1 Personal Insights: How Healthy Are You?

1.2 Wellness Clinic

1.3 Ethics in Research

1.4 Chapter 1 Review

References

1. "Constitution of the World Health Organization." *Chronicle of the World Health Organization*. Geneva, Switzerland: WHO, 1947.
2. Gordon, James. Personal interview. Institute of Noetic Sciences with William Poole. *The Heart of Healing*. Atlanta:

Turner Publishing, 1993. Hales, Dianne, and Robert Hales. *Caring for the Mind*. New York: Bantam Books, 1995.
3. Cunningham, Alastair. "Pies, Levels and Languages: Why the Contribution of Mind to Health Has Been Underesti-

mated." *Advances: The Journal of Mind-Body Health,* Vol. 11, No. 2, Spring 1995. Smith, Roger. "Does Spirit Matter?" *Advances: The Journal of Mind-Body Health*, Winter 1992.

4. Cool, Lisa Collier. "Faith and Healing." *American Health*, November 1997.

5. Harris, T. George. "Harvard's Healing Prayer." *Spirituality & Health*, Vol. 1, No. 1, May 1998.

6. Scott, Robert Owens. "The Most Important Health Factor Your Doctor Isn't Talking About." *Spirituality & Health*, preview issue, Fall 1996.

7. Cool, "Faith and Healing."

8. Benson, Herbert. *Timeless Healing*. New York: Scribner's, 1996.

9. "Health: That's What Friend & Family Are For." *Facts of Life: An Issue Briefing for Health Reporters from the Center for Advancement of Health*, Vol. 2, No. 6, November–December 1997.

10. Woloshin, S., et al. "Perceived Adequacy of Tangible Social Support and Health Outcomes in Patients with Coronary Artery Disease." *Journal of General Internal Medicine*, October 1997.

11. Cohen, Sheldon et al. "Social Ties and Susceptibility to the Common Cold." *Journal of the American Medical Association*, June 25, 1997.

12. "Births and Deaths, United States: 1996." National Center for Health Statistics, released September 11, 1997.

13. Ibid.

14. Crose, Royda. *Why Women Live Longer Than Men*. San Francisco: Jossey-Bass, 1997.

15. Commonwealth Fund Commission on Women's Health. "Women's Health-Related Behaviors and Use of Clinical Preventive Services." Los Angeles: UCLA Center for Health Policy Research, 1995.

16. Haseltine, Florence. *Women's Health Research*. Washington, DC: American Psychiatric Press, 1997.

17. *Healthy People 2000 Midcourse Review* and *Development of Healthy People 2010 Objectives*. Office of Disease Prevention and Health Promotion, Department of Health and Human Services.

18. Clements, Mark, and Dianne Hales. "How Healthy Are We?" *Parade Magazine*, September 7, 1997.

19. Blendon, Robert, et al. "How White and African Americans View Their Health and Social Problems." *Journal of the American Medical Association*, Vol. 273, No. 4, January 25, 1995.

20. Voelker, Rebecca. "Speaking the Languages of Medicine and Culture." *Journal of the American Medical Association*, Vol. 273, No. 21, June 7, 1995.

21. Beckham, Edgar. "Diversity Opens Doors to All." *New York Times Education Supplement*, January 5, 1997.

22. Goldsmith, Marsha. "Polished or Tarnished, the Golden Door." *Journal of the American Medical Association*, Vol. 273, No. 21, June 7, 1995. Sullivan, Mary. "Improved Health for Women and Minorities Is of Major Importance to NIH." *NIH News & Features*, Spring 1995.

23. "Births and Deaths, United States: 1996."

24. Ibid.

25. Legato, Marianne. *Gender-Specific Aspects of Human Biology for the Practicing Physician*. Armonk, NY: Futura Publishing, 1997.

26. Ibid.

27. Ibid.

28. Marchand, Lorraine. "Minorities Benefit from Diabetes Research." *NIH News & Features*, Spring 1995.

29. "Study Details Health of Chinese-Americans." *American Medical News*, May 18, 1992.

30. Department of Health and Human Services.

31. Ibid.

32. Douglas, Kathy, et al. "Results from the 1995 National College Health Risk Behavior Study." *Journal of American College Health*, Vol. 46, September 1997.

33. Winkelby, Marilyn, et al. "Education Is a Better Predictor of Health Than Wealth." *American Journal of Public Health*, June 1992.

34. Georgiou, Constance, et al. "Among Young Adults, College Students and Graduates Practiced More Healthful Habits and Made More Healthful Food Choices Than Did Nonstudents." *Journal of the American Dietetic Association*, Vol. 97, No. 7, July 1997.

35. Bandura, Albert. *Self-Efficacy in Changing Societies*. Cambridge, Eng: Cambridge University Press, 1995.

36. O'Brien, William, et al. "Predicting Health Behaviors Using Measures of Optimism and Perceived Risk." *Health Values*, Vol. 19. No. 1, January–February 1995.

37. Chen, William. "Enhancement of Health Locus of Control Through Biofeedback Training." *Perceptual and Motor Skills*, Vol. 80, No. 2, April 1995.

38. Steenbarger, Brett, et al. "Prevention in College Health: Counseling Perspectives." *Journal of American College Health*, Vol. 43, January 1995.

39. Jones, Laurie. "Does Prevention Save Money?" *American Medical News*, January 9, 1995. Knapp, Jane. "A Call to Action: Institute of Medicine Report on Emergency Medical Services for Children." *Pediatrics*, Vol. 98, No. 2, July 10, 1995.

40. Ibid.

41. Pyeritz, Reed, personal interview.

42. Toriello, Helga, personal interview.

43. "African American College Students' Health Behaviors and Perceptions of Related Health Issues." *Journal of American College Health*, Vol. 42, No. 5, March 1994.

CHAPTER 2

MANAGING STRESS

After studying the material in this chapter, you should be able to:

Define stress and stressors and **use** the general adaptation syndrome to explain how stress relates to health.

List some personal causes of stress, especially those felt by students, and **discuss** how their effects can be prevented or minimized.

List the major social stressors and **explain** how these can cause stress.

Describe the symptoms of stress-related adjustment disorders.

Explain the relationship of stress to heart disease, high blood pressure, the immune system, and digestive disorders.

Explain how you can improve your resistance to stress, and **describe** some techniques to help manage stress.

You know about stress. You live with it every day: the stress of passing exams, preparing for a career, meeting people, facing new experiences. Everyone, regardless of age, gender, race, or income, has to deal with stress—as an individual and as a member of society.

Yet stress in itself isn't necessarily bad. An individual's response to stress, not the stressful situation itself, is what matters most. Stress always involves an interaction between a life situation and a person's ability to cope. Perhaps one of the best ways to think of it is captured by the Chinese word for crisis, which consists of two characters— one means danger; the other, opportunity. Stress involves both.

By learning to anticipate stressful events, to manage day-to-day stress, and to prevent stress overload, you can find alternatives to running endlessly on a treadmill of alarm, panic, and exhaustion. The stress-management skills in this chapter provide a good start. As you organize your time, release tension, and build up internal resources, you will begin to experience the sense of control and confidence that makes stress a challenge rather than an ordeal.

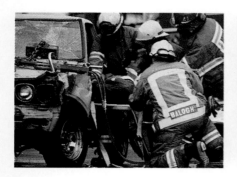 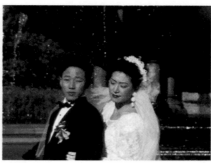

Types of stressors. An automobile accident is an example of an acute stressor. Getting married is an example of a positive stressor.

What Is Stress?

People use the word "stress" in different ways: as an external force that causes a person to become tense or upset, as the internal state of arousal, and as the physical response of the body to various demands. Dr. Hans Selye, a pioneer in studying physiological responses to challenge, defined **stress** as "the nonspecific response of the body to any demand made upon it." In other words, the body reacts to **stressors**—the things that upset or excite us—in the same way, regardless of whether they are positive or negative. A stressor may be a bomb threat in a crowded stadium, a pop quiz, or a parent's announcement of a divorce or remarriage, but the body's response is always the same.

Some of life's happiest moments—births, reunions, weddings—are enormously stressful. We weep with the stress of frustration or loss; we weep, too, with the stress of love and joy. Selye coined the term **eustress** for positive stress in our lives (*eu* is a Greek prefix meaning "good"). Eustress challenges us to grow, adapt, and find creative solutions in our lives. **Distress** refers to the negative effects of stress that can deplete or even destroy life energy. Ideally, the level of stress in our lives should be just high enough to motivate us to satisfy our needs and not so high that it interferes with our ability to reach our fullest potential.

The key to coping with stress is realizing that your *perception* and *response* to a stressor are crucial. Changing the way you interpret events or situations—a skill called *reframing*—makes all the difference. An event, such as a move to a new city, is not stressful in itself. A move becomes stressful if you see it as a traumatic upheaval rather than an exciting beginning of a new chapter in your life.

To get a sense of your own stress level, ask yourself the following questions about the preceding week of your life:

- How often have you felt out of control?
- How often have you felt confident that you'd be able to handle personal problems?
- How often have you felt things were generally going your way?
- How often have you felt that things were piling up so high you'd never be able to catch up?

Think through your answers. If the experiences of being out of control or overwhelmed outnumbered those of confidence and control, it's time to develop a stress-management plan and put it into action.

Theories of Stress

There are many biological theories of stress. The best known may be the **general adaptation syndrome (GAS),** developed by Hans Selye, who postulated that our bodies constantly strive to maintain a stable and consistent physiological state. This is called **homeostasis.** Stressors, whether in the form of physical illness or a demanding job, disturb this state and trigger a nonspecific physiological response. The body attempts to restore homeostasis by means of an **adaptive response.**

Selye's general adaptation syndrome (GAS), which describes the body's response to a stressor—whether threatening or exhilarating—consists of three distinct stages:

1. *Alarm.* When a stressor first occurs, the body responds with changes that temporarily lower resistance. Levels of certain hormones may rise; blood pressure may increase (see Figure 2-1). The body quickly makes internal adjustments so it can cope with the stressor and return to normal activity.

2. *Resistance.* If the stressor continues, the body mobilizes its internal resources to try to sustain homeostasis. For example, if a loved one is seriously hurt in an accident, we initially respond very intensely and feel great anxiety. During the subsequent stressful period of recuperation, we struggle to carry on as normally as possible, but this requires considerable effort.

3. *Exhaustion.* If the stress continues long enough, we cannot keep up our normal functioning. Even a small amount of additional stress at this point can cause a breakdown.

Another theory—the cognitive-transactional model of stress, developed by Richard Lazarus—looks at the relation between stress and health. As he sees it, stress can have a powerful impact on health. Conversely, health can affect a person's resistance or coping ability. Stress, according to Lazarus, is "neither an environmental stimulus, a characteristic of the person, nor a response, but a relationship between demands and the power to deal with them without unreasonable or destructive costs."[1] Thus, an event may be seen as stressful by one person but not by another, or it may seem stressful on one occasion but not on another. For instance, one student may think of speaking in front of the class as extremely stressful, while another relishes the chance to do so—except on days when he's not well-prepared. Other researchers have confirmed that self-perceptions play a role in the relation between stress and psychological well-being and that self-esteem also may be important, particularly for college students.[2]

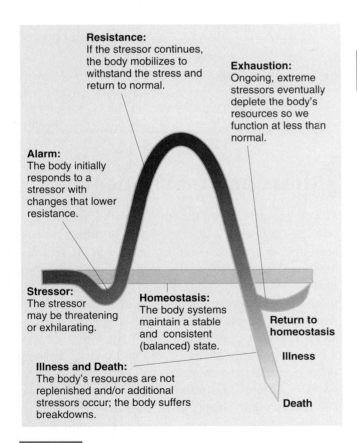

Figure 2-1 The three stages of Selye's General Adaptation Syndrome (GAS): Alarm, resistance, exhaustion.

Strategies for Prevention

Putting Stress in Perspective

In *Stress Without Distress*, Hans Selye offers these guidelines:

✔ Admit that there is no perfection. But in each category of achievement something is tops; be satisfied to strive for that.

✔ Do not underestimate the delight of real simplicity.

✔ Whatever situation you meet in life, consider first whether it is really worth fighting for.

✔ Try to keep your mind on the pleasant aspects of life and on actions that improve your situation. Nothing paralyzes your efficiency more than frustration; nothing helps it more than success.

✔ Even after the greatest defeats, combat the depressing thought of being a failure by taking stock of all your past achievements, which no one can deny you.

✔ When faced with a task that is very painful yet indispensable to achieve your aim, don't procrastinate.

✔ Finally, do not forget that there is no ready-made success formula that would suit everybody.

The Challenge of Change

Life never stops changing. In childhood, we must leave our parents when we begin school and learn how to make friends on our own. As teenagers, we must come to terms with the physical transformation of our bodies and with new responsibilities and freedoms. As young adults, we must set goals and directions for our lives and establish close supportive relationships. After you graduate, you will face a never-ending series of changes as you become an employee, homeowner, spouse, parent. By anticipating these potential stressors, you can plan ways to cope and reduce their impact.

Some of us are more vulnerable to life changes and crises than are others. The stress of growing up in families troubled by alcoholism, drug dependence, or physical, sexual, or psychological abuse may have a lifelong impact—particularly if these problems are not recognized and dealt with. Other early experiences, positive and negative, also can affect our attitude toward stress—and our resilience to it. Our general outlook on life, whether we're optimistic or pessimistic, can determine whether we expect the worst and feel stressed or anticipate a challenge and feel confident. The when, where, what, how, and why of stressors also affect our reactions. The number and frequency of changes in our lives, along with the time and setting in which they occur, have a great impact on how we'll respond.

Stressors can be *acute* (such as a parent's death), *sequential* (such as the series of lifestyle changes that occur after a baby's birth), *intermittent* (such as monthly bills or weekly tests), or *chronic* (such as living in a dangerous, high-crime neighborhood). (See Figure 2-2.) Our level of ongoing stress affects our ability to respond to a new day's stressors. Each of us has a breaking point for dealing with stress. A series of too-intense pressures or too-rapid changes can push us closer and closer to that point. That's why it's important to anticipate potential stressors and plan how to deal with them.

Stress experts Thomas Holmes, M.D., and Richard Rahe, M.D., devised a scale to evaluate individual levels of stress and potential for coping, based on *life-change units* that estimate each change's impact. The death of a partner or parent ranks high on the list, but even changing apartments is considered a stressor. People who accumulate more than 300 life-change units in a year are more likely to suffer serious health problems. Scores on the scale, however, represent "potential stress"; the actual impact of the life change depends on the individual's response. (See Self-Survey: "Student Stress Scale.")

In ongoing research, Holmes has evaluated variations in life events among many groups, including college students, medical students, football players, pregnant women, alcoholics, and heroin addicts. Heroin addicts and alcoholics have the highest totals of life-change units, followed by college students. In general, younger people experience more life changes than do older people; factors such as gender, education, and social class also have a strong impact.[3] Marriage seems to promote greater stability and fewer changes.

If you score high on the Student Stress Scale, think about the reasons your life has been in such turmoil. Are there any steps you could take to make your life more stable? Of course, some changes, such as your parents' divorce or a friend's accident, may be beyond your control. Even then, you can respond in ways that may protect you from disease. One of the best is letting out negative feelings, such as anger, frustration, or sorrow, by either talking or writing them down.

Strategies for Prevention

Adapting to Change: The Three R's

✔ *Recover.* Everyone needs time to regain a sense of balance. After a transition, trauma, setback, or loss, allow yourself time to get in touch with how you're feeling.

✔ *Refocus.* Change creates a mixed array of feelings, and you need to sort these out. Think through what has happened, why, and where it might lead.

✔ *Regenerate.* Take extra good care of yourself. Rest, eat nutritiously, exercise regularly. Draw on your personal sources of support, such as faith, family, and friends.

Stress and the Student

You've probably heard that these are the best years of your life, but being a student—full-time or part-time, in your late teens, early twenties, or later in life—can be extremely stressful. You may feel pressure to perform well to qualify for a good job or graduate school. To meet steep tuition payments, you may have to juggle part-time work and coursework. You may feel stressed about choosing a major, getting along with a difficult roommate, passing a particularly hard course, or living up to your parents' and teachers' expectations. If you're an older student, you may have children, housework, and homework to balance. Your days may seem so busy and your life so full that you worry about coming apart at the seams. One thing is for certain: You're not alone.[4]

According to surveys of students at colleges and universities around the country and the world, stress

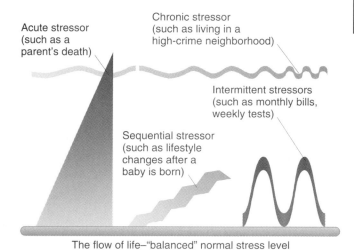

Figure 2-2

The varieties of stress. Individuals react differently to stress, and life presents stress in a variety of levels and intensities.

Self-Survey

Student Stress Scale

The Student Stress Scale, an adaptation of Holmes and Rahe's Life Events Scale for college-age adults, provides a rough indication of stress levels and possible health consequences.

In the Student Stress Scale, each event, such as beginning or ending school, is given a score that represents the amount of readjustment one has to make as a result of the change. In some studies, using similar scales, people with serious illnesses have been found to have high scores.

To determine your stress score, add up the number of points corresponding to the events you have experienced in the past twelve months.

1. Death of a close family member	100
2. Death of a close friend	73
3. Divorce of parents	65
4. Jail term	63
5. Major personal injury or illness	63
6. Marriage	58
7. Getting fired from a job	50
8. Failing an important course	47
9. Change in the health of a family member	45
10. Pregnancy	45
11. Sex problems	44
12. Serious argument with a close friend	40
13. Change in financial status	39
14. Change of academic major	39
15. Trouble with parents	39
16. New girlfriend or boyfriend	37
17. Increase in workload at school	37
18. Outstanding personal achievement	36
19. First quarter/semester in college	36
20. Change in living conditions	31
21. Serious argument with an instructor	30
22. Getting lower grades than expected	29
23. Change in sleeping habits	29
24. Change in social activities	29
25. Change in eating habits	28
26. Chronic car trouble	26
27. Change in number of family get togethers	26
28. Too many missed classes	25
29. Changing colleges	24
30. Dropping more than one class	23
31. Minor traffic violations	20

Total Stress Score _____

Here's how to interpret your score: If your score is 300 or higher, you're at high risk for developing a health problem. If your score is between 150 and 300, you have a fifty-fifty chance of experiencing a serious health change within two years. If your score is below 150, you have a one-in-three chance of a serious health change.

Making Changes
Coping with Life Changes

If you're going through a lot of change, you can take steps to minimize harmful effects. Here are some suggestions:
- Review the Student Stress Scale often so you're familiar with different life events and the amount of stress they can cause.
- When change occurs, think about its meaning and your feelings about it.
- Try to come up with different ways of adjusting to the change.
- Don't rush into action; take time to make a careful decision.
- Pace yourself. Even if you have a lot to do, stick to a reasonable schedule that allows you some time off to relax.
- Look at each change as a part of life's natural flow, rather than as a disruption in the way things should be.

Source: Mullen, Kathleen, and Gerald Costello. *Health Awareness Through Discovery.*

levels are consistently high and stressors are remarkably similar.[5] Among the most common are:
- Test pressures.
- Financial problems.
- Frustrations, such as delays in reaching goals.
- Problems in friendships and dating relationships.
- Daily hassles.
- Academic failure.
- Pressures as a result of competition, deadlines, and the like.
- Changes, which may be unpleasant, disruptive, or too frequent.

Campus life can be rather overwhelming at first, especially as a freshman with everything to learn.

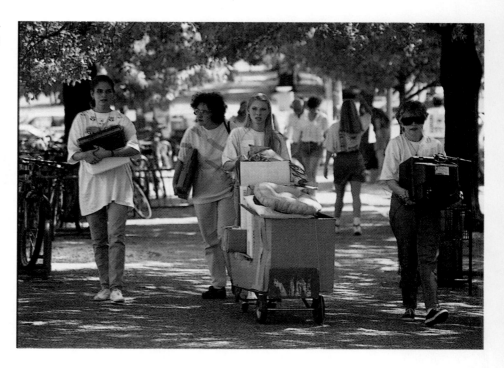

• Losses, whether caused by the breakup of a relationship or the death of a loved one.

   During their first year at school the self-esteem of college freshmen typically falls, but students recover their self-confidence in their second year. They become more positive, introspective, and independent and have a stronger sense of their own intellectual ability. It may well be that as students acclimate to college, they experience less stress and therefore view themselves more positively.[6]

   In some studies, certain groups of students, such as women and Asian Americans, report higher levels of stress and more intense reactions to stressors.[7] Students say they react to stress in various ways: physiologically (by sweating, stuttering, trembling, or developing physical symptoms); emotionally (by becoming anxious, fearful, angry, guilty, or depressed); behaviorally (by crying, eating, smoking, being irritable or abusive); or cognitively (by thinking about and analyzing stressful situations and strategies that might be useful in dealing with them). Social support makes a big difference.[8] Students with a truly supportive network of friends and family available to them report greater satisfaction and less psychological distress. This is particularly true of certain cultures, such as Hispanic, that place great value on the family.[9]

Strategies for Prevention

Reaching Out for Support

✔ If you move away from home to go to college, stay in touch with at least one friend. It's worth the effort to keep people you cherish in your life.

✔ Try different forms of "networking"—e-mail, online, chat rooms, campus clubs, support groups.

✔ Check in with siblings. The bossy big sister and devilish little brother have done the same thing you did: They've grown up. Get to know each other as adults who share memories of the past as well as plans for the future.

✔ Make time for friends. Even half an hour for a quiet lunch or a cup of coffee with a friend can keep a relationship close.

✔ Be the kind of friend you'd like to have. If you listen when your friends need to talk, if you're considerate and caring, they will be, too.

Test Stress

For many students, midterms and final exams are the most stressful times of the year. Studies at various colleges and universities found that the incidence of colds and flu soared during finals. The reason seems to be that

Pulsepoints

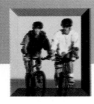

Top Ten Stress Busters

1. Strive for balance. Review your commitments and plans, and if necessary, scale down.

2. Get the facts. When faced with a change or challenge, seek accurate information, which can bring vague fears down to earth.

3. Talk with someone you trust. A friend or a health professional can offer valuable perspective as well as psychological support.

4. Sweat away stress. Even when your schedule gets jammed, carve out 20 or 30 minutes several times a week to walk, swim, bicycle, jog, or work out at the gym.

5. Express yourself in writing. Keeping a journal is one of the best ways to put your problems into perspective.

6. Take care of yourself. Get enough sleep. Eat a balanced diet. Limit your use of sugar, salt, and caffeine, which can compound stress by leading to fatigue and irritability. Watch your alcohol intake. Drinking can cut down on your ability to cope.

7. Set priorities. Making a list of things you need to do and ranking their impor-

tance helps direct your energies so you're more efficient and less stressed.

8. Help others. One of the most effective ways of dealing with stress is to find people in a worse situation and do something positive for them.

9. Cultivate hobbies. Pursuing a personal pleasure can distract you from the stressors in your life and help you relax.

10. Master a form of relaxation. Whether you choose meditation, yoga, mindfulness, or another technique, practice it regularly.

stress depresses the levels of the protective immune cells that ward off viruses. Students who don't come down with infections during exams often feel the impact of test stress in other ways. Many suffer headaches, upset stomachs, skin flareups, or insomnia.[10]

Test stress affects different people in different ways. Sometimes students become so preoccupied with the possibility of failing that they can't concentrate on studying. Others, including many of the best and brightest students, freeze up during tests and can't comprehend multiple-choice questions or write essay answers, even if they know the material.

The students most susceptible to exam stress are those who believe they'll do poorly and who see tests as extremely threatening. Unfortunately, such negative thoughts often become a self-fulfilling prophecy. As they study, these students keep wondering, "What good will studying do? I never do well on tests." As their fear increases, they try harder, pulling all-nighters. Fueled by caffeine, munching on sugary snacks, they become edgy and find it harder and harder to concentrate. By the time of the test, they're nervous wrecks, scarcely able to sit still and focus on the exam.

Can you do anything to reduce test stress and feel more in control? Absolutely. One way is to defuse stress through relaxation. In a study by researchers Janice

Kiecolt-Glaser and Ron Glaser of Ohio State University, one group of students was taught relaxation techniques—such as controlled breathing, meditation, progressive relaxation, and guided imagery (visualization)—a month before finals. The more the students used these "stress busters," the higher were their levels of immune cells during the exam period. The extra payoff was that they felt calmer and in better control during their tests.[11] (See Pulsepoints: "Top Ten Stress Busters.")

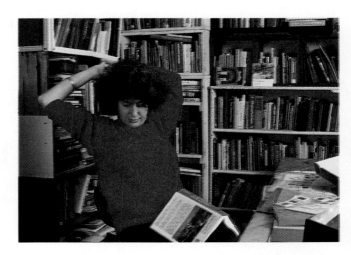

A stretch break and a few deep breaths will help make your studying more effective and will help keep your stress level down.

Strategies for Prevention

Defusing Test Stress

✔ *Plan ahead.* A month before finals, map out a study schedule for each course. Set aside a small amount of time every day or every other day to review the course materials.

✔ *Be positive.* Instead of dwelling on any past failures, focus on how well you will do when you are well prepared and confident. Picture yourself taking your final exam. Imagine yourself walking into the exam room feeling confident, opening up the test booklet, and seeing questions for which you know the answers.

✔ *Take regular breaks.* Get up from your desk, breathe deeply, stretch, and visualize a pleasant scene. You'll feel more refreshed than you would if you chugged another cup of coffee.

✔ *Practice.* Some teachers are willing to give practice finals to prepare students for test situations, or you and your friends can make up tests for each other.

✔ *Talk to other students.* Chances are that many of them share your fears about test taking and may have discovered some helpful techniques of their own. Sometimes talking to your adviser or a counselor can also help.

✔ *Be satisfied with doing your best.* You can't expect to ace every test; all you can and should expect is your best effort. Once you've completed the exam, allow yourself the sweet pleasure of relief that it's over.

Minority Stressors

Regardless of your race or ethnic background, college may bring culture shock. You may never have encountered such a degree of diversity in one setting. You probably will meet students with different values, unfamiliar customs, entirely new ways of looking at the world—experiences you may find both stimulating and stressful.

If you're a minority student, you may feel a double burden. In addition to academic demands, financial worries, and the usual campus stressors, many students from racial and cultural minority groups report extra stressors that can be, as one researcher put it, "both the cause and the effect of academic difficulty."[12] Various reports have shown that African-American and non-Asian minority students at predominantly white colleges have lower grade point averages, experience higher attrition rates, and are less likely to graduate within five years or to enter graduate programs than are white students or minority students at institutions that are not predominantly white. They also experience college as more stressful and report greater feelings of not belonging.[13]

All minority students share some common stressors. In one study of minority freshmen entering a large, competitive university, Asian, Latino, Filipino, African-American, and Native-American students all felt more sensitive and vulnerable to the college social climate, to interpersonal tensions between themselves and nonminority students and faculty, to experiences of actual or perceived racism, and to racist attitudes and discrimination (discussed later in this chapter, under Societal Stressors). Despite scoring above the national average on the SAT, the minority students in this study did not feel accepted as legitimate students and sensed that others viewed them as unworthy beneficiaries of affirmative action initiatives. While most said that overt racism was rare and relatively easy to deal with, they reported subtle pressures that undermined their academic confidence and their ability to bond with the university. Balancing these stressors, however, was a strong sense of ethnic identity, which helped buffer some stressful effects.[14]

The roots of stress are complex and different for members of various minority groups. For instance, some African-American students tend to view white campuses as hostile, alienating, and socially isolating and to report greater estrangement from the campus community and heightened discomfort in interactions with faculty and peers.[15] Although their rates of depression are similar to those of Caucasian students, they often report higher levels of anxiety.[16] Latino students have identified three major types of stressors in their college experiences: academic (related to exam preparation and faculty interaction), social (related to ethnicity and interpersonal competence), and financial (related to their economic situation).[17]

Diversity exists within as well as among particular cultural groups, and this, too, can create stress. With more than 30 different cultures represented in the Asian-American community, for instance, there are divisions along class, ethnic, and generational lines. Some Asian students who recently immigrated to the United States report feeling ostracized by students of similar ancestry who are second- or third-generation Americans. While they take pride in being truly bicultural and bilingual, the newcomers feel ambivalent about mainstream American culture. "My parents stress the importance of traditions; my friends tell me to get with it and act like an American," says one Asian-born student who has spent five years in the United States. "I feel trapped between cultures."

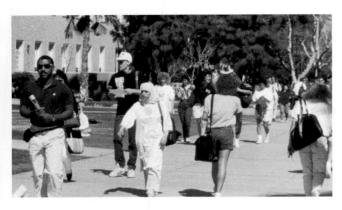

On campus, minority students often feel the stresses of college life as well as the stress of discrimination, however subtle.

Preparing for the Future

In addition to their here-and-now concerns, college students face another source of stress: concern about establishing careers after graduation. For today's students, the outlook is brighter than in the past decade. By 2005, according to the Bureau of Labor Statistics, employment will grow by 26 million jobs.[18]

More so than ever, preparation means education—and it does pay off. In the course of their careers, college graduates earn 77% more than those without degrees, reports economist John Sargent of the Bureau of Labor Statistics, who notes that "the occupations that require the most education—and, coincidentally, have the highest earnings—will be growing the fastest in the next ten years." At least a third of the fastest-growing fields, including health care and computer sciences, generally require a bachelor's degree.

Strategies for Prevention

Preparing for the World of Work

✔ Take school seriously. Whatever you do, you're going to need to know how to express yourself effectively, work with figures, and master basic skills.

✔ Develop specialized skills. Familiarize yourself with different computer systems and software. Learn a language or study abroad, if possible.

✔ Acquire a range of experiences. By volunteering and participating in extracurricular activities, you can learn valuable skills—how to work as part of a team, motivate others, plan a major event.

✔ Get a part-time or summer job. Work experience shows that you're reliable, gives you references, and helps you discover what type of work suits you best.

✔ Become an intern or "temp." Paid or unpaid internships and temporary jobs provide a good opportunity to gain experience, make contacts, and utilize your skills.

Other Personal Stressors

At every stage of life, you will encounter challenges and stressors. Among the most common are those related to work, overwork, illness, and disability.

Job Stress

More so than ever, many people find that they are working more and enjoying it less. In 1969, the average American laborer worked 1786 hours a year, according to Harvard economist Juliet Schor, Ph.D., author of *The Overworked American: The Unexpected Decline of Leisure*. Twenty years later the annual average was up to 1949 hours per worker, the equivalent of an extra month a year.[19] By 1994, American blue-collar workers were putting in 2007 hours a year, while other workers in other nations were reducing their hours on the job. According to sociologist John Robinson, Ph.D., director of the Americans' Use of Time Project at the University of Maryland, working parents are under the most severe time pressure in society today: Men and women between the ages 30 and 50—the peak time for parenting—have less free time than do younger or older individuals.[20] Meanwhile, the technological wizardry that was supposed to make life easier—cellular phones, modems, faxes, laptop computers—has simply extended the boundaries of where and when we work. As a result, more people are caught up in an exhausting cycle of overwork, which causes stress, which makes work harder, which leads to more stress.[21]

Yet work in itself is not hazardous to health. Attitudes about work and habits related to how we work are the true threats. In fact, a job—stressful or not, enjoyable or not—can be therapeutic for survivors of heart attacks. According to a recent study sponsored by the National Institute of Mental Health, 90% of heart attack patients who returned to work showed decreased emotional distress—compared to increased distress among those who chose not to return to their jobs. "Even in patients who previously disliked their jobs, we found that resumption of employment substantially enhanced their psychological well-being," explains researcher Kathryn Rost of the University of Arkansas.[22]

Workaholism and Burnout

People who become obsessed by their work and careers can turn into *workaholics,* so caught up in racing toward the top that they forget what they're racing toward and why. In some cases they throw themselves into their work to mask or avoid painful feelings or difficulties in their own lives. One consequence is **burnout**, a state of physical, emotional, and mental exhaustion brought on by constant or repeated emotional pressure. Particularly in the helping professions, such as social work or nursing, men and women who've dedicated themselves to others may realize they have nothing left in themselves to give.[23]

The early signs of burnout include exhaustion, sleep problems or nightmares, increased anxiety or nervousness, muscular tension (headaches, backaches, and the like), increased use of alcohol or medication, digestive problems, such as nausea, vomiting, or diarrhea, loss of interest in sex, frequent body aches or pain, quarrels with family or friends, negative feelings about everything, problems concentrating, job mistakes and accidents, and feelings of depression, hopelessness, and helplessness. The best way to avoid burnout is learning to cope well with smaller, day-to-day stresses. Then, tiny frustrations won't smolder into a blaze that may be impossible to put out.[24]

Strategies for Prevention

Preventing Burnout

✔ Develop healthy lifestyle habits, which will enhance your resistance to stress and ability to cope.

✔ Learn to recognize situations that you cannot change so that you don't waste energy trying to change them.

✔ Draw a line between your personal life and your professional responsibilities. Don't let problems with one affect the other.

✔ Practice at least one stress-management technique (exercise, meditation, relaxation, and so on) regularly.

✔ Develop positive outlets (such as exercise) instead of negative addictions (such as smoking or drinking).

Illness and Disability

Just as the mind can have profound effects on the body, the body can have an enormous impact on our emo-

tions. Whenever we come down with the flu or pull a muscle, we feel under par. When the problem is more serious or persistent—a chronic disease like diabetes, for instance, or a lifelong hearing impairment—the emotional stress of constantly coping with it is even greater.

A common source of stress for college students is a learning disability, which affects one of every ten Americans.[25] Most learning-disabled have average or above-average intelligence, but they rarely live up to their ability in school. Some have only one area of difficulty, such as reading or math. Others have problems with attention, writing, communicating, reasoning, coordination, social competence, and emotional maturity—all of which may make it difficult, if not impossible, for them to find and keep jobs. Special training and a better understanding of what's wrong can make an enormous difference.

Learning disorders can be hard to recognize in adults, who often become adept at covering up or compensating for their difficulties. However, someone with a learning disability may be

- Unable to engage in a focused activity such as reading.
- Extremely distractible, forgetful, or absent-minded.
- Easily frustrated by waiting, delays, or traffic.
- Disorganized, unable to manage time efficiently and complete tasks on time.
- Hot-tempered, explosive, constantly irritated.
- Impulsive, making decisions with little reflection or information.
- Easily overwhelmed by ordinary hassles.
- Clumsy, with a poor body image and poor sense of direction.
- Emotionally immature.
- Physically restless.

Individuals with several of these characteristics should undergo diagnostic tests to evaluate their skills and abilities and to determine whether remedial training, available through state offices of vocational rehabilitation, can help. (See Personal Voices: "Living with a Learning Disability.")

Societal Stressors

Not all stressors are personal. Centuries ago the poet John Donne observed that no man is an island. Today, on an increasingly crowded and troubled planet, these

Personal Voices   Living with a Learning Disability

When Tom was growing up, no one knew about learning disabilities. His kindergarten teacher wrote "M.R." (for mentally retarded) on his permanent record, so his teachers wrote him off. The other kids called him "dummy" and "blockhead" and laughed at him because he couldn't read or write well. He just thought he was stupid. It wasn't until he was 27 years old that he finally found out that he's not.

If he's tested orally, Tom's IQ is 135, which is very high, but his brain doesn't work the way others do. "Imagine taping a piece of paper to your forehead and then trying to write your name on it with your left hand," Tom explains. "That's what I have to deal with 24 hours a day." He has dyslexia (a reading disability), dysgraphia (a handwriting disorder), attention deficits, and vision and hearing impairments. "I can't make sense of information the first time I hear it—or the second. I can't write the letters in a word all the same size. I can't spell. My learning disabilities are never going to go away or get better, but over the years, I've found ways to cope."

What makes it hard for people like Tom is that learning disabilities are invisible. "When I say I can't do something, people don't understand that I'm not saying I don't want to," Tom explains. "Telling me to write down a phone message, for instance, is like telling a blind person to get in a car and drive. There are things I cannot do, no matter how much I'd like to."

From the moment Tom gets up in the morning, he has to be completely organized. "The only way I can process information is one step at a time, so I try to prepare as much as I can in a quiet place. I've never been able to make change, so if I'm taking a bus, I count out the exact fare and put it in one pocket and the same amount for the return trip in another. I avoid writing checks in public because it takes me so long to remember how to spell "eleven" or "twelve." I carry a little cheat sheet in my wallet, but I'm embarrassed to use it."

Reading is torture for Tom. Anything with small print, like a telephone directory, is a blur. "But if I call information for a number, I can't get it after listening to the recording twice. It took three tries for me to get my driver's license. Even now if someone honks at me, I get flustered. Since I can't judge how fast cars are coming at me, I'll drive miles out of my way to avoid a left turn."

Tom barely made it through high school. "I bounced back and forth between special-education courses and mainstream classes. In the "dumb-bunny" courses, I'd get straight A's. But if I went into an average class, I couldn't keep up. Lots of teachers passed me just because I was quiet and didn't make trouble. If I'd been able to take my tests orally—like many learning disabled ("LD") kids today—I might have been an A student. Instead I met with failure after failure, which destroyed my self-esteem."

Finding and keeping a job after graduation was difficult. "If I had to take a written test or fill out a job application, I never got hired. I ended up doing things like bathing dogs in a local kennel." At age 26, Tom took an entrance exam for the Air Force and passed by one point.

"I was elated. This was my first chance to be on my own, to be part of something. When I left for basic training, I was determined to make it. But right away, there were problems. I couldn't stay in step and march with the others. The drill sergeant would yell, "Don't you know the difference between left and right?" I didn't. I couldn't take notes in classes or pass the exams. I was heartbroken when I was sent home."

When he sought his old tutor's advice, he learned about new diagnostic tests for learning disabilities in adults. They showed that he had multiple disabilities in the way he perceived and processed information. "It was such a relief to realize that I wasn't stupid. Today LD kids are diagnosed at an early age and given special accommodations. That wasn't true a generation ago; we fell through the cracks."

For almost two years, Tom worked on vision and hearing therapy, basic academic tutoring, sensorimotor exercises, and counseling with a psychotherapist who has a background in learning disabilities. Today he is working for a bachelor's degree at an alternative university where students work independently and do not have to attend lectures or take written tests. He also works at part-time jobs to support himself. "Unfortunately, the kind of work I can handle without too much stress—like putting together materials for shrink-wrapping at a mailing house—isn't stimulating or rewarding. But one of my LD friends passed along some advice: It's okay to spend ten minutes feeling sorry for yourself, but make sure you spend the next forty-five minutes doing something about it. That's what I'm trying try to do."

D.H.

words seem truer than ever. Problems such as discrimination and violence can no longer be viewed only as economic or political issues. Directly or indirectly, they affect the well-being of all who inhabit the earth—now and in the future. Even more mundane stressors, such as traffic, can lead to outbursts of anger that have come to be known as "road rage".[26]

Discrimination

Discrimination can take many forms—some as subtle as not being included in a conversation or joke, some as blatant as threats scrawled on a wall, some as violent as brutal beatings. Because it can be hard to deal with individually, discrimination is a particularly sinister form of

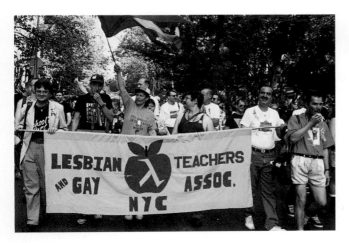

Community action can challenge the hateful assumptions that lead to discrimination, a stressor in its blatant and its subtle forms.

stress. By banding together, however, those who experience discrimination can take action to protect themselves, challenge the ignorance and hateful assumptions that fuel bigotry, and promote a healthier environment for all.

In the last decade, there have been reports of increased intolerance among young people and greater tolerance of expressions and acts of hate on college campuses. To counteract this trend, many schools have set up programs and classes to educate students about each other's different backgrounds and to acknowledge and celebrate the richness diversity brings to campus life. Educators have called on universities to make campuses less alienating and more culturally and emotionally accessible, with programs and policies targeted not only at minority students but also at the university as a whole.

Violence

The deliberate use of physical force to abuse or injure is a leading killer of young people in the United States—and a potential source of stress in all our lives. Chances are that you or someone you know has been the victim of a violent crime, and awareness of our own vulnerability adds to the stress of daily living. As studies have documented, the increased crime rate in inner-city communities results in stress, which leads to various health and mental problems among minority Americans.[27] (Chapter 17 discusses violence, abuse, and other threats to personal safety.)

A Personal Stress Survival Guide

Although stress is a very real threat to emotional and physical well-being, its impact depends not just on what happens to you, but on how you handle it. If you tried to predict who would become ill based simply on life-change units or other stressors, you'd be correct only about 15% of the time.

Some individuals are particularly prone to worry and constantly dwell on the negative aspects of what's happening or what may happen. Both psychological counseling, which teaches "reframing techniques" to develop a more positive viewpoint, and medications, including the serotonin-boosting agents described in Chapter 4, can make a difference in lowering their levels of chronic stress.[28] The inability to feel in control of stress, rather than stress itself, is often the most harmful.

In studying individuals who manage stress so well that they seem "stress-resistant," researchers have observed that these individulas share many of the following traits:

- They respond actively to challenges. If a problem comes up, they look for resources, do some reading or research, and try to find a solution rather than giving up and feeling helpless. Because they've faced numerous challenges, they have confidence in their abilities to cope.

- They have personal goals, such as getting a college degree or becoming a better parent.

- They rely on a combination of planning, goal setting, problem solving, and risk taking to control stress.

- They use a minimum of substances such as nicotine, caffeine, alcohol, or drugs.

- They regularly engage in some form of relaxation, from meditation to exercise to knitting, at least 15 minutes a day.

- They tend to seek out other people and become involved with them.

In order to achieve greater control over the stress in your life, start with some self-analysis: If you're feeling overwhelmed, ask yourself: Are you taking an extra course that's draining your last ounce of energy? Are you staying up late studying every night and missing morning classes? Are you living on black coffee and jelly doughnuts? While you may think that you don't have time to reduce the stress in your life, some simple changes can often ease the pressure you're under and help you achieve your long-term goals.

One of the simplest, yet most effective, ways to work through stress is by putting your feelings into words that only you will read. The more honest and open you are as you write, the better. In studies at Southern Methodist University, psychologist James Pennebaker, Ph.D., found that college students who wrote in their journals about traumatic events felt much better afterward than those who wrote about superficial topics. Recording your experiences and feelings on paper or audiotape may help decrease stress and enhance well-being.[29]

Since the small ups and downs of daily life have an enormous impact on psychological and physical well-being, getting a handle on daily hassles will reduce your stress load. The positive strategies described in Chapter 3 can help.

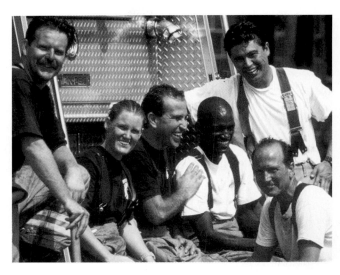

Humor is a positive coping mechanism, especially for individuals in high-stress professions.

Strategies for Change

How to Cope with Stress

✔ Recognize your stress signals. Is your back bothering you more? Do you find yourself speeding or misplacing things? Force yourself to stop whenever you see these early warnings and say, "I'm under stress; I need to do something about it."

✔ Keep a stress journal. Focus on intense emotional experiences and "autopsy" them to try to understand why they affected you the way they did. Re-reading and thinking about your notes may reveal the underlying reasons for your response.

✔ Try "stress-inoculation." Rehearse everyday situations that you find stressful, such as speaking in class. Think of how you might handle the situation, perhaps by breathing deeply before you talk.

✔ Put things in proper perspective. Ask yourself: Will I remember what's made me so upset a month from now? If you had to rank this problem on a scale of 1 to 10, with worldwide catastrophe as 10, where would it rate?

✔ Think of one simple thing that could make your life easier. What if you put up a hook to hold your keys so that you didn't spend five minutes searching for them every morning?

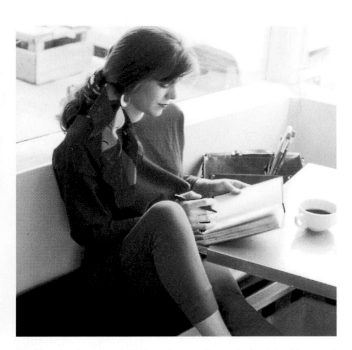

No time to de-stress? Writing in your journal about feelings and difficulties is a simple and very effective way to keep stress from building up.

Positive Coping Mechanisms

After a perfectly miserable, aggravating day, a teacher comes home and yells at her children for making too much noise. Another individual, after an equally stressful day, jokes about what went wrong during the all-time most miserable moment of the month. Both of these people are using defense mechanisms—actions or behaviors that help protect their sense of self-worth. The first is displacing anger onto someone else; the second uses humor to vent frustration.

Under great stress, we all may turn to negative defense mechanisms to alleviate anxiety and eliminate conflict. These can lead to maladaptive behavior, such as rationalizing overeating by explaining to yourself that you need the extra calories to cope with the extra stress in your life. **Coping mechanisms** are healthier, more mature and adaptive ways of dealing with stressful situations. While they also ward off unpleasant emotions, they usually are helpful rather than harmful. The most common are:

- Sublimation, the redirection of any drives considered unacceptable into socially acceptable channels. For example, someone who is furious with a friend or relative may go for a long run to sublimate anger.

- Religiosity, in which one comes to terms with a painful experience, such as a child's death, by experiencing it as being in accord with God's will.

- Humor, which counters stress by focusing on comic aspects. Medical students, for instance, often make jokes in anatomy lab as a way of dealing with their anxieties about working with cadavers.

- Altruism, which takes a negative experience and turns it into a positive one. For example, an HIV-positive individual may talk to teenagers about AIDS prevention.

Managing Time

Every day you make dozens of decisions, and the choices you make about how to use your time directly affect your stress level. If you have a big test on Monday and a term paper due Tuesday, you may plan to study all weekend. Then, when you're invited to a party Saturday night, you go. Although you set the alarm for 7:00 A.M. on Sunday, you don't pull yourself out of bed until noon. By the time you start studying, it's 4:00 P.M., and anxiety is building inside you.

How can you tell if you've lost control of your time? The following are telltale symptoms of poor time management:

- Rushing.

- Chronic inability to make choices or decisions.

- Fatigue or listlessness.

- Constantly missed deadlines.

- Not enough time for rest or personal relationships.

- A sense of being overwhelmed by demands and details and having to do what you don't want to do most of the time.

One of the hard lessons of being on your own is that your choices and your actions have consequences. Stress is just one of them. But by thinking ahead, being realistic about your workload, and sticking to your plans, you can gain better control over your time and your stress levels.

Overcoming Procrastination

Putting off until tomorrow what should be done today is a habit that creates a great deal of stress for many students. The three most common types of procrastination are: putting off unpleasant things, putting off difficult tasks, and putting off tough decisions. Procrastinators are most likely to delay by wishing they didn't have to do what they must or by telling themselves they "just can't get started," which means they never do.

People procrastinate, not because they're lazy, but to protect their self-esteem and make a favorable impression. "Procrastinators often perceive their worth as based solely on task ability, and their ability is determined only by how well they perform on completed tasks," notes psychologist Joseph Ferrari, Ph.D. "By never completing the tasks, they are never judged on their ability, thus allowing them to maintain an illusion of competence."[30]

To get out of a time trap, keep track of the tasks you're most likely to put off, and try to figure out why you don't want to tackle them. Think of alternative ways to get tasks done. If you put off library readings, for instance, figure out if the problem is getting to the library or the reading itself. If it's the trip to the library, arrange to walk over with a friend whose company you enjoy.

Develop daily time-management techniques, such as a "To Do" list. Rank items according to priorities: A, B, C, and schedule your days to make sure the A's get accomplished. Try not to fixate on half-completed projects. Divide large tasks, such as a term paper, into smaller ones, and reward yourself when you complete a part.

Do what you like least first. Once you have it out of the way, you can concentrate on the tasks you do enjoy. You also should build time into your schedule for interruptions, unforeseen problems, unexpected events, and so on, so you aren't constantly racing around. Establish ground rules for meeting your own needs (including getting enough sleep and making time for friends) before saying yes to any activity. Learn to live according to a three-word motto: Just do it!

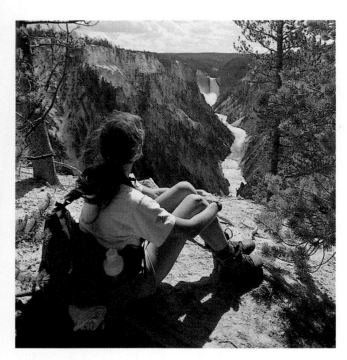

Spending time outdoors is a good way to leave behind daily tensions.

Relaxation Techniques

Relaxation is the physical and mental state opposite that of stress. Rather than gearing up for fight or flight, our bodies and minds grow calmer and work more smoothly. We're less likely to become frazzled and more capable of staying in control. The most effective relaxation techniques include progressive relaxation, visualization, meditation, mindfulness, and biofeedback.

Progressive relaxation works by intentionally increasing and then decreasing tension in the muscles. While sitting or lying down in a quiet, comfortable setting, you tense and release various muscles, beginning with those of the hand, for instance, and then proceeding to the arms, shoulders, neck, face, scalp, chest, stomach, buttocks, genitals, and so on, down each leg to the toes. Relaxing the muscles can quiet the mind and restore internal balance.[31]

Visualization, or **guided imagery**, involves creating mental pictures that calm you down and focus your mind. As we note in Chapter 20, some people use this technique to promote healing when they are ill. The Glaser study showed that elderly residents of retirement homes in Ohio who learned progressive relaxation and guided imagery enhanced their immune function and reported better health than did the other residents. Visualization skills require practice and, in some cases, instruction by qualified health professionals.[32]

Meditation has been practiced in many forms over the ages, from the yogic techniques of the Far East to the Quaker silence of more modern times. Meditation helps a person reach a state of relaxation, but with the goal of achieving inner peace and harmony. There is no one right way to meditate, and many people have discovered how to meditate on their own, without even knowing what it is they are doing. Among college students, meditation has proven especially effective in increasing relaxation.[33] Most forms of meditation have common elements: sitting quietly for 15 to 20 minutes once or twice a day, concentrating on a word or image, and breathing slowly and rhythmically. If you wish to try meditation, it often helps to have someone guide you through your first sessions. Or try tape recording your own voice (with or without favorite music in the background) and playing it back to yourself, freeing yourself to concentrate on the goal of turning the attention within.

Mindfulness is a modern-day form of an ancient Asian technique that involves maintaining awareness in the present moment. You tune in to each part of your body, scanning from head to toe, noting the slightest sensation. You allow whatever you experience—an itch, an ache, a feeling of warmth—to enter your awareness. Then you open yourself to focus on all the thoughts, sensations, sounds, and feelings that enter your awareness. Mindfulness keeps you in the here-and-now, thinking about what is rather than about "what if" or "if only."

Biofeedback, discussed in Chapter 20, is a method of obtaining feedback, or information, about some physiological activity occurring in the body. An electronic monitoring device attached to a person's body detects a change in an internal function and communicates it back to the person through a tone, light, or meter. By paying attention to this feedback, most people can gain some control over functions previously thought to be beyond conscious control, such as body temperature, heart rate, muscle tension, and brain waves. Biofeedback training consists of three stages:

1. Developing increased awareness of a body state or function.

2. Gaining control over it.

3. Transferring this control to everyday living without use of the electronic instrument.

The goal of biofeedback for stress reduction is a state of tranquility, usually associated with the brain's production of alpha waves (which are slower and more regular than normal waking waves). After several train-

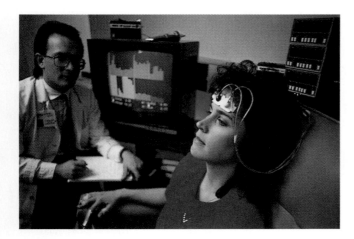

Biofeedback training uses electronic monitoring devices to teach conscious control over heart rate, body temperature, and muscle tension. Once the technique is learned, the electronic feedback is unnecessary.

ing sessions, most people can produce alpha waves more or less at will.[34]

Stress Overload

Excessive, unmanaged stress can affect every aspect of your life, jeopardizing your physical well-being, your psychological health, your behavior, and your performance at school or work. Monitor yourself for any of the following clues that your body, mind, and behavior may provide—and don't ignore them.

The Toll on the Mind

Life happens: Cars crash. Loved ones leave. Money runs out. Such stressors always take a toll on an individual, and it's normal to feel sad, tense, overwhelmed, angry, or incapable of coping with the ordinary demands of daily living. Usually such feelings and behaviors subside with time. The stressful event fades into the past, and those whose lives it has touched adapt to its lasting impact. But sometimes individuals remain extremely distressed and unable to function as they once did.

Adjustment Disorders

The term **adjustment disorder** refers to an out-of-the-ordinary response to a stressful event or situation. Any event or combination of circumstances can lead to an adjustment disorder. The stressor does not have to be extreme; even a seemingly minor event—such as learning that an ex-boyfriend or girlfriend has married—may cause great psychological pain.[35]

Specific developmental events, such as leaving home, getting married, having a child, losing a job, or retirement, can trigger adjustment disorders. Although any one at any age can have difficulty adapting to a life crisis, most people who seek treatment for adjustment disorders are in their twenties.

The symptoms of adjustment disorders vary. After being fired, a store clerk may feel jumpy all the time, unable to sleep, irritable, and angry. A student whose boyfriend suddenly breaks up with her may find it hard to concentrate during lectures. A person identified as HIV-positive may seek out new sex partners and not use safe-sex practices.

The problem for individuals reeling from the impact of a life crisis is trying to figure out which feelings are normal and which are not. The two key signs of an adjustment disorder are distress and impairment: Individuals feel extremely upset or cannot work or relate to others the way they once did, and their symptoms persist for more than three to six months after a stressful event.[36]

There is no specific remedy for an adjustment disorder, although the goal is always the same: improving an individual's ability to adapt. Ordinarily, time helps ease the pain or difficulty of coping with a stressful situation. When the impact of a crisis is more intense, supportive counseling or brief psychotherapy (described in Chapter 4) can help an individual understand the significance of what has happened, put it into perspective, and deal with it in a healthier way.

Strategies for Prevention

Recognize the Warning Signals of Stress Overload

✔ Experiencing physical symptoms, including chronic fatigue, headaches, indigestion, diarrhea, and sleep problems.

✔ Having frequent illness or worrying about illness.

✔ Self-medicating, including nonprescription drugs.

✔ Having problems concentrating on studies or work.

✔ Feeling irritable, anxious, or apathetic.

✔ Working or studying longer and harder than usual.

✔ Exaggerating, to yourself and others, the importance of what you do.

✔ Becoming accident-prone.

✔ Breaking rules, whether it's a curfew at home or a speeding limit on the highway.

✔ Going to extremes, such as drinking too much, over-spending, or gambling.

Posttraumatic Stress Disorder

In the past, **posttraumatic stress disorder (PTSD)** was viewed as a psychological response to out-of-the-ordinary stressors, such as captivity or combat. However, these are hardly the only experiences that can forever change the way people view themselves and their world. With the recent surge in violent crime and in natural disasters, thousands of individuals have experienced or witnessed traumatic events.[37] Children, in particular, are likely to develop PTSD symptoms when they live through a traumatic event or witness a loved one or friend being assaulted. Sometimes an entire community, such as the residents of a town hit by a devastating flood or hurricane, develops symptoms.

In a survey of more than 400 undergraduates, 84% listed at least one traumatic event of sufficient intensity potentially to elicit posttraumatic stress disorder. One third had experienced four or more such events. The students who had these experiences—which included witnessing violence or death, child abuse, and sexual assault—reported higher levels of depression, anxiety, and other psychological symptoms.[38]

A history of childhood sexual abuse can greatly increase the likelihood of developing PTSD.[39] An episode that repeats the abuse, such as a sexual assault

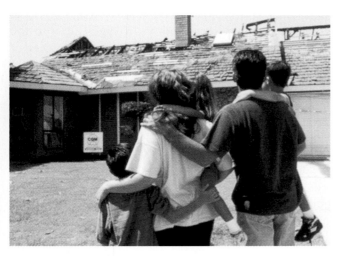

Posttraumatic stress disorder symptoms occur when we live through traumatic events. Survivors, the injured, and family members can experience mild to extreme symptoms following such traumas.

or rape, can trigger an intense reaction as individuals "reexperience" the initial trauma of their youth.[40] Adolescents who are dependent on alcohol also are particularly susceptible to PTSD.[41]

In PTSD, individuals reexperience their terror and helplessness again and again in their dreams or intrusive thoughts. To avoid this psychic pain, they may try to avoid anything associated with the trauma. Some enter a state of emotional numbness and no longer can respond to people and experiences the way they once did, especially when it comes to showing tenderness or affection. Those who've been mugged or raped may be afraid to venture out by themselves.

The sooner trauma survivors receive psychological help, the better they are likely to fare. Often talking about what happened with an empathic person or someone who's shared the experience as soon as possible—preferably before going to sleep on the day of the event—can help an individual begin to deal with what has occurred. Group sessions, ideally beginning soon after the trauma, allow individuals to share views and experiences. Behavioral, cognitive, and psychodynamic therapy (described in Chapter 4) can help individuals suffering PTSD.

The Toll on the Body

While stress can sometimes be the spice of life, it also can be the kiss of death. Just as it can undermine psychological contentment, it can erode physical well-being. Many medical researchers believe that stress may be the greatest single contributor to disease (see Figure 2-3). According to the American Institute of Stress, 75 to 90% of all visits to physicians involve stress-related complaints.

The Cardiovascular System

In the 1970s, cardiologists Meyer Friedman, M.D., and Ray Rosenman, M.D., suggested that excess stress may be the most important factor in the development of heart disease. They compared their patients to individuals of the same age with healthy hearts and developed two general categories: Type A and Type B. (The Type C cancer-prone personality is discussed in Chapter 13.)

Hardworking, aggressive, and competitive, Type A's never have time for all they want to accomplish, even though they usually try to do several tasks at once. Type B's are more relaxed, though not necessarily less ambitious or successful. (Of course, people who are extremely Type B may never accomplish anything.) Type-A

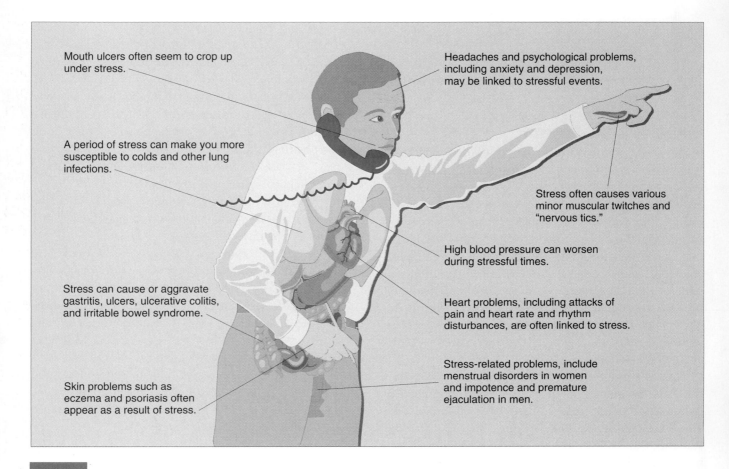

Mouth ulcers often seem to crop up under stress.

A period of stress can make you more susceptible to colds and other lung infections.

Stress can cause or aggravate gastritis, ulcers, ulcerative colitis, and irritable bowel syndrome.

Skin problems such as eczema and psoriasis often appear as a result of stress.

Headaches and psychological problems, including anxiety and depression, may be linked to stressful events.

Stress often causes various minor muscular twitches and "nervous tics."

High blood pressure can worsen during stressful times.

Heart problems, including attacks of pain and heart rate and rhythm disturbances, are often linked to stress.

Stress-related problems, include menstrual disorders in women and impotence and premature ejaculation in men.

Figure 2-3 Long-term, unmanaged stress can affect any and every part of the body and result in chronic, often serious disease.

behavior has been found to be the major contributing factor in the early development of heart disease.

The degree of danger associated with Type-A behavior remains controversial. According to a 22-year followup study of 3000 middle-aged men by researchers at the University of California, Berkeley, both smoking and high blood pressure proved to be much greater threats than Type-A behavior with respect to heart attack risk. Of all the personality traits linked with Type-A behavior, the one that has emerged as most sinister is chronic hostility or cynicism. People who are always mistrustful, angry, and suspicious are twice as likely to suffer blockages of their coronary arteries.[42]

"If you're racing around because you're a go-getter—you're enthusiastic, you're positive—the evidence is that it doesn't hurt you," says behavioral medicine specialist Redford Williams, M.D., of Duke University. On the other hand, hostile Type A's react to anger with an excessive surge of adrenaline. In Williams' studies, they also were more overweight, consumed more alco-

hol, smoked more cigarettes, and drank more caffeine. "Our findings suggest that hostile Type A's autonomic nervous system is balanced differently," he says.[43]

Mental stress also has been implicated in myocardial ischemia (inadequate blood and oxygen flow to the heart muscle). In one study, 22% of episodes of ischemia occurred during times of high mental stress but low physical activity. Even low levels of mental stress and negative emotions, including feelings of frustration, tension, and sadness, can double the number of episodes of ischemia in individuals with coronary artery disease.[44] Positive emotions lower this risk. Recognizing the importance of reducing stress in vulnerable individuals, cardiologists often recommend stress-management training in addition to conventional therapies.[45]

Stress reduction, including biofeedback and relaxation techniques, can help reduce the risk. Social support also helps lower cardiovascular reactivity. In a study of 90 college students, students given support from a confederate before and during the time they gave a speech showed smaller increases in systolic blood pressure than those who faced the stress of public speaking without support.[46]

The Immune System

The powerful chemicals triggered by stress dampen or suppress the immune system—the network of organs, tissues, and white blood cells that defend against disease. Impaired immunity makes the body more susceptible to many diseases, including infections (from the common cold to tuberculosis) and disorders of the immune system itself.

Traumatic stress, such as losing a loved one through death or divorce, can impair immunity for as long as a year. Even minor hassles take a toll. Under exam stress, students experience a dip in immune function and a higher rate of infections. Ohio State University researchers found a significant drop in the immune cells that normally ward off infection and cancer in medical students during exam periods.[47]

Certain uplifts, including humor and altruism, may buffer the harmful effects of stress. In studies of college students, watching videotapes of comedians bolstered immune function. Altruism may be good for the body as well as the soul. Students who provided services to others or who watched a tape of Mother Teresa caring for the poor showed a temporary boost in immunity.[48]

The Digestive System

Do you ever get butterflies in your stomach before giving a speech in class or before a big game? The digestive system is, as one psychologist quips, "an important stop on the tension trail." To avoid problems, pay attention to how you eat: Eating on the run, gulping food, or overeating result in poorly chewed foods, an overworked stomach, and increased abdominal pressure. The combination of poor eating habits and stress can add up to real pain in the stomach.

Some simple strategies can help you avoid stress-related stomach aches. Many people experience dry mouth or sweat more under stress. By drinking plenty of water, you replenish lost fluids and prevent dehydration. Fiber-rich foods counteract common stress-related problems, such as cramps and constipation. It's also important not to skip meals. If you do, you're more likely to feel fatigued and irritable.

Be wary of overeating under stress. Some people eat more simply because they scarf down meals too quickly. Others reach for snacks to calm their nerves or comfort themselves. Watch out for caffeine. Coffee, tea, and cola drinks can make your strained nerves jangle even more. Also avoid sugary snacks. They'll send your blood sugar levels on a roller coaster ride—up one minute, down the next.

Other Stress Symptoms

Stress can affect any organ system in the body, causing painful symptoms or a flareup of chronic conditions such as asthma. By interfering with our alertness and ability to concentrate, stress also increases the risk of accidents at home, at work, and on the road.

Headaches are one of the most common stress-related conditions. The most common type, tension headache, is caused by involuntary contractions of the scalp, head, and neck muscles. **Migraine headache** is the result of constriction (narrowing), then dilation (widening) of blood vessels within the brain; chemicals leak through the vessel walls, inflame nearby tissues, and send pain signals to the brain. Surveys of college women show that Type-A behavior can trigger both types of headache.

Stress also can be a culprit. The best strategy is preventive: doing a "relaxercise" a day, such as progressive relaxation or biofeedback, described in this chapter. Breathing and relaxation techniques, usually coupled with medication, also can relieve headaches after they strike.[49]

Stress also is closely linked to skin conditions. If you break out the week before an exam, you know firsthand that skin can be extremely sensitive to stress. Among the other skin conditions worsened by stress are acne, psoriasis, herpes, hives, and eczema. With acne, increased touching of the face, perhaps while cramming for a test, may be partly responsible. Other factors, such as temperature, humidity, and cosmetics and toiletries, may also play a role.

Making This Chapter Work for You
Meeting the Challenge of Stress

- Stress is the physiological and psychological response to any demand placed on us, or our bodies, whether positive or negative.

- Eustress, or positive stress, challenges us to grow, adapt, and find creative solutions in our lives. Distress refers to the negative effects of stress that can deplete or even destroy life energy.

- Theories of stress include Hans Selye's general adaptation syndrome, which consists of three distinct stages: alarm, resistance, and exhaustion. The genetic-constitutional perspective looks at the role of predisposing factors, which can influence resistance and make us more or less susceptible to stress. The cognitive-transactional model of stress, developed by Richard Lazarus, looks at the interrelation between stress and health.

■ Common student stressors on campus include test pressures, financial problems, personal frustrations, problems in friendships and dating relationships, daily hassles, academic failure, competitive pressure, unpleasant or disruptive changes, and personal losses. Adjusting to college life is stressful in itself.

■ Minority students encounter additional stressors, including a hostile or unfriendly social climate, interpersonal tensions between themselves and nonminority students and faculty, experiences of actual or perceived racism, and more subtle racist attitudes and discrimination.

■ Jobs are a major source of stress for Americans. Two problems related to job stress are workaholism, characterized by excessive devotion to work, and burnout, a state of physical, emotional, and mental exhaustion brought on by constant or repeated emotional pressure.

■ Chronic illness and disability, including learning disabilities, can be major sources of stress in an individual's life.

■ Social stressors—such as discrimination and violence—also are a threat to physical and psychological well-being.

■ Stress-management techniques, which include better time management, overcoming procrastination, and increased appreciation of leisure time, can help reduce distress and enhance feelings of control over daily stress.

■ Techniques such as progressive relaxation, visualization, meditation, mindfulness, and biofeedback can help soothe both body and mind and reduce the harmful effects of stress.

■ Stress can affect psychological well-being and cause adjustment disorders and posttraumatic stress disorder. Prompt recognition and treatment can help overcome these problems.

■ Stress overload can contribute to heart disease, high blood pressure, immune disorders, digestive problems, and other ailments.

College is a perfect time to learn and practice the art of stress reduction. You can start applying the techniques and concepts outlined in this chapter immediate-

Health Online

Biobehavioral Institute of Boston's Stress Audit
http://www.bbinst.org/stressaudit/stress3.cgi

The Behavioral Institute of Boston's Stress Audit is a comprehensive assessment of your stress levels in many areas of life, including job, family, social, financial, and emotional stress. After you take the survey, the Stress Audit will tell you how you compare with the general population in each area of stress. It will also analyze your general susceptibility to stress, the sources of stress in your life, and the symptoms of stress you now show. You will also get some advice on how to lower your vulnerability to stress.

Think about it ...

• According to the Stress Audit, how does your stress level compare with that of the general population? What might you do to reduce your stress in areas where it is especially high?

• Why do you think the things in the Susceptibility to Stress inventory are especially important?

• If you were to design a new inventory for this site on School Stress, what might you include?

ly. You may want to begin by doing some relaxation or awareness exercises. They can give you the peace of mind you need to focus more effectively on larger issues, goals, and decisions.

You needn't see stress as a problem to solve on your own. Reach out to others. As you build friendships and intimate relationships, you may find that some irritating problems are easier to put into perspective. Don't be afraid to laugh at yourself and to look for the comic or absurd aspects of a situation. In addition, you might try some simple approaches that can help boost your stress resistance and resilience, including the following:

- *Focusing.* Take a strain inventory of your body every day to determine where things aren't feeling quite right. Ask yourself, "What's keeping me from feeling terrific today?" Focusing on problem spots, such as stomach knots or neck tightness, increases your sense of control over stress.

- *Reconstructing stressful situations.* Think about a recent episode of distress; then write down three ways it could have gone better and three ways it could have gone worse. This should help you see that the situation wasn't as disastrous as it might have been, and help you find ways to cope better in the future.

- *Self-improvement.* When your life feels out of control, turn to a new challenge. You might try volunteering at a nursing home, going for a long-distance bike trip, or learning a foreign language. As you work toward your new goal, you'll realize that you still can cope and achieve.

- *Exercise.* Regular physical activity can relieve stress, boost energy, lift mood, and keep stress under control.

If stress continues to be a problem in your life, you may be able to find help through support groups or counseling. Your school may provide counseling services or referrals to mental health professionals; ask your health instructor or the campus health department for this information. Remember that each day of distress robs you of energy, distracts you from life's pleasures, and interferes with achieving your full potential.

 ## Key Terms

The terms listed here are used within the chapter. Page numbers are included for each term. A definition of each term is given in the green Glossary pages at the end of this book.

adaptive response *42*
adjustment disorder *56*
biofeedback *55*
burnout *50*
coping mechanisms *54*
distress *42*
eustress *42*

general adaptation syndrome (GAS) *42*
guided imagery *55*
homeostasis *42*
meditation *55*
migraine headache *59*
mindfulness *55*

posttraumatic stress disorder (PTSD) *57*
progressive relaxation *55*
stress *42*
stressor *42*
visualization *55*

 ## Review Questions

1. What is stress? What causes stress? What is the general adaptation syndrome?
2. How are stress and heart disease related? stress and the immune system? stress and the digestive system?
3. What are the characteristics of a stress-resistant personality?
4. Name some social stressors. How can the effects of these be minimized or prevented?
5. Differentiate between Type-A and Type-B behaviors. What type of behavior do you exhibit? How do these behaviors affect your health?
6. How can you manage stress in your life more effectively?

Critical Thinking Questions

1. Studies have shown that meditation and relaxation techniques can have a positive impact on health. In fact, insurance companies will now pay for medical care that includes these techniques. Critics condemn these practices as unsound, or at least as lacking sufficient scientific proof to warrant their use. Others consider meditation to be too "self-indulgent." What do you think: How valuable are these techniques, and for whom?

2. Identify three stressful situations in your life and describe how you might attempt to decrease or eliminate the stressors associated with them. Identify three examples of eustress.

3. Can you think of any ways in which your behavior or attitudes might create stress for others? What changes could you make to avoid doing so?

4. What advice might you give an incoming freshman at your school about managing stress in college? What techniques have been most helpful for you in dealing with stress?

Connections to Personal Health Interactive

To enhance your understanding of the material covered in this chapter, check out the following study aids on the **Personal Health Interactive CD-ROM**. *Each numbered icon within the chapter corresponds to an appropriate activity listed here.*

2.1 Personal Insights: How Stressed Are You?
2.2 Chapter 2 Review

References

1. Lazarus, R., and R. Launier, "Stress-Related Transactions Between Person and Environment." in *Perspectives in Interactional Psychology*. New York: Plenum, 1978.

2. Goldman, Cristin, and Eugene Wong. "Stress and the College Student." *Education*, Vol. 117, No. 4, Summer 1997.

3. Gadzella, Bernadette. "Student-Life Stress Inventory: Identification of and Reactions to Stressors." *Psychological Reports*, Vol. 74, No. 2, April 1994.

4. Wagner, Betsy. "Living on the Edge." *Life Management*. 3rd ed. Guilford, CT: Dushkin Publishing Group, 1995.

5. Gerdes, Eugenia, and Guo Ping. "Coping Differences Between College Women and Men in China and the United States." *Genetic, Social and General Psychology Monographs,* Vol. 120, No. 2, May 1994. Puccio, Gerard, et al. "Person-Environment Fit: Using Commensurate Scales to Predict Student Stress." *British Journal of Educational Psychology,* Vol. 63, No. 3, November 1993.

6. Goldman and Wong, "Stress and the College Student."

7. Demakis, George, and Dan McAdams. "Personality, Social Support, and Well-Being Among First-Year College Students." *College Health Journal*, Vol. 28, No. 2, June 1994.

8. Neville, Helen, et al. "Relations Among Racial Identity Attitudes, Perceived Stressors, and Coping Styles in African American College Students." *Journal of Counseling and Development*, Vol. 75, No. 4, March–April 1997.

9. Solberg, V. Scott, and Pete Villarreal. "Examination of Self-Efficacy, Social Support and Stress as Predictors of Psychological and Physical Distress Among Hispanic College Students." *Hispanic Journal of Behavioral Sciences*, Vol. 19, No. 2, May 1997.

10. "College-Age Freedom Can Trigger Illness." *USA Today Magazine*, Vol. 125, No. 2610, December 1996.

11. Glaser, Ronald, and Janice Kiecolt-Glaser. *Handbook of Human Stress and Immunity*. San Diego: Academic Press, 1994. Hornig-Rohan, Mary. "Stress, Immune-Mediators, and Immune-Mediated Disease," *Advances: The Journal of Mind-Body Health,* Vol. 11, No. 2, Spring 1995.

12. Saldana, Delia. "Acculturative Stress: Minority Status and Distress." *Hispanic Journal of Behavioral Sciences,* Vol. 16, No. 2, May 1994.

13. Ibid.

14. Smedley, Brian, et al. "Minority Status Stresses and the College Adjustment of Ethnic Minority Freshmen." *Journal of Higher Education,* Vol. 64, No. 5, July–August 1993.

15. Ibid.

16. Launier, Raymond. "Stress Balance and Emotional Life Complexes in Students in a Historically African American College." *Journal of Psychology*, Vol. 131, No. 2, March 1997.

17. Solberg, V., et al. "Social Support, Stress and Hispanic College Adjustment: Test of a Diathesis Stress Model." *Hispanic Journal of Behavioral Sciences,* Vol. 16, No. 3, August 1994. Solberg, V., et al. "Development of the Col-

lege Stress Inventory for Use with Hispanic Populations."
Hispanic Journal of Behavioral Sciences, Vol. 15, No. 4,
November 1993.

18. U.S. Bureau of Labor Statistics, personal inquiry.

19. Schor, Juliet. *The Overworked American: The Unexpected
Decline of Leisure.* New York: Basic Books, Harper-
Collins, 1992.

20. John Robinson, personal interview.

21. Kline, Marsha, and David Snow. "Effects of a Worksite
Coping Skills Intervention on the Stress, Social Support
and Health Outcomes of Working Mother." *Journal of
Primary Prevention,* Vol. 15, No. 2, Winter 1994.

22. Rost, Kathryn, and G. Richard Smith. "Work Buffers Emotional Stress of First Heart Attack. "*Archives of Internal
Medicine,* February 1992.

23. Davis, Susan. "Burnout." *American Health,* December
1994.

24. Kagan, Norman, et al. "Stress Reduction in the Workplace: The Effectiveness of Psychoeducational Programs."
Journal of Counseling Psychology, Vol. 42, No. 1, January
1995.

25. Gallegos, Daniel Joseph. "A Comparative Study of College Students With and Without Learning Disabilities on
Levels of Stress and Coping." *Dissertation Abstracts International,* Vol. 54, No. 2, August 1993.

26. Hennessy, Dwight, and David Weisenthal. "The Relation-
ship Between Traffic Congestion, Driver Stress and Direct
Versus Indirect Coping Behaviors." *Ergonomics,* Vol. 40,
No. 3, March 1997.

27. Wakhisi, Tsitis. "Crime: A Leading Health Hazard for
Minorities." *Crisis,* Vol. 101, No. 8, November–December
1994.

28. Hallowell, Edward, and Annie Paul. "Why Worry?" *Psychology Today*, Vol. 30, No. 6, November–December
1997.

29. Pennebaker, James. "Putting Stress into Words: Health,
Linguistic and Therapeutic Implications." *Behavioral
Research,* Vol. 31, No. 6, 1993. Pitariua, Horia, and Frank
Landy. "Some Personality Correlates of Time Urgency."
Revue Roumaine de Psychologie, Vol. 37, No. 1,
January–June 1993.

30. Ferrari, Joseph. "Self-Destructive Motivation—Personality,
Social, and Clinical Perspectives." Presentation, American
Psychological Association, August 1992.

31. Benson, Herbert, and Michael McKee. "Relaxation and
Other Alternative Therapies." *Patient Care,* Vol. 27, No.
20, December 15, 1993.

32. Kiecolt-Glaser, Janice, and Ronald Glaser. "Stress and the
Immune System: Human Studies." *Review of Psychiatry*
(Vol. 11). Washington, D.C.: American Psychiatric Press,
1992.

33. Janowiak, John. "The Effects of Meditation on College
Students' Self-Actualization and Stress Management." *Dissertation Abstracts International,* Vol. 53, No. 10, April
1993.

34. Benson and McKee, "Relaxation and Other Alternative
Therapies."

35. Greenberg, William, et al. "Adjustment Disorder as an
Admission Diagnosis." *American Journal of Psychiatry,*
Vol. 152, No. 3, March 1995.

36. Hales, Dianne, and Robert E. Hales. *Caring for the Mind:
The Comprehensive Guide to Mental Health.* New York:
Bantam Books, 1995.

37. Breslau, Naomi, et al. "Risk Factors for PTSD-Related
Traumatic Events: A Prospective Analysis." *American
Journal of Psychiatry,* Vol. 152, No. 4, April 1995.

38. Vrana, Scott, and Dean Lauterbach. "Prevalence of Trau-
matic and Post-Traumatic Psychological Symptoms in a
Nonclinical Sample of College Students." *Journal of
Traumatic Stress,* Vol. 7, No. 2, April 1994. Nemiah, John.
"A Few Intrusive Thoughts on Posttraumatic Stress Disor-
der." *American Journal of Psychiatry,* Vol. 152, No. 4,
April 1995.

39. Rodriguez, Ned, et al. "Posttraumatic Stress Disorder in
Adult Female Survivors of Childhood Sexual Abuse: A
Comparison Study." *Journal of Consulting and Clinical
Psychology,* Vol. 675, No. 1, February 1997.

40. Briggs, Lynne, and Peter Joyce. "What Determines Posttraumatic Stress Disorder Symptomatology for Survivors
of Childhood Sexual Abuse?" *Child Abuse and Neglect,*
Vol. 21, No. 6, June 1997.

41. Deykin, E. Y., and S. L., Buka. "Prevalence and Risk Fac-
tors for Post-Traumatic Stress Disorder Among Chemically
Dependent Adolescents." *American Journal of
Psychiatry,* June 1997.

42. Bruehl, Stephen, et al. "Coping Styles, Opioid Blockade
and Cardiovascular Response to Stress." *Journal of
Behavioral Medicine,* Vol. 17, No. 1, February 1994.

43. Williams, Redford, and Virginia Williams. *Anger Kills.*
New York: Times Books, 1993.

44. Gullette, Elizabeth, et al. "Effects of Mental Stress on
Myocardial Ischemia During Daily Life." *Journal of the
American Medical Association,* Vol. 277, No. 19, May 21,
1997.

45. Mittleman, Murray, and Malcolm Maclure. "Mental Stress
During Daily Life Triggers Myocardial Ischemia." *Journal
of the American Medical Association,* Vol. 277, No. 19,
May 21, 1997.

46. Lepore, Stephen, et al. "Social Support Lowers Cardiovascular Reactivity to an Acute Stressor." *Psychosomatic
Medicine,* Vol. 55, No. 6, November–December 1993.

47. Glaser and Kiecolt-Glaser, *Handbook of Human Stress
and Immunity.*

48. Giles, Dwight, and Janet Eyler. "The Impact of a College
Community Service Laboratory on Students' Personal,
Social and Cognitive Outcomes." *Journal of Adolescence,*
Vol. 17, No. 4, August 1994.

49. Eller, Daryn. "Workouts That Fight Stress." *American
Health,* May 1994.

CHAPTER 3

FEELING GOOD

After studying the material in this chapter, you should be able to:

Explain the goal of psychological health and **list** some characteristics of psychologically healthy people.

Discuss the relationship of needs, feelings, values, and goals to psychological health.

Define self-esteem and **list** some strategies for boosting it, as well as some strategies for improving a negative mood.

Discuss the concept of emotional intelligence and how it can help individuals find meaning in life, achieve a sense of control, and maintain a desired energy level.

List healthy and unhealthy coping mechanisms, and **explain** ways to create more positive and effective coping mechanisms in your own life.

Explain the value of sleep.

You wake up, and the world seems new. You feel energetic, alert, eager for whatever the day will hold. You have a smile on your face and a spring in your step. The reason: You are in peak psychological health.

In every culture and country, psychologically healthy men and women generally share certain characteristics: They value themselves and strive toward happiness and fulfillment. They establish and maintain close relationships with others. They accept the limitations as well as the possibilities that life has to offer. And they feel a sense of meaning and purpose that makes the gestures of living worth the effort required.

Feeling good does not depend on money, success, recognition, or status. At any age, at any level of education and achievement, regardless of disability or disease, it is possible to find happiness and fulfillment in life. Achieving the highest possible level of psychological well-being, like achieving peak physical well-being, depends primarily on assuming responsibility for yourself. This chapter will help you accomplish this by offering insight into your needs, values, and feelings—and by providing guidance on how to manage your moods, pursue happiness, find meaning in life, and connect with others.

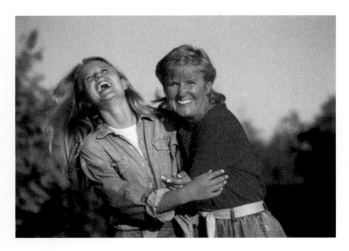

Peak psychological health. Psychologically healthy people value themselves, find meaning and purpose in life, and build close relationships with others.

What Is Psychological Health?

"A sound mind in a sound body is a short but full description of a happy state in this world," the philosopher John Locke wrote in 1693. More than 300 years later his statement still rings true. Both physical and psychological well-being are essential to total wellness.

Psychological health encompasses both our emotional and mental states—that is, our feelings and our thoughts. **Emotional health** generally refers to feelings and moods, both of which are discussed later in this chapter. Characteristics of emotionally healthy persons that psychologist Deane Shapiro identified in an analysis of major studies of emotional wellness include the following:

- Determination and effort to be healthy.
- Flexibility and adaptability to a variety of circumstances.
- Development of a sense of meaning and affirmation of life.
- An understanding that the self is not the center of the universe.
- Compassion for others.
- The ability to be unselfish in serving or relating to others.
- Increased depth and satisfaction in intimate relationships.
- A sense of control over the mind and body that enables the person to make health-enhancing choices and decisions.[1]

Mental health describes our ability to perceive reality as it is, to respond to its challenges, and to develop rational strategies for living. The mentally healthy person doesn't try to avoid conflicts and distress but can cope with life's transitions, traumas, and losses in a way that allows for emotional stability and growth. The characteristics of mental health include:

- The ability to function and carry out responsibilities.
- The ability to form relationships.
- Realistic perceptions of the motivations of others.
- Rational, logical thought processes.

There is considerable overlap between psychological and **spiritual health**, which (as defined in Chapter 1) involves our ability to identify our basic purpose in life and to experience the fulfillment of achieving our full potential. However, many people consider the two separate. "We like to think that emotional problems have to do with the family, childhood, and trauma—with personal life but not with spirituality," observes Thomas Moore, author of *Care of the Soul*, "Yet it is obvious that the soul, seat of the deepest emotions, can benefit greatly from the gifts of a vivid spiritual life and can suffer when it is deprived of them."[2]

In addition, **culture** helps to define psychological health. While, in one culture, men and women may express feelings with great intensity, shouting in joy or wailing in grief, in another culture such behavior might be considered abnormal or unhealthy. In our diverse society, many cultural influences affect Americans' sense of who they are, where they came from, and what they believe. One of the best ways to appreciate the influence of a culture—whether your own or a different one—is by becoming aware of, and taking the time to observe, the rituals that are characteristic of that culture. (See Spotlight on Diversity: "Connecting with Your Roots").

Strategies for Prevention

Tips for Psychological Fitness

✔ Recognize and express your feelings. Pent-up emotions tend to fester inside, building into anger or depression.

✔ Don't brood. Rather than merely mulling over a problem, try to find solutions that are positive and useful.

✔ Take one step at a time. As long as you're taking some action to solve a problem, you can take pride in your ability to cope.

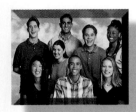

Spotlight on Diversity
Connecting with Your Roots

Every society has created holidays or rituals of celebration that serve valuable purposes: They bring people together, strengthen the bonds among them, reinforce the values and beliefs they share, and provide a sense of belonging, meaning, and purpose. In the United States, all Americans celebrate the fourth of July. For Christians, Christmas may be the most widely celebrated—and most commercialized—holiday. For Jews, Channukah is a time of special rejoicing. Other cultures in our society have special days in which people can reconnect with their roots and reaffirm their sense of who they are. These dates include:

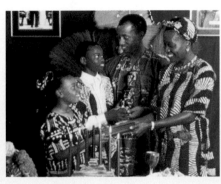

Special holidays, such as Kwanzaa, give people a chance to celebrate and remember the traditions that have helped make them who they are today.

- Kwanzaa. This Swahili word means "first fruits of the harvest." Created in 1966 as an alternative to Christmas for African Americans, Kwanzaa—observed from December 26 to January 1—is not a religious holiday, but a cultural one that focuses on seven ancient but timeless principles: unity, self-determination, collective work and responsibility, cooperative economics, purpose, creativity, and faith.
- American Indian Day. In 1915, the American Indian Association set aside the second Saturday in May (since expanded to the entire weekend) to pay tribute to the hundreds of thousands of Native Americans killed in wars over the centuries. Celebrations include pow-wows, dances, speeches, and religious ceremonies.
- Cinco de Mayo. This term—Spanish for the fifth of May—refers to the anniversary of the 1862 Battle of Puebla, in

which Mexican forces defeated French invaders, a victory that boosted morale and showed the determination of the Mexican people. In Mexico, May 5 is a national holiday. In the United States, Mexican Americans celebrate it with festivities, such as parades and dances.
- Chinese New Year. Celebrated on the first new moon after the sun enters Aquarius (somewhere between January 21 and February 20), the Chinese New Year is a special event commemorated differently by various Chinese nationalities. Traditional Chinese believe that during this night deities and the spirits of their ancestors return to earth for a family reunion. To pay homage to them, they observe customs such as settling old debts, making clothing and foods, and preparing festivities to bid the old year farewell and the new one welcome. Oranges and fish are traditional gifts, while shops, restaurants, and homes hang red pieces of paper with the word "fu," which means happiness, blessings, or good fortune.
- Book Hok Nam. The Laotian new year occurs on the twelfth day of the Lao fifth month, usually around April 13 or 14, and the celebration lasts five days. Traditional activities include cleaning the images of the Lord Buddha in temples, visiting parents and employers to wish them luck in the new year, and buying and releasing fish, small birds, turtles, snails, or crabs to ensure good luck.

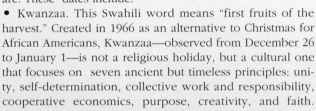

✔ Get involved with others. Reach out and communicate your feelings to someone you trust, either a friend or, if necessary, a professional.

Knowing Yourself

Who are you? Probably the first answer that comes to mind is your name, because that's the way you introduce yourself to others. Of course, you are identified by numbers, too: social security, student I.D., draft registration, driver's license, and credit cards. You also play

many roles: To a special few, you're a son, daughter, partner, spouse, parent, or friend. To others, you're a student, voter, taxpayer, worker, colleague, or consumer. You are part of certain cultural and ethnic groups and may practice a certain religion. But when you're all alone, eye-to-eye with yourself in the mirror, who is the person you see? Who is the real you? (See Self-Survey: "Well-Being Scale")

You may spend a lifetime searching for the answer—the most important journey you'll ever make. If you fail to find your true identity, it doesn't matter much what else you find. You can gain insight into your own personality and behavior by learning about your feelings, needs, and values.

Self-Survey

Well-Being Scale

Part I

The following questions contain statements and their opposites. Notice that the statements extend from one extreme to the other. Where would you place yourself on this scale? Place a circle on the number that is most true for you at this time. Do not put your circles between numbers.

Life Purpose and Satisfaction

1. During most of the day, my energy level is — very low　1　2　3　4　5　6　7　very high

2. As a whole, my life seems — dull　1　2　3　4　5　6　7　vibrant

3. My daily activities are — not a source of satisfaction　1　2　3　4　5　6　7　a source of satisfaction

4. I have come to expect that every day will be — exactly the same　1　2　3　4　5　6　7　new and different

5. When I think deeply about life — I do not feel there is any purpose to it　1　2　3　4　5　6　7　I feel there is a purpose to it

6. I feel that my life so far has — not been productive　1　2　3　4　5　6　7　been productive

7. I feel that the work* I am doing — is of no value　1　2　3　4　5　6　7　is of great value

8. I wish I were different than who I am. — agree strongly　1　2　3　4　5　6　7　disagree strongly

9. At this time, I have — no clearly defined goals for my life　1　2　3　4　5　6　7　clearly defined goals for my life

10. When sad things happen to me or other people — I cannot feel positive about life　1　2　3　4　5　6　7　I continue to feel positive about life

11. When I think about what I have done with my life, I feel — worthless　1　2　3　4　5　6　7　worthwhile

12. My present life — does not satisfy me　1　2　3　4　5　6　7　satisfies me

13. I feel joy in my heart — never　1　2　3　4　5　6　7　all the time

14. I feel trapped by the circumstances of my life. — agree strongly　1　2　3　4　5　6　7　disagree strongly

15. When I think about my past — I feel many regrets　1　2　3　4　5　6　7　I feel no regrets

16. Deep inside myself — I do *not* feel loved　1　2　3　4　5　6　7　I feel loved

17. When I think about the problems that I have — I do not feel hopeful about solving them　1　2　3　4　5　6　7　I feel very hopeful about solving them

*The definition of work is not limited to income-producing jobs. It includes childcare, housework, studies, and volunteer services.

Part II

Self-Confidence During Stress (answer according to how you feel during stressful times)

1. When there is a great deal of pressure being placed on me — I get tense　1　2　3　4　5　6　7　I remain calm

2. I react to problems and difficulties — with a great deal of frustration　1　2　3　4　5　6　7　with no frustration

3. In a difficult situation, I am confident
that I will receive the help that I need.   disagree strongly   1   2   3   4   5   6   7   agree strongly

4. I experience anxiety   all the time   1   2   3   4   5   6   7   never

5. When I have made a mistake   I feel extreme dislike   1   2   3   4   5   6   7   I continue to like myself
for myself

6. I find myself worrying that
something bad is going to happen
to me or those I love   all the time   1   2   3   4   5   6   7   never

7. In a stressful situation   I cannot concentrate easily   1   2   3   4   5   6   7   I can concentrate easily

8. I am fearful   all the time   1   2   3   4   5   6   7   never

9. When I need to stand up for myself   I cannot do it   1   2   3   4   5   6   7   I can do it easily

10. I feel less than adequate
in most situations   agree strongly   1   2   3   4   5   6   7   disagree strongly

11. During times of stress, I feel
isolated and alone.   agree strongly   1   2   3   4   5   6   7   disagree strongly

12. In really difficult situations   I feel *unable* to respond   1   2   3   4   5   6   7   I feel able to respond
in positive ways   in positive ways

13. When I need to relax   I experience no peace—   1   2   3   4   5   6   7   I experience a peacefulness—
only thoughts and worries   free of thoughts and worries

14. When I am in a frightening
situation   I panic   1   2   3   4   5   6   7   I remain calm

15. I worry about the future   all the time   1   2   3   4   5   6   7   never

Scoring

The number you circled is you score for that question. Add your scores in each of the two sections and divide each sum by the number of questions in the section.

- Life Purpose and Satisfaction: _____ ÷ 17 = _____.___
- Self-Confidence During Stress:_____ ÷ 15 = _____.___
- Combined Well-Being:
(add scores for both) _____ ÷ 32 = _____.___

Each score should range between 1.00 and 7.00 and may include decimals (for example 5.15).

Interpretation:

VERY LOW: 1.00 TO 2.49

MEDIUM LOW: 2.50 TO 3.99

MEDIUM HIGH: 4.00 TO 5.49

VERY HIGH: 5.50 to 7.00

These scores reflect the strength with which you feel these positive emotions. Do they make sense to you? Review each scale and each question in each scale. Your score on each item gives you information about the emotions and areas in your life where your psychological resources are strong, as well as the areas where strength needs to be developed.

If you notice a large difference between the LPS and SCDS scores, use this information to recognize which central attitudes and aspects of your life most need strengthening. If your scores on both scales are very low, talk with a coun-

selor or a friend about how you are feeling about yourself and your life.

SOURCE: Copyright 1989, Dr. Jared Kass. *Inventory of Positive Psychological Attitudes*, See Credits.

Making Changes ....

Boosting Your Self-Esteem

- Use affirmations, positive statements that help reinforce the most positive aspects of your personality and experience. Every day, you can boost your sense of esteem by saying positive things about you to yourself, such as "I am a loving, caring person," or "I am honest and open in expressing my feelings." You may want to write some affirmations of your own on index cards and flip through them occasionally.

- List the things you would like to have or experience. Construct the statements as if you were already enjoying the situations you list, beginning each sentence with "I am." For example, "I am feeling great about doing well in my classes," or "I am enjoying the opportunity to meet new people." Visualize each desired situation; and get in the habit of repeating this process several times each day.

- When your internal critic—the negative inner voice we all have—starts putting you down, tune it out. Force yourself to think of a situation that you handled well or something about yourself that you're especially proud of.

Your Feelings

Feelings are the emotional equivalents of body temperature or blood pressure, vital signs that indicate what's going on inside us. Some feelings serve as signals leading us toward pleasure, goodness, and love and away from harm and hurt. They run the gamut from the joy of finding love, which fills us with warmth and excitement, to the cold, bleak despair of losing a cherished partner or parent.

Often words aren't sufficient to express our emotions, which tend to be vague and hard to pin down enough to describe to others. Sometimes our bodies "do the talking": We cry in anguish, we laugh in delight, we sigh in sadness, we grimace in anger. Sometimes we cut ourselves off from our feelings, if only because their intensity scares us. We can't always explain why we feel the way we do—and we may not want to admit, even to ourselves, that we're just as capable of having negative feelings as we are of positive ones.

Feelings can affect us physically as well as psychologically. Negative feelings, such as frustration and anger, can actually undermine our health, whereas love, happiness, and other positive emotions can enhance and protect our well-being. Paying attention to feelings can help us keep in tune with, and respond to, our deepest needs.

Strategies for Change
. . . .
Getting in Touch with Your Emotions

✔ Keep a psychological journal. Rather than making notes about the who, where, when, and how of your life, write down what you're feeling and, if possible, why.

✔ Reflect on what happens each day or week, and identify the most meaningful parts. If you experience an intense emotion—positive or negative—describe the circumstances and the effects of the experience.

✔ If you find yourself worrying about a particular person or situation, record your concerns in detail. Try to discern the underlying reasons for your concern.

Your Needs

Newborns are unable to survive on their own. They depend on others for the satisfaction of their physical needs for food, shelter, warmth, and protection, as well as their less tangible emotional needs. In growing to maturity, children take on more responsibility and become more independent. No one, however, becomes totally self-sufficient. As adults, we easily recognize our basic physical needs, but we often fail to acknowledge our emotional needs. Yet they, too, must be met if we are to be as fulfilled as possible.

The humanist theorist Abraham Maslow believed that human needs are the motivating factors in personality development. First, we must satisfy basic physiological needs, such as those for food, shelter, and sleep. Only then can we pursue fulfillment of our higher needs—for safety and security, love and affection, and self-esteem. Few individuals reach the state of **self-actualization**, in which one functions at the highest possible level and derives the greatest possible satisfaction from life. (See Figure 3-1.)

Your Values and Morals

Your **values** are the criteria by which you evaluate things, people, events, and yourself; they represent what's most important to you. In a world of almost dizzying complexity, values can provide guidelines for making decisions that are right for you. If understood and applied, they help give life meaning and structure.

Social psychologist Milton Rokeach distinguished between two types of values. *Instrumental* values represent ways of thinking and acting that we hold important, such as being loving or loyal. *Terminal* values represent goals, achievements, or ideal states that we strive toward, such as happiness.[3] Both instrumental and terminal values form the basis for your attitudes and your behavior.

There can be a large discrepancy between what people say they value and what their actions indicate about their values. That's why it's important to clarify your own values, making sure you understand what you believe so that you can live in accordance with your beliefs. To do so, follow these steps:

1. Carefully consider the consequences of each choice.

2. Choose freely from among all the options.

3. Publicly affirm your values by sharing them with others.

4. Act out your values.[4]

Values clarification is not a once-in-a-lifetime task, but an ongoing process of sorting out what matters most to you. If you believe in protecting the environment, do

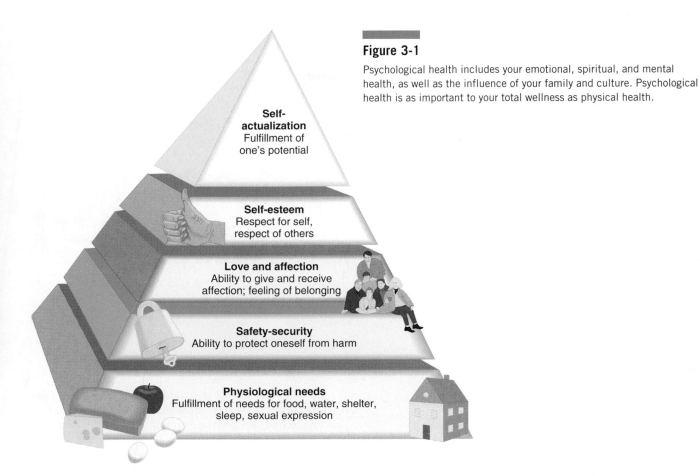

Figure 3-1

Psychological health includes your emotional, spiritual, and mental health, as well as the influence of your family and culture. Psychological health is as important to your total wellness as physical health.

Self-actualization
Fulfillment of one's potential

Self-esteem
Respect for self, respect of others

Love and affection
Ability to give and receive affection; feeling of belonging

Safety-security
Ability to protect oneself from harm

Physiological needs
Fulfillment of needs for food, water, shelter, sleep, sexual expression

you shut off lights, or walk rather than drive, in order to conserve energy? Do you vote for political candidates who support environmental protection? Do you recycle newspapers, bottles, and cans? Values are more than ideals we'd like to attain; they should be reflected in the way we live day by day.

The values of society are in a state of constant change: Because of an increasing focus on individuality, organizations are now placing more emphasis on creativity, flexibility, and responsiveness. Because of greater value given to enriching life experiences, interest in the arts, travel, and lifelong education is growing. In health behavior, values are shifting from an emphasis on curing illness to greater commitment to promoting wellness—as seen in the decline in smoking.[5]

The values of college students also change over the decades. In the 1960s, many young people sought to dedicate their lives to peace, saving the environment, and challenging traditional ways of doing things. By the 1980s, students tended to focus more on practical considerations and chose majors that would lead to lucrative careers. Today educators report another shift, this time toward greater concern about quality of life, community action, environmental advocacy, and helping people in need. This trend is reflected in the popularity of courses that deal with finding meaning in life.

Strategies for Change

Being True to Yourself

✔ Take the tombstone test: What would you like to have written on your tombstone? In other words, how would you like to be remembered? Your honest answer should tell you, very succinctly, what you value most.

✔ Describe yourself, as you are today, in a brief sentence. Ask friends or family members for their descriptions of you. How would you have to change to become the person you want to be remembered as?

✔ Try the adjective test: Choose three adjectives that you'd like to see associated with your reputation. Then list what you've done or can do to earn such descriptions.

Like our value system, our **moral** judgments—our sense of right and wrong—change throughout our life. According to Lawrence Kohlberg's theory of moral development, we develop a sense of morality as we grow.[6] As children, we behave in certain ways because we fear punishment or expect something in return. As adolescents, we may base our judgments on peer approval above all else. At the next stage of moral development, we become more concerned about laws and authority figures, so we may work hard to please a boss or not speed to avoid getting a ticket. As our moral development continues, we make decisions based on personal honor and self-respect and on our commitment to principles of respect for others and doing the right thing. At the very highest levels, justice becomes a primary value.

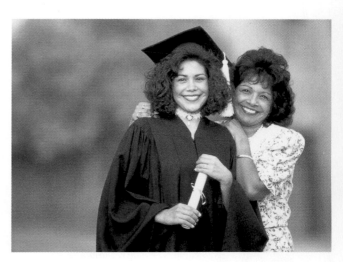

There can be great satisfaction in achieving a goal for which you worked long and hard.

Your Goals

We define ourselves not only by what we are now, but also by what we might become in the future. Career goals, in particular, have a tremendous impact. When you choose a vocation, you make a decision that affects how you spend your days, how you occupy your mind, whom you meet, and how you interact with them. College is an ideal time to think about careers, to imagine yourself in different jobs, and to prepare yourself for the type of work that most appeals to you.

Sometimes your aspirations may exceed your reach—but in stretching toward a dream, you will attain more of your potential. It is important, however, to be realistic about your abilities and opportunities. You may be the best basketball player on your block, but are you good enough to play professionally? Would it be more realistic to plan a career in coaching?

Don't underestimate your potential, but be honest. Look beyond yourself to your environment. What are the opportunities in the field that interest you most? Do you need a graduate degree? What about your financial obligations? Would you be able to get financial aid? Can you work days and study in the evenings? What about your family's involvement? Chart out a step-by-step plan to meet your goal, and remember: The first steps toward meeting any goal are the most important. If you're uncertain of which interests to pursue, look into internship programs or volunteer jobs that might give you a better sense of whether you'd be happy working in a particular field.

Boosting Self-Esteem

I am me.

In all the world there is no one else exactly like me. There are persons who have some parts like me, but no one adds up exactly like me. Therefore, everything that comes out of me is authentically mine because I alone chose it.

I own everything about me—my body, including everything it does; my mind, including all its thoughts and ideas; my eyes, including the images of all they behold; my feelings, whatever they may be—anger, joy, frustration, love, disappointment, excitement; my mouth, and all the words that come out of it, polite, sweet, or rough, correct or incorrect; my voice, loud or soft; and all my actions, whether they be to others or to myself. . . .

I own me, and therefore I can engineer me.

I am me, and I am okay.

Virginia Satir, *Peoplemaking*

After reading this declaration of **self-esteem**, think about how you feel about the person you are. Put down this book for a few minutes and draw a picture of how you see yourself. Don't worry about style or skill; simply try to capture your self-image on paper. Then analyze what you've drawn. How big is the figure you've sketched? Does it fill the page or occupy just one small corner? Is it active or still, smiling or frowning, attractive or awkward? Your drawing may hold clues to how you feel about yourself. Stop and think: What do you like about yourself? What do you dislike? What makes you unique? What gives you your greatest sense of satisfaction and pride?

Each of us wants and needs to feel significant as a human being with unique talents, abilities, and roles in life. A sense of self-esteem, of belief or pride in ourselves, gives us confidence to dare to attempt to achieve at school or work and to reach out to others to form friendships and close relationships. Self-esteem is the little voice that whispers, "You're worth it. You can do it. You're okay."

Self-esteem is based, not on external factors like wealth or beauty, but on what you believe about yourself. It's not something you're born with; self-esteem develops over time. It's also not something anyone else can give to you, although those around you can either help boost or diminish your self-esteem.

The seeds of self-esteem are planted in childhood when parents provide the assurance and appreciation youngsters need to push themselves toward new accomplishments: crawling, walking, forming words and sentences, learning control over their bladder and bowels. Two pillars of childhood self-esteem, say experts in child development, are confidence and competence. "Kids need to feel lovable and unconditionally loved to feel good about themselves," says therapist Stephanie Marston, author of *The Magic of Encouragement;* "...the other pillar of self-esteem is feeling capable and knowing you make a contribution to the family and later to the world."[7]

Adults, too, must consider themselves worthy of love, friendship, and success if they are to be loved, to make friends, and to achieve their goals. Low self-esteem is more common in people who have been abused as children and in those with psychiatric disorders, including depression, anxiety, alcoholism, and drug dependence.[8] Feeling one did not receive love and encouragement as a child can also lead to poor self-esteem. Adults with poor self-esteem may unconsciously enter relationships that reinforce their self-perceptions and may prefer and even seek out people who think poorly of them.

Increasingly, educators, business managers, and health caregivers are realizing that self-esteem is critical in making teenagers less destructive, employees more productive, and welfare recipients more self-sufficient. Hundreds of schools have added self-esteem materials to their curricula, and major corporations have added self-esteem training to their employee programs. Although such efforts have their critics, programs that encourage a reality-based sense of one's worth have won respect and acceptance.

One of the most useful techniques for bolstering self-esteem is developing the habit of positive thinking and talking.[9] While negative observations, such as constant criticisms or reminders of the most minor of faults,

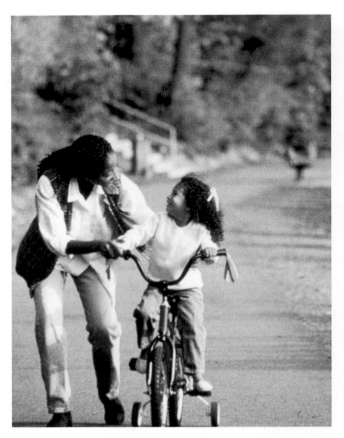

Children need opportunities to learn and succeed so that they can develop a sense of competence and self-worth.

can undermine self-image, positive affirmations—compliments, kudos, encouragements—have proven effective in enhancing self-esteem and psychological well-being. Individuals who fight off negative thoughts fare better psychologically than those who collapse when a setback occurs or who rely on others to make them feel better. (See Personal Voices: "Mei-Lin's Struggle for Self-Esteem.")

Strategies for Change

How to Feel Better About Yourself

✔ To make sure you're sending yourself the right messages, tune into the unspoken commentary playing in your head.

✔ If you spot a self-put-down (e.g., "What a klutz!" or "I screwed up again!"), scream (silently) "STOP!" or "DELETE!" Then give yourself a compliment to replace the criticism.

Personal Voices Mei-Lin's Struggle for Self-Esteem

Mei-Lin's parents were hoping for a boy when she was born. Instead, they got a daughter. When her brother was born fourteen months later, everyone focused on him. Throughout her childhood, Mei-Lin felt second-best, nowhere near as special as her beloved younger brother. The only way in which she felt superior was academically, but even straight A's at school didn't win the attention she craved at home.

High school was devastating for Mei-Lin's self-esteem. Whereas other girls giggled and flirted happily with boys, Mei-Lin couldn't think of anything to say. She pulled her hair back into a long braid; wore her reading glasses everywhere; and, once again, felt invisible. Her grades were consistently high, but she rarely spoke up in class. "No one cares about my opinion," she explained to a teacher who asked why she stayed so quiet when she obviously knew the material well.

Mei-Lin won a scholarship to a highly competitive private college in a faraway state. She was terrified and thrilled, all at the same time. As she hugged her family good-bye, she realized that at least they had accepted her as she was. Would anyone else ever do that? Mei-Lin didn't think so. Probably most of the other students were smarter. Surely the outgoing, popular girls wouldn't want anything to do with her. Boys probably wouldn't even notice her.

Mei-Lin kept to herself once she got to college, spending weekends at the library and taking on extra-credit projects. The only friend she made during her first semester was her roommate. Yolanda was everything Mei-Lin was not: sure of herself, upbeat, friendly. People seemed to buzz around her constantly. Yet Yolanda genuinely wanted to spend time with Mei-Lin. She'd wait to have breakfast with her, give her hilarious minute-by-minute accounts of her dates, and make plans for the two of them to go to a concert or movie.

"Well, she has to like me," Mei-Lin told herself. "She has to live with me." At the end of their first semester, Yolanda told Mei-Lin that there was a really terrific person she ought to get to know better.

"Who?" Mei-Lin asked.

"You," was the answer. Yolanda ticked off some of the qualities that made Mei-Lin special: her kindness, her intelligence, her sensitivity, her sense of humor. At Yolanda's insistence, Mei-Lin joined a group of students going to a concert one Friday night. When they started arguing about music—one of Mei-Lin's passions—she found herself speaking up often. And, to her delight, the other students wanted to hear what she had to say. As she headed back to the dorm, one of the young men quietly asked for her phone number.

Mei-Lin began to look at herself in a new light. When Yolanda suggested that she wear her hair loose, Mei-Lin looked in the mirror and realized that she wasn't as mousy as she'd always felt. When students in her dorm included her in their activities, she saw that they truly enjoyed her company. When she made the dean's list, she allowed herself to savor her academic achievement. As she acknowledged her strengths, she found it easier to accept her weaknesses, including her shyness and lack of athletic ability.

When Mei-Lin returned home the summer after her freshman year, her family and friends were amazed. "You've really blossomed," her mother said. Although Mei-Lin enjoyed the compliments, she realized that their words weren't what had made her feel good about herself. She had learned a lot from the really terrific person Yolanda had introduced her to. Above all, she'd learned to know and like herself.

✔ If you hear your mind replaying the same negative observations again and again, try to trace them back to their source. Did they come from your parents, teachers, siblings? Say, "That's what they think, but it's not necessarily true."

✔ Make a list of the qualities you like best about yourself. Replay the list in your mind when you're feeling down about yourself.

✔ Spend more time doing those activities you know you do best. For example, if you are a good cook, prepare a meal for someone; if you are good at writing, write a letter to someone.

✔ Separate what you do, especially any mistakes you make, from who you are. Instead of saying, "I'm so stupid," tell yourself, "That wasn't the smartest move I ever made, but I'll learn from it."

Emotional Intelligence

Once a person's "IQ"—or intelligence quotient—was considered the leading determinant of achievement. However, psychologists have determined that another "way of knowing," dubbed **emotional intelligence**, may make an even greater difference in a person's personal and professional success. In his international bestseller on what some call "EQ" (for emotional quotient), psychologist Daniel Goleman, Ph.D., identified five components of emotional intelligence: self-awareness, altruism, personal motivation, empathy, and the ability to love and be loved by friends, partners, and family members. People who possess high emotional intelligence are the people who truly succeed in work as well as play, building flourishing careers and lasting, meaningful relationships.[10]

Emotional intelligence isn't fixed at birth, and increasingly its precepts are being taught as part of the curriculum at primary and secondary schools. Even corporations are hiring consultants to boost employees' EQ, since it's been shown to directly affect teamwork, confidence, and productivity.[11] Emotions can be our allies, explains Dr. Jeanne Segal, helping us form loving and meaningful relationships, while making us well-rounded and profoundly sensitive beings. If repressed, they can be our enemies, oppressing us like well-armored dictators. By listening to our body's messages, we can incorporate both emotional and rational intelligence in our daily lives.[12]

Managing Your Moods

Feelings come and go within minutes. A **mood** is a more sustained emotional state that colors our view of the world for hours or days. According to surveys by psychologist Randy Larsen, Ph.D., of the University of Michigan, bad moods descend upon us an average of three out of every ten days. "A few people—about 2%—are happy just about every day," he says. "About 5% report bad moods four out of every five days."[13]

"Mood is now recognized as a central element of human behavior, and mood management is basic to many of our common daily activities," observes psychologist Robert Thayer of California State University, who reports that more than a dozen research laboratories are studying neurobiology and mood regulation.[14] These scientists have found that people in various countries use many different methods to change their moods: listening to music, talking to a friend, going for a walk, keeping busy, trying to rectify a problem, eating, praying, shopping.[15]

There are gender differences in mood management: Men typically try to distract themselves (a partially successful strategy) or use alcohol or drugs (an ineffective tactic). Women are more likely to talk to someone (which can help) or to ruminate on why they feel bad (which doesn't help).[16] Learning effective mood-boosting, mood-regulating strategies can help both men and women pull themselves up and out of an emotional slump. (See Pulsepoints: "Ten Ways to Pull Yourself Out of a Bad Mood").

Problem-Oriented Methods

The most effective way to banish a sad or bad mood is by changing what caused it in the first place—if you can figure out what made you upset and why. "Most bad moods are caused by loss or failure in work or intimate relationships," says Larsen. "The questions to ask are: What can I do to fix the failure? What can I do to remedy the loss? Is there anything under my control that I can

---

Pulsepoints

Ten Ways to Pull Yourself Out of a Bad Mood

1. Accentuate the positive. Think of the parts of your life that are going well rather than mulling over what's not.

2. Review past successes. Remind yourself of what you've accomplished before to motivate yourself to accomplish more in the future.

3. Pray. In a Gallup poll of 1007 Americans, religious practices rated as the most effective way of relieving depression.

4. Listen to music. While many forms of distraction help, at least temporarily, this is one of the most popular and effective mood boosters.

5. Treat yourself. Indulgences—big or small, expensive or not— can bring you up when you're feeling down. The reason: They make you feel special.

6. Volunteer. A third of Americans— some 89 million people—give of themselves through volunteer work. By doing the same, you may feel better too.

7. Exercise. In various studies around the world, physical exertion ranks as one of the best ways to change a bad mood, raise energy, and reduce tension.

8. Act happy. Putting on a happy face doesn't make problems disappear, but it does improve mood.

9. Focus on the future. Although you can't rewrite the past, you can learn from it. Resolve to try harder and do better the next time around.

10. Set a limit on self-pity. Tell yourself, "I'm going to feel sorry for myself this morning, but this afternoon, I've got to get on with my life."

change? If there is, take action and solve it." Rewrite the report. Ask to take a make-up exam. Apologize to the friend whose feelings you hurt. Tell your parents you feel bad about the argument you had.

If there's nothing you can do, accept what happened and focus on doing things differently next time. "In our studies, resolving to try harder actually was as effective in improving mood as taking action in the present," says Larsen. You also can try to think about what happened in a different way and put a positive spin on it. This technique, known as *cognitive reappraisal,* or "reframing," helps you look at a setback in a new light: What lessons did it teach you? What would you have done differently? Could there be a silver lining or hidden benefit?

Emotion-Oriented Methods

If you can't identify or resolve the problem responsible for your emotional funk, the next-best solution is to concentrate on altering your negative feelings. For example, try setting a quick, achievable goal that can boost your spirits with a small success. Clean out a closet; sort through the piles of paper on your desk; write the letter to your aunt you've been putting off for weeks.

Another good option is to get moving. In a recent review of studies of mood regulation, California State University psychologists ranked exercise as the single most effective strategy for banishing bad feelings.[17] Numerous studies have confirmed that aerobic work-

outs, such as walking or jogging, significantly improve mood. Even nonaerobic exercise, such as weight-lifting, can boost spirits; improve sleep and appetite; reduce anxiety; irritability; and anger; and produce feelings of mastery and accomplishment.

Although it's tempting to pull away from others when you're in a slump, it's better not to withdraw. "It's never a good idea to sulk by yourself when you're feeling down," says Larsen. "Pretend to be extraverted if you have to, but do spend time with other people." As he notes, friends often can help improve your mood by giving you good feedback. But be wary of seeking out companions solely for a gripe-and-groan session. You might end up feeling worse rather than better.

Taking your mind off your troubles, rather than mulling over what's wrong, is one of the most often used mood boosters, but it's only partly successful. Simple distractions—watching television, for instance, or reading—work only temporarily. Activities that engage the imagination, on the other hand, seem to have more lasting effects. Listening to music, for instance, is one of the most popular and effective ways of distracting people from their troubles and changing their bad moods (see Table 3-1).

What Doesn't Work

Giving in to a bad mood and resigning yourself to feeling out of sorts practically guarantees that you won't feel better soon. Negative expectations tend to be self-fulfill-

---

TABLE 3-1   MOOD-BOOSTERS: WHAT WORKS AND WHAT DOESN'T

These are the most common ways that college students use to feel happier, release anger, or enhance feelings of well-being. Some work better than others.

Most Effective	Partly Effective	Not Effective
Taking action to solve a problem	Socializing	"Venting"
Reappraising what happened	Distracting yourself	Blaming others
Thinking about other successes		Being alone
Rewarding yourself		Giving up
Resolving to try harder		
Making "downward" comparisons (to less fortunate individuals)		

SOURCE: Based on research by psychologist Randy Larsen, Ph.D., of the University of Michigan.

ing, and individuals who expect to feel bad do indeed report greater unhappiness.[18] "Venting" or "letting it all out" also does little good. "Screaming or crying only serves to reinforce a negative emotion," says Larsen. "In our studies, people who vented their emotions were more likely to remain just as upset hours afterward."

Thinking again and again about faults, failings, or misfortunes not only perpetuates a bad mood but can also contribute to depression. Individuals who ruminate in this way are less likely to engage in distracting pleasant activities—even if they believe they would enjoy them.[19] Yet, despite their low mood, they are convinced that they should perform at a high level.[20]

Turning to alcohol or drugs to escape sorrows may offer temporary relief, but once the buzz is gone, so is the good mood. And you may end up thinking even less of yourself because of your reliance on chemical crutches. Similarly, if you console yourself with ice cream, chocolate, or other tasty treats, you may be setting yourself up for another slump the next time you step on the scale.

Pursuing Happiness

Psychologist David Myers, author of *The Pursuit of Happiness: Who Is Happy—and Why*, defines happiness as "a sense of well-being, a feeling that life as a whole is going well."[21] This state depends not on big achievements, but on little pleasures. As recent studies have shown, happiness tends to be highest when people combine frequent good experiences—the daily joys of having a caring partner, a productive job, or enjoyable hobbies—with occasional very intense pleasures, such as a special vacation or a promotion.[22]

There is no one route to happiness—nor are there any barriers to achieving it. "Happiness doesn't depend on how old you are or how much money you make, whether you're male or female, or what race you belong to," says Myers. "It does depend on certain personality traits, whether your work suits your skills, whether you have close relationships and an active religious faith."

Happiness also depends on cultural contexts. In studies comparing Western and Chinese views of happiness, individuals in the West define happiness as an internal state, one that relies on internal contentment, while the Chinese place greater emphasis on interpersonal or external satisfaction.[23] Age, gender, and person-

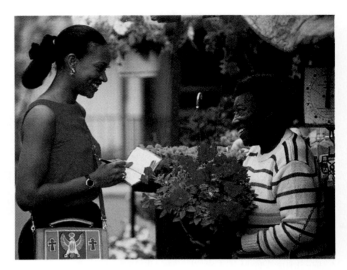

Happiness and optimism go hand in hand. Small rewards can keep your spirits high and remind you that you are special.

ality factors, such as extraversion, dutifulness, and achievement, also affect an individual's sense of happiness.[24]

The best predictors of happiness are the characteristics of good psychological health: high self-esteem, optimism, extraversion, and a sense of being in control. In addition to these four key traits, happy people are more likely to have healthy and fit bodies; realistic goals and expectations, supportive friendships; an intimate, sexually warm marriage; and a faith that provides support, purpose, and acceptance.

Happiness is not just a state of mind but quite literally a state of brain. By means of sophisticated imaging techniques, neuroscientists have discovered differences in brain chemistry and activity when people are experiencing happiness, sadness, and other moods. In both women and men, happiness activates a specific region in the frontal cortex (described in Chapter 4).[25] However, there are differences in the impact of sadness on the brains of women and men, with a much larger area of the female brain being affected than that of the male brain.[26]

Happiness affects brain functions as well as the brain itself. Studies in which individuals had to recognize or name certain words found differences in basic information processing, depending on their perceived happiness.[27] It also matters whether people link their feelings of happiness to positive or negative life events. In a study of 89 college students, the "linkers" were most likely to see their happiness as contingent on attaining important goals in life.[28]

Becoming Optimistic

The dictionary defines **optimism** as "an inclination to anticipate the best possible outcome." In *Healthy Pleasures*, Robert Ornstein and David Sobel redefine it psychologically as "the tendency to seek out, remember, and expect pleasurable experiences. It is an active priority of the person, not merely a reflex that prompts us to look on the sunny side."[29]

For various reasons—because they believe in themselves, because they trust in a higher power, because they feel lucky—optimists expect positive experiences from life. When bad things happen, they tend to see setbacks or losses as specific, temporary incidents. In their eyes, a disappointment is "one of those things" that happens every once in a while, rather than the latest in a long string of disasters. And rather than blaming themselves ("I always screw things up," pessimists might say), optimists look at all the different factors that may have caused the problem.

"What you expect is what you get," say Ornstein and Sobel, who suggest a simple test of your optimism level: Write down as many as you can of the wonderful experiences you expect to have in the future. Then describe the difficult, trying things you think might happen. How many positive experiences did you list? How many negative ones? Two years after a group of elderly men and women took this test, the optimists who had listed more positive than negative expectations reported fewer physical symptoms of ill health, fewer colds, fewer days off from work, more energy, and a greater sense of psychological well-being.

Individuals aren't born optimistic or pessimistic; in fact, researchers have documented changes over time in the ways that individuals view the world and what they expect to experience in the future. "We have a choice about how we think," asserts psychologist Martin Seligman, Ph.D., author of *Learned Optimism*. "We can choose to change the habits of pessimism into optimism." The key is disputing the automatic negative thoughts that flood our brains and choosing to believe in our own possibilities. "Optimism is a set of learned skills," says Seligman. "Once learned, these skills persist because they feel so good to use. And reality is usually on our side."[30]

Savoring Pleasures

"Treating yourself is one of the best ways to cheer yourself up," says psychologist Larsen of the University of Michigan. "A night out is fun in itself, but it also imparts an important message: You're worth it. As adults we all need occasional reminders that we are special and deserve some special things."

This doesn't mean you have to break the bank. When you're feeling low, even simple indulgences, like sleeping in a few extra minutes or eating your lunch out in the sun, can make you feel better. If you're feeling down, plan a reward for yourself every day, and make it a habit to include small pleasures—such as sharing a joke with a friend or taking time to watch a splendid sunset—in your daily routine.[31]

Looking on the Light Side

Humor, which enables us to express fears and negative feelings without causing distress to ourselves or others, is one of the healthiest ways of coping with life's ups and downs. Laughter stimulates the heart, alters brain wave patterns and breathing rhythms, reduces perceptions of pain, decreases stress-related hormones, and strengthens the immune system. Even in cases of critical or fatal illnesses, humor can help people live with greater joy until they die.

Joking and laughing are ways of expressing honest emotions, of overcoming dread and doubt, and of connecting with others. They also can defuse rage. After all, it's almost impossible to stay angry when you're laughing. To tickle your funny bone, try keeping a file of favorite cartoons or jokes. Go to a comedy club instead of a movie. And when you see or hear something that makes you laugh out loud, don't keep it to yourself—multiply the mirth by sharing it with a friend.

Strategies for Prevention

....

How to Be Happy

✔ Make time for yourself. It's impossible to meet the needs of others without recognizing and fulfilling your own.

✔ Invest yourself in closeness. Give your loved ones the gift of your time and caring.

✔ Work hard at what you like. Search for challenges that satisfy your need to do something meaningful.

- ✔ Be upbeat. If you always look for what's wrong about yourself or your life, you'll find it—and feel even worse.
- ✔ Organize but stay loose. Be ready to seize an unexpected opportunity to try something different.
- ✔ Despite inevitable highs and lows, strive for a sense of balance.

Finding Meaning in Life

"What's it all about?" It's the question almost everyone asks sooner or later. Whether dreams come true or die, whether we achieve our goals or not, we find ourselves confronting difficult questions about the purpose of our lives. We're especially likely to ask such questions when bad things happen or when we face daunting difficulties—circumstances that are an unavoidable part of life. Many people find answers through loving relationships, spiritual development, and acts of charity and good will.

Loving and Being Loved

"One can live magnificently in this world if one knows how to work and how to love, to work for the person one loves and to love one's work," Leo Tolstoy wrote. You may not think of love as a basic need like food and rest, but it is essential for both physical and psychological well-being.

Although being loved is enough to get us started in a healthy life, as mature individuals we need to express love as well as to receive it, to be able to form a union with another person while retaining our own identity and integrity. We evolve toward this state of loving, beginning from the infant's total self-concern and gradually learning to love others and to find fulfillment by fulfilling the needs of others. Since relationships are so vital to our well-being, Chapter 8 is devoted to exploring our ties to friends, parents, partners, spouses, and children.

Caring for the Soul

As discussed in Chapter 1, spiritual development is part of total health. "The soul needs an intense, full-bodied spiritual life as much as and in the same way that the body needs food," observes psychologist Thomas Moore in *Care of the Soul*. "Just as the mind digests ideas and produces intelligence, the soul feeds on life and digests it, creating wisdom and character out of the fodder of experience."[32]

For years, spiritual matters were rarely recognized or discussed by mental health professionals. Until 1982, fewer than 3% of the articles published in leading psychiatry journals focused on spirituality or religiousity. Since then dozens of scientific studies have found that spiritual beliefs and activities—such as prayer or meditation—positively affect psychological well-being and may even speed recovery from medical illness.[33] How? "Faith provides a support community, a sense of life's meaning, a reason to focus beyond self, and a timeless perspective on life's temporary ups and downs," observes psychologist David Meyers.

Doing Good

Altruism—helping or giving to others—enhances self-esteem, relieves physical and mental stress, and protects psychological well-being. Hans Selye, the father of stress research, described cooperation with others for the self's sake as altruistic egotism, whereby we satisfy our own needs while helping others satisfy theirs. This concept is essentially an updated version of the golden rule: Do unto others as you would have them do unto you. The important difference is that you earn your neighbor's love and help by offering them love and help.

Giving helps those who give as well as those who receive. People involved in community organizations, for instance, consistently report a surge of well-being called *helper's high*, which they describe as a unique sense of calmness, warmth, and enhanced self-worth.[34] College students who provided community service as part of a semester-long course reported changes in attitude (including a decreased tendency to blame people for their misfortunes), self-esteem (primarily a belief that they can make a difference), and behavior (a greater commitment to do more volunteer work).[35]

The options for giving of yourself are limitless: Volunteer to serve a meal at a homeless shelter. Collect donations for a charity auction. Teach in an illiteracy program. Perform the simplest act of charity: pray for others. "Whenever I hear of someone with a problem, I say three prayers for them," one woman reports; "It makes me feel better—and I hope it helps them, too."

Feeling in Control

Although no one has absolute control over destiny, there is a great deal that we can do to control how we think, feel, and behave. By assessing our life situations realistically, we can make plans and preparations that allow us to make the most of our circumstances. By doing so, we gain a sense of mastery. In nationwide surveys, Americans who feel in control of their lives report greater psychological well-being than those who do not, as well as "extraordinarily positive feelings of happiness."[36]

Developing Autonomy

One goal that many people strive for is **autonomy**, or independence. Both family and society influence our ability to grow toward independence. Autonomous individuals are true to themselves. As they weigh the pros and cons of any decision, whether it's using or refusing drugs or choosing a major or career, they base their judgment on their own values, not those of others. Their ability to draw on internal resources and cope with challenges has a positive impact on both their psychological well-being and their physical health, including recovery from illness.[37] Those who've achieved autonomy may seek the opinions of others, but they do not allow their decisions to be dictated by external influences. Because of this, it is said that their **locus of control**—that is, where they view control as originating—is *internal* (from within themselves) rather than *external* (from others).

Becoming Assertive

Being **assertive** means recognizing your feelings and making your needs and desires clear to others. Unlike aggression, a far less healthy means of expression, assertiveness usually works. You can change a situation you don't like by communicating your feelings and thoughts in nonprovocative words, by focusing on specifics, and by making sure you're talking with the person(s) who is directly responsible.

Becoming assertive isn't always easy. Many people have learned to cope by being passive and not communicating their feelings or opinions. Sooner or later they become so irritated, frustrated, or overwhelmed that

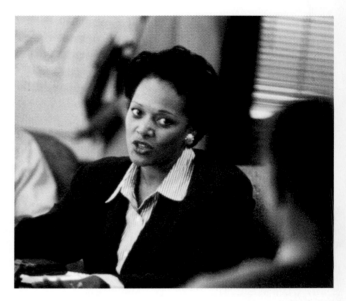

Practicing assertiveness allows you to express yourself without aggression, to communicate and accomplish your goals.

they explode in an outburst—which they think of as being assertive. However, such behavior is so distasteful to them that they'd rather be passive. But assertiveness doesn't mean screaming or telling someone off. You can communicate your wishes calmly and clearly.

Even at its mildest, assertiveness can make you feel better about yourself and your life. The reason: When you speak up or take action, you're in the pilot seat. And that's always much less stressful than taking a back seat and trying to hang on for dear life.

Strategies for Change

Asserting Yourself

✔ Remind yourself that as an individual, you have certain rights—including the right to make mistakes, to change your mind, to say "I don't understand" or "I don't know."

✔ Don't expect an instant transformation. Assertiveness is a skill that takes time and practice to acquire.

✔ Decide what's really important and what's not before speaking up and setting limits.

✔ Don't think you have to be obnoxious in order to be assertive. It's most effective to state your needs and preferences without any sarcasm or hostility.

Boosting Energy

Do you drag through the day? Do you feel that you're running on empty? Sometimes the causes of fatigue are psychological, and a lack of energy can be a symptom of a mental disorder, such as depression.[38] However, often fatigue stems from a lack of any one of three energy essentials: exercise, good nutrition, or sleep.

Exercise

While you may think that working out will wear you down, regular aerobic activities such as walking, jogging, cycling, or swimming in fact have the opposite effect. Daily workouts promote alertness and relax body and mind so that you sleep better and feel more energetic. Exercise also produces gradual psychological changes. As they condition their bodies, individuals who exercise release anger and anxiety and feel better about their bodies and lives. Seeing for themselves that they're capable of change, exercisers may feel more competent and confident about other aspects of their lives.

Almost any form of physical activity—from walking to weight-lifting—can help. (See Figure 3-2.) While even a single session does some good, a regular regimen of daily exercise is better.[39] Individuals who regularly engage in aerobic activity report higher energy levels, better mood, and lower likelihood of depression.[40] (Chapter 5 provides a complete discussion of exercise and its benefits.)

Eating Right

Both your body and mind need good nutrition to run efficiently. To keep energy levels up, try five small meals throughout the day rather than three large ones. Always start with a healthy breakfast. Take time to eat nutritious

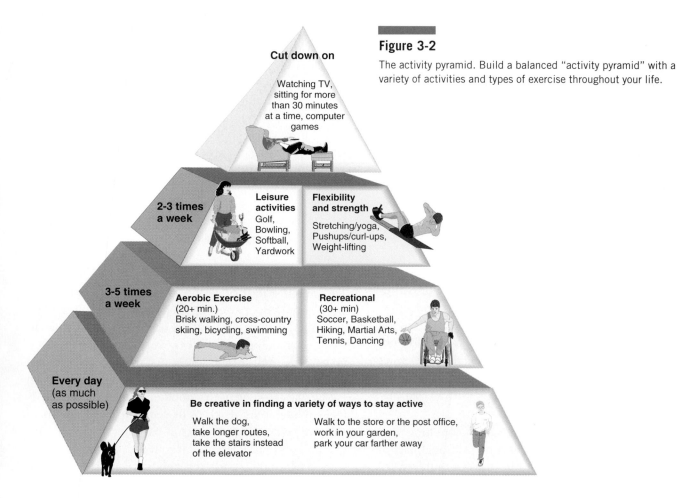

Figure 3-2

The activity pyramid. Build a balanced "activity pyramid" with a variety of activities and types of exercise throughout your life.

Cut down on

Watching TV, sitting for more than 30 minutes at a time, computer games

2-3 times a week

Leisure activities
Golf, Bowling, Softball, Yardwork

Flexibility and strength
Stretching/yoga, Pushups/curl-ups, Weight-lifting

3-5 times a week

Aerobic Exercise (20+ min.)
Brisk walking, cross-country skiing, bicycling, swimming

Recreational (30+ min)
Soccer, Basketball, Hiking, Martial Arts, Tennis, Dancing

Every day (as much as possible)

Be creative in finding a variety of ways to stay active

Walk the dog, take longer routes, take the stairs instead of the elevator

Walk to the store or the post office, work in your garden, park your car farther away meals. If you wolf down a hamburger and fries in the car on your way to class, or munch on chips and pretzels as you study, you're setting yourself and your stomach up for some problems. If you're physically uncomfortable because of poor eating habits, you'll be psychologically ill at ease as well—unable to concentrate on tasks at hand, to relax, or to enjoy the people around you.[41] (Chapter 6 provides detailed information on eating right for life.)

Getting Enough Sleep

You stay up late cramming for a final. You drive through the night to visit a friend at another campus. You get up for an early class during the week but stay in bed until noon on weekends. And you wonder: "Why am I so tired?" The answer: You're not getting enough sleep— and you're not alone. According to the National Commission on Sleep Disorders Research, one out of every three Americans has problems sleeping. And even those who aren't having difficulty don't log as much sleep time as they'd like. Over the last century, we have cut our average nightly sleep time by more than 20%.[42]

Whenever we fail to get adequate sleep, we accumulate what researchers call a *sleep debt.* With each night of too little rest, our body's need for sleep grows until it becomes irresistible. "We don't tend to have a good handle on our amount of sleep debt," says psychiatrist William Dement, M.D., of Stanford University, a pioneer in sleep research. "So when we finally go bankrupt, it happens fast. People can go from feeling wide awake to falling asleep in five seconds. If you are behind the wheel of a car, you could end up dead."[43] According to the Department of Transportation, each year 200,000 sleep-related accidents claim more than 5000 lives, cause hundreds of thousands of injuries, and incur billions in indirect costs.[44]

The only solution to sleep debt is the obvious one: paying it back. Individuals who add an hour or two to their nightly sleep time are more alert, more productive, and less likely to have accidents. And because sleepy people tend to be irritable and edgy, those who get more rest also tend to be happier, healthier, and easier to get along with.

Sleep Basics

We spend a third of our lives sleeping—more time than we spend working, loving, or playing. Although sleepers may look quiet and seem unresponsive to the world around them, their brains and bodies are going through a series of profound changes. Scientists differentiate between certain periods of the night when the eyes dart rapidly back and forth beneath closed lids, called **rapid-eye-movement (REM) sleep**, and quieter, non-REM sleep stages. Most adults spend 20 to 25 percent of the night in REM sleep, when our most vivid dreaming takes place.

Each night as you fall asleep, you go through the same sequence of sleep stages: Your body begins to slow down, and muscular tension decreases. As you enter stage 1 of non-REM sleep, your brain waves become smaller, pinched, and irregular. Mundane thoughts flit through your mind; if awakened from this twilight zone, you might deny having slept at all. As you enter stage 2, your brain waves become larger, with occasional bursts of activity. Your eyes become unresponsive, so that even if your eyelids were gently lifted, you wouldn't see. In stage 3, your brain waves are much slower and about five times larger than in stage 1. In stage 4, the most profound state of unconsciousness, your brain waves form a slow, jagged pattern; and you would be very difficult to arouse. (See Figure 3-3.)

The full journey to the depths of tranquility takes more than an hour. Then you begin your ascent—not to consciousness but to REM sleep. The muscles of your middle ear vibrate. Your brain waves resemble the patterns of waking more than of deep sleep. The muscles of your face, limbs, and trunk are slack. Your pulse and breathing quicken, and your brain temperature and blood flow increase. Your eyes dart back and forth. If wakened, you're likely to report a fantasylike dream.

Your body repeats this sequence four or five times a night. In an eight-hour night's rest, you spend two hours in REM sleep; over the course of a lifetime, you'll spend five or six years dreaming and three times that amount in the quieter stages of sleep.

How Much Sleep Is Enough?

There's no one formula for how long a good night's sleep should be. Expecting all people to need the same amount of rest would be as absurd as expecting them to eat the same amount of food every day. Normal sleep times range from five to ten hours; the average is seven and a half. About one or two people in a hundred can get by with just five hours; another small minority needs twice that amount. Each of us seems to have an innate sleep *appetite* that is as much a part of our genetic programming as hair color and skin tone.

To figure out your sleep needs, keep your wake-up time the same every morning and vary your bedtimes.

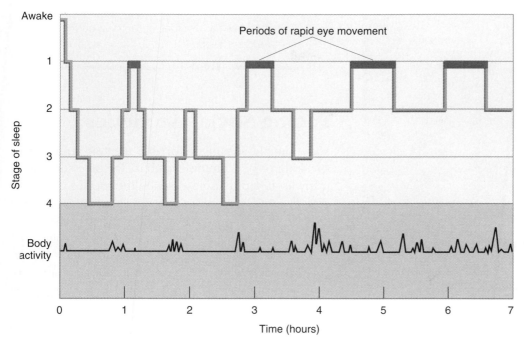

Periods of rapid eye movement

Figure 3-3

A sleep cycle. During the first hour or so sleep becomes deeper, then the level ascends to a period of REM sleep (indicated by thick bars). The sleep cycle is repeated, with some variations, throughout the night.

Are you groggy after six hours of shut-eye? Does an extra hour give you more stamina? What about an extra two hours? Since too much sleep can make you feel sluggish, don't assume that more is always better. Listen to your body's signals, and adjust your sleep schedule to suit them.

Strategies for Change

How to Sleep Like a Baby

✔ Keep regular hours for going to bed and getting up in the morning. Stay as close as possible to this schedule on weekends as well as weekdays.

✔ Develop a sleep ritual—such as stretching, meditation, yoga, prayer, or reading a not-too-thrilling novel—to ease the transition from wakefulness to sleep.

✔ Don't drink coffee late in the day. The effects of caffeine can linger for up to eight hours. And don't smoke. Nicotine is an even more powerful stimulant—and sleep saboteur—than caffeine.

✔ Don't rely on alcohol to get to sleep. Alcohol disrupts normal sleep stages; so you won't sleep as deeply or as restfully as you normally would.

✔ Don't nap during the day if you're having problems sleeping through the night.

Connecting with Others

At every age, people who feel connected to others tend to be healthier physically and psychologically. College students are no exception: Those who have a supportive, readily available network of relationships are less psychologically distressed and more satisfied with life.[45] (See Chapter 8 for a comprehensive discussion of communication, friendship, and intimacy.)

The opposite of *connectedness* is **social isolation**, a major risk factor for illness and early death. Individuals with few social contacts face two to four times the mortality rate of others. The reason may be that their social isolation weakens the body's ability to ward off disease. Medical students with higher-than-average scores on a loneliness scale had lower levels of protective immune cells.[46] The end of a long-term relationship—through separation, divorce, or death—also dampens immunity.[47]

It is part of our nature as mammals and as human beings to crave relationships. But invariably we end up alone at times. Solitude is not without its own quiet joys—time for introspection, self-assessment, learning from the past, and looking toward the future. Each of us can cultivate the joy of our company, of being alone without crossing the line and becoming lonely.[48]

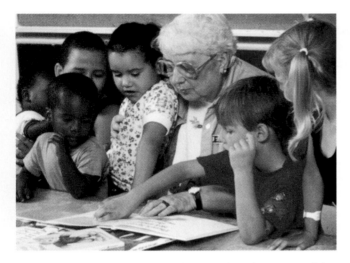

Volunteering is a rewarding way of connecting with others, giving of yourself, and feeling connected to your community.

Overcoming Loneliness

More so than many other countries, we are a nation of loners. Recent trends—longer work hours, busy family schedules, frequent moves, high divorce rates—have created even more lonely people. Only 23% of Americans say they're never lonely. Loneliest of all are those who are divorced, separated, or widowed and those who live alone or solely with children. Among single adults who have never been married, 42% feel lonely at least sometimes. However, loneliness is most likely to cause emotional distress when it is a chronic rather than an episodic condition.[49]

To combat loneliness, people may join groups, fling themselves into projects and activities, or surround themselves with superficial acquaintances.[50] Others avoid the effort of trying to connect, sometimes limiting most of their personal interactions to chat groups on the Internet. But the true keys to overcoming loneliness are developing resources to fulfill our own potential and learning to reach out to others. In this way, loneliness can become a means to personal growth and discovery.[51]

Strategies for Prevention

How to Avoid Feeling Lonely

✔ Learn to be by yourself. Enjoying your own company helps make you the sort of person others enjoy.

✔ Pursue some interests on your own—hiking in the woods, perhaps, or joining a singing group.

✔ Keep in touch with old friends, even when miles or years may separate you.

✔ Give of yourself as a volunteer. Nothing warms the spirit more than reaching out to those who need you.

Facing Social Anxieties

Many people are uncomfortable meeting strangers or speaking or performing in public. In some surveys, as many as 40% of people describe themselves as shy, or *socially anxious.*[52] Some shy people—an estimated 10 to 15% of children—are born with a predisposition to social anxieties.[53] Others become shy because they don't learn proper social responses or because they experience rejection or shame. As a result, normal apprehension intensifies in situations in which they might be watched or criticized by others. They feel extremely self-conscious, embarrassed, and nervous. When attention is on them alone, they may tremble, breathe very rapidly (hyperventilate), sweat, or develop a dry mouth or nausea.

Social anxieties often become a problem in late adolescence. Students may develop symptoms when they go to a party at a fraternity or sorority or are called on in class. Some experience symptoms when they try to perform any sort of action in the presence of others, even such everyday activities as eating in public, using a public restroom, or writing a check. In a severe form of social anxiety, called **social phobia**, individuals typically fear and avoid various social situations. In performance anxiety—a subtype of social phobia—the main fear is of performing in front of others. The key difference between these problems and normal shyness and self-consciousness is the degree of distress and impairment that individuals experience.

If you're shy, you can overcome much of your social apprehensiveness on your own, in much the same way as you might set out to stop smoking or lose weight. For example, you can improve your social skills by pushing yourself to introduce yourself to a stranger at a party or to chat about the weather or the food selections with the person next to you in a cafeteria line. Gradually you'll acquire a sense of social timing and a verbal ease that will take the worry out of close encounters with others.

Those with more disabling social anxiety may do best with professional guidance, which has proven highly effective. One common technique used by experts is role playing, in which individuals act out situations that normally produce butterflies in the stomach, such as returning a defective product to a store or calling for a date.[54] With practice and time, most individuals are able to emerge from the walls that shyness has built around them and take pleasure in interacting with others.

Strategies for Change
Developing Social Skills

✔ If you want to get to know someone you see on campus or at work, write down what you want to say, and rehearse on your own or with a friend.

✔ Use a mirror to practice making eye contact and smiling. Talk into a tape-recorder to improve your speaking voice and volume.

✔ Observe and copy the behavior of people who handle social situations well, perhaps those who make clear what they want without being obnoxious.

✔ Every two weeks, invite someone to accompany you on an inexpensive outing, such as a visit to a museum.

✔ When you're with others, focus on them and what they're saying. Try not to think about how you look or what you're saying.

Getting Along with Difficult People

Sooner or later we all have to deal with relatives, friends, roommates, colleagues, or bosses who annoy, attack, blame, manipulate, or infuriate us. Some simply have habits or behaviors that "push our buttons," grating on our nerves and clashing with our way of doing things. Others consistently irritate almost everyone they encounter. What makes them so difficult to deal with?

"Chances are that the most frustrating people in your life have personality disorders," says psychiatrist John Oldham, M.D., coauthor of *The Personality Self-Portrait*, who notes that the difference between ordinary orneriness or eccentricity and **personality disorders** is a matter of degree.[55] These common conditions are not difficulties that people *have*—like depression or anxiety—but fundamental problems with who they *are*: how they feel, how they see themselves, how they relate to others.

"A lot of people have some rough edges, but 10 to 15% of men and women have so many that they're always running into difficulties—and always have been, ever since they were teenagers or young adults," says Oldham. "They have problems getting along in every work situation. They get into relationship after relationship that doesn't work out. There's always fireworks or static in their lives."

These extremely difficult people don't just make themselves miserable; they exasperate everyone around them. Since you can't avoid them, you have to know how to cope with them—and the first step is understanding. "They aren't being difficult on purpose; they really can't help themselves," explains Allen Frances, M.D., chairman of psychiatry at Duke University Medical Center. This realization may help friends and family members, who are often confused and hurt by the difficult people in their lives. "The best approach, he says, is "not to try to get them to change, but to try to understand why they're difficult and find ways to work around them."[56]

It can help to keep some emotional distance and not take annoying behavior personally. Most obnoxious behavior has more to do with the other person's insecurities than with you. When difficult people behave badly, they typically blame others for "making" them do so. A personality disorder may be an explanation for obnoxious, inconsiderate, annoying behavior, but it's not an excuse. Respect your own rights as a person, and expect others to do the same.

If you need to confront a difficult person for any reason, simply state how you feel or what you observe without judging. Exquisitely sensitive to rejection or disapproval, many such individuals overreact to any comment that could be construed as a criticism or challenge. You also can try to give them some of what they need. You don't have to cave in, but be pragmatic. If a friend or coworker is always suspicious, keep plans out in the open so it's clear that you're not hiding anything. If all else fails, you may have to write off a difficult person. Some individuals are so incorrigibly deceitful, manipulative, or destructive that a healthy relationship with them is impossible. Even if they feign remorse and swear to behave better, they actually feel little, if any, guilt.

Making This Chapter Work for You
A Guide to Psychological Wellness

■ Emotional health and mental health are both components of psychological health, our ability to be in touch with our feelings, to perceive reality as it is, and to work toward personal fulfillment.

■ The psychologically healthy person is reasonable, self-aware, productive, realistic, and has an appreciation of self and life and the capacity to love others and maintain relationships.

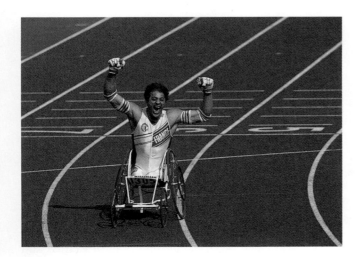

The characteristics of psychological health include a feeling of self-worth, an acceptance of life's possibilities, and a sense of fulfillment. We may not be in touch with these feelings all the time, but when we are, we also feel joy that we're alive.

- According to humanist theorist Abraham Maslow, we must first satisfy basic physiological needs—such as those for food, shelter, and sleep—before striving to fulfill higher needs for security, love and affection, and *self-actualization*, the state of functioning at the highest possible level and deriving the greatest possible satisfaction from life.

- Our attitudes and behavior are based on two types of values. Instrumental values represent ways of thinking and acting that we hold important, such as being loving or loyal. Terminal values represent goals, achievements, or ideal states toward which we strive.

- Self-esteem is belief or pride in ourselves, based on a sense of self-respect and acceptance that develops over time. Positive thinking and self-talk, through which we send complimentary or encouraging messages to ourselves, are the most useful techniques for bolstering self-esteem.

- While we all tend to experience bad moods, it is possible to manage, or *regulate*, mood through a variety of strategies. The most effective focus on the problem that caused the bad mood; others aim at dispelling negative feelings.

- Happiness is a sense of subjective well-being that tends to be highest when people combine frequent good experiences with occasional very intense pleasures. It is not based on wealth, beauty, or fame, but on characteristics such as high self-esteem, optimism, and the ability to form close relationships.

- Optimism involves the conscious decision to seek out and expect positive experiences from life. Along with savoring life's pleasures, large and small, and looking for the humor in daily living, it is a key to finding happiness and achieving good psychological health.

- We find meaning and fulfillment in life in various ways, including the experiences of loving and being loved, of developing our own spirituality, and of reaching out to help others.

- Autonomy (a sense of independence) and assertiveness (making your needs and desires clear to others) are keys to a feeling of mastery and being in control of one's life.

- The essential requirements for feeling energetic are regular exercise, good nutrition, and adequate sleep. A good night's sleep consists of cycles of both REM (rapid-eye-movement) sleep and quiet, deep (non-REM) sleep. Many Americans do not get adequate sleep and consequently are not functioning at their best.

- Social isolation is a major risk factor for illness and early death. While loneliness and social anxieties—fears of interacting with others or being observed by others—are common, they can be overcome.

- Many people who are difficult to get along with suffer from personality disorders, long-standing conditions that reflect their lack of flexibility in adapting to new situations. Since these people are not likely to change, it is best to find ways to work around their often irritating personality characteristics.

Like physical health, psychological well-being is not a fixed state of being, but a process. The way you live every day affects how you feel about yourself and your world. Here are some basic guidelines that you can rely on to make the most of the process of living:

- **Accept yourself.** As a human being, you are, by definition, imperfect. Come to terms with the fact that you are a worthwhile person despite your mistakes.

- **Respect yourself.** Recognize your abilities and talents. Acknowledge your competence and achievements, and take pride in them.

- **Trust yourself.** Learn to listen to the voice within you, and let your intuition be your guide.

- **Love yourself.** Be happy to spend time by yourself. Learn to appreciate your company and to be glad you're you.

Health Online

What's Your Emotional Intelligence Quotient?
http://www.utne.com/lens/bms/9bmseq.html

This ten-item self-quiz will help you assess your level of emotional intelligence and compare it to the national average. The site, sponsored by the *Utne Reader* magazine, also includes links to other pages on emotional intelligence and features a chat room dedicated to discussion of the issue and scores on this quiz.

Think about it ...

- In what ways might emotional intelligence be more important than IQ?

- Have you ever known a person who seemed to have a high IQ but low emotional intelligence? How did this affect the person?

- If your emotional intelligence score is lower than you would like, what might you do to learn emotional skills? What, if anything, should society do to teach emotional intelligence to children?

■ **Stretch yourself.** Be willing to change and grow, to try something new and dare to be vulnerable.

■ **Look at challenges as opportunities for personal growth.** "Every problem brings the possibility of a widening of consciousness," psychologist Carl Jung once noted. Put his words to the test.

■ **Think of not only where but also who you want to be a decade from now.** The goals you set, the decisions you make, the values you adopt now will determine how you feel about yourself and your life as you enter the 21st century.

 ## Key Terms

The terms listed here are used within the chapter. Page numbers are included for each term.
A definition of each term is given in the green Glossary pages at the end of this book.

altruism *79*
assertive *80*
autonomy *80*
culture *66*
emotional health *66*
emotional intelligence *74*
locus of control *80*

mental health *66*
mood *75*
moral *72*
optimism *78*
personality disorder *85*
rapid-eye-movement (REM)
  sleep *82*

self-actualization *70*
self-esteem *72*
social isolation *83*
social phobia *84*
spiritual health *66*
values *70*

 ## Review Questions

1. What are the characteristics of an emotionally healthy person?

2. What are some common emotional needs? feelings? values? goals? How do they relate to psychological health?

3. What are the components of emotional and mental well-being? Why are they important?

4. What is the sequence of sleep stages? How can an individual's sleep needs be determined?

5. What are coping mechanisms? Which ones are positive? What are defense mechanisms? How do they differ? How can you create more positive and effective coping mechanisms for yourself?

6. How do personality disorders differ from mental disorders such as depression and anxiety? If you experienced difficulty working with a person who had a personality disorder, what might you do?

Critical Thinking Questions

1. A growing number of schools, from kindergarten through college, are adding courses on emotional intelligence. Supporters argue that learning to understand and respect feelings is as important as learning math or science. Critics contend that mastering basic academics is most important. What do you think? Can emotional intelligence be taught? How would you rate your "emotional I.Q."?

2. Are you aware of your ability to view life positively or negatively? Which way do you most often describe your life? What could you do to become more psychologically healthy?

3. What are some things you can do to achieve happiness? Of these, which have you done before? Have you been successful? Can you think of other ways to achieve happiness not mentioned in the text?

Connections to Personal Health Interactive

To enhance your understanding of the material covered in this chapter, check out the following study aids on the **Personal Health Interactive CD-ROM**. *Each numbered icon within the chapter corresponds to an appropriate activity listed here.*

3.1 Your Ideal Self
3.2 Personal Alertness Inventory
3.3 Personal Insights: How Good Do You Feel?

3.4 Dream Journal
3.5 Chapter 3 Review

References

1. Shapiro, Deane, and Walsh, Roger. *Beyond Health and Normalcy*. New York: Van Nostrand Reinhold, 1983.
2. Moore, Thomas. *Care of the Soul*. New York: Harper Perennial, 1994.
3. Rokeach, M. *Understanding Human Values: Individual and Society*. New York: Free Press, 1979.
4. Ibid.
5. Plummer, Joseph. "Changing Values: The New Emphasis on Self-Actualization." *Life Management,* 3rd ed. Guilford, CT: Dushkin Publishing Group, 1995.
6. Kohlberg, L. *The Psychology of Moral Development*. San Francisco: Harper & Row, 1983.
7. Stephanie Marston, personal interview.
8. Butler, Andrew, et al. "A Comparison of Self-Esteem Lability and Low Trait Self-Esteem as Vulnerability Factors for Depression." *Journal of Personality and Social Psychology*, Vol. 66, No. 1, January 1994.
9. Lightsley, Owen. "Positive Automatic Cognitions as Moderators of the Negative Life Event-Dysphoria Relationship." *Cognitive Therapy and Research*, Vol. 18, No. 4, August 1994. Lightsley, Owen. "'Thinking Positive' as a Stress Buffer: The Role of Positive Automatic Cognitions in Depression and Happiness." *Journal of Counseling Psychology*, Vol. 41, No. 3, 1994.
10. Goleman, Daniel. *Emotional Intelligence*. New York: Bantam Books, 1997.
11. Simmons, Steve, and John C. Simmons, Jr. *Measuring Emotional Intelligence: The Groundbreaking Guide to Applying the Principles of Emotional Intelligence*. New York: Summit, 1997.
12. Segal, Jeanne. *Raising Your Emotional Intelligence: A Practical Guide*. New York: Henry Holt, 1997.
13. Randy Larsen, personal interview.
14. Thayer, Robert, et al. "Self-Regulation of Mood: Strategies for Changing a Bad Mood, Raising Energy and Reducing Tension." *Journal of Personality and Social Psychology*, Vol. 67, No. 5, 1994. George, Mark, et al. "Brain Activity During Transient Sadness and Happiness in Healthy Women." *American Journal of Psychiatry*, Vol. 152, No. 3, March 1995. Robinson, Robert. "Mapping Brain Activity Associated with Emotion." *American Journal of Psychiatry*, Vol. 152, No. 3, March 1995.
15. Larsen, Randy. "Emotion Regulation in Everyday Life: An Experience Sampling Study." Presented at the American

Psychological Association, Toronto, 1993. Korotkov, David, and Edward Hannah. "Extraversion and Emotionality as Proposed Superordinate Stress Moderators." *Personality and Individual Differences*, Vol. 16, No. 5, May 1994.

16. Larsen, Randy, interview.

17. Thayer, "Self-Regulation of Mood."

18. Catanzo, Salvatore, and Gregory Greenwood. "Expectancies for Negative Mood Regulation, Coping and Dysphoria Among College Students." *Journal of Counseling Psychology*, Vol. 41, No. 1, 1994.

19. Lyubomirsky, Sonja, and Susan Nolen-Hoeksema. "Self-Perceptuating Properties of Dysphoric Rumination." *Journal of Personality and Social Psychology*, Vol. 63, No. 2, 1993.

20. Cervone, Daniel, et al. "Mood, Self-Efficacy, and Performance Standards: Lower Moods Induce Higher Standards for Performance." *Journal of Personality and Social Psychology*, Vol. 67, No. 3, September 1994.

21. Myers, David. *The Pursuit of Happiness: Who Is Happy— and Why*. New York: William Morrow, 1992.

22. Reich, John, et al. "The Road to Happiness." *Psychology Today*, July–August 1994.

23. Lu, Luo, and Jian Bin Shih. "Sources of Happiness: A Qualitative Approach." *Journal of Social Psychology*, Vol. 137, No. 2, April 1997.

24. Furnham, Adrian, and Helen Cheng. "Personality and Happiness." *Psychological Reports*, Vol. 80, No. 3, June 1997. Lu, Luo, et al. "Personal and Environmental Correlates of Happiness." *Personality & Individual Differences*, September 1997.

25. Lane, Richard, et al. "Neuroanatomical Correlates of Happiness, Sadness, and Disgust." *American Journal of Psychiatry*, Vol. 154, No. 7, July 1997.

26. George, Mark, et al. "Gender Differences in Regional Cerebral Blood Flow During Transient Self-Induced Sadness or Happiness." *Biological Psychiatry*, November 1996.

27. Niedenthal, Paula, et al. "Being Happy and Seeing 'Happy': Emotional State Mediates Visual Word Recognition." *Cognition & Emotion*, Vol. 11, No. 4, July 1997.

28. McIntosh, William, et al. "Goal Beliefs, Life Events, and the Malleability of People's Judgments of Their Happiness." *Journal of Social Behavior & Personality*, Vol. 12, No. 2, June 1997.

29. Ornstein, Robert, and David Sobel. *Healthy Pleasures*. Reading, MA: Addison-Wesley, 1990.

30. Seligman, Martin. *Learned Optimism: The Skill to Conquer Life's Obstacles, Large and Small*. New York: Alfred A. Knopf, 1991.

31. Brami, Elisabeth, and Philippe Bertran. *Little Moments of Happiness*. New York: Stewart Tabori & Chang, 1997.

32. Moore, *Care of the Soul*.

33. Benson, Herbert. *Timeless Healing*. New York: Scribner's, 1996.

34. George, Jennifer, and Arthur Brief. "Feeling Good-Doing Good: A Conceptual Analysis of the Mood at Work— Organizational Spontaneity Relationship." *Psychological Bulletin*, Vol. 112, No. 2, 1992.

35. Giles, Dwight, and Janet Eyler. "The Impact of a College Community Service Laboratory on Students' Personal,

Social and Cognitive Outcomes." *Journal of Adolescence*, Vol. 17, No. 4, August 1994.

36. Larsen, Randy, interview.

37. Stone, Arthur, et al. "Psychological Coping: Its Importance for Treating Medical Problems." *Mind/Body Medicine*, Vol. 1. No. 1, March 1995.

38. "Psychiatric Disorders and Medical Care Utilization Among People in the General Population Who Report Fatigue." *Journal of General Internal Medicine*, Vol. 8, August 1993.

39. "Mood Alterations with a Single Bout of Physical Activity." *Perceptual and Motor Skills*, Vol. 72, 1991.

40. Maroulakis, Emmanuel, and Vannis Zervas. "Effects of Aerobic Exercise on Mood of Adult Women." *Perceptual and Motor Skills*, Vol. 76, 1993.

41. Christensen, Larry, and Clare Redig. "Effect of Meal Composition on Mood." *Behavioral Neuroscience*, Vol. 107, No. 2, 1993.

42. Hales, Dianne, and Robert E. Hales. "Sleep Disorders." in *Caring for the Mind: The Comprehensive Guide to Mental Health*. New York: Bantam Books, 1995.

43. William Dement, personal interview.

44. Hales and Hales, "Sleep Disorders."

45. Demakis, George, and Dan McAdams. "Personality, Social Support and Well-Being Among First-Year College Students." *College Student Journal*, Vol. 28, No. 4, June 1994. Liange, Belle, and Anne Bogat. "Culture, Control and Coping: New Perspectives on Social Support." *American Journal of Community Psychology*, Vol. 22, No. 1, February 1994. Forgas, Joseph. "Sad and Guilty? Affective Influences on the Explanation of Conflict in Close Relationships." *Journal of Personality and Social Psychology*, Vol. 66, No. 1, 1994.

46. Schwartz, Richard. "Loneliness." *Harvard Review of Psychiatry*, Vol. 5, No. 2, July–August 1997.

47. "Health: That's What Friend & Family Are For." *Facts of Life: An Issue Briefing for Health Reporters from the Center for Advancement of Health*, Vol. 2, No. 6, November–December 1997.

48. Bucholz, Ester. *The Call of Solitude: Alonetime in a World of Attachment*. New York: Simon & Schuster, 1997.

49. Rokach, Ami, and Heather Brock. "Loneliness and the Effects of Life Changes." *Journal of Psychology*, Vol. 131, No. 3, May 1997.

50. Nurmi, Jari-Erik, and Katarina Salmela-Aro. "Social Strategies and Loneliness." *Personality & Individual Differences*, Vol. 23, No. 2, August 1997.

51. Rokach, Ami. "Relations of Perceived Causes and the Experience of Loneliness." *Psychological Reports*, Vol. 80, No. 3, June 1997.

52. Mannuzza, Salvatore, et al. "Generalized Social Phobia." *Archives of General Psychiatry*, Vol. 52, No. 3, March 1995.

53. Potts, Nicholas, and Jonathan Davidson. "Epidemiology and Pharmacotherapy of Social Phobia." *Psychiatric Times*, February 1995. Morris, Lois. "Social Anxiety." *American Health*, January–February 1995.

54. Ross, Jerilyn. *Triumph over Fear*. New York: Bantam Books, 1994.

55. John Oldham, personal interview.

56. Allen Frances, personal interview.

CHAPTER 4

CARING FOR THE MIND

After studying the material in this chapter, you should be able to:

Identify the major psychological problems experienced by members of our society.

Describe the symptoms and risk factors associated with depression, anxiety disorders, attention disorders, and schizophrenia.

List strategies to help prevent suicide.

Discuss behaviors indicating the need for professional help and how to find such help.

Explain why neuropsychiatrists consider the brain to be the last frontier in their research.

List and briefly **explain** a variety of modern approaches used by professional therapists.

We all live through bad days, sad times, crushing setbacks, heart-breaking losses. We may eat too much, sleep too little, reach too often for a drink or drug. At some point in life, one of every three people develops an emotional disorder. Young adulthood—the years from the late teens to the mid-twenties—is a time when many serious disorders, including bipolar illness (manic depression) and schizophrenia, often develop. The saddest fact is not that so many feel so bad, but that so few realize they can feel better. Only one out of every five men and women who could use treatment ever seeks help. Yet 80 to 90% of those treated for psychological problems recover, most within a few months.[1]

The problems of the mind can be far more perplexing than the ailments of the body. If the problem were an aching knee or a queasy stomach, we might know—or could easily find out—its cause, what we can do about it, whether to see a doctor. But because psychological pain can't be seen, touched, X-rayed, or biopsied, we can't always be sure how serious distress is. Yet, if ignored, emotional aches and pains can become more severe and more difficult to overcome—and can increase the risk and cost of physical illness.

By learning about psychological disorders, you may be able to recognize early warning signals in yourself or your loved ones so you can deal with potential difficulties or seek professional help for more serious problems.

What Is Mental Well-Being?

Mental health is not an absence of distress, but rather the capacity to think rationally and logically and to cope with life's transitions, stresses, traumas, and losses in a way that allows for emotional stability and growth. As described in Chapter 3, mentally healthy individuals value themselves, perceive reality as it is, accept their limitations and possibilities, carry out their responsibilities, establish and maintain close relationships, pursue work that suits their talent and training, and feel a sense of fulfillment that makes the efforts of daily living worthwhile (see Figure 4-1).

The borders between mental health and illness are not well marked, however. Where does eccentricity end and abnormality begin? When does sadness deepen into depression? When does stress intensify into endless **anxiety**? How does fantasy lose touch completely with reality? Where is the line between everyday ups and downs and serious problems that urgently need attention?

There are no clear answers. Our view of mental illness is fuzzy. According to Laurie Flynn, executive director of the National Alliance of the Mentally Ill (NAMI):

> On any given day almost everyone has a mental health problem—whether it's the stress of modern living, grief, or getting along with others. But these are not mental illnesses. They don't disable. They don't require medication. No one would identify themselves as mentally ill because of

them. Someone who is stressed out and someone with schizophrenia may both need help, but one has a problem of everyday living and the other has a serious medical disease.[2]

(See Self-Survey: "Is Something Wrong?")

What Is a Mental Disorder?

While lay people may speak of "nervous breakdowns" or "insanity," these are not scientific terms. The U.S. government's official definition states that a serious mental illness is "a diagnosable mental, behavioral, or emotional disorder that interferes with one or more major activities in life, like dressing, eating, or working."[3]

The mental health profession's standard for diagnosing a mental disorder is the pattern of symptoms, or diagnostic criteria, spelled out for the almost 300 disorders in the American Psychiatric Association's *Diagnostic and Statistical Manual,* 4th edition *(DSM-IV).* It defines a **mental disorder** as "a clinically significant behavioral or psychological syndrome or pattern that occurs in an individual and that is associated with present distress (a painful symptom) or disability (impairment in one or more important areas of functioning) or with a significantly increased risk of suffering death, pain, disability, or an important loss of freedom."[4]

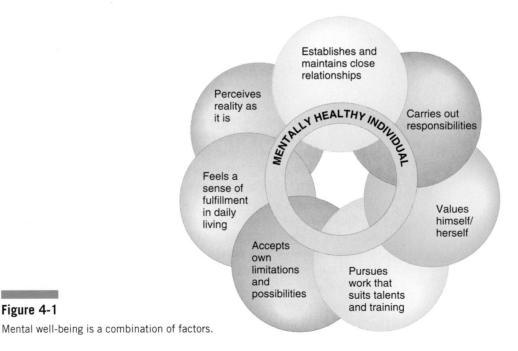

Figure 4-1

Mental well-being is a combination of factors.

Self-Survey

Is Something Wrong?

Which of the following apply to you? Think about how you've been feeling over the past month, and check all that apply. Be honest with yourself.

- feel depressed or sad for several weeks ❑

- lack energy or feel tired all the time ❑

- take no joy or pleasure in normally enjoyable activities ❑

- think or talk about suicide ❑

- experience extreme mood swings ❑

- feel helpless or hopeless ❑

- feel excessively anxious ❑

- abuse alcohol or drugs ❑

- show a marked change in personality ❑

- feel unable to cope with problems and daily activities ❑

- show marked changes in eating or sleeping patterns ❑

- feel extremely angry, hostile, or violent ❑

- express bizarre or grandiose ideas ❑

- be unable to control or stop destructive behavior, like gambling or drinking ❑

- develop troubling physical symptoms that have no known medical cause ❑

- see things, experience sensations, or hear voices that don't exist ❑

. . . .

The more of these boxes that describe what you (or someone close to you) have been experiencing in recent weeks, the more reason you have to be concerned that something may be wrong. This chapter provides information on common mental disorders, as well as guidance on finding and evaluating a therapist and advice on coping with everyday problems.

Psychological symptoms don't mean that you're "crazy," but they do indicate you need help in sorting out your life. Just as your body sometimes breaks down under the normal strain of day-to-day living, your mind also is vulnerable to dysfunction. Seeking help is the first step to feeling better and finding solutions to your problems. If you are struggling with a problem, you may want to schedule an appointment with a mental health professional at your school's counseling or student health-services facility.

Making Changes . . . .

Deciding If You Need Help

If you are still unsure about whether to seek help, the following questions may help in making the decision:

- Are emotional problems getting in the way of your work, relationships, or other aspects of your personal life?

- Have you been feeling less happy, less confident, and less in control than usual for a period of several weeks or longer?

- Have you reached the point of being so unhappy that you want to do something about it?

- Have close, trusted friends or family members commented on changes in your behavior and personality?

- Have your own efforts to deal with a problem failed to resolve the situation?

- Is dealing with everyday problems more of a struggle than it used to be?

- Do you feel emotionally "stuck" and helpless to change your own behavior or the circumstances you are in?

The key question to ask yourself is not, "Am I mentally ill?" or "Do I have serious problems?" but "Could I use some help right now?" If the answer is yes, do it. Therapy may turn out to be a catalyst and tool for change or a source of support when you need it most. At the very least, the psychological equivalent of a checkup can make sure that a problem isn't more serious than you may have realized.

How Common Are Mental Disorders?

Individuals with mental and emotional problems often feel terribly alone, as if no one else experiences or understands the misery they feel. Yet, as careful epidemiologic studies conducted in recent years have shown, mental disorders are much more common than had long been assumed. During any given year, 30% of Americans suffer from at least one mental disorder.[5] This statistic comes from the National Comorbidity Survey, which was based on face-to-face interviews with 8098 men and women from ages 15 to 54 who were representative of the entire population of the United States. According to these findings, the most common single mental disorder is major **depression**, while the anxiety disorders are the most prevalent group of mental illnesses. Other common problems are alcohol dependence and abuse, drug dependence and abuse, and dysthymia (chronic mild depression).

According to the survey, many individuals suffer from several mental disorders: 14% reported three or more disorders during their lifetime while an additional 13% had at least two mental disorders. Yet only 42% of those with a lifetime history of one or more mental disorders ever received any professional care. Just one in every four (26%) obtained treatment from a mental health professional.[6]

How Mental Health Affects Physical Health

Mental disorders affect not just the mind, but also the body. Depression can have an impact on treatment and recovery from many physical conditions, including asthma, stroke, heart disease, and cancer. Individuals recovering from heart attacks, for example, have a much greater risk of dying if they develop major depression. Anxiety can lead to intensified asthmatic reactions, skin conditions, and digestive disorders. As discussed in Chapter 2, stress can play a role in hypertension, heart attacks, and sudden cardiac death. Research into the relationship between the mind, the central nervous system, and the immune system has spawned a new scientific field, **psychoneuroimmunology**, which explores the intricate connections between the mind and the body.[7]

Not acknowledging and addressing psychological distress can contribute to major health problems, including high blood pressure, heart disease, cancer, and immune-related disorders. By some estimates, as many as 60% of those who seek help from physicians suffer primarily from a psychological problem. Treating mental health problems leads not only to improved health but also to lower health-care costs. According to various studies, mental health care has reduced annual medical costs by 9.5 to 21%. Psychiatric treatment reduces hospitalizations, cuts medical expenses, and reduces work disability. The American Psychiatric Association's Commission on Psychotherapy by Psychiatrists estimates that every dollar spent on psychotherapy may save four dollars in medical costs.[8]

The Last Frontier

The brain represents the sum of human knowledge, emotion, memory, and experience. It enables us to think and talk, to remember and anticipate, to work and play, to express our needs and control our desires. It has been called the last and the greatest biological frontier—more complex and more challenging than anything else in the entire universe. Some describe the spongy mass of gray and white matter within the skull as an enlightened machine that combines the analytic ability of a computer, the organizational skills of a filing system, and the communications network of a telephone switchboard. Yet no machine or invention, however sophisticated, can crack a joke, dream of daffodils, believe in a hereafter, or fall in love.

The brain has intrigued scientists for centuries, but only recently have its explorers made dramatic progress in unraveling its mysteries. Leaders in **neuropsychiatry**—the field that brings together the study of the brain and the mind—remind us that 95% of what is known about brain anatomy, chemistry, and physiology has been learned in the last decade. These discoveries have reshaped our understanding of the organ that is central to our identity and well-being and have fostered great hope for more effective therapies for the more than 1000 disorders—psychiatric and neurologic—that affect the brain and nervous system.

Inside the Brain

Each human brain contains hundreds of billions of nerve cells, or **neurons**, and support cells called **glia**.

Most are present at birth, when the brain weighs less than a pound. In the first six years of life—the period when we acquire more knowledge more rapidly than ever again—the brain reaches its full weight of about 3 pounds (see Figure 4-2).

The neurons are the basic working units of the brain. Like snowflakes, no two are exactly the same. Each consists of a cell body containing the **nucleus**; a long fiber, called the **axon**, which can range from less than an inch to several feet in length; an **axon terminal**, or ending; and multiple branching fibers called **dendrites**. The glia serve as the scaffolding for the brain, separate the brain from the bloodstream, assist in the growth of neurons, speed up the transmission of nerve impulses, and engulf and digest damaged neurons.

As the master control center for the body, the brain is constantly receiving information from the senses and relaying messages to various parts of the body. Some of these messages travel through the spinal cord, which extends from the neck about two-thirds of the way

down the backbone. Other signals are carried by nerves that connect the brain directly with certain parts of the body.

Historically, scientists have focused on the anatomy or structures of the brain in their attempts to understand how it functions and why it sometimes malfunctions. Modern neuropsychiatrists have shifted much of their attention to biochemical processes within the brain, particularly those involved in communication between neurons.

Communication Within the Brain

Neurons "talk" with each other by means of electrical and chemical processes (see Figure 4-3). An electric charge, or impulse, travels along an axon to the terminal, where packets of chemicals called **neurotransmitters** are stored. When released, these messengers flow out of the axon terminal and cross a **synapse**, a spe-

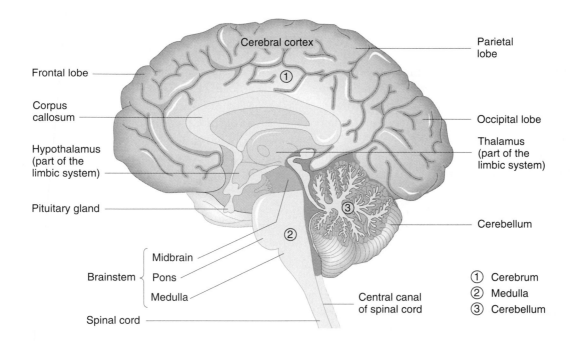

Figure 4-2

The brain. The three major parts of the brain are the cerebrum, cerebellum, and brainstem. The cerebrum is divided into two hemispheres—the left which regulates the right side of the body and the right, the left side. The cerebellum plays the major role in coordinating movement, balance, and posture. The brainstem contains centers that control breathing, blood pressure, heart rate, and other "autonomic" physiological functions.

Figure 4-3

The neuron is the basic working unit of the brain. Neurotransmitters released across the synapse transmit the chemical nerve impulse from one neuron to another.

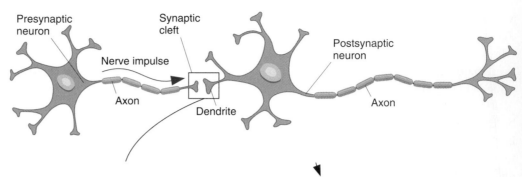

Presynaptic neuron

Synaptic cleft

Postsynaptic neuron

Nerve impulse

Axon

Dendrite

Axon

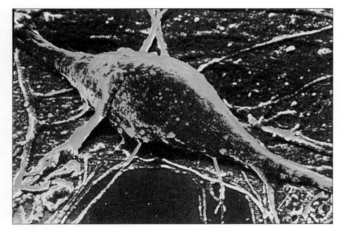

Neuron, magnified 3100 times.

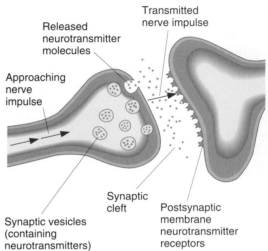

Transmitted nerve impulse

Released neurotransmitter molecules

Approaching nerve impulse

Synaptic cleft

Synaptic vesicles (containing neurotransmitters)

Postsynaptic membrane neurotransmitter receptors

cialized site at which the axon terminal of one neuron comes extremely close to a dendrite from another neuron. On the surface of the dendrite are **receptors**, protein molecules designed to bind with neurotransmitters. It takes only about a ten-thousandth of a second for a neurotransmitter and a receptor to come together—a union that neuropsychiatrist Richard Restak, M.D., author of *Receptors*, has lyrically compared to an embrace between two lovers. Neurotransmitters that do not connect with receptors may remain in the synapse until they are reabsorbed by the cell that produced them—a process called **reuptake**—or broken down by enzymes.[9]

A malfunction in the release of a neurotransmitter, in its reuptake or elimination, or in the receptors or secondary messengers may result in abnormalities in thinking, feeling, or behavior. Some of the most promising and exciting research in neuropsychiatry is focusing on correcting such malfunctions. Serotonin and its receptors, for instance, have been shown to affect mood, sleep, behavior, appetite, memory, learning, sexuality,

and aggression and to play a role in several mental disorders.

The discovery of a possible link between low levels of serotonin and some cases of major depression has already led to the development of more precisely targeted **antidepressant** medications that boost serotonin to normal levels. In the next decade, neuropsychiatric research may yield a new generation of breakthrough medications for an ever-growing number of mental disorders.[10]

Anxiety Disorders

The most common type of mental illness, anxiety disorders may involve inordinate fears of certain objects or situations (**phobias**), episodes of sudden, inexplicable terror (**panic attacks**), chronic distress (**generalized anxiety disorder**, or **GAD**), or persistent, disturbing thoughts and behaviors (**obsessive compulsive disorder**). Over a lifetime, according to the National Comorbidity Survey, as many as one in four Americans may experience an **anxiety disorder**. Only one of every four of these individuals is ever correctly diagnosed and treated. Yet most who do get treatment, even for severe and disabling problems, improve dramatically.

Phobias

Phobias—the most prevalent type of anxiety disorder—are out-of-the-ordinary, irrational, intense, persistent fears of certain objects or situations. In the course of a lifetime, about 11% of adults develop such acute terror that they go to extremes to avoid whatever it is that they fear, even though they realize that these feelings are excessive or unreasonable. The most common phobias involve animals, particularly dogs, snakes, insects, and mice; the sight of blood; closed spaces (*claustrophobia*); heights (*acrophobia*); air travel and being in places or situations from which they perceive it would be difficult or embarrassing to escape (*agoraphobia*).

Although various medications have been tried, none is effective by itself in relieving phobias. The best approach is behavior therapy, which consists of gradual, systematic exposure to the feared object (a process called *systematic desensitization*). Numerous studies have proven that exposure—especially in-vivo exposure, in which individuals are exposed to the actual source of their fear rather than simply imagining it—is highly effective; medical hypnosis—the use of induction of an altered state of consciousness—also can help.[11]

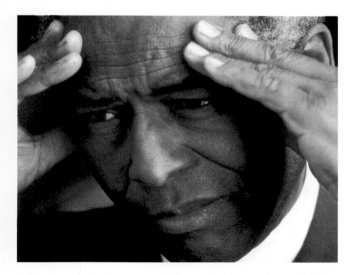

Most panic attacks occur during normal everyday activities. Observing someone having a panic attack, you may get no indication that the person is experiencing a high degree of distress.

Panic Attacks and Panic Disorder

Individuals who have had panic attacks describe them as the most frightening experiences of their lives. Without reason or warning, their hearts race wildly. They may become light-headed or dizzy. Because they can't catch their breath, they may start breathing rapidly and hyperventilate. Parts of their bodies, such as their fingers or toes, may tingle or feel numb. Worst of all is the terrible sense that something horrible is about to happen: that they will die, lose their minds, or have a heart attack. Most attacks reach peak intensity within ten minutes. Afterward individuals live in dread of another one. **Panic disorder** develops when attacks recur or apprehension about them becomes so intense that individuals cannot function normally.

About one-third of all young adults experience at least one panic attack between the ages of 15 and 35. Full-blown panic disorder occurs in about 1.6% of all adults in the course of a lifetime and usually develops before age 30. Women are more than twice as likely as men to experience panic attacks, although no one knows precisely why. Parents, siblings, and children of individuals with panic disorders also are more likely to develop them than are others.

The two primary treatments for panic disorder are cognitive-behavioral therapy, which teaches specific strategies for coping with symptoms like rapid breathing, and medication. Treatment helps as many as 90% of those with panic disorder either improve significantly or recover completely, usually within six to eight weeks. Individuals who receive cognitive-behavioral therapy as well as medication are less likely to suffer relapses than those taking medication alone.[12]

Strategies for Change
··
Recognizing Panic

The characteristic symptoms of panic attacks are:

✔ Palpitations, pounding heart, or accelerated heart rate.

✔ Sweating.

✔ Trembling or shaking.

✔ Sensations of shortness of breath or smothering.

✔ Feeling of choking.

✔ Chest pain or discomfort.

✔ Nausea or abdominal distress.

✔ Feeling dizzy, unsteady, lightheaded, or faint.

✔ Feelings of unreality or being detached from oneself.

✔ Fear of losing control or going crazy.

✔ Fear of dying.

✔ Numbness or tingling sensations.

✔ Chills or hot flushes.

Generalized Anxiety Disorder

The hallmark of a generalized anxiety disorder (GAD) is excessive or unrealistic apprehension that causes physical symptoms and lasts for six months or longer. Unlike fear, which helps us recognize and avoid real danger, GAD is an irrational or unwarranted response to harmless objects or situations of exaggerated danger. The most common symptoms are faster heart rate, sweating, increased blood pressure, muscle aches, intestinal pains, irritability, sleep problems, and difficulty concentrating.

Chronically anxious individuals worry—not just some of the time, and not just about the stresses and strains of ordinary life—but constantly, about almost everything: their health, families, finances, marriages, potential dangers. Treatment for GAD may consist of a combination of psychotherapy, behavioral therapy, and antianxiety drugs.[13]

Obsessive-Compulsive Disorder

As many as 1 in 40 Americans has a type of anxiety called obsessive-compulsive disorder (OCD). Some of these individuals suffer only from an *obsession*, a recurring idea, thought, or image that they realize, at least initially, is senseless. The most common obsessions are repetitive thoughts of violence (e.g., killing a child), contamination (becoming infected by shaking hands), and doubt (wondering whether one has performed some act, such as having hurt someone in a traffic accident). Most people with OCD also suffer from a *compulsion*, repetitive behavior performed according to certain rules or in a stereotyped fashion. The most common compulsions involve handwashing, cleaning, hoarding useless items, counting, or checking (e.g., making sure a door is locked dozens of times).[14]

Individuals with OCD realize that their thoughts or behaviors are bizarre, but they cannot resist or control them. Eventually, the obsessions or compulsions consume a great deal of time and significantly interfere with normal routine, job functioning, or usual social activities or relationships with others. A young woman who must follow a very rigid dressing routine may always be late for class, for example; a student who must count each letter of the alphabet as he types may not be able to complete a term paper.

OCD is believed to have biological roots. It may be a result of gene abnormalities, head injury, or even an autoimmune reaction after childhood infection with strep bacteria.[15] Treatment may consist of cognitive therapy to correct irrational assumptions, behavioral techniques such as progressively limiting the amount of time someone obsessed with cleanliness can spend washing and scrubbing, and medication. About 70 to 80% of those with OCD improve with treatment.[16]

Depressive Disorders

Comparing everyday "blues" to a **depressive disorder** is like comparing a cold to pneumonia. Major depression can destroy a person's joy for living. Food, friends, sex, or any form of pleasure no longer appeals. It is impossible to concentrate on work and responsibilities. Unable to escape a sense of utter hopelessness, depressed individuals may fight back tears throughout the day and toss and turn through long, empty nights. Thoughts of death or suicide may push into their minds.

But there is good news: Depression is a treatable disease; psychotherapy is remarkably effective for mild depression. In more serious cases, antidepressant medication can lead to dramatic improvement in 75 to 80% of depressed patients.[17]

Major Depression

The simplest definition of **major depression** is sadness that does not end. The incidence of major depression has soared over the last two decades, especially among young adults. The National Comorbidity Survey found that major depression is the most widespread mental disorder, affecting 10.3% of Americans in any given year. Unfortunately, fewer than one out of every three depressed people ever seeks treatment.

Most cases of major depression can be treated successfully, usually with psychotherapy, medication, or both. Psychotherapy alone works in more than half of mild-to-moderate episodes of major depression. Two specific psychotherapies—cognitive-behavioral therapy and interpersonal therapy (described later in this chapter)—have proved as helpful as antidepressant drugs in treating mild cases of depression, although they take longer than medication to achieve results.[18]

Antidepressant medications work for more than half of those with moderate-to-severe depression and may be useful in treating mild depression in individuals who do not improve with psychotherapy alone (see the section on psychiatric drug therapy, later in this chapter). These prescription drugs generally take three or four weeks to produce significant benefits and may not have their full impact for up to eight weeks. Combined treatment with psychotherapy and medication helps individuals with severe chronic or recurrent major depression as well as those who do not fully improve with medication or psychotherapy alone.

In individuals who cannot take antidepressant medications because of medical problems, or who do not improve with psychotherapy or drugs, *electroconvulsive therapy (ECT)*—the administration of a controlled electrical current through electrodes attached to the scalp—remains the safest and most effective treatment. About 50% of depressed individuals who do not get better with antidepressant medication and psychotherapy improve after ECT.[19]

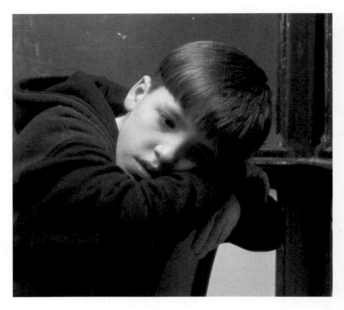

An increasing number of children suffer from bouts of depression, experiencing feelings of overwhelming hopelessness, helplessness, and sadness.

Strategies for Change

Recognizing Major Depression

The characteristic symptoms of major depression include:

- ✔ Feeling depressed, sad, empty, discouraged, tearful.
- ✔ Loss of interest or pleasure in once-enjoyable activities.
- ✔ Eating more or less than usual and either gaining or losing weight.
- ✔ Having trouble sleeping or sleeping much more than usual.
- ✔ Feeling slowed down or restless and unable to sit still.
- ✔ Lack of energy.
- ✔ Feeling helpless, hopeless, worthless, inadequate.
- ✔ Difficulty concentrating, forgetfulness.
- ✔ Difficulty thinking clearly or making decisions.
- ✔ Persistent thoughts of death or suicide.
- ✔ Withdrawal from others, lack of interest in sex.
- ✔ Physical symptoms (headaches, digestive problems, aches and pains).

Manic Depression (Bipolar Disorder)

Manic depression, or **bipolar disorder**, consists of mood swings that may take individuals from *manic* states of feeling euphoric and energetic to depressive states of utter despair. In episodes of full mania, they may become so impulsive and out of touch with reality that they endanger their careers, relationships, health, or even survival. One percent of the population—about 2 million American adults—suffer from this serious but treatable disorder, which affects both genders and all races equally.

The characteristic symptoms of manic depression include mood swings (from happy to miserable, optimistic to despairing, etc.); changes in thinking (thoughts speeding through one's mind; unrealistic self-confidence; difficulty concentrating; delusions; hallucinations); changes in behavior (sudden immersion in plans and projects; talking very rapidly and much more than usual; excessive spending; impaired judgment; impulsive sexual involvement); and changes in physical condition (less need for sleep; increased energy; fewer health complaints than usual). During "manic" periods, individuals may make grandiose plans or take dangerous risks.[20] But they often plunge from this highest of highs to a horrible low depressive episode, in which they may feel sad, hopeless, and helpless, and develop other symptoms of major depression. The risk of suicide is very real. (See Personal Voices: "Life on the Edge.")

Professional therapy is essential in treating bipolar disorders. Medication—lithium carbonate or an anticonvulsant drug—is the keystone of treatment, although psychotherapy plays a critical role in helping individuals understand their illness and rebuild their lives. Most individuals continue taking medication indefinitely after remission of their symptoms because the risk of recurrence is high.

Other Forms of Depression

In **seasonal affective disorder (SAD)**, annual episodes of depression usually begin at the same time each year, most often from the beginning of October through November, and end in March or April, with the coming of spring. January and February, often cloudy and dark, are usually the worst months. According to National Institute of Mental Health (NIMH) estimates, some 10 million Americans have SAD. Although the gloomy gray days of winter can dampen anyone's spirits, these indi-

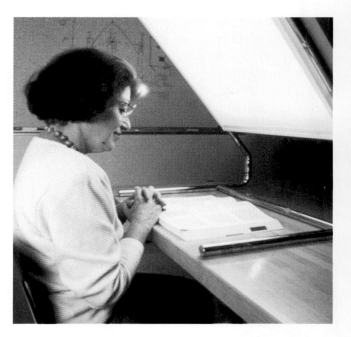

People with seasonal affective disorder (SAD), a form of depression, can be treated with bright-light therapy.

viduals feel helpless, guilt-ridden, and hopeless and have difficulty thinking and making decisions. Typically, they eat more and gain weight. In particular, many crave rich carbohydrates. They spend many more hours asleep, yet feel chronically exhausted.

SAD often improves with a specialized treatment: exposure to bright light, known as *phototherapy*. Since the first reports on this approach in 1980, numerous studies have confirmed improvement in people with SAD who sit in front of a specially designed light box every day during winter months.[21] For severe forms of seasonal depression, therapists may combine phototherapy with antidepressant medications.

Dysthymia is the clinical term for chronic mild depression. Dysthymia, which usually develops in childhood, adolescence, or early adult life, occurs equally in boys and girls, but in adults it is more common among women. Individuals with this disorder experience symptoms of depression most of the day, and more days than not, for a period of at least two years. They also may have low self-esteem, eat and sleep more or less than usual, lack energy, have problems concentrating or making decisions, and feel a sense of hopelessness. Their symptoms, however, are less intense than those of major depression. Psychotherapy, antidepressant medication, or a combination of both may be effective in treating dysthymia. Aerobic exercise seems to be an especially helpful form of adjunctive, or additional, therapy.

Personal Voices Life on the Edge

Jack was a golden boy. He started reading when he was 4, staged magic shows when he was 6, skied the expert runs when he was 8. He captivated other youngsters with his daredevil exploits. As a teenager, he was a star athlete and an honor student—although he was always testing the limits, showing up late for practices or skipping classes.

"Jack likes to live on the edge," his mother would say, with a mix of exasperation and indulgence. She worried that someday he'd go over the edge. Over the years, she'd seen a side of him few others ever did—sudden rages, bleak depressions, frenzied bursts of activity. She would wait until Jack calmed down and then try to talk with him, but by then he was back to his usual charming self.

When he was in college, Jack set out to make his first million. As a design project, he developed a lightweight mesh backpack for hikers and bikers. Borrowing a girlfriend's sewing machine, he stayed up all night putting together a prototype. He hounded sporting goods manufacturers until they agreed to see him. His presentations were so creative and persuasive that three companies bid on manufacturing rights. By the time he turned 21, Jack had set up his own company, which he dubbed "Primo!"—the first.

Jack's schoolwork suffered as his business thrived. He would cut classes and buy others' notes to study for tests. During one finals week, he seemed to be running on sheer adrenalin. Night after night, he stayed up writing papers and cramming for tests. Chugging coffee and chain-smoking, he'd talk nonstop to anyone who would listen, his mind flitting from one subject to the next. Even though he was sure he'd aced every course, Jack barely passed, and he was put on academic probation.

By the time grades were posted, Jack's spirits had plummeted. He retreated to his room and lay there, unable to get up, unwilling to talk with anyone. He felt that he'd been found out, that the faculty had finally discovered what no one else had even suspected: that he was a fake, a fast-talking fraud who wasn't as smart or capable as most people thought. This dark time didn't pass as quickly as others had in the past, and Jack's worried friends called his parents, who packed his things and drove their pale, subdued son home for the summer.

Jack didn't return to college for his final year. Instead he had a plan to develop an entire line of sporting accessories and market them by sponsoring adventure trips—white-water rafting, sky-diving, skiing, biking crosscountry, mountain climbing. Fired up with enthusiasm, Jack rounded up backers for his venture. Primo's first line of sportsgear, produced in eye-jolting neon colors, was a smash. But Jack had overestimated his production capabilities, and he couldn't keep up with retailers' demands. Some nights he'd go to the warehouse himself and package orders.

Staff members coming to work in the morning would find him trying to pack six cartons at once, racing back and forth and babbling to himself.

When Jack's investors forced him to turn over the day-to-day management of Primo to experienced executives, he threw himself into planning the adventure excursions and decided to hire a video crew to do a documentary as he personally undertook each one. Borrowing against his company's assets, he spent a fortune on an elaborate launch, which included skydivers and a catered party for a thousand. Jack was so wired that day that many thought he was high on coke. When he became incoherent, his friends took him to the hospital. Tests revealed no drugs, but a consulting psychiatrist came up with the diagnosis: bipolar disorder.

During his first week on a psychiatric ward, Jack remembers "I could feel myself slipping in and out of reality." By the time of his discharge two weeks later, Jack was definitely back in touch. "I had to survey the wreckage of my life: the money I'd spent, the company I'd almost bankrupted, a whole string of relationships that had never amounted to anything." With the help of psychotherapy and ongoing treatment with drugs to control mood swings, Jack is building a new life, one he describes as "saner, with highs that are not quite so high and lows that aren't quite so low and a feeling, finally, of being in control."

Suicide

Suicide is not in itself a psychiatric disorder, but it can be the tragic consequence of emotional and psychological problems. Every year 30,000 Americans—among them many young people who seem to have "everything to live for"—commit suicide. Ten times this many individuals attempt to take their own lives.

In the last thirty years, reported suicides among young adults between the ages of 15 and 24 have tripled. According to a 1995 report by the Centers for Disease Control and Prevention, suicide has become an increasingly serious problem among the nation's youth, with big increases among children between the ages of 10 and 14 and among young African-American men. College students commit suicide at about half the rate of young people their age who are not in school. Suicide rates at highly competitive schools are not significantly different from those at less rigorous ones. However, college students do think about suicide and, in lesser numbers, make specific plans for taking their own lives (see

CAMPUS FOCUS: SUICIDE

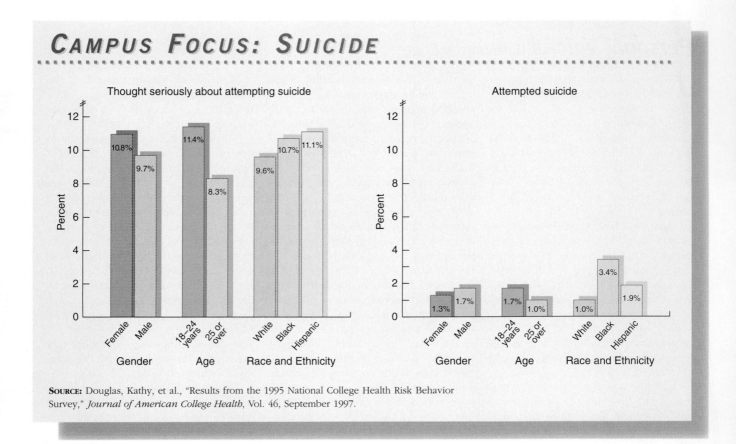

Thought seriously about attempting suicide

Attempted suicide

SOURCE: Douglas, Kathy, et al., "Results from the 1995 National College Health Risk Behavior Survey," *Journal of American College Health*, Vol. 46, September 1997.

Campus Focus: "College Students and Suicide"). In the National College Health Risk Behavior Study, 10.3% of students had thought seriously about attempting suicide, 6.7% had made specific plans for suicide, 1.5% had attempted suicide, and 0.4% had required medical attention because of a suicide attempt.[22]

Among all young people under age 25, firearms-related deaths account for 65% of suicides. Among those aged 15 through 19, firearm-related suicides account for 81% of the increase in the overall suicide rate since 1980. Other stresses that may contribute to the soaring suicide rates among the young are psychological problems, mental disorders, drug abuse, school pressures, social difficulties, concern and confusion about sexual orientation, and family problems.[23]

At all ages, men commit suicide three times more frequently than women, but women attempt suicide much more often than men. Elderly men are ten times more likely to take their own lives than older women; teenage boys kill themselves more than twice as often as girls. The suicide rate is generally higher for whites than other races, although it is rising among young African

Americans in inner-city neighborhoods, who commit suicide twice as often as white men of their age. Native Americans have a suicide rate five times higher than that of the general population.

But suicide is not inevitable. Appropriate treatment can help as many as 70 to 80% of those at risk for suicide. Among young people, early recognition and treatment for depressive disorders and alcohol and drug use could save thousands of lives each year.[24]

Strategies for Prevention
....
Helping to Prevent Suicide

If someone you know has talked about suicide, behaved unpredictably, or suddenly emerged from a severe depression into a calm, settled state of mind, don't rule out the possibility that he or she may attempt suicide.

✔   Encourage your friend to talk. Ask concerned questions. Listen attentively. Show that you take the person's feelings seriously and truly care.

✔ Don't offer trite reassurances. List reasons to go on living, try to analyze the person's motives, or try to shock or challenge him or her.

✔ Suggest solutions or alternatives to problems. Make plans. Encourage positive action, such as getting away for a while to gain a better perspective on a problem.

✔ Don't be afraid to ask whether your friend has considered suicide. The opportunity to talk about thoughts of suicide may be an enormous relief, and—contrary to a long-standing myth—will not fix the idea of suicide more firmly in a person's mind.

✔ Don't think that people who talk about killing themselves never carry out their threat. Most individuals who commit suicide give definite indications of their intent to die.

✔ If you feel that you aren't making any headway, suggest that both you and your friend talk to an expert.

✔ Stay close until you can get help. If you must leave your friend alone, negotiate with him or her. Have your friend promise that he or she won't do anything to harm himself or herself without first calling you. If your friend does call, get to him or her as soon as possible. Call for help immediately.

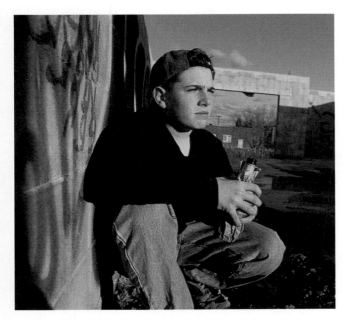

Suicide rates for young adults have risen dramatically in the last three decades. A sense of helplessness can lead to thoughts of suicide, and alcohol and drug use may increase depression and confuse thinking.

Why Do People Want to Kill Themselves?

Why? This question haunts partners, parents, children, relatives, friends, coworkers. There may never be a good enough explanation for what happened. Usually a suicide attempt is a desperate cry for help, a last attempt at communication. To people who take their own lives, death seems the best, if not the only, solution—not only for themselves, but also for their families and friends.

Many of those who kill themselves suffer from mental disorders. Some cannot cope any more; cannot think rationally; or feel ashamed, lonely, or helpless. Those with debilitating or terminal diseases may think of suicide as a welcome end to their struggle with infirmity and pain. Older individuals, who are faced with the loss of their own good health, of the people they love most, or of the activities that gave them decades of satisfaction, may see suicide as an alternative to a future without hope. (Physician-assisted suicide is discussed in Chapter 19.)

Understanding suicide in the young is especially hard. According to some experts, many teens have a sense of immortality and do not believe, in their heart of hearts, that death is final; others may not be able to see any other way out of whatever difficulties they find themselves in. Sometimes pressure to succeed or an overreaction to what seems a major failure can drive young people to kill themselves.

Substance abuse may play a major role. Naturally impulsive, young people who drink or take drugs may be especially likely to act without thinking and take their lives in a burst of rage or frustration. Those who first turned to drugs or alcohol as a way of easing their anxiety or escaping pressures may feel increasingly desperate as they realize that their problems haven't gone away or that they are losing control over their drinking or drug use.

More than half of all young people who attempt suicide may be clinically depressed. Often they feel that no one needs them or cares. Many have suffered a loss: the end of a romance or friendship, the death of a loved one, their parents' separation or divorce. According to studies comparing adolescents who attempt suicide, and those considered at risk, with normal teens, youths who try to kill themselves feel more hopeless and are more likely to say that life just isn't worth living.

In some circumstances, the thought of suicide seems to capture the imagination of young people. When one

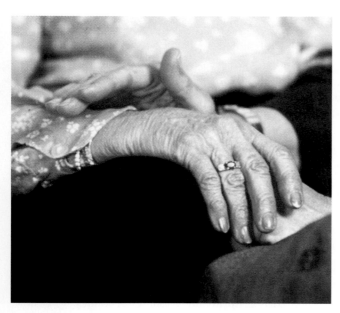

Depression and suicidal thoughts are closely linked. Educating close friends and relatives about depression prepares them to offer help and comfort during difficult times.

suicide occurs in a community, it can spark a cluster of similar teen deaths. Studies of the impact of television movies on teen suicides have produced conflicting results, but some therapists feel that teens, who are especially prone to the effects of peer influence, may feel inspired to kill themselves after watching televised movies that portray suicide victims sympathetically.

What Leads to Suicide?

Researchers have looked for explanations for suicide by studying everything from phases of the moon to seasons (suicides peak in the spring in most young people and adults) to birth order in the family. They have found no conclusive answers. A constellation of influences—mental disorders, personality traits, biologic and genetic vulnerability, medical illness, and psychosocial stressors—may combine in ways that lower an individual's threshold of vulnerability. No one factor in itself may ever explain fully why a person chooses death.

Mental Disorders

As many as 95% of those who commit suicide have a mental disorder. Two in particular—depression and alcoholism—account for two-thirds of all suicides. Suicide also is a risk for those with other disorders, including schizophrenia and personality disorders.

Substance Abuse

Many of those who commit suicide drink beforehand, and their use of alcohol may lower their inhibitions. Since alcohol itself is a depressant, it can intensify the despondency suicidal individuals are already feeling. Alcoholics who attempt suicide often have other risk factors, including major depression, poor social support, serious medical illness, and unemployment. Drugs of abuse also can alter thinking and lower inhibitions against suicide.

Hopelessness

The sense of utter hopelessness and helplessness may be the most common contributing factors in suicide. When hope dies, individuals view every experience in negative terms and come to expect the worst possible outcomes for their problems. Given this way of thinking, suicide often seems a reasonable response to a life seen as not worth living.

Family History

One out of every four people who attempt suicide has a family member who also tried to commit suicide. While a family history of suicide is not in itself considered a predictor of suicide, two mental disorders that can lead to suicide—depression and bipolar disorder (manic depression)—do run in families.

Physical Illness

People who commit suicide are likely to be ill or to believe that they are. About 5% actually have a serious physical disorder, such as AIDS or cancer. While suicide may seem to be a decision rationally arrived at in persons with serious or fatal illness, this may not in fact be the case. Depression, not uncommon in such instances, can warp judgment. When the depression is treated, the person may no longer have suicidal intentions.

More than 80% of those who commit suicide have seen a physician about a medical complaint within the six months preceding suicide. To help general physicians identify people at risk of suicide, researchers at Johns Hopkins University developed a set of four crucial questions:

- Have you ever had a period of two weeks or more when you had trouble falling asleep, staying asleep, waking up too early, or sleeping too much?

- Have you ever had two weeks or more during which you felt sad, blue, depressed or when you lost interest and pleasure in things you usually cared about or enjoyed?

- Has there been a period of two weeks or more when you felt worthless, sinful, or guilty?
- Has there ever been a period of time when you felt that life was hopeless?

Anyone who answers yes to these questions should be referred immediately to a mental health professional.

Brain Chemistry

Investigators have found abnormalities in the brain chemistry of individuals who complete suicide, especially low levels of a metabolite of the neurotransmitter serotonin. There are indications that individuals with a deficiency in this substance may have as much as a ten times greater risk of committing suicide than those with higher levels.[26]

Access to Guns

For individuals already facing a combination of predisposing factors, access to a means of committing suicide, particularly to guns, can add to the risk. Unlike other methods of suicide, guns almost always hit their mark. States with stricter gun-control laws have much lower rates of suicides than states with more lenient laws.

Other Factors

Individuals who kill themselves often have gone through more major life crises—job changes, births, financial reversals, divorce, retirement—in the previous six months, compared with others. Long-standing, intense conflict with family members or other important people may add to the danger. In some cases, suicide may be an act of revenge that offers the person a sense of control—however temporary or illusory. For example, a husband whose wife has had an affair may rationalize that he can get back at her, and have the final word, by killing himself. Others may feel that, by rejecting life, they are rejecting a partner or parent who abandoned or betrayed them.

Strategies for Prevention

If You Start Thinking About Suicide

At some point, the thought of ending it all—the disappointments, problems, bad feelings—may cross your mind. This

experience isn't unusual. But if the idea of taking your life persists or intensifies, you should respond as you would to other warnings of potential threats to your health—by getting the help you need:

✔ Talk to a mental health professional. If you have a therapist, call immediately. If not, call a suicide hot line.

✔ Find someone you can trust and talk with honestly about what you're feeling. If you suffer from depression or another mental disorder, educate trusted friends or relatives about your condition so they are prepared if called upon to help.

✔ Write down your more uplifting thoughts. Even if you are despondent, you can help yourself by taking the time to retrieve some more positive thoughts or memories. A simple record of your hopes for the future and the people you value in your life can remind you of why your own life is worth continuing.

✔ Avoid drugs and alcohol. Most suicides are the results of sudden, uncontrolled impulses, and drugs and alcohol can make it harder to resist these destructive urges.

✔ Go to the hospital. Hospitalization can sometimes be the best way to protect your health and safety.

Attention Disorders

Little more than a decade ago mental health professionals assumed that what is now termed **attention deficit/hyperactivity disorder (ADHD)**—the most common psychiatric diagnosis in childhood—was strictly kids' stuff. They were wrong. A half to two-thirds of youngsters with ADHD do not outgrow their restless, reckless ways at puberty. In all, 1 to 2% of adult men and women—at least 5 million Americans—have problems sustaining attention or controlling their movements and impulses.[27]

ADHD—a term that has replaced *minimal brain dysfunction* and *hyperactivity*—refers to a spectrum of difficulties in controlling motion and sustaining attention. Adults with ADHD have one or more of three primary symptoms: hyperactivity, impulsivity, and distractibility. Rather than scooting around a room, they may tap their fingers or jiggle their feet. Some appear calm and organized but cannot concentrate long enough to finish reading a paragraph or follow a list of directions. Others, on a whim, go on buying sprees or take wild dares.

There is no specific test for detecting attention disorders, and diagnosis, based on the patient's history and a therapist's interview, can be difficult. Adults with ADHD receive the same medications that children do—stimulant drugs that, paradoxically, can aid concentration and reduce restlessness. Medication often makes it possible for adults with ADHD to benefit from other treatments, such as psychotherapy, general counseling, vocational rehabilitation, and academic tutoring.[28]

Strategies for Change

Recognizing an Attention Disorder

Recognizing ADHD can be the first step in getting help for a person with this disorder, who may have no idea that this is a treatable condition. The characteristic symptoms of ADHD in adults are:

✔ Feelings of restlessness, fidgeting, squirming; difficulty waiting.

✔ Extreme distractibility, forgetfulness, absent-mindedness, irritation when stuck in traffic.

✔ Disorganization, inability to finish tasks, switching from task to task haphazardly; inability to remain still or engage in a focused activity such as reading.

✔ Difficulty in solving problems or managing time.

✔ Hot temper, explosive outbursts, constant irritation; low tolerance of stress, easily overwhelmed by ordinary hassles; frequent mood swings.

✔ Impulsiveness, making decisions with little reflection or information, abruptly beginning and ending relationships, recklessness.

✔ Clumsiness, poor body image, poor sense of direction.

✔ Immaturity.

Schizophrenia

Schizophrenia, one of the most debilitating mental disorders, profoundly impairs an individual's sense of reality. As the National Institute of Mental Health (NIMH) puts it, schizophrenia, which is characterized by abnormalities in brain structure and chemistry, destroys "the inner unity of the mind" and weakens "the will and drive that constitute our essential character." It affects every aspect of psychological functioning, including the ways in which people think, feel, view themselves, and relate to others.

Individuals with schizophrenia may hear, see, or feel things that do not exist—a voice telling them to jump from a bridge, a statue crying tears of blood, a spaceship beaming a light upon them. Frightened and vulnerable, they may devote all their energy to warding off the demons within. Unable to take care of themselves, they may look messy and disheveled. They often move in unusual ways, such as rocking or pacing, or repeat certain gestures again and again. They may believe that someone or something, such as the devil, is putting thoughts into their heads or controlling their actions. Some think they are reincarnations of Christ or Napoleon. About a third attempt to take their own lives, often in response to a command they hear inside their heads.

Schizophrenia is most likely to occur between the ages of 17 and 24. One-half to 1% of the population—about 1 in every 150 people—suffers from this disorder. According to NIMH's epidemiological data, the total lifetime prevalence for schizophrenia in the United States ranges from 1 to 1.9%. This means that between 2.5 million and 4.75 million Americans may have schizophrenia at any one time.

Schizophrenia typically consists of several stages. During the *prodromal phase,* a period ranging from months to years, individuals withdraw from social interactions, pay less attention to keeping clean or dressing appropriately, or act in peculiar ways. In the acute, or *active phase,* individuals develop "positive symptoms." They may experience delusions and become convinced that space aliens have taken control of their bodies or hallucinate and hear voices mocking them. Some talk nonstop, rambling on without making any clear point; others repeatedly shake their heads, tap their feet, or assume odd postures or positions. After positive symptoms subside, individuals enter the *residual phase,* which is characterized by "negative" symptoms, such as general apathy, flattened emotions, or inappropriate emotional reactions (for example, laughing when someone is hurt).

For centuries, the quest for a cure for this frightening and often tragic disease led to desperate methods, including spraying a strong stream of water at a patient's spine, injecting the patient with horse serum, and administering huge doses of vitamins. Today, for the vast majority of individuals with schizophrenia, antipsychotic drugs are the foundation of treatment.[29] They make most people with schizophrenia feel more comfortable and in control of themselves, help organize chaotic thinking, and reduce or eliminate delusions or

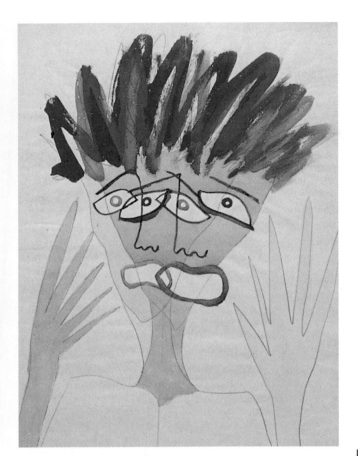

"My Head Is Going Round and Round." This drawing by a patient suffering from schizophrenia expresses the anxiety and agitation that may occur with this brain abnormality.

hallucinations, allowing fuller participation in normal activities. Those who do not improve significantly on medication almost invariably do even worse without it.

Most of the antipsychotic drugs have a similar mode of action. While some may act more quickly than others, almost all are equally effective. But they can have problematic side effects, including uncontrollable facial tics, tongue tremors, and jaw movements known as tardive dyskinesia. Nearly one-third of individuals given conventional antipsychotics continue to have residual symptoms, such as apathy. In the past, little, if anything, could be done to relieve these negative symptoms. However, new antipsychotics, such as risperidone, olanzapine, and clozapine, can relieve such symptoms and help individuals who do not improve with standard medications or who develop intolerable side-effects.[30]

Some individuals with schizophrenia recover completely. However, many thousands—perhaps as many as 200,000—live on the street or in homeless shelters.

Strategies for Change

Recognizing the Signs of Schizophrenia

The characteristic symptoms of schizophrenia include:

✔ Hallucinations.

✔ Delusions.

✔ Inability to think in a logical manner.

✔ Talking in rambling or incoherent ways.

✔ Making odd or purposeless movements or not moving at all.

✔ Repeating others' words or mimicking their gestures.

✔ Showing few, if any, feelings; responding with inappropriate emotions.

✔ Lacking will or motivation to complete a task or accomplish something.

✔ Functioning at a much lower level than in the past at work, in interpersonal relations, or in taking care of themselves.

Overcoming Problems of the Mind

An estimated 34 million Americans currently receive professional psychotherapy or counseling; millions more need such help. Yet many people do not seek treatment because they see psychological problems as a sign of weakness rather than illness. They also may not realize that scientifically proven therapies can bring relief, often in a matter of weeks or months.

Because an individual's perception of a problem is "culture-specific"—that is, influenced by his or her cultural, social, and religious beliefs—those who've immigrated to the United States from other countries may treat symptoms of psychological distress in different ways. For instance, Asian-American college students tend to seek medical care for physical symptoms, such as aches, pains, or sleep problems, but forego counseling for a mental disorder, because it is more appropriate in their native cultures to do so.[31]

Where to Turn

As a student, your best contact for identifying local services may be your health education instructor or depart-

Pulsepoints

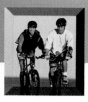

Ten Ways to Help a Troubled Friend or Relative

1. Take your loved one seriously. Troubled individuals need to know you are willing to listen without lecturing or criticizing them.

2. Don't try to treat the problem yourself. Well-intentioned comments (like "You'll feel better after a good rest") may make matters worse.

3. Encourage openness and honesty. Discussing troubling issues frankly can help a person realize that he or she is facing very real difficulties and may require some assistance to work through them.

4. Seek out information. The more you know, the more insight you'll have. Educate yourself about mental disorders and their treatments.

5. Maintain as normal a relationship as possible. Acknowledge the person's pain, but try to preserve your usual ways of relating to each other.

6. Give and expect respect. Psychological distress may explain hurtful behavior, but it does not excuse it.

7. Resist the temptation to "overfunction." If you take on his or her responsibilities, the person will feel even more helpless and inadequate.

8. Foster the will to be well. Talk in positive terms about the future, though not at the expense of honesty about current feelings and fears.

9. Live your own life. Though it may be difficult, you must pursue your own interests for the sake of your own psychological well-being.

10. Be patient. Recovery can take time. Don't be discouraged by temporary setbacks. The mind, like the body, heals slowly and cannot be rushed.

---

ment. The health instructors can tell you about general and mental health counseling available on campus, school-based support groups, community-based programs, and special emergency services. On campus, you can also turn to the student health services or the office of the dean of student services or student affairs.

Within the community, you may be able to get help through the city or county health department and neighborhood health centers. Local hospitals often have special clinics and services; and there are usually local branches of national service organizations, such as United Way or Alcoholics Anonymous, other 12-step programs, and various support groups. You can call the psychiatric or psychological association in your city or state for the names of licensed professionals. (Check the telephone directory for listings.) Your primary physician may also be able to help.

The telephone book is another good resource. Special programs are often listed either by the nature of the service, by the name of the neighborhood or city, or by the name of the sponsoring group. In some places, the city's name may precede a listing: the New York City Suicide Hot Line, for instance. In addition to suicide-prevention programs, other listings usually include crisis intervention, violence prevention, and child-abuse prevention programs; drug-treatment information; shelters for battered women; senior citizen centers; and self-help and counseling services. Many services have special hot lines for coping with emergencies. Others provide information as well as counseling over the phone. (See Pulsepoints: "Ten Ways to Help a Troubled Friend or Relative.")

Types of Therapists

Many people refer to anyone in the mental health field as a "psychotherapist," but this is not an official designation, and anyone can advertise as one. Only professionally trained individuals who have met state licensing requirements are certified as psychiatrists, psychologists, or social workers. Before selecting any of these mental health professionals, be sure to check the person's background and credentials.

The most common types of mental health professionals are psychiatrists, psychologists, social workers, psychiatric nurses, and marriage and family therapists. **Psychiatrists** are licensed medical doctors (M.D.s) who complete medical school; a year-long internship (including at least four months of internal medicine and usually two months of neurology); and a three-year residency that provides training in various forms of psychotherapy (including couples, family, and group therapy), psychopharmacology (the study of drugs that affect the mind), and both outpatient and inpatient treatment of mental disorders. They can prescribe medications and make medical decisions. *Board-certified* psychiatrists have passed oral and written examinations following completion of residency training. Child psychiatrists undergo additional academic and clinical training to work with children and adolescents; geriatric psychiatrists have special expertise in the problems of older men and women.

Psychologists complete a graduate program (including clinical training and internships) in human psychology but do not study medicine and cannot prescribe medication. They must be licensed in most states in order to practice independently. An increasing number have a doctorate (either a Ph.D. or Psy.D.) plus postdoctoral training, and are trained in a variety of psychotherapeutic techniques rather than in one particular school or theory. Some have additional training in working with children and families.

Certified social workers or licensed clinical social workers (LCSWs) usually complete a two-year graduate program and have specialized training in helping people with mental problems in addition to conventional social work. Some have doctoral degrees. Most states certify or license social workers as an independent profession and require two years of supervised postgraduate clinical work and a qualifying examination.

Psychiatric nurses have nursing degrees and have passed a state examination. They usually have special training and experience in mental health care, although no specialty licensing or certification is required.

Marriage and family therapists, licensed in some but not all states, usually have a graduate degree, often in psychology, and at least two years of supervised clinical training in dealing with relationship problems. Psychiatrists, psychologists, and clinical social workers may specialize in marriage and family counseling or devote much of their practices to helping couples and families.

Other therapists include pastoral counselors, members of the clergy who offer psychological counseling; hypnotherapists, who use hypnosis for problems such as smoking and obesity; stress-management counselors, who teach relaxation methods; and alcohol and drug counselors, who help individuals with substance abuse problems. Anyone can use these terms to describe themselves professionally, and there are no licensing requirements.

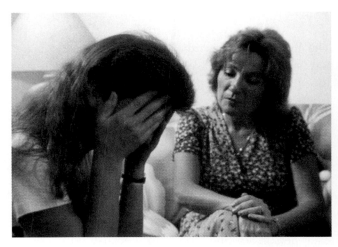

A therapist's education, title, and qualifications may vary. The qualities of compassion and caring are also important in choosing the right therapist.

Strategies for Change

Choosing a Therapist

In making your final choice of a therapist, here are some considerations and questions to keep in mind:

✔ Do you feel you could work well together? Will the therapist treat you as a whole person, rather than an illness, and help you deal with the impact your problem may have on your personal development, your relationships, and your life?

✔ Do you feel the therapist shows genuine concern, takes you seriously, treats you with respect, and shares or accepts your values? Regardless of his or her qualifications or reputation, a therapist who is not understanding and caring probably is not the right choice.

✔ Is your therapist willing to explore all treatment options to find what works best for you? Will this include medication as well as specific psychotherapeutic techniques?

✔ If the therapist is not a physician and medication may be necessary, who will work with you to weigh the side effects of specific drugs against their benefits? Who will prescribe and monitor your medication?

✔ Will your therapist be supportive if you want a second opinion about treatment? Will he or she work with you to evaluate others' recommendations?

✔ Remember that you are choosing someone in whom you may confide your most intimate secrets and fears. Of course, you want a competent therapist with the right training, knowledge, skills, and experience. But you also must choose someone you can trust.

Options for Treatment

The term **psychotherapy** refers to any type of counseling based on the exchange of words in the context of the unique relationship that develops between a mental health professional and a person seeking help. The process of talking and listening can lead to new insight, relief from distressing psychological symptoms, changes in unhealthy or maladaptive behaviors, and more effective ways of dealing with the world.

Most mental health professionals today are trained in a variety of psychotherapeutic techniques and tailor their approach to the problem, personality, and needs of each person seeking their help. Because skilled therapists may combine different techniques in the course of therapy, the lines between the various approaches often blur.

Because insurance companies and health-care plans often limit the duration of psychotherapy, many mental health professionals are adopting a *time-limited* format in order to make the most of every session, regardless of the length of treatment. Brief or short-term psychotherapy typically focuses on a central theme, problem, or topic and may continue for several weeks to several months. The individuals most likely to benefit are those who are interested in solving immediate problems rather than changing their characters, can think in psychological terms, and are motivated to change.

Psychodynamic Psychotherapy

For the most part, today's mental health professionals base their assessment of individuals on a **psychodynamic** understanding that takes into account the role of early experiences and unconscious influences in *actively* shaping behavior. (This is the *dynamic* in psychodynamic.) Psychodynamic treatments work toward the goal of providing greater insight into problems and bringing about behavioral change. Therapy may be brief, consisting of 12 to 25 sessions, or may continue for several years. According to current thinking, psychotherapy can actually rewire the network of neurons within the brain in ways that ease distress and improve functioning in many areas of daily life.[32] Classical psychoanalysis, developed by Sigmund Freud, is a complex, lengthy process that deals with long-repressed feelings and issues. Less widely used than briefer forms of psychotherapy, it remains an option best suited for mentally healthy, high-functioning individuals who want to explore distressing patterns in their lives, such as a series of failed relationships.

Interpersonal Therapy (IPT)

Interpersonal Therapy (IPT), originally developed for research into the treatment of major depression, focuses on relationships in order to help individuals deal with unrecognized feelings and needs and improve their communication skills. IPT does not deal with the psychological origins of symptoms but rather concentrates on current problems of getting along with others. The supportive, empathic relationship that is developed with the therapist, who takes an even more active role than in psychodynamic psychotherapy, is the most crucial component of this therapy. The emphasis is on the here and now and on interpersonal—rather than intrapsychic—issues. Individuals with major depression, chronic difficulties developing relationships, dysthymia, or bulimia (see Chapter 6 on eating disorders) are most likely to benefit. IPT usually consists of 12 to 16 sessions.

Cognitive-Behavioral Therapy

This approach, which focuses on inappropriate or inaccurate thoughts or beliefs, aims to help individuals break out of a distorted way of thinking. The techniques of **cognitive therapy** include identification of an individual's beliefs and attitudes, recognition of negative thought patterns, and education in alternative ways of thinking. Individuals with major depression or anxiety disorders are most likely to benefit, usually in 15 to 25 sessions.

Behavior therapy strives to substitute healthier ways of behaving for maladaptive patterns used in the past. Its premise is that distressing psychological symptoms, like all behaviors, are learned responses that can be modified or unlearned. Some therapists believe that changing behavior also changes how people think and feel. As they put it, "Change the behavior, and the feelings will follow." Behavior therapies work best for disorders characterized by specific, abnormal patterns of acting—such as alcohol and drug abuse, anxiety disorders, and phobias—and for individuals who want to change bad habits.

Psychiatric Drug Therapy

Medications that alter brain chemistry and relieve psychiatric symptoms have brought great hope and help to millions of people. Thanks to the recent development of a new generation of more precise and effective **psychiatric drugs**, success rates for treating many common and disabling disorders—depression, panic disorder,

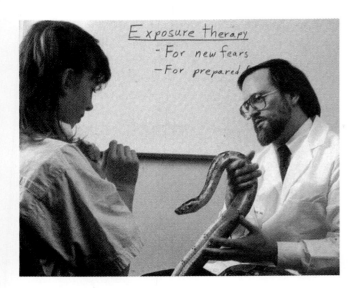

Systematic desensitization is one of the behavior therapies used to treat phobias.

schizophrenia, and others—have soared. Often used in conjunction with psychotherapy, sometimes used as the primary treatment, these medications have revolutionized mental health care.

At some point in their lives, about half of all Americans will take a psychiatric drug. The reason may be depression, anxiety, a sleep difficulty, an eating disorder, alcohol or drug dependence, impaired memory, or another disorder that disrupts the intricate chemistry of the brain.

In the last decade alone, the number of available psychiatric drugs has doubled. These medications are now among the most widely prescribed drugs in the United States. Three of the top ten prescription drugs sold in this country are serotonin-boosting antidepressants—best known by their trade names Prozac, Paxil, and Zoloft—that are used to treat a variety of problems, including obsessive-compulsive disorder, premenstrual syndrome and attention deficits, as well as depression. An estimated 14 million Americans have used Prozac, the best known antidepressant; each week physicians write 170,000 new prescriptions for this drug. Overall, Americans spend $4.3 billion on antidepressant medications every year; by the year 2000, this figure is expected to surpass $6 billion. [33]

Psychiatric medications affect every aspect of a person's physical, mental, and emotional functioning. Some take effect immediately; others take several weeks to relieve symptoms; a few continue to exert their effects even after an individiual discontinues their use. When

taken appropriately, psychiatric agents can alleviate tremendous suffering and reduce the financial and personal costs of mental illness by lessening the need for hospitalization and by restoring an individual's ability to function normally, to work, and to contribute to society. But they do have side-effects and must be used with care. This is especially true for their use in children, during or immediately after pregnancy, or in the elderly.

Strategies for Prevention

What You Need to Know About Psychiatric Drugs

These are some of the questions consumers should ask prior to beginning drug therapy:

✔ Why is it necessary to take this medication? What specific symptoms will it relieve? Are there other possible benefits?

✔ What are the possible side effects and risks? Do I have to take it before or after eating? Will it affect my ability to drive, operate machinery, or work?

✔ How long will it be before the medication begins to help? How can I tell if the drug is working?

✔ Is there any danger from skipping a dose? What are the risks of overdosing? Does this medicine interact with any other medications? Can I drink alcohol while taking this medication? Are there any foods or substances I should avoid?

✔ How long will I have to take this medication? Is there a danger that I'll become addicted? What are the odds that this medicine will help me? What if this drug doesn't work?

Does Treatment Work?

According to the National Mental Health Advisory Council and the American Psychiatric Association, treatments for severe mental disorders—such as major depression, bipolar (manic-depressive) illness, panic disorder, and schizophrenia—are as or more effective than those available in other branches of medicine, including surgery. Treatments tailored to each individual's condition and needs can help 80 to 90% of those suffering from depression and bipolar disorder and 70 to 80% of those with panic disorder. More than 60% of those with schizophrenia can be relieved of acute symptoms with proper therapy, and advances in medication are pushing this percentage ever higher.[34]

Making This Chapter Work for You

Preventing and Solving Psychological Problems

■ Mental health is not an absence of distress, but rather the capacity to think rationally and logically and to cope with life's transitions, stresses, traumas, and losses in a way that allows for emotional stability and growth.

■ As defined by the American Psychiatric Association's *Diagnostic and Statistical Manual,* 4th edition *(DSM-IV),* a mental disorder is "a clinically significant behavioral or psychological syndrome or pattern that occurs in an individual and that is associated with present distress (a painful symptom) or disability (impairment in one or more important areas of functioning) or with a significantly increased risk of suffering death, pain, disability, or an important loss of freedom."

■ During any given year, 30% of Americans suffer from at least one mental disorder. According to the National Comorbidity Survey, the most common single mental disorder is major depression, while the anxiety disorders are the most prevalent group of mental disorders. Only 42% of those with a lifetime history of one or more mental disorders ever receive any professional care.

■ Psychological distress can contribute to major health problems, including high blood pressure, heart disease, cancer, and immune-related disorders. Treating mental disorders often reduces medical care costs.

■ The brain contains hundreds of billions of nerve cells, or neurons, which are the basic working units of the brain. Each consists of a cell body containing the nucleus; a long fiber, called the axon, which can range from less than an inch to several feet in length; an axon terminal, or ending; and multiple branching fibers, called dendrites.

■ Communication with the brain involves a process called neurotransmission, in which an electric charge or impulse travels along a neuron's axon to the terminal, where packets of chemicals, called neurotransmitters, are released. They cross a synapse, a space between two neurons, to connect with specialized receptors on another neuron.

■ The most common type of mental disorders, anxiety disorders may involve episodes of sudden, inexplicable terror (panic attacks), inordinate fears of certain objects or situations (phobias), chronic distress (generalized anxiety disorder, or GAD), or persistent, disturbing thoughts and behaviors (obsessive-compulsive disorder).

■ Major depression, the most widespread mental disorder, has increased among young adults. Symptoms include a sense of helplessness or hopelessness, lack of energy, sleep disturbances, and loss of interest in food, sex, and work. Depression can be successfully treated with psychotherapy, drug therapy, or a combination.

■ Other forms of depression include manic depression (or bipolar disorder), characterized by extreme mood swings; seasonal affective disorder, which develops only at certain times of the year; and dysthymia, chronic mild depression. All can be effectively treated by different therapies.

■ The number of suicides is growing, especially among young people. As many as 50% of college students say they think about suicide, while 8 to 15% act on these thoughts. The degree of hopelessness is a key variable in determining which students actually attempt to take their own lives.

■ Many factors may contribute to suicide: depression, other mental disorders, substance abuse, feelings of loss or failure, physical illness, family history, altered brain chemistry, and access to guns. If the danger of suicide is recognized and individuals receive professional help, suicide can be prevented.

■ Attention disorders are common among adults, affecting 1 to 2% of men and women. Their three primary symptoms are hyperactivity, impulsivity, and distractibility, and they often interfere with school and work performance. Medication is highly effective for adults, as it is for children with attention disorders.

■ Schizophrenia profoundly impairs an individual's sense of reality. Individuals in the active phase of schizophrenia develop positive symptoms, such as hallucinations and delusions. In the residual phase, individuals suffer symptoms, such as general apathy or inappropriate emotional reactions. Although there is no cure for schizophrenia, powerful antipsychotic drugs can reduce confusion, anxiety, delusions, and hallucinations.

■ There are many types of mental health professionals—psychiatrists, psychologists, licensed social workers, psychiatric nurses, and marriage and family therapists—and many options for treatment of mental disorders. Options for treatment include psychodynamic psychotherapy, interpersonal therapy, cognitive-behavioral therapy, and psychiatric drugs.

■ Treatment can help 80 to 90% of those suffering from depression and bipolar disorder and 70 to 80% of those with panic disorder. More than 60% of those with schizophrenia can be relieved of acute symptoms with proper therapy, and advances in medication are pushing this percentage ever higher.

There is a primary rule in evaluating your own emotional mental health: If your problems are interfering with the way you function, it's time to seek help. If you feel less happy, less confident, and less in control for a prolonged period, or if others comment on changes in your behavior and personality, ask for help. "Seeing a therapist is giving yourself the opportunity to create options," says one psychotherapist, "and that may be the greatest gift we can give to ourselves or the people who love us."

Health Online

New York University Department of Psychiatry Online Screening
http://www.med.nyu.edu/Psych/public.html

This site features online screening tests for depression, anxiety, male and female sexual disorders, attention deficit disorder, and personality disorders. There is also information on the diagnosis of psychological problems, their treatment, and self-help options. While it certainly can't take the place of evaluation by a mental health professional, the screening tests at this site may give you a sense of whether or not you should seek professional help for a problem.

Think about it ...

• According to these tests, do you have any warning signs of possible psychological problems? Are these in areas you have felt you had problems with in the past?

• Do you think online screening tests like this might help people with symptoms of psychological problems seek professional help?

• If you were to design a screening test for mental wellness instead of illness, what criteria might you include?

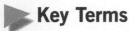 Key Terms

The terms listed here are used within the chapter. Page numbers are included for each term.
A definition of each term is given in the green Glossary pages at the end of this book.

antidepressant   *96*

anxiety   *92*

anxiety disorders   *96*

attention deficit/hyperactivity
   disorder (ADHD)   *105*

axon   *95*

axon terminal   *95*

behavior therapy   *110*

bipolar disorder   *100*

certified social worker   *109*

cognitive therapy   *110*

dendrites   *95*

depression   *94*

depressive disorders   *98*

dysthymia   *100*

generalized anxiety disorder
   (GAD)   *96*

glia   *94*

interpersonal therapy (IPT)   *110*

licensed clinical social worker
   (LCSW)   *109*

major depression   *99*

marriage and family
   therapist   *109*

mental disorder   *92*

neurons   *94*

neuropsychiatry   *94*

neurotransmitters   *95*

nucleus   *95*

obsessive-compulsive disorder
   (OCD)   *96*

panic attack   *96*

panic disorder   *97*

phobia   *96*

psychiatric drugs   *110*

psychiatric nurse   *109*

psychiatrists   *108*

psychodynamic   *110*

psychologists   *109*

psychoneuroimmunology   *94*

psychotherapy   *110*

receptors   *96*

reuptake   *96*

schizophrenia   *106*

seasonal affective disorder
   (SAD)   *100*

synapse   *95*

 Review Questions

1. What is mental health? What is a mental disorder? What are some factors that can cause psychological problems to develop?

2. Define and give examples of the following disorders: anxiety, depression, schizophrenia. What are the risk factors for each disorder? How can individuals with these types of disorders be helped?

3. Why do some individuals attempt suicide? What puts a person at higher risk? How can someone who is suicidal be helped?

4. How can you tell if you need professional help in overcoming a psychological problem? Who can help, and what types of therapy might you try?

5. What role do psychiatric drugs play in the treatment of psychological illnesses?

6. Is it possible to recover fully from a psychological illness?

 Critical Thinking Questions

1. Your friend Danny hasn't been himself lately. He's often tired and withdrawn, and isn't interested in any of the things that excited him last term. He broke up with his girlfriend, but that was months ago, and you don't know why he's still so upset. He's started skipping classes, and when you ask what's up, he just shrugs and says, "Nothing." When you suggest he talk with a counselor, Danny blows up and tells you to forget it. What can you do to help? What are your responsibilities when you notice that a friend or acquaintance is depressed or possibly suicidal? Why is the stigma of emotional problems so great in our society?

2. Paula went to a therapist when she was feeling depressed and was given a prescription for an antidepressant called fluoxetine (trade name Prozac). Her therapist recommended the drug because it causes fewer side effects than other medications. However, Paula later read in a news magazine that

some patients, claiming that Prozac had made them violent or suicidal, had sued the drug's manufacturers. Their suits didn't win in court, but Paula was less certain about taking the prescribed medication. What do you think she should do? How would you weigh the risks and benefits of taking a psychiatric drug?

3. Research has indicated that many homeless men and women are in need of outpatient psychiatric care, often because they suffer from chronic mental illnesses or alcoholism. Yet government funding for the mentally ill is inadequate, and homelessness itself can make it difficult, if not impossible, for people to gain access to the care they need. How do you feel when you pass homeless individuals who seem disoriented or out of touch with reality? Who should take responsibility for their welfare? Should they be forced to undergo treatment at psychiatric institutions?

 ## Connections to Personal Health Interactive

 near right

To enhance your understanding of the material covered in this chapter, check out the following study aids on the **Personal Health Interactive CD-ROM** *. Each numbered icon within the chapter corresponds to an appropriate activity listed here.*

4.1 Recovery from Mental Illness
4.2 Personal Insights: How Healthy Is Your Mind?
4.3 Lobes of the Cerebral Cortex, Saggital View of the Brain, and The Synapse

4.4 Suicide Notes
4.5 Personal Voices: Schizophrenia
4.6 Applied Psychologists
4.7 Chapter 4 Review

References

1. Hales, Robert, and Stuart Yudofsky. *The American Psychiatric Press Textbook of Psychiatry*. 3rd ed. Washington, DC: American Psychiatric Press, 1998.
2. Laurie Flynn, personal interview.
3. Hales, Dianne, and Robert Hales. *Caring for the Mind: The Comprehensive Guide to Mental Health*. New York: Bantam Books, 1995.
4. American Psychiatric Association. *Diagnostic and Statistical Manual of Mental Disorders*. 4th ed. Washington, DC: American Psychiatric Association, 1994. Andreasen, Nancy. "The Validation of Psychiatric Diagnosis: New Models and Approaches." *American Journal of Psychiatry*, Vol. 152, No. 2, February 1995.
5. Kessler, Ronald, et al. "Lifetime and 12-Month Prevalence of *DSM-III-R* Psychiatric Disorders in the United States: Results from the National Comorbidity Study." *Archives of General Psychiatry*, Vol. 51, No. 1, January 1994.
6. Ibid.
7. Hales and Hales, *Caring for the Mind*.
8. Simon, Gregory, et al. "Health Care Costs Associated with Depressive and Anxiety Disorders in Primary Care." *American Journal of Psychiatry*, Vol. 152, No. 3, March 1995.
9. Lamberg, Lynne. "Psychotherapy Reduces Disability, Saves Money." *Journal of the American Medical Association*, Vol. 278, No. 1, July 2, 1997.
10. Hales, Robert, and Stuart Yudofsky. *The American Psychiatric Press Textbook of Neuropsychiatry*. 2nd ed. Washington, DC: American Psychiatric Press, 1997.
11. "Hypnosis: More Than a Suggestion," *Harvard Health Letter*, Vol. 22, No. 12, October 1997.
12. Sanderson, William. "Cognitive Behavior Therapy." *American Journal of Psychotherapy*, Vol. 51, No. 2, Spring 1997.
13. Wickelgren, Ingrid. "When Worry Rules Your Life: Can Simple Anxiety Be a Mental Illness?" *Health*, Vol. 11, No. 8, November–December 1997.
14. Leckman, James, et al. "Symptoms of Obsessive-Compulsive Disorder." *American Journal of Psychiatry*, Vol. 35, No. 7, July 1997.
15. Brown, Phyllida. "Over and Over and Over ..." *New Scientist*, Vol. 155, No. 2093, August 2, 1997.
16. Jones, Mairwen K., et al. "The Cognitive Mediation of Obsessive-Compulsive Handwashing." *Behaviour Research and Therapy*, Vol. 35, No. 9, September 1997.

Amir, Naden, et al. "Strategies of Thought Control in Obsessive-Compulsive Disorder." *Behaviour Research and Therapy*, Vol. 35, No. 9, September 1997.

17. Klien, Donald, and Michael Thase. "Medication vs. Psychotherapy for Depression." *American Society for Clinical Psychopharmacology*, Vol. 8, No. 2, Fall 1997.

18. Wood, Alison, et al. "Controlled Trial of Brief Cognitive-Behavioral Intervention in Adolescent Patients with Depressive Disorders." *Journal of Child Psychology and Psychiatry and Allied Disciplines*, Vol. 37, No. 6, September 1996.

19. Jacobs, Dourglas, et al. "Reevaluation of Depression." *Mind / Body Medicine*, Vol. 1. No. 1, March 1995. Katon, Wayne, et al. "Collaborative Management to Achieve Treatment Guidelines: Impact on Depression in Primary Care." *Journal of the American Medical Association*, Vol. 273, No. 13, April 5, 1995. Brown, Diane, et al. "Major Depression in a Community Sample of African Americans." *American Journal of Psychiatry*, Vol. 152, No. 3, March 1995.

20. Daly, Ian. "Mania." *Lancet,* Vol. 349, No. 9059, April 19, 1997.

21. Sato, Toru. "Seasonal Affective Disorder and Phototherapy: A Critical Review." *Professional Psychology, Research and Practice*, Vol. 28, No. 2, April 1997.

22. Douglas, Kathy, et al. "Results from the 1995 National College Health Risk Behavior Study." *Journal of American College Health*, Vol. 46, September 1997.

23. Clum, George, and Greg Febbraro. "Stress, Social Support and Problem-Solving Appraisal/Skills: Prediction of Suicide Severity Within a College Sample." *Journal of Psychopathology and Behavioral Assessment*, Vol. 16, No. 1, March 1994.

24. Leutwyler, Kristin. "Suicide Prevention." *Scientific American*, Vol. 276, No. 3, March 1997.

25. Hillard, James. "Predicting Suicide." *Psychiatric Services*, March 1995, Vol. 46, No. 3, March 1995.

26. Cooper-Patrick, Lisa, et al. "Preventing Suicide by Asking the Right Questions." *Journal of the American Medical Association*, December 13, 1994.

27. Biederman, Joseph, et al. "High Risk for Attention Deficit Hyperactivity Disorder Among Children of Parents with Childhood Onset of the Disorder." *American Journal of Psychiatry*, Vol. 152, No. 3, March 1995. Faigel, Harris. "Attention Deficit Disorder in College Students." *Journal of American College Health*, Vol. 43, No. 4, January 1995. Heiligenstein, Eric, and Richard Keeling. "Presentation of Unrecognized Attention Deficit Hyperactivity Disorder in College Students." *Journal of American College Health*, Vol. 43, No. 5, March 1995.

28. Farley, Dixie. "Attention Disorder: Overcoming the Deficit." *FDA Consumer*, Vol. 31, No. 5, July–August 1997.

29. Rose, Verna. "APA Practice Guidelines for the Treatment of Patients with Schizophrenia." *American Family Physician*, Vol. 56, No. 4, September 15, 1997.

30. Amadio, Patricia, et al. "New Drugs for Schizophrenia: An Update for Family Physicians." *American Family Physician*, Vol. 56, No. 4, September 15, 1997. Patlak, Margie. "Schizophrenia: Drugs, Therapy Can Turn Life Around for Some." *FDA Consumer*, Vol. 31, No. 6, September–October 1997.

31. Lippincott, Joseph, and John Mierzwa. "Propensity for Seeking Counseling Services: A Comparison of Asian and American Undergraduates." *Journal of College Health*, Vol. 43, March 1995.

32. Vaughan, Susan. *The Talking Cure: The Science Behind Psychotherapy*. New York: G. P. Putnam's Sons, 1997.

33. Vallone, Doris. "Antidepressants and Anxiolytics." *RN*, Vol. 60, No. 7, July 1997.

34. Hales, Robert. *The Psychiatric Pill Book*, in preparation. Davidson, Jonathan, et al. "Panel Discussion on the Antidepressants." *American Society for Clinical Psychopharmacology*, Vol. 8, No. 2, Fall 1997.

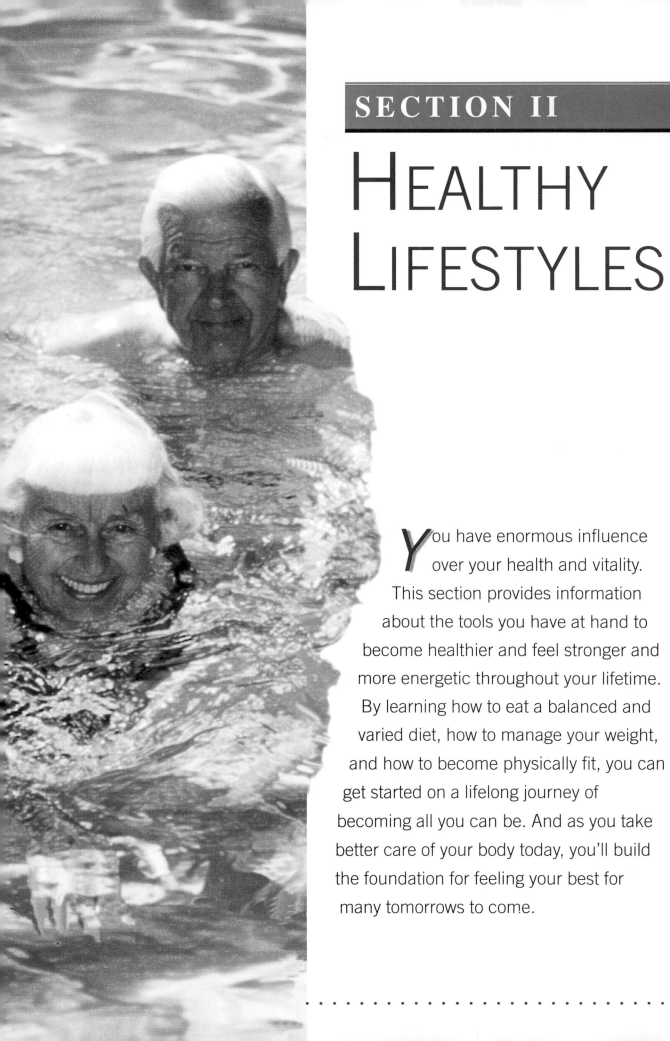

HEALTHY LIFESTYLES

You have enormous influence over your health and vitality. This section provides information about the tools you have at hand to become healthier and feel stronger and more energetic throughout your lifetime. By learning how to eat a balanced and varied diet, how to manage your weight, and how to become physically fit, you can get started on a lifelong journey of becoming all you can be. And as you take better care of your body today, you'll build the foundation for feeling your best for many tomorrows to come.

CHAPTER 5

THE JOY OF FITNESS

After studying the material in this chapter, you should be able to:

List and **explain** the components of physical fitness.

Explain the benefits of exercise as a strategy for health prevention.

Compare and **contrast** aerobic exercises and strength or muscular exercises.

List the potential health effects of using anabolic steroids.

Discuss the different fitness needs of men and women.

Plan a personal exercise program, and **list** nutritional and safety strategies that you should also pursue.

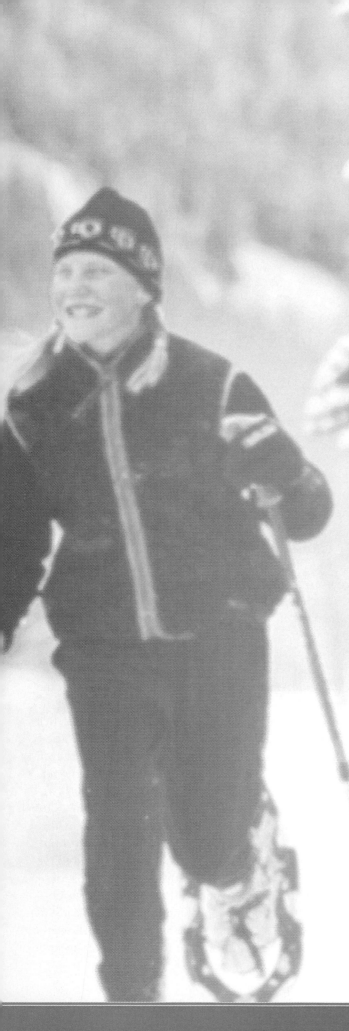

D on't just sit there: Do something! This is the latest message from fitness experts to a nation of couch potatoes.[1] Don't worry about fancy equipment, special clothes, personal trainers: Just get moving. Walk rather than ride. Take the stairs, not the elevator. Bend. Twist. Reach. Wherever you go, whenever you can, put your body to use. You might just save your life.

What has happened to yesteryear's slogans, such as "Go for the burn" and "No pain, no gain"? The nation's top fitness experts have conceded that they simply weren't working——and, in some cases, were even unsafe. Sixty percent of Americans move so little during the course of a day that they qualify as inactive or barely active. Among certain groups, such as women, as many as 70% do not get any regular exercise.[2] On the whole, Americans are fatter, less fit, and far more prone to health problems than they were a decade ago. And we are paying a high price for our sedentary ways: Physical inactivity contributes to approximately one in every four deaths from chronic disease in the United States.[3]

To protect your health, you don't have to turn into a jock or a fitness fanatic. All you have to do is become more active. This chapter can help. It presents current exercise recommendations, explores common barriers to active lifestyles, describes types of exercise, and provides guidelines for getting into shape and exercising safely.

The three basic components of physical fitness. (a) Flexibility. (b) Cardiovascular fitness. (c) Muscular strength and endurance.

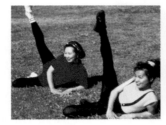

(a)

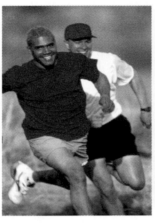

(b)

(c)

What Is Physical Fitness?

The simplest, most practical definition of **physical fitness** is the ability to respond to routine physical demands, with enough reserve energy to cope with a sudden challenge. You can consider yourself fit if you meet your daily energy needs; can handle unexpected extra demands; have a realistic but positive self-image; and are protecting yourself against potential health problems, such as heart disease.

Fitness consists of three basic components: flexibility, cardiovascular or aerobic fitness, and muscular strength and endurance. Other factors, such as body composition and agility, also may be considered in assessing overall fitness. However, if you focus on the three basic components of physical fitness, your body will operate at maximum capacity for as many years as you live.

Flexibility is the range of motion around specific joints—for example, the stretching you do to touch your toes or twist your torso. Flexibility depends on many factors: your age, gender, and posture; bone spurs; and how fat or muscular you are. As children develop, their flexibility increases until adolescence. Then a gradual loss of joint mobility begins and continues throughout adult life. Both muscles and connective tissue, such as tendons and ligaments, shorten and become tighter if

not used at all or not used through their full range of motion.

Cardiovascular fitness refers to the ability of the heart to pump blood through the body efficiently. It is achieved through **aerobic exercise**—any activity, such as brisk walking or swimming, in which the amount of oxygen taken into the body is slightly more than, or equal to, the amount of oxygen used by the body. In other words, aerobic exercise involves working out strenuously without pushing to the point of breathlessness. **Anaerobic exercise** is any activity in which the amount of oxygen taken in by the body cannot meet the demands of the activity; there is thus an oxygen deficit that must be made up later. An example of an anaerobic exercise is sprinting the quarter-mile, which leaves even the best-trained athletes gasping for air. In *nonaerobic exercise*, there is frequent rest between activities, as happens in bowling, softball, and doubles tennis. The body easily takes in all the oxygen needed for these activities, so your heart and lungs don't really get a workout.

Strength—the absolute maximum weight that we can lift, push, or press in one effort—is what most of us equate with muscular fitness. However, **endurance**—the ability to keep lifting, pushing, or pressing—is just as important. It's not enough to be able to hoist a shovelful of snow; you've got to be able to keep shoveling until the entire driveway is clear.

Physical **conditioning** (or training) refers to the gradual building up of the body to enhance one or more of the three main components of physical fitness: flexibility, cardiovascular or aerobic fitness, and muscular strength and endurance.

What Exercise Can Do for You

If exercise could be packed into a pill, it would be the single most widely prescribed and beneficial medicine in the nation. Why? Because nothing can do more to help your body function at its best (Figure 5-1). With regular activity, your heart muscles become stronger and pump blood more efficiently. Your heart rate and resting pulse slow down. Your blood pressure may drop slightly from its normal level.

Regular physical activity thickens the bones and can slow the loss of calcium that normally occurs with age. Exercise increases flexibility in the joints and improves digestion and elimination. It speeds up metabolism, so the body burns up more calories and body fat decreases. It heightens sensitivity to insulin (a great benefit for diabetics) and may lower the risk of developing diabetes. In addition, exercise enhances clot-dissolving substances in the blood, helping to prevent strokes, heart attacks, and pulmonary embolisms (clots in the lungs). Regular, vigorous exercise can actually extend the lifespan. (See Pulsepoints: "Ten Reasons to Work Out.")

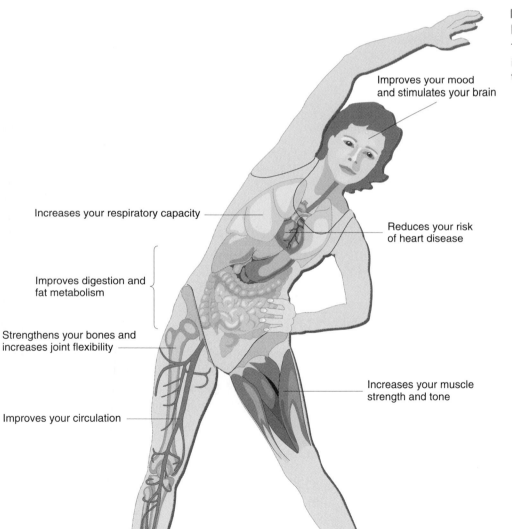

Figure 5-1

The benefits of exercise. Exercise improves your body and mind more than you might expect.

Improves your mood and stimulates your brain

Increases your respiratory capacity

Reduces your risk of heart disease

Improves digestion and fat metabolism

Strengthens your bones and increases joint flexibility

Increases your muscle strength and tone

Improves your circulation

Pulsepoints   Ten Simple Changes to Improve Your Health

1. Improve cardiovascular fitness. Regular activity strengthens the heart so it pumps blood more efficiently.

2. Tone muscles. With exercise, muscles become firmer, function more smoothly, and are capable of withstanding much more strain.

3. Reduce stress. Working out releases tensions and enhances your ability to deal with daily challenges.

4. Improve mood. Exercise may be the single most effective strategy for changing a bad mood. It also works wonders for reducing anxiety and depression.

5. Burn calories. Exercise speeds up metabolism, so the body uses more calories during and after a workout.

6. Increase flexibility. Exercise stretches and lengthens muscles and increases flexibility in the joints.

7. Enhance strength and stamina. Muscle workouts improve the circulation of blood in the tissues and increase the body's ability to do sustained work.

8. Keep bones strong. Regular physical activity (especially weight-bearing activities) thickens the bones, possibly

preventing the slow loss of calcium that normally occurs with age.

9. Lower the risk of disease. Exercise helps prevent many serious health problems, including high blood pressure, strokes, heart attacks, and certain cancers.

10. Put more life in your years—and possibly more years in your life. Physical activity slows the aging process, so you remain healthier and more active for a longer time. And if you work out often and vigorously enough, you can actually extend your lifespan.

A Hardier Heart and Stronger Lungs

Officials at the Centers for Disease Control and Prevention (CDC) have identified insufficient exercise as one of the leading preventable causes of coronary death in this country. Sedentary people are about twice as likely to die of a heart attack as people who are physically active.[4] (See Chapter 12 for a detailed discussion of exercise and the prevention of heart disease.) In addition to its effects on the heart, exercise makes the lungs more efficient. They take in more oxygen, and their vital capacity (ability to take in and expel air) is increased, providing more energy for you to use.

Better Bones

Weak and brittle bones are common among people who don't exercise. **Osteoporosis**, a condition in which bones lose their mineral density and become increasingly soft and susceptible to injury, affects a great many older people. Women, in particular, are more vulnerable because their bones are less dense to begin with. (See Chapter 18 for more on osteoporosis prevention.)

Brighter Mood

Exercise makes people feel good from the inside out. As discussed in Chapters 2 and 3, exercise boosts mood, increases energy, reduces anxiety, improves concentration and alertness, and enables people to handle stress better.[5] During long workouts, some people experience what is called "runner's high," which may be the result of increased levels of mood-elevating brain chemicals called **endorphins**.

Protection Against Certain Cancers

Exercise reduces the risk of colon and rectal cancers, possibly by enhancing digestion and elimination. In women, exercise also may help reduce the risk of cancer of the breast and reproductive organs.[6]

Lower Weight

Aerobic exercise burns off calories during your workout, because as your body responds to the increased demand from your muscles for nutrients, your metabolic rate rises. Moreover, this surge persists for as long as

12 hours after exercise, so you continue to use up more calories than usual even after you've stopped sweating. In addition, aerobic exercise suppresses appetite, so you aren't as tempted to eat. It also helps dieters lose fat rather than lean muscle tissue when they cut back on calories.[7] (See Chapter 7 for information on exercise and weight control.)

A More Active Old Age

Exercise slows the changes that are associated with advancing age: loss of lean muscle tissue, increase in body fat, and decrease in work capacity. In addition to lowering the risk of heart disease and stroke, exercise also helps older men and women retain the strength and mobility needed to live independently. Male and female runners over age 50 have much lower rates of disability and much lower health care costs than less active seniors.[8] (See Chapter 18 for more information on aging and exercise.)

How Much Exercise Do You Need?

Whatever your age, gender, or health status, you can benefit from exercise. As large, long-term studies have shown, increasing activity, even in middle age, can reduce the danger of dying before one's expected time.[9] Even light exercise (any activity that increases oxygen consumption less than three times the level burned by the body at rest) can improve physical and emotional well-being. The more active you are, the more benefits you gain (see Figure 5-2).

Moderate Exercise

The CDC and the American College of Sports Medicine currently call for a minimum of 30 minutes a day of moderate physical activity at least five times a week.[10] "Moderate" refers to any activity that increases oxygen consumption to three to six times the amount used by the body at rest.

In terms of health benefits, 30 minutes of moderate-intensity exercise, either in one sustained period or in shorter bursts of activity, is the equivalent of a brisk two-mile walk. Almost any form of exertion—gardening,

dancing, housework, playing actively with children—can help lower your risk of many chronic health problems, including heart disease, high blood pressure, diabetes, osteoporosis, colon cancer, anxiety, and depression.

"An active lifestyle does not require a regimented, vigorous exercise program," the experts who drafted the new recommendations have stated. "Instead, small changes that increase daily physical activity will enable individuals to reduce their risk of chronic disease and may contribute to enhanced quality of life." According to the CDC, if every currently sedentary American were to devote half an hour a day to some moderate activity, there would be an annual decline of 250,000 deaths a year. In a recent study of unfit men, moderate exercise led to a 40% decline in death from all causes.[11] (See Personal Voices: "Turning Back the Clock.")

Strategies for Prevention

The Least You Should Do

How can you make sure you meet the minimum of 30 minutes of physical activity? Here are some ideas:

✔ Walk, skate, or bicycle instead of driving or taking a bus.

✔ Take the stairs whenever and wherever you can.

✔ While watching television, do calisthenics, lift free weights, or ride a stationary bicycle.

✔ Play ball with friends or children.

✔ Dance—either with friends or by yourself as you listen to music at home.

Vigorous Exercise: Adding Years to Your Life

Although becoming more active can improve your overall health, it won't necessarily make you physically fit. To achieve your optimal fitness level—to function at your physiological best—you should follow the recommendations of the American College of Sports Medicine and regularly engage in both aerobic activities for the cardiovascular system and strength-training exercises for the muscles. Aerobic activities should be performed for 20 to 60 minutes three to five times a week; strength workouts, two to three times a week.

Getting the Benefits of Exercise: How Much and How Long?

Light Exercise:

Activities that increase oxygen consumption to less than three times the level burned by the body at rest. Some health benefits can be expected.

- Walking slowly (strolling)
- Stationary cycling (low to moderate pedaling, low resistance)
- Swimming (slowly treading water)
- Golf, using a powered cart
- Bowling
- Fishing while sitting
- Power boating
- Home care (like carpet sweeping)
- Mowing the lawn (using a riding mower)
- Home repair (like carpentry)

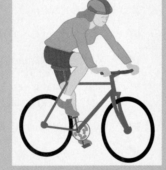

Moderate Exercise:

Activities that increase oxygen consumption to three to six times the level burned by the body at rest. The Centers for Disease Control and the American College of Sports Medicine recommend that every adult do 30 minutes or more of activities like these on most days, and preferably every day. Many studies suggest that these activities have life-prolonging value.

- Walking briskly (3 to 4 miles an hour)
- Cycling for pleasure or transportation (up to 10 miles an hour)

- Swimming, using moderate effort
- Conditioning exercises and general calisthenics
- Racket sports (like table tennis)
- Fishing (standard and casting)
- Canoeing (leisurely, 2 to 3.9 miles an hour)
- Home care (like general cleaning)
- Mowing the lawn (using a power mower)
- Home repair (like painting)

Hard or Vigorous Exercise:

Activities that raise oxygen consumption to more than six times the level burned by the body at rest, with examples of the duration and frequency that a new study suggests may be associated with the biggest reduction in death rates.

- Walking briskly uphill or with a load; 4 to 5 miles an hour for 45 minutes a day, 5 times a week
- Fast cycling or racing (more than 10 miles an hour); 1 hour, 4 times a week
- Swimming (fast treading or crawl); swimming laps 3 hours a week
- Cardiovascular exercise (stair-climbing machine or ski machine); 2 to 3 hours a week
- Racket sports (singles tennis or racquetball); an hour of singles tennis three days a week
- Fishing (wading in a rushing stream)
- Canoeing (more than 4 miles an hour)
- Moving furniture (picking up heavy furniture)
- Mowing the lawn (using a hand mower)

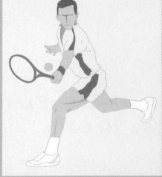

Source: *New York Times*, April 23, 1995.

Figure 5-2
Getting the Benefits of Exercise.

In addition to producing more health benefits, only vigorous exercise (defined as any activity that raises metabolic rate to six times or more above the resting rate) offers an added reward: a longer life. In a 1995 study that followed 17,300 men for more than 20 years, those who burned up 1500 calories in vigorous exercise—the equivalent of walking briskly or jogging for about 15 miles a week—had a 25% lower death rate than those who expended less than 150 calories a week.[12] The more active the men were—up to an activity level of 3000 calories a week—the longer they were likely to live. Smoking history, body weight, and age did not affect the relationship between physical activity and risk of death.

Personal Voices Turning Back the Clock

At age 30, Jamal looked in the mirror and realized he no longer was the boy he used to be. With a big frame for his six-feet-two-inch-tall body, he'd never really thought about his weight—until it ballooned up to 240 pounds. "I hated to admit it, but I had a waist problem," he says. He also found that walking up a single flight of stairs left him breathless. "I thought, 'If I'm out of shape now, where will I be ten or twenty years down the road?'"

Jamal stopped and took a hard look, not just at his weight and fitness, but at his lifestyle. "It wasn't a pretty picture," he recalls. "I'd been a jock in high school and college. For a few years after graduation, I'd played softball and hand-ball pretty regularly. But life has a way of getting busy, and I didn't have time—or make time—for regular exercise. I decided it was time to change. I resolved that, since there are 24 hours in a day, I should spend one of them on my body."

Starting with a slow jog a few mornings a week, Jamal worked up to four miles five times a week. Three days a week he lifted weights, working different muscle groups every day to get maximum benefits. He also took up boxing at a local gym. The results were dramatic. His weight dropped to 200 pounds, with a waist measure of 33 inches. His blood pressure, which had been climbing, stabilized at 120 over 80.

Jamal changed what went into his body as well as what he did to exercise it. "My diet was terrible," he explains. "I lived on fried chicken, mashed potatoes with gravy, eggs—stuff loaded with fat and cholesterol." Now he mainly eats vegetables, cereals, turkey, chicken and fish. "I avoid sugars. If something has more than two grams of fat in it, I rarely eat it," he declares.

Today Jamal describes himself as better than ever: "I'm stronger now than I was in high school. I've got loads of energy. I don't feel old in any way. In fact, I feel like I turned back the clock and bought myself another ten years."

Strategies for Prevention

How to Add Years to Your Life

To exercise at a vigorous enough level to burn up 1500 calories a week, you could:

✔ Walk at a rate of three to four miles an hour five times a week.

✔ Jog at a rate of six to seven miles an hour for three hours a week.

✔ Rollerblade for two and a half hours a week.

✔ Cycle for an hour four times a week.

✔ Swim laps for three hours a week.

✔ Play singles tennis for an hour three days a week.

Making The Commitment

Most people are aware of the tremendous benefits of physical fitness and say they'd like to be in better shape, but they do not—or cannot—commit themselves to a regular exercise program. Women are less likely to work out regularly than men. As noted in Campus Focus: College Students and Physical Activity, on page 126, 43.7% of male college students but only 33% of female students engage in vigorous physical activity regularly. However, the percentages participating in moderate physical activity are about equal: 19.3% of women and 19.7% of men. A significant percentage of students do not exercise at all.[13]

Many roadblocks get in the way of good intentions to exercise: lack of time, lack of affordable, accessible, or safe places to exercise, scheduling difficulties, injuries or other physical limitations, bad weather, or a dislike of working up a sweat. In a 1997 survey of 2993 women, lack of discipline was the primary reason inactive women didn't exercise more. Other significant barriers include a lack of confidence in their abilities, lack of skills, or self-consciousness. Active women report that the key to their success is building exercise into their schedules every day.[14]

If you aren't as active as you wish you could be or know you should be, college may be an ideal time to start. And this course may help—now and in the future. In one study that compared college alumni who had taken a health and physical education course with others who had not, those who'd taken the course were more likely to engage in aerobic exercise. They also, not coincidentally, are less likely to smoke and have lower intakes of dietary fat, cholesterol, and sodium.[15]

CAMPUS FOCUS: COLLEGE STUDENTS AND PHYSICAL ACTIVITY

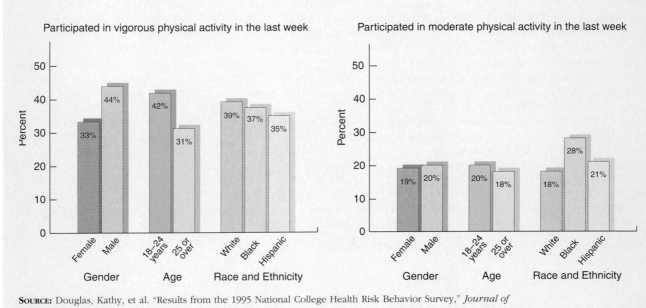

SOURCE: Douglas, Kathy, et al. "Results from the 1995 National College Health Risk Behavior Survey," *Journal of American College Health*, Vol. 46, September 1997.

Getting Started

Most people don't need to see a doctor before beginning a gradual, sensible exercise program. However, you should seek medical advice if you match any of the following descriptions:

- You've had a heart attack; your doctor has told you that you have heart trouble or a heart murmur; or your father, mother, brother, or sister had a heart attack before age 50.

- You often have pains or pressure in your left or mid-chest area or in your left neck, shoulder, or arm during or right after exercise, or you feel faint or have spells of dizziness, or you experience extreme breathlessness after mild exertion (such as a short walk at a moderate pace).

- Your doctor has told you that you have high blood pressure that is not under control or bone or joint problems, such as arthritis.

- You have a medical condition, such as diabetes, that might need special attention in an exercise program.

- You should also check with your doctor if you are over 40 and haven't been exercising two or three times a week.

Starting Young

According to recent estimates, 20 to 30% of American school children are overweight. Two–thirds cannot meet minimum fitness standards. One of every five will develop clinical symptoms of heart disease before age 16. Half of all grade-school youngsters don't get enough exercise to develop healthy cardiorespiratory systems. Half of all girls between ages 6 and 17 and one-third of all boys in this age range cannot run a mile in less than ten minutes.[16]

Today's out-of-shape children don't move as much as they should—mainly because they don't have to. "Exercise isn't built into kids' lives," observes Lyle Micheli, director of Sports Medicine at Boston Children's Hospital.[17] They ride rather than walk to school, play

Self-Survey

Are You Ready to Exercise?

Mark each statement **true** or **false**.

1. I don't want to exercise. _____
2. I have thought about exercising, but no particular type appeals to me. _____
3. I have thought about exercising, but I haven't made any plans to do so yet. _____
4. I have thought about exercising and plan to try it in the next month. _____
6. I have thought about exercising and tried it within the past year, but I gave up. _____
7. I have thought about exercising and have tried some small bits. _____
8. I have actually chosen some type of exercise. _____
9. I have actually started working out regularly. _____
10. I almost always work out regularly. _____

Scoring

The last question to which you answered true is your score (i.e., if you answered True to question 8 and False to questions 9 and 10, your score is eight).

What Your Score Means

1: "I Don't Want to Exercise." At this point, you should gather as much information as possible about yourself and your attitude about fitness (from the comfort of an armchair, of course). Talk to family members and active friends or rent an inspiring sports movie. Don't be afraid to complain about how much you hate to exert yourself; complaining can raise your exercise awareness, the first step to increasing physical activity.

2 to 5: "I'm Thinking About It." You know what you need to do to get into shape but you can't quite convince yourself to make the effort. Adopting a fitness role model—someone you know or someone you'd like to know—can inspire you to get moving. Pick some activity you enjoy and watch a pro: Go to the ballet, the circus or a basketball game. Then try imagining yourself in a new, active role, doing a pirouette, say, or making a free throw. A bit of creative visualization can help move you from contemplation to action.

6 to 7: "I'm Getting Ready." You're making small changes in your behavior, like actually trying some of the moves in a TV aerobics program or walking to work on nice days. Continue to fantasize about yourself as a fit person, then set concrete exercise goals.

8 to 9: "I'm Getting Started." You've gotten off the couch and begun moving your body in some kind of vigorous fashion. Don't try to do too much too soon, or you risk injuring yourself and rejoining the ranks of the sedentary. Reinforce your good habits by telling lots of people about your new regimen (that way, you'll be less likely to slack off). Make things easier for yourself by joining a gym that's on the way to work or laying out your exercise clothes the night before.

10: "I'm Keeping On." For the most part, you've learned to overcome roadblocks to exercise—injury, vacation, or the flu—and to persevere. But if you do occasionally fall off the fitness wagon (and who doesn't?), don't beat yourself up. Just use the motivational tricks that got you working out in the first place.

Making Changes
Psyching Yourself Up to Work Out

- Set goals. People who keep their eyes on a prize—whether it's lowering blood pressure or improving their time on a 10K run—are more likely to stick with an exercise plan.
- Go for twelve. The most noticeable fitness gains come in the first six to twelve weeks of an exercise program. If you stick with it that long, you're more likely to keep working out.
- Alternate athletic activities. If you mainly jog, try step aerobics as a change of pace. Switching activities breaks the monotony and also gives muscles you've been using time to recover.
- Keep a log. If you chart your mood and energy levels on days with or without exercise, you'll probably see the emotional payoff of being physical.
- If you don't feel like exercising, tell yourself you'll just work out for ten minutes. Chances are that when you reach that point you'll want to continue.
- Reward yourself. An occasional new running shirt or jacket can feel well earned after you've reached a certain milestone in your shape-up regimen.

SOURCE: *American Health*, November 1994.

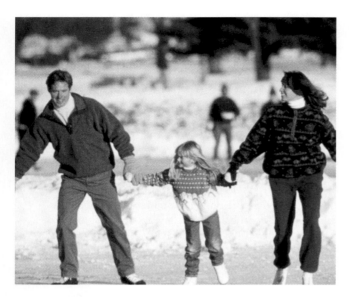

Encouraging children to be physically active gives them an advantage in aerobic fitness and endurance—and establishes the fitness habit for life.

computer games rather than kickball, and spend endless hours in front of the television. And the more hours of TV they watch, the chubbier children tend to be.

Although the fitness of today's youth could definitely use improvement, the situation is far from hopeless. Youngsters have the capacity to make greater gains in aerobic fitness and muscular strength and endurance than do adults. Health promotion programs based on a realistic assessment of children's interests and motivations for getting physical have the potential to change activity patterns in childhood or adolescence—and to lay the foundation for greater fitness throughout life.[18]

Women: On the Sidelines

Lack of exercise is especially common among women. Even though research has shown definite health benefits for women—including a lower risk of osteoporosis, certain cancers, and heart disease—approximately 70% of women are sedentary or irregularly active. In a 1995 study of 55,506 women age 18 and older, only 27% reported following a regular exercise program. Younger women are more active than older women; white women are more likely to be active than Latin or African-American women. The women with the least education and the lowest incomes were less likely to

report regular activity than high school and college graduates, or those earning $50,000 or more per year.[19]

In a study of African-American college freshmen enrolled in a personal health course, 54% of the men, but only 15% of the women, were moderately to highly active.[20] Young women say they exercise as a means of gaining recognition or controlling their weight. As women get older, they're more likely to exercise for the sake of health, fitness, or stress management.[21] But family matters can get in their way. In a study of 1113 urban women between the ages of 20 and 49, mothers were much less active—even though they viewed exercise as just as beneficial as did the women without children.[22]

Misconceptions about exercise also can keep women from exercising. Some fear that working out will bulk up their muscles. Nevertheless, because of lower testosterone levels, the average woman's muscles won't become as bulky as a man's, regardless of how much iron she pumps. While even well-trained women tend to lag behind men in upper body strength, in other aspects of fitness, such as reaction times, women often outscore men. In many fitness categories, there are greater differences among individuals of the same gender than there are between the two genders, with some women outperforming almost all men.[23]

Exercise physiologists have found no significant differences with respect to physical capabilities (such as oxygen intake or ability to work to exhaustion) throughout a woman's menstrual cycle. Indeed, many women report fewer menstrual cramps as they become more active, and women who exercise—even marathon runners—are no more likely than others to suffer menstrual irregularities.[24]

Flexibility

By simplest definition, *flexibility* refers to your ability to go through the complete range of motion that your joints allow in a comfortable, fluid fashion. Some people seem to be born more flexible than others. Other factors that affect flexibility include age, gender, posture, and how fat or muscular you are.

Of all the components of fitness, flexibility is the one most likely to be overlooked—until problems start. Unused muscles hold more tension, which can lead to muscle strain. And muscles shorten and tighten if they aren't used. If you spend a lot of time sitting in front of a computer, for instance, the hamstring muscles in your legs get shorter, and that can lead to lower back pain.

Everyone needs to work on overall flexibility, regardless of general fitness or activity level. But if you exercise, flexibility can be critical. Stiffness in one area (the shoulders, for instance) can increase the risk of injury in others (such as the knees and ankles during a run). Different sports require flexibility in different parts of the body. For swimming, flexible shoulders are crucial; for tennis and golf, the lower back has to be limber. Cyclists should be sure to stretch their quadriceps (front thigh muscles) and calves, while runners should concentrate on their hamstrings and feet.

Keep in mind that warming up and stretching are not the same thing. A warm-up involves getting the heart beating, breaking a sweat, and readying the body for more vigorous activity. Stretching, on the other hand, is a specific activity intended to elongate muscles and keep joints limber, not simply a prelude to some other activity, such as a game of tennis or a three-mile run.

Stretching and warming up can prevent the soreness that occurs in surrounding connective tissue when muscle fibers are injured. Stretching actually may be more important after your workout. It helps move lactic acid out of your muscles, increases your range of motion, decreases soreness, and helps get blood, oxygen, and other nutrients to the muscle tissues.[25]

An extra benefit of stretching is that, like a body yawn, it loosens you up and relieves tension. Even a brief stretch break during the day can be relaxing. However, although stretching is one of the safest activities, it's important that you do it properly so you don't end up hurting instead of helping yourself. Always practice *static,* or passive, stretching—moving gradually into a stretch that you hold for a short time (6 to 60 seconds). An example of such a stretch is letting your hands slowly slide down the front of your legs (keeping your knees in a soft, unlocked position) until you reach your toes and holding this final position for several seconds before slowly straightening up.

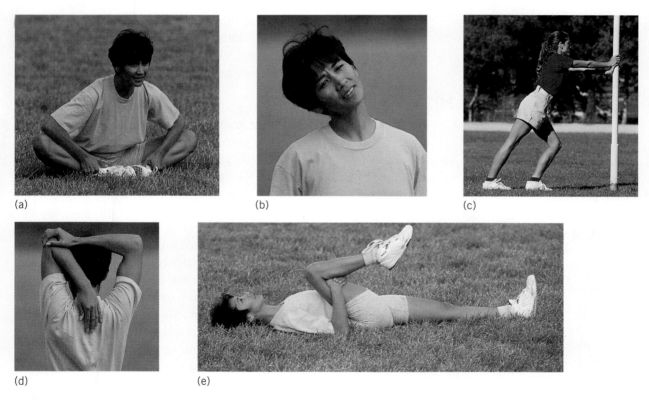

(a)   (b)   (c)

(d)   (e)

Some simple stretching exercises. (a) *Foot pull for the groin and thigh muscles.* Sit on the ground and bend your legs so that the sole of your feet touch. Pull your feet closer as you press on your knees with your elbows. Hold for 10 seconds; repeat. (b) *Lateral head tilt.* Gently tilt your head to each side. Repeat several times. (c) *Wall stretch for the Achilles tendon.* Stand 3 feet from a wall or post with your feet slightly apart. Keeping your heels on the ground, lean into the wall. Hold for 10 seconds; repeat. (d) *Triceps stretch for the upper arm and shoulder.* Place your right hand behind your neck and grasp it above the elbow with your left hand. Gently pull the elbow back. Repeat with the left elbow. (e) *Knee-chest pull for lower back muscles.* Lying on your back, clasp one knee and pull it toward your chest. Hold for 15–30 seconds; repeat with the other knee.

Ballistic stretching, by comparison, is characterized by rapid bouncing or jerking movements, such as a series of up-and-down bobs as you try again and again to touch your toes with your hands. These bounces can stretch muscle fibers too far, causing the muscle to contract rather than stretch; they can also tear ligaments and weaken or rupture tendons, the strong fibrous cords connecting muscles to bones.

To avoid problems, think of the muscle as a rubber band. If you abruptly stretch it out and release it, a rubber band snaps back. If you stretch it too hard or too far, it can break. But if you pull it gently, hold it, and gently release it, the rubber band stretches with far less strain. That's how you want to stretch your muscles.

Always move slowly into a stretch position. You should never feel pain, although you will feel a slight tugging as you extend your stretch. Reach to this point of discomfort and then back off slightly, relaxing and allowing your muscles to adjust. You should hold this stretch until the feeling of tension diminishes. Concentrate on the feeling of the stretch itself, not on the flexibility you want to attain. Perform stretching exercises regularly. "Use it or lose it" is the motto to keep in mind when it comes to flexibility.

Strategies for Change

Safe Stretching

Before you begin, increase your body temperature by slowly marching or running in place. Sweat signals that you're ready to start stretching.

✔ Don't force body parts beyond their normal range of motion. Stretch to the point of tension, back off, and hold for ten seconds to a minute.

✔ Do a minimum of five repetitions of each stretch, with equal repetitions on each side.

✔ Don't hold your breath. Continue breathing slowly and rhythmically throughout your stretching routine. To strengthen muscles, tighten the muscles opposite the ones you're stretching. For example, when you're stretching your hamstrings, the major muscles in the backs of your thighs, you should tighten your quadriceps, the major muscles in the front of your thighs.

✔ Don't do any stretches that require deep knee bends or full squats. These positions can harm your knees and lower back.

Cardiovascular or Aerobic Fitness

Your heart and lungs need regular work to reach peak efficiency. If you haven't been exercising regularly, even mild forms of exertion, such as climbing stairs, can seem rigorous. As you get in shape, however, your body will be able to handle greater challenges with ease.

Your Target Heart Rate

The best way you can be sure you're working hard enough to condition your heart and lungs but not overdoing it is to use your pulse, or heart rate, as a guide. One of the easiest places to feel your pulse is in the carotid artery in your neck. Tilt your head back slightly and to one side. Use your middle finger or forefinger, or both, to feel for your pulse. (Do not use your thumb; it has a beat of its own.) To determine your heart rate, count the number of pulses you feel for 10 seconds and multiply that number by six, or count for 30 seconds and multiply that number by two. Learn to recognize the pulsing of your heart when you're lying or sitting down. On your fitness record, make note of your **resting heart rate**.

Start taking your pulse during, or immediately after, exercise, when it's much more pronounced than when you're at rest. Three minutes after heavy exercise, take your pulse again. The closer that reading is to your resting heart rate, the better your condition. If it takes a long time for your pulse to recover and return to its resting level, your body's ability to handle physical stress is poor. As you continue working out, however, your pulse will return to normal much more quickly.

You don't want to push yourself to your maximum heart rate; yet you must exercise at about 60% to 85% of that maximum to get cardiovascular benefits from your training. This range is called your **target heart rate**. If you don't exercise intensely enough to raise your heart rate at least this high, your heart and lungs won't benefit from the workout. If you push too hard, on the other hand, and exercise at or near your absolute maximum heart rate, you run the risk of placing too great a burden on your heart.

Table 5-1 lists target heart rates for various ages. The following formulas can also be used to calculate your maximum and target heart rates (in beats per minute). For men, the formula is as follows:

TABLE 5-1   TARGET HEART RATE

	Men			Women		
Age	Average Maximum Heart Rate (100%)	Target Heart Rate (60–85%)		Average Maximum Heart Rate (100%)	Target Heart Rate (60–85%)	
20	200	120	170	205	123	174
25	195	117	166	200	120	170
30	190	114	162	195	117	166
35	185	111	157	190	114	162
40	180	108	153	185	111	157
45	175	105	149	180	108	153
50	170	102	145	175	105	149
55	165	99	140	170	102	145
60	160	96	136	165	99	140
65	155	93	132	160	96	136
70	150	90	128	155	93	132

$$220 - Age = \begin{array}{c} \text{Maximum} \\ \text{Heart} \\ \text{Rate} \end{array} \times .60 \begin{array}{c} \text{(Target} \\ \text{Zone for} \\ \text{Beginners)} \end{array} = \begin{array}{c} \text{Target} \\ \text{Heart} \\ \text{Rate} \end{array}$$

Example for a 20-year-old man:

$$220 - 20 = 200 \begin{array}{c} \text{Maximum} \\ \text{Heart} \\ \text{Rate} \end{array} \times .60 = 120 \begin{array}{c} \text{Target} \\ \text{Heart} \\ \text{Rate} \end{array}$$

For women, the formula is as follows:

$$225 - Age = \begin{array}{c} \text{Maximum} \\ \text{Heart} \\ \text{Rate} \end{array} \times .60 \begin{array}{c} \text{(Target} \\ \text{Zone for} \\ \text{Beginners)} \end{array} = \begin{array}{c} \text{Target} \\ \text{Heart} \\ \text{Rate} \end{array}$$

Example for a 20-year-old woman:

$$225 - 20 = 205 \begin{array}{c} \text{Maximum} \\ \text{Heart} \\ \text{Rate} \end{array} \times .60 = 123 \begin{array}{c} \text{Target} \\ \text{Heart} \\ \text{Rate} \end{array}$$

In the initial stages of training, aim for the lower end of your target zone (the 60% calculated above), and gradually build up to 75% of your maximum heart rate. After six months or more of regular exercise, you can push up to 85% of your maximum heart rate if you wish, though you don't have to work that hard just to stay in shape. As long as you use your target heart rate as your guide, your exercise intensity should be just right.

Walking

More men and women—an estimated 65 million in all, according to the National Sporting Goods Association—are taking to their feet. Some, casualties of high-intensity sports, can no longer withstand the wear-and-tear of rigorous workouts. Others want to shape up, slim down, or ward off heart disease and other health problems. The good news for all is that walking may well be the perfect exercise.

According to recent studies, walking at an easy to moderate pace for 40 to 60 minutes is actually better than exercising hard for just 20 minutes. While both approaches enhance fitness, walking is less likely to lead to injuries.[26] Walking develops cardiovascular fitness, builds up endurance, burns fat, and strengthens muscles in the lower body. Another bonus is stress reduction. Since you can do it during a break or at lunch time, walking builds relaxation into your day.[27]

If you're an exercise novice, start with a ten-minute walk every other day. As you get into better condition, you'll go further. In about four to six weeks, you should be able to manage a mile in 20 minutes. For maximum cardiovascular benefits, the American College of Sports Medicine suggests walking at least 20 to 30 minutes three or four times a week. A simple way of determining whether you're moving at a good pace is this rule of thumb: If you can sing as you walk, you're going too slow; if you can't talk, you're going too fast.

Treadmills are a good alternative to outdoor walks—and not just in bad weather. They keep you moving at a certain pace, they're easier on the knees, and they allow you to exercise in a climate-controlled, pollution-free environment—a definite plus for many city dwellers.

Waterwalking in a pool or at a lake or beach is another alternative—and an excellent exercise. Because of the water's resistance, you don't have to walk as fast in water as you would on land to burn the same number of calories. Walking two miles per hour in thigh-high water is equivalent to three miles per hour on land.

In race-walking, or striding (as its noncompetitive form is called), you must keep your lead foot on the ground as your trailing leg pushes off, and your knee remains straight as your body passes over that leg. As a result, one foot is always supporting the body, so the maximum impact per step is much lower than when you run and the injury rate is low.

Because their stride is shorter, race-walkers have to stretch their hips forward and backward, which is good for flexibility. Because of the extra effort, they can get an added bonus: they burn up more calories than they would running at the same speed over the same distance.

Strategies for Change

Putting Your Best Foot Forward

✔ Walk very slowly for five minutes, and then do some simple stretches.

✔ Maintain good posture. Focus your eyes ahead of you, stand erect, and pull in your stomach.

✔ Use the heel-to-toe method of walking. The heel of your leading foot should touch the ground before the ball or toes of that foot do. When you push off with your trailing foot, bend your knee as you raise your heel. You should be able to feel the action in your calf muscles.

✔ Pump your arms back and forth to burn 5 to 10% more calories and get an upper-body workout as well.

✔ End your walk the way you started it—let your pace become more leisurely for the last five minutes.

Jogging and Running

The difference between jogging and running is speed. You should be able to carry on a conversation with someone on a long jog or run; if you're too breathless to talk, you're pushing too hard.

If your goal is to enhance aerobic fitness, long, slow, distance running is best. If you want to improve your speed, try *interval training*, which consists of repeated hard runs over a certain distance, with intervals of relaxed jogging in between. Depending on what suits you and what your training goals are, you can vary the distance, duration, and number of fast runs, as well as the time and activity between them. Interval training is usually done on a track and should not be attempted unless you're in top shape.

If you have been sedentary, it's best to launch a walking program before attempting to jog or run. Start by walking for 15 to 20 minutes three times a week at a comfortable pace. Continue at this same level until you no longer feel sore or unduly fatigued the day after exercising. Then increase your walking time to 20 to 25 minutes, speeding up your pace as well.

When you can handle a brisk-minute walk, alternate fast walking with slow jogging. Begin each session walking, and gradually increase the amount of time you spend jogging. If you feel breathless while jogging, slow down and walk. Continue to alternate in this manner until you can jog for ten minutes without stopping. If you gradually increase your jogging time by one or two minutes with each workout, you'll slowly build up from 10 to 20 or 25 minutes per session. For optimal fitness, you should jog at least three times a week.

Strategies for Change

Running Right

✔ As you run, keep your back straight and your head up. Run tall, with your buttocks tucked in. Look straight ahead. Hold your arms slightly away from your body. Your elbows should be bent slightly so that your forearms are almost parallel to the ground. Move your arms rhythmically to propel yourself along.

✔ Have your heels hit the ground first. Land on your heel, rock forward, and push off the ball of your foot. if this is difficult, try a more flat-footed style.

✔ Avoid running on the balls of your feet; this produces soreness in the calves because the muscles must contract for a longer time. To avoid shin splints (a dull ache in the lower shins), stretch regularly to strengthen the shin muscles and to develop greater flexibility in your ankles.

✔ Avoid running on hard surfaces and making sudden stops or turns.

✔ Breathe through your nose and mouth to get more volume. Learn to "belly breathe": When you breathe in, your belly should expand; when you breathe out, it should flatten. if your breathing becomes labored, try exhaling with resistance through pursed lips so that your body utilizes more oxygen per breath.

✔ When you approach a hill, shorten your stride. Lift your knees higher; pump your arms more. If the hill is really steep, lean forward. When you start downhill, lean forward, and run as if you were on a flat surface. Don't lean back, because doing so could strain your knees and the muscles in your legs.

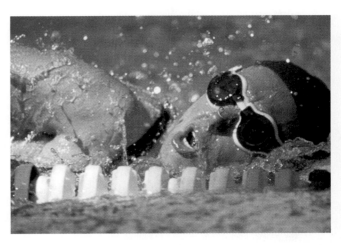

Swimming is good exercise for people of all ages—particularly for cardiovascular fitness and flexibility.

Swimming

More than 100 million Americans dive into the water every year. What matters for our heart's health, however, is getting a good workout, not just getting wet. Swimming is an excellent exercise for cardiovascular fitness and also rates fairly high for weight control, muscular function, and flexibility. However, it's not as effective as activities such as walking and running for building strong bones and preventing osteoporosis.

For aerobic conditioning, you have to swim laps, using a freestyle, butterfly, breast-, or backstroke. (The sidestroke is too easy.) You've also got to be a good enough swimmer to keep churning through the water for at least 20 minutes. Your heart will beat more slowly in water than on land, so your heart rate while swimming is not an accurate guide to exercise intensity. You should try to keep up a steady pace that's fast enough to make you feel pleasantly tired, but not completely exhausted, by the time you get out of the pool.

Swimming is good for people of all ages, particularly those over 50 or with physical handicaps. Swimming facilities are available in nearly all communities. Check your college gym; your local YWCA, YMCA, or JCC; your city recreation department; and other schools in your area.

Strategies for Change
....
Smart Swimming

✔ Start by swimming 50 yards and rest when you feel breathless.

✔ Try to swim 100 yards, rest for a minute, and then swim another 100 yards.

✔ Increase your distance slowly. See if you can work up to 700 yards in 18 minutes.

✔ Stick to the crawl, the butterfly, the breaststroke, or the backstroke.

Cycling

Bicycling, indoors and out, can be an excellent cardiovascular conditioner, as well as an effective way to control weight—provided you aren't just along for the ride. If you coast down too many hills, you'll have to ride longer up hills or on level ground in order to get a good workout. Half of all bikes now sold in the United States are mountain bikes, sturdy cycles with knobby tires that allow bikers to climb up and zoom down dirt trails and explore places traditional racing bikes couldn't go. However, an 18-speed bike can make pedaling too easy, unless you choose gears carefully. To gain aerobic benefits, mountain bikers have to work hard enough to raise their heart rates to their target zone and keep up that intensity for at least 20 minutes.

Using a one-wheel stationary cycle with a tension-control knob, you can adjust the amount of effort required; start with low resistance, then increase the tension until you're working at your target heart rate. You can put the cycle in front of a television set or look out the window if you feel the need for some scenery—or you can read or simply meditate while pedaling.

Strategies for Change
Smart Cycling

✔ If you're not used to cycling, start slowly. Work up from 5 minutes of steady pedaling (interrupted by rest periods if necessary) to 10, 15, 20, and 25 minutes. Limit your rides to 5–10 minutes the first week. Increase your time and speed gradually to avoid sore thigh muscles. Rest when you feel breathless.

✔ Keep your elbows slightly bent to allow for a more relaxed upper body. Change your hand positions periodically to avoid numbness.

✔ Monitor your heart rate to make sure you're working within your target range.

✔ When riding outdoors, be sure to wear a helmet. Look for proof that it conforms to either the Snell or ANSI standard for head protection.

✔ Make yourself visible. Wear reflective clothing if you can. If you cannot, remember that drivers see bright pink, yellow, and orange most easily.

✔ Always follow the rules of the road—stick to the right, stop at stop signs, heed one-way signs, and so on.

Crosscountry Skiing

One of the most effective forms of aerobic exercise, crosscountry or Nordic skiing, has become an increasingly popular winter sport. Thanks to machines that simulate the moves of Nordic skiing, it's now possible to "ski" in any season. Because almost every muscle in the body gets a workout, crosscountry skiing is excellent for all-around conditioning. Using the poles works the arms, shoulders, back, and abdomen, while the kick-and-glide action of skiing involves virtually all the muscles of the legs, thighs, and abdomen. Also, as exercisers breathe faster and more deeply, their rib, abdominal, and shoulder muscles get a workout. Another plus: The risk of joint and ligament injury while crosscountry skiing is lower than for many other impact-aerobic activities (and much lower than for downhill skiing).

Other Aerobic Activities

Because variety is the spice of an active life, many people prefer different forms of aerobic exercise. All can provide many health benefits. Among the popular options:

- *Skipping rope.* This is essentially a form of stationary jogging with some extra arm action thrown in. It is excellent both as a heart conditioner and as a way of losing weight. Always warm up before starting and cool down afterward. To alleviate boredom, try skipping to music, and vary the steps: both feet together, alternating left and right feet, or jumping up and down on one leg,

- *Aerobic dancing.* This activity combines music with kicking, bending, and jumping. A typical class (you can also dance at home to a video or TV program) consists of stretching exercises and sit-ups, followed by aerobic dances and cool-down exercises. A particular benefit of aerobic dance is that people get enjoyment and stimulation from the music; they're also able to move their bodies without worrying about skill and technique. "Soft," or low-impact, aerobic dancing doesn't put as much strain on the joints as "hard," or high-impact, routines.

- *Step training or bench aerobics.* This low-impact workout combines step, or bench, climbing with music and choreographed movements. Basic equipment consists of a bench 4 to 12 inches high. The fitter you are, the higher the bench—but the higher the bench, the greater the risk of knee injury. A 40-minute step workout is equivalent to running at seven miles an hour in terms of oxygen uptake and calories burned.

- *Stair-climbing.* An estimated 4 million Americans are stepping up to fitness, according to the American Sports Data Institute. You could run up the stairs in an office building or dormitory, but most people use stair-climbing machines available in home models and at gyms and health clubs. On most versions of these machines, exercisers push a pair of pedals up and down—much easier on the feet and legs than many other activities.

- *Rollerblading.* In-line skating can increase aerobic endurance and muscular strength and is less stressful on joints and bones than running or high-impact aerobics. Rollerbladers can adjust the intensity of their workout by varying the terrains. (Obviously, they'll have to work harder while going up hills, and less so on the slide down.) They can also buy special training wheels and weights to increase resistance and make muscles work harder. One caution: Protective gear, including a helmet, knee and elbow pads, and wrist guards, is essential.

Muscular Strength and Endurance

Although aerobic workouts condition your insides (heart, blood vessels, and lungs), they don't exercise many of the muscles that shape your outsides and provide power when you need it. Strength workouts are important because they enable muscles to work efficiently and reliably. Conditioned muscles function more smoothly and contract somewhat more vigorously and with less effort. With exercise, muscle tissue becomes firmer and can withstand much more strain—the result of toughening the sheath protecting the muscle and developing more connective tissue within it (see Figure 5-3).

Muscular strength and endurance are critical for handling everyday burdens, such as cramming a 20-pound suitcase into an overhead luggage bin or hauling a trunk down from the attic. Prolonged exercise prepares the muscles for sustained work by improving the circulation of blood in the tissue. The number of tiny blood vessels, called capillaries, increases by as much as 50% in regularly exercised muscles; and existing capil-

Strength workouts increase circulation

The heart's right half pumps oxygen-poor blood to capillary beds in lungs. There, O_2 diffuses into blood and CO_2 diffuses out. The oxygenated blood flows into the heart's left half where it is then pumped to capillary beds throughout the body

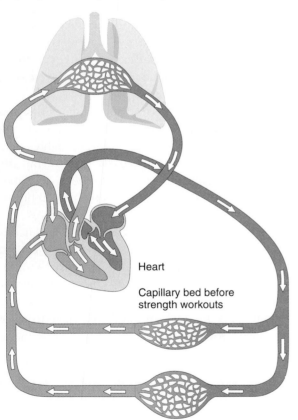

Heart

Capillary bed before strength workouts

Capillary bed after 8–12 weeks of strength workouts (extra capillaries develop, circulation increases)

Strength workouts build muscles

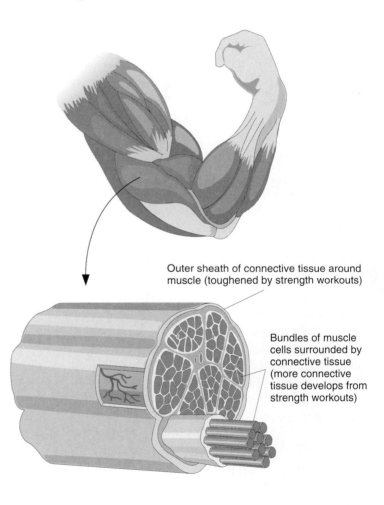

Outer sheath of connective tissue around muscle (toughened by strength workouts)

Bundles of muscle cells surrounded by connective tissue (more connective tissue develops from strength workouts)

Figure 5-3

Strength training in combination with aerobic exercise develops muscles, burns fat, and increases blood circulation and oxygen supply to body tissues.

laries open wider so that the total circulation increases by as much as 400%, thus providing the muscles with a much greater supply of nutrients. This increase occurs after about eight to twelve weeks in young persons, but takes longer in older individuals. Inactivity reverses the process, gradually shutting down the extra capillaries that have developed.

The latest research on fat-burning shows that the best way to reduce your body fat is to add muscle-strengthening exercise to your workouts.[28] Muscle tissue is your very best calorie-burning tissue, and the more you have, the more calories you burn, even when you are resting. You don't have to become a serious body builder. Using handheld weights (also called free weights) two or three times a week is enough. Just be sure you learn how to use them properly because you can tear or strain muscles if you don't practice the proper weight-lifting techniques.

A balanced workout regimen of muscle-building and aerobic exercise does more for you than just burn fat. It gives you more endurance by promoting better distribution of oxygen to your tissues and increasing the blood flow to your heart.

Exercise and Muscles

Your muscles never stay the same. If you don't use them, they atrophy, weaken, or break down. If you use them rigorously and regularly, they grow stronger. The only way to develop muscles is by demanding more of them than you usually do. This is called **overloading**. As you train, you have to increase the number of repetitions or the amount of resistance gradually and work the muscle to temporary fatigue. That's why it's important not to quit when your muscles start to tire. Some exercise enthusiasts believe that the experience of pain—the "burn"—signals that exercise is paying off; however, others contend that it means you're pushing too hard and risking injury.

You need to exercise differently for strength than for endurance. To develop strength, you do a few repetitions with heavy loads. As you increase the load, object, or weight your muscles must move, you increase your strength. To increase endurance, you do many more repetitions with lighter loads. If your muscles are weak and you need to gain strength in your upper body, you may have to work for weeks to do a half-dozen regular pushups. Then you can start building endurance by

doing as many pushups as you can before collapsing in exhaustion.[29]

Isometric exercises are those in which you push or pull against an immovable object, with each muscle contraction being held for five to eight seconds and being repeated five to ten times daily. Isometric exercises seem to raise blood pressure in some people, which can be dangerous; they're not generally used to develop muscle strength.

Isotonic exercises are those in which the muscle moves a moderate load several times, as in weight-lifting or calisthenics. The kind of isotonic exercise best for producing muscular strength involves high resistance and a low number of repetitions. On the other hand, you can develop the greatest flexibility, coordination, and endurance with isotonic exercises that incorporate lower resistance and frequent repetitions.

For isotonic exercise, you can use free weights (such as barbells and dumbbells) or Nautilus or Universal equipment, found in most gyms and health clubs. Nautilus and Universal weight-training machines use the principle of progressive resistance. The Universal equipment is a system of cables, pulleys, and weights. Nautilus machines have a special cam (a pulley with an off-center axis) that adjusts the resistance for exercise in all positions.

Isokinetic exercises that use special machines provide resistance to overload muscles throughout the entire range of motion. These exercises are highly effective in strengthening specific muscle groups; but the sophisticated mechanical devices are expensive, elaborate, and generally available only at commercial fitness clubs.

Muscular training is highly specific, which means that you have to exercise certain muscles for certain results. If you want to build up your leg muscles to run a marathon, pushups won't help—just as running a marathon won't develop your upper body. If you're training with specific goals in mind, you have to tailor your exercise program to make sure you meet them.

Designing a Muscle Workout

A workout with weights should exercise your body's primary muscle groups: the *deltoids* (shoulders), *pectorals* (chest), *triceps* and *biceps* (back and front of upper arms), *quadriceps* and *hamstrings* (front and back of thighs), *gluteus maximus* (buttocks), and *abdomen* (see Figure 5-4). Various machines and free-weight routines focus on each muscle group, but the principle is always the same: Muscles contract as you raise and lower a weight, and you repeat the lift-and-lower routine until the muscle group is tired.

A weight-training program is made up of both **sets** (set numbers of repetitions of the same movement) and **reps** (the single performance of exercises, such as lifting 75 pounds once). You should allow your breath to return to normal before moving on to each new set. Pushing yourself to the limit builds strength.

Maintaining proper breathing techniques during weight training is crucial. To breathe correctly, inhale when muscles are relaxed, and exhale when you push or lift. Don't ever hold your breath because oxygen flow helps prevent muscle fatigue and injury.

Remember that your muscles need sufficient time to recover from a weight-training session. Allow no less than 48 hours, but no more than 96 hours, between training sessions, so that your body can recover from the workout and so that you'll avoid overtraining. Workouts on consecutive days do more harm than good, because the body can't recover that quickly. Two or three thirty-minute training sessions a week should be sufficient for building strength and endurance. Indeed, you can obtain 70% to 80% as much improvement by strength training twice a week as three times a week. However, your muscles will begin to atrophy if you let more than three or four days pass without exercising them. For total fitness, you may want to schedule aerobic workouts for your days off from weight training.[30]

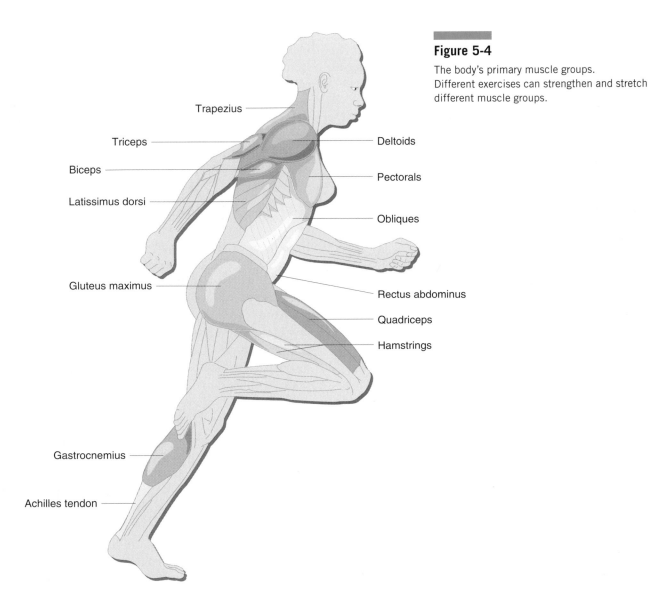

Figure 5-4

The body's primary muscle groups. Different exercises can strengthen and stretch different muscle groups.

Trapezius

Triceps

Biceps

Latissimus dorsi

Gluteus maximus

Gastrocnemius

Achilles tendon

Deltoids

Pectorals

Obliques

Rectus abdominus

Quadriceps

Hamstrings

Strategies for Prevention

Working with Weights

If you plan to work with free weights, here are some guidelines for using them safely and effectively:

✔ Don't train alone—for safety's sake. Work with a partner so you can serve as spotters for each other and help motivate each other as well.

✔ Always warm up and stretch before weight training; also be sure to stretch after training.

✔ Begin with relatively light weights (50% of the maximum you can lift), and increase the load slowly until you find the weight that will cause muscle failure at anywhere from eight to twelve repetitions. (Muscle failure is the point during a workout at which you can no longer perform or complete a repetition through the entire range of motion.)

✔ In the beginning, don't work at maximum intensity. Increase your level of exertion gradually over two to six weeks to allow your body to adapt to new stress without soreness.

✔ Always train your entire body, starting with the larger muscle groups. Don't focus only on specific areas, although you may want to concentrate on your weakest muscles.

✔ Always use proper form. Unnecessary twisting, lurching, lunging, or arching can cause serious injury. Remember, quality matters more than quantity. One properly performed set of lifts can produce a greater increase in strength and muscle mass than many sets of improperly performed lifts.

Pumping Steroids

Anabolic steroids, synthetic derivatives of the male hormone testosterone, are approved for medical use in treating severe burns and injuries. However, some competitive athletes seeking an extra edge, those trying to transform their bodies and look strong, and the "fighting elite"—gang members, police, and bouncers who want to increase their size and strength—use steroids, usually in dangerous forms and doses, to gain weight and strength. (See Chapter 14 for a further discussion of steroid abuse.)

Some users inject high doses of steroids intended only for horses. Others, in a practice called "stacking," take several different steroids at the same time. Steroids do increase weight and muscle strength; but they have dangerous side effects on the liver, reproductive organs, and the mind (see Chapter 14 on substance abuse). Long-term use also reduces levels of beneficial high-density lipoproteins, thereby increasing the risk of heart disease.[31]

In addition, the sharing of needles to inject steroids could result in transmission of HIV from an infected person to others. Anabolic steroids also have profound psychological effects. Long-term, high-dose use may lead to a preoccupation with steroid use, difficulty stopping despite side effects, drug craving, and withdrawal symptoms (including depression).

Some athletes and bodybuilders are experimenting with alternatives to steroids, including human growth hormone (HGH) and gamma hydroxybutyrate (GHB). Neither substance is safe, and they should never be taken in the mistaken belief that they can add bulk to muscles. The use of HGH, an injectable form of the hormone that produces normal growth, carries the risk of hepatitis or HIV infection from tainted needles, as well as other medical complications. GHB, a substance naturally found in the central nervous system, can cause sudden sleepiness, short-term coma, vomiting, dizziness, headache, nausea, vomiting, and seizures.

Total Fitness

No one single exercise can stretch and strengthen your muscles and also enhance your cardiovascular fitness. That's why **cross-training** (alternating two or more different types of fitness activities) and **aerobic circuit training** (combining aerobic and strength exercises to build both cardiovascular fitness and muscular strength and endurance) have become increasingly popular:

- *Cross-training.* The pioneers of contemporary cross-training were triathletes, who run, swim, and cycle. Depending on the specific sports, cross-training can yield various benefits. Alternating aerobic workouts with weight-lifting, for example, can increase speed and performance. Alternating running with a low-impact aerobic exercise, such as swimming, lessens the risk of knee, ankle, or shin injuries. Cross-training also helps exercisers avoid boredom and offers the pleasures of variety.

There's no one cross-training combination that's right for everyone. To plan a program, first identify your fitness goals: Do you want to control your weight, get stronger, feel better about yourself, improve your general health, and improve your performance in a particular competitive sport? Your unique fitness goals will dictate the cross-training program that's right for you.

*   *Aerobic circuit training.* Done individually or in a group at a gym or health club, aerobic circuit training generally involves weight-training equipment (such as free weights or Nautilus or Universal machines) and aerobic stations (treadmills, stationary bikes, stair-climbing machines, or cross-country skiing machines). By alternating weight and aerobic stations and moving quickly from one station to the next, exercisers can get a total-body workout. Some aerobic circuit trainers have reported significant improvements in aerobic capacity as well as enhanced toning and shaping of muscles.

Nutrition for Exercise

A balanced diet that follows the Food Guide Pyramid described in Chapter 6 can supply everything most exercisers need to perform well. However, endurance athletes whose workouts last an hour or more do best with a diet high in complex carbohydrates, which help keep the level of sugar in the blood steady and increase the amount of available glycogen, the body's fuel reserve, which is stored in the liver. This prevents sudden drops in blood glucose, weakness, and lightheadedness.

Because muscles are made of protein, many exercisers think that more protein will make their muscles stronger. Yet heavy workouts don't significantly increase your body's need for protein, and high-protein diets don't lead to high performance. In fact, the American Dietetic Association has warned that too much protein can actually impair athletic performance by placing an excessive burden on the kidneys and liver.

If you're interested in high-octane nutrition to enhance your athletic performance, you may be tempted to try "body building" or "high-energy" foods, drugs, or dietary supplements, such as amino acids. Don't. You'll be wasting a lot of money, and you might end up feeling worse, rather than better, because of a nutritional imbalance.

What you do need before and during a workout is water. On a hot day, some athletes lose 2 pounds during a training session; that amounts to a quart of sweat. And as their bodies become dehydrated, their hearts find it more difficult to satisfy the demands of their muscles for oxygen and nutrients.

Water works best to prevent dehydration, because it's absorbed more quickly than any athletic drink or beverage containing sugar, sodium, potassium, or other ingredients. The American Dietetic Association dictates "plain cool water" as the fluid of choice for "most persons undertaking moderate exercise in moderate temperature conditions."

Although you may have heard a great deal about salt tablets, stay away from them. They're unnecessary and potentially dangerous. You do lose some salt in sweat, but the loss is minimal—and more than made up for by the huge amounts of sodium most Americans get in their daily diet.

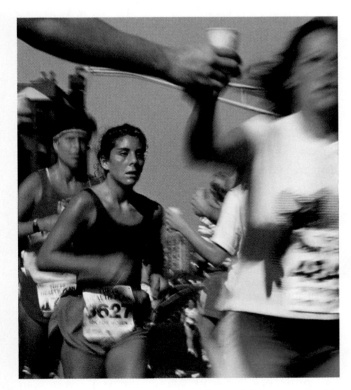

Water for your workout. Plain water before and during a workout is the best way to prevent dehydration.

Sports Safety

Whenever you work out, you don't want to risk becoming sore or injured. Starting slowly when you begin any new fitness activity is the smartest strategy. Keep a simple diary to record the time and duration of each workout. Get accustomed to an activity first and then begin to work harder or longer. In this way, you strengthen your musculoskeletal system so you're less likely to be injured, you lower the cardiovascular risk, and you build the exercise habit into your schedule.

Even seasoned athletes should "listen to their bodies." If you develop aches and pains beyond what you might expect from an activity, stop. Never push to the point of fatigue. If you do, you could end up with sprained or torn muscles.

Preventing Injuries

According to the American Physical Therapy Association, the most common exercise-related injury sites are the knees, feet, back, and shoulders, followed by the ankles and hips. **Acute injuries**—sprains, bruises, and pulled muscles—are the result of sudden trauma, such as a fall or collision. **Overuse injuries**, on the other hand, are the result of overdoing a repetitive activity, such as running. When one particular joint is overstressed—such as a tennis player's elbow or a swimmer's shoulder—tendinitis, an inflammation at the point where the tendon meets the bone, can develop. Other overuse injuries include muscle strains and aches and stress fractures, which are hairline breaks in a bone, usually in the leg or foot.

To prevent injuries and other exercise-related problems before they happen, use common sense and take appropriate precautions.

Strategies for Prevention
. . . .
Protecting Yourself

✔ Many exciting, exhilarating sports—including kayaking, skiing, hang gliding, and windsurfing—entail some risks. If you choose these activities, your responsibility is to learn the basics for safe participation. The fundamental principles include:

✔ Get proper instruction and, if necessary, advanced training from knowledgeable instructors.

✔ Make sure you have good equipment and keep it in good condition. Know how to check and do at least basic maintenance on the equipment yourself. Always check your equipment prior to each use (especially if you're renting it).

✔ Always make sure that stretching and exercises are preventing, not causing, injuries.

✔ Use reasonable protective measures, including wearing helmets when cycling.

✔ For some sports, such as boating, always go with a buddy.

✔ Take each outing seriously—even if you've dived into this river a hundred times before, even if you know this mountain like you know your own backyard. Avoid the unknown under adverse conditions (e.g., hiking unfamiliar terrain during poor weather or kayaking a new river when water levels are unusually high or low) or when accompanied by a beginner whose skills may not be as strong as yours.

✔ Never combine alcohol or drugs with any sport.

Thinking of Temperature

Prevention is the wisest approach to heat problems. Always dress appropriately for the weather and be aware of the health risks associated with temperature extremes.

Heeding Heat

Always wear as little as possible when exercising in hot weather. Choose loose-fitting, lightweight, white or light-colored clothes. Cotton is good because it absorbs perspiration. Never wear rubberized or plastic pants and jackets to sweat off pounds. These sauna suits will cause you to lose water only—not fat—and, because they don't allow your body heat to dissipate, they can be dangerous. On humid days, carry a damp washcloth to wipe off perspiration and cool yourself down. Be sure to drink plenty of fluids while exercising (especially water), and watch for the earliest signs of heat problems, including cramps, stress, exhaustion, and heatstroke. (See Chapter 17 for a further discussion of safety precautions.)

Coping with Cold

Protect yourself in cold weather (or cold indoor gyms) by covering as much of your body as possible, but don't overdress. Wear one layer less than you would if you were outside but not exercising. Don't use warm-up clothes of waterproof material because they tend to trap heat and keep perspiration from evaporating. Make sure your clothes are loose enough to allow movement and exercise of the hands, feet, and other body parts, thereby maintaining proper circulation. Choose dark colors that absorb heat. And because 40% or more of your body heat is lost through your head and neck, wear a hat, turtleneck, or scarf. Make sure you cover your hands and feet as well; mittens provide more warmth and protection than gloves.

Toxic Workouts

If you live in a large city, you may have to consider the risks of exercising in polluted air. On smoggy days, avoid a noontime workout. Exposure to ground-level ozone, produced as sunlight reacts with exhaust fumes, can irritate the lungs and constrict bronchial tubes. An ozone level of 0.12 part per million causes, on the average, a 13% decline in lung capacity. This level is the maximum considered safe under the Clean Air Act, but it is often surpassed in New York, Los Angeles, and other urban areas.

Overtraining

About half of all people who start an exercise program drop out within six months. One common reason is that they **overtrain**, pushing themselves to work too intensely too frequently. Signs of overdoing it include persistent muscle soreness, frequent injuries, unintended weight loss, nervousness, and an inability to relax. If you're pushing too hard, you may find yourself unable to complete a normal workout, or have difficulty recovering afterward.

If you develop any of the symptoms of overtraining, reduce or stop your workout sessions temporarily. Make gradual increases in the intensity of your workouts. Allow 24 to 48 hours for recovery between workouts. Make sure you get adequate rest. Check with a physical education instructor, coach, or trainer to make sure your exercise program fits your individual needs.

Evaluating Fitness Products and Programs

Just as you have to be a good health-care consumer (see Chapter 20), you should be a smart fitness consumer as well. Whatever activity you choose—even one as simple as walking—you'll find plenty of products to choose from. Make sure you judge them according to function, not fanciness or form.

How to Buy Athletic Shoes

For many aerobic activities, good shoes are the most important purchase you'll make. Take the time to choose well. Here are some basic guidelines:

- Shop for shoes in the late afternoon, when your feet are most likely to be somewhat swollen—just as they will be after a workout.
- For walking shoes, look for a shoe that's lightweight, flexible, and roomy enough for your toes to wiggle, with a well-cushioned, curved sole; good support at the heel; and an upper made of a material that breathes (allows air in and out).
- For running shoes (see Figure 5-5), look for good

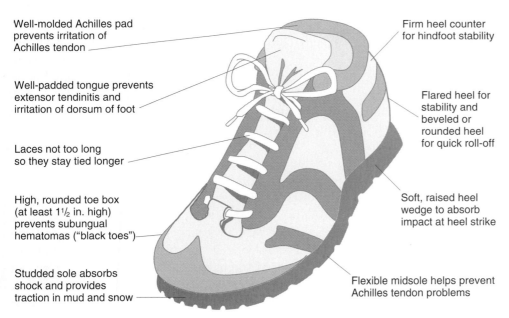

Well-molded Achilles pad prevents irritation of Achilles tendon

Well-padded tongue prevents extensor tendinitis and irritation of dorsum of foot

Laces not too long so they stay tied longer

High, rounded toe box (at least 1½ in. high) prevents subungual hematomas ("black toes")

Studded sole absorbs shock and provides traction in mud and snow

Firm heel counter for hindfoot stability

Flared heel for stability and beveled or rounded heel for quick roll-off

Soft, raised heel wedge to absorb impact at heel strike

Flexible midsole helps prevent Achilles tendon problems

Figure 5-5

What to look for when you buy athletic shoes.

Source: Canadian Podiatric Sports Medicine Academy.

cushioning, support, and stability. You should be able to wiggle your toes easily, but the front of your foot shouldn't slide from side to side, which could cause blisters. Your toes should not touch the end of the shoe because your feet will swell with activity. Allow about half an inch from the longest toe to the tip of the shoe.

- For racquetball shoes, look for reinforcement at the toe for protection during foot drag. The sole should allow minimal slippage. There should be some heel elevation to lessen strain on the back of the leg and Achilles tendon. The shoe should have a long "throat" to ensure greater control by the laces.

- For tennis shoes, look for reinforcement at the toe. The sole at the ball of the foot should be well padded, because that's where most pressure is exerted. The sides of the shoe should be sturdy, for stability during continuous lateral movements. The toe box should allow ample room and some cushioning at the tips. A long throat ensures greater control by the laces.

Don't wear wet shoes for training. Let wet shoes air-dry, because a heater will cause them to stiffen or shrink. Use powder in your shoes to absorb moisture, lessen friction, and prevent fungal infections. Break in new shoes for several days before wearing them for a long-distance run or during competition.

Exercise Equipment

Always try out equipment before buying it. If you decide to purchase a stationary bicycle, for instance, read all the product information. Ask someone in your physical education department or at a local gym for recommendations. Try out a bicycle at the gym. Make sure any equipment you purchase is safe and durable.

Think about your fitness goals. If you're primarily interested in aerobic fitness, try out stationary bicycles, stair-climbing machines, rowing machines, treadmills, and crosscountry skiing machines. Spend five to ten minutes working at moderate intensity. How do your movements on this particular piece of equipment feel to you—awkward or fluid, extremely difficult or surprisingly easy?

If you're considering strength-training equipment, remember that free weights are your least expensive option. The best resistance machines are also the most expensive, with prices soaring over $1000. Would you use one often enough to justify that cost? Or would an annual health-club membership be more cost-effective?

Your exercise style is also an important consideration. Are you going to find sitting at a stationary bicycle for 30 minutes too boring? Are you motivated enough to hoist free weights on your own several times a week? The best home exercise equipment will do you no good unless you use it.

Fitness Facilities

If you decide to join a gym or health club, find out exactly what facilities and programs it offers. The club should be located close to home, campus, or work and should be open at convenient hours. Think about your schedule and when you'll have time to work out. Visit the club at the times you're most likely to use it: during peak hours, you might have to wait half an hour for a turn on the Nautilus machines.

A club should have facilities for a complete workout, including both aerobic and muscle workouts: exercycles, rowing machines, treadmills, stair-climbing machines, stationary bicycles, a running track, aerobics classes, a swimming pool, strength-training equipment, and, if that's what you're looking for, racquetball and squash courts and a large gym for basketball and volleyball.

Find out whether all facilities are available to all members at all times. Some clubs reserve the pool for families only or kids' lessons at certain times. Ask if you can try out the club before joining. Find out what the membership includes. Will you end up paying extra for lockers, towels, classes, and the like? Are student discounts offered? Beware of long-term memberships; many clubs go out of business or change ownership often. Pay attention to cleanliness and to the atmosphere and people. Do the members seem to be significantly older or younger, or in much better or worse shape, than you are? You're more likely to work out regularly in a place, and with people, you like.[32]

Many people find that working with a trained professional—either one-on-one or in a class—provides incentive, prevents injury, and makes exercise more enjoyable. Before signing up, always check out the qualifications of instructors or trainers. Ask to observe some classes. Do they always begin with a warm-up and end with a cool-down? Do instructors move around and give personalized attention? Do they watch for signs of overexertion or jerky, dangerous movements? Do they stress safety principles? Does their approach suit your personality and goals? The answers to these questions will help you find the class that's right for you.

Making This Chapter Work for You
Shaping Up

- A physically fit person has enough energy to meet routine physical demands, with enough reserve energy to cope with unexpected challenges. Fitness itself has three basic components: flexibility, cardiovascular fitness, and muscular strength and endurance.

- The preventive benefits of physical activity include a healthier heart, greater lung capacity, increased metabolism, stronger bones, better mood and mental health, protection against certain forms of cancer, lower weight, and a more active old age.

- Habitual inactivity increases death rates from all causes, especially heart disease. But increasing activity level, even in middle age, can reduce the risk of an early death. Even light exercise can improve physical and emotional well-being, but moderate to rigorous activity produces greater benefits.

- The CDC and the American College of Sports Medicine currently recommend a minimum of 30 minutes a day of moderate physical activity at least five days a week. This can take almost any form—gardening, walking, dancing, housework, playing actively with children—and can help lower the risk of many chronic health problems, including heart disease, high blood pressure, diabetes, osteoporosis, colon cancer, anxiety, and depression.

- To achieve optimal fitness and function at your physiological best, the American College of Sports Medicine recommends a regular program of both aerobic activities for the cardiovascular system and strength-training exercises for the muscles. Aerobic activities should be performed for 20 to 60 minutes three to five times a week; strength workouts, two to three times a week.

- Only vigorous exercise has been proven to extend the lifespan. In a 1995 study, men who burned up 1500 calories in vigorous exercise—the equivalent of walking briskly or jogging for about 15 miles a week—had a 25% lower death rate than those who expended less than 150 calories a week.

- Although they may be aware of exercise's potential benefits, many Americans remain inactive. Among the most common obstacles to exercise are: a lack of time; a lack of affordable, accessible, or safe places to exercise; scheduling difficulties; injury or other physical limitations; bad weather; a dislike of rigorous exertion; and a lack of confidence in individual physical abilities.

- The seeds for a sedentary life may be sown in childhood, and many of today's youngsters are inactive, overweight, and unfit. Adult women are less likely to exercise than men. They may not have the same fitness goals, or they may refrain from exercising because of misconceptions about its safety or effects.

- Different types of exercise produce different benefits. Stretching can improve flexibility. Aerobic exercises, which cause the heart and lungs to work harder and more efficiently, improve cardiovascular fitness. Building up strength and endurance through strength workouts ensures muscular fitness. A complete fitness program should include exercises for flexibility, aerobic fitness, and muscular strength.

- Among the many options for aerobic exercise are brisk walking; race-walking; jogging or running; swimming; indoor and outdoor cycling; crosscountry skiing, skipping rope; aerobic dancing; low-impact aerobics; and various new activities, such as stair-climbing, rollerblading, and step training.

- A weight-training program for muscular fitness should exercise the body's primary muscle groups. One particularly dangerous shortcut to building up muscles is the use of anabolic steroids, which can damage the cardiovascular system, liver, reproductive organs, and mental abilities.

- To get the most of physical activity, you need to eat a balanced diet, use common sense to prevent injuries, protect yourself from heat and cold, and avoid potential risks—such as pollution and overtraining.

Even though fitness products and facilities can make exercise more appealing, getting physical doesn't mean joining a health club, buying designer sportswear, or working out on expensive bodybuilding equipment. All

Health Online

Cool Tools   http://www.e2consult.com/tools.htm

This site will help you with your fitness program by calculating your target heart rate and your energy expenditure during exercise. You can also take the Rockport One Mile Walking Test and calculate your results here. In addition, there are tips for those who would like to start a fitness program but don't know how to begin.

Think about it ...

- How might the information you get from this site help you plan your personal fitness program? How might it help a dedicated athlete?

- This site is maintained by E2 Consulting, a health and fitness software company. Does that information detract from or enhance your impression of the reliability of this site in any way?

you need, other than some good shoes for your feet, is a genuine desire to make the most of your body and a strategy for getting started.

Becoming more active is, above all else, a matter of making a commitment to make more of your body. Here are some guidelines to get you going:

- Add a new sport or physical activity you genuinely enjoy to your schedule.

- Carve out time for this activity. Write "Running" or "Tennis" (or whatever) on your calendar.

- Always try to exercise at the same time of day. For instance, you could jog in the morning before breakfast or in the evening before dinner.

- Get someone to go out with you, if that helps.

- As you aim for optimal fitness, start out slowly and proceed gradually, and be aware that there will be plateaus in your progress. Some days you'll exercise more slowly than others; that's okay. Some days you

may not be able to exercise at all because of illness or bad weather; that, too, is okay. Just keep in mind that when you start exercising regularly again, you should build up slowly to reach your prior fitness level.

- Be sure you don't overwork your body so that it becomes fatigued or injured. If your muscles persistently feel sore and stiff, if you have headaches, continuing fatigue, loss of appetite or weight, or cessation of menstruation; or if you develop emotional symptoms, such as depression or a lack of interest in your sport, you may be exercising too hard.

After a few months of leading a more active life, stop and take stock. Think of how much more energy you have at the end of the day. Ask if you're feeling any less stressed, despite the push and pull of daily pressures. Focus on the unanticipated rewards of exercise. Savor the exhilaration of an autumn morning's walks; the thrill of feeling newly toughened muscles bend to your will; or the satisfaction of a long, smooth stretch after a stressful day. Enjoy the pure pleasure of living in the body you deserve.

Key Terms

The terms listed here are used within the chapter. Page numbers are included for each term.
A definition of each term is given in the green Glossary pages at the end of this book.

acute injuries *140*	**endurance** *120*	**overuse injuries** *140*
aerobic circuit training *138*	**flexibility** *120*	**physical fitness** *120*
aerobic exercise *120*	**isokinetic** *136*	**rep (or repetition)** *137*
anaerobic exercise *120*	**isometric** *136*	**resting heart rate** *130*
cardiovascular fitness *120*	**isotonic** *136*	**sets** *137*
conditioning *121*	**osteoporosis** *122*	**strength** *120*
cross-training *138*	**overloading** *136*	**target heart rate** *130*
endorphins *122*	**overtrain** *141*	

 Review Questions

1. Why should you exercise? What are some of the benefits of exercise?

2. Define physical fitness. What are the three basic components of physical fitness, and how does each contribute to good health?

3. How does exercise help prevent heart disease? cancer? osteoporosis? weight gain?

4. How do you calculate your target heart rate? What kinds of activities should you engage in to reach and maintain that rate?

5. What are anabolic steroids? Why do some individuals use them? What are some of the health risks associated with steroid use?

6. What are some of the elements to consider in designing an exercise program? Design an exercise program for yourself. What are your goals, and how will you stick to them?

Personal Health
5.2
INTERACTIVE

 Critical Thinking Questions

1. Some exercise advocates have called for mandatory physical fitness training in schools and fitness requirements that students would have to meet in order to be promoted or graduate. Do you agree? Should schools focus solely on educating students' brains, or should physical fitness be a significant part of their education as well? Do you feel that your education has provided you with the information you need to stay fit throughout your life? Why or why not?

2. Shelley knows that exercise is good for her health, but figures that she can keep her weight down by dieting and worry about her heart and health when she gets older. "I look good. I feel okay. Why should I bother exercising?" she asks. What would you say in reply?

3. When he started working out, Jeff simply wanted to stay in shape. But he felt so pleased with the way his body looked and responded that he kept doing more. Now he runs ten miles a day (longer on weekends), lifts weights, and works out on Nautilus equipment almost every day, and plays racquetball or squash whenever he gets a chance. Is Jeff getting too much of a good thing? Is there any danger in his fitness program? What would be a more reasonable approach?

Connections to Personal Health Interactive

To enhance your understanding of the material covered in this chapter, check out the following study aids on the **Personal Health Interactive CD-ROM**. *Each numbered icon within the chapter corresponds to an appropriate activity listed here.*

5.1 Personal Insights: How Fit Are You?
5.2 Chapter 5 Review

 # References

1. Pate, Russell, et al. "Physical Activity and Public Health: A Recommendation from the Centers for Disease Control and Prevention and the American College of Sports Medicine." *Journal of the American Medical Association,* Vol. 273, No. 5, February 1, 1995.

2. Centers for Disease Control and Prevention. "Prevalence of Recommended Levels of Physical Activity Among Women." *Morbidity and Mortality Weekly Report*, Vol. 44, No. 6, February 17, 1995.

3. Centers for Disease Control and Prevention.

4. Franklin, Barry, and James Wappes. "Heart Health for a Lifetime." *Physician and Sports Medicine*, Vol. 28, No. 11, November 1997.

5. Martinsen, Egil, and Thoms Stephens. "Exercise and Mental Health in Clinical and Free-Living Populations." *Advances in Exercise Adherence.* Champaign, Ill: Human Kinetics Publishers, 1994. Chollar, Susan. "The Psychological Benefits of Exercise." *American Health*, June 1995. Grabmeier, Jeff. "Exercise to Beat the Blahs." *American Health*, May 1995.

6. Brown, Harriet. "The Other Reward of Exercise; to a Better Mood and Leaner Limbs You Can Add a Lower Cancer Risk." *Health,* Vol. 8, No. 4, July–August 1994.

7. Pinkowish, Mary. "Exercising to Keep Weight Off." *Patient Care*, Vol. 31, No. 19, November 30, 1997.

8. Fries, James, et al. "Older Runners." *Annals of Internal Medicine*, October 1994. Welty, Ellen. "Fitness Through the Ages: Stay in Shape—in Your 20s, 30s, 40s and Beyond." *American Health*, July–August 1994. "Inactivity Increases Chance of Stroke in Older Men." *American Journal of Epidemiology*, Vol. 28, No. 9, November 1994.

9. Blair, Steven, et al. "Changes in Physical Fitness and All-Cause Mortality: A Prospective Study of Healthy and Unhealthy Men." *Journal of the American Medical Association*, Vol. 273, No. 14, April 12, 1995. Paffenbarger, Ralph, et al. "The Association of Changes in Physical-Activity Level and Other Lifestyle Characteristics with Mortality Among Men." *New England Journal of Medicine*, Vol. 328, No. 8, February 25, 1993.

10. Pate, et al., "Physical Activity and Public Health."

11. Blair, Steven, et al. "Physical Fitness and All-Cause Mortality: A Prospective Study of Healthy Men and Women." *Journal of the American Medical Association*, November 3, 1989.

12. Lee, I-Min, et al. "Exercise Intensity and Longevity in Men: The Harvard Alumni Health Study." *Journal of the American Medical Association*, Vol. 273, No. 14, April 19, 1995.

13. Douglas, Kathy, et al. "Results from the 1995 National College Health Risk Behavior Survey." *American Journal of College Health*, Vol. 46, September 1997.

14. "Factors Affecting Women's Motivation for Physical Activity." *Melpomene Journal*, Vol. 16, No. 3, November 1997.

15. Pearman, Silas, et al. "The Impact of a Required College Health and Physical Education Course on the Health Status of Alumni." *American Journal of College Health*, Vol. 46, September 1997.

16. U.S. Public Health Service. "Physical Activity in Children." *American Family Physician*, Vol. 50, No. 6, November 1, 1994. Davis, Kathryn, et al. "North Carolina Children and Youth Fitness Study." *Journal of Physical Education, Recreation & Dance*, Vol. 65, No. 8, October 1994.

17. Michele, Lyle. Personal interview.

18. Douthitt, Vicki. "Psychological Determinants of Adolescent Exercise Adherence." *Adolescence*, Vol. 29, No. 115, Fall 1994.

19. Centers for Disease Control and Prevention. "Prevalence of Recommended Levels of Physical Activity Among Women." *Morbidity and Mortality Weekly Report*, Vol. 44, No. 6, February 17, 1995.

20. Kelley, George, and Kristi Kelley. "Physical Activity Habits of African-American College Students." *Research Quarterly for Exercise and Sport*, Vol. 65, No. 3, September 1994.

21. "Incentives for Exercise in Younger and Older Women." *Journal of Sport Behavior*, Vol. 17, No. 2, June 1994. Cash, Thomas, et al. "Why do Women Exercise?" *Perceptual and Motor Skills*, Vol. 78, No. 2, April 1994.

22. "Women and Exercise Participation: The Mixed Blessings of Motherhood." *Health Care for Women International,* July–August 1994.

23. Kase, Lori Miller. "The Weaker Sex?" *American Health,* December 1994.

24. Shangold, Mona, et al. "Evaluation and Management of Menstrual Dysfunction in Athletes." *Journal of the American Medical Association,* March 23/30, 1990.

25. "To Stretch or not Stretch?" *Tufts University Health and Nutrition Letter,* Vol. 15, No. 18, December 1997.

26. Dolgener, Forrest, et al. "Validation of the Rockport Fitness Walking Test in College Males and Females." *Research Quarterly for Exercise and Sport,* Vol. 65, No. 2, June 1994.

27. "Improving Your Walking Workout." *University of California, Berkeley Wellness Letter,* Vol. 13, No. 3, December 1997. Early, Tracy. "Test Your Walking I.Q." *Current Health,* Vol. 24, No. 3, November 1997.

28. Artunian, Judy. "Burning Body Fat." *Current Health,* Vol. 21, No. 3, November 1994.

29. Durnin, J. "Low Body Mass Index, Physical Work Capacity and Physical Activity Levels." *European Journal of Clinical Nutrition,* Vol. 48, No. 3, November 15, 1994.

30. Stanten, Michele. "Weights or Aerobics: Which Comes First?" *Prevention,* Vol. 49, No. 12, December 1997.

31. Sachtleben, Thomas, et al. "Serum Lipoprotein Patterns in Long-Term Anabolic Steroid Users." *Research Quarterly for Exercise and Sport,* Vol. 68, No. 1, March 1997.

CHAPTER 6

NUTRITION FOR LIFE

After studying the material in this chapter, you should be able to:

List and **define** the basic nutrients necessary for a healthy body.

Describe the Food Guide Pyramid and **explain** its significance for nutrition.

Explain current recommendations for healthy eating, and **use** the nutritional information provided on the new food labels to make healthy choices.

Compare the advantages and disadvantages of various alternative diets and ethnic foods.

Explain the contributions of good nutrition to the prevention of heart disease and cancer.

Explain the importance of food safety to personal health.

Develop a personal plan for nutritional choices that promotes good health.

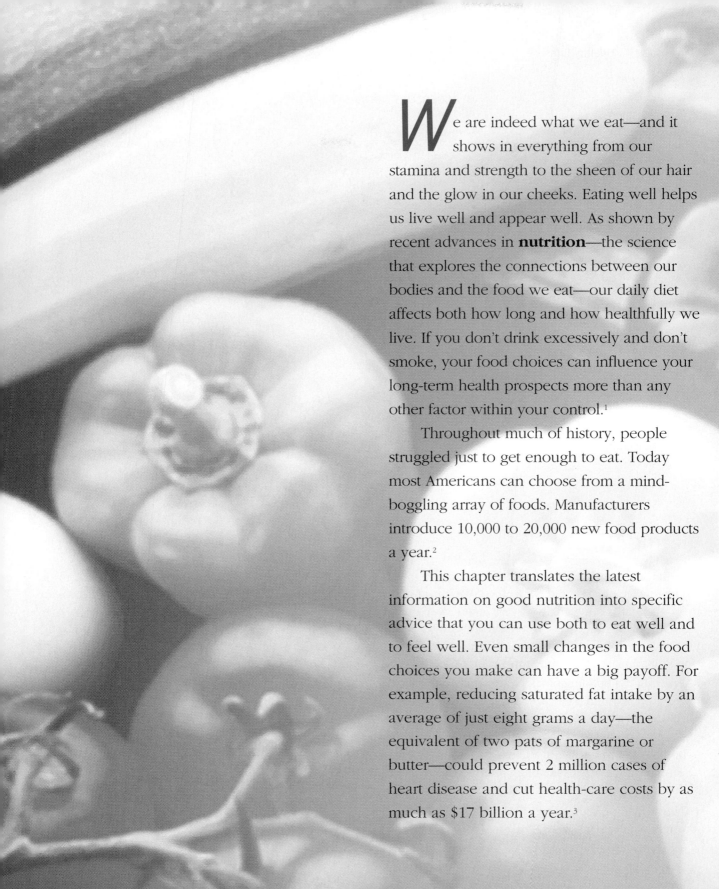

We are indeed what we eat—and it shows in everything from our stamina and strength to the sheen of our hair and the glow in our cheeks. Eating well helps us live well and appear well. As shown by recent advances in **nutrition**—the science that explores the connections between our bodies and the food we eat—our daily diet affects both how long and how healthfully we live. If you don't drink excessively and don't smoke, your food choices can influence your long-term health prospects more than any other factor within your control.[1]

Throughout much of history, people struggled just to get enough to eat. Today most Americans can choose from a mind-boggling array of foods. Manufacturers introduce 10,000 to 20,000 new food products a year.[2]

This chapter translates the latest information on good nutrition into specific advice that you can use both to eat well and to feel well. Even small changes in the food choices you make can have a big payoff. For example, reducing saturated fat intake by an average of just eight grams a day—the equivalent of two pats of margarine or butter—could prevent 2 million cases of heart disease and cut health-care costs by as much as $17 billion a year.[3]

Figure 6-1

Digestive system. The organs of the digestive system break down food into nutrients the body can use.

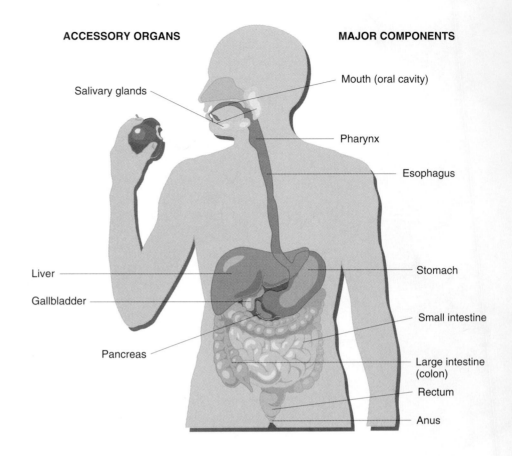

ACCESSORY ORGANS

Salivary glands

Liver

Gallbladder

Pancreas

MAJOR COMPONENTS

Mouth (oral cavity)

Pharynx

Esophagus

Stomach

Small intestine

Large intestine (colon)

Rectum

Anus

Eating Right

We are faced with more choices than our great-great-grandparents could ever have imagined. We must figure out how much of which foods we need every day.

We all need the same essential **nutrients** to form muscles, bones, and other tissues and to provide energy for work and play. These nutrients include:

- *Proteins*, the building blocks of the body needed for growth, maintenance, and replacement of body cells.

- *Carbohydrates*, organic compounds that provide our bodies and brains with glucose—their basic fuel. Simple carbohydrates are often referred to as sugars; complex carbohydrates as starches.

- *Fats*, which provide energy and serve as carriers for certain vitamins.

- *Vitamins*, organic substances needed in very small amounts by the body to perform a variety of functions.

- *Minerals*, naturally occurring inorganic substances that are needed in small amounts for certain essential functions in the body.

- *Water*, the often-forgotten but essential substance

that helps in digestion, elimination, and maintenance of bodily fluids and temperature.

Nutrients reach our body's structures through the process of digestion (see Figure 6-1). Each of the organs of the digestive system contributes to the process by either mechanically or chemically breaking down foods into small molecules capable of being absorbed into body cells.

Nutritionists have conducted thousands of studies to determine the types and amounts of nutrients that individuals of different ages, genders, sizes, and levels of activity need in order to feel and perform at their best. Epidemiological studies assess the dietary habits and health status of a particular population, while metabolic studies examine the effects of different nutrients in animal or human metabolism.

Strategies for Change

....
Dietary Guidelines

Based on nutritional research, the United States Department of Agriculture (USDA) has compiled the RDA (Recommended Daily Allowances) tables. The USDA has also developed the following guidelines for all Americans older than age 2 to help ensure lifelong optimal health and lower the risk of chronic diseases:

✔ *Eat a variety of foods.* Choosing among different types of foods every day helps ensure that you get the protein, vitamins, and minerals you need.

✔ *Maintain a healthy weight.* Excess pounds can increase your risk of high blood pressure, heart disease, stroke, certain cancers, and the most common kind of diabetes. (See Chapter 7 for more on weight management.)

✔ *Choose a diet low in fat, saturated fat, and cholesterol.* Fat contains more than twice the calories of an equal amount of protein or carbohydrates, and increases your risk of heart disease and certain types of cancer.

✔ *Choose a diet with plenty of vegetables, fruits, and grain products.* These foods provide vitamins, minerals, fiber, and complex carbohydrates.

✔ *Use sugars only in moderation.* Sugars, or simple carbohydrates, provide few nutrients for their calories and can contribute to tooth decay. (Simple and complex carbohydrates are discussed later in this chapter.)

✔ *Use salt and sodium only in moderation.* Excessive sodium intake, as discussed in Chapter 12 on cardio

vascular illness, may increase your risk of high blood pressure. The Food and Drug Administration recommends that all adults restrict sodium to no more than 2400 milligrams a day.

✔ *If you drink alcoholic beverages, do so only in moderation.* Alcohol, which has a very low *nutrient density* (nutritional value compared to calories), can lead to dependence and other health problems. (See Chapter 15 for a thorough discussion of alcohol consumption.)

The Food Guide Pyramid

The USDA's Food Guide Pyramid (see Figure 6-2), adopted in 1992, replaced the traditional Basic Four Food Groups—meats, milk products, fruits and vegetables, breads and cereals—with five categories. These categories are not considered nutritional equals. For the sake of good health, you need some food from all the groups every day, but in different amounts.

"The idea of the pyramid is to get people to eat more of the foods at its base (grains, fruits, and vegeta-

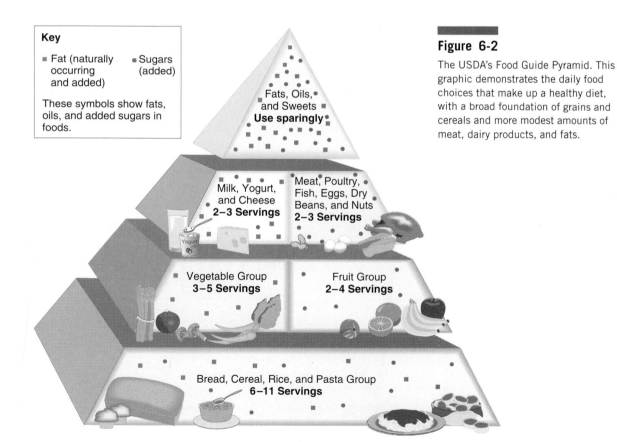

Key

■ Fat (naturally occurring and added)   ● Sugars (added)

These symbols show fats, oils, and added sugars in foods.

Fats, Oils, and Sweets
Use sparingly

Milk, Yogurt, and Cheese
2–3 Servings

Meat, Poultry, Fish, Eggs, Dry Beans, and Nuts
2–3 Servings

Vegetable Group
3–5 Servings

Fruit Group
2–4 Servings

Bread, Cereal, Rice, and Pasta Group
6–11 Servings

Figure 6-2

The USDA's Food Guide Pyramid. This graphic demonstrates the daily food choices that make up a healthy diet, with a broad foundation of grains and cereals and more modest amounts of meat, dairy products, and fats.

bles) and fewer of those toward the top (meat, milk products, sugars, and fats)," says Ann Shaw, Ph.D., a nutritionist with the federal Agriculture Research Service.[4] Foods in one group cannot substitute for those in another. Although the new guide doesn't ban any foods from plates or palates, the pyramid clearly advises less of some favorites, including meat. "Your maximum daily protein intake should be 5 to 7 ounces, with no more than half of that coming from red meat," says Shaw. "We're trying to get people to eat fewer servings of meat and to eat smaller ones—the size of a deck of cards, not half the dinner plate."

The foods that should take center stage at meal time are grain products. "They've been staples of the American diet for years," Shaw notes, "But we used to view them as fillers that we ate to satisfy our appetites and fill us up. Now we recognize their value as a source of nutrients, fiber, and energy." College students generally do not eat well-balanced diets. According to the National College Health Risk Behavior Survey, only 25% of undergraduate women and 28% of undergraduate men eat five or more servings of fruit or vegetables every day. Yet 84.9% of the women and 69.6% of the men have two or more servings of high-fat foods.[5] (See Campus Focus: "Nutrition on Campus.")

Although following the pyramid may seem complicated at first, it doesn't have to be. Simple changes in what you eat can transform a lopsided eating plan into a well-balanced one. (See Self-Survey: "Rate Your Diet.")

Breads, Cereals, Rice, and Pasta (6–11 servings a day)

These foods are the foundation of a healthy diet because they are a good source of complex **carbohydrates**. Both **simple** and **complex carbohydrates** (starches) have 4 calories per gram. Sugars provide little more than a quick spurt of energy, whereas complex carbohydrates are rich in vitamins, minerals, and other nutrients. Less than 25% of the daily calories in a typical American diet comes from complex carbohydrates; ideally, they should account for 50% to 60%.

A typical serving in this category might be one slice

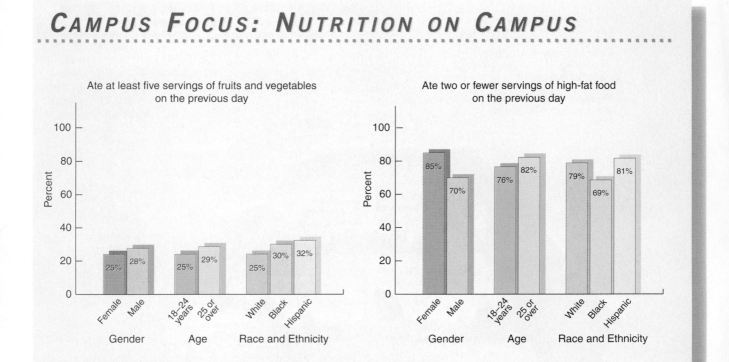

CAMPUS FOCUS: NUTRITION ON CAMPUS

SOURCE: Douglas, Kathy, et al. "Results from the 1995 National College Health Risk Behavior Survey." *American Journal of College Health*, Vol. 46, September 1997

Self-Survey

Rate Your Diet

Step 1

For a week write down everything you eat and drink for meals and snacks. Include the approximate amount eaten (i.e., ½ cup, 1 large, 12 oz. can, etc.).

	Mon	**Tues**	**Wed**	**Thurs**	**Fri**	**Sat**	**Sun**
Grains							
Vegetables							
Fruits							
Milk, yogurt, cheese							
Meat, poultry, dry beans, eggs, nuts							
Fats, oil, sweets, cheese							

Step 2: Are You Getting Enough Vegetables, Fruits, and Grains?

How often do you eat:	Seldom/never	1–2 times a week	3–5 times a week	Almost daily
At least 3 servings of vegetables a day?				
Starchy vegetables like potatoes, corn, or peas?				
Foods made with dry beans, lentils, or peas?				
Dark green or deep yellow vegetables (broccoli, spinach, collards, carrots, sweet potatoes, squash)?				
At least two servings of fruit a day?				
Citrus fruits and 100% fruit juices (oranges, grapefruit, tangerines)?				
Whole fruit with skin or seeds (berries, apples, pears)?				
At least six servings of breads, cereals, pasta, or rice a day?				

The best answer for each of the above is "almost daily." Use your food diary to see which foods you should be eating more often.

Step 3: Are You Getting Too Much Fat?

How often do you eat:	Seldom/never	1–2 times a week	3–5 times a week	Almost daily
Fried, deep-fat fried, or breaded food?				
Fatty meats, such as sausages, luncheon meat, fatty steaks or roasts?				
Whole milk, high-fat cheeses, ice cream?				
Pies, pastries, rich cakes?				
Rich cream sauces and gravies?				
Oily salad dressings or mayonnaise?				

Butter or margarine on vegetables,
rolls, bread, or toast? _____

Ideally, you should be eating these foods no more than one or two times a week. If your
food diary indicates that you're eating them more frequently, your fat intake may well be too high.

Step 4: Are You Getting Too Much Sodium?

How often do you eat:	Seldom/never	1–2 times a week	3–5 times a week	Almost daily
Cured or processed meats, such as ham, sausage, frankfurters, or luncheon meats?				
Canned vegetables or frozen vegetables with sauce?				
Frozen TV dinners, entrees, or canned or dehydrated soups?				
Salted nuts, popcorn, pretzels, corn chips, or potato chips?				
Seasoning mixes or sauces containing salt?				
Processed cheese?				
Salt added to table foods before you taste them?				

Ideally, you should be eating these high-sodium items no more than one or two times a week.
If your food diary indicates that you're eating them more frequently, your sodium intake may
well be too high.

Making Changes ....
How to Improve Your Diet

- Follow the Food Guide Pyramid in planning your daily meals.

- Read food nutritional labels carefully. Always check fat and sodium content.

- Rethink your meal choices. Have cereal or whole-grain toast instead of eggs for breakfast, salad in place of a burger for lunch, rice or pasta dishes rather than meats as a main course for dinner.

- Include a green or orange food at both lunch and dinner. Add extra vegetables to every recipe that calls for them.

- Serve fresh fruit or vegetable salsas instead of sauces for meat, poultry or fish.

- Peel and slice fruit at home and take it along to work in a plastic bag for a snack.

- Rather than sipping a soda at your desk or drinking gatorade after working out, choose water or 100% fruit juice instead.

- Use herbs and spices as seasonings for vegetables and meats instead of salt.

SOURCE: Adapted from materials prepared by the USDA Human Nutrition Information Service.

of bread, and one ounce of ready-to-eat cereal (or one-half cup of cooked cereal, rice, or pasta). Although many people think of these foods as fattening, it's actually what you put on them, such as butter on a roll or cream sauce on pasta, that adds extra calories.

Here are suggestions for getting more grains in your diet:

- Add brown rice or barley to soups.

- Check labels of rolls and bread, and choose those with at least 2 to 3 grams of fiber per slice. Grain products made with white or refined wheat flour have had most of their fiber-rich bran mechanically removed. However, if fiber has been added, some white breads may actually have more fiber than multigrain breads.

- Go for pasta power. Pasta has 210 calories per

cooked cup and only 9 calories from fat. Like whole-grain breads, whole-grain pastas may provide more nutrients than those made with refined flour.

Vegetables (3–5 servings a day)

Naturally low in fat and high in fiber, vegetables provide crucial vitamins (such as A and C) and minerals (such as iron and magnesium). As discussed later in this chapter and in Chapter 13, numerous studies linking diet to cancer have found "extraordinarily consistent scientific evidence" supporting the protective role of certain vegetables as well as fruits in preventing cancers of the lung, stomach, colon, bladder, pancreas, esophagus, mouth, larynx, cervix, ovary, endometrium, and breast. These benefits are so great that some have dubbed the switch to more produce as a "nutrition revolution."[6]

A serving in this category consists of one cup of raw leafy vegetables, one-half cup of other vegetables (either cooked or raw), three-quarters cup of vegetable juice, or one potato or ear of corn. Since different types of vegetables provide different nutrients, it's best to eat a variety. Dark green vegetables are especially good sources of vitamins and minerals; certain greens (such as collards, kale, turnip, and mustard) provide calcium and

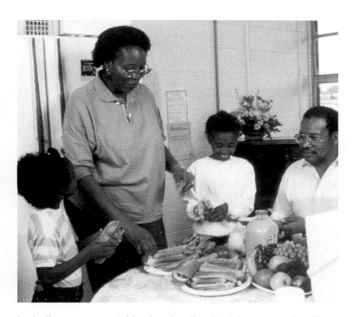

Including more vegetables in your diet doesn't mean eating like a rabbit—order the vegetable pizza instead of the pepperoni next time, and add extra vegetables to your sandwiches and soups.

iron. Winter squash, carrots, and the plant family that includes broccoli, cabbage, kohlrabi, and cauliflower (the **crucifers**) are high in fiber, rich in vitamins, and excellent sources of **indoles**, chemicals that help lower cancer risk.

Here are ways to increase your vegetable intake:

- Make or order sandwiches with extra tomatoes or other vegetable toppings.
- Add extra vegetables whenever you're preparing soups, sauces, and so on.
- If you can't find fresh vegetables, use frozen. They contain less salt than canned veggies.
- Use raw vegetables for dipping, instead of chips.

Fruit (2-4 servings a day)

Like whole grains and vegetables, fruits are excellent sources of vitamins, minerals, and fiber. Along with vegetables, fruits may protect against cancer; those who eat little produce have a cancer rate twice that of people who eat the most fruits and vegetables.[7] A serving consists of a medium apple, banana, or orange; a half-cup of chopped, cooked or canned fruit; or three-quarters of a cup of fruit juice.

Try the following suggestions to get more fruit into your daily diet:

- Carry a banana, apple, or package of dried fruit with you as a healthy snack.
- Eat fruit for dessert or a snack. Try poached pears, baked apples, or fresh berries.
- Start the day with a daily double: a glass of juice and a banana or other fruit on cereal.
- Add citrus fruits (such as slices of grapefruit, oranges, or apples) to green salads, rice, grains, and chicken, pork, or fish dishes.
- Squeeze fresh lemon or lime juice over seafood, fruit salads, or vegetable dishes.

Meat, Poultry, Fish, Dry Beans, Eggs, and Nuts (2–3 servings a day)

These foods are excellent sources of **protein**, which forms the basic framework for our muscles, bones, blood, hair, and fingernails and is essential for growth and repair. In addition, meat, poultry, fish, dry beans, eggs, and nuts supply phosphorus, iron, zinc, vitamin B-6, niacin, and other vitamins and minerals.

A serving in this category consists of 2 or 3 ounces of lean, cooked meat, fish, or poultry (roughly the size of an average hamburger or the amount of meat on half a medium chicken breast). An egg or one-half cup of cooked dry beans can substitute for 1 ounce of lean meat. Thus, one day's total protein intake might include an egg at breakfast, a serving of beans or 2 ounces of sliced chicken in a sandwich at lunch, and 3 ounces of fish for dinner.

To pick the best protein, try these recommendations:

- Choose the leanest meats, such as beef round or sirloin, pork tenderloin, or veal. Broil or roast instead of fry. Trim fat before cooking, which can lower the fat content of the meat you eat by more than 10%. Marinate low-fat cuts to increase tenderness.
- Cook stews, boiled meat, or soup stock ahead of time; refrigerate; and remove the hardened fat before using. Drain fat from ground beef after cooking.
- Watch out for processed chicken and turkey products; for example, bolognas and salamis made from turkey can contain 45% to 90% fat.
- Select small chickens when you shop: They're leaner than large ones. Broiler-fryers are lowest in fat, followed by roasters. Remove skin before eating poultry.
- Choose fish as a leaner alternative to meat. It's high in protein, and packed with vitamins and minerals. Fatty acids help lower the risk of cardiovascular disease.[8]
- Substitute bean-based dishes, such as chili or lentil stew, for meat entrees.

Milk, Yogurt, and Cheese (2–3 servings a day)

Most milk products are high in calcium, riboflavin, protein, and vitamins A and B-12. The Food Guide Pyramid recommends two servings of milk, yogurt, or cheese for most adults and three for women who are pregnant or breast-feeding. In addition, teenagers and young adults up to age 24 should also get three servings of milk products a day. Dairy products, such as milk and yogurt, are the best calcium sources, but be sure you choose products that are lowfat, or preferably nonfat. A serving in

this category consists of an 8-ounce cup of milk, one cup of plain yogurt, 1½ ounces of hard cheese, or one tablespoon of cheese spread. An 8-ounce glass of non-fat milk is a more nutritious choice than a tablespoon of a high-fat cheese spread.

To make sure you get more milk with less fat, try the following:
- Gradually switch from whole milk to 2%-fat (reduced fat) milk, then to 1%-fat (low-fat) milk, then to nonfat (skim) milk.
- Substitute fat-free sour cream or nonfat plain yogurt for sour cream.
- Use part-skim or low-fat cheeses whenever possible.
- Note that cottage cheese is lower in calcium than most cheeses. Thus, one cup of cottage cheese counts as only one-half serving of milk.

Fats, Oils, and Sweets

The Food Guide Pyramid places fats, oils, and sweets at the very top so that Americans will realize they should use them only in very small amounts. These foods supply calories but little or no vitamins or minerals.

Added sugars include sweeteners used in processing or at the table (such as jams, jellies, syrups, corn sweetener, molasses, fruit-juice concentrate, and the sugar in candy, cake, and cookies). These foods often are hidden in favorites—such as soft drinks (9 teaspoons of sugar per can), low-fat fruit yogurt (7 teaspoons per cup), fruit pie (6 teaspoons per serving), and catsup (a teaspoon in every tablespoon).

Try the following:
- Avoid temptation by not keeping a stash of cookies or candies.
- Put a small, child-sized spoon in the sugar bowl.
- When you crave a sweet, reach for nature's candy: fruit.
- If you want a daily sweet, have it as dessert, when you'll eat less of it, rather than as a snack.
- Drink fruit juices and water instead of sugar-laden soft drinks.

Water

The Food Guide Pyramid doesn't include water, but that doesn't mean it isn't important. Water makes up 85% of the blood, 70% of the muscles, and about 75% of the brain.[9] It carries nutrients, maintains temperature, lubricates joints, helps with digestion of food, and helps rid your body of waste through urine. Although we can live for several weeks without food, we would die after a few days without water. A loss of 5% of the body's water causes dizziness, fatigue, headache, and weakness; a 15% to 20% loss can be fatal. Water is an important element in the production of sweat, which evaporates from the skin to cool the body.

You lose about 64 to 80 ounces of water a day—the equivalent of eight to ten 8-ounce glasses—through urine, perspiration, bowel movements, and normal exhalation.[10] You lose water more rapidly if you're ill, live in a dry climate, are at a high altitude, drink a lot of coffee or alcohol (which increase urination), skip a meal, exercise, or travel on an airplane. Drink water before and during exercise to prevent dehydration. A general guideline is to drink one or two 8-ounce glasses of water 30 minutes to an hour before exercising and half to three-quarters of a glass of water every 10 to 20 minutes during a workout.

To keep up your water supply, try these tips:

- Don't substitute soft drinks, coffee, tea, or alcoholic beverages for water.
- Take regular water breaks to prevent mild dehydration. Keep a water bottle or pitcher nearby whenever possible.
- Respond quickly to thirst, which is a good but not

foolproof indicator of dehydration. If you're ill, exercising, or at a high altitude, you need more fluid than usual, even if you don't feel thirsty.

- Check your urine. Dark yellow urine means your kidneys had to concentrate waste material into a smaller volume of water, while pale urine is a sign of good hydration.

The Payoffs of the Pyramid

The benefits of following the Food Guide Pyramid are many. By heeding its recommendations for eating a nutritious variety of foods, you'll be able to lower fat, increase fiber, get more vitamins and minerals, and possibly protect yourself from many illnesses.

Less Fat

Fats are a concentrated form of energy, providing 9 calories per gram—more than twice the amount in carbohydrates or proteins. A high-fat diet can lead to obesity and increase the risk of heart disease, certain cancers, and other health problems. (See Pulsepoints: "Top Ten Ways to Cut Fat.")

Pulsepoints

Top Ten Ways to Cut Fat

1. Eat less meat. Rather than making meat the heart of a meal, think of it as a flavoring ingredient.

2. Forget frying. Instead, steam, boil, bake, or microwave vegetables or meats.

3. Switch to reduced-fat and nonfat dairy products. Rather than buying whole-fat dairy products, choose skim milk, fat-free sour cream, and low- or nonfat yogurts.

4. Season with herbs and spices. Avoid using fatty sauce, butter, or margarine over your vegetables, pastas, or other dishes.

5. Avoid high-fat fast foods. Hot dogs, fried foods, packaged snack foods, and pastries are most likely to be high in fat.

6. Say no to ice cream. As a tasty treat, try frozen ices and nonfat frozen yogurt instead.

7. Read labels carefully. Remember that "cholesterol-free" doesn't necessarily mean fat-free. Avoid products that contain highly saturated coconut oil, palm oil, or lard.

8. Check the numbers. When buying prepared foods, choose items that con-

tain no more than 3 grams of fat per 100 calories.

9. Remove all visible fat. When you do serve meat, make sure to choose lean cuts and trim fat before and/or after cooking.

10. Think small. Remember that a dinner-size serving of meat should be about the size of a deck of cards or the palm of your hand. As you cut back on meat portions, serve larger amounts of fresh fruits and vegetables, grains, and beans.

Forms of Fat

Fat can be saturated or unsaturated. **Saturated fats**, found mainly in meat, lard, butter, and "tropical" vegetable oils (such as coconut and palm), are most dangerous because they can increase the risk of heart disease and certain cancers, including those of the colon and breast. **Unsaturated fats**, which are usually liquid at room temperature, include polyunsaturates, such as those in oils derived from corn, soybeans, sunflowers, sesame, and cotton plants, and monounsaturates, such as those in olive and canola oils. Monounsaturated fats may be most healthful because they lower the levels of harmful forms of cholesterol (see next section). Polyunsaturates in liquid oils can do the same, although they may also reduce beneficial cholesterol forms.

A 1998 report on more than 60,000 women in Sweden found that those who ate diets high in monounsaturated fats had a significantly reduced risk of breast cancer, while those whose daily diets included polyunsaturated fats had a strongly increased breast cancer risk. These results were similar to those of previous studies that had documented the benefits of olive oil, but this study showed a more clear-cut link between polyunsaturated fats and breast cancer than earlier research.[11]

Although Americans have long been advised to curtail dietary fat, particularly saturated fat, a 1997 report suggested that the type of fat—not the quantity eaten—may have a greater impact on heart health. Based on data from 80,000 nurses followed for 14 years, researchers concluded that most dangerous of all may be so-called **trans fats**, formed when liquid vegetable oils are processed to make hard or semisoft table spreads and cooking fats. Trans fats also are found in beef and dairy foods.[12]

In both animals and humans, trans fats may interfere with the metabolism of polyunsaturated fatty acids, which prevent the buildup of plaque in the arteries. They also reduce protective high-density lipoproteins (the "good" cholesterol discussed in Chapter 12 on heart disease) and increase levels of triglycerides, another potentially harmful form of fat. Some researchers believe that, on a gram-for-gram basis, trans fats are riskier than saturated fats.[13]

When you do use them, which fats should you choose? Olive oil, which is high in monounsaturated fats, is one of the best vegetable oil for salads and cooking. It has been used for thousands of years in countries around the Mediterranean, which have relatively low levels of heart disease. Canola oil is lowest in saturated fat and can be used for baking, stir-frying, and salad dressings.

In 1998, products made of Olean (also known by its generic name, olestra), the first calorie-free fat replacement ingredient that can be used to fry foods, entered the national marketplace. Because the ingredients of Olean are processed in a special way, the body doesn't break them down and so Olean doesn't add fat or calories to foods. On the basis of more than 150 research studies, the FDA approved Olean for use in savory snacks, such as chips and crackers, and many medical organizations, including the American Dietetic Association, have supported its use as one way to reduce fat and calories in the diet. However, some participants in early tests have reported gastrointestinal side effects, and consumer advocacy groups, such as the Center for Science in the Public Interest, have warned that fat replacement products may pose potential risks that could outweigh their benefits.[14]

The Cholesterol Connection

Dietary fats can increase blood levels of **cholesterol**, a lipid (fat) known mainly for its role in the development of heart disease (discussed in Chapter 12). In the body, cholesterol is essential for the production of many hormones, the formation of the outer membranes protecting our body cells, and the functioning of the liver. However, when blood cholesterol levels become too high, the excess cholesterol can build up within the arteries (a condition called *atherosclerosis*). Foods high in saturated fat raise blood cholesterol levels more than any other foods, even those high in cholesterol.[15] Cutting back on fats, a strategy that has been proven healthful for adults, also is a safe and beneficial means of lowering high cholesterol levels in children over the age of 2.[16] (See Table 6-1.)

More Fiber

The increased servings of grains, fruits, and vegetables called for in the Food Guide Pyramid provide an added benefit: more of the indigestible leaves, stems, skins, seeds, and hulls of grains and plants containing dietary **fiber**. *Insoluble fibers*—cellulose, lignin, and some hemicellulose—increase bulk in feces, prevent constipation and diverticulosis (a painful inflammation of the bowel), and may lower the risk of colon cancer, heart disease, and stroke.[17] Whole grains also may help prevent chronic diseases, such as diabetes.[18] Good sources of insoluble fiber are wheat and corn bran (the outer layer), leafy greens, and the skins of fruits and root vegetables. *Soluble fibers*—pectin, gums, and some hemi-

TABLE 6-1 PERCENTAGE OF FAT CALORIES IN FOODS

Type of food	Less Than 15% of Calories from Fat	15%–30% of Calories from Fat	30%–50% of Calories from Fat	More Than 50% of Calories from Fat
Fruits and Vegetables	Fruits, plain vegetables, juices, pickles, sauerkraut		French fries, hash browns	Avocados, coconuts, olives
Bread and Cereals	Grains and flours, most breads, most cereals, corn tortillas, pita, matzoh, bagels, noodles and pasta	Corn bread, flour tortillas, oatmeal, soft rolls and buns, wheat germ	Breakfast bars, biscuits and muffins, granola, pancakes and waffles, donuts, taco shells, pastries, croissants	
Dairy Products	Nonfat milk, dry curd cottage cheese, nonfat cottage cheese, nonfat yogurt	Buttermilk, low-fat yogurt, 1% milk, low-fat cottage cheese,	Whole milk, 2% milk, creamed cottage cheese	Butter, cream, sour cream, half & half, most cheeses, (including part-skim and lite cheeses)
Meats		Beef round; veal loin, round, and shoulder; pork tenderloin	Beef and veal, lamb, fresh and picnic hams	All ground beef, spareribs, cold cuts, beef, hot dogs, pastrami
Poultry	Egg whites	Chicken and turkey (light meat without skin)	Chicken and turkey (light meat with skin, dark meat without skin), duck and goose (without skin)	Chicken/turkey (dark meat with skin), chicken/turkey hot dogs and bologna, egg yolks, whole eggs
Seafood	Clams, cod, crab, crawfish, flounder, haddock, lobster, perch, sole, scallops, shrimp, tuna (in water)	Bass and sea bass, halibut, mussels, oyster, tuna (fresh)	Anchovies, catfish, salmon, sturgeon, trout, tuna (in oil, drained)	Herring, mackerel, sardines
Beans and Nuts	Dried beans and peas, chestnuts, water chestnuts		Soybeans	Tofu, most nuts and seeds, peanut butter
Fats and Oils	Oil-free and some lite salad dressings			Butter, margarine, all mayonnaise (including reduced-calorie), most salad dressings, all oils
Soups	Bouillons, broths, consomme	Most soups	Cream soups, bean soups, "just add water" noodle soups	Cheddar cheese soup, New England clam chowder
Desserts	Angel food cake, gelatin, some new fat-free cakes	Pudding, tapioca	Most cakes, most pies	
Frozen Desserts	Sherbert, low-fat frozen yogurt, sorbet, fruit ices	Ice milk	Frozen yogurt	All ice cream
Snack foods	Popcorn (air popped), pretzels, rye crackers, rice cakes, fig bars, raisin biscuit cookies, marshmallows, most hard candy, fruit rolls	Lite microwave popcorn, Scandinavian "crisps," plain crackers, caramels, fudge, gingersnaps, graham crackers	Snack crackers, popcorn (popped in oil), cookies, candy bars, granola bars	Most microwave popcorn, corn and potato chips, chocolate, buttery crackers

SOURCE: American Heart Association/USDA.

cellulose—lower blood cholesterol and may help control blood sugar levels.[19] Good sources of soluble fiber are oats, beans, barley, and the pulp of many fruits and vegetables, such as apples and citrus fruits. Foods rich in fiber also have higher levels of many other beneficial components, such as vitamins that may protect against cancer and heart disease.

Despite the benefits of fiber, few Americans eat enough. The National Cancer Institute recommends that a person consume 20 to 35 grams a day, but the average intake is about 11 to 13 grams. More servings of fruit and vegetables could make a big difference in fiber intake. One apple or half a grapefruit can add 2 grams of fiber to your diet. (See Table 6-2 for good fiber sources.)

If you have not been eating a high-fiber diet, increase grains, fruits, and vegetables gradually. A sudden increase in fiber intake can result in intestinal gas, bloating, cramps, and diarrhea—the consequences of fermentation of fiber and sugars in the colon. Try to spread out your fiber intake throughout the day and increase total consumption gradually to avoid these effects. An extremely high-fiber diet may block absorption of some minerals, such as zinc, iron, and calcium, but most nutritionists feel that high-fiber foods are rich enough in nutrients to compensate for any such losses. Individuals taking fiber pills or powders, which contain no nutrients, are more likely to suffer mineral deficiencies.

Knowing What You Eat

For years, many manufacturers advertised products as "nutritious," "healthy," or otherwise good for you, but offered little or no proof to back up such claims. Today, thanks to the Nutrition Labeling and Education Act, enacted in 1994, food manufacturers must provide information about fat, calories, and ingredients in large type on packaged food labels that must show how a food item fits into a daily diet of 2000 calories. The law also restricts nutritional claims for terms such as *healthy*, *low fat*, or *high fiber.*[20]

In evaluating food labels and claims, keep in mind that, while individual foods vary in their nutritional value, what matters is your total diet. If you eat too much of any one food—regardless of what its label states—you may not be getting the variety and balance of nutrients that you need.

TABLE 6-2 SOURCES OF DIETARY FIBER

Amount of Total Fiber	Good Sources of Insoluble Fiber	Good Sources of Soluble Fiber
More than 5 grams	High-fiber wheat-bran cereal (1 oz)	Pinto, kidney, navy beans(dried, cooked, 1/2 cup)
2–5 grams	Lentils (dried, cooked, 1/2 cup)	Oat bran, oatmeal (dry, 1 oz)
	Whole wheat crackers (6)	Barley (dry, 1 oz)
	Banana (medium)	Berries (1/2 cup)
	Potato (medium, with skin)	Apple, pear (medium, with skin)
	Buckwheat groats (dry, 1 oz)	Orange, grapefruit (medium)
	Shredded-wheat cereal (1 oz)	Figs, prunes (dried, 3)
	Brown rice (cooked, 1/2 cup)	Okra, cabbage, peas, turnips,
	Brussels sprouts, broccoli,	sweet potato (cooked, 1/2 cup)
	spinach (cooked, 1/2 cup)	Chick-peas, split peas, lima
	Wheat germ (3 Tbsp)	beans (cooked, 1/2 cup)
	Whole wheat flour (1 oz)	Carrots (cooked, 1/2 cup)
1–2 grams	Whole wheat bread (1 slice)	Peach, nectarine (medium)
	Pasta (cooked, 1 cup)	Apricots (2)
	Rye bread (1 slice)	
	Corn (1/2 cup)	
	Low-fiber wheat cereal (1 oz)	
	Cauliflower (cooked, 1/2 cup)	

SOURCE: Wellness Letter, April 1992.

Figuring Out Food Labels

As Figure 6-3 shows, the "Nutrition Facts" on food labels present a wealth of information—if you know what to look for. The label focuses on those nutrients most clearly associated with disease risk and health: total fat, saturated fat, cholesterol, sodium, total carbohydrate, dietary fiber, sugar, and protein.

- *Calories.* Calories are the measure of the amount of energy that can be derived from food. Science defines a **calorie** as the amount of energy required to raise the temperature of one gram of water by one degree Celsius. In the laboratory, the caloric

content of food is measured in 1000-calorie units called *kilocalories*. The "calorie" referred to in everyday usage is actually the equivalent of the laboratory kilocalorie.

The label lists two numbers for calories: calories per serving and calories from fat per serving. This allows consumers to calculate how many calories they'll consume and to determine the percentage of fat in an item.

- *Serving size.* Rather than the tiny portions manufacturers sometimes used in the past to keep down the number of calories per serving, the new labels reflect more realistic portions. Serving sizes, which have been defined for approximately 150 food cate-

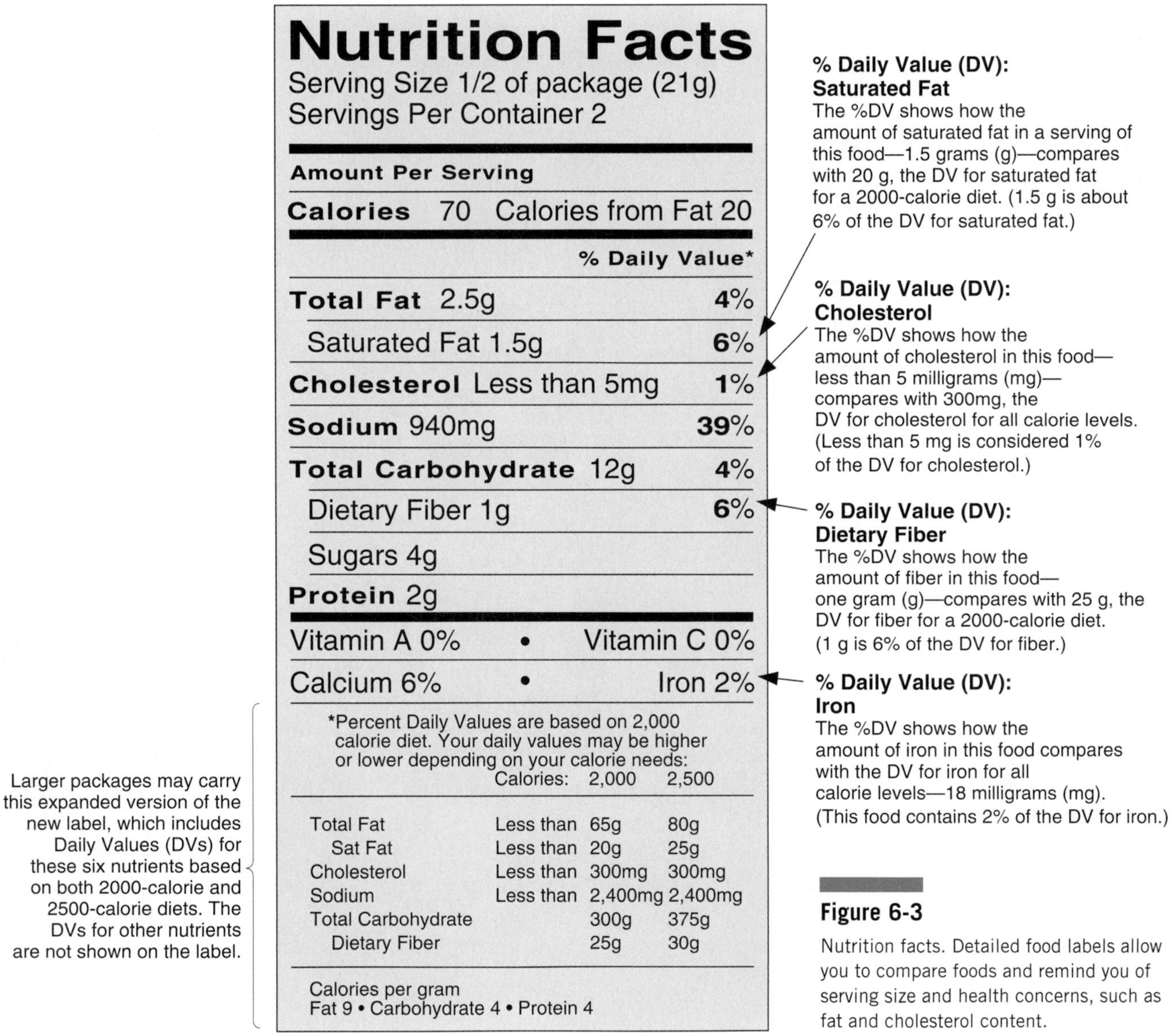

Larger packages may carry this expanded version of the new label, which includes Daily Values (DVs) for these six nutrients based on both 2000-calorie and 2500-calorie diets. The DVs for other nutrients are not shown on the label.

Nutrition Facts
Serving Size 1/2 of package (21g)
Servings Per Container 2

Amount Per Serving

Calories 70   Calories from Fat 20

% Daily Value*

Total Fat 2.5g	**4%**
Saturated Fat 1.5g	**6%**
Cholesterol Less than 5mg	**1%**
Sodium 940mg	**39%**
Total Carbohydrate 12g	**4%**
Dietary Fiber 1g	**6%**
Sugars 4g	
Protein 2g	

Vitamin A 0%	•	Vitamin C 0%
Calcium 6%	•	Iron 2%

*Percent Daily Values are based on 2,000 calorie diet. Your daily values may be higher or lower depending on your calorie needs:

		Calories:	2,000	2,500
Total Fat	Less than		65g	80g
Sat Fat	Less than		20g	25g
Cholesterol	Less than		300mg	300mg
Sodium	Less than		2,400mg	2,400mg
Total Carbohydrate			300g	375g
Dietary Fiber			25g	30g

Calories per gram
Fat 9 • Carbohydrate 4 • Protein 4

**% Daily Value (DV):
Saturated Fat**
The %DV shows how the amount of saturated fat in a serving of this food—1.5 grams (g)—compares with 20 g, the DV for saturated fat for a 2000-calorie diet. (1.5 g is about 6% of the DV for saturated fat.)

**% Daily Value (DV):
Cholesterol**
The %DV shows how the amount of cholesterol in this food— less than 5 milligrams (mg)— compares with 300mg, the DV for cholesterol for all calorie levels. (Less than 5 mg is considered 1% of the DV for cholesterol.)

**% Daily Value (DV):
Dietary Fiber**
The %DV shows how the amount of fiber in this food— one gram (g)—compares with 25 g, the DV for fiber for a 2000-calorie diet. (1 g is 6% of the DV for fiber.)

**% Daily Value (DV):
Iron**
The %DV shows how the amount of iron in this food compares with the DV for iron for all calorie levels—18 milligrams (mg). (This food contains 2% of the DV for iron.)

Figure 6-3

Nutrition facts. Detailed food labels allow you to compare foods and remind you of serving size and health concerns, such as fat and cholesterol content.

gories, must be the same for similar products (for example, different brands of potato chips) and for similar products within a category (for example, snack foods such as pretzels, potato chips, and popcorn). This makes it easier to compare the nutritional content of foods.

- *Daily Values (DVs).* DVs refer to the total amount of a nutrient that the average adult should aim to get or not exceed on a daily basis. The DVs for cholesterol, sodium, vitamins, and minerals are the same for all adults. The DVs for total fat, saturated fat, carbohydrate, fiber, and protein are based on a 2000 calorie daily diet—the amount of food ingested by many American men and active women.

- *Percent Daily Values (%DV).* The goal for a full day's diet is to select foods that together add up to 100% of the DVs. The %DVs show how a particular food's nutrient content fits into a 2000-calorie diet.   Individuals who consume (or should consume) fewer than 2000 total calories a day have to lower their DVs for total fat, saturated fat, and carbohydrates—for example, if their caloric intake is 10% less than 2000 calories, they would lower the DV by 10%. Similarly, those who consume more than 2,000 calories should adjust the DVs upward.

- *Calories per gram.* The bottom of the food label lists the number of calories per gram for fat, carbohydrates, and protein.

What Should You Look For?

Different people may zero in on different figures on the food label—for example, calories if they're watching their weight, specific ingredients if they have **food allergies**. Among the useful items to check are the following:

- *Calories from fat.* Get into the habit of calculating the percentage of fat calories in a food before buying or eating it.

- *Total fat.* Since the average person munches on 15 to 20 food items a day, it's easy to overload on fat. Saturated fat is a figure worthy of special attention because of its reported link to several diseases (discussed later in this chapter).

- *Cholesterol.* Cholesterol is made by and contained in products of animal origin only. Many high-fat products, such as potato chips, contain 0% cholesterol because they're made from plants and are cooked in

vegetable fats. However, the vegetable fats they contain can be processed and made into saturated fats that are more harmful to the heart than cholesterol itself.

- *Sugars.* There is no DV for sugars because health experts have yet to agree on a daily limit. The figure on the label includes naturally present sugars, such as lactose in milk and fructose in fruit, as well as those added to the food, such as table sugar, corn syrup, or dextrose.

- *Fiber.* A "high-fiber" food has 5 or more grams of fiber per serving. A "good" source of fiber provides at least 2.5 grams. "More or added" fiber means at least 2.5 grams more per serving than similar foods—10% more of the DV for fiber.

- *Calcium.* "High" equals 200 milligrams (mg) or more per serving. "Good" means at least 100 mg, while "more" indicates that the food contains at least 100 mg more calcium—10% more of the DV—than the item usually would have.

- *Sodium.* Since many foods contain sodium, most of us routinely get more than we need. It's important to read labels carefully to avoid excess sodium, which can be a health threat.[21]

- *Vitamins.* A DV of 10% of any vitamin makes a food a "good" source; 20% qualifies it as "high" in a certain vitamin.

Nutrition labeling for fresh produce, fish, meat, and poultry remains voluntary. Packages too small for a full-sized label must provide an address or phone number so that consumers can obtain information from the manufacturer.[22]

Vitamins and Minerals

Vitamins and **minerals** are nutrients that are essential to regulating growth, maintaining tissue, and releasing energy from foods. Vitamins help put proteins, fats, and carbohydrates to use. Together with the enzymes in the body, they help produce the right chemical reactions at the right times. They're also involved in the manufacture of blood cells, as well as hormones and other compounds.

Some vitamins are produced within the body. Vitamin D, for example, is manufactured in the skin after exposure to sunlight, and then changed to an active form through processes in the liver and then kidney.

However, most vitamins must be ingested. Vitamins such as A, D, E, and K are *fat-soluble*—absorbed through the intestinal membranes and stored in the body. The B vitamins and vitamin C are *water-soluble*—absorbed directly into the blood and then used up or washed out of the body in urine and sweat. They must be replaced daily. (See Table 6-3.)

The elements carbon, oxygen, hydrogen, and nitrogen make up 96% of our body weight. The other 4% consists of minerals, which help build bones and teeth, aid in muscle function, and help our nervous systems transmit messages. We need daily about a tenth of a gram (100 mg) or more of each of the *major minerals*: sodium, potassium, chloride, calcium, phosphorus, and magnesium. We also need daily about a hundredth of a gram (10 mg) or less of each of the *trace minerals*: iron (more than that for premenopausal women), zinc, selenium, molybdenum, iodine, cobalt, copper, manganese, fluoride, and chromium (see Table 6-4). Scientists are studying the health benefits of copper, chromium, and other minerals, but it is not yet known whether deficiencies increase the risk of disease or whether higher amounts are protective.[23]

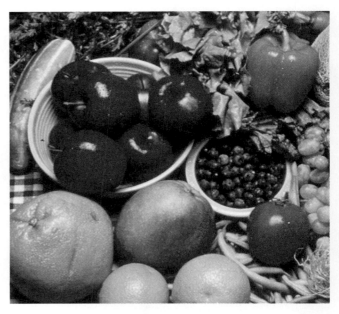

Antioxidant salad. Believe it or not, it's easy to get your daily antioxidant fix directly from food. Just eat an orange for breakfast and half a carrot for lunch and you'll have all the vitamin A (1000 retinal equivalents) and vitamin C (60 milligrams) you need for the day.

Antioxidants: The Promise of Prevention

Antioxidants are substances that prevent the harmful effects caused by oxidation within the body. There has been great general and scientific interest in the antioxidant vitamins, particularly vitamin C, vitamin E, and beta carotene (a form of Vitamin A). The proven health benefits of these vitamins are many. Vitamin C speeds healing, helps prevent infection, and prevents scurvy. Vitamin E helps prevent heart disease by stopping the oxidation of low-density lipoprotein (the harmful form of cholesterol), strengthens the immune system, and may help prevent Alzheimer's disease, cataracts, and some forms of cancer. Beta carotene aids eyesight and resistance to infection and keeps skin, hair, teeth, gums, and bones healthy.[24]

Antioxidants also may prevent damage to our cells caused by *free radicals* (oxygen molecules formed by normal metabolic processes) as well as by smog, smoke, radiation, and cancer-promoting chemicals. These free radicals act like biological terrorists in the body, damaging or killing healthy cells so they cannot perform their usual functions. For example, free radicals may alter a cell's DNA (deoxyribonucleic acid), the basic genetic blueprint, in ways that could lead to uncontrolled cell growth—that is, to cancer. They also may play a role in the buildup of cholesterol in the arteries.[25]

Some epidemiological studies have shown that people with the highest intake of various antioxidants have a lower incidence of heart disease, certain cancers, cataracts, and infectious illnesses.[26] However, in other studies, large amounts of antioxidants in the diet have had no effect or have possibly increased the incidence of disease. Some researchers contend that not smoking and receiving appropriate treatment for high blood pressure and high cholesterol can be far more beneficial than taking antioxidant vitamins.[27]

Large-scale studies now underway should give a clearer idea of the potential of antioxidants. In one study, 22,000 physicians are taking either beta carotene or a placebo and being followed to see if they have a lower rate of cancer. Because there currently is no conclusive scientific evidence for the effectiveness of antioxidants, or for the safety of taking large amounts of these substances over many years, the FDA does not recommend antioxidant supplements.

TABLE 6-3 KEY INFORMATION ABOUT THE VITAMINS

Vitamin	Major Dietary Sources	Major Functions	Signs of Severe, Prolonged Deficiency	Signs of Extreme Excess
Fat-Soluble				
A	Fat-containing and fortified dairy products; liver; provitamin carotene in orange and deep green fruits and vegetables	Antioxidant; retinoic acid affects gene expression; needed for epithelial cells and all new cell synthesis; still under intense study	Night blindness; dry, scaling skin; increased susceptibility to infection	Damage to liver, bone; headache, irritability, vomiting, hair loss, blurred vision; some fetal defects; yellowed skin
D	Fortified and full-fat dairy products, egg yolk (diet often not as important as sunlight exposure)	Promotes absorption and use of calcium and phosphorus	Rickets (bone deformities) in children; osteomalacia (bone softening) in adults	Calcium deposition in tissues leading to cerebral, cardiovascular, and kidney damage
E	Vegetable oils and their products; nuts, seeds	Antioxidant to prevent cell membrane damage; still under intense study	Possible anemia and neurological effects	Generally nontoxic, but may worsen clotting defect in vitamin K deficiency
K	Green vegetables; tea; dairy products; produced internally by intestinal bacteria	Aid in formation of certain proteins, especially those for blood clotting	Defective blood coagulation, causing severe bleeding on injury	Liver damage and anemia from high doses of the synthetic form menadione
Water-Soluble				
Thiamin (B-1)	Pork, legumes, peanuts, enriched or whole-grain products	Coenzyme used in energy metabolism	Nerve changes; sometimes edema; heart failure; beriberi	Generally nontoxic, but repeated injections may cause shock reaction
Riboflavin (B-2)	Dairy products, meats, eggs, enriched grain products, green leafy vegetables	Coenzyme used in energy metabolism	Skin lesions	Generally nontoxic
Niacin	Nuts, meats; provitamin tryptophan in most proteins	Coenzyme used in energy metabolism	Pellagra (multiple vitamin deficiencies including niacin)	Flushing of face, neck, hands; potential liver damage
B-6	High-protein foods in general; bananas, potatoes, avocados	Coenzyme used in amino acid metabolism	Nervous, skin, and muscular disorders; anemia	Unstable gait, numb feet, poor coordination
Folic acid	Green vegetables, orange juice, nuts, legumes, grain products	Coenzyme used in DNA and RNA metabolism; single carbon utilization; needed for hemoglobin synthesis	Megaloblastic anemia; pernicious anemia when due to inadequate intrinsic factor; nervous system damage	Thought to be nontoxic
Pantothenic acid	Animal products and whole grains; widely distributed in foods	Coenzyme used in energy metabolism	Fatigue, numbness, and tingling of hands and feet	Generally nontoxic; occasionally causes diarrhea
Biotin	Widely distributed in foods	Coenzyme used in energy metabolism	Scaly dermatitis	Thought to be nontoxic
C (ascorbic acid)	Fruits and vegetables, especially broccoli, cabbage, cantaloupe, cauliflower, citrus fruits, green pepper, kiwi fruit, strawberries	Functions in synthesis of collagen; is an antioxidant; aids in detoxification; improves iron absorption; still under intense study	Scurvy; petechiae (minute hemorrhages around hair follicles); weakness; delayed wound healing; impaired immune response	Gastrointestinal upsets, confounds certain lab tests

Source: Shils, M. E., and V. R. Young, eds. *Modern Nutrition in Health and Disease.* Philadelphia: Lea & Febiger, 1988.

TABLE 6-4   KEY INFORMATION ABOUT MANY ESSENTIAL MINERALS

Mineral	Major Dietary Sources	Major Functions	Signs of Severe, Prolonged Deficiency	Signs of Extreme Excess
Major Minerals				
Calcium	Milk, cheese, dark green vegetables, legumes	Bone and tooth formation; blood	Stunted growth; perhaps less bone mass clotting; nerve transmission	Depressed absorption of some other minerals; perhaps kidney damage
Magnesium	Whole grains, green leafy vegetables	Component of enzymes	Neurological disturbances	Neurological disturbances
Sodium	Salt, soy sauce, cured meats, pickles, canned soups, processed cheese	Body water balance; nerve function	Muscle cramps; reduced appetite	High blood pressure in genetically predisposed individuals
Potassium	Meats, milk, many fruits and vegetables, whole grains	Body water balance; nerve function	Muscular weakness; paralysis	Muscular weakness; cardiac arrest
Trace Minerals				
Iron	Meats, eggs, legumes, whole grains, green leafy vegetables	Components of hemoglobin, myoglobin, and enzymes	Iron deficiency anemia, weakness, impaired immune function	Acute: shock, death Chronic liver damage; cardiac failure
Iodine	Marine fish and shellfish, dairy products, iodized salt, some breads	Component of thyroid hormones	Goiter (enlarged thyroid)	Iodide goiter
Fluoride	Drinking water, tea, seafood	Maintenance of tooth (and maybe bone) structure	Higher frequency of tooth decay	Acute: gastrointestinal distress Chronic: mottling of teeth; skeletal deformation
Zinc	Meats, seafood, whole grains	Component of enzymes	Growth failure; scaly dermatitis; reproductive failure; impaired immune function	Acute: nausea; vomiting; diarrhea Chronic: adversely affects copper metabolism, anemia; and immune function
Selenium	Seafood, meat, whole grains	Component of enzymes functions in close association with vitamin E	Muscle pain; maybe heart muscle deterioration	Nausea and vomiting; hair and nail loss

SOURCE: Shils, M. E. "Magnesium." In Shils, M. E., and V. R. Young, eds., *Modern Nutrtion in Health and Disease.* Philadelphia: Lea & Febiger, 1988. Fairbanks, V. F., and E. Beutler. "Iron." In Shils and Young, eds., *Modern Nutrition.* Solomons, N. W. "Zinc and Copper." In Shils and Young, eds., *Modern Nutrition.* Underwood, E. J. *Trace Elements in Human and Animal Nutrition.* New York: Academic Press, 1977.

Do You Need Supplements?

An estimated 100 million Americans spend $6.5 billion a year on vitamins and minerals, according to the Council for Responsible Nutrition in Washington, D.C., a trade group for the vitamin supplement industry. So many people are taking supplements to prevent cancer, protect their hearts, lengthen their lives, or enhance their energy that some say "vitamania" is sweeping the country.[28]

Despite such widespread enthusiasm, medical experts express concern about the safety of dietary supplements, which are not covered by government regulation. According to the Dietary Supplement Health and Education Act of 1994, the difference between a dietary supplement and a drug depends largely on the use of the product. A product is considered a drug if the maker claims that the substance is intended for diagnosis, prevention, treatment, or cure of a disease. Dietary supplements are meant to do exactly that—to supplement a person's diet, and no more.[29]

Many health experts feel that the best way to make sure your body gets the vitamins and minerals it needs is to follow the Food Guide Pyramid and eat a wide variety of foods. If you rely on vitamin/mineral pills and fortified foods to make up for poor nutrition, you may shortchange yourself. However, supplements can benefit people whose diets do not provide adequate nutrients. For instance, supplements of the antioxidant selenium may help lower the risk of lung, colorectal, and prostate cancers in people living in areas with low soil selenium.[30] Selenium may also prevent these cancers in individuals with a history of skin cancer.[31,32]

In addition to antioxidants, substances known as **phytochemicals** (chemicals that exist naturally in plants) may have disease-fighting properties. For example, indoles, from crucifers such as broccoli and cabbage, may protect against breast and prostate cancer. Coumarins in citrus fruit and tomatoes may stimulate anticancer enzymes. Capsaicin in hot peppers may protect DNA from carcinogens (see Table 6-5). With its emphasis on a variety of healthful foods, the Food Guide Pyramid can ensure that you get a good mix of these potentially beneficial substances. However, for certain people for whom it is difficult to obtain adequate amounts of critical nutrients from diet alone, supplements may be recommended.

Folic Acid

Beginning in 1998, food manufacturers began adding folic acid, or folate, a B vitamin, to America's food. The primary reason is that insufficient levels of folic acid increase the risk of neural tube defects (abnormalities of the brain and spinal cord), such as spina bifida, in which a piece of the spinal cord protrudes from the spinal column.

Folic acid, or folate, also has other benefits, including the synthesis of oxygen-carrying **hemoglobin** in the blood. It also may help prevent cervical and other cancers by strengthening the chromosomes. Elderly men and women often have low folate, and scientists are studying whether supplements might reduce their incidence of coronary artery disease.[33]

Calcium

Calcium, the most abundant mineral in the body, builds strong bone tissue throughout our lives and plays a vital role in heart and brain functioning. Adequate calcium is especially critical for pregnant or nursing women, who need it to meet the additional needs of their babies' bodies. (See Chapter 10 for a complete discussion of diet and pregnancy.) Calcium may also help control high blood pressure and prevent colon cancer in adults.

TABLE 6-5 SOME FOODS RICH IN ANTIOXIDANTS AND PHYTOCHEMICALS

Antioxidant	Food	Phytochemical	Food
Beta carotene	Apricots, Asparagus, Brussels sprouts, Cantaloupe, Carrot, Peach, Romaine lettuce, Spinach, Sweet potato	Capsaicin	Hot peppers
		Coumarins	Citrus fruit, Tomatoes
		Flavonoids	Berries, Carrots, Citrus fruit, Peppers, Tomatoes
Selenium	Lean meat, 100% whole wheat bread, Nonfat milk, Skinless chicken, 100% whole-grain cereal, Seafood	Genistein	Beans, Peas, Lentils
		Indoles	Broccoli, Cabbage family
Vitamin C	Asparagus, Broccoli, Brussels sprouts, Cabbage, Collard greens, Grapefruit, Green pepper, Orange juice, Strawberries, Tomato juice	Isothiocyanates	Broccoli, Cabbage, Mustard, Horseradish
		Ligands	Barley, Flaxseed, Wheat
		Lycopene	Pink grapefruit, Tomatoes
Vitamin E	Almonds, 100% whole wheat bread, Wheat germ, 100% whole-grain cereal, Safflower oil	S-allycysteine	Chives, Garlic, Onions
		Triterpenoids	Citrus fruit, Licorice root

Adequate calcium intake during the teens and twenties may be crucial to prevent osteoporosis, the bone-weakening disease that strikes one out of every four women over the age of 60 (see Chapter 18 for further discussion of osteoporosis). Dietary calcium can significantly increase the bone density of children, safeguarding against osteoporosis in later life. Research has shown that elderly men and women who consume adequate calcium can keep their bones strong and prevent fractures.[34]

In 1994, the federal Consensus Development Conference on Optimal Calcium Intake issued revised recommendations on daily calcium intake for different age and gender groups. They are:

- 1200 to 1500 mg for teenagers and young adults.
- 1000 mg for women aged 25 to 50.
- 1000 to 1500 mg for postmenopausal women aged 51 to 64.
- 800 mg for men under 65.
- 1500 mg for men and women 65 and older.
- 800 mg for children under age 10.

Although calcium-rich foods should provide the bulk of calcium intake, the federal panel noted that calcium-fortified foods and supplements may be needed to ensure adequate calcium intake.[35] The best supplements are calcium citrate and calcium carbonate, which should be taken in doses of no more than 500 mg with meals. Calcium supplements from bone meal or dolomite may be contaminated with lead or other heavy metals; these are so full of other substances that, taken on a daily basis, they can cause significant gastrointestinal distress. Intake of more than 2000 mg of calcium daily may be toxic.

Iron

Iron is an essential ingredient of hemoglobin, the protein that makes the blood red and carries oxygen to all our tissues. Because oxygen is needed to convert food into energy, too little iron—and thus too little hemoglobin—can trigger an internal energy crisis. Getting enough iron can be a big problem for women, whose iron stores are drained by menstruation, pregnancy, and nursing. Half of all women of childbearing age get less than the RDA of 15 mg, and 5% suffer from iron-deficiency anemia.

The symptoms of iron deficiency are sensitivity to cold, chronic fatigue, edginess, depression, sleeplessness, and susceptibility to colds and infections. To boost

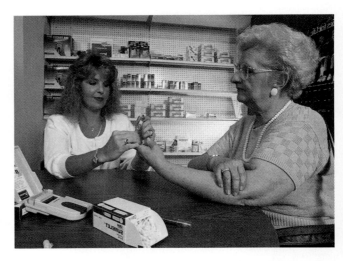

Women are more susceptible to anemia than men. A healthy diet that includes whole-grain cereals, broccoli, and foods rich in vitamin C is a good strategy for boosting iron stores.

your iron, use the following strategies. Don't take supplements unless you've had a blood test that indicates you should. Excess iron can cause severe constipation and other complications.

Strategies for Prevention
Getting More Iron in Your Diet

✔ Eat vegetables and starches high in iron: whole-grain cereals (such as bran flakes), broccoli, soybeans, and red kidney beans.

✔ To increase the amount of iron your body absorbs from these plant foods, eat foods high in vitamin C at the same meal.

✔ Eat iron-rich lean red meats two or three times a week. Oysters are also a good iron source.

✔ Don't drink tea with your meal, because the tannin in it may interfere with iron absorption.

Multivitamin Supplements

Even though there's little proof that multivitamin supplements can help them, many people figure that taking them certainly can't hurt. As they see it, supplements serve as a nutritional insurance policy, something to fall back on in case they don't get everything they need from whole foods. For the most part, this is true. "If you have a good diet and you take a multivitamin supplement, there's probably no danger," says nutritionist Ann Shaw. "But if you take megadoses of a single vitamin or several different vitamins, you could run into problems."[36]

As scientists note, most health benefits and dangers stem from more than one source, so it's unlikely that changing any one nutrient will in itself produce great benefits—and may, by interfering with the complex balance of nutrients, do harm. This is particularly true for the **fat-soluble vitamins**, primarily A and D, which can build up in our bodies and cause serious complications, such as damage to the kidneys, liver, or bones. Large doses of water-soluble vitamins, including the B vitamins, also may be harmful. Excessive intake of vitamin B-6 (pyridoxine), often used to relieve premenstrual bloating, can cause neurological damage, such as numbness in the mouth and tingling in the hands. (An excessive amount in this case is 250 to 300 times the recommended dose.) High doses of vitamin C can produce stomach aches and diarrhea. Niacin, often taken in high doses to lower cholesterol, can cause jaundice, liver damage, and irregular heartbeats as well as severe, uncomfortable flushing of the skin.

Large doses of vitamins can be especially dangerous for individuals with certain health conditions. Excessive intake of vitamin C or D may precipitate the formation of kidney stones in the urinary tract. Too much vitamin B-6 may inhibit milk production in breastfeeding mothers. In individuals suffering from epilepsy, folate may interfere with their drug therapy.

Strategies for Prevention

Who Should Take Multivitamin Supplements?

If you belong to any of the following groups, check with your doctor about the potential pluses of adding vitamins or vitamin-rich foods to your daily diet:

✔ Pregnant, breast-feeding, and menopausal women.

✔ People at risk for heart attack, especially smokers.

✔ Strict vegetarians.

✔ People with chronic illnesses that may interfere with appetite or the body's use of nutrients.

✔ Individuals taking medications that affect appetite or digestion.

✔ The elderly.

▌The Way We Eat

For centuries, Native Americans ate a diet of corn, beans, fish, game, wild greens, wild fruits, squash, and tomatoes. Over time the United States—a nation of immigrants—has imported a wide variety of ethnic cuisines. Although many people think of foods such as hamburgers, steak, potatoes, and cheesecake or ice cream as "all-American" favorites, in most cities across the country, it is possible to taste dozens of different cultural cuisines.

Dietary Diversity

Whatever your cultural heritage, you have probably sampled Chinese, Mexican, Indian, Italian, and Japanese foods. If you belong to any of these ethnic groups, you may eat these cuisines regularly. Each type of ethnic cooking has its own nutritional benefits and potential drawbacks (see Table 6-6). In addition, different foods or eating rituals may have special religious or cultural significance (see Spotlight on Diversity: "Food for the Soul").

The African-American Diet

African-American cuisine traces some of its roots to food preferences from West Africa (for example, peanuts, okra, and black-eyed peas), as well as to traditional American foods, such as fish, game, greens, and sweet potatoes. Cajun cuisine, most closely associated with New Orleans, blends both African and French traditions in dishes such as gumbos (thick spicy soups), sausage, red beans, and seafood. African-American cooking uses many nutritious vegetables, such as collard greens and sweet potatoes, as well as legumes. However, some dishes include high-fat food products such as peanuts and pecans or involve frying, sometimes in saturated fat.

The Chinese Diet

The mainland Chinese diet, which is plant-based, high in carbohydrates, and low in fats and animal protein, is considered one of the healthiest in the world. However, Chinese food is prepared differently in America. Chinese restaurants here serve more meat and sauces than are generally eaten in China. According to laboratory tests of typical take-out dishes from Chinese restaurants, many have more fats and cholesterol than hamburger or egg dishes from fast-food outlets.

TABLE 6-6 DIET AND LIFE EXPECTANCY

Nutritionists in various countries have different ideas about what constitutes a healthful diet. Putting science aside, here's a look at eating habits and longevity in several developed countries around the world.

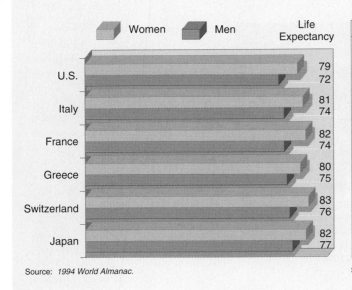

Women	Men	Life Expectancy
U.S.		79 / 72
Italy		81 / 74
France		82 / 74
Greece		80 / 75
Switzerland		83 / 76
Japan		82 / 77

Source: *1994 World Almanac.*

Country	Traditional Diet
U.S.	High in meat, fat, sugar, processed foods. Low in seafood, grains, fresh fruits and vegetables.
Italy	High in cheese, olive oil, meat, grains, wine. Low in processed foods.
France	High in butter, cheese, wine. Low in meat, processed foods.
Greece	High in olives, olive oil, yogurt, seafood, cheese, nuts. Low in meat, processed foods.
Switzerland	High in animal fat, cheese and meat. Low in seafood.
Japan	High in seafood, soy products, rice. Low in fat, cheese, meat.

Source: *American Health,* December 1994.

To eat healthfully when you choose Chinese cuisine, select boiled, steamed, or stir-fried dishes, mix entrees with steamed rice, and lift food out of a container with chopsticks or a fork and transfer it to serving bowls to leave excess sauce behind.[37] Order wonton soup rather than egg rolls or pork spareribs. To avoid the cholesterol in egg yolks, steer away from items made with lobster or egg foo yung sauces. If you are prone to high blood pressure, watch out for the high sodium content of soy and other sauces, and of a seasoner called MSG (monosodium glutamate). Some people are sensitive to MSG, and most restaurants offer some MSG-free dishes or will leave out MSG on request.

The Japanese Diet

The traditional Japanese diet is very low in fat, which may be why the incidence of heart disease is low in Japan. Dietary staples include soybean products, fish, vegetables, noodles, and rice. A variety of fruits and vegetables are also included in many dishes. However, Japanese cuisine is high in salted, smoked, and pickled foods. Watch out for deep-fried dishes such as tempura, and salty soups and sauces (which you can ask for on the side). Ask for broiled entrees in a restaurant or non-fried dishes made with tofu, a soybean curd protein, which has no cholesterol.

The Italian Diet

Even babies like spaghetti, a food that's both good tasting and good for you because it's rich in complex carbohydrates. Olive oil, another essential of Italian kitchens, is healthful because it's rich in monounsaturated fats.[38] But not all Italian dishes are equally healthful: The cooking of northern Italy features much more beef, butter, and cream. Epidemiological studies have shown that residents of this region have a much greater incidence of heart disease than their southern neighbors. The Mediterranean cuisine of southern Italy consists mainly of pasta, vegetables, fruit, and fish. Best bets for a nutritious meal include cioppino (fish soup); minestrone (vegetable soup); pasta primavera (with vegetables); or pasta with marinara (tomato, onion, and garlic), marsala (wine), or white or red clam sauces. Limit high-fat foods, such as fettucini alfredo, ravioli, and cannelloni.

The French Diet

Traditional French cuisine, which includes rich, high-fat sauces and dishes, has never been considered healthful.

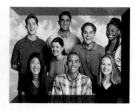

Spotlight on Diversity
Food for the Soul

Eating has always been more than a biological necessity. Throughout history, men, women, and children have gathered to thank their gods for the gift of food and to break bread together as an act of connection and celebration. Every culture and religion includes eating rituals in its teachings and practices. Here are some examples:

• **Judaism**. Families celebrate Passover with a Seder, a commemorative meal that features unleavened bread, wine, and bitter herbs. Orthodox Jews heed the law of Moses, which prohibits eating many foods, including pork and shellfish; they say a prayer of gratitude before and after meals. It also is customary for practicing Jews to fast on Yom Kippur, the annual Day of Atonement.

• **Christianity**. "Give us this day our daily bread," Christians ask in their best-known prayer, the "Our Father." In the Eucharist, a central part of Christian religious services, priests and ministers take a wafer of bread and a cup of wine and consecrate them as the body and blood of Jesus Christ. Roman Catholics avoid meat on Fridays and during the pre-Easter season of Lent. Certain Protestant sects also follow strict dietary rules. Seventh-Day Adventists, for instance, abstain from alcohol and all stimulants including coffee.

• **Hinduism**. As they worship Lakshmi, the goddess of prosperity, Hindu families place offerings of rice, fruit, and other foods before her statue and pour ghee, or clarified butter, over it. Vegetarianism is part of Hindu philosophy,

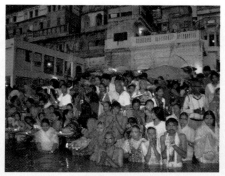

In many cultures, food is more than a mere source of sustenance; it is often associated with religious celebration and a sense of community, as well as deeper symbolic meaning.

based on the ethical principle of ahimsa (nonviolence or nonkilling) and the belief that meat, fish, and eggs are dominated by "inflaming" energy that can interfere with spiritual development. Alcohol is viewed as a source of "dissipating" energy, while foods such as grains, beans, milk, fruits, and nuts are chosen to promote physical and spiritual harmony and balance.

• **Zen Buddhism**. Its followers are strict vegetarians who eat no meat, fish, eggs, cheese, or other animal products. Their diet consists mainly of rice, grains, beans, and bean products, such as tofu, and vegetables. The preparation of meals is valued as an act of love and compassion, and fasting as a way toward moral and spiritual development.

• **Shinto**. The native religion of Japan views food not just as a gift from the gods but as a deity in itself. Ancient myths speak of rice as a goddess, who is still enshrined and revered throughout Japan. In modern Japan, many people routinely say "Itadakimasu," which means "I humbly receive this gift," before eating.

Even though they were created with the soul rather than the body in mind, eating rituals can benefit physical as well as spiritual health. Rather than frantically preparing and scarfing down meals—as happens all too often in our fast-paced, secular world—a simple observance, such as a moment of silence before eating, can force us to pause and think about what we're about to do. Such steps allow us to slow down, refocus, relax, and enjoy a meal more.

Yet nutritionists have been stumped to explain the so-called French paradox. Despite a diet high in saturated fats, the French have one of the lowest rates of coronary artery disease in the world. Is their lifestyle less stressful? Is there some beneficial ingredient in the wines they drink with their meals?

No one knows exactly, but nutritionists note there are some healthful aspects of the French way of eating: The French eat more fresh fruits and vegetables than Americans. They get less of their fat from red meat. They

snack less. And they consume more than half of their daily calories by 2:00 P.M.—unlike Americans, who usually eat their biggest meal late in the day.[39]

The Mexican Diet

The cuisine served in Mexico features rice, corn, and beans, which are low in fat and high in nutrients.[40] However, the dishes Americans think of as Mexican are far less healthful. Burritos, for example, especially when topped with cheese and sour cream, are very high in fat.

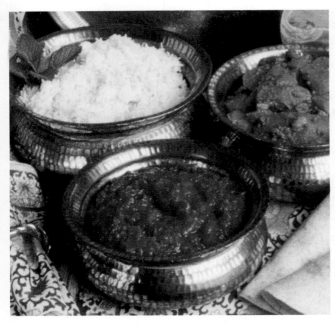 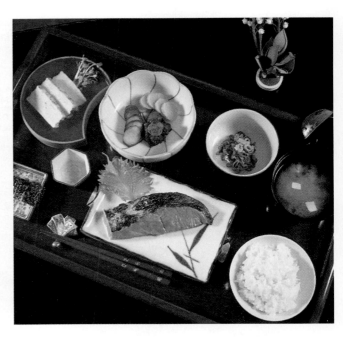

All-American diversity. The rice and beans of Mexico are healthy and high in protein, but too much cheese can cancel some of the benefits. The Japanese diet is high in seafood and rice and low in fats, cheese, and meat.

Although guacamole has a high fat content, it contains mostly monounsaturated fatty acids, a better form of fat.

When eating at Mexican restaurants, ask that cheese and sour cream be served on the side. Avoid refried beans, which are usually cooked in lard. Hold back on guacamole, quesadillas, and enchichaladas. Nutritious choices include rice, beans, and shrimp or chicken tostadas on unfried corn meal tortillas.

The Indian Diet

Many Indian dishes highlight healthful ingredients such as vegetables and legumes (beans and peas). However, many also use "ghee" (a form of butter) or coconut oil, which is rich in harmful saturated fats. The best advice in an Indian restaurant is to ask how each dish is prepared. Good choices include daal or dal (lentils), karbi or karni (chickpea soup), and chapati (tortilla-like bread). Hold back on bhatura (fried bread), coconut milk, and samosas (fried meat or vegetables in dough).

The Southeast Asian Diet

A rich variety of fruits and vegetables—bamboo shoots, bok choy, cabbage, mangoes, papayas, cucumbers—provides a sound nutritional basis for this diet. In addition, most foods are broiled or stir-fried, which keeps fat low. However, coconut oil and milk, used in many

sauces, are high in fat. The use of MSG and pickled foods means the sodium content is high. At Thai or Vietnamese restaurants, choose salads (larb is a chicken salad with mint) or seafood soup (po tak).

Vegetarian Diets

Not all vegetarians avoid all meats. Some, who call themselves "lact-ovo-pesco-vegetarians," eat dairy products, eggs, chicken and fish, but not red meat. **Lacto-vegetarians** eat dairy products as well as grains, fruits and vegetables; **ovo-lacto-vegetarians** also eat eggs. Pure vegetarians, called **vegans**, eat only plant foods; often they take vitamin B-12 supplements, because that vitamin is normally found only in animal products. If they select their food with care, vegetarians can get sufficient amounts of protein, vitamin B-12, iron, and calcium without supplements (see Figure 6-4).

The key to getting sufficient protein from a vegetarian diet is understanding the concept of **complementary proteins**. Meat, poultry, fish, eggs, and dairy products are **complete proteins** that provide the nine essential **amino acids**—substances containing carbon, hydrogen, oxygen, and nitrogen that the human body cannot produce itself. **Incomplete proteins**, such as legumes or nuts, may have relatively low levels of one

Figure 6-4

Vegetarian Food Guide Pyramid. This version of the Food Guide Pyramid has been modified for use by vegetarians. Compare it to the Food Guide Pyramid shown in Figure 6-2.

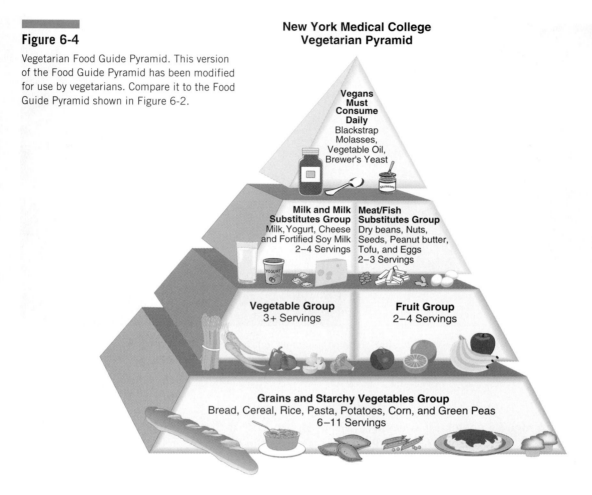

**New York Medical College
Vegetarian Pyramid**

Vegans Must Consume Daily
Blackstrap Molasses, Vegetable Oil, Brewer's Yeast

Milk and Milk Substitutes Group
Milk, Yogurt, Cheese and Fortified Soy Milk
2–4 Servings

Meat/Fish Substitutes Group
Dry beans, Nuts, Seeds, Peanut butter, Tofu, and Eggs
2–3 Servings

Vegetable Group
3+ Servings

Fruit Group
2–4 Servings

Grains and Starchy Vegetables Group
Bread, Cereal, Rice, Pasta, Potatoes, Corn, and Green Peas
6–11 Servings

or two essential amino acids, but fairly high levels of others. By combining complementary protein sources, you can make sure that your body makes the most of the nonanimal proteins you eat. Many cultures rely heavily on complementary foods for protein. In Middle Eastern cooking, sesame seeds and chick-peas are a popular combination; in Latin American dishes, beans and rice, or beans and tortillas; in Chinese cuisine, soy and rice.

Vegetarian diets have proven health benefits. Studies show that vegetarians' cholesterol levels are low, and vegetarians are seldom overweight. As a result, they're less apt to be candidates for heart disease than those who consume large quantities of meat. Vegetarians also have lower incidences of breast, colon, and prostate cancer; high blood pressure; and osteoporosis. When combined with exercise and stress reduction, vegetarian diets have led to reductions in the buildup of harmful

plaque within the blood vessels of the heart. (See Chapter 13 for a further discussion of the connections between diet and heart disease.)

Fast Food: Nutrition on the Run

Not all fast foods are junk foods—that is, high in calories, sugar, salt, and fat, and low in nutrients. But while it's not all bad, fast food has definite disadvantages. A meal in a fast-food restaurant may cost twice as much as the same meal prepared at home and may provide half your daily calorie needs. The fat content of many items is extremely high. A Burger King Whopper with cheese contains 723 calories and 48 grams of fat, 18 grams from saturated fat. A McDonald's Sausage McMuffin with egg has 517 calories and 33 grams of fat, 13 grams from saturated fat. Many fast-food chains have switched from beef tallow or lard to unsaturated vegetable oils for frying, but the total fat content of the foods remains the same (see Table 6-7).

In response to criticism by health professionals and consumers in general, many fast-food outlets have also added lighter menu items, such as salads, grilled chicken sandwiches on whole-grain buns, and nonfat yogurt. Some have reduced sodium in their products, removed

additives from fish breading, and taken MSG out of sausages.

At regular restaurants or cafeterias, with a little extra attention, you can usually get a better nutritional value for the calories you consume. For example, you can request that your entree be baked or broiled without fat. You can also ask that fresh vegetables be steamed without salt or butter. When possible, ask for luncheon rather than dinner-sized portions. Or order appetizers

TABLE 6-7 SOME POPULAR SNACK FOODS

Snack Food [a]	Calories	Grams of Fat [b]	Milligrams of Sodium
Chex Mix	182	7	432
Corn chips (plain)	230	14	269
Cheese puffs or twists	236	15	447
Popcorn (air-popped)	31	trace	0
(oil-popped with added salt)	55	3	97
(caramel coated, with peanuts)	171	3	126
(caramel coated, without peanuts)	152	5	72
(cheese flavor)	58	4	98
Popcorn cakes (1 cake)	38	trace	29
Pork skins (plain)	116	7	391
(barbecue flavor)	114	7	567
Potato chips (plain)	152	10	168
(barbecue)	139	9	213
(cheese flavor)	140	8	225
(light)	134	6	139
(sour cream and onion)	150	10	177
Potato sticks	188	12	90
Pretzels (with added salt)	162	2	729
Rice cakes (plain, 1 cake)	35	trace	29
Tortilla chips (plain)	178	9	188
Trail mix[c]	693	44	343
Almonds (dry roasted)	810	71	15
(oil roasted)	970	91	16
Cashews (oil roasted)	748	63	22
Mixed nuts (dry roasted)	814	70	16
(oil roasted)	876	80	16
Peanuts (oil roasted with added salt)	837	71	624
Pistachios (dry roasted)	776	68	8

[a] All values listed are for one cup—a mere handful or two—unless otherwise indicated.
[b] Someone following an 1800-calorie diet should average no more than 60 grams of fat a day.
[c] Contains raisins, oil-roasted peanuts, dried sunflower seed kernels, dates, oil-roasted cashews, oil-roasted almonds, dried coconut, and oil-roasted pumpkin seed kernels.
SOURCES: *USDA Handbooks* 8–19 and 8–12.

and side dishes instead of an entree, for instance, tomato soup, a salad, and vegetables. Ask for your salad dressing on the side, request low-calorie dressing if available, or make your own dressing with lemon juice or vinegar.

Strategy for Prevention
A Guide to Fast Foods

✔ For breakfast, avoid croissants or muffins stuffed with eggs or meat; they pack as many as 700 calories. Better options include plain scrambled eggs (150–180 calories), pancakes without butter or syrup (400 calories), and English muffins (185 calories each).

✔ For lunch or dinner, if you want meat, go for plain hamburgers (no cheese), which average 275 to 350 calories. An even better choice is roast beef, which is lower in fat and calories.

✔ Be wary of fast-food fish. With frying oil trapped in the breading and creamy tartar sauce on top, fried-fish sandwiches supply more calories (425–500) and fat than regular hamburgers.

✔ Avoid fried chicken; the coatings tend to retain grease. If you want bite-sized chicken, select bites made of chicken breast, not processed chicken (which contains fatty, ground-up skin).

✔ Ask for unsalted items; they are available. (Many chains have also reduced the amount of sodium used in cooking.)

✔ If you sample the salad bar, steer clear of mayonnaise, bacon bits, oily vegetable salads, and rich dressings.

Food Safety

Increasingly, Americans are concerned not just with whether the food they eat is nutritious, but whether it's safe. Many unsuspected safety hazards have been identified by **food toxicologists**, specialists who detect toxins (potentially harmful substances) and treat the conditions they produce.

Pesticides, Processing, and Irradiation

Plants and animals naturally produce compounds that act as pesticides to aid in their survival. The vast majority of the pesticides we consume are therefore natural, not added by farmers or food processors. As discussed in depth in Chapter 21, *commercial* pesticides save billions of dollars of valuable crops from pests, but they also may endanger human health and life.

Fearful of potential risks in pesticides, many consumers are purchasing **organic** foods. The term *organic* refers to foods produced without the use of commercial chemicals at any stage. Some independent certifying groups certify foods as organic if they have no detected residues of pesticides, even though pesticides may have been used in their cultivation. Foods that are truly organic are cleaner and have much lower levels of residues than standard commercial produce. There's no guarantee that the organic produce you buy at a grocery or health-food store is more nutritious than other produce. However, buying organic foods is one way in which you can work toward a healthier environment.

Irradiation is the use of radiation, either from radioactive substances or from devices that produce X rays, on food. It doesn't make the food radioactive. Its primary benefit is to prolong the shelf life of food. Like the heat in canning, irradiation can kill all the microorganisms that might grow in a food, and the sterilized food can then be stored for years in sealed containers at room temperature without spoiling. Are irradiated foods safe to eat? The best available answer is a qualified yes, because we don't have complete data yet. Most of the research conducted so far has focused on low-dose irradiation to delay ripening and destroy insects. In 1997 the FDA approved the irradiation of red meat as a means of eliminating dangerous bacteria that could cause food poisoning. Irradiation had previously been approved for poultry, where it was used to kill disease-causing bacteria like Salmonella and fruits and vegetables, where it is used in low doses to kill funguses and molds.[41]

Some consumers are concerned about the potentially harmful effects of giving animals antibiotics (to prevent infection) and hormones (such as bovine somatotropin, to increase milk production in cows). Conclusive scientific studies have not been done, but several state legislatures have considered restricting the use or sale of milk produced by cows that have been given hormones. There also has been controversy over the labeling of such products. Consumers argue that they have a right to know whether hormones have been used; manufacturers contend they need not divulge this information.

Genetically engineered foods—custom built to improve quality or remove unwanted traits—may become an important part of our diets in the future. By modifying the genetic makeup of plants, engineers will be able to produce apples that resist insects, raspberries that last longer, and potatoes that absorb less fat in cooking. Will these items be as tasty and healthful as foods grown the old-fashioned way? And will they have unforeseen health hazards? That's yet to be seen.

Additives: Risks versus Benefits

Additives are substances added to foods to lengthen storage time, change taste in a way the manufacturer thinks is better, alter color, or otherwise modify them to make them more appealing. The average American takes in approximately 160 pounds of food additives per year: over 140 pounds of sweeteners, 15 pounds of table salt, and 5 to 10 pounds of all others.

Additives provide numerous benefits. Sodium and calcium propionate, sodium benzoate, potassium sorbate, and sulfur dioxide prevent the growth of bacteria, yeast, and mold in baked goods. BHA (butylated hydroxyanisole), BHT (butylated hydroxytoluene), propyl gallate, and vitamin E protect against the oxidation of fats (rancidity). Other additives include leavening agents, emulsifiers, stabilizers, thickeners, dough conditioners, and bleaching agents.

Some additives can pose a risk to eaters. For example, nitrites—used in bacon, sausages, and lunch meats to inhibit spoilage, prevent botulism, and add color—can react with other substances in your body or in food to form potentially cancer-causing agents called *nitrosamines*. In the last decade, the food industry has reduced the amount of nitrite used to cure foods, so there should be less danger than in the past. Sulfites, used to prevent browning, can produce severe, even fatal, allergic reactions in sensitive individuals. The FDA has required the labeling of sulfites in packaged foods and has banned the use of sulfites on fresh fruits and vegetables, including those in salad bars.

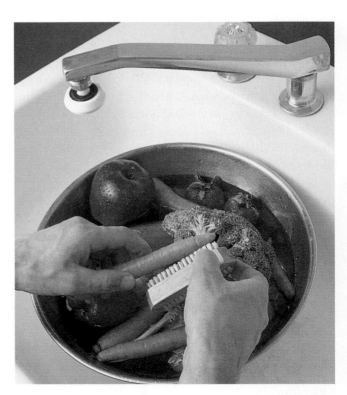

Clean food from a clean kitchen. Wash produce thoroughly in fresh water to remove dirt and any pesticide residue, scrubbing when necessary to clean off soil.

Food-borne Infections

Someone in the United States is stricken with food poisoning approximately every second of every day, says the Council for Agricultural Sciences and Technology. Every year as many as 35 million Americans suffer from food poisoning; some 9000 die as a result. In a study of food-borne illnesses, the General Accounting Office estimated that such illnesses cost the economy some $22 billion annually. The World Health Organization describes food as "the major source of exposure to disease-causing agents—biological and chemical—from which no one in either the developing or developed countries is spared."[42] (See Chapter 11 for an in-depth discussion of infectious illnesses.)

Food-borne infections generally produce nausea, vomiting, and diarrhea from twelve hours to five days after infection. The symptoms and severity depend on the specific microorganism and the victim's overall health. Although the illnesses tend to be short term and not usually severe, they can be fatal to those whose immune systems are impaired or whose general health is poor. (See Table 6-8.)

Salmonella is a bacterium that contaminates many foods, particularly undercooked chicken, eggs, and sometimes processed meat. Eating contaminated food can result in Salmonella poisoning, which causes diarrhea and vomiting. The Centers for Disease Control and Prevention (CDC) estimates that there are approximately 40,000 reported cases of Salmonella poisoning a year; the actual number of cases could be anywhere from 400,000 to 4 million. Another bacterium, *Campylobacter jijuni*, may cause even more stomach infections than Salmonella. Found in water, milk, and some foods, *Campy-*

lobacter poisoning causes severe diarrhea and has been implicated in causing stomach ulcers.

Bacteria can also cause illness by producing toxins in food. *Staphlycoccus aureus*, the most common cause of food–borne intoxication, occurs when cooked foods are cross-contaminated with the bacteria from raw foods and not stored properly. Staph infections cause nausea and abdominal pain anywhere from thirty minutes to eight hours after ingestion.

Bacteria account for two-thirds of food–borne infections, and thousands of suspected cases of infection with *Escherichia coli*, or **E. coli** bacteria in undercooked or inadequately washed food have been reported. (See Chapter 11 on infectious diseases.) In one outbreak in

TABLE 6-8 COMMON CULPRITS

	Source	Symptoms	Onset	Prevention
Bacterial				
Campylobacter Jejuni	Bacteria on poultry, cattle, and sheep that can contaminate the meat or milk of these animals.	Diarrhea, abdominal cramping, fever and/or bloody stools.	2 to 5 days.	Cook foods thoroughly; drink pasteurized milk.
Escherichia coli (E.coli)	Water, raw or undercooked meat and cross-contaminated foods.	Watery or bloody diarrhea, abdominal cramps, or vomiting.	10 to 72 hours.	Cook foods thoroughly; wash hands well.
Salmonella	Raw or undercooked meat, poultry or eggs, and unpasteurized milk.	Nausea, abdominal cramps, diarrhea, fever, and/or headache.	5 hours to 4 days.	Cook foods thoroughly; wash hands well.
Staphylococcus aureus	Food left too long at room temperature, including meat, poultry, or egg products, tuna, potato salad, and cream-filled pastries. Unlike other bacteria, staphylococci grow well in foods that are high in sugar or salt; any food can be contaminated by infected food handlers.	Vomiting, nausea, diarrhea, abdominal pain, and/or cramps.	30 minutes to 8 hours.	Cook foods thoroughly; refrigerate leftovers immediately; wash your hands before and after handling food.
Nonbacterial				
Hepatitis A virus	Oysters, clams, mussels, or scallops that come from waters polluted with untreated sewage, and improper food handling with unwashed hands.	Weakness, appetite loss, nausea, vomiting, and fever; jaundice may develop.	15 to 50 days.	Buy seafood from reputable markets; wash hands well.
Trichinella spiralis	(causes trichinosis) A parasite found in raw or undercooked pork or carnivorous animals.	Muscle pain, swollen eyelids, and/or fever; can be fatal.	8 to 15 days.	Cook meat thoroughly.

SOURCE: USDA.

Washington State in 1995, the failure of fast-food restaurants to cook hamburger meat to a temperature high enough to kill *Escherichia coli* bacteria led to the hospitalization of 151 people and three deaths.[43]

An uncommon but sometimes fatal form of food poisoning is **botulism**, caused by the *Clostridium botulinum* organism. Improper home-canning procedures are the most common cause of this potentially fatal problem.

Strategies for Prevention
....
Protecting Yourself from Food Poisoning

✔ Clean food thoroughly. Wash produce thoroughly. Wash utensils, plates, cutting boards, knives, blenders, and other cooking equipment with very hot water and soap after preparing raw meat, poultry, or fish to avoid contaminating other foods or the cooked meat.

✔ Drink only pasteurized milk. Raw or unpasteurized milk increases the danger of microbial infections.

✔ Don't eat raw eggs. Since raw eggs can be contaminated with Salmonella, don't use them in salad dressings, eggnog, or other dishes.

✔ Cook chicken thoroughly. About a third of all poultry sold contains harmful organisms. Thorough cooking eliminates any danger.

✔ Cook pork to an internal temperature of 170°F to kill parasites called Trichina occasionally found in the muscles of pigs.

✔ Keep foods hotter than 140°F or colder than 40°F. The temperatures in between are a danger zone. if you must leave foods out—perhaps at a buffet or picnic—don't let them stay in the temperature danger zone for more than two hours. After that time, throw the food away.

✔ Refrigerate leftovers as soon as possible and use them within three days. If frozen, use leftovers within two to three months.

Food Allergies

A woman nibbles on a strawberry and collapses. A boy develops hives immediately after eating a peanut butter sandwich. A baby vomits after swallowing some regular milk. In each case, the body has responded as if the food being consumed were a threatening invader and has mobilized its internal forces to fight against it.

Physicians disagree as to which foods are the most common triggers of food allergies. Cow's milk, eggs, seafood, wheat, soybeans, nuts, seeds, and chocolate have all been identified as culprits. The symptoms they provoke vary. One person might sneeze if exposed to an irritating food; another might vomit or develop diarrhea; others might suffer headaches, dizziness, hives, or a rapid heartbeat. Symptoms may not develop for up to 72 hours, making it hard to pinpoint which food was responsible. (See Chapter 11 for a further discussion of allergies.)

If you suspect that you have a food allergy, see a physician with specialized training in allergy diagnosis. Medical opinion about the merits of many treatments for food allergies is divided. Once you've identified the culprit, the wisest and sometimes simplest course is to avoid it.

Nutritional Quackery

The American Dietetic Association describes nutritional quackery as a growing problem for unsuspecting consumers. Yet, because so much nutritional nonsense is garbed in scientific-sounding terms, it can be hard to recognize bad advice when you get it. One basic rule: If the promises of a nutritional claim sound too good to be true—they probably are (Table 6-9).

If you seek the advice of a nutrition consultant, check his or her credentials and professional associations carefully. Because licensing isn't required in all states, almost anyone can call him- or herself a nutritionist, regardless of qualifications. Be wary of diplomas from obscure schools and organizations that allow anyone who pays dues to join. (One physician obtained a membership for his dog!) Registered dietitians (R.D.s), who have bachelor's degrees from approved programs and specialized training (including an internship), and who pass a certification examination, are usually members of the American Dietetic Association (ADA), which sets the standard for quality in diets. Nutrition experts with M.D.s or Ph.D.s generally belong to the ADA, the American Institute of Nutrition, or the American Society of Clinical Nutrition; all have stringent membership requirements.

Consumers should be wary of any nutritional supplements sold in health stores or through health and bodybuilding magazines that contain ingredients that

TABLE 6-9 NUTRIENTS FROM A TO ZINC

The Nutrient	The Claims	The Truth
Amino acids	Increase muscle mass.	There is no solid evidence that amino acid supplements promote muscle building. Very little is known about the side effects of taking high doses of single or combination amino acid supplements.
Beta carotene (converted into vitamin A in the body)	Reduces your risk of cancer; stimulates the immune system.	The evidence that beta carotene and other antioxidant supplements prevent disease comes from several animal and human studies that suggest beta carotene may reduce cancer risk. Further studies are necessary before conclusive proof is available.
B complex Vitamins	Provide energy; help relieve stress and may help reduce heart disease risk.	Though B vitamins assist in energy production, only food actually provides energy. There is no evidence that B vitamins relieve stress. In a single recent study, vitamins B12 and B6 and folic acid were linked to a lower risk of heart disease and stroke. Long thought to be nontoxic, some B vitamins such as B6 and niacin may have serious side effects when taken in very high doses. For example, large doses of B6 have been linked to neurological disorders.
Vitamin C	Prevents colds, certain cancers, and heart disease.	Research suggests that vitamin C supplements can lessen the severity of colds but not prevent them. Observational studies have shown that vitamin C may help prevent cancer and heart disease, but too few clinical trials have been conducted to substantiate those results.
Calcium	Prevents osteoporosis and colon cancer and reduces high blood pressure.	Calcium plays a critical role in preventing osteoporosis, but it is only one of several factors, including heredity and availability of other nutrients, such as vitamin D. Results of research on calcium's role in preventing colon cancer are still preliminary. The mineral may play a role in regulating blood pressure among some people, but there is currently no way of knowing who might benefit from a supplement.
Chromium picolinate	Reduces body fat, builds muscle and improves overall fitness.	There is no scientific evidence that chromium supplements affect body fat, muscle mass, or fitness levels. Regular, large doses of chromium may aggravate diabetes.
Vitamin E	Reduces the risk of heart disease and cancer.	Medical experts believe vitamin E may protect against oxidation of LDL cholesterol, a process that can lead to blocked arteries. Research has shown that supplements of at least 100 IU may protect against heart disease. Very few side effects have been reported, even in doses as high as 3200 IU. (High doses of vitamin E supplements should not be used by anyone taking anticoagulation medication, however.) There is observational evidence that vitamin E supplments help prevent cancer, but clinical studies have proved inconsistent.
Niacin	Helps lower cholesterol.	Research has clearly shown that niacin, in the form of nicotinic acid, is an effective and inexpensive alternative to cholesterol-lowering drugs. Dosage should be prescribed by a doctor. Niacin may produce side effects, such as flushing and itching and gastrointestinal distress, and time-released niacin can be toxic to the liver.
Zinc	Boosts immunity, wards off colds, and improves sex drive.	Some studies have found that zinc taken at the onset of a cold can lessen its severity and that it can improve immune function in elderly people. High doses of zinc, however, may *suppress* immune function. There is no evidence that zinc supplements affect sexual performance.

SOURCE: *American Health,* July–August 1995.

have not been tested and proven safe. The FDA, alarmed by unproven claims for various vitamins and minerals, has begun clamping down on manufacturers who make unproven claims for these products, such as claiming that particular substances can delay or prevent aging.

Strategies for Prevention
....
Becoming a Smart Nutrition Consumer

✔ Don't believe everything you read. A quick way to spot a bad diet book is to look in the index for a diet to prevent or treat rheumatoid arthritis (none exists). If you find one, don't buy the book.

✔ Before you try any new nutritional approach, check with your doctor or a registered dietitian or call the ADA consumer hot line.

✔ Don't believe ads or advisers basing their nutritional recommendations on hair analysis, which is not accurate in detecting nutritional deficiencies.

✔ Be wary of anyone who recommends megadoses of vitamins or nutritional supplements, which can be dangerous. High doses of Vitamin A, which some people take to clear up acne, can be toxic.

✔ Question personal testimonies about the powers of some magical-seeming pill or powder, and be wary of "scientific articles" in journals that aren't reviewed by health professionals.

Making This Chapter Work for You
A Food Guide for the Twenty-First Century

■ Nutrition—the science that explores the connections between our bodies and the food we eat—has shown that our daily diet affects our long-term health prospects more than any other factor within our control.

■ Official nutrition advice is based on research, including epidemiological studies, which assess the dietary habits and health status of a particular population, and metabolic studies, which examine the effects of different nutrients in animal or human metabolism.

■ Health officials recommend that Americans reduce fat intake, eat more grains, fruits, and vegetables, and consume only moderate amounts of salt, sugar, and alcohol.

■ The USDA's Food Guide Pyramid reflects scientific recognition of the health benefits of complex carbohydrates (plant-based foods such as whole grains, vegetables, and fruits), which should form the core of our daily diet. Americans should eat fewer servings of animal products, such as dairy products, meats, poultry, and eggs. Added fats and sugars should be used sparingly.

■ The benefits of following the Food Guide Pyramid include less dietary fat, increased fiber, and more vitamins and minerals.

■ Saturated fats, found in meat and animal products, can increase the risk of heart disease and certain cancers, including those of the colon and breast. When converted to liquid form in vegetable oils, polyunsaturated fats form potentially harmful substances known as trans fatty acids. Monounsaturates, the most beneficial form of fat, are found in olive and canola oils. Dietary fats, especially saturated ones, can increase blood levels of cholesterol.

■ Fiber (found in whole grains, vegetables, and fruit) helps keep the intestines healthy and aids elimination; prevents diverticulosis; is low in calories; and may lessen the risks of certain illnesses, such as heart disease, colon cancer, and diabetes.

■ The Nutrition Labeling and Education Act requires food manufacturers to provide substantial information about fat, calories, and ingredients. Food labels must state serving size, calories per serving, fat per serving, daily values (the total amount of a nutrient that the average adult should not exceed on a daily basis), and percent daily values (an indication of how a particular food's nutrition content fits into a 2000-calorie diet).

■ Vitamins and minerals may play an important role in preventing disease. Certain antioxidant vitamins (particularly vitamin C, vitamin E, and beta carotene, a form of Vitamin A) may prevent damage to our cells by free radical oxygen molecules.

■ Most people eating a balanced diet don't need vitamin supplements. However, certain people may benefit from a supplement of folic acid, calcium, iron, or a multivitamin.

Health Online

■ Because of its rich cultural diversity, American diets include foods from many different countries, including China, Mexico, India, Italy, France, and Japan. Each type of cuisine has its own nutritional benefits and potential drawbacks.

■ An increasing number of people are cutting down on meats or adopting a vegetarian diet, which may or may not include dairy products, fish, or poultry.

■ Because of their concern about pesticides, some Americans prefer organic foods, even though there's no guarantee that these foods haven't been exposed to existing contaminants in the air, water, or soil.

■ Food safety has become an increasingly important issue because of the possible dangers of food-borne illnesses, additives, antibiotics and hormones in meat, pesticides, and irradiation.

■ Food allergies and nutritional gimmicks can also endanger health. In each case, you have to seek out available information, weigh the risks versus the benefits, and make the choices that seem best for your health.

After reading this chapter, you may well conclude that eating isn't simple anymore. You're right. Every time you grill bacon for breakfast, grab a quick cheeseburger for lunch, or heat up a burrito for dinner, you're making a choice that could have a long-term negative impact on your health. But responsibility for wise food choices extends beyond the individual. In studies of interventions designed to promote better nutrition, simple changes—such as adding more salads in a cafeteria or giving out informational literature in a supermarket— have led to healthful changes in individuals' food choices and eating habits. The more you learn about what you eat, the more likely you are to choose wisely and eat well.

While we must eat to live, eating can also bring a special joy and satisfaction to living. Here are some guidelines for eating for physical and psychological well-being:

- Eat with people whom you like.

- Talk only of pleasant things while eating.

- Eat slowly. Focus on the taste of each food you're eating.

- When you eat, eat—don't write, work, or talk on the phone.

- Eat because you're hungry, not to change how you feel.

- After eating, take time to be quiet and rest.

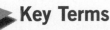

Key Terms

The terms listed here are used within the chapter. Page numbers are included for each term.
A definition of each term is given in the green Glossary pages at the end of this book.

additives   *175*

amino acids   *171*

antitoxidants   *163*

botulism   *177*

calorie   *161*

carbohydrates   *152*

cholesterol   *158*

complementary proteins   *171*

complete proteins   *171*

complex carbohydrates   *152*

crucifers   *155*

E. coli   *176*

fat-soluble vitamins   *168*

fiber   *158*

food allergies   *162*

food toxicologists   *174*

hemoglobin   *166*

incomplete proteins   *171*

indoles   *155*

irradiation   *174*

lacto-vegetarians   *171*

minerals   *162*

nutrients   *150*

nutrition   *149*

organic   *174*

ovo-lacto-vegetarians   *171*

phytochemicals   *166*

protein   *155*

saturated fat   *158*

simple carbohydrates   *152*

trans fats   *158*

unsaturated fat   *158*

vegans   *171*

vitamins   *162*

Review Questions

1. List at least six guidelines for a healthy diet. Why are these important?

2. What nutrients are necessary to maintain a healthy body? Give examples of good sources of each.

3. What food groups make up the Food Guide Pyramid? How many servings of each should you eat each day? How many do you eat?

4. How can diet help prevent cancer? reduce the risk of heart disease?

5. What types of people would benefit from vitamin supplements? What are the dangers of taking megadoses of vitamins or minerals?

6. What are the advantages of using pesticides and food additives? What dangers are associated with the use of pesticides? With additives? Do you think it's a good idea to eat organic foods? Why or why not?

Critical Thinking Questions

1. Scientists are using genetic engineering to develop foods, such as tomatoes that won't bruise easily, cows that will produce more milk, or corn that will grow larger ears. Some consumer advocates argue that these items shouldn't be put on the market because they haven't been studied carefully enough. What do you think of these foods? Would you eat them?

2. Which alternative or ethnic diet do you think has the best-tasting food? Which is the most healthy? Why?

3. Is it possible to meet nutritional requirements on a limited budget? Have you ever been in this situation? What would you recommend to someone who wanted to eat healthfully on $30 a week?

4. Consider the number of times a week you eat fast food. How much money would you have saved if you had eaten home-prepared meals? What different foods from the bottom levels of the Food Guide Pyramid might you have eaten instead?

Connections to Personal Health Interactive

To enhance your understanding of the material covered in this chapter, check out the following study aids on the **Personal Health Interactive CD-ROM**. *Each numbered icon within the chapter corresponds to an appropriate activity listed here.*

6.1 Personal Insights: How Nutritious Is Your Diet?

6.2 Point of View: Dietician

6.3 Chapter 6 Review

 References

1. Center for Science in the Public Interest, American Cancer Society, et al. *Prescription: Good Nutrition.* Washington, DC: Center for Science in the Public Interest, 1994.
2. Henkel, John. "Genetic Engineering: Fast Forwarding to Future Foods." *FDA Consumer*, Vol. 29, No. 3, April 1995.
3. Center for Science in the Public Interest.
4. Ann Shaw. Personal interview.
5. Douglas, Kathy, et al. "Results from the 1995 National College Health Risk Behavior Survey." *Journal of American College Health*, Vol. 46, September 1997.
6. "Nutrition Revolution." *University of California, Berkeley Wellness Letter*, Vol. 13, No. 12, September 1997.
7. "More Evidence for Antioxidants." *Harvard Women's Health Watch*, Vol. 2, No. 5, January 1995.
8. Uauy-Dagach, Ricardo, and Alfonso Valenzuela. "Marine Oils: The Health Benefits of n-3 Fatty Acids." *Nutrition Reviews*, Vol. 54, No. 11, November 1996. Nair, Sudheera, et al. "Prevention of Cardiac Arrhythmia by Dietary (n-3) Polyunsaturated Fatty Acids and Their Mechanisms of Action." *Journal of Nutrition*, Vol. 127, No. 3, March 1997.
9. Conkling, Winifred. "Water: How Much Do We Need?" *American Health*, May 1995.
10. Ibid.
11. Wolk, Alijca. "Dietary Fat Intake and the Risk of Breast Cancer in Women." *Archives of Internal Medicine*, January 1998.
12. Hu, Frank, et al. "Dietary Fat Intake and the Risk of Coronary Heart Disease in Women." *New England Journal of Medicine*, Vol. 337, No. 21, November 20, 1997.
13. Brody, Jane. "Making Sense of Latest Twist on Fat in the Diet." *New York Times*, November 25, 1997.
14. "What the Experts Say about Olean." Procter & Gamble Press Information, February 1998.
15. Callaway, Wayne. "Reexamining Cholesterol and Sodium Recommendations." *Nutrition Today*, Vol. 29, No. 5, September–October 1994.
16. The Writing Group for the DISC Collaborative Research Group. "Efficacy and Safety of Lowering Dietary Intake of Fat and Cholesterol in Children with Elevated Low-Density Lipoprotein Cholesterol." *Journal of the American Medical Association*, Vol. 273, No. 18, May 10, 1995.
17. Elash, Anita. "Powerful Grains and Beans." *Maclean's*, Vol. 110, No. 43, October 27, 1997.
18. Hunter, Beatrice. "The Neglected Wholegrains." *Consumers' Research Magazine*, Vol. 80, No. 7, July 1997. Maki, Kevin, et al. "Fiber Intake and Risk of Developing Non-Insulin-Dependent Diabetes Mellitus." *Journal of the American Medical Association*, Vol. 277, No. 22, June 11, 1997. Salmeron, Jorge, et al. "Dietary Fiber, Glycemic Load, and Risk of Non-Insulin-Dependent Diabetes Mellitus in Women." *Journal of the American Medical Association*, Vol. 277, No. 6, February 12, 1997.
19. Mee, Karen, and David Gee. "Apple Fiber and Gum Arabic Lowers Total and Low-Density Lipoprotein Cholesterol Levels in Men with Mild Hypercholesterolemia." *Journal of the American Dietetic Association*, Vol. 97, No. 4, April 1997.
20. Byrd-Bredbenner, Carol. "Designing a Consumer Friendly Nutrition Label." *Journal of Nutrition Education*, Vol. 26, No. 4, July–August 1994. Lytle, Victoria. "What's Behind the New Food Labels?" *NEA Today*, Vol. 13, No. 2, September 15, 1994. DeVries, Jonathon, and Amy Nelson. "Meeting Analytical Needs for Nutrition Labeling." *Food Technology,* Vol. 48, No. 7, July 1994. Mermelstein, Neil H. "Nutrition Labeling Regulatory Update." *Food Technology*, Vol. 48, No. 7, July 1994.
21. Kurtzweil, Paula. "Scouting for Sodium: and Other Nutrients Important to Blood Pressure." *FDA Consumer*, Vol. 28, No. 7, September 1994.
22. "Changes in Meat and Poultry Nutrition Labeling Regulations: Implications for Nutrition Educators." *Journal of Nutrition Education*, Vol. 26, No. 1, January–February 1994.
23. Mertz, Walter. "A Balanced Approach to Nutrition for

Health: The Need for Biologically Essential Minerals and Vitamins." *Journal of the American Dietetic Association,* Vol. 94, No. 11, November 1994.

24. Butler, Robert. "Vitamin E Supplements." *Geriatrics*, Vol. 52, No. 7, July 1997.

25. Norvell, C. "Have You Had Your Antioxidants Today?"

26. Blumberg, Jeffrey. "Do Antioxidants Reduce Disease?" *American Health*, May 1994.

27. Horton, Richard. "Reversing Risk In Coronary Disease." *Lancet*, Vol. 344, No. 8935, November 26, 1994.

28. Brody, Jane. "In Vitamin Mania, Millions Take a Gamble on Health." *New York Times*, October 26, 1997.

29. Lewis, Ricki. "Dietary Supplements: What Are the Risks?" *The 1998 World Book Health & Medical Annual.* Chicago: World Book, 1998.

30. Fleet, James. "Dietary Selenium Repletion May Reduce Cancer Incidence in People at High Risk Who Live in Areas with Low Soil Selenium." *Nutrition Reviews*, Vol. 55, No. 7, July 1997.

31. Barone, Jeanine. "Foods:The Best Source for Nutrients." *The 1998 World Book Health & Medical Annual.* Chicago: World Book, 1998.

32. "Selenium May Prevent Some Cancers in Patients with History of Skin Cancer." *Geriatrics*, Vol. 52, No. 2, February 1997.

33. Powers, Mike. "The Folate Debate." *Human Ecology Forum*, Vol. 25, No. 2, July–August 1997.

34. Prince, Richard. "Diet and the Prevention of Osteoporotic Fracture." *New England Journal of Medicine*, Vol. 227, No. 10, September 4, 1997.

35. National Institutes of Health Consensus Development Panel on Optimal Calcium Intake. "Optimal Calcium Intake." *Journal of the American Medical Association,* Vol. 272, No. 24, December 28, 1994. Denny, Sharon. "Getting the Facts About Food Myths." *Current Health*, Vol. 21, No. 3, November 1994.

36. Ann Shaw. Personal interview.

37. Liebmann-Smith, Richard. "Moo Shu Porky." *American Health*, November 1993.

38. Simopoulos, Artemis P. "The Mediterranean Food Guide: Greek Column Rather Than Egyptian Pyramid." *Nutrition Today,* Vol. 30, No. 2, April 1995.

39. Englebardt, Stanley. "Eat, Drink, and Go Back to Work." *American Health*, June 1994.

40. Block, Gladys, et al. "Sources of Energy and Six Nutrients in Diets of Low-Income Hispanic-American Women and Their Children: Quantitative Data from HHANES, 1982–1984." *Journal of the American Dietetic Association,* Vol. 95, No. 2, February 1995.

41. Kolata, Gina. "F.D.A., Saying Process Is Safe, Approves Irradiating Red Meat." *New York Times*, December 3, 1997.

42. Gavzer, Bernard. "We Can Make Our Food Safer." *Parade*, October 19, 1997.

43. Stoeckle, Mark, and Douglas R. Gordon. "Infectious Diseases." *Journal of the American Medical Association,* Vol. 273, No. 13, June 7, 1995.

CHAPTER 7

EATING PATTERNS AND PROBLEMS

After studying the material in this chapter, you should be able to:

Describe three different methods for determining your ideal body weight.

Identify several factors that influence food consumption.

Identify and **describe** the symptoms and dangers associated with abnormal eating behaviors and eating disorders.

Define obesity and **describe** its relationship to genetics, lifestyle, and major health problems.

Explain how health problems are created by fad diets.

Design a personal plan for sensible weight management.

America is turning into the land of the large. According to federal statistics, 35% of all Americans aged 20 and older are **obese**; that is, they weigh at least 20% more than they should. Even children are getting heavier. The percentage of youngsters aged 6 to 11 who are overweight increased from 11% in the late 1970s to 14% in the mid-1990s.[1]

Ironically, as average weights have increased, the quest for thinness has become a national obsession. In a society in which slimmer is seen as better, anyone who is less than lean may feel like a failure. Individuals—especially young women—who are overweight or embarrassed by their appearance often assume that they would be happier, sexier, or more successful in thinner bodies. And so they diet. At any given time, 33% to 40% of women and 20% to 24% of men are trying to lose weight. Another 28% of all adults are trying to maintain a weight loss—usually without success.[2]

This chapter explores our national preoccupation with slimness; examines unhealthy eating patterns and eating disorders; explains what obesity is and why excess pounds are dangerous; shows why fad diets don't work; and tells how to control weight safely, sensibly, and permanently. (See Self-Survey.)

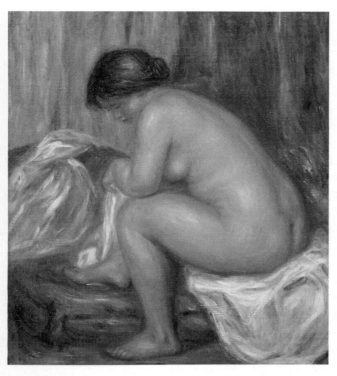

The body beautiful. "Thinner is better" is not the worldwide standard, and in past centuries more flesh rather than less was considered healthy and beautiful. This painting by Renoir, from the late 1880s, shows a more rounded feminine ideal.

Body Image

Throughout most of history, bigger was better. The great beauties of centuries past, as painted by such artistic masters as Rubens and Renoir, were soft and fleshy, with rounded bellies and dimpled thighs. Many developing countries still regard a full figure, rather than a thin one, as the ideal standard for health and beauty. "Fattening huts," in which brides-to-be eat extra food to plump up before marriage, still exist in some African cultures. Among certain Native Americans of the Southwest, if a girl is thin at puberty, a fat woman places her foot on the girl's back so she will magically gain weight and become more attractive.

On the eve of the 21st century in the United States, men and women are paying more attention to their body image than ever before. "We've become a nation of appearance junkies and fitness zealots driven to think, talk, strategize, and worry about our bodies with the same fanatical devotion we applied to putting a man on the moon," says psychologist Judith Rodin, Ph.D.[3] Such self-absorption can affect self-esteem and confidence and lead to a preoccupation with weight and potentially dangerous forms of dieting.[4]

Even though studies show that men don't necessarily consider the slimmest women the most attractive, young women—especially white women—grow up thinking that thin is better.[5] African-American women often have more positive attitudes toward their bodies, feeling more satisfied with their weight and seeing themselves as more attractive.[6] However, there are no significant differences between African-American and white women *dieters* in terms of self-esteem and body dissatisfaction.[7]

A preoccupation with weight and appearance, in and of itself, can be harmful. "The quest for the perfect body is, like most wars, a costly one—emotionally and physically, to say nothing of financially," notes psychologist Rodin, who argues that "what your body really needs is moderate exercise, healthy foods, sensual pleasures, and relaxation. Give it those, and it will respond by treating you better." And, in the process, you'll feel better about yourself.

What Should You Weigh?

Many factors determine what you weigh: heredity, eating behavior, food selection, amount of daily exercise. For any individual of a given height, there is no single best weight, but a range of healthy weights. The traditional weight tables prepared by the insurance industry relate weight and height to how long policyholders live, not to their health, vitality, or appearance. The 1990 government recommendations for healthy body weights allowed higher weights for men and women over age 35. However, recent studies have shown that men and women whose weights rise as they age face increased risks to their health and longevity.

Given the different interpretations and views of ideal body weight, many specialists in eating disorders rely on standardized tables that give healthy ranges of **Body-Mass Index (BMI)**, a standard index assessing the ratio of a person's weight to height (Figure 7-1). A body mass below 19 indicates the slimness end of the spectrum, while one above 29 represents obesity. Individuals with a Body Mass Index below 19 have been shown to have the lowest long-term health risks, while the relative risk of premature death increases as body mass increases (Table 7-1).

Another way of assessing weight is by measuring body fat. The lowest health risks are associated with a body fat percentage of weight below 20 for men and 25 for women. Body fat may be assessed in different ways. **Skin calipers**, which pinch skin folds at the arms, waist, and back, are the most widely used, although they may be less accurate than other techniques. Proper use of these instruments by trained personnel is critical in getting a precise reading. **Hydrostatic weighing**—weighing a person in water to distinguish buoyant fat from denser muscle—is far more precise. Other methods include whole-body counting, which measures the total amount of K-40, a naturally occurring form of potassium found primarily in lean tissue; imaging methods, such as computerized tomography (CT) and magnetic resonance imaging (MRI); ultrasonography, which uses high-frequency sound waves; and bioelectrical impedance assessment (BIA), which measures the resistance of the body to a flow of alternating electric current.

The distribution of weight and the location of fat storage also are important. Fat at the hips, which is more common in women and more difficult to lose than abdominal fat, is stored primarily for special purposes, such as extra energy needs during pregnancy and nursing. Abdominal fat seems more dangerous. The bigger the waist and belly, the higher the risk of various diseases, such as diabetes, heart disease, and stroke. Figure 7-2 illustrates how to calculate your waist-to-hip ratio.

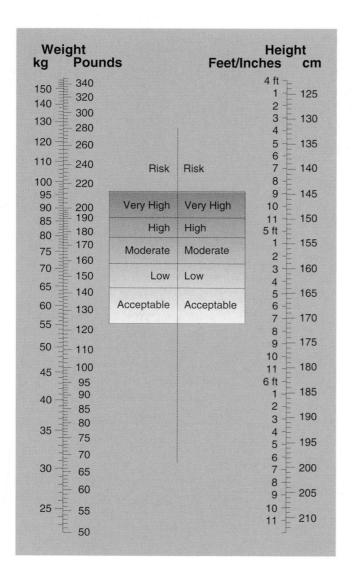

Figure 7-1

Calculating your body mass index (BMI) and risk. To find out if your current level of body fat increases your health risks, draw a straight line from your weight to your height. Your level of risk is determined by where you cross the center line. Beware, too, that at the bottom of the "acceptable" range, health risks begin to increase again.

TABLE 7-1 DO YOU WEIGH TOO MUCH?

Thinner is usually better, but obesity can be fatal, according to a Harvard study of 115,000 women published in the *New England Journal of Medicine*. Figuring out where you stand requires calculating a single number—your body-mass index—so that those with different heights can be compared.

Calculating Your Body-Mass Index

A. Multiply your weight in pounds by .45 to get kilograms.

B. Convert your height to inches and multiply this number by .0254 to get meters.

C. Multiply your height number by itself.

D. Divide this into your weight in kilograms.

A woman 5 feet 4 inches tall weighing 110 pounds:

A.
$$110 \times .45 = 49.5$$

B. 5'4" = 64"
$$64 \times .0254 = 1.6256$$

C.
$$1.6256 \times 1.6256 = 2.64257536$$

D.
$$\frac{49.5}{2.64257536} = 18.7$$

would have a body-mass of 19. If she weighed 140 pounds, her body-mass index would be 24, and if she weighed 186 pounds, her index would be 32.

A woman 5 feet 7 inches tall weighing 160 pounds:

A.
$$160 \times .45 = 72$$

B. 5'7" = 67"
$$67 \times .0254 = 1.7018$$

C.
$$1.7018 \times 1.7018 = 2.8961232$$

D.
$$\frac{72}{2.8961232} = 24.9$$

would have a body-mass index of 24.9. If she weighed 180 pounds, her index would be 28, and if she weighed 195 pounds, her body-mass index would be 30.3.

Where You Stand

The study found that middle-aged women whose body-mass indexes were below 19 had the lowest risk of premature dealth.

19 and below	Lowest risk
19 to 24.9	20 percent higher
25 to 26.9	30 percent higher
27 to 28.9	60 percent higher
Over 29	100 percent higher

SOURCES: *New England Journal of Medicine*, Dr. Thomas P. Bersot, Gladstone Institute of Cardiovascular Disease.

Strategies for Change

Rethinking Your Weight Goals

Regardless of what you weigh, chances are that in your mind's eye you're fatter than you are in reality—or fatter than you want to be. Stop looking at your bathroom scale or in your mirror, and look inside. Answer these questions as honestly as you can:

✔ If you could choose your weight, what would it be? Why? At what weight do you have enough energy to make it through an average day, yet not feel hungry all the time?

✔ What's the weight range that's best for your height and body-frame size? How does this compare with what you consider your ideal weight? (See Table 7-2 for a formula to use in calculating your ideal weight.)

✔ What do you think is a realistic weight for you to strive for? Have you ever gotten to, and stayed at, this weight? If you had to choose between the weight that was best for your health and the one you thought most attractive, which would you choose? Why?

✔ Is there a middle weight for which you could strive?

Calories: How Many Do You Need?

Calories are the measure of the amount of energy that can be derived from food. Science defines a **calorie** as the amount of energy required to raise the temperature

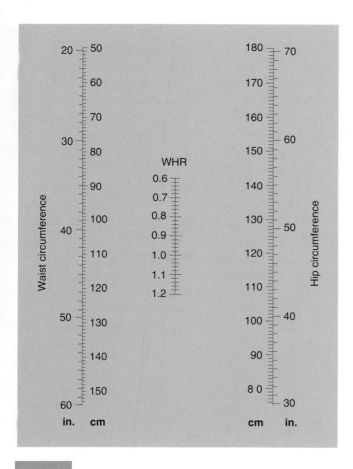

Figure 7-2
Determining waist-to-hip ratio (WHR). Use a straightedge to draw a
line from your waist circumference (left) to your hip circumference
(right). The point at which the line crosses the center column is
your WHR.

Sources: Data from Gray, G. A., and D. S. Gray. "Obesity: Part 1:
Pathenogensis." *Western Journal of Medicine*, Vol. 149, 1988. In Christian,
Janet, and Janet Greger. *Nutrition for Living*, 4th ed. Redwood City, CA:
Benjamin Cummings, 1994.

of 1 gram of water by one degree Celsius. In the laboratory, the caloric content of food is measured in 1000-
calorie units called *kilocalories*. The calorie referred to in
everyday usage is actually the equivalent of the laboratory kilocalorie. (The Hales Health Almanac at the back
of this book contains calorie counts for many foods.)

The number of calories you need every day
depends on your gender, age, size, and activity level. An
"average" adult woman—with a median height of 5'4"
and a weight of 138 pounds—generally needs 1900 to
2200 calories. An average man—with a median height of
5'10" and a weight of 174 pounds—generally consumes
2300 to 2900 calories. How many calories you need
depends on your gender, age, body-frame size, weight,

percentage of body fat, and your **basal metabolic rate
(BMR)**—the number of calories needed to sustain your
body at rest.

Your activity level also affects your calorie requirements. Regardless of whether you consume fat, protein,
or carbohydrates, if you take in more calories than
required to maintain your size and don't work them off

**TABLE 7-2 CALCULATING YOUR
IDEAL WEIGHT**

Here are two widely used formulas for calculating your
ideal weight, based on body-fat percentages of less than
20% for men and less than 26% for women. For men, the
first formula is as follows:

Height (in inches) × 4 − 128 = Ideal Weight

If you have a large frame, add 10% to the total. Thus, a 6'
tall man with a large frame would make the following
calculations:

72 × 4 = 288
288 − 128 = 160
160 × 0.10 = 16
160 + 16 = 176 pounds, Ideal Weight

For women, the formula is slightly different:

Height (in inches) × 3.5 − 108 = Ideal Weight

A 5' 4" woman with a medium frame would perform
these calculations:

64 × 3.5 = 224
224 − 108 = 116 pounds, Ideal Weight

The second, even simpler formula for men is to allow
106 pounds for the first 5 feet of height, and to add 6
pounds for each additional inch thereafter. Thus, for a 6'
man, the calculations would be as follows:

106 + (12 × 6) = 106 + 72 = 178 pounds, Ideal Weight

The second formula for women is to allow 100 pounds
for the first 5 feet of height, and to add 5 pounds for
each additional inch thereafter. For a 5' 4" woman, the
calculations would be as follows.

100 + (4 × 5) = 100 + 20 = 120 pounds, Ideal Weight

Notice that the results from applying these two formulas
don't match perfectly: this underscores the fact that there
is a range of at least 5–10 pounds in the ideal weight for
every height.

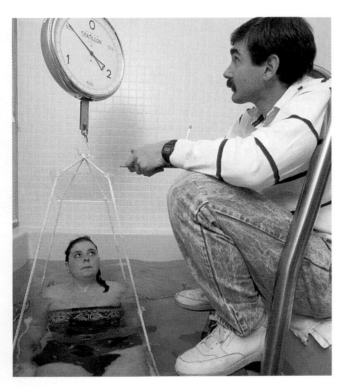

Measuring body fat. The most accurate way of measuring body fat is hydrostatic weighing in an immersion tank.

in some sort of physical activity, your body will convert the excess to fat (Table 7-3).

Hunger, Satiety, and Set Point

Why do you wake up starving or feel your stomach rumbling during a late afternoon lecture? The simple answer is **hunger**: the physiological drive to consume food. More than a dozen different signals may influence and control our desire for food. Researchers at the National Institutes of Health have discovered appetite receptors within the hypothalamus region of the brain that specifically respond to hunger messages carried by chemicals. Hormones, including insulin and stress-related epinephrine (adrenaline), may also stimulate or suppress hunger. Even the size of our fat cells may affect how hungry we feel. (Many overweight people have fat cells two to two-and-a-half times larger than normal.)

Appetite—the psychological desire to eat—usually begins with the fear of the unpleasant sensation of hunger. We learn to avoid hunger by eating a certain amount of food at certain times of the day, just as dogs in the laboratory learn to avoid electric shocks by jump-

ing at the sound of a warning bell. But appetite is easily led into temptation. In one famous experiment, psychologists bought bags of high-calorie goodies—peanut butter, marshmallows, chocolate-chip cookies, and salami—for their test rats. The animals ate so much on this "supermarket diet" that they gained more weight than any laboratory rats ever had before. The snack-food diet that fattened up these rats was particularly high in fats. Biologists speculate that creamy, buttery, or greasy foods may cause internal changes that increase appetite and, consequently, weight.

We stop eating when we feel satisfied; this is called **satiety**, a feeling of fullness and relief from hunger. According to the **set-point theory**, each individual has an unconscious control system for regulating appetite and satiety to keep body fat at a predetermined level, or *set point*. If our fat stores fall too low, our appetite gnaws at us, so we eat more. Conversely, appetite subsides if we overeat.

From this perspective, diets are doomed to fail because they pit the dieter against tireless internal enemies: the set point and its enforcer, appetite. The only

TABLE 7-3   HOW MANY CALORIES DO YOU NEED DAILY?

Desirable Weight (lb)	High Activity	Medium Activity	Low Activity
Women			
99	1700	1500	1300
110	1850	1650	1400
121	2000	1750	1550
128	2100	1900	1600
132	2150	1950	1650
143	2300	2050	1800
154	2400	2150	1850
165	2550	2300	1950
Men			
121	2400	2150	1850
132	2550	2300	1950
143	2700	2400	2050
154	2900	2600	2200
165	3100	2800	2400
176	3250	2950	2500
187	3300	3100	2600

CAMPUS FOCUS: EATING BEHAVIORS ON CAMPUS

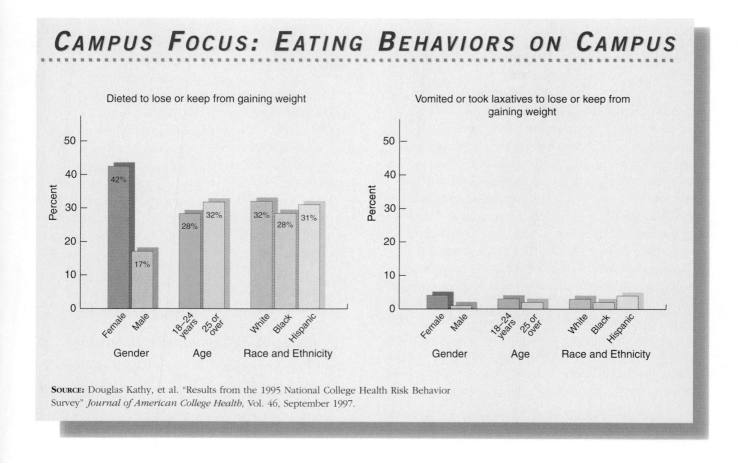

SOURCE: Douglas Kathy, et al. "Results from the 1995 National College Health Risk Behavior Survey" *Journal of American College Health*, Vol. 46, September 1997.

effective alternative is lowering, or resetting, the set point. And the safest, most effective way to do so is through physical activity, which dampens appetite in the short run and lowers the set point for the long term. Moderate activity not only works up an appetite but also helps work it off.

Unhealthy Eating Behavior

Sooner or later many people *don't* eat the way they should. They may skip meals, thereby increasing the likelihood that they'll end up with more body fat, a higher weight, and a higher blood cholesterol level. Others live on "diet" foods, but consume so much of them that they gain weight anyway. Yet others engage in more extreme forms of what health professionals call "disordered eating." They continuously go on and off diets, eat compulsively, or binge on high-fat treats. Such behaviors can be warning signs of potentially serious eating disorders that should not be ignored.[9]

College students—particularly women—are at risk for unhealthy eating behaviors. As Campus Focus: Eating Behaviors on Campus shows, about one in five undergraduates is overweight. Among women, 42.1% have dieted to lose or keep from gaining weight; 16.7% of the men have done the same. Seven % of undergraduate women have taken diet pills; 4.2% have vomited or used laxatives for weight control.[10]

The prevalence of disordered eating symptoms and eating disorders has increased dramatically in the last 20 years. In some studies as many as 64% of college women have reported at least one unhealthy eating behavior. One reason may be the pressure some young women feel to attain what some have called the "Super Woman" ideal. As they try to excel in multiple roles, they diet, induce vomiting, or restrict food intake for the sake of meeting their idealized standards for appearance.[11] Sorority women, some researchers have found, may have an even greater fear of becoming fat. They tend to be more dissatisfied with their bodies and are more concerned with weight and dieting than college women in general.[12]

Extreme Dieting

As members of a National Institutes of Health (NIH) Technology Assessment Conference Panel observed, there is a health paradox when it comes to dieting in America: "On the one hand, many people who do not need to lose weight are trying to. On the other hand, most who do need to lose weight are not succeeding."[13] Only one of every ten women who diet does so for health reasons; the others do so to look better or feel better about themselves. Yet dieting itself can do more harm than good, causing serious vitamin and mineral deficiencies and, in some cases, increasing a person's relative risk of dying by about 1.5 to 2.5 times.[14]

"Extreme" dieters go beyond cutting back on calories or increasing physical activity and become preoccupied with what they eat and weigh. Although their weight never falls below 85% of normal, their weight loss is severe enough to cause uncomfortable physical consequences, such as weakness and sensitivity to cold. Technically, these dieters do not have *anorexia nervosa* (discussed later in the chapter), but they are at increased risk for it.

Extreme dieters may think they know a great deal about nutrition, yet many of their beliefs about food and weight are misconceptions or myths. For instance, they may eat only protein because they believe complex carbohydrates, including fruits and breads, are fattening. When they're anxious, angry, or bored, they focus on food and their fear of fatness. Dieting and exercise become ways of coping with any stress in their lives.

Sometimes nutritional education alone can help change this eating pattern. However, many avid dieters who deny that they have a problem with food may need counseling (which they usually agree to only at their family's insistence) to correct dangerous eating behavior and prevent further complications.

Compulsive Overeating

Individuals who eat compulsively cannot stop putting food in their mouths. They eat fast; they eat a lot; they eat even when they're full; and they may eat round the clock rather than at set meal times—often in private because of embarrassment over how much they consume.

Some mental health professionals describe compulsive eating as a food addiction that is much more likely to develop in women. According to Overeaters Anonymous (OA), an international support agency, many women who eat compulsively view food as a source of comfort against feelings of inner emptiness, low self-esteem, and fear of abandonment.

Recovery from compulsive eating can be challenging because people with this problem cannot give up entirely the "substance" they abuse. Like everyone else, they must eat. However, they can learn new eating habits and ways of dealing with underlying emotional problems. An OA survey found that most of its members joined to lose weight but later felt the most important effect was their improved emotional, mental, and physical health. As one woman put it, "I came for vanity but stayed for sanity."

Strategies for Change

Recognizing Compulsive Overeating

The following behaviors may signal a potential problem:

✔ Turning to food when depressed or lonely, when feeling rejected, or as a reward.

✔ A history of failed diets and anxiety when dieting.

✔ Thinking about food throughout the day.

✔ Eating quickly and without pleasure.

✔ Frequent talking about food, or refusing to talk about food.

✔ Fear of not being able to stop eating once you start. Continuing to eat even when you're no longer hungry.

Binge Eating

Binge eating—the rapid consumption of an abnormally large amount of food in a relatively short time—often occurs in compulsive eaters. Individuals with a binge-eating disorder typically eat a larger-than-ordinary amount of food during a relatively brief period, feel a lack of control over eating, and binge at least twice a week for at least a six-month period. During most of these episodes, individuals experience at least three of the following:

• Eating much more rapidly than usual.

• Eating until they feel uncomfortably full.

• Eating large amounts of food when not feeling physically hungry.

- Eating large amounts of food throughout the day with no planned mealtimes.

- Eating alone because they are embarrassed by how much they eat and by their eating habits.

It is not clear whether dieting leads to binge eating—or vice versa.[15] Binge-eaters may spend up to several hours eating, and consume 2000 or more calories-worth of food in a single binge—more than many people eat in a day. After such binges, they usually do not induce vomiting, use laxatives, or rely on other means (such as exercise) to control weight. They simply get fatter. As their weight climbs, they become depressed, anxious, or troubled by other psychological symptoms to a much greater extent than others of comparable weight.[16]

About 2% of Americans—some 5 million in all—may have binge-eating disorder.[17] It is most common among young women in college and, increasingly, in high school. Persons who binge-eat may require professional help to change their behavior. Treatment includes education, behavioral approaches, cognitive therapy, and psychotherapy. As they recognize the reasons for their behavior and begin to confront the underlying issues, individuals usually are able to resume normal eating patterns.

Food Cravings

A food craving is an intense desire for a specific food. Some individuals may crave certain substances because of a nutritional need. Pregnancy is one period during which this can occur. For instance, a pregnant woman may want pickles because her body needs salt to maintain a proper balance of fluids. Cravings also may be based on brain chemistry. Some researchers speculate that certain foods stimulate the release of specific neurotransmitters in the brain.

Most food cravings are normal. Some women crave sweets before or during their menstrual periods. The association of a place with a particular food can induce a craving, such as a yearning for a hot dog at a ballpark—a perfectly normal behavior. The most craved foods are chocolate and ice cream, followed by fatty and spicy foods and sweets.[18] However, some cravings may be symptoms of undetected illnesses. A constant thirst, for instance, may be an early sign of diabetes; sometimes a desire for ice is a symptom of anemia.

Eating Disorders

Just a few decades ago there was no official psychiatric diagnosis for behaviors that are now collectively called **eating disorders**, the most common of which are anorexia nervosa and bulimia nervosa. Even though these problems involve food, researchers increasingly view them as "dieting disorders" that affect and are affected by a person's body image and that can threaten psychological and physical well-being.[19] (Table 7-4 lists the medical complications of eating disorders.)

TABLE 7-4   MEDICAL COMPLICATIONS OF EATING DISORDERS

Related to Weight Loss

Loss of fat and muscle mass, including heart muscle

Increased sensitivity to cold

Irregular heartbeats

Bloating, constipation, abdominal pain

Amenorrhea (absence of menstruation)

Growth of fine babylike hair over body

Abnormal taste sensations

Osteoporosis

Depression

Sudden death

Related to Purging

Abnormal levels of crucial chemicals

Inflammation of the salivary glands and pancreas

Erosion of the esophagus and stomach

Severe abdominal pain

Erosion and decay of dental enamel, particularly of front teeth

Fatigue and weakness

Seizures

SOURCES: Hales, Robert, et al. *American Psychiatric Press Textbook of Psychiatry*, 3rd ed. Washington, DC: American Psychiatric Press, 1998.

If someone you know has an eating disorder, let your friend know you're concerned and that you care. Don't criticize or make fun of his or her eating habits. Encourage your friend to talk about other problems and feelings, and suggest that he or she talk to the school counselor or someone at the mental health center, the family doctor, or another trusted adult. Offer to go along if you think that will make a difference.

Anorexia Nervosa

Although *anorexia* means loss of appetite, most individuals with **anorexia nervosa** are, in fact, hungry all the time. For them, food is an enemy—a threat to their sense of self, identity, and autonomy. In the distorted mirror of their mind's eye, they see themselves as fat or flabby even at a normal or below-normal body weight.

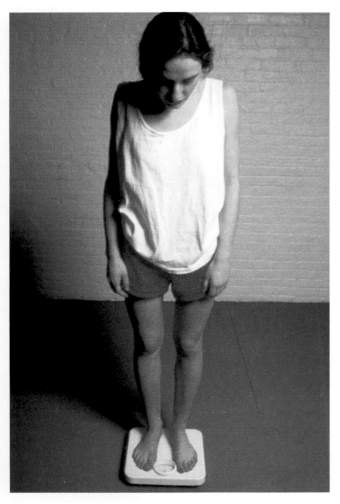

Anorexia nervosa is complex in its causes, and successful treatment usually involves medical, nutritional, and behavioral therapy.

Some simply feel fat; others think that they are thin in some places and too fat in others, such as the abdomen, buttocks, or thighs.

The incidence of anorexia nervosa has increased in the last three decades in most developed countries. An estimated 0.5 to 1% of young women in their late teens and early twenties develop anorexia. According to the American Psychiatric Association (APA)'s Work Group on Eating Disorders, cases are increasing among males, minorities, women of all ages, and possibly preteens. Anorexia usually develops between the ages of 10 and 30; the average age at onset is 17. Ninety % of all individuals with anorexia nervosa are women.[20]

In the *restricting* type of anorexia, individuals lose weight by avoiding any fatty foods, and by dieting, fasting, and exercising.[21] Some start smoking as a way of controlling their weight.[22] In the *binge eating/purging* type, they engage in binge eating, purging (through self-induced vomiting, laxatives, diuretics, or enemas), or both. Obsessed with an intense fear of fatness, they may weigh themselves several times a day, measure various parts of their body, check mirrors to see if they look fat, and try on different items of clothing to see if they feel tight.

The causes of anorexia nervosa are complex; genetic, biochemical, and developmental factors may play a role.[23] Its consequences are serious: Menstrual periods stop in women; testosterone levels decline in men. Adolescents with this disorder do not undergo normal sexual maturation, such as breast development, and may not reach their anticipated height. Even individuals who look and feel reasonably healthy may have subtle or hidden abnormalities, including heart irregularities and arrhythmias that can increase their risk of sudden death. Women who do not menstruate for six months or more may develop osteoporosis and suffer irreversible weakening and thinning of their bones as a result.[24]

Even when they realize that they are jeopardizing their health, people with anorexia tend to fear that treatment will make them worse—that is, fatter. They need repeated reassurance that they will not become overweight and that they can and will find healthier ways of coping with life.

According to current practice guidelines, treatment of anorexia nervosa includes medical therapy (such as "refeeding" to overcome malnutrition) and behavioral, cognitive, psychodynamic, and family therapy (described in Chapter 4). Antidepressant medication sometimes can help, particularly when there is a personal or family history of depression. Most people who get help do return to normal weight, but it can take a long time for their eating behaviors to become normal and for them to deal with troubling body image issues.[25]

Strategies for Change

••••••••••••••••••••••••••••••••••••

Recognizing Anorexia Nervosa

The characteristics of anorexia nervosa include:

✔ A refusal to maintain normal body weight.

✔ An intense fear of gaining weight or becoming fat, even though underweight.

✔ A distorted body image, so that the person feels fat even when emaciated.

✔ In women, the absence of at least three menstrual cycles.

Bulimia Nervosa

Individuals with **bulimia nervosa** go on repeated eating binges and rapidly consume large amounts of food, usually sweets, stopping only because of severe abdominal pain or sleep, or because they are interrupted. Those with *purging* bulimia induce vomiting or take large doses of laxatives to relieve guilt and control their weight. In *non-purging* bulimia, individuals use other means, such as fasting or excessive exercise, to compensate for binges.[26]

According to the DSM-IV, 1 to 3% of adolescent and young American women develop bulimia. Among female college students, 4 out of 100 are bulimic.[27] Some experiment with bingeing and purging for a few months and then stop when they change their social or living situation. Others—an estimated 1 to 3% of adolescent and young adult females—develop longer-term bulimia. Among males, this disorder is about one-tenth as common. The average age for developing bulimia is 18.[28]

Many factors, including psychological, developmental, and biochemical influences, can contribute to bulimia nervosa.[29] This disorder often begins after a rigid diet of several weeks to a year that may have altered brain chemistry in such a way as to disrupt the normal mechanisms for appetite and satiety. Because they're so distressed when they break their diet and binge, dieters

may begin to purge. Once they realize that vomiting reduces the anxiety triggered by gorging, they no longer fear overeating and fall into a regular binge–purge habit. (See Personal Voices: "I'm Not 'Pudge' Anymore.")

Bulimia may continue for many years, with binges alternating with periods of normal eating. Often dentists are the first to detect bulimia because they notice damage to teeth and gums, including erosion of the enamel from the stomach acids in vomit. Repeated vomiting can lead to other complications as it robs the body of essential nutrients and fluids, causes dehydration and electrolyte imbalances, and impairs the ability of the heart and other muscles to function. Bulimia can trigger cardiac arrhythmias and, occasionally, sudden death.[30]

Most mental health professionals treat bulimia with a combination of nutritional counseling, psychodynamic, cognitive-behavioral therapy, individual or group psychotherapy, and medication. The drug most often prescribed is an antidepressant medication such as Prozac or fluoxetine, which increases levels of the neurotransmitter serotonin. About 70% of those who complete treatment programs reduce their bingeing and purging, although flareups are common in times of stress.

Strategies for Prevention

••••••••••••••••••••••••••••••••••••

Recognizing Bulimia Nervosa

The characteristics of bulimia nervosa include:

✔ Repeated binge eating.

✔ A feeling of lack of control over eating behavior.

✔ Regular reliance on self-induced vomiting, laxatives, or diuretics.

✔ Strict dieting or fasting, or vigorous exercise, to prevent weight gain.

✔ A minimum average of two bingeing episodes a week for at least three months.

✔ A preoccupation with body shape and weight.

▌Obesity

Obesity is characterized by excess fat in the body and a body weight of 20% or more above the ideal weight for a person of that height and gender. *Mild obesity* refers to a body weight that is 20% to 40% above the ideal weight; *moderate obesity,* to a body weight that is 41% to

Personal Voices "I'm Not 'Pudge' Anymore"

Nina's childhood nickname was "Pudge." "I loved sweets," she recalls, "And I ate so many of them that I looked like the Campbell's soup kid, with chubby cheeks that everyone loved to pinch." As Nina entered her teens, her friends all suddenly seemed to develop thin, shapely bodies. "It's just baby fat," her mother would say when Nina worried about her formless figure. "It'll melt off as you get older and taller."

Nina couldn't wait that long. She went on a strict low-fat, low-calorie diet. Every day she portioned out what she would eat into tiny servings. Within a month, she'd shed 20 pounds. Everyone complimented Nina on her new figure, including boys who'd never looked at her before. But as Nina returned to her old eating habits, her weight climbed back up. By the time she went away to college, she'd lost and gained the same 20 pounds several times.

During her frantic first semester on her own, Nina never seemed to stop eating. Someone at the dorm was always calling for pizza. Parents would send care packages stuffed with goodies. At the library, Nina would munch on candy bars during study breaks. During Christmas break, her mother baked all her favorites, and Nina came back to school determined to diet. She tried a slow, sensible approach, but it was frustrating watching others eat the treats Nina loved. "How can you eat so much and stay so skinny?" she asked one of the girls on her floor. "Come on," her friend said, "I'll show you my secret." She led her to the bathroom, where she leaned over a toilet, expertly stuck her index finger down her throat and threw up.

Soon Nina was doing the same things. All week long she thought about what she'd eat in what she thought of as her "Friday night pig-out." She'd hoard chips and cookies, steal extra pieces of cake from the cafeteria and buy a half-gallon of ice cream at the local store. If asked to go out with friends on Fridays, she'd say no. She couldn't imagine how she'd make it through the week without having her binge to look forward to. Alone in her room, she would eat, and eat, and eat as fast as she could, hardly even taking time to chew. She stopped only when it was physically impossible to put another bite in her mouth. Feeling bloated and disgusted, she'd go to the bathroom and force herself to vomit. Almost always she'd feel better immediately.

Nina kept bingeing and purging throughout her years at college. Her dentist was the first one to suspect a problem. "I've seen the same kind of erosion of tooth enamel and gum irritation in lots of young women with bulimia," she told Nina. "Take my advice: Go talk with a therapist." Nina, who'd been troubled by feelings of anxiety and depression, decided to talk to one of the counselors at the student health center. That's where she learned about eating disorders.

The counselor recommended a therapist who used a cognitive-behavioral approach. As part of her homework, Nina had to record everything she ate, whether she induced vomiting, and how she felt at the time. Together with the therapist, she reviewed this record and identified the situations that had triggered bingeing or purging. She then developed a plan to avoid high-risk circumstances, such as not staying in on Fridays, and instead arrange to go out with others. She also came up with a list of alternative ways of coping, such as calling or visiting a friend when she felt like bingeing. The therapists also taught Nina some basic stress-management and relaxation techniques and had her write out the negative consequences of her behavior, such as wasting money on food bought for binges. They drew up a contract in which Nina agreed to reduce her binges; as a reward, she would be able to spend the money that usually went for food on other kinds of treats for herself. Nina also worked on reexamining her beliefs about her body, her self-worth, her relationships with other people, and the role of food in her life.

Within three months, Nina was able to reduce greatly her bingeing-and-purging-pattern. But five years after graduation, a man she'd been seeing for three years broke up with her. Depressed and distressed, she returned to the comfort of "pigging out." Knowing she needed help, she consulted a psychiatrist, who prescribed medication as well as brief psychotherapy to deal with the underlying issues. Within a month, Nina was bingeing much less often, although she now realizes that when times get tough, she's likely to be tempted to bury her troubles with food. "But I'm not 'Pudge' anymore. I've learned there are better ways to cope with stress."

100% above the ideal weight; and *severe obesity,* to a body weight that is 100% or more above the ideal weight for a person of that height and gender.

Although more people in certain regions of the country are likely to be heavy, obesity affects all racial and ethnic groups. A third of white American women are obese—as are nearly 50% of African-American and Mexican-American women. In some Native American communities, up to 70% of all adults are dangerously overweight.[31]

Weight problems can start at an earlier age. Obesity in children has increased by more than 50% in the last 20 years. As many as 27% of children and 21% of teens are heavier than they should be.[32] Childhood obesity increases the risk of adult heart disease, diabetes, and osteoporosis.[33]

Adding extra pounds over the years is another danger, according to two 1995 studies by Harvard University researchers. One, which followed 115,818 women for 14 years, found that those who gained 11 to 17 pounds had a 25% greater risk of a heart attack than women who gained 10 pounds or less. Those who put on 18 to 24 pounds increased their heart attack risk by 65%, while those who gained more than 40 pounds nearly tripled their risk. Women with body weight in the upper-normal range and those who gain even modest amounts of weight during adulthood may have an increased risk of heart disease. The second study found that even a modest weight gain increases the likelihood of earlier death in women.[34]

Men who put on pounds over the years face similar risks. Studies have shown that overweight middle-aged men have a higher risk of dying from all causes, especially from heart disease and certain cancers, than those who are normal weight or underweight. Among men who have smoked, the risk of dying is almost two times higher for those with the highest body weight than for those with the lowest body weight. Men who weigh 20% less than the average for American men have the lowest risk of dying from all causes.[35]

What Causes Obesity?

Are some people fated to be fat? Scientists have identified a gene for a protein that signals the brain to halt food intake or to step up metabolic rate to make use of extra calories. If this gene is defective or malfunctions, it could contribute to weight problems. The discovery of a genetic predisposition to excess weight could explain, at least in part, why children with obese parents tend to be obese themselves, especially if both parents are obese.[36] A protein named leptin also may play a role. When laboratory mice are injected with high doses of leptin, they initially decrease their food intake, increase their metabolic rate, and become much thinner. Eventually, the body adapts to the high levels of leptin and becomes resistant to its effects.[37]

Yet genes are not the sole culprits. As scientists now realize, obesity is a complex and serious disorder with multiple causes.[38] These include

- *Developmental factors.* Some obese people have a high number of fat cells, others have large fat cells,

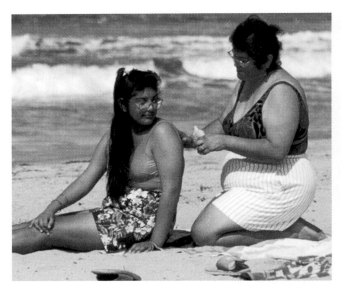

Obesity tends to run in families, so heredity may play a role in your weight. But environment and behavior also play roles: If you choose to eat high-calorie, high-fat foods, you're likely to become overweight.

and the most severely obese have both more *and* larger fat cells. Whereas the size of fat cells can increase at any time in life, the number is set during childhood, possibly as the result of genetics or over-feeding at a young age.

- *Social determinants.* In affluent countries, people in lower socioeconomic classes tend to be more obese. For reasons unknown, those in the upper classes, who can afford as much food as they want, tend to be leaner. Education may be one factor; another is that a healthy, nonfattening diet with plenty of fresh fruits and vegetables is more expensive.

- *Physical activity.* Obesity tends to go with a sedentary lifestyle. In those countries where many people tend to work at physically demanding jobs, obesity is rare. Physical activity prevents obesity by increasing caloric expenditure, decreasing food intake, and increasing metabolic rate.

- *Emotional influences.* Obese people are neither more nor less psychologically troubled than others. Psychological problems, such as irritability, depression, and anxiety, are more likely to be the result of obesity than the cause. However, emotions do play some role in weight problems. Just as some people reach for a drink or a drug when they're upset, others cope by overeating, bingeing, or purging.[39]

- *Lifestyle*. People who watch more than three hours of TV a day are twice as likely to be obese as those who watch less than an hour. Even those who log between one and two hours are fatter than those who watch just one. Researchers don't know if TV watching causes obesity or if obese people watch more TV, but they have found that heavy TV viewers are not just fat, but far less physically active or fit.

The Dangers of Obesity

Obesity has long been singled out as a major health threat that increases the risk of many chronic diseases. Obese people have three times the normal incidence of high blood pressure and diabetes. Very heavy women have a threefold higher risk of heart attack and chronic chest pain than very lean women. Excess weight in women has been linked with an increased incidence of high blood pressure, ovarian cancer, and breast cancer. Obese men have an increased chance of heart disease and cancer of the colon, rectum, and prostate. If overweight individuals have surgery, they're more likely to develop complications. Even relatively small amounts of excess fat—as little as 5 pounds—can add to the dangers in those already at risk for hypertension and diabetes.

Moreover, in our calorie-conscious and thinness-obsessed society, obesity can be a heavy psychological burden and is often seen as a sign of failure, laziness, or inadequate willpower. As a result, overweight men and women often blame themselves for becoming heavy, and feel guilty and depressed as a result. In fact, the psychological problems once considered the cause of obesity may be its consequence.[40]

Does obesity lead to a shorter life? The answer is far from clear—and intensely controversial. A 1998 analysis of 62,116 men and 262,019 women who had never smoked and had no history of heart disease, stroke, or cancer found an association between greater body-mass index and higher death rates. However, the relative risk of being heavy declined with age, disappearing altogether by the time people reached age 74.[41]

In responding to such findings, some experts have argued that the data linking overweight and death are "limited, fragmentary, and inconclusive" and that doctors may campaign against obesity because of a tendency to "medicalize behavior" they do not approve of. In some cases, they note, the means to which individuals turn in their attempts to lose weight may be riskier than any dangers posed by the excess pounds they carry.[42] However, other experts counter that obesity indirectly contributes to as many as 318,000 deaths a year.[43] What is even less clear is the actual danger of being mildly to moderately overweight.[44]

Strategies for Change

Building Better Body Image

Here are some ways of improving your body esteem if you're overweight:

✔ Don't put off special plans until you reach a certain magical weight: do what you want to do now.

✔ Start being the person you want to be—your body will catch up with you.

✔ Focus on the parts of your body you like. Maybe you have beautiful brown eyes or powerful shoulders.

✔ Don't put yourself down or joke about your weight.

✔ Treat yourself with the respect you'd like to receive from others.

✔ Try new activities. Don't let weight loss be the center of your life. Take up folk dancing, sailing, gardening, or some other hobby. And the more active your new interest, the better.

Overcoming Weight Problems

Each year an estimated 80 million Americans go on a diet, but no matter how much weight they lose, 95% gain it back within five years.[45] At any given time, more than 25% of adults in this country are trying to lose weight, while millions of others are trying to keep off the weight they lost. Most dieters cut back on food, not because they want to *feel* better, but because they want to *look* better. Individuals who drastically reduce their food intake and make weight loss a major part of their lives may be jeopardizing their physical and psychological well-being.

The best approach to obesity depends on how overweight a person is. For extreme obesity, medical treatments, including surgery, may be necessary to overcome the danger to a person's health and life. People who are moderately or mildly obese can lose weight through different approaches, including behavioral modification

Pulsepoints

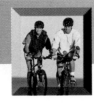

Top Ten Ways to Lose Weight

1. Take charge of your weight. Successful dieters often simply decide that they no longer are going to be fat.

2. Make a commitment. Join a group, such as an on-campus support group.

3. Bite and write. As an exercise, for a week, record every morsel that goes into your mouth. Reread your diary to find out what, how much, when, and where you eat—and why.

4. Don't skip meals. People who eat three meals a day burn off 10% more calories than meal skippers.

5. Snack sensibly. Avoid high-fat snack foods. Reach for plain popcorn, rice cakes, vegetables, and fruit instead.

6. Eat at a moderate pace. Slow down and savor each bite. And avoid that second helping—the "little bit more" you don't really need.

7. Narrow your options. While you should eat an assortment of food, be wary of too many tempting tastes at one meal. We eat more when offered many different foods at once.

8. Graze, don't gorge. Spread calorie intake over the day rather than stuffing yourself at any one meal. Potential pay-

offs include better performance, greater stamina, and less likelihood of a weight gain.

9. Get a buddy. If you want to lose weight, don't go it alone. Dieters who double up with a friend or spouse lose more weight and are more likely to keep it off.

10. Move it and lose it. Don't lie down when you can sit; don't sit when you can stand; don't stand when you can walk; don't walk when you can run. The more active you are, the more calories you use up.

(monitoring food intake, altering eating style, avoiding eating "triggers," and similar strategies); cognitive therapy (changing thoughts or beliefs that lead to overeating); and social support (participating in groups such as Overeaters Anonymous).[46] The keys to overcoming obesity are acknowledging biological limits, addressing individual differences, altering unrealistic expectations, and individualizing treatment. (See Pulsepoints: "Top Ten Ways to Lose Weight.") Although research is still at very preliminary stages, there have been reports of various drugs that, at least in laboratory animals, have led to reductions in body fat.

Severe Obesity

A body weight that is more than 100% over the ideal is a life-threatening condition. Because of the medical dangers they face, some severely obese men and women, as a last resort, may undergo surgery to reduce the volume of their stomachs and to tighten the passageway from the stomach to the intestine. Others opt for a "gastric bubble," a soft, polyurethane sac placed in the stomach to make the person feel full while following a low-calorie diet. It is not yet clear whether people who lose weight with this bubble will be able to keep it off.

In a federally sponsored four-year study of prescription appetite suppressants ("diet drugs"), individuals

who initially weighed an average of 200 pounds took medications in addition to dieting, exercising, receiving counseling, and learning behavior-modification skills (such as handling stressful situations in which they might overeat). They lost an average of more than 30 pounds and kept the weight off as long as they took the drugs, which for some was three and a half years. When they stopped taking the drugs, however, their weight crept back up—even though they continued dieting, exercise, and behavior modification. Medical and nutritional experts disagree about the safety of long-term use of appetite suppressants. Some argue that their benefits outweigh any risks; others consider them potentially hazardous.

Moderate Obesity

For people with a body weight that is 41% to 100% over the ideal, doctors recommend a supervised diet, behavior modification, and physical activity. In addition to cutting down on daily calories, patients keep careful records of when, what, and why they eat; learn good nutrition; and work with a nutritional counselor.

Mild Obesity

Rather than going on low-calorie diets, people with a body weight 20% to 40% over the ideal should cut back

Self-Survey

Do You Know How to Lose Weight?

When it comes to weight control, willpower isn't enough: A sound knowledge of exercise, nutrition, and healthy eating behavior is essential. To test your weight-loss know-how, try this quiz, which was developed by Dr. Kelly Brownell, director of the Yale University Center for Eating and Weight Disorders.

Instructions:

In each section, mark the statements True or False.

Section I: Nutrition

1. The calorie is a measure of the amount of fat in a food. _____
2. If you eat an equal number of servings from each of the five food groups in the Food Guide Pyramid, you'll get a balanced diet. _____
3. The recommended daily intake of dietary fat is 30% or less of total calories. _____
4. Carbohydrates aren't as important as other nutrients are, and they should make up only about 30% of your daily diet. _____
5. One gram of fat contains more than twice the calories of one gram of carbohydrate or protein. _____

Section II: Behavior

1. Keeping a daily record of what you eat is essential for weight loss. _____
2. Ordering à la carte at restaurants is a better idea than ordering package meals. _____
3. It's best to take all of what you'll eat in one serving so that you won't need additional helpings. _____
4. When you're trying to lose weight, it's a good idea to go food shopping when you're hungry so you can test your willpower. _____
5. Controlling how much you eat at a special event is easier if you eat a low-calorie snack before you go. _____

Section III: Exercise

1. Walking one mile burns almost as many calories as running one mile. _____
2. Exercise can help keep you from losing muscle tissue when you're trying to lose weight. _____
3. Climbing stairs requires more energy per minute—and therefore burns more calories per minute—than many more popular forms of exercise, such as swimming or jogging. _____
4. No exercise can help you lose fat in specific parts of the body. _____
5. Exercise must be done in specific amounts—say, at least 30 minutes at a stretch—to help you lose weight. _____

Section IV: Myths

1. The most important factor in weight reduction is dis-covering the psychological roots of your weight problem. _____
2. There's no such thing as a slow or underactive metabolism. _____
3. Since excess dietary fat has been linked to heart disease and other health problems, it's best to eliminate all fat from your diet. _____
4. Eating quickly helps you enjoy food more because your taste buds get more stimulation. _____
5. The calorie level necessary to lose weight is the same for all people. _____

Answers

Section I: Nutrition

1. **False**. The calorie is a measure of the energy your body gets from a food. Fat supplies some of the calories in some foods, but so do carbohydrates and protein.
2. **False**. You should eat the following every day: two to three servings of dairy products; two to three servings of meat, poultry or other high-protein foods (fish, beans, eggs, and nuts); two to four servings of fruit; three to five servings of vegetables; and six to eleven servings of breads and cereals (including rice and pasta).
3. **True**. If you follow the Food Guide Pyramid, you should be able to keep your fat calories under 30%.
4. **False**. Carbohyrates should make up the largest portion of your daily diet (between 55% and 60% of total calories).
5. **True**. One gram of fat contains nine calories, while one gram of carbohydrate or protein contains only four calories.

Section II: Behavior

1. **True**. People who have lost weight and kept it off generally report that record keeping was one key to their success.
2. **True**. If you order a package meal—say, a hamburger with french fries and coleslaw—you'll probably end up with more calories than you want or need.
3. **False**. It's best to take one portion at a time, because it interrupts the tendency to eat without thinking and gives you time to consider whether you really need more food.
4. **False**. Shopping on an empty stomach is asking for trouble. You'll do less impulse buying if you shop *after* eating.

5. **True**. Eating a low-calorie food before you go will take the edge off your hunger and help you resist the high-calorie snacks, such as chips and nuts, typically served at parties.

Section III: Exercise

1. **True**. How far you go is more important than how fast you go, so walking helps with weight control.
2. **True**. Exercise can prevent muscle loss while maximizing fat loss. For weight loss, exercise combined with dieting is preferable to dieting alone.
3. **True**. Climbing stairs is an excellent way to burn calories.
4. **True**. You can reduce fat in general, but you cannot dictate where it will come off.
5. **False**. Any amount of exercise helps, so do what you can.

Section IV: Myths

1. **False**. Psychological problems are at the root of some, but not all, cases of overweight. And there's no evidence that uncovering these causes helps with weight loss.
2. **False**. There are wide variations in metabolic rate—how fast calories are used by the body for energy—among different people.
3. **False**. Fat plays an important role in the body, including protecting vital organs and preventing excessive heat loss, so it shouldn't be totally eliminated from your diet.
4. **False.** Your taste buds catch nothing but a blur if the food shoots past. If you slow down, the food will taste better, and you may feel more satisfied and therefore eat less.
5. **False**. There are large differences in how much weight people lose when they have the same caloric intake. Some women, for example, lose weight on 2,000 calories a day while others don't lose any on 1,000.

Scoring

Give yourself one point for each correct answer and total the points for each section.

Section I: Nutrition

5 You're a nutrition nabob! With so many food facts at your fingertips, controlling your weight should be no heavy task.

3 or 4 Your food choices could use a dash more nutriton know-how if you want to keep your weight at a palatable level.

1 or 2 You need to be enlightened on food if you want to scale down.

Section II: Behavior

5 You ain't misbehavin': Your eating and food shopping

habits are right on target.

3 or 4 You may want to brush up on your p's and q's: Some of your habits may be hindering your efforts.

1 or 2 If you don't break your bad habits, you'll always be fighting the battle of the bulge.

Section III: Exercise

5 You've got a leg up on controlling your weight.

3 or 4 You should work out the kinks in your workout to help keep your weight in check.

1 or 2 Shape up, or you'll never like the shape of things to come!

Section IV: Myths

5 It's no myth that you know what you're talking about.

3 or 4 Watch out: If you don't separate food fact from food fiction, you may be led astray.

1 or 2 When it comes to weight control, don't believe everything you read.

Making Changes
Long-Term Weight Management

If you decide to change your eating habits in order to lower your weight, try following these steps:

- *Establish your goals.* Subtract your target weight from your actual weight and calculate how long it will take you to lose the difference, based on a weekly loss of 1½ pounds.
- *Never say diet.* Going on a diet implies going off a diet sooner or later.
- *Be realistic.* Trying to shrink to an impossibly low weight dooms you to defeat. Start off slowly and make steady progress. If your weight creeps up 5 pounds, go back to the basics of your program. Take into account normal fluctuations, but watch out for an upward trend. If you let your weight continue to creep up, it may not stop until you have a serious weight problem—again.
- *Recognize that there are no quick fixes.* Ultimately, quick-loss diets are very damaging physically and psychologically because when you stop dieting and put the pounds back on you feel like a failure.
- *Note your progress.* Make a graph, with your initial weight as the base, to indicate your progress. View plateaus or occasional gains as temporary setbacks rather than disasters.
- *Adopt the 90% rule.* If you practice good eating habits 90% of the time, a few indiscretions won't make a difference. In effect, you should allow for occasional cheating, so that you don't have to feel guilty about it.
- *Try, try again.* Remember, dieters don't usually keep weight off on their first attempt. The people who eventually succeed try various methods until they find the plan that works for them.

SOURCE: *American Health,* November 1994:29–31.

moderately on their food intake and concentrate on developing healthy eating and exercise habits. Many moderately to mildly overweight people turn to national organizations such as Weight Watchers, or to other commercial weight-loss groups. Most of these programs offer behavior-modification techniques, inspirational lectures, and carefully designed nutritional programs, but dropout rates are high. As many as half the members drop out in six weeks.

Strategies for Change

Evaluating a Diet

If you hear about a new diet that promises to melt away fat, don't try it until you get answers to the following questions:

✔ Does it include a wide variety of nutritious foods?

✔ Does it provide at least 1200 calories a day?

✔ Is it designed to reduce your weight by one-half to two pounds per week?

✔ Does it emphasize moderate portions?

✔ Does it use foods that are easy to find and prepare?

✔ Can you follow it wherever you eat—at home, work, restaurants, or parties?

✔ Is its cost reasonable?

If the answer to any of these questions is no, don't try the diet; then ask yourself one more question: Is losing weight worth losing your well-being?

A Practical Guide to Weight Management

Even experienced dieters who've tried dozens of ways of losing weight often know little about the most effective ways to shed pounds and keep them off. (See Self-Survey: "Do You Know How to Lose Weight?") In studies of successful dieters, those who were highly motivated, who monitored their food intake, increased their activity, set realistic goals, and received social support from others were most likely to lose weight. Another key to long-term success is tailoring any weight-loss program to an individual's gender, lifestyle, and cultural, racial, and ethnic values.[47]

A Customized Weight-Loss Plan

"If there's one thing we've learned in decades of research into weight management, it's that the one-diet-fits-all approach doesn't work," says clinical psychologist David Schlundt, Ph.D., of Vanderbilt University.[48] The key is recognizing the ways you tend to put on weight and developing strategies to overcome them. Here are some examples:

- Do you simply like food and consume lots of it? If so, keep a diary of everything you put in your mouth and tally up your daily total in calories and fat grams. The numbers may stun you. Look for where most of the calories come from—probably high-fat foods such as whole milk, chocolate, cookies, fried foods, potato chips, steaks—and cut down on how much and how often you eat them.

- Do you eat when you're bored, sad, frustrated, or worried? If so, you may be especially susceptible to "cues" that trigger eating. "People get in the habit of using food to soothe bad feelings or cope with boredom," says Schlundt. "Sometimes the real issue is a self-esteem or body-image problem." Dealing with these concerns is generally more helpful in the long run than dieting.

- Do you "graze," nibbling on snacks rather than eating regular meals? If so, limit yourself to low-calorie, low-fat foods, like carrots, celery, grapes, or air-popped popcorn. Take sips of water regularly to freshen your mouth. Even if you're only having a few crackers or carrots, put them on a plate, and try to eat in the same place, preferably while seated. This helps you break the habit of putting food in your mouth without thinking.

Diet Traps to Avoid

Whatever your eating style, there are only two effective strategies for losing weight: eating less and exercising more. Unfortunately, most people search for easier alternatives that almost invariably turn into dietary dead ends. The following are among the most common traps to avoid.

Diet Foods

According to the Calorie Control Council, 90% of Americans choose some foods labeled "light".[49] But even though these foods keep growing in popularity, Americans' weights keep rising. There are several reasons: Many people think choosing a food that's lower in calories, fat-free, or "light" gives them a license to eat as much as they want. What they don't realize is that many foods that are low in fat are still high in sugar and calories. And too much of any food, even one with zero fat and relatively few calories per serving, can sabotage a diet and lead to weight gain.

What about the artificial sweeteners and fake fats that appear in many diet products? Nutritionists caution to use them in moderation, and not to substitute them for basic foods, such as grains, fruits, and vegetables (see Chapter 6).

The Yo-Yo Syndrome

On-and-off-again dieting, especially by means of very-low-calorie diets (under 800 calories a day), can be self-defeating and dangerous. Some studies have shown that "weight cycling" may make it more difficult to lose weight or keep it off. Repeated cycles of rapid weight loss followed by weight gain may even change food preferences. Chronic crash dieters often come to prefer foods that combine sugar and fat, such as cake frosting.[50]

There is a way to avoid weight cycling and overcome its negative effects: exercise. Researchers at the University of Pennsylvania found that when overweight women who also exercised went off a very-low-calorie diet, their metabolisms did not stay slow but bounced back to the appropriate level for their new, lower body weights.[51] The reason may be exercise's ability to preserve muscle tissue. The more muscle tissue you have, the higher your metabolic rate.

Very-Low-Calorie Diets

Any diet that promises to take pounds off fast can be dangerous. For reasons that scientists don't fully understand, rapid weight loss is linked with increased mortality. Most risky are very-low-calorie diets that provide fewer than 800 calories a day. Whenever people cut back drastically on calories, they immediately lose several pounds because of a loss of fluid. As soon as they return to a more normal way of eating, they regain this weight.

On a very-low-calorie diet, as much as 50% of the weight you lose may be muscle (so you'll actually look flabbier). Because your heart is a muscle, it may become so weak that it no longer can pump blood through your body. In addition, your blood pressure may plummet,

causing dizziness, lightheadedness, and fatigue. You may develop nausea and abdominal pain. You may lose hair. If you're a woman, your menstrual cycle may become irregular, or you may stop menstruating altogether. As you lose more water, you also lose essential vitamins, and your metabolism slows down. Even reaction time slows, and crash dieters may not be able to respond as quickly as usual.[52]

Once you go off an extreme diet—as you inevitably must—your metabolism remains slow, even though you're no longer restricting your food intake. The human body appears to alter its energy use to compensate for weight loss. In a 1995 study, researchers found that individuals who'd lost 10% of their weight on a liquid-formula diet burned fewer calories than before their diet. These metabolic changes may make it harder for people to maintain a reduced body weight after dieting.[53]

Diet Pills and Products

In their search for a quick fix to weight problems, millions of people have tried often-risky remedies. In the 1920s, some women swallowed patented weight-loss capsules that turned out to be tapeworm eggs. In the 1960s and 1970s, addictive amphetamines were common diet aids. In the 1990s, new appetite suppressants known as fen-phen ("fen" referring to fenfluramine [Pondimin] or dexfenfluramine [Redux], appetite depressants, and the "phen" referring to phentermine, a type of amphetamine) became popular. An estimated 6 million Americans, most of them women, took fen-phen, which helped control cravings by boosting the brain chemical serotonin.[54] In September 1997, fen-phen was taken off the market after these agents were linked to heart valve problems.[55]

The search for the perfect diet drug continues—with plenty of economic incentives for drug makers. By some estimates, the potential market for weight-loss pills totals at least $5 billion. Other diet products, including diet sodas and low-fat foods, also are a very big business. Yet people who use these products aren't necessarily sure to slim down. In fact, people who consume such products often gain weight because they think that they can afford to add high-calorie treats to their diet.

Liquid Diets

Liquid diets, such as Optifast, Medifast, and other programs, supply 420 to 800 calories a day and include sufficient protein to preserve muscle tissue. For several months, dieters on these plans eat no solid food, consuming only the special liquid formula and water. These extreme diets, generally reserved for those at least 40% or more overweight, do result in rapid loss, but they can be hazardous.

Today's liquid diets contain more protein, carbohydrates, vitamins, and minerals than the formulas that led to at least 58 deaths in the late 1970s. However, programs that rely solely on liquid formulas should be supervised by a doctor or hospital that provides weekly screening of blood pressure, heart function, electrolyte levels, urine content, and potassium—all indicators of how the body is coping without real food. The side effects of liquid diets include dry skin, hair loss, constipation, gum disease, sensitivity to cold, and mood swings. Only 10% to 20% of those who enroll in liquid-diet programs manage to stay within ten pounds of their target weight a year and a half after entering the program.

Strategies for Prevention
··
Protecting Yourself from Diet Hucksters

The National Council Against Health Fraud cautions dieters to watch for warnings of dangerous or fraudulent programs, including:

✔ Promises of very rapid weight loss.

✔ Claims that the diet can eliminate "cellulite" (a term used to refer to dimply fatty tissue on the arms and legs).

✔ "Counselors" who are really salespersons pushing a product or program.

✔ No mention of any risks associated with the diet.

✔ Unproven gimmicks, such as body wraps, starch blockers, hormones, diuretics, or "unique" pills or potions.

✔ No maintenance program.

Exercise: The Best Solution

You may think that exercise will make you want to eat more. Actually, it has the opposite effect. The combination of exercise and cutting back on calories may be the most effective way of taking weight off and keep it off.

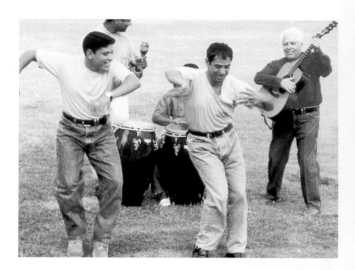

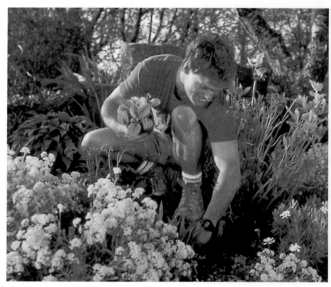

Exercise isn't just tennis or jogging. You can increase your daily exercise by such simple changes as taking the stairs instead of the escalator. Walking, gardening, hiking, and other not-so-strenuous activities can provide enjoyment as well as exercise.

As recent research has shown, exercise keeps your metabolic rate up while you're dieting—and afterward. Exercise, along with a healthy diet, can lead to weight losses of up to 10 pounds.[56]

Exercise has other benefits: it increases energy expenditure, it builds up muscle tissue, and it burns off fat stores.[45] Exercise also may reprogram metabolism so that individuals burn up more calories during and after a workout. (See Chapter 5 for a complete discussion of exercise.)

Once you start an exercise program, keep it up. Individuals who've started an exercise program during or after a weight-loss program are consistently more successful in keeping off most of the pounds they've shed.[57]

Strategies for Change
Working Off Weight

✔ *Get moving.* Take the stairs instead of the elevator. Get off the bus a few blocks from your home and walk the rest of the way.

✔ *Walk.* Most people find it hard to make excuses for not walking 15 minutes every day. Once you start, increase gradually so that you go farther and faster.

✔ *Exercise daily.* You're more likely to lose and keep weight off if you exercise regularly. Try to burn 1800 to 2000 calories a week through exercise—the equivalent of 18 to 20 miles of walking or jogging.

✔ *Get physical.* There are more ways to burn calories than traditional exercise activities: Dancing, hiking, gardening can all help you get in shape. Check your campus bulletin boards and newspapers for information on rock-climbing, kayaking, skiing, and other fun forms of working out.

Making This Chapter Work for You
Weighing in for a Healthy Future

■ According to recent government statistics, the percentage of obese men and women—those weighing more than 20% over their ideal weight—has risen from 25% to 33% in the last decade. Some 58 million Americans weigh at least 20% more than their ideal body weight.

■ At any given time, 33% to 40% of adult women and 20% to 24% of adult men are trying to lose weight; another 28% of both women and men are trying to maintain a weight loss.

■ Weight has become a central preoccupation in many people's lives. However, an obsession with appearance can be dangerous to physical and psychological well-being. People who want to look or be thinner may develop unhealthy eating behaviors, such as extreme dieting and bingeing, that can undermine their health and diminish their self-esteem.

■ Many factors determine what a person should weigh: heredity, eating behavior, food selection, amount of daily exercise. For any individual of a given height, there is no single best weight, but a range of healthy weights. Many specialists on eating disorders rely on standardized tables that give healthy ranges of body-mass index (BMI), a standard index for assessing the ratio of a person's weight to height.

■ Health experts generally advise keeping body fat below 20% of weight for men and 25% for women. The most common ways of measuring an individual's body fat include skin calipers (which pinch skin folds at the arms, waist, and back) and hydrostatic immersion testing (which weighs a person in water to distinguish buoyant fat from denser muscle).

■ A person's waist-hip ratio can indicate health risks. Abdominal fat seems more dangerous than fat stored on the hips, thighs, and buttocks. The bigger the waist and belly, the higher the risk of various diseases, such as diabetes, heart disease, and stroke.

■ The number of calories you need every day depends on your gender, age, size, and activity level. An "average" adult woman—with a median height of 5'4" and a weight of 138 pounds—generally needs 1900 to 2200 calories. An average man—with a median height of 5'10" and a weight of 174 pounds—generally needs 2300 to 2900 calories.

■ Hunger, the physiological drive to consume food, stimulates our appetite or desire for food. We stop eating when we achieve a state of satisfaction called satiety. According to the set-point theory, each individual has an unconscious control system for regulating appetite and satiety to keep body fat at a predetermined level, or set point.

■ Unhealthy eating behaviors, such as extreme or chronic dieting, compulsive overeating, and binge eating (the rapid consumption of an abnormally large amount of food in a relatively short time) can be early warning signals of more serious eating disorders.

■ The eating disorders anorexia nervosa and bulimia nervosa are most common among young women.

■ The causes of anorexia nervosa are complex; genetic, biochemical, and developmental factors may play a role. Its consequences include extreme weight loss, cessation of menstrual periods in women, decline in testosterone levels in men, heart irregularities, and arrhythmias that can increase the risk of sudden death. Because of their fear of fatness, many people with this disorder resist seeking help. A combination of medical therapy and psychotherapy can lead to recovery.

■ Individuals with bulimia nervosa go on repeated eating binges and rapidly consume large amounts of food, usually sweets. Those with purging-type bulimia induce vomiting or take large doses of laxatives to control their weight. Individuals with nonpurging bulimia use other means, such as fasting or excessive exercise, to compensate for binges. Complications include damaged tooth enamel, dehydration, electrolyte imbalance, cardiac arrhythmias, and even sudden death. Most mental health professionals treat bulimia with a combination of nutritional counseling, psychotherapy, and medication.

■ People gain weight whenever they take in more calories than they burn off. About a third of adults in the United States are obese. Many different factors contribute to obesity, including heredity, environment, culture, and development. Mild obesity refers to being 20% to 40% above his or her ideal weight. An individual who is 41% to 100% above his or her ideal weight is moderately obese, and a person who is more than 100% above his or her ideal weight is severely obese.

■ Obese people are at risk for developing high blood pressure, diabetes, heart disease, certain kinds of cancer, and other life-threatening conditions. Severely obese people can be treated by stomach reduction surgery and long-term medications; moderately and mildly obese individuals do best with diet, exercise, and behavior modification.

■ In studies of successful dieters, those who were highly motivated, who monitored their food intake, set realistic goals, and received social support from others were most likely to lose weight.

■ Many people fall into diet traps, such as an overreliance on low or reduced fat and other "light" foods, a pattern of off-and-on or yo-yo dieting, very-low-calorie diets, appetite suppressants, diet aids (such as gum, powders, or potions, and low- or no-calorie soft drinks and snacks), and liquid diets.

■ Exercise in combination with diet is the most effective means of losing excess pounds and keeping them off. Exercise increases energy expenditure, builds up muscle tissue and burns off fat stores. Exercise also may reprogram your metabolism so that you burn up more calories during and after a workout.

If you are overweight, the insight and information in this chapter can help you set up an effective weight-loss program. But losing weight is only the first step. You also have to keep off the pounds you've shed. Here are some ways to do so:

■ *Become a slow eater.* Your brain needs 20 minutes to register that you're full. Eat at a moderate pace, chew each bite thoroughly, and pause regularly throughout your meal. Always wait before taking second helpings.

■ *Develop alternative pleasures.* Learn to indulge your other senses. Listen to music. Soak in a bubble bath. Take up hiking, gardening, yoga.

■ *Treat your taste buds.* If you're giving up or cutting down on rich foods, try highly spiced dishes, such as a hot Indian curry or a spicy Mexican entree, as a main course.

■ *Develop strategies for social occasions.* Always eat something that's filling and low in calories before a party. Decide in advance which items you'll eat and which you won't—pretzels and carrot sticks, but not chips, for instance.

■ *Set a danger zone.* Don't let your weight climb more than 3 or 4 pounds above your ideal weight. If you do, take action immediately rather than waiting until you gain an additional 5 or 10 pounds.

Health Online

Healthy Body Calculator   http://www.dietitian.com/ibw/ibw.html

The Healthy Body Calculator allows you to input your age, gender, height, activity level, and frame size and then determines your healthy weight range. You can also enter your weight goal, information about your nutrient intake, and your waist-to-hip ratio for more detailed results.

Think about it ...

- According to the Healthy Body Calculator, are you within your healthy weight range?
  If not, are you willing to take steps to change your weight?

- What are three things you could do each day to become more physically active?
  And what three specific changes could you make to your diet to make it healthier?

- Do you have any older relatives or friends who are overweight?
  Have they suffered any physical problems that might be related to their weight?

 ## Key Terms

The terms listed here are used within the chapter. Page numbers are included for each term.
A definition of each term is given in the green Glossary pages at the end of this book.

anorexia nervosa *196*	**bulimia nervosa** *197*	**obese** *240*
appetite *192*	**calorie** *190*	**obesity** *197*
basal metabolic rate (BMR) *191*	**eating disorders** *195*	**satiety** *192*
binge eating *194*	**hunger** *192*	**set-point theory** *192*
body-mass index *188*	**hydrostatic weighing** *189*	**skin calipers** *189*

 ## Review Questions

1. What is a calorie? How many calories are needed to maintain a healthy body?

2. What is the set-point theory? Why does the set point make it difficult to diet? How can this problem be overcome?

3. What are the symptoms of anorexia? of bulimia? How can each of these eating disorders be overcome?

4. How much overweight does a person have to be to be considered obese? What role do genetics, lifestyle, and overeating play in determining whether an individual becomes obese?

5. What is the best way to lose weight? What are some of the dangers associated with dieting?

6. What is your ideal weight? How does your actual weight compare? What changes, if any, do you need to make in your lifestyle to achieve and maintain your ideal weight?

Critical Thinking Questions

1. Ask your friends—particularly your women friends—how they feel about their bodies. Chances are they'll mention something they hate: their hair, their hips, their height, and, most often of all, their weight. What do you think leads to such dissatisfaction? What can individuals do to feel better about the way they look?

2. Different cultures have different standards for body weight and attractiveness. Within our society, even men and women often seem to follow different standards. What influences have shaped your personal feelings about desired weight?

3. If you could choose skin calipers or hydrostatic immersion testing, which would you select to determine your body fat? Explain the reasons for your choice.

Connections to Personal Health Interactive

To enhance your understanding of the material covered in this chapter, check out the following study aids on the **Personal Health Interactive CD-ROM***. Each numbered icon within the chapter corresponds to an appropriate activity listed here.*

7.1 Personal Insights: Do You Like to Eat?

7.2 Personal Voices: Anorexia Nervosa

7.3 Diet Tips

7.4 Career: Dietician

7.5 Chapter 7 Review

References

1. Dortch, Shannon. "America Weighs In." *American Demographics*, Vol. 19, No. 6, June 1997.

2. NIH Task Force on the Prevention and Treatment of Obesity: Weight Cycling. *Journal of the American Medical Association*, Vol. 272, 1994, p. 1196

3. Rodin, Judith. "Cultural and Psychosocial Determinants of Weight Concerns." *Annals of Internal Medicine*, October 1, 1993.

4. Rumpel, Catherine, and Tamara Harris. "The Influence of Weight on Adolescent Self-Esteem." *Journal of Psychosomatic Research*, Vol. 38, No. 6, August 1994. Tordjman, Sylvie, et al. "Preliminary Study of Eating Disorders Among French Female Adolescents and Young Adults." *International Journal of Eating Disorders*, Vol. 16, No. 3, November 1994. Stice, Eric, and Heather Shaw. "Adverse Effects of the Media Portrayed Thin Ideal on Women and Linkages to Bulimic Symptomatology." *Journal of Social and Clinical Psychology,* Vol. 13, No. 3, Fall 1994.

5. Alley, Thomas, and Katherine Scully. "The Impact of Actual and Perceived Changes in Body Weight on Women's Physical Attractiveness." *Basic & Applied Social Psychology*, Vol. 15, No. 4, December 1994. Levine, Michael, et al. "The Relation of Sociocultural Factors to Eating Attitudes and Behaviors Among Middle School Girls." *Journal of Early Adolescence*, Vol. 14, No. 4, November 1994 .

6. Allison, David, et al. "Weight-Related Attitudes and Beliefs of Obese African-American Women." *Journal of Nutrition Education*, Vol.27, No. 1, January–February 1995. Stevens, June, et al. "Attitudes toward Body Size and Dieting." *American Journal of Public Health*, Vol. 84, No. 8, August 1994.

7. Caldwell, Marcia, et al. "Relationship of Weight, Body Dissatisfaction, and Self-Esteem in African American and White Female Dieters." *International Journal of Eating Disorders*, Vol. 22, No. 2, September 1997.

8. Carr-Nangle, Rebecca, et al. "Body Image Changes over the Menstrual Cycle in Normal Women." *International Journal of Eating Disorders*, Vol. 16, No. 3, November 1994. Hetherington, Marion. "Aging and the Pursuit of Slimness: Dieting and Body Satisfaction Through Life." *Appetite*, Vol. 23, No. 2, October 1994.

9. Hunter, Beatrice Trum. "Eating Disorders: Perilous Compulsions." *Consumers' Research Magazine*, Vol. 80, No. 9, September 1997.

10. Douglas, Kathy, et al."Results from the 1995 National College Health Risk Behavior Survey." *Journal of American College Health*, Vol. 46, September 1997.

11. Hart, Kathleen, and Maureen Kenny. "Adherence to the Super Woman Ideal and Eating Disorder Symptoms among College Women." *Sex Roles: A Journal of Research*, Vol. 36, No. 7–8, April 1997.

12. Schulken, Ellen, et al. "Sorority Women's Body Size Perceptions and Their Weight-Related Attitudes and Behaviors." *Journal of American College Health*, Vol. 46, September 1997.

13. NIH Technology Assessment Panel. "Methods for Voluntary Weight Loss and Control." *Annals of Internal Medicine,* June 1, 1992.

14. Blair, Stephen, et al. "Body Weight Change, All-Cause Mortality, and Cause-Specific Mortality in the Multiple Risk Factor Intervention Trial." *Annals of Internal Medicine*, October 1, 1993.

15. Bulik, Cynthia, et al. "Initial Manifestations of Disordered Eating Behavior: Dieting versus Binging." *International Journal of Eating Disorders*, Vol. 22, No. 2, September 1997.

16. Antony, Martin, et al. "Psychopathology Correlates of Binge Eating and Binge Eating Disorder." *Comprehensive Psychiatry*, Vol. 35, No. 5, September–October 1994. Nangle, Douglas, et al. "Binge Eating Disorder and the Proposed DSM-IV Criteria: Psychometric Analysis of the Questionnaire of Eating and Weight Patterns." *International Journal of Eating Disorders*, Vol. 16, No. 2, September 1994.

17. American Psychiatric Association. *Diagnostic and Statistical Manual of Mental Disorders,* 4th ed. Washington, DC: American Psychiatric Association, 1994.

18. Rodin, Judy, et al. "Food Cravings in Relation to Body Mass Index, Restraint and Estradiol Levels: A Repeated Measures Study in Healthy Women." *Appetite*, December 1991.

19. Beumont, Pierre, et al. "Diagnoses of Eating or Dieting Disorders: What May We Learn from Past Mistakes?" *International Journal of Eating Disorders*, Vol. 16, No. 4, December 1994. Fairburn, Christopher, and Sarah Beglin. "Assessment of Eating Disorders: Interview or Self-Report Questionnaire?" *International Journal of Eating Disorders*, Vol. 16, No. 4, December 1994.

20. American Psychiatric Association (APA), Work Group on Eating Disorders.

21. Fernstrom, Madelyn, et al. "Twenty-Four-Hour Food Intake in Patients with Anorexia Nervosa and in Healthy Control Subjects." *Biological Psychiatry*, Vol. 36, No. 10, November 1994.

22. Ogden, Jane, and Pauline Fox. "Examination of the Use of Smoking for Weight Control in Restrained and Unrestrained Eaters." *International Journal of Eating Disorders*, Vol. 16, No. 2, September 1994.

23. Walters, Ellen, and Kenneth Kendler. "Anorexia Nervosa and Anorexic-Like Syndromes in a Population-Based Female Twin Sample." *American Journal of Psychiatry*, Vol. 152, No. 1, January 1995.

24. Hersen, Michel, and Samuel M. Turner. "Eating Disorders." In *Diagnostic Interviewing*, 2nd ed. New York: Plenum Press, 1994. Garner, David, and Lionel Rosen. "Eating Disorders." In *Handbook of Aggressive and Destructive Behavior in Psychiatric Patients*. New York: Plenum Press, 1994.

25. Hales, Dianne, and Robert E. Hales. *Caring for the Mind: The Comprehensive Guide to Mental Health*. New York: Bantam Books, 1995.

26. van der Ster Wallin, G., et al. "Binge Eating Versus Nonpurged Eating in Bulimics: Is There a Carbohydrate Craving After All?" *Acta Psychiatrica Scandinavica*, Vol. 89, No. 6, June 1994.

27. Taibbi, Robert. "Anorexia and Bulimia." *Current Health*, Vol. 20, No. 8, April 1994.

28. American Psychiatric Association.

29. Leal, Linda, et al. "The Relationship Between Gender, Symptoms of Bulimia, and Tolerance for Stress." *Addictive Behaviors*, Vol. 20, No. 1, January–February 1995. Boumann, Christine, et al. "Risk Factors for Bulimia Nervosa: A Controlled Study of Parental Psychiatric Illness and Divorce." *Addictive Behaviors*, Vol. 19, November–December 1994. Weiss, Lillie, et al. "Bulimia Nervosa: Definition, Diagnostic Criteria, and Associated Psychological Problems." In *Understanding Eating Disorders: Anorexia Nervosa, Bulimia Nervosa, and Obesity*. Philadelphia: Taylor & Francis, 1994.

30. Sansone, Randy, and Lori Sansone. "Bulimia Nervosa: Medical Complications." In *Understanding Eating Disorders: Anorexia Nervosa, Bulimia Nervosa, and Obesity*. Philadelphia: Taylor & Francis, 1994.

31. Centers for Disease Control and Prevention. Polednak, Anthony. "Weight/Height Ratio in Hispanic Adults Surveyed by Telephone." *Health Values*, Vol. 19, No. 2, March–April 1995.

32. Mellin, Laurel. "Treating Pediatric Obesity." *Clinical Profile*, Vol. 7, No. 2, Spring 1995.

33. Gutin, Bernard. "Childhood Obesity and the Risk of Chronic Disease." Presentation at the Sports Science Institute Conference, June 1997.

34. Willett, Walter, et al. "Weight, Weight Change, and Coronary Heart Disease in Women: Risk Within the 'Normal' Weight Range." *Journal of the American Medical Association*, Vol. 273, No. 6, February 8, 1995.

35. Lee, I-Min, et al. "Exercise Intensity and Longevity in Men: The Harvard Alumni Health Study." *Journal of the American Medical Association*, Vol. 273, No. 15, April 19, 1995. Blair, Steven, et al. "Changes in Physical Fitness and All-Cause Mortality: A Prospective Study of Healthy and Unhealthy Men." *Journal of the American Medical Association*, Vol. 273, No. 14, April 12, 1995. Lee, I-Min, et al. "Body Weight and Mortality: A 27-Year Follow-Up of Middle-Aged Men." *Journal of the American Medical Association*, Vol. 270, No. 23, December 15, 1993. Lee, I-Min, and Ralph Paffenbarger, Jr. "Change in Body Weight and Longevity." *Journal of the American Medical Association*, Vol. 268, No. 15, October 21, 1992. .

36. Magid, Barry. "Is Biology Destiny After All?" *Journal of Psychotherapy Practice & Research*, Vol. 4, No. 1, Winter 1995.

37. Spector, Rosanne. "Researchers Discover New Target for Obesity Drugs." *Stanford University Medical News*, October 1, 1997.

38. Brownell, Kelly, and Thomas Wadden. "Etiology and

Treatment of Obesity: Understanding a Serious, Prevalent, and Refractory Disorder." *Journal of Consulting and Clinical Psychology*, August 1992.

39. Zwaan, Martina de, et al. "Eating Related and General Psychopathology in Obese Females with Binge Eating Disorder." *International Journal of Eating Disorders*, Vol. 15, No 1, January 1994. Telch, Christy, and Stewart Agras. "Obesity, Binge Eating and Psychopathology: Are They Related?" *International Journal of Eating Disorders*, Vol. 15, No. 1, January 1994. Webber, Eleanor. "Psychological Characteristics of Binging and Nonbinging Obese Women." *Journal of Psychology,* Vol. 128, No. 3, May 1994. Karlsson, Jan, et al.

40. "Predictors and Effects of Long-Term Dieting on Mental Well-Being and Weight Loss in Obese Women." *Appetite*, Vol. 23, No. 1, August 1994. Ross, Catherine. "Overweight and Depression." *Journal of Health and Social Behavior*, Vol. 35, No. 1, March 1994.

41. Stevens, June, et al. "The Effect of Age on the Association Between Body-Mass Index and Mortality." *New England Journal of Medicine*, Vol. 338, No. 1, January 1, 1998.

42. Kassirer, Jerome, and Marcia Angell. "Losing Weight: An Ill-fated New Year's Resolution?" *New England Journal of Medicine*, Vol. 338, No. 1, January 1, 1998.

43. Kolata, Gina. "The Fat's in the Fire, Again." *New York Times*, January 11, 1998.

44. Gaesser, Glenn, and Michael Fumento. "Are the Health Risks of Obesity Exaggerated?" *Insight on the News*, Vol. 13, No. 41, November 10, 1997.

45. Horowitz, Janice, and Lawrence Mondi. "Fat Times." *Time*, January 16, 1995.

46. Foster, Gary, and Philip Kendall. "The Realistic Treatment of Obesity: Changing the Scales of Success." *Clinical Psychology Review*, Vol. 14, No. 8, 1994. Sperry, Len. "Helping People Control Their Weight: Research and Practice." In *Addictions: Concepts and Strategies for Treatment*. Gaithersburg, MD: Aspen Publishers, 1994.

47. "Weight Loss Programs and Weight Maintenance." *American Family Physician*, Vol. 55, No. 7, November 15, 1997.

48. David Schlundt. Personal interview.

49. Margolis, Dawn. "The Lowfat Trap." *American Health*, May 1995.

50. Brownell, K. D., and Judy Rodin. "Medical, Metabolic, and Psychological Effects of Weight Cycling." *Archives of Internal Medicine*, June 27, 1994.

51. Ibid.

52. "Cutting Calories Too Much Can Slow Reaction Time." *Tufts University Health & Nutrition Letter*, Vol. 14, No. 6, August 1997. Raloff, Janet. "Dieting Impairs Reaction Time." *Science News*, Vol. 151, No. 21, May 24, 1997.

53. Rudolph L., et al. "Changes in Energy Expenditure Resulting from Altered Body Weight." *New England Journal of Medicine*, Vol. 332, No. 10. March 9, 1995. Roust, L. R., et al. "Effects of Isoenergetic, Low-Fat Diets on Energy Metabolism in Lean and Obese Women." *American Journal of Clinical Nutrition*, October 1994. Sintsova, N. "Adaptation to Low-Calorie Diet in Obese Patients." *Human Physiology*, September–October 1993.

54. "The Painful Business of Losing Weight. "*The Economist*, Vol. 344, No. 8032, August 30, 1997.

55. Kolata, Gina. "How Fen-Pehn, a Diet 'Miracle,' Rose and Fell." *New York Times*, September 23, 1997. Cowley, Geoffrey, and Karen Springen. "After Fen-Phen." *Newsweek*, Vol. 130, No. 13, September 29, 1997.

56. Parr, Richard. "Exercising to Lose 10 to 20 Pounds." *Physician and Sportsmedicine*, Vol. 25, No. 4, April 1997.

57. Linkowish, Mary Desmond. "Winning at Losing: Some Optimism about Weight-loss Maintenance." *Patient Care*, Vol. 31, No. 17, October 30, 1997.

58. Katoh, Junichi, et al. "Effects of Exercise on Weight Reduction in Middle-Aged Obese Women." *Current Therapeutic Research*, Vol. 55, No. 9, September 1994.

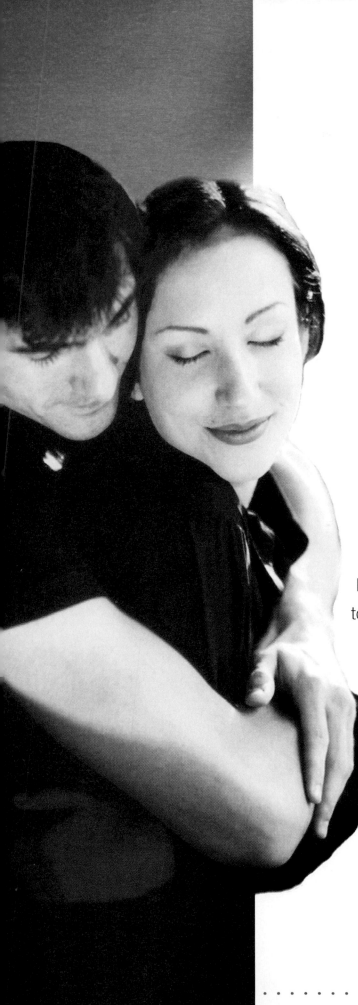

RESPONSIBLE SEXUALITY

*O*ur most special relationships are those that bring us closer to others—our friends, partners, spouses, parents, and children. Such intimacy is the most rewarding and often the most demanding of human involvements. The giving of ourselves to another—sharing thoughts, feelings, experiences, and sexual pleasure—touches the essence of what it means to be human. This section provides a comprehensive philosophical and practical view of relating to others. Each of the chapters focuses on the unique form of personal responsibility involved in every close relationship: a responsibility that looks beyond the self to those we care for and love.

COMMUNICATING AND RELATING

After studying the material in this chapter, you should be able to:

Define friendship and **explain** how friendship grows.

Compare and **contrast** the behavioral expectations for friendship, dating, and mature love.

Describe the typical progress of a relationship from dating to mature love.

List and **explain** three living arrangements today's adults might choose.

Explain how some of the problems likely to affect long-term relationships can be prevented.

Name some of the major issues facing parents in the world today.

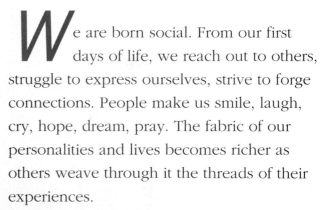

We are born social. From our first days of life, we reach out to others, struggle to express ourselves, strive to forge connections. People make us smile, laugh, cry, hope, dream, pray. The fabric of our personalities and lives becomes richer as others weave through it the threads of their experiences.

How we feel about ourselves affects how others feel about us. But we also must be able to communicate our feelings and needs. Relationships begin with signals: yes, no, and maybe. From the first, we should try to make our signals clear (Figure 8-1). As we progress to messages, we should try to respond honestly and naturally and to express our feelings as precisely as we can. As individuals and as part of society, we need to care about others and to know that others care about us, to feel for others and have others feel for us, to share what we know and to learn from what others know.

Sending clear messages through words, gestures, expressions, and behaviors is the essence of good communication. The more effectively we communicate, the more likely we are to create good relationships built on honesty, understanding, and mutual trust. Such relationships can infuse our lives with a richness no solitary pleasure can match.

This chapter discusses the social needs we all share, the ways some of us respond to those needs, and the possibilities that exist for coming together from our solitude to warm ourselves in each other's glow of life.

Figure 8-1

Relationships begin with signals. The more effective our signals—verbal as well as gestures and expressions—the more likely we are to build good relationships.

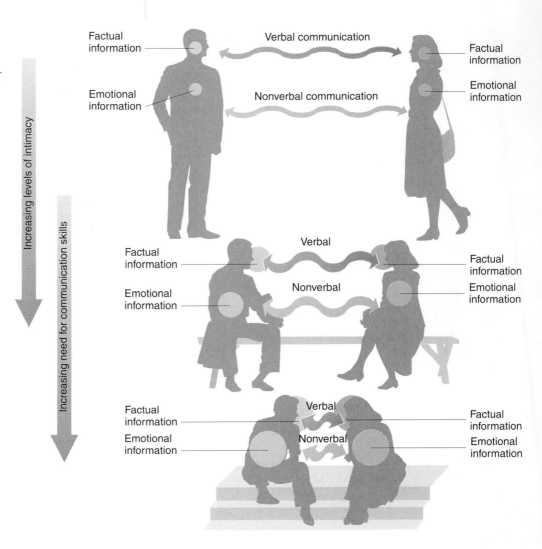

Increasing levels of intimacy

Increasing need for communication skills

Factual information — Verbal communication — Factual information

Emotional information — Nonverbal communication — Emotional information

Factual information — Verbal — Factual information

Emotional information — Nonverbal — Emotional information

Factual information — Verbal — Factual information

Emotional information — Nonverbal — Emotional information

Personal Communication

Getting to know someone is one of life's greatest challenges and pleasures. When you find another person intriguing—as a friend, as a teacher, as a colleague, as a possible partner—you want to find out as much as you can about him or her and to share more and more information about yourself. Roommates may talk for endless hours. Friends may spend years getting to know each other. Partners in committed relationships may delight in learning new things about each other.

Communication stems from a desire to know and a decision to tell. Each of us chooses what information about ourselves we want to disclose and what we want to conceal or keep private. But in opening up to others, we increase our own self-knowledge and understanding.

Communicating Feelings

A great deal of daily communication focuses on facts: on the who, what, where, when and how. Information is easy to convey and comprehend. Emotions are not. Some people have great difficulty saying "I appreciate you" or "I care about you," even though they are genuinely appreciative and caring. Others find it hard to know what to say in response and how to accept such expressions of affection.

Some people feel that relationships shouldn't require any effort, that there's no need to talk of responsibility between people who care about each other. Yet responsibility is implicit in our dealings with anyone or anything we value—and what can be more valuable than those with whom we share our lives? Friendships and other intimate relationships always demand an emotional investment, but the rewards they yield are great.

Sometimes people convey strong emotions with a kiss or a hug, a pat or a punch, but such actions aren't precise enough to communicate exact thoughts. Stalking out of a room and slamming the door may be clear signs of anger, but they don't explain what caused the anger or suggest what to do about it. You must learn how to communicate all feelings clearly and appropriately if you hope to become truly close to another person.

As two people build a relationship, they must sharpen their communication skills, so that they can discuss all the issues they may confront. They must learn how to communicate anger as well as affection, hurt as well as joy—and they must listen as carefully as they speak. If and when love grows, they will find themselves as concerned with the other as with the self.

Strategies for Change

How to Enhance Communication

✔ *Use "I" statements.* Describe what's going on with you. Say, "I worry about being liked" or "I get frustrated when I can't put my feelings into words." Avoid generalities such as "You never think about my feelings," or "Nobody understands me."

✔ *Gently ask how the other person feels.* If your friend or partner describes thoughts rather than feelings, ask for more adjectives. Was he or she sad, excited, angry, hurt?

✔ *Become a very good listener.* When another person talks, don't interrupt, ask why, judge, or challenge. Nod your head. Use your body language and facial expression to show you're eager to hear more.

✔ *Respect confidences.* Treat a friend's or partner's secrets with the discretion they deserve. Consider them a special gift entrusted to your care.

Gender Differences in Communication

Every man and every woman is unique, but researchers who've carefully observed each gender have observed differences in the way many—but not necessarily all—

men and women use language. There are complex reasons why men and women may use words in different ways. Deborah Tannen, Ph.D., a professor of linguistics at Georgetown University and author of *You Just Don't Understand: Women and Men in Conversation,* theorizes that men and women communicate for different reasons. In many public situations, men speak to convey information, to challenge others, to achieve status in a group, or to put themselves in a "one-up" situation. Many women, on the other hand, feel more comfortable with private conversations among friends and family. They talk to achieve and nurture intimacy, to promote closeness and equality in a group, and to build better connections to others.[1]

In an analysis of more than 125 studies in various cultures, psychologist Judith Hall, Ph.D., of Northeastern University, author of *Nonverbal Sex Differences,* found differences, starting at third grade, in each gender's awareness of nonverbal messages. In general, girls and women proved to be consistently more accurate than boys and men at interpreting unspoken messages in gestures, facial expressions, and tone of voice. Whether looking at photographs or watching videotapes or actual interactions, women showed significantly greater skill than men in figuring out how the people they observed were feeling. Even in experiments in which words were deliberately garbled or did not betray any feelings, women were able to intuit the emotional content of a conversation.[2]

The existence of gender differences in communication styles does not mean that one gender's preference is right, wrong, better, or worse than the other's. However, recognition of the fact that the sexes use language differently can help both men and women avoid jumping to erroneous conclusions and overcome potential obstacles to their mutual understanding and acceptance.

Nonverbal Communication

More than 90% of communication may be nonverbal. While we speak with our vocal cords, we communicate with our facial expressions, tone of voice, hands, shoulders, legs, torsos, posture. "Body language is a very elementary level of communication that people react to without realizing why," observes Albert Mehrabian, Ph.D., a professor of psychology at the University of California, Los Angeles (UCLA) and author of *Silent Messages.* "It's the building block upon which more advanced verbal forms of communication rest."[3]

Self-Survey

How Strong Is the Communication and Affection in Your Relationship?

Effective, caring communication and loving affection markedly enhance a couple's relationship. The following self-test may help you to assess the degree of good communication, love, and respect in your intimate relationship. If you agree or mostly agree with a statement, answer yes. If you disagree or mostly disagree, answer no. You may wish to have your partner respond to this assessment as well. If so, mark your answers on a separate sheet.

1. My partner seeks out my opinion.	Yes	No
2. My partner cares about my feelings.	Yes	No
3. I don't feel ignored very often.	Yes	No
4. We touch each other a lot.	Yes	No
5. We listen to each other.	Yes	No
6. We respect each other's ideas.	Yes	No
7. We are affectionate toward one another.	Yes	No
8. I feel my partner takes good care of me.	Yes	No
9. What I say counts.	Yes	No
10. I am important in our decisions.	Yes	No
11. There's lots of love in our relationship.	Yes	No
12. We are genuinely interested in one another.	Yes	No
13. I love spending time with my partner.	Yes	No
14. We are very good friends.	Yes	No
15. Even during rough times, we can be empathetic.	Yes	No
16. My partner is considerate of my viewpoint.	Yes	No
17. My partner finds me physically attractive.	Yes	No
18. My partner expresses warmth toward me.	Yes	No
19. I feel included in my partner's life.	Yes	No
20. My partner admires me.	Yes	No

Scoring: A preponderance of yes answers indicates that you enjoy a strong relationship characterized by good communication and loving affection. If you answered yes to fewer than seven items, it is likely that you are not feeling loved and respected and that the communication in your relationship is decidedly lacking.

SOURCE: Gottman, John. *Why Marriages Succeed or Fail.* New York: Simon & Schuster, 1994. See Hyde and DeLameter, 1997, 6th ed., p. 272

Making Changes ....
Getting Along Better with Your Partner

- Before you say anything to your partner, ask yourself three things: Is it true? Is it kind? Is it necessary?
- Never miss the opportunity to compliment or say something encouraging to or about your partner.
- Have a forgiving view of people. Believe that most are trying to do the best they can.

- Keep an open mind: Discuss, don't argue. Remember that it's possible to disagree without being disagreeable.
- Let your virtues speak for themselves.
- Forget about counting to 10: Count to 100 or 1000 before doing or saying anything that could make matters worse.
- If your partner criticizes you, try to see if there's any truth to the comment. If so, make changes. If not, ignore it and live so that no one will believe the negative remarks.
- Cultivate your sense of humor. Laughter is the shortest distance between two people.
- Seek not so much to be consoled, as to console; not so much to be understood, as to understand; not so much to be loved, as to love.

SOURCE: Adapted from *Currents.* San Bruno, CA: Bay Pacific Health Plan, Summer 1990. Survey from *Low Is Not Enough* by Aaron Beck. Copyright © 1988 by Aaron Beck, M.D. Reprinted by permission of HarperCollins Publishers, and in Canada, Arthur Pine Associates, New York.

In fact, learning to interpret what people *don't* say can reveal more than what they *do* say. "Understanding nonverbal communication is probably the best tool there is for a good life of communicating, be it personally or professionally," says Marilyn Maple, Ph.D., an educator at the University of Florida. "It's one of the most practical skills you can develop. When you can consciously read what others are saying unconsciously, you can deal with issues before they become problems."[4]

Culture has a great deal of influence over body language. In some cultures, for example, establishing eye contact is considered hostile or challenging; in others, it conveys friendliness. A person's sense of personal space—the distance they feel most comfortable in keep-

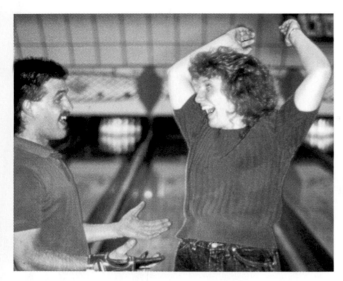

Body language. Cultural influences aside, people who have good self-esteem are comfortable with themselves and the world.

ing from others—also varies in different societies. Nonverbal messages also reveal something important about the individual. "Nonverbal messages come from deep inside of you, from your own sense of self-esteem," says Maple. "To improve your body language, you have to start from the inside and work out. If you're comfortable with yourself, it shows. People who have good self-esteem, who give themselves status and respect, who know who they are, have a relaxed way of talking and moving and always come across best."

Strategies for Change
···
Getting Your Signals Straight

✔ *Tune into your body talk.* Notice details about the way you speak, gesture, and move. If possible, watch yourself on videotape. Analyze the emotions you're feeling at the time and think of how they may be influencing your body language.

✔ *Learn to establish good eye contact, but don't glare or stare.* If you sense that someone feels uncomfortable with an intense eye grip, shift your focus so that your gaze hits somewhere between the eyes and the chin, rather than pupil-to-pupil.

✔ *Avoid putting up barriers.* If you fold your arms across your chest, you'll look defensive or uninterested in contact. Crossing your legs or ankles also can seem like a way of keeping your distance.

✔ *Identify the little things you characteristically do when you're tense.* Some people pat their hair or pick at their ears; others rub their necks, twist a ring or watch, twirl a lock of hair, or play with a pen. Train yourself to become aware of what you're doing (have a friend give you a signal, if necessary) and to control your mannerisms.

Forming Relationships

We first learn how to relate in our families, as children. Our relationships with parents and siblings change dramatically as we grow toward independence. Relationships between friends also change as they move or develop different interests; between lovers, as they come to know more about each other; between spouses, as they pass through life together; and between parents and children, as youngsters develop and mature. But throughout life, close relationships, tested and strengthened by time, allow us to explore the depths of our souls and the heights of our emotions.

I, Myself, and Me

The way each of us perceives himself or herself affects all the ways we reach out and relate to others. If we feel unworthy of love, others may share that opinion. Self-esteem and self-love (discussed in Chapter 3) provide a positive foundation for our relationships with others. Self-love doesn't mean vanity or preoccupation with our own needs; rather, it is a genuine concern and respect for ourselves so that we remain true to our own feelings and beliefs. We can't know or love or accept others until we know and love and accept ourselves, however imperfect we may be.

If we're lacking in self-esteem, our relationships may suffer. According to research on college students by psychologists at the University of Texas, individuals with negative views of themselves seek out partners (friends, roommates, dates) who are critical and rejecting—and who confirm their low opinions of their own worth.[5]

Friendship

Friendship has been described as "the most holy bond of society." Every culture has prized the ties of respect, tolerance, and loyalty that friendship builds and nurtures. An anonymous writer put it well:

A friend is one who knows you as you are,
Understands where you've been,
Accepts who you've become,
And still gently invites you to grow.

Friends can be a basic source of happiness, a connection to a larger world, a source of solace in times of trouble. Although we have different friends throughout life, often the friendships of adolescence and young adulthood are the closest we ever form. They ease the normal break from parents and the transition from childhood to independence.

Friendship transcends all boundaries of distance and differences and enhances feelings of warmth, trust, love, and affection between two people. It is a common denominator of human existence that cuts across major social categories: In every country, culture, and language, human beings make friends. Friendship is both a universal and a deeply satisfying experience.

"Wishing to be friends," Aristotle wrote, "is quick work, but friendship is a slowly opening fruit." The qualities that make a good friend include honesty, acceptance, dependability, empathy, and loyalty. More than anything else, good friends are there when we need them. They see us at our worst but never lose sight of our best. They share our laughter and tears, our triumphs and tragedies.

Personal Health
8.2
INTERACTIVE

Strategies for Change
·······································
Being a Good Friend

✔ *Be willing to open up.* The more you share, the deeper the bond between you and your friend will become.

✔ *Be sensitive to your friend's feelings.* Keep in mind that, like you, your friend has unique needs, desires, and dreams.

✔ *Express appreciation.* Be generous with your compliments. Let your friends know you recognize their kindnesses.

✔ *Know that friends will disappoint you from time to time.* They, too, are only human. Accept them as they are. Admitting their faults need not reduce your respect for them.

✔ *Talk about your friendship.* Evaluate the relationship periodically. If you have any gripes or frustrations, air them.

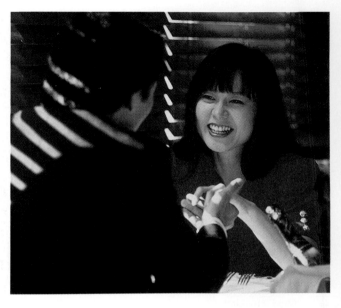

Dating refers to any occasion during which two people share their time. Your dating experiences can help you explore your social and sexual identity.

Dating

A date is any occasion during which two people share their time. It can be a Friday night dance, a bicycle ride, a dinner for two, or a walk in the park. Friends and lovers go on dates; so do complete strangers. Some men date other men; some women date other women. We don't expect to love, or even like, everyone we date. Yet the people you date reveal something about the sort of person you are.

While in school, you may go out with people you meet in class or on campus. However, with more people remaining single longer, the search for a good date has become more complex. Singles bars have become less popular because of the dangers of excessive drinking and casual sex. Cafes, laundromats, health clubs, and bookstores have become more acceptable as places to meet new people. Personal ads and "cyberspace"—the electronic web linking people through computers—are alternative ways to meet potential dates.

Dating can do more than help you meet people. By dating, you can learn how to make conversation, get to know more about others as well as yourself, and share feelings, opinions, and interests. In adolescence and young adulthood, dating also provides an opportunity for exploring your sexual identity. Some people date for months and never share more than a good-night kiss. Others may fall into bed together before they fall in love or even "like."

It's often difficult to sort out your emotional feelings about someone you're dating from your sexual desires. The first step to making responsible sexual decisions is respecting your sexual values and those of your partner. If you care about the other person—not just his or her body—and the relationship you're creating, sex will be an important, but not the all-important, factor while you're dating. (Chapter 9 discusses sexual decision making and etiquette.)

Sexual Attraction

What draws two people to each other and keeps them together: chemistry or kismet, survival instincts or sexual longings? "Probably it's a host of different things," reports sociologist Edward Laumann, Ph.D., coauthor of *Sex in America*, a landmark survey of 3432 men and women conducted by the National Opinion Research Center at the University of Chicago.[6] "But what's remarkable is that most of us end up with partners much like ourselves—in age, race, ethnicity, socioeconomic class, education."

Why? "You've got to get close for sexual chemistry to occur," says Laumann. "Sparks may fly when you see someone across a crowded room, but you only see a preselected group of people—people enough like you to be in the same room in the first place. This makes sense because initiating a sexual relationship is very uncertain. We all have such trepidations about being too fat, too ugly, too undesirable. We try to lower the risk of rejection by looking for people more or less like us."

In the University of Chicago survey, most men and women chose sexual and marital partners of the same race, the same or similar religion and socioeconomic class, and within five years of their own age. More than 75% selected partners of similar education levels.[7] Physical attractiveness also plays a role in sexual attraction—at least for men, who consistently place more emphasis on looks than do women.[8] In his cross-cultural research, psychologist David Buss, Ph.D., author of *The Evolution of Desire*, found that men in 37 sample groups drawn from Africa, Asia, Europe, North and South America, Australia, and New Zealand rated youth and attractiveness as more important in a possible mate than did women. Women placed greater value on potential mates who were somewhat older, had good financial prospects, and were dependable and hardworking. Many said physical appearance did matter—not as much as financial responsibility and dependability.[9]

The reason for this gender difference could be evolutionary. Throughout time, men have sought fertile females of "high reproductive value." Two outward signs of female fertility are youth and a more subtle factor: waist-to-hip ratio. When researchers analyzed the physical dimensions of the women considered most attractive by men in various studies, those with the slimmest waists and roundest hips were consistently rated as most desirable.[10]

From an evolutionary perspective, women have had to look for mates who could provide greater security for their offspring. For them, a man's power, wealth, and status—which require more time to assess—mattered more than appearance. But today's women may have different criteria: In a survey of over 1500 *Psychology Today* readers, women said a man's ability to empathize or talk about feelings, his intelligence, and his sense of humor mattered most—far more than his facial appearance and body build. Women also indicated that they usually accept the way their men look, even if they fail to match up to their ideal.[11]

Intimate Relationships

The term **intimacy**—the open, trusting sharing of close, confidential thoughts and feelings—comes from the Latin word for *within*. Intimacy doesn't happen at first sight, or in a day or a week or a number of weeks. Intimacy requires time and nurturing; it is a process of revealing rather than hiding, of wanting to know another and to be known by that other. (See Figure 8-2 for the elements of love.) Although intimacy doesn't require sex, an intimate relationship often includes a sexual relationship, heterosexual or homosexual.

All of our close relationships, whether they're with parents or friends, have a great deal in common. We feel we can count on these people in times of need. We feel that they understand us and we understand them. We give and receive loving emotional support. We care about their happiness and welfare. However, when we choose one person above all others to share a life with, there is something even deeper and richer—something we call romantic love.

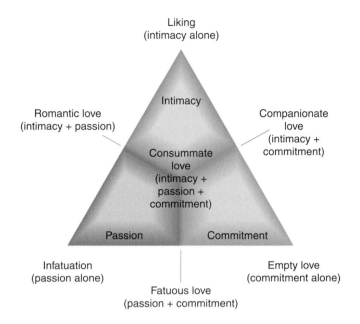

Figure 8-2

Sternberg's love triangle: (a) the three components of love and (b) the various kinds of love as reflected in different combinations of the three components. *Note:* Non-love is the absence of all three components.

Romantic Love

Falling in love is an intense, dizzying experience (Figure 8-3). A person not only enters our life but takes possession of it as well. We are intrigued, flattered, delighted—but is this love, or a love of loving? At the time you're experiencing it, you may not care. You're in such a state of giddy elation that it doesn't matter, at least for the moment, whether it stems from a strong sexual attraction, a fear of loneliness, loneliness itself, or a hunger for approval.

"We use the word love in such a sloppy way that it can mean almost nothing or absolutely everything," observes Diane Ackerman, Ph.D., author of *A Natural History of Love*, who notes that "love" is such a small word to convey "an idea so immense and powerful that it has altered the flow of history, calmed monsters, kindled works of art, cheered the forlorn, turned tough guys to mush, consoled the enslaved, driven strong women mad, glorified the humble, fueled national scandals, bankrupted robber barons, and made mincemeat of kings."[12]

We like to think of this powerful force, this source of both danger and delight, as something that defies analysis. However, in recent years, as scientists have attempted to study love objectively, they have provided new perspectives on its nature.

An Anthropological View

When you first fall in love, you may be sure that no one else has ever known the same dizzying, wonderful feelings. Yet, while every romance may be unique, romantic love is anything but. In a comprehensive study of societies around the world, anthropologists William Jankowiak of the University of Nevada-Las Vegas and Edward Fischer of Tulane University found evidence of romantic love in at least 147 of the 166 cultures they studied. The experience of an "intense attraction that involves the idealization of the other, within an erotic context, with the expectation of enduring for some time in the future," they concluded, "constitutes a human universal, or at the least, a near-universal."[13]

Another anthropologist, Helen Fisher, Ph.D., author of *Anatomy of Love: The Natural History of Monogamy, Adultery and Divorce*, describes romantic love "as a very primitive, basic human emotion, as basic as fear, anger or joy." As she explains, it pulled men and women of prehistoric times into the sort of partnerships that were essential to child rearing. But after about four years—just "long enough to rear one child through infancy," says Fisher—romantic love seemed to wane, and primitive couples tended to break up and find new partners. This "four-year itch" may well have endured through the centuries, contends Fisher, who notes that divorce statistics from most of the 62 cultures she has studied still show a pattern of restlessness four years into a marriage.[14]

A Biochemical View

The heart is the organ we associate with love, but the brain may be where the action really is. According to research on **neurotransmitters** (messenger chemicals within the brain), love sets off a chemical chain reaction that causes our skin to flush, our palms to sweat, and our lungs to breathe more deeply and rapidly. The "love chemicals" within the brain—dopamine, norepinephrine and phenylethylamine (PEA—have effects similar to those of amphetamines, stimulant drugs that intensify physiological reactions (see Chapter 14).[15]

Infatuation may indeed be a natural high, but like other highs, this rush doesn't last—possibly because the body develops tolerance for love-induced chemicals, just as it does with amphetamines. However, as the initial lovers' high fades, other brain chemicals may come

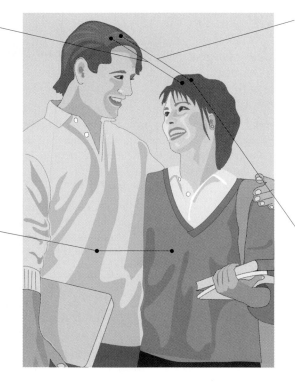

Imprinting
Evolution, genetics, psychological experience, even smells can trigger romantic reactions to another person.

Attachment
During this attachment stage, chemicals flow into the brain, and produce a sense of security, peace, and calm.

Attraction
Your brain is revved up by neurochemicals that produce feelings of euphoria and elation. The attraction lasts 2–3 years and then starts to wane.

"Cuddle" chemicals
The brain's pituitary gland secretes oxytocin which produces feelings of relaxed satisfaction and attachment.

Figure 8-3

Love can't just be chemistry! It's still a mystery, but scientists and other researchers have offered some new perspectives as they aim to analyze this thing called love.

into play: the endorphins, morphinelike chemicals that can help produce feelings of well-being, security, and tranquility. These feel-good molecules may increase in partners who develop a deep attachment.

Strategies for Change

Is It Infatuation, "Like," or Love?

A romantic relationship shows definite promise if:

✔ You feel at ease with your new partner.

✔ You feel good about your new partner both when you're together and when you're not.

✔ Your partner is open with you about his or her life—past, present, and future.

✔ You can say no to each other without feeling guilty.

✔ You feel cared for, appreciated, and accepted as you are.

✔ Your partner really listens to what you have to say.

Mature Love

Social scientists have distinguished between passionate love—characterized by intense feelings of elation, sexual desire, and ecstasy—and companionate love, which is

characterized by friendly affection and deep attachment. (See Self-Survey: "How Strong is the Communication and Affection in Your Relationship?") Often relationships begin with passionate love and evolve into a more companionate love. Sometimes the opposite happens and two people who know each other well discover that their friendship has "caught fire" and the sparks have flamed an unexpected passion.

Mature love is a complex combination of sexual excitement, tenderness, commitment, and—most of all—an overriding passion that sets it apart from all other love relationships in one's life. This passion isn't simply a matter of orgasm, but also entails a crossing of the psychological boundaries between oneself and one's lover. You feel as if you're becoming one with your partner while simultaneously retaining a sense of yourself. (For other characteristics of mature, healthy love, see Pulsepoints: "Ten Characteristics of a Good Relationship.")

When Love Ends

Breaking up is indeed hard to do. Sometimes two people grow apart gradually, and both of them realize that they must go their separate ways. More often, one person falls out of love first. It hurts to be rejected; it also hurts to inflict pain on someone who once meant a great

Pulsepoints — Ten Characteristics of a Good Relationship

1. Trust. Partners are able to confide in each other openly, knowing their confidences will be respected.

2. Togetherness. In a healthy relationship, two people create a sense of both intimacy and autonomy. They enjoy each other's company but also pursue solitary interests.

3. Expressiveness. Partners in healthy relationships say what they feel, need, and desire.

4. Staying power. Couples in committed relationships keep their bond strong through tough times by proving that they will be there for each other.

5. Security. Because a good relationship is strong enough to absorb conflict and anger, partners know they can express their feelings honestly. They also are willing to risk vulnerability for the sake of becoming closer.

6. Laughter. Humor keeps things in perspective—always crucial in any sort of ongoing relationship or enterprise.

7. Support. Partners in good relationships continually offer each other encouragement, comfort, and acceptance.

8. Physical affection. Sexual desire may fluctuate or diminish over the years, but partners in loving, long-term relationships usually retain some physical connection.

9. Personal growth. In the best relationships, partners are committed to bringing out the best in each other and have the other's best interests at heart.

10. Respect. Caring partners are aware of each other's boundaries, need for personal space, and vulnerabilities. They do not take each other or their relationship for granted.

---

deal to you. In surveys, college students say it's more difficult to initiate a breakup than to be rejected. Those who decided to end a relationship reported greater feelings of guilt, uncertainty, discomfort, and awkwardness than those with whom they broke up.[16]

While the pain does ease over time, it can help both parties if they end their relationship in a way that shows kindness and respect. Your basic guideline should be to think of how you would like to be treated if someone were breaking up with you. Would it hurt more to find out from someone else? Would it be more painful if the person you cared for lied to you or deceived you, rather than admitted the truth? Saying, "I don't feel the way I once did about you; I don't want to continue our relationship," is hard, but it's also honest and direct.

Strategies for Change

Dealing with Rejection

✔ Remind yourself of your own worth. You are no less attractive, intelligent, interesting, or lovable because someone ends his or her relationship with you.

✔ Accept the rejection as a statement of the other person's preference rather than trying to debate or defend yourself.

✔ Think of other people who value or have valued you, who accept and even see as appealing the same characteristics the rejecting person viewed as undesirable.

✔ Don't withdraw from others. Although you may not want to risk further rejection, it's worth the gamble to get involved again. The only individuals who've never been rejected are those who've never reached out to connect with another.

Living Arrangements

Today's adults have many choices to explore regarding how and with whom they might live: returning to one's primary family, staying single, living with one or more friends, living in a long-term relationship with a lover of the same or opposite sex, or getting married. Increasingly, men and women in their twenties are spending more time considering all their options before committing themselves to an exclusive relationship.

Living with Parents

According to the Census Bureau, young adults between the ages of 18 and 24 are more likely to be living in their parents' homes in the 1990s than young people were in the 1970s. One in eight adults between the ages of 25 and 34 is still living with parents—compared with one in eleven in 1980. Their reasons include the high cost of housing and the low incomes most men and women earn in their early twenties. People also are getting married later in life. In 1997, the median age for a first-time groom was 27 years; for a first-time bride, 24.5 years—significantly older than in decades past.[17]

Single Life

One in four Americans over 18 has never married—compared to one in six in 1970. In young adulthood, single men outnumber single women; after age 40, however, there are more single women than single men. Perhaps because there are so many singles, more and more Americans are living alone. Approximately one quarter of the households in the nation are one-person homes, and approximately 10% of today's young men and women will never marry.[18] Being single no longer marks a transition phase between living with parents and living with a spouse, but is an accepted, appealing lifestyle for millions of men and women.

The number-one reason people remain single is not being able to find the right person, according to psychologist Florence Kaslow, Ph.D., director of the Florida Couples and Family Institute. For women, the next two reasons for staying single are their careers and independence. For men, independence and resolving personal issues are the second and third reasons for not marrying. Most of the women and all of the men in her study said that they would like to get married—someday.[19]

Only 5% of bachelors over age 40 ever marry. Never-married men in this age group tend to avoid emotional intimacy, fear conflict, and shy away from challenges in life, according to a study of 30 lifelong bachelors. In general, the men didn't hate women, but they seemed reluctant to get involved, make demands, or assert their needs in relationships.[20]

Increasing numbers of single people, including those living alone or with heterosexual or homosexual partners, claim that they are discriminated against in housing, credit, insurance, membership groups, and medical services. Those who oppose the concept of singles' rights say that extending spousal benefits to singles or "domestic partners" would erode the institution of marriage and cause a bureaucratic mess. Despite such opposition, the campaign for singles' rights is winning increasing support.

Strategies for Change

How to Stay Single and Satisfied

✔ Fill your life with meaningful work, experiences, and people.

✔ Build a network of supportive friends who care for and about you.

✔ Try not to spend holidays alone.

✔ Be open to new experiences that can expand your feelings about yourself and your world.

✔ Don't miss out on a special event because you don't have someone to accompany you: Go alone.

✔ Volunteer to help others less fortunate, or become involved in church and social organizations.

Living Together

Although couples have always shared homes in informal relationships without any official ties, "living together," or **cohabitation**, has become more common, increasing by 80% in the last two decades. There are about seven unmarried couples for every 100 married ones. Often young people live together in a trial marriage, getting to know each other better to see whether they're compatible—although this does not necessarily lead to a more successful marriage. People who have been married and divorced may be content just sharing their lives with one another.

Unmarried couples aren't very different from married couples: They share, they talk, they quarrel. They're also gaining legal recognition; some U.S. cities have "domestic partnership" laws that grant a variety of spousal rights—such as insurance benefits and bereavement leave—to partners, heterosexual or homosexual, who live together. Couples counselors in some cities say that more than half of the partners they see aren't married. Men and women who live together are equally likely to split up or to marry.

More than half of all marriages now follow cohabitation. Some argue that living together should enhance the chance of long-term happiness in marriage because it allows two people to assess their compatibility. Others contend that couples who live together are less committed to each other and their relationship. According to some reports, couples who live together show more signs of incompatibility or sexually disloyalty and report being less happy than married pairs. If they do marry, they face a higher risk of divorce than couples who did not live under the same roof before their nuptials.[21]

Committed Relationships

Even though men and women today may have more sexual partners than in the past, most still yearn for an intense, supportive, exclusive relationship, based on mutual commitment and enduring over time. In our society, most such relationships take the form of heterosexual marriages, but partners of the same sex or heterosexual partners who never marry also may sustain long-lasting, deeply committed relationships. These couples are much like married people: They make a home, handle daily chores, cope with problems, celebrate special occasions, plan for the future—all the while knowing that they are not alone, that they are part of a pair that adds up to far more than just the sum of two individual souls.

Marriage

Like everything which is not the involuntary result of fleeting emotion but the creation of time and will, any marriage,

happy or unhappy, is infinitely more interesting and significant than any romance, however passionate.

W. H. Auden

Contemporary marriage has been described as an institution that everyone on the outside wants to enter and everyone on the inside wants to leave. About 90% of all American adults marry—for as long as they both love, if not live. According to the Census Bureau, the marriage rate has dropped dramatically, with a lower percentage of couples tying the knot in the 1990s than in previous decades.[23] This trend may reflect a variety of new social forces, such as increases in cohabitation and divorce.

Not too long ago, marriage was often a business deal, a contract made by parents for economic or political reasons when the spouses-to-be were still very young. Today, in some countries, it is still culturally acceptable to arrange marriages in this manner. Even in America, certain ethnic groups, such as Asians who have recently immigrated to the United States, plan marriages for their children. In such arrangements, the marriage partners are likely to have similar values and expectations. However, the newlyweds also start out as strangers who may not even know whether they like—let alone love—each other. Sometimes arranged marriages do lead to loving unions; sometimes they trap both partners in loneliness and longing.

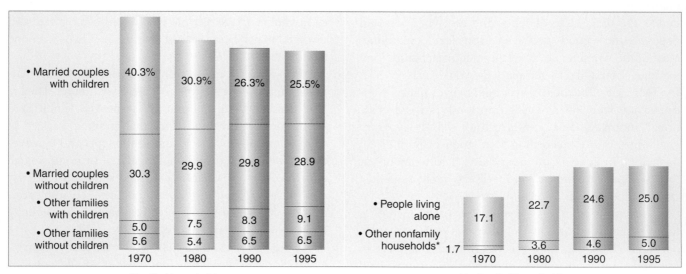

Family Households

Nonfamily Households

*Unrelated people sharing a home—for example, boarders or roommates—or unmarried couples living together.

Figure 8-4

The Changing American Household. More Americans are living alone, and there are fewer married couples with children at home.

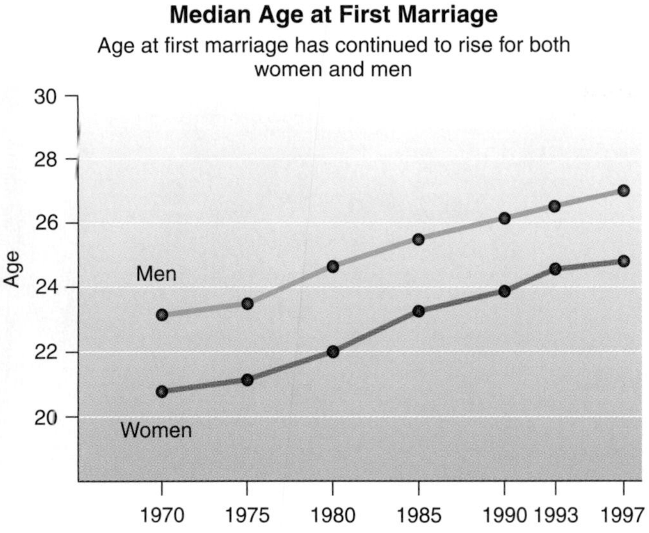

Median Age at First Marriage
Age at first marriage has continued to rise for both women and men
30
28
26
24
22
20
Age
Men
Women
1970
1975
1980
1985
1990
1993
1997

Figure 8-5

SOURCE: Bureau of the Census. *Marital Status and Living Arrangements: March 1993, 1994, 1997.*

Most of today's marriages aren't arranged, but even in this day and age, partners often marry because they have to: one out of every six brides is pregnant on her wedding day. Other young couples marry as a way to escape from their parents' homes and authority. But most people say they marry for one far-from-simple reason: love.

Preparing for Marriage

With more than half of all marriages ending in divorce, there's little doubt that modern marriages aren't made in heaven. Are some couples doomed to divorce even before they swap "I do's"? Could counseling before a marriage increase its odds of success? According to recent research findings, the answer to both questions is yes.[24]

Finding Mr. or Ms. Right

Generally, men and women marry people from the geographical area they grew up in and from the same social background. Differences in religion and race can add to the pressures of marriage, but they also can enrich the relationship if they aren't viewed as obstacles. Generally speaking, in our culturally diverse society, interracial and crosscultural marriages are becoming more common and widely accepted. According to the Census Bureau, there are four times as many interracial couples today than there were in 1970, with as many as 1 marriage out of every 50 crossing racial lines.

Some of the things that appeal to us in a date become less important when we select a mate; others become key ingredients in the emotional cement holding two people together. According to psychologist Robert Sternberg of Yale University, the crucial ingredients for commitment are the following:

- Shared values.
- A willingness to change in response to each other.
- A willingness to tolerate flaws.
- A match in religious beliefs.
- The ability to communicate effectively.

The single best predictor of how satisfied one will be in a relationship, according to Sternberg, is not how one feels toward a lover, but the difference between how one would like the lover to feel and how the lover actually feels. Feeling that the partner you've chosen loves too little or too much is, as he puts it, "the best predictor of failure."[25]

Premarital Assessments

There are scientific ways of predicting marital happiness. One is a premarital assessment inventory called PREPARE that uses 125 items to identify strengths and

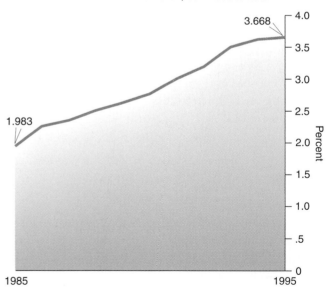

The Rise in Unmarried Couples
The number of unmarried couples in the U.S., both with and without children, continues to rise.
3.668
1.983
4.0
3.5
3.0
2.5
2.0
1.5
1.0
.5
0
Percent
1985
1995

Figure 8-6

SOURCE: Census Bureau.

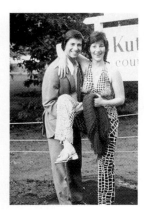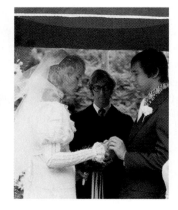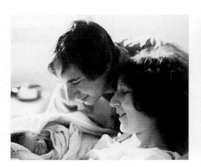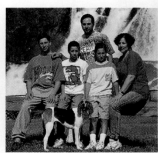

A relationship is just as alive as the individuals who create it. It grows if there is caring, it can blossom if there is emotional nourishment, and it endures if there is commitment.

weaknesses in 11 aspects of a relationship: realistic expectations, personality issues, communication, conflict resolution, financial management, leisure activities, sex, children, family and friends, egalitarian roles, and religious orientation. In longitudinal studies in which couples took the assessment prior to marriage and then were interviewed three years after they married, the PREPARE inventory was about 80% accurate in predicting which couples would divorce and which would have happy marriages.[26] Couples who become aware of potential conflicts by means of the inventory may be able to resolve them through professional counseling. In some cases, they may want to reconsider or postpone their wedding.

Other signs of a rocky relationship have been identified by psychologist John Gottman, Ph.D., author of *Why Marriages Succeed or Fail* and *What Predicts Divorce*, who analyzed the behavior of 2000 couples in 20 different studies.[27] Among the common predictors of marital discord, unhappiness, and separation that he identified are:

- A high level of arousal during a discussion.

- Defensive behaviors such as making excuses and denying responsibility for disagreements.

- A wife's expressions of contempt.

- A husband's stonewalling (showing no response when a wife expresses her concerns).

By looking for such behaviors, Gottman has been able to predict with better than 90% accuracy whether a couple will separate within the first few years of marriage.

Strategies for Prevention

When to Think Twice About Getting Married

Don't get married if:

✔ You or your partner is constantly asking the other such questions as "Are you sure you love me?"

✔ You spend most of your time together disagreeing and quarreling.

✔ You're both still very young (under the age of 20).

✔ You're really looking in the relationship for a mother or father, not an equal.

✔ Your boyfriend or girlfriend has behaviors (such as non-stop talking), traits (such as bossiness), or problems (such as drinking too much) that really bother you and that you're hoping will change after you're married.

✔ Your partner wants you to stop seeing your friends, quit a job you enjoy, or change your life in some other way that diminishes your overall satisfaction.

Types of Marriage

Sociologists have categorized marriages as traditional or companion-oriented. In **traditional marriages**, the couples assume prescribed societal roles. In **companion-oriented marriages**, the partnership and its rewards—rather than the roles of fathering, mothering, and breadwinning—are primary. Psychologist Judith Wallerstein, Ph.D., author of *The Good Marriage,* has expanded the current view of successful marriage through interviews with 50 couples who'd been married from 10 to 40 years. In addition to traditional and companionate unions, she found **romantic marriages**, in which sexual passion never seems to die, and **rescue marriages**, in which one partner suffered a traumatic childhood and sees marriage as a way of healing. Regardless of type, a marriage can succeed, she asserts, if it fulfills basic tasks, such as providing a sense of intimacy and autonomy and providing a safe haven that is strong enough to absorb inevitable conflicts.[28]

Issues in Marriage and Other Committed Relationships

No two people can live together in perfect harmony all the time. Some of the issues that crop up in any long-term relationship include the following:

Unrealistic Expectations

Partners may think that their significant others should always be as attractive, charming, and tolerant as they were when they were dating. They may assume that their partners will always agree with them or will automatically see their point of view; or they may believe that their one true love will always be able to

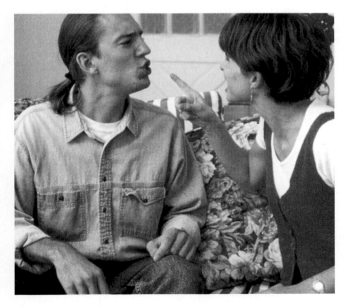

Fighting fairly. You can learn to argue effectively, without attacking others or damaging relationships.

meet all their needs. Because no one could ever live up to such expectations, the partners are doomed to disappointment.

Settling Differences

Contrary to what you may assume, arguments can be good for the health of a relationship. According to the National Institute of Mental Health, couples who learn how to fight fairly and effectively have a 50% lower divorce rate than those who haven't mastered the art of disagreeing. Results of a study of 150 couples from pre-marriage through the first ten years of marriage (the highest risk period for divorce) led researchers to conclude that "nondestructive" arguing lowers the likelihood for physical violence, helps couples stay together longer, and benefits children by preparing them to build good intimate relationships as adults.[29]

Strategies for Change

How to Fight Fairly

The art of arguing is a skill, like bicycle riding, that anyone can master with time, patience, and plenty of practice. Here are some basic ground rules:

✔ Learn to listen. Rather than thinking about what you're going to say next, tune in to your partner. Think before you open your mouth. Taking a few deep breaths gives you time to weigh your words.

✔ Use the speaker/listener technique. When one person has the floor, the other listens. Start sentences with "I'll," not "You." Instead of attacking with a statement such as "You're jealous and immature," say, "I feel hurt when you quiz me about my old relationships."

✔ Make sure you're arguing about the right issue. Are you angry simply because your partner is never on time? Or because you don't seem to be the top priority?

✔ Don't embarrass each other by fighting in front of others.

✔ Don't attack each other so viciously that one of you is backed into a corner. Be fair. Whenever there's a cheap shot, one of you should stop the fight by crying "Foul!"

✔ Avoid generalizations such as "You always interrupt me." Focus on the issue at hand.

✔ If you can't come to terms on a particular issue, agree to disagree, or to keep talking in the future.

Money

Money may make the business world go around, but it has the opposite effect on relationships: It knocks them off their tracks, brings them to a halt, twists them upside down. However, even though almost all couples quarrel about money, they rarely fight over how much they have. What matters more—whether they make $10,000 or $100,000 a year—is what money means to both partners. How does each person use money to meet emotional needs? Who decides how the money is spent? Who keeps track? Until they resolve these issues, couples may quarrel over money as long as they're together.

Strategies for Change

How to Avoid Fighting over Money

✔ Understand that having different money values or expectations doesn't make one of you right and the other wrong.

✔ Recognize the value of unpaid work. A partner who's finishing school or taking care of the children is making an important contribution to the family and its future.

✔ Go over your finances together, so you have a firm basis in reality for what you can and can't afford.

✔ Talk about the financial goals you hope to attain five years from now. Set priorities to meet them.

✔ Also, set aside money for each of you to spend without asking or answering to the other; even a small amount can make each partner feel more independent.

Sex

Like every other aspect of a relationship, sex evolves and changes over the course of marriage. The redhot sexual chemistry of the early stages of intimacy invariably cools down. Even so, the happiest couples have sex more often than unhappily married pairs do.[30]

What matters most isn't quantity alone, but the quality of sexual activity and intimacy. (Chapter 9 presents guidelines for making sex better.) Are both partners satisfied with their sexual relationship? Does one partner always initiate sex? Do the partners talk about their preferences and pleasures? Sexuality, like personality, is dynamic and changes throughout life. Do the partners acknowledge and adapt to these changes? Do they feel sufficiently at ease with each other to discuss anxieties about sex? The answers to these questions can determine how sexually gratifying a marriage is for both spouses.

Extramarital Affairs

How faithful are American mates? The answer depends on the questions researchers ask and whom they ask. In face-to-face interviews with 3432 Americans, aged 18 to 59, University of Chicago researchers found that 25% of men and 15% of women had had affairs, and that 94% of the married subjects had been monogamous in the last year.[31] Another survey of 1049 Americans, aged 18 to 65, found that one out of six had had an extramarital relationship—19% of the men and 15% of the women.[32]

High or low, numbers are little comfort when affairs do occur. A husband or wife who learns about a spouse's affair typically feels a devastating sense of betrayal as well as deep feelings of shame, fear of abandonment, depression, and anger. Two crucial questions determine whether a marriage can survive: Do the spouses still feel a serious commitment to each other? And do they love each other and want to grow old together?

Two-Career Couples

Two-career couples now make up about two-thirds of families with children under age 18. More than 60% of women with children work—a dramatic increase from the 1960s, when only 30% of mothers worked outside the home. Two careers can bring pressure to a relationship: Both individuals may come home tired and irritable; both may have to spend a great deal of time on their jobs; both may have to travel or work on weekends. It becomes even more important for partners to discuss their problems openly.

Couples pursuing individual careers sometimes face difficult choices. What happens, for example, if the husband is offered a promising job in another city? Does the wife quit her job, pack up, and move? What if she's offered a promising job elsewhere? Does her husband automatically pack up and go? Some couples resolve such dilemmas by working in different cities and spending weekends together. Others try to alternate career and home priorities. However imperfect these arrangements may be, they work for some couples.

The working couples most likely to stay together are those who are not tightly tied to traditional gender roles. Because neither spouse has very narrow expectations of what the other should or shouldn't be doing, both are free to pursue individual interests outside the home.

Strategies for Prevention
Handling Dual-Career Stress

✔ Plan your weekends. List your priorities, and take turns selecting what you'll do.

✔ Keep dating. Block out a time at least once a week to enjoy each other's company and to talk about your concerns and feelings.

✔ Spend a night or, if possible, a weekend alone at least once every three months.

✔ You both know what it's like to deal with office politics, angry bosses, and rush-hour traffic. Empathize with and reassure each other.

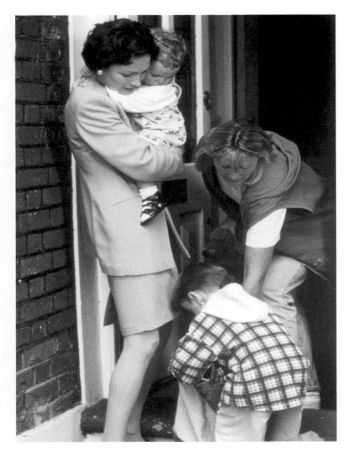
Two-career couples cope with balancing family and work in various and sometimes imperfect ways.

✔ Accept help without imposing your standards. Whoever does the shopping or washes the car shouldn't have to do it the other's way. Just be grateful you didn't have to do it yourself.

The Rewards of Marriage

Despite its problems, marriage endures because it is a fulfilling way for two people to live. As researchers have proven, good marriages make people happy and healthy. A 1995 report to the Population Council of America, based on the National Survey of Families and Households, a sampling of 13,000 adults, found that marriage offers dramatic benefits over single life and cohabitation: Married people enjoy better health, more money, and more satisfying sex lives.[33]

Marriage seems especially beneficial for men. Married men have lower rates of alcohol and drug abuse, depression, and risk-taking behavior than divorced men. They have sex twice as often as most single men and report higher levels of satisfaction with their sex lives than either single or cohabiting men. They earn more money—possibly because they have more incentive to do so. Women get less dramatic benefits from marriage. Their wages usually go down, especially after they have children; they spend more time on housework; and their sexual satisfaction is the same as that of unmarried women. However, both spouses benefit when they pool their money and invest in better medical care, safer surroundings, better foods, a healthier lifestyle, and other things that raise their standard of living and lower their level of stress.[34]

Couples Therapy

According to the Association of Family and Marital Therapists, at least one of every five couples in this country needs professional counseling—and increasing numbers are seeking help. Some 4.6 million couples—married or not—now turn to the 50,000 licensed family therapists in the United States, a dramatic increase over the 1.2 million who sought help in 1980.[35] The relationships of about two-thirds of those who get counseling do improve, according to both the couples' own judgments and objective measures of satisfaction.[36]

A well-trained counselor can spot destructive behavior patterns and help couples see their situations in a new light. Therapy often helps stop spouses from hurting each other so badly that they can't stay together. If nothing else, it can help both partners decide whether to continue or end the relationship.

Strategies for Prevention

Making the Most of a Committed Relationship

✔ Focus on what's right with your partner. Be kinder to your partner. Don't take for granted the nice things your spouse does.

✔ Learn to negotiate for what you want. One effective approach is offering your mate what he or she wants in return.

✔ Look for the problem behind the problem. Often an affair or a lack of sexual interest is merely a symptom; the real question is why this problem has developed.

✔ Keep your perspective. Uncapped toothpaste tubes or food not prepared exactly to your taste may be annoying, but are they worth a fight?

✔ Rather than thinking of all the things your partner is or isn't doing, look for things you can do to make your marriage better.

Divorce

More than 1.2 million marriages end in divorce every year. The divorce rate soared in the 1960s and 1970s but peaked at a rate of 5.3 per 1000 in 1981. Since then it has slowly declined (see Figure 8-7). In 1996 there were about 1.17 million divorces and about 2.33 million marriages.[37] However, the U.S. divorce rate remains the highest in the world—even though divorce is becoming more common everywhere.

More than one in every five men and women who have ever been married have been divorced. Increasingly, therapists and family counselors are urging couples to try to work out their differences—for their own and their children's sake. As many people have discovered, divorce hurts.

Even after their hopes for happiness with one spouse end, men and women still yearn to mesh two personalities, two life histories, and two persons' dreams

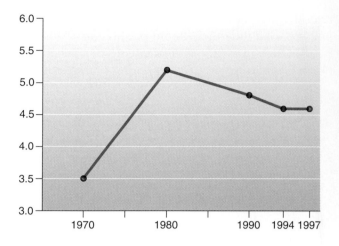

Figure 8-7

The Divorce Rate. The divorce rate—the number of divorces in a given year per 1000 persons in the population—has declined slightly in recent years.

SOURCE: Bureau of the Census. The rate for 1994 is for the 12 months ending with September 1994.

into a marriage. Eighty percent of divorced men and women remarry, and the remarriage rate increases with the number of times an individual has been divorced. The remarriage rate after a second divorce is 90%, after a third divorce, it's even higher.

Family Ties

The structure of the family is undergoing profound change. In the United States, 52% of families currently have no children under age 18 living at home; by the year 2010, 59% may be childfree. The average household size is expected to decline from 2.62 members in 1995 to 2.53 in 2010.[38]

Diversity Within Families

The "all-American" **family**—as portrayed on television and in movies—is typically white and middle-class. But families of different cultures—Italian to Indian to Indonesian—reflect different traditions, beliefs, and values. Within African-American families, for instance, traditional gender roles are often reversed, with women serving as head of the household, a kinship bond uniting several households, and a strong religious commitment or orientation. In Chinese-American families, both spouses may work and see themselves as breadwinners, but the wife may not have an equal role in decision making. In Latino families, wives and mothers are acknowledged and respected as healers and dispensers of wisdom. At the same time, they are expected to defer to their husbands, who see themselves as the strong, protective, dominant head of the family. As time passes and families from different cultures become more integrated into American life, traditional gender roles and decision-making patterns often change, particularly among the youngest family members.

American families also are diverse in other ways. An unmarried career woman may be raising a child on her own. A lesbian couple may be parents of a child that one partner conceived through artificial insemination. Three of every ten households consist of blended families, formed when one or both of the partners getting married bring children from a previous union. In the future, social scientists predict, American families will become even more diverse, or pluralistic. But even as norms or expectations about the configurations of families have changed, values or ideas about the intents and purposes of families have not. American families of every type still support each other and strive toward values such as commitment and caring.

One of the main functions of the family is to serve as a training ground for living. We use our experiences in the family to learn how to behave with other individuals. Therefore, if parents behave lovingly and with respect toward each other and their children, their children learn how to have loving and healthy relationships with others. If children are victims of abusive parents at home, however, they may become someone else's victim—or abuser—elsewhere. (See Chapter 17 for a discussion of domestic violence.)

Becoming Parents

Parenting is a 24-hour-a-day, 7-day-a-week, 52-week-a-year job, with no sabbaticals or sick leaves and no opportunity to renegotiate the contract. Having a child is an experience that deeply affects, involves, and changes a man and a woman.

When Baby Makes Three

New parents are likely to feel proud one moment and anxious the next. The infant may fascinate them both, but the adjustment to a baby-centered life can cause

resentment. The husband who feels that his wife is more concerned with the baby than with him often feels jealous, which in turn makes him feel guilty. The mother, still recovering from childbirth, may feel overwhelmed by new responsibilities and the daunting physical demands of caring for a newborn.

Experts in family development, who have been studying the changes a baby brings to a marriage, note that marital satisfaction invariably declines, if only slightly, while the number of separations and divorces rises after a baby's arrival. However, couples who stick together as partners through the process of becoming parents can keep their marriages strong.

As Children Grow

Parenting by choice rather than by chance has revolutionized the hows, whos, whats, and whens of having children. Yet the basic job of parents—meeting the needs of their children—remains the same. Children have tangible needs for food, shelter, and protection that must be met, or their physical welfare will be at risk. Children also have intangible needs—psychological and emotional—that must be met, or their ability to have fruitful lives and satisfying relationships may be in jeopardy.

A child's greatest need is for love—the feeling of being wanted and cared for, of being special, and of realizing that the parents like the child for him- or herself. According to a study that followed 379 kindergarten-aged children for 36 years, warm, loving parenting—the kind that supplies plenty of hugs, kisses, and cuddles—has more influence on adult social adjustment than any other parental or childhood factor. The individuals whose mothers and fathers were openly affectionate were able to sustain long and relatively happy marriages, raise children, develop close friendships, and enjoy varied activities outside their marriage.[39]

Children have other needs, too. They need security—assurance that their parents will be there when needed most; protection; confidence; and a feeling of belonging. They need role models to learn behavior from and a sense of clear limits and controls. Parents are responsible for establishing values of what is right or wrong and for guiding by example as well as with words.

With each year that passes in a child's life, the conflict between independence and dependence becomes more intense. Children are drawn into the larger world outside the family and home, and their parents are torn between clinging to them and pushing them out of the nest. It's not enough to set rules; parents must also advise a child on how to make decisions within those rules.

The teen years—the transition from childhood to adulthood—are, for parents and children, the best and worst of times. Children becoming teenagers develop more responsibility, a greater sense of self, and more independence. Simultaneously, they may rebel, challenging and testing their parents. Setting limits—such as curfews and dating guidelines—may set off a confrontation instead of being a simple matter of stating policy. A teen's emerging sexuality may be difficult for the parents to acknowledge and accept. (Chapter 9 discusses adolescent sexuality.)

Siblings

The ways in which siblings relate as children often affect their interactions with each other—and with others, including their mates—when they grow up. Sibling rivalry, for instance, though normal, can lead to unhealthy ways of relating to others. For example, siblings who had to compete fiercely for parental attention or affection may remain competitive throughout life, doing anything necessary in order to come out on top. And youngsters who feel that their parents clearly prefer another child in the family may come to think that they're inadequate or somehow unworthy of love.

Siblings typically grow more distant during adolescence, as they focus on developing their own identities. This separation continues during early adulthood. However, in middle age, most adults report positive relationships with siblings. Some are bound by loyalty, even if they don't feel friendly toward a brother or sister. Others socialize with siblings but are closer to friends. In old age, sisters and brother-sister pairs have more positive relationships than brothers; elderly African Americans tend to have more positive relationships with their siblings than do elderly whites.[40]

Working Parents

Throughout the world, mothers have taken on increased economic responsibility for their families. As a result, they are working longer hours at home and on the job. In the United States, nearly half of employed married women contribute half or more of their family's income. As Figure 8-8 shows, many more women with young children are working either full or part time. Of all

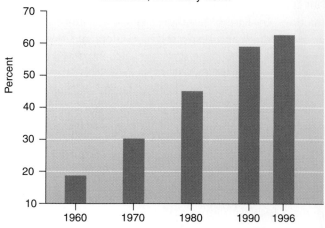

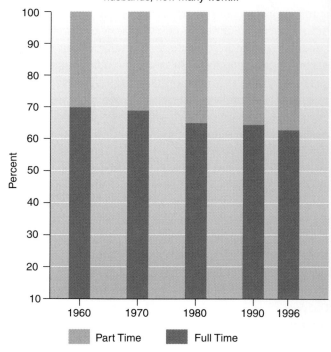

Figure 8-8 Working Mothers. An increasing number of women with young children work full or part time.

SOURCE: Bureau of Labor Statistics

women who work, 16.8% have children under six years of age.

Partly out of necessity and partly because they want to, many men are taking on more family responsibilities, including about a third of child care. However, fathers' involvement takes different forms than it does

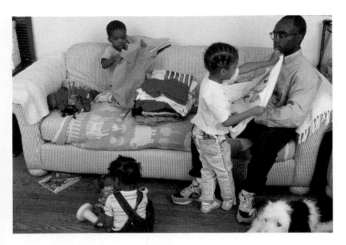

Dads' changing roles. Sharing parenting duties can take many forms, but those who do share equitably may be the happiest.

for mothers. "Women do basic maintenance: feeding, bathing, day-in-and-day-out chores, while fathers do trips to the zoo and special outings," observes Arlie Hochschild, Ph.D., professor of sociology at the University of California, Berkeley, and author of *The Second Shift.* "But the most pervasive difference is that women assume mental responsibility for children." Yet, she notes, the happiest couples are those who share parenting duties as equitably as possible.[41]

Children of Divorce

Each year divorce separates more than a million children from their parents. The breakup of a marriage has an enormous impact on many aspects of a child's life, including his or her standard of living. Very young children may become more babyish, irritable, and dependent. Preschool or young school-age children may blame themselves, feeling that "Daddy left because I was bad." School-age children may feel lonely, helpless, and depressed; they may develop illnesses or have problems in their friendships. Preteens may experiment with alcohol, drugs, and sex. For teenagers, divorce may make separating from the family and establishing an adult identity even harder.

Long-term studies show that the impact of divorce on children varies. According to one of the largest and most comprehensive studies of children of divorce, most youngsters fare well academically. In an analysis of data collected on 1700 children, ages 5 to 8, from divorced households, the key factor in their academic achieve-ment was not the absence of their father but the education of their mothers. The children of more highly educated moms consistently did better in school than those whose mothers had less formal education.[42]

Psychologically, divorce can take a greater toll. According to various reports, 15% to 20% of all children whose parents divorce may require professional therapy. Psychologist Judith Wallerstein, who pioneered in the study of children of divorce, reports that virtually all of the youngsters whom she has seen or studied have suffered some emotional scars as a result of the breakup of their parents' marriage.[43]

Strategies for Change

Helping Children of Divorce

✔ Don't give youngsters everything they want just to get them to like you more than the other parent.

✔ Be honest, but spare your children the gory details.

✔ Don't use children as bullets. Don't fight in front of them.

✔ Let children know it's okay for them to love both their parents.

✔ Spend time with the children. Give them a chance to talk about how they feel.

✔ Let them know that you love them and that they are not responsible for the breakup.

One-Parent and Blended Families

Almost a quarter of all white families, more than half of all African-American families, and about a third of all Latino families are headed by a single parent. Like two-parent families, one-parent families are all different. An educated divorced woman in her thirties with one school-age child has many more options and opportunities than a young, unskilled, never-married woman with three preschoolers. However, at every economic level, the amount of time single parents spend with their children is not significantly different from that spent by parents in two-parent families.

Each year about half a million children become part of new, **blended families** when their parents remarry. Over the years many studies have found significant differences in family and relationship processes in these families. However, improved communication and problem solving can help blended families work through their problems.[44]

Children can also be encouraged to spend time with members of the extended family or friends to experience other role models.

Dysfunctional Relationships

Relationships that don't promote healthy communication, honesty, and intimacy are sometimes called **dysfunctional**. Individuals with addictive behaviors or dependence on drugs or alcohol (see Chapters 14 and 15), and the children or partners of such people, are especially likely to find themselves in such relationships.

Often partners have magical, unrealistic expectations (e.g., they expect that a relationship with the right person will make their life okay), and one person uses the other almost as if he or she were a mood-altering drug. The partners may compulsively try to get the other to act the way they want. Both persons may not trust or may deceive each other. Often they isolate themselves from others, thus trapping themselves in a recurring cycle of pain.

Dysfunctional families exist in every economic, social, educational, religious, and racial group. They inflict emotional pain on children through destructive behaviors, such as physical, emotional, verbal, or sexual abuse; physical or emotional neglect; and alcoholism or drug use. Although alcohol or drugs do not in themselves create dysfunctional families, they can push parents over a psychological brink. The results can be emotionally devastating. The children of alcoholics, drug users, and parents with other addictive behaviors are prone to learning disabilities, eating disorders, compulsive achievement, and addiction.

Codependence

As used by contemporary therapists, the term **codependence** (or coaddiction) refers to the tendency of the spouses, partners, parents, and friends of individuals with addictive behaviors to allow or *enable* their loved ones to continue their self-destructive habits. Codependent individuals focus on their loved ones, even to the extent of giving up their own lives. They change who they are and what they feel in order to please others, feel responsible for meeting others' needs, have low self-esteem, and frequently have compulsions of their own. However, codependent behaviors need to be evaluated in the context of an individual's culture. For exam-

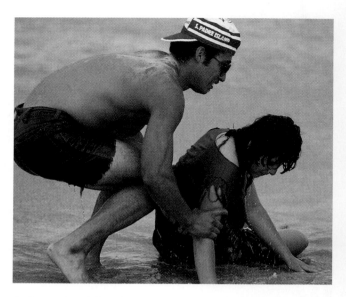

Caring and enabling. Codependence involves family members in covering for those with substance abuse problems, which in turn allows substance abusers to continue their behavior.

ple, the emphasis on family values and support that is part of the value system of many Latinos would not be considered codependent behavior.

Codependents Anonymous, founded in 1986 for men and women whose common problem is an inability to maintain functional relationships, is one of the fastest-growing support programs in the country. Other self-help groups for codependents include Al-Anon (for adult family members of alcoholics), Alateen (for the teenaged children of addicts), Nar-Anon (for people in relationships with individuals who abuse drugs), O-Anon (for those whose family members have eating disorders), and Gam-Anon (for those living with people who have gambling problems). Local chapters of these groups can be found in the white pages of the telephone book. Through such groups, codependent individuals can learn how to leave behind guilt feelings, how to become less judgmental and moralistic, how to understand their powerlessness over their loved one's problem, and how to do what needs to be done for themselves as well as the addict.

Strategies for Prevention
....
Are You Codependent?

Read through the following list of characteristics of codependence and check any that apply to you:

CHAPTER 8 Communicating and Relating 235

✔ I find myself covering for another person's alcohol or drug use, eating or work habits, gambling, sexual escapades, or general behavior.

✔ I spend a great deal of time talking about and worrying about other people's behavior/problems/future instead of living my own life.

✔ I have marked or counted bottles, searched for a hidden stash, or in other ways monitored someone else's behavior.

✔ I find myself taking on more responsibility at home or in a relationship, even though I resent it.

✔ I ignore my own needs in favor of meeting someone else's.

✔ I'm afraid that if I get angry, the other person will leave or not love me.

✔ I worry that if I leave a relationship or stop controlling the other person, that person will fall apart.

✔ I spend less time with friends and more with my partner/parent/child in activities that I wouldn't normally choose.

✔ My self-esteem depends on what others say and think of me, or on my possessions or job.

✔ I grew up in a family in which there was little communication, in which expressing feelings wasn't acceptable, and in which there were either rigid rules or none at all.

If you identify with more than three of these statements, you may be codependent. There are many useful books on codependence at libraries and bookstores. You may also wish to visit a support group on campus or in your area or talk with a counselor.[45]

Enabling

Experts on the subject of addiction first identified traits of codependence in spouses of alcoholics, who followed a predictable pattern of behavior: While intensely trying to control the drinkers, the codependent mates would act in ways that allowed the drinkers to keep drinking. For example, if an alcoholic found it hard to get up in the morning, his wife would wake him up, pull him out of bed and into the shower, and drop him off at work. If he was late, she made excuses to his boss. The husband was the one with the substance-abuse problem, but without realizing it, his wife was enabling him to continue drinking. In fact, he might not have been able to keep up his habit without her unintentional cooperation.

The different styles or components of enabling include the following:

- *Shielding.* Codependents may cover up for abusers, preventing them from experiencing the full impact of the harmful consequences of their behavior—for example, by dropping off a paper or report so that the addicted person can avoid a missed deadline.
- *Controlling.* A codependent may try to control the significant other—for instance, by withholding sex or using sex as a reward for cutting down on an addictive behavior.
- *Taking over responsibilities.* The codependent may take over such household chores as shopping or running errands.
- *Rationalizing.* Codependents try to rationalize their partners' addiction by telling themselves that a compulsive behavior pattern, like workaholism, is making the person more successful, or that drinking helps him or her relax.
- *Cooperating.* Sometimes codependents become involved in the person's compulsion, perhaps placing bets for a gambler or buying alcohol for a drinker.
- *Rescuing.* The codependent may become overprotective—for example, by allowing the user to use drugs at home to avoid the risk of an accident or arrest.

Codependence progresses just as an addiction does, and codependents excuse their own behavior with many of the same defense mechanisms used by addicts, such as rationalization ("I cut class so I could catch up on my reading, not to keep an eye on my partner") and denial ("He likes to gamble, but he never loses more than he can afford"). In time, just as an addict's world becomes smaller and smaller, codependents lose sight of everything but their loved one. They feel that if they can only "fix" this person, everything will be fine.

Making This Chapter Work for You
Building Better Relationships

■ Sending clear messages through words, gestures, expressions, and behaviors is the essence of good communication. Effective communication helps create good relationships built on honesty, understanding, and mutual trust.

■ Men and women use language in different ways.

Men tend to speak to convey information, to challenge others, to achieve status in a group, or to put themselves in a "one-up" situation. Women, on the other hand, tend to talk to achieve and nurture intimacy, to promote closeness and equality in a group, and to build better connections to others.

- Nonverbal communication refers to the unspoken messages people send with their gestures, expressions, and body movements.

- A genuine concern and respect for ourselves helps us remain true to our own feelings and beliefs and enhances the likelihood that we will seek out healthy, positive relationships.

- Friendships are among the most cherished bonds among people. In today's society, friends often become our extended family, providing acceptance, warmth, and loyalty.

- Dating provides opportunities to get to know other people, to practice social skills, and to explore one's sexuality.

- Sexual attraction usually involves many different factors, including similarity in age, race, ethnicity, socioeconomic class, education, physical attractiveness, power, wealth, and status.

- Romantic love is characterized by intense passion. This type of bond, which anthropologists have found in almost all societies, may help pull men and women into the sort of partnerships needed to care for children. From a biochemical view, infatuation may trigger a rise in certain neurotransmitters that create a natural high that is very pleasurable—but not long-lasting.

- Mature love combines sexual excitement, tenderness, a sincere commitment to bringing out the best in each other, the encouragement of mutual growth, a willingness to risk vulnerability, and the ability to enjoy solitude or separateness from one's partner.

- Increasingly, young adults are spending longer periods of time living on their own, with their parents, or with a partner, before deciding about marriage.

- If they do marry, most couples do so for love. The older and more similar two people are, the more likely they are to have a successful marriage. Premarital assessments can identify behavior patterns that can predict the likelihood of divorce.

- Even happily married couples must contend with many complex issues and pressures, including dual careers, money, sex, and day-to-day disagreements.

- For all its challenges, marriage provides many rewards. Married people are more likely to be healthier, to live longer, and to be better able to cope with stress than are single people.

- Divorce rates have remained fairly stable, and more people are seeking help to make their marriages work. However, more marriages around the world are ending in divorce.

- Parenthood is among the most demanding, difficult, and gratifying responsibilities a person will ever have. Today more fathers are actively involved with their children, and more mothers have careers. Both parents must work together to meet the physical and psychological needs of growing children.

- The number and percentage of traditional two-parent families has fallen, while the number of single-parent homes has skyrocketed.

- The response of children to the divorce of their parents depends on their age and on the amount of fighting before and after the divorce.

- Dysfunctional relationships do not promote healthy communication, honesty, and intimacy and can be emotionally destructive, especially for children.

Throughout life, each of us is responsible for keeping up our end of a relationship—with friends, dates, partners, spouses, and children. This means that again and again we must struggle toward understanding. Here are some guidelines that may help:

- Develop the habit of asking the other people in your life about their feelings, thoughts, interests, and desires. Never assume.

- With friends, partners, and families, function as a team. Work at making decisions and solving problems together.

- Give the people you care about daily doses of the four A's: attention, acceptance, approval, and affection.

- Don't play games, such as trying to make a friend jealous, getting even, or proving someone wrong.

- Be polite. Politeness is a way of saying "I care about you," and it means more than an expensive gift.

- Give as much of yourself as you can. The more time you can give to the people who mean the most to you, the closer you'll become. You won't have to wonder what you're getting out of your relationships; you'll discover that the getting comes with the giving.

Health Online

The Marriage Toolbox   http://www.marriagetools.com/

This site contains lots of online advice for creating and maintaining a loving marriage or repairing one with problems. In addition to stories, advice, and reflections on marriage, there is a place for you to create an online journal about your experiences with relationships.

Think about it ...

- Do you think love is enough to sustain a marriage, or does it take more?
  What other qualities might be important?

- You probably know people in happy and not-so-happy marriages. Can you list five ways of communicating that you see in the happy marriages and five others in the less happy ones?

- What do you think is the ideal age for a person to get married?
  What would you like to have accomplished before marriage?

 ## Key Terms

The terms listed here are used within the chapter. Page numbers are included for each term.
A definition of each term is given in the green Glossary pages at the end of this book.

blended family   *233*
codependence   *234*
cohabitation   *223*
companion-oriented
  marriage   *226*

dysfunctional   *234*
family   *230*
intimacy   *219*
neurotransmitters   *220*
rescue marriage   *227*

romantic marriage   *227*
traditional marriage   *226*

 ## Review Questions

1. What are the characteristics of a friendship? How does friendship develop and grow? Can you describe the different stages?

2. How does a relationship progress from dating to mature love? Define each stage and describe the steps involved.

3. What kinds of living arrangements might today's adults choose? Name three different types of living arrangements and explain how they differ from one another.

4. What are some issues that might surface in a long-term relationship over time? Explain how these issues might affect the relationship and some methods for successful coping.

5. What kinds of pressures are found in dual-career families? What can couples who both work do to resolve some of the pressures of parenting?

6. What are some expectations of being a parent? Are there any factors that might challenge those expectations? How might some of these issues be resolved?

Critical Thinking Questions

1. Increasing numbers of single people, including those living alone or with heterosexual or homosexual partners, claim that they are discriminated against in housing, credit, insurance, membership groups, and medical services. Those who oppose the concept of singles' rights say that extending spousal benefits to singles or domestic partners would erode the institution of marriage and cause a bureaucratic mess. Do you think marital status should determine how individuals are treated? Why or why not?

2. While our society has become more tolerant, marriages between people of different religious and racial groups still face special pressures. What issues might arise if a Christian marries a Jewish or Muslim man or woman? What about the issues facing partners of different races? How could these issues be resolved? What are your own feelings about mixed marriages? Would you date someone of a different religion or race? Why or why not?

3. What are your personal criteria for a successful relationship? Develop a brief list of factors you consider important, and support your choices with examples or experiences from your own life.

Connections to Personal Health Interactive

To enhance your understanding of the material covered in this chapter, check out the following study aids on the **Personal Health Interactive CD-ROM**. *Each numbered icon within the chapter corresponds to an appropriate activity listed here.*

8.1 Personal Insights: Do People Understand You?
8.2 Likeable Personality Traits
8.3 Culture and Conflict
8.4 Punishment and Parenting
8.5 Chapter 8 Review

References

1. Tannen, Deborah. *You Just Don't Understand: Women and Men in Conversation.* New York: Ballantine, 1990.

2. Hall, Judith. Personal interview.

3. Mehrabian, Albert. Personal interview.

4. Maple, Marilyn. Personal interview.

5. Swann, William, et al. "Socialization Patterns of Depressed and Non-Depressed College Students." *Journal of Abnormal Psychology,* Vol. 104, 1992.

6. Laumann, Edward. Personal interview.

7. Laumann, Edward, et al. *The Social Organization of Sexuality.* Chicago: University of Chicago Press, 1994.

8. Sprecher, Susan, et al. "Mate Selection Preferences." Sex Roles, June 1994. Feingold, Alan. "Sex Differences in the Effects of Similarity and Physical Attractiveness."*Basic & Applied Social Psychology,* September 1991; "Gender Differences in Effects of Physical Attractiveness on Romantic Attraction." *Journal of Personality & Social Psychology,* November 1990.

9. Buss, David. *The Evolution of Desire.* New York: Basic Books, 1994.

10. Singh, Devendra. "Adaptive Significance of Female Physical Attractiveness: Role of Waist-to-Hip Ratio." *Journal of Personality and Social Psychology,* Vol. 65, No. 2, August 1993. "Is Thin Really Beautiful and Good?" *Personality & Individual Differences,* January 1994. "Adaptive Significance of Female Physical Attractiveness." *Journal of Personality and Social Psychology,* August 1993. "Body Shape and Women's Attractiveness." *Human Nature,* 1993. Cohn, Lawrence, and Nancy Adler. "Female and Male Perceptions of Ideal Body Shapes." *Psychology of Women Quarterly,* March 1992.

11. "The Beefcaking of America." *Psychology Today,* November/December 1994.

12. Ackerman, Diane. *A Natural History of Love.* New York: Vintage Books, 1995.

13. Jankowiak, William, and Edward Fischer.

14. Fisher, Helen. Personal interview.

15. Ackerman, *A Natural History of Love.*

16. Baumeister, R., et al. "Unrequited Love: On Heartbreak, Anger, Guilt, Scriptlessness and Humiliation." *Journal of Personality and Social Psychology*, Vol. 64, 1993.

17. Bureau of the Census.

18. Ibid.

19. Kaslow, Florence. "The Thirty-Something Women: Companionship, Children, and Career Choices." American Psychological Association Meeting, Boston, August 1990.

20. Waehler, Charles. "Personality Characteristics of Never-Married Men." American Psychological Association Meeting, San Francisco, August 1991.

21. Bureau of the Census.

22. Steinhauer, Jennifer. "Big Benefits in Marriage, Studies Say." *New York Times*, April 10, 1995. Demaris, Alfred, and K. Vaninadha Rao. "Premarital Cohabitation and Subsequent Marital Stability in the United States: A Reassessment." *Journal of Marriage and the Family,* February 1992.

23. Bureau of the Census.

24. Gottman, John. *Why Marriages Succeed or Fail.* New York: Simon & Schuster, 1994.

25. Sternberg, Robert. Personal interview.

26. Larsen, A., and Olson, D. "Predicting Marital Satisfaction Using PREPARE: A Replication Study." *Journal of Marital and Family Therapy*, Vol. 15, 1989.

27. Gottman, J. *Why Marriages Succeed or Fail.* Gottman, J. *What Predicts Divorce?* Gottman, John, et al. "Predictors of Divorce." *Journal of Family Psychology*, Vol. 1, No. 1, 1992.

28. Wallerstein, Judith. *The Good Marriage.* New York: Random House, 1995.

29. Greeley, Andrew. "Faithful Attraction." *Psychology Today,* March 1990.

30. Robinson, John, and Geoffrey Godbey. "No Sex, Please …We're College Graduates." *American Demographics*, February 1998.

31. Laumann et al., *The Social Organization of Sexuality.*

32. Clemens, Mark. "Sex in America." *Parade*, August 7, 1993.

33. Steinhauer, Jennifer. "Big Benefits in Marriage, Studies Say." *New York Times*, April 10, 1995.

34. Ibid.

35. Gleick, Elizabeth. "Should This Marriage Be Saved?" *Time*, February 17, 1995.

36. Association of Family and Marital Therapists. Personal interview.

37. Statisical Summary. *Pediatrics*, December 1997.

38. McLeod, Ramon. "U.S. Growth Rate of New Households at 146-Year Low." *San Francisco Chronicle*, May 3, 1996.

39. Franz, Carol, David McClelland, and Joel Weinberger. "Childhood Antecedents of Conventional Social Accomplishment in Midlife Adults: A 36 Year Prospective Study." *Journal of Personality and Social Psychology*, April 1991.

40. Klagsbrun, Francine. *Mixed Feelings: Love, Hate, Rivalry and Reconciliation Among Brothers and Sisters.* New York: Bantam Books, 1992.

41. Abelson, Reed. "When Waaa Turns to Why." *New York Times*, November 11, 1997.

42. Mott, Frank. Director of the Center for Human Resources Research, Ohio State University. Personal interview.

43. Wallerstein, Judith, and Sandra Blakeslee. *Second Chances.* New York: Ticknor & Fields, 1989.

44. Bray, James. "Longitudinal Changes in Stepfamilies: Impact on Children's Adjustment." American Psychological Association Meeting, Washington, DC, August 1992.

45. Blau, Melinda. "No Life to Live." *American Health*, May 1990.

CHAPTER 9

PERSONAL SEXUALITY

After studying the material in this chapter, you should be able to:

Explain the major factors that influence sexual identity and gender identity in our society, and **indicate** how these differ in some other cultures.

Describe the male and female reproductive systems and the functions of the individual components of each system.

Describe some conditions or issues unique to women's sexual health and men's sexual health.

Describe some methods for preventing infection from HIV and other sexually transmitted diseases.

List the common concerns of men and women about sexual performance difficulties.

Human **sexuality**—the quality of being sexual—is as rich, varied, and complex as life itself. Along with our **sex**, or biological maleness or femaleness, it is an integral part of who we are, how we see ourselves, and how we relate to others. Of all of our involvements with others, sexual **intimacy**, or physical closeness, can be the most rewarding. But while sexual expression and experience can provide intense joy, they also can involve great emotional turmoil.

You are ultimately responsible for your sexual health and behavior. You make decisions that affect how you express your sexuality, how you respond sexually, and how you give and get sexual pleasure. Yet most sexual activity involves another person. Therefore, your decisions about sex—more so than those you make about nutrition, drugs, or exercise—have important effects on other people. Recognizing this fact is the key to responsible sexuality.

Sexual responsibility means learning about your body, your partner's body, your sexual development and preferences, and the health risks associated with sexual activity. This chapter is an introduction to your sexual self and an exploration of sexual issues in today's world. It provides the information and insight you can use in making decisions and choosing behaviors that are responsible for all concerned.

Becoming Male or Female

Physiological maleness or femaleness, or biological sex, is indicated by the sex chromosomes, hormonal balance, and genital anatomy. **Gender** refers to the psychological and sociological, as well as the physical, aspects of being male or female. You are born with a certain *sexual identity* based on your sexual anatomy and appearance; you, your parents, and society mold your *gender identity*.

Are You an X or a Y?

Biologically, few absolute differences separate the sexes: Males alone can make sperm and contribute the chromosome that causes embryos to develop as males; females alone are born with sex cells (eggs or ova), menstruate, give birth, and breast-feed babies. But the process of becoming male or female is a long and complex one.

In the beginning, all human embryos have undifferentiated sex organs. Only after several weeks do the sex organs differentiate, becoming either male or female **gonads** (testes or ovaries), the structures that produce the future reproductive cells of an individual. This initial differentiation process depends on genetic instructions in the form of the sex chromosomes, referred to as X and Y. If a Y (or male) chromosome is present in the embryo, about seven weeks after conception, it signals the sex organs to develop into testes. If a Y chromosome isn't present, an embryo begins developing ovaries in the eighth week. From this point on, the sex hormones produced by the gonads, not the chromosomes, play the crucial role in making a male or female.

The Role of Hormones

In Greek, *hormone* means "set into motion"—and that's exactly what our **hormones** do. These chemical messengers, produced by various organs in the body, including the sex organs, and carried to target structures by the bloodstream, arouse cells and organs to specific activities and influence the way we look, feel, develop, and behave.

The group of organs that produce hormones is referred to as the **endocrine system**. Except for the sex organs, males and females have identical endocrine systems. Directing the endocrine system is the *hypothala-*

mus, a pea-sized section of the brain. The pituitary gland, directly beneath the hypothalamus, turns the various glands on and off in response to messages from it.

The ovaries produce the sex hormones most crucial to women, **estrogen** and **progesterone**. The primary sex hormone in men is **testosterone**, which is produced by the testes and the adrenal glands. However, both men and women have small amounts of the hormones of the opposite sex. Estrogen, in fact, is crucial to male fertility and gives sperm what researchers describe as their "reproductive punch." [1]

The sex hormones begin their work early in an embryo's development. As soon as the testes are formed, they start releasing testosterone, which stimulates the development of other structures, such as the penis. The absence of testosterone in an embryo causes female genitals to form. (If the testes of a genetic male don't produce testosterone, the fetus will develop female genitals. Similarly, if a genetic female is exposed to excessive testosterone, the fetus will have ovaries but will also develop male genitals.)

As puberty begins, the pituitary gland initiates the changes that transform boys into men and girls into women. When a boy is about 14 years old and a girl about 12, their brains stimulate the hypothalamus to secrete a hormone called *gonadotropin releasing hormone (GnRH)*. This substance causes the pituitary gland to release hormones called **gonadotropins**. These, in turn, stimulate the gonads to make sex hormones. (See Figure 9-1.)

The gonadotropins are *follicle-stimulating hormone (FSH)* and *luteinizing hormone (LH)*. In girls, these hormones travel to the ovary and stimulate the production of estrogen. As estrogen increases, a girl's **secondary sex characteristics** develop. Her breasts become fuller, her external genitals enlarge, and fat is deposited on her hips and buttocks. Estrogen keeps her hair thick and skin smooth. She begins menstruating because she has begun ovulating, the process that prepares her body to conceive and carry a baby.

According to biologist Martha McClintock of the University of Chicago, the maturing of the adrenal glands also brings about the first flicker of sexual desire. After years of being oblivious to physical charms, boys and girls suddenly look around a crowded classroom and, as McClintock puts it, start to "notice—with a capital N" that someone, whether of the same or the other sex, looks particularly good to them. They feel a zing that may not be sexual in the adult sense but definitely

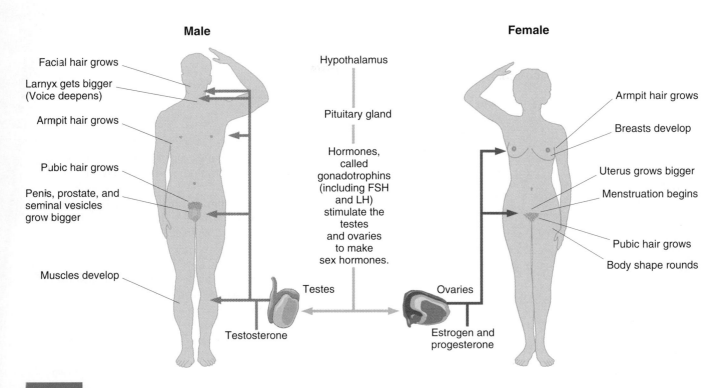

Figure 9-1

Puberty. The body's endocrine system produces hormones that trigger body changes in males and females. Additional body changes include growth spurts and changes to the skeleton.

carries a charge. A year and a half to two years later, as the reproductive glands churn out much greater amounts of sex hormones, desire kicks in. In the University of Chicago analysis, this happened at a mean age of 11.9 for girls and 11.2 for boys, with first sexual activity beginning more than three years later for girls (at age 15.2) and two years later for boys (at age 13.1).[2]

In addition to the adrenals, a girl's ovaries also begin to mature—again, at an earlier age than many had assumed. In a 1997 analysis of growth charts from 17,077 girls from ages 3 to 12, researchers at the University of North Carolina at Chapel Hill found that, by age 8, 15 % of white girls and 48 % of African-American girls show signs of sexual development. (The reasons for this racial discrepancy are not known.) The mean ages for breast development are 8.87 years for African-American girls and 9.96 years for white girls; for pubic hair, they are 8.78 years and 10.51 years, respectively. African-American girls begin menstruating at 12.16 years; white girls, at 12.88 years.[3]

In boys, the gonadotropins stimulate the testes to produce testosterone, which triggers the development of male secondary sex characteristics. Their voices deepen,

hair grows on their faces and bodies, their penises become thicker and longer, and their muscles become stronger.

The sex hormones released during puberty change the growth pattern of childhood, so that a boy or girl may now spurt up 4 to 6 inches in a single year. The skeleton matures very rapidly until, at the end of puberty (usually around age 18), the growth centers at the ends of the bones close off. Estrogen causes girls' bones to stop growing at an earlier age than boys' bones.

Gender Differences

As scientists have documented, men and women do think, act, and react in different ways. *Brain scans* by high-resolution imaging equipment indicate that male and female brains are different. There are also gender differences in sensory skills. Throughout life, a woman's senses of hearing, taste, and smell are more acute than a man's, while men have sharper vision. In tests of physical power, most men can outmuscle most women, but when it comes to precision tasks, such as working door

Self-Survey

How Much Do You Know About Sex?

Mark each of the following statements True or False:

1. Men and women have completely different sex hormones.
2. Premenstrual syndrome (PMS) is primarily a psychological problem.
3. Circumcision diminishes a man's sexual pleasure.
4. Sexual orientation may have a biological basis.
5. Masturbation is a sign of emotional immaturity.
6. Only homosexual men engage in anal intercourse.
7. Despite their awareness of AIDS, many college students do not practice safe sex.
8. After age 60, lovemaking is mainly a fond memory, not a regular pleasure of daily living.
9. Doctors advise against having intercourse during a woman's menstrual period.
10. Only men ejaculate.
11. It is possible to be infected with HIV during a single sexual encounter.
12. Impotence is always a sign of emotional or sexual problems in a relationship.

Answers:

1. False. Men and women have the same hormones, but in different amounts.
2. False. PMS has been recognized as a very real physiological disorder that may be caused by a hormonal deficiency, abnormal levels of thyroid hormone, changes in brain chemicals, or social and environmental factors, such as stress.
3. False. Sex therapists have not been able to document differences in sensitivity to stimulation between circumcised and uncircumcised men.
4. True. Researchers have documented structural differences in the brains of homosexual men and women.
5. False. Throughout a person's life, masturbation can be a form of sexual release and pleasure.
6. False. As many as one in every four married couples under age 35 have reported that they occasionally engage in anal intercourse.
7. True. In one recent study, more than a third of college students had engaged in vaginal or anal intercourse at

least once in the previous year without using effective protection from conception or sexually transmitted diseases (STDs).
8. False. More than a third of American married men and women older than 60 make love at least once a week as do 10% of those older than 70.
9. False. There's no medical reason to avoid intercourse during a woman's menstrual period.
10. False. Stimulation of the Grafenberg spot in a woman's vagina may lead to a release of fluid from her urethra during orgasm.
11. True. Although the risk increases with repeated sexual contact with an infected partner, an individual can contract HIV during a single sexual encounter.
12. False. Many erection difficulties have physical causes.

Making Changes ....
Informing Yourself About Sex

Your score on this self-survey may indicate that you know a lot more—or less—about sex than you thought you did. Part of sexual responsibility is being informed about sexuality, including reproductive anatomy, sexual orientation, the range of sexual behaviors, and ways of protecting yourself from sexually transmitted diseases.

How can you get good information about sex? If you have questions about sexual biology or behavior, you can usually get accurate and understandable answers from college-level human sexuality textbooks. If you're concerned about birth control or protection from sexually transmitted diseases, your college health clinic and your local Planned Parenthood clinic are excellent resources. For questions regarding your own sexual and reproductive health and organs, visit a health care professional for a thorough examination.

Knowledge about sex can help free you from misconceptions that could be dangerous to your health. And there's an added psychological benefit as well: The more you know, the less confused you'll feel about your own sexuality.

latches or inserting pegs in a pegboard, women have proven more adept.[4]

Are such differences signs that men and women are born different? Or do we become different because of our environment and experiences? This question—one of the most controversial in the behavioral sciences—is far too complex for an either-or answer. "You can't pull

apart nature and nurture," says Diane Halpern, Ph.D., a psychology professor at California State University in San Bernardino and author of *Sex Differences in Cognitive Ability*. "There are things that men, on average, excel at, and things that women, on average, excel at. But the fact that there are differences doesn't mean that one is good and one is bad or that there's a winner or a

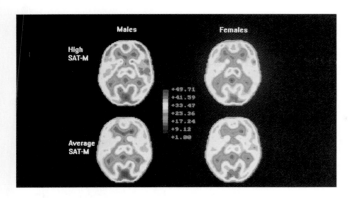

The two photos above are actual brain scans of a male and a female subject. Notice the differences in the highlighted areas.

drivers, engineers, pilots, coal miners, physicians, and executives.

An alternative to both male and female sexual type-casting is the concept of **androgyny**, a word that literally translates (from the Greek) as "man woman." Androgynous individuals combine aspects of both masculinity and femininity into their personalities and lifestyles. They act in ways that seem appropriate to a given relationship or situation—instead of in ways that seem appropriately masculine or feminine. Such behaviors can enhance compatibility and satisfaction in a relationship.[6]

loser."[5] In fact, the real issue may not be what makes for gender differences, but what difference—if any—the differences make.

Sexual Stereotypes

Being male is not the same as being masculine, and being female is not the same as being feminine. Today more men and women are breaking out of traditional stereotypes. Men are acknowledging their feelings and fears and taking on what were formerly women's jobs—becoming nurses and secretaries at work, and doing the grocery shopping and laundry at home. Although there still aren't any female linebackers in the National Football League (and no one expects that there will be), women have taken their places among astronauts, truck

Strategies for Prevention

Avoiding Sexual Stereotyping

✔ Language counts. Do you always say "he" for a doctor and "she" for a nurse? By changing your language you can help eliminate sexual stereotypes.

✔ Think of ten different ways to complete this sentence: "A real man…" Do the same with the sentence beginning, "A real woman…" Then complete a sentence starting with "A real person…"

✔ List some of the attributes you admire in someone of the other sex. How do those attributes compare with the attributes you value in yourself or your same-sex friends?

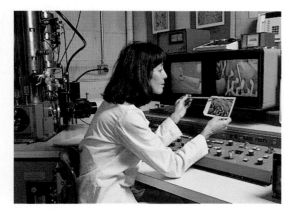

Not too long ago, we might have assumed that this woman is a laboratory assistant instead of the scientist she is. And we probably would have assumed that this man is a doctor instead of a nurse. In today's world, it's more common that interest and hard work—rather than sex-role stereotypes—define job success.

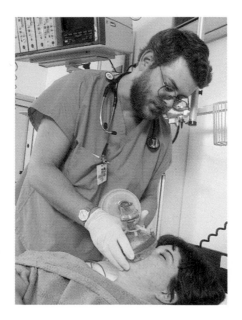

Women's Sexual Health

Only recently has medical research devoted major scientific investigations to issues in women's health. In fact, until 1993, the National Institutes of Health routinely excluded women from experimental studies because of concerns about menstrual cycles and pregnancy. In clinical settings, women are more likely to have their symptoms dismissed as psychological and not to be referred to a specialist than are men with identical complaints. Some physicians are suggesting the creation of a new medical specialty (distinct from obstetrics and gynecology) that would be devoted to women's health to provide more comprehensive care and overcome the current gender gap in health services.[7]

Female Sexual Anatomy

As illustrated in Figure 9-2a, the **mons pubis** is the rounded, fleshy area over the junction of the pubic bones. The folds of skin that form the outer lips of a woman's genital area are called the **labia majora**. They cover soft flaps of skin (inner lips) called the **labia minora**. The inner lips join at the top to form a hood over the **clitoris**, a small elongated erectile organ, and the most sensitive spot in the entire female genital area. Below the clitoris is the **urethral opening**, the outer opening of the thin tube that carries urine from the bladder. Below that is a larger opening, the mouth of the **vagina**, the canal that leads to the primary internal organs of reproduction. The **perineum** is the area between the vagina and the anus (the opening to the rectum and large intestine).

At the back of the vagina is the **cervix**, the opening to the womb, or **uterus** (see Figure 9-2b). The uterine walls are lined by a layer of tissue called the **endometrium**. The **ovaries**, about the size and shape of almonds, are located on either side of the uterus, and contain egg cells called **ova** (singular, **ovum**). Extending outward and back from the upper uterus are the **fallopian tubes**, the canals that transport ova from the ovaries to the uterus. When an egg is released from an ovary, the fingerlike ends of the adjacent fallopian tube "catch" the egg and direct it into the tube.

The Menstrual Cycle

As shown in Figure 9-3, the hypothalamus monitors hormone levels in the blood and sends messages to the pituitary gland to release follicle stimulating hormone (FSH) and luteinizing hormone (LH). In the ovary, these hormones stimulate the growth of a few of the immature eggs, or ova, stored in every woman's body. Usually, only one ovum matures completely during each monthly cycle. As it does, it increases its production of the female sex hormone estrogen, which in turn triggers the release of a larger surge of LH.

At midcycle, the increased LH hormone levels trigger **ovulation**, the release of the egg cell, or ovum. Estrogen levels drop, and the remaining cells of the follicle then enlarge, change character, and form the **corpus luteum**, or yellow body. In the second half of the menstrual cycle, the corpus luteum secretes estrogen and larger amounts of progesterone. The **endometrium** (uterine lining) is stimulated by progesterone to thicken and become more engorged with blood in preparation for nourishing an implanted, fertilized ovum.

If the ovum is not fertilized, the corpus luteum disintegrates. As the level of progesterone drops, **menstruation** occurs; the uterine lining is shed during the course of a menstrual period. If the egg is fertilized and pregnancy occurs, the cells that eventually develop into the placenta secrete *human chorionic gonadotropin (HCG)*, a messenger hormone that signals the pituitary not to start a new cycle. The corpus luteum then steps up its production of progesterone. Many women experience physical or psychological changes, or both, during their monthly cycles. Usually the changes are minor, but more serious problems can occur.

Premenstrual Syndrome (PMS)

Women with **premenstrual syndrome (PMS)** experience bodily discomfort and emotional distress for up to two weeks, from ovulation until the onset of menstruation. Three to 15% of these women develop very severe symptoms. In some studies, as many as 40% to 45% of women have reported at least one premenstrual symptom.

Once dismissed as a psychological problem, PMS has been recognized as a very real physiological disorder that may be caused by a hormonal deficiency; abnormal levels of thyroid hormone; an imbalance of estrogen and progesterone; changes in brain chemicals; or social and environmental factors, particularly stress. Because there are no consistent or objective ways of diagnosing premenstrual complaints, it's hard to know precisely how many women are affected.

The most common symptoms of PMS are mood changes, anxiety, irritability, difficulty concentrating, forgetfulness, impaired judgment, tearfulness, digestive symptoms (diarrhea, bloating, constipation), hot flashes, palpitations, dizziness, headache, fatigue, changes in

A. External structure

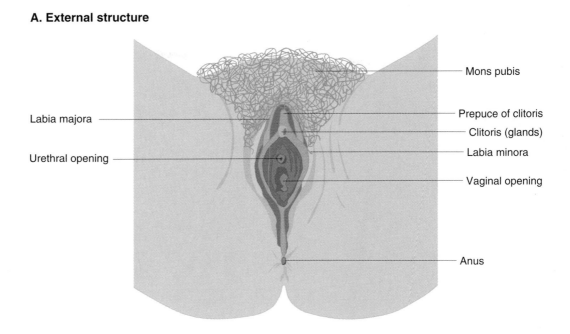

Figure 9-2

The female sex organs and reproductive structure.

Mons pubis
Prepuce of clitoris
Clitoris (glands)
Labia minora
Vaginal opening
Anus
Labia majora
Urethral opening

B. Internal structure

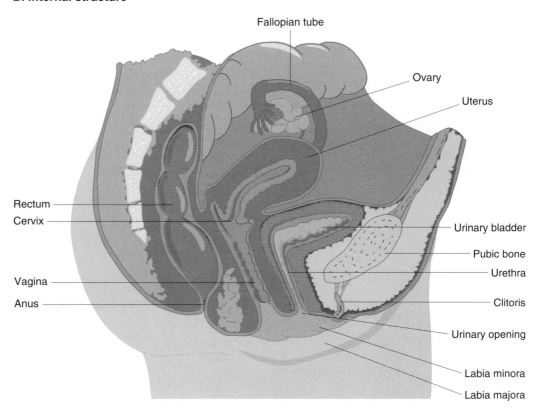

Fallopian tube
Ovary
Uterus
Rectum
Cervix
Vagina
Anus
Urinary bladder
Pubic bone
Urethra
Clitoris
Urinary opening
Labia minora
Labia majora

appetite, cravings (usually for sweets or salt), water retention, breast tenderness, and insomnia. For a diagnosis to be made, women—using a self-rating symptom scale or calendar—must report troubling premenstrual symptoms in the period before menstruation in at least two successive menstrual cycles.[8]

Treatments for PMS depend on specific symptoms. Diuretics (drugs that speed up fluid elimination) can relieve water retention and bloating. Relaxation techniques have led to a 60% reduction in anxiety symptoms. Sleep deprivation, or the use of bright light to adjust a woman's circadian or daily rhythm, also has

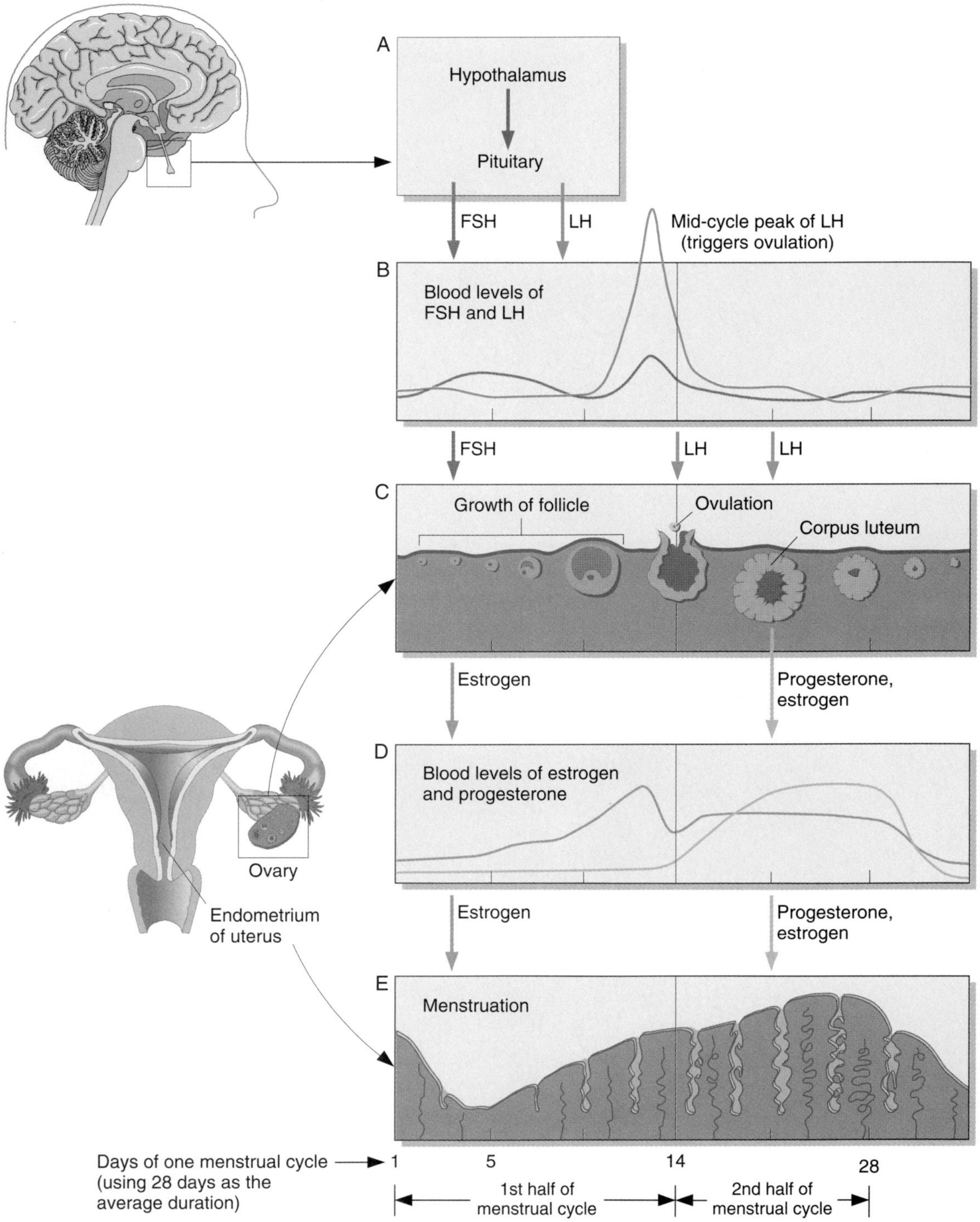

Figure 9-3

The menstrual cycle. Levels of the gonadotrophins (FSH and LH) rise and then fall to stimulate the cycle. These changes affect the levels of the hormones estrogen and progesterone, which in turn react with LH and FSH. As a result, the lining of the uterus prepares to receive a fertilized egg while the ovarian follicle matures and then ruptures, releasing the ovum (eggs) into the fallopian tube. If a fertilized egg is deposited, pregnancy begins. But if the egg is not fertilized, progesterone production decreases and the uterine lining is shed (menstruation). At this point both estrogen and progesterone levels have dropped, so the pituitary responds by producing FSH, and the cycle begins again.

proven beneficial. Behavioral approaches, such as exercise or charting cycles, help by letting women know when they're vulnerable. Psychiatric drugs that boost the neurotransmitter serotonin, such as the antidepressants Prozac and Zoloft, also have provided significant relief for symptoms such as tension, depression, irritability, and mood swings.[9]

Premenstrual Dysphoric Disorder (PMDD)

Premenstrual dysphoric disorder, which is not related to PMS, occurs in an estimated 1% to 3% of all menstruating women. It is characterized by regular symptoms of depression (depressed mood, anxiety, mood swings, diminished interest or pleasure) during the last week of the menstrual cycles. Women with PMDD cannot function as usual at work, school, or home. They feel better a few days after menstruation begins.

PMDD remains controversial, primarily for political reasons. Some women's advocacy groups oppose labeling women with menstruation-linked symptoms as mentally ill. Others contend that a diagnosis of PMDD simply recognizes the distress some women experience and may make it easier for them to obtain needed help.

Strategies for Prevention

Preventing Premenstrual Problems

✔ *Get plenty of exercise.* Physically fit women usually have fewer problems both before and during their periods.

✔ *Eat frequently and nutritiously.* In the week before your period, your body doesn't regulate the levels of sugar, or glucose, in your blood as well as it usually does.

✔ *Swear off salt.* If you stop using salt at the table and while cooking, you may gain less weight premenstrually, feel less bloated, and suffer less from headaches and irritability.

✔ *Cut back on caffeine.* Coffee, colas, diet colas, chocolate, and tea can increase breast tenderness and other symptoms.

✔ *Don't drink or smoke.* Some women become so sensitive to alcohol's effects before their periods that a glass of wine hits with the impact of several stiff drinks. Nicotine worsens low blood sugar problems.

✔ *Watch out for sweets.* Premenstrual cravings for sweets are common, but try to resist. Sugar may pick you up, but later you'll feel worse than before.

Menstrual Cramps

Dysmenorrhea is the medical name for the discomforts—abdominal cramps and pain, back and leg pain, diarrhea, tension, water retention, fatigue, and depression—that can occur during menstruation. About half of all menstruating women suffer from dysmenorrea. The cause seems to be an overproduction of bodily substances called *prostaglandins,* which typically rise during menstruation.

Women who produce excessive prostaglandins have more severe menstrual cramps. During a cramp, the uterine muscles may contract too strongly or frequently, and temporarily deprive the uterus of oxygen, causing pain. Medications that inhibit prostaglandins can reduce menstrual pain, and exercise can also relieve cramps.

Amenorrhea

Women may stop menstruating—a condition called **amenorrhea**—for a variety of reasons, including a hormonal disorder, drastic weight loss, strenuous exercise, or change in environment. "Boarding-school amenorrhea" is common among young women who leave home for school. Distance running and strenuous exercise also can lead to amenorrhea. The reason may be a drop in body fat from the normal 18%–22% to 9%–12%. To be considered amenorrhea, a woman's menstrual cycle is typically absent for three or more consecutive months. Prolonged amenorrhea can have serious health consequences, including a loss of bone density that may lead to stress fractures or osteoporosis.

In recent years scientists have discovered that the menstrual cycle actually begins in the brain with the production of gonadotropin-releasing hormone (GnRH). Each month a surge of GNRH sets into motion the sequence of steps that lead to ovulation, the potential for conception, and, if conception doesn't occur, menstruation. This understanding has led to the development of chemical mimics, or analogues, of GnRH—usually administered by nasal spray—that trigger ovulation in women who don't ovulate or menstruate normally.

Toxic Shock Syndrome (TSS)

This rare, potentially deadly bacterial infection primarily strikes menstruating women under the age of 30 who use tampons. Both *Staphylococcus aureus* and group A

Streptococcus pyogenes can produce toxic shock syndrome (TSS). Symptoms include a high fever; a rash that leads to peeling of the skin on the fingers, toes, palms, and soles; dizziness; dangerously low blood pressure; and abnormalities in several organ systems (the digestive tract and the kidneys) and in the muscles and blood. Treatment usually consists of antibiotics and intense supportive care; intravenous administration of immunoglobulins that attack the toxins produced by these bacteria also may be beneficial. (See Chapter 11 for more on TSS.)

Strategies for Prevention
....
Preventing Toxic Shock

Menstruating women should follow these guidelines to reduce their risk of TSS:

✔ Use sanitary napkins instead of tampons.

✔ If you do use tampons, check the labels for information on absorbency (which the FDA has required manufacturers to provide), and avoid superabsorbent brands.

✔ Change tampons three or four times during the day.

✔ Use napkins during the night or for some time during each day of menstrual flow.

Perimenopause and Menopause

As the baby-boom generation ages, more people are focusing their attention on the major changes that occur in a woman's middle years. In the next decade, the number of women between the ages of 45 and 54 will increase by half, from 13 million to 19 million. Thus, a large segment of the population will be entering **perimenopause**, the period from a woman's first irregular cycles to her last menstruation. **Menopause**, defined as the complete cessation of menstrual periods for 12 consecutive months, officially arrives, generally at age 51 or 52. About 9% to 15% of women breeze through this transition with only trivial symptoms. Another 9% to 15% are virtually disabled. The majority fall somewhere in between these extremes.

Estrogen, the dominant hormone of a woman's reproductive years, begins its slow decline at about age 35. Dwindling levels of estrogen subtly affect many aspects of a woman's health, from her mouth (where dryness, unusual tastes, burning, and gum problems can

develop) to her skin (which may become drier, itchier, and overly sensitive to touch). The drop in estrogen levels also may cause hot flashes (bursts of perspiration that last from a few seconds to 15 minutes), which often happen at night, disturbing sleep and causing fatigue. With less estrogen to block them, a woman's androgens, or male hormones, may have a greater impact, causing acne, hair loss, and, according to some anecdotal reports, surges in sexual appetite. (Other women, however, report a drop in sexual desire.)

At the same time, a woman's clitoris, vulva, and vaginal lining begin to shrivel, sometimes resulting in pain or bleeding during intercourse. Since the thinner genital tissues are less effective in keeping out bacteria and other pathogens, urinary tract infections may become more common. Some women develop breast or ovarian cysts, which usually go away on their own.

Eventually, a woman's ovaries don't respond at all to her pituitary hormones. After the last ovulatory cycle, progesterone is no longer secreted, and estrogen levels decrease rapidly. Although considerable controverssry has surrounded its use, *hormone-replacement therapy (HRT)* can reduce some of the side effects of estrogen reduction, including vaginal dryness, hot flashes, bladder problems, short-term memory loss, and mood swings. (See Chapter 18 for a more extensive discussion of menopause and the usefulness of HRT.)

Men's Sexual Health

Because the male reproductive system is simpler in many ways than the female, it's often ignored—especially by healthy young men. However, just like women, men should make regular self-exams (including checking their penises, testes, and breasts, as described in Chapter 13) part of their routine.

Male Sexual Anatomy

The visible parts of the male sexual anatomy are the **penis** and **scrotum**, the pouch that contains the **testes** (see Figure 9-4). The testes manufacture testosterone and **sperm**, the male reproductive cells. Immature sperm are stored in the **epididymis**, a collection of coiled tubes adjacent to each testis.

The penis contains three hollow cylinders loosely covered with skin. The two major cylinders, the *corpora cavernosa,* extend side by side through the length of the penis. The third cylinder, the *corpus spongiosum,* sur-

A. External structure

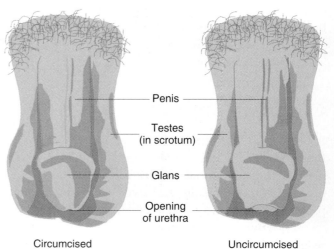

Penis

Testes
(in scrotum)

Glans

Opening
of urethra

Circumcised   Uncircumcised

B. Internal structure

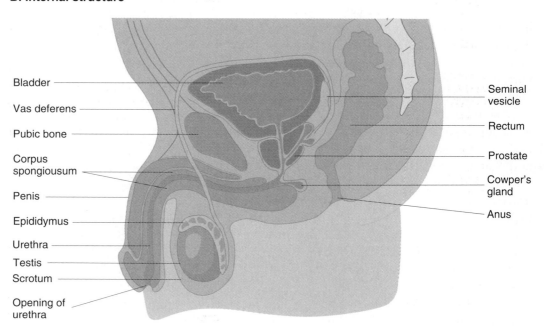

Bladder

Vas deferens

Pubic bone

Corpus
spongiousum

Penis

Epididymus

Urethra

Testis

Scrotum

Opening of
urethra

Seminal
vesicle

Rectum

Prostate

Cowper's
gland

Anus

rounds the **urethra**, the channel for both seminal fluid and urine (see Figure 9-4).

When hanging down loosely, the average penis is about 3¾ inches long. During erection, its internal cylinders fill with so much blood that they become rigid, and the penis stretches to an average length of 6¼ inches. About 90% of all men have erect penises measuring between 5 and 7 inches in length. There is no relation, however, between penis size and female sexual satisfaction; a woman's vagina naturally adjusts during intercourse to the size of her partner's penis.

Inside the body are several structures involved in the production of seminal fluid, or **semen**, the liquid in which sperm cells are carried out of the body during ejaculation. The **vas deferens** are two tubes that carry sperm from the epididymis into the urethra. The **seminal vesicles**, which make some of the seminal fluid, join with the vas deferens to form the **ejaculatory ducts**. The **prostate gland** produces some of the seminal fluid, which it secretes into the urethra during ejaculation. The **Cowper's glands** are two pea-sized structures on either side of the urethra (just below where it emerges from the prostate gland) and connected to it via tiny ducts. When a man is sexually aroused, the Cowper's glands often secrete a fluid that appears as a droplet at the tip of the penis. This fluid is not semen, although it occasionally contains sperm.

Circumcision

In its natural state, the tip of the penis is covered by a fold of skin called the foreskin. About 60% of baby boys in the United States undergo **circumcision**, the surgical removal of the foreskin. However, increasingly more parents are opting for the natural look.

"For Jewish and Muslim parents, circumcision is a religious choice," says pediatric surgeon Mary Brandt of Baylor College of Medicine in Houston. "But for other cases, it's mostly a matter of choice, and many parents are declining the procedure." Parents who choose not to have their sons circumcised should not attempt to retract the foreskin, cautions Brandt. This could lead to infection, bleeding, or scarring. As a boy gets older, gradual retraction of the foreskin during bath time helps it dilate, with full retraction possible by age two to four.[10]

The most common medical benefit of circumcision is that it prevents the accumulation of oils and secretions under the foreskin, which could cause swelling or infection. Some studies have found that uncircumcised baby boys and sexually active men are more likely to develop urinary tract infections (UTIs) than are circumcised males. However, careful washing of the genitals and good general hygiene can lower this risk. In an analysis of data on 1410 men, uncircumcised men were no more likely to contract sexually transmitted diseases than circumcised ones.[11]

The disadvantages of circumcision include risks associated with anesthesia and surgery, bleeding, and possible infection. Because of concern about pain, increasing numbers of physicians apply a topical painkiller or inject a local anesthetic agent into the penis to reduce or eliminate pain.[12] There is little consensus on what impact the presence or absence of a foreskin has on sexual functioning or satisfaction.[13] Circumcision provides clear medical benefits, but parents should also carefully consider the risks it involves.

Prostate Problems

The chestnut-sized prostate gland, which surrounds the urethra at the base of the bladder, is a common source of concern. The most common problem in younger men is infection, or **prostatitis**, which can cause fever, pain during bowel movements, pain during a rectal exam, and pus in the urine. Infrequent sexual activity is one cause of prostatitis, and occasional bursts of sexual activity between long periods of abstinence are also likely to produce this problem. Prostatitis is usually treated with antibiotics, such as sulfa medications.

After age 40, the prostate enlarges; this condition, called **benign prostatic hypertrophy**, occurs in every man. By age 50, half of all men have some enlargement of the gland; after 70, three-quarters do. As it expands, the prostate tends to pinch the urethra, decreasing urinary flow and creating a sense of urinary urgency, particularly at night. Other warning signs of prostate problems include difficult urination, blood in the urine, painful ejaculation, or constant lower-back pain.

The drug Proscar (generic name, finasteride), which shrinks an enlarged prostate, has provided an alternative to corrective surgery for many men. Other drugs are being tried experimentally. Another alternative is "thermal therapy," which heats the prostate to alleviate urinary problems caused by prostate enlargement. Gentler and safer than surgery, it seems to be equally effective.[14]

The older a man gets, the more likely he is to develop prostate cancer, which now affects one in every eleven American men and claims 30,000 lives each year (see Chapter 13). Second only to lung cancer in terms of mortality, prostate cancer is more common in African Americans than in white Americans. Scientists have developed a screening test that measures levels of a protein called *prostate-specific antigen (PSA)* in the blood. The test, designed to detect prostate cancer at its earliest, most curable stage, is not precise and often indicates cancer where none exists. Men over age 50 should also receive annual rectal examinations, in which a doctor inserts a (gloved) finger into the rectum and feels the prostate for abnormal growths that may indicate cancer.

Midlife Changes

Although men don't experience the dramatic hormonal upheaval that women do at midlife, they do experience a decline by as much as 30% to 40% in their primary sex hormone, testosterone, between the ages of 48 and 70. This drop may cause a range of symptoms, including decreased muscle mass, greater body fat, loss of bone density, flagging energy, lowered fertility, and impaired virility. Some researchers are experimenting with testosterone supplements, which, in tests with young men, have been shown to increase lean body mass and decrease body fat—at least temporarily. However, other researchers warn that, particularly in older men, excess testosterone might raise the risk of prostate cancer and heart disease.

While the production of testosterone diminishes with age, sexual ability and enjoyment do not. However, men should expect some differences in their sexual response as they grow older, including the following:

- A need for more time and arousal to achieve erection.
- A longer time before ejaculation.
- A briefer orgasm.
- A decrease in the force of expulsion of the semen at orgasm.
- A smaller volume of ejaculate.
- A more rapid loss of erection after orgasm.
- A lengthening of the time after ejaculation until a man is again capable of intercourse and orgasm.

Responsible Sexual Decision Making

"The new openness about sex and the greater threat of physical danger from sex suggest a need for increased responsibility, better communication, and more respect for individuals," state the student authors of *Sexual Etiquette 101*.[15] As they note, today's students are confronting many difficult issues as they make choices about their sexual lives. Sexual decision making always takes place within the context of an individual's values (discussed in Chapter 3) and perceptions of right and wrong behavior. Making sexually responsible decisions means considering all the possible consequences of sexual behavior for both yourself and your partner. It must always take into account, not just personal preferences and desires, but the very real risks of unwanted pregnancy, sexually transmitted diseases (STDs) and long-term medical consequences (such as impaired fertility). You also must consider the emotional consequences of a sexual relationship—not just for yourself but also for your partner.

The following sections may help ensure that the sexual decisions you make are responsible ones.

Informing Yourself

Most people grow up with a lot of myths and misconceptions about sex. (See Self-Survey: "How Much Do You Know About Sex?") Rather than relying on what peers say or what you've always thought was true, find out the facts. This textbook is a good place to start. The student health center and the library can provide additional materials on sexual identity, orientation, behavior, and health, as well as on options for reducing your risk of acquiring sexually transmitted diseases (discussed in Chapter 11) or becoing pregnant.

Talking About Sex

Many—if not most—people feel awkward or embarrassed discussing sex. Yet few topics are more important to bring up. Honest, open, caring communication is the key to a satisfying sexual relationship. Ideally, you should spend time talking about other personal subjects, getting to know a potential sexual partner, and enjoying each other's company before sex becomes the major focus of what you say or do together. (The communication skills described in Chapter 8 can help.)

Prior to any sexual activity that involves a risk of sexually transmitted infection or pregnancy, both partners should talk about their prior sexual histories (including number of partners and exposure to STDs) and other high-risk behavior, such as the use of injection drugs. They should also discuss the issue of birth control and which methods might be best for them to use. If you know someone well enough to consider having sex with that person, you should be able to talk about such sensitive subjects. If a potential partner is unwilling to talk or hedges on crucial questions, you shouldn't be engaging in sex.

Styles of communicating vary among white Americans, African Americans, Hispanic Americans, and Asian Americans. While white and African Americans may openly discuss sex with partners, Hispanic American couples generally do not discuss their sexual relationship. Asian Americans also are less inclined to discuss sex and to value nonverbal, indirect, and intuitive communication over explicit verbal interaction.[16]

Deciding to Abstain

If practiced for the sake of avoiding pregnancy, **abstinence** is defined as refraining from intercourse. If practiced to prevent the transmission of STDs, it means no exchange of body fluids. Individuals who abstain from sexual activity, not just for a weekend or a summer vacation but as a lifestyle choice, are described as celibate. (Celibacy is discussed later in this chapter.)

Abstinence is one sexual choice—the most risk-free in relation to sexually transmitted diseases (STDs). Deciding to abstain may also be a social choice, to wait until you are in a committed, permanent, monogamous relationship.

Because engaging in sexual intercourse is never 100% risk-free, abstinence is the safest possible option, especially for young people. Realizing this, increasing numbers of adolescents and young adults are choosing to remain virgins until they enter a committed, permanent, monogamous relationship. Rather than saying "no" to sex, they are saying, "not yet." The principle behind this decision is simple. As one essayist put it, "The more you indulge in anything, good or bad, but especially bad—in drugs, casual sex, violence, idiot music, stupidity, driving 90 m.p.h., bad manners, rage—the more you lose. The more you abstain, the more you gain."[17]

Although many people assume that most young people are sexually active, this is not the case. According to the Centers for Disease Control, more than 40% of high school students are virgins, while more than 60% report not having had sex within the last three months. You don't have to be a virgin to decide to abstain from sex. Many individuals who were sexually active in the past are choosing abstinence because the risk of medical complications associated with STDs increases with the number of sexual partners a person has.[18]

"Having sex" refers to the motions two people go through to achieve sexual pleasure; "making love" is a profound sharing of emotion and experience. Which do you want? Here are some other questions to consider as you think about the significance of becoming sexually intimate with a partner:

- What role do I want relationships and sex to have in my life at this time?

- What are my values as they pertain to sexual relationships? Do I believe that intercourse should be reserved for a permanent partnership or committed relationship?

- Will a decision to engage in sex enhance my positive feelings about myself or my partner? Do I have questions about my sexual orientation or the kinds of people who attract me?

- Do I and my partner both want to have sex? Is my partner pressuring me in any way? Am I pressuring my partner? Am I making this decision for myself or my partner?

- Have my partner and I discussed our sexual histories and risk factors? Have I spoken honestly about any STDs I've had in the past? Am I sure that neither my partner nor I have a sexually transmitted infection?

- Have we taken precautions against unwanted pregnancy and STDs?

The Right to Say No

Whether couples are on a first date or have been married for years, each partner always has the right *not* to have sex. Unfortunately, "no" sometimes seems to mean different things to men and women. In a 1994 survey by University of Chicago researchers, 22.8% of the women said they had been forced to do something sexually that they did not want to, usually by their spouse or someone they knew well or loved. Yet only 2.8% of the men felt that they had ever forced a woman to perform a sexual act. Why the discrepancy? The researchers speculate that men don't perceive their behavior as coercive, even when women feel pressured into unwanted sexual activities.[19]

Heeding basic rules of sexual etiquette (see Pulsepoints: "Ten Top Rules of Sexual Etiquette") can help couples avoid such situations. At some campuses, such as Antioch College in Ohio, freshmen must attend workshops on sexual consent and adhere to a campus policy that requires "willing and verbal consent" for each sexual act. (Chapter 17 also discusses sexual coercion.)

Personal Health
9.4
INTERACTIVE

Strategies for Change
....
How to Say No to Sex

✔ First of all, recognize your own values and feelings. If you believe that sex is something to be shared only by people who've already become close in other ways, be true to that belief.

Pulsepoints

Top Ten Rules of Sexual Etiquette

1. Be sure sexual activity is consensual. Coercion can take many forms: physical, emotional and verbal. All cause psychological damage and undermine trust and respect.

2. No means no. At any point in a relationship, whether the couple is dating or married, either individual has the right to say "no."

3. In sexual situations, always think ahead. For the sake of safety, think about potential dangers—parking in an isolated area, going into a bedroom with someone you hardly know, and the like—and options to protect yourself.

4. Be aware of your own and your partner's alcohol and drug intake. The use of such substances impairs judgment and reduces the ability to say no. While under their influence, you may engage in sexual behavior you'll later regret.

5. Be prepared. If there's any possibility that you may be engaging in sex, be sure you have the means to protect yourself against unwanted pregnancy and sexually transmitted diseases (STDs).

6. Communicate openly. If you or your partner cannot talk openly and honestly about your sexual histories and contraception, you avoid having sex. For the sake of protecting your sexual health, you have to be willing to ask—and answer—questions that may seem embarrassing.

7. Share responsibility in a sexual relationship. Both partners should be involved in protecting themselves and each other from STDs and, if heterosexual, unwanted pregnancy.

8. Respect sexual privacy. Revealing sexual activities violates the trust between two partners. Bragging about a sexual conquest demeans everyone involved.

9. Do not sexually harass others. Pinches, pats, sexual comments or jokes, and suggestive gestures are offensive and disrespectful. (See Chapter 15 for more on harassment.)

10. Be considerate. A public display of sexual affection can be extremely embarrassing to others. Roommates, in particular, should be sensitive and discrete in their sexual behavior.

SOURCE: Adapted from: Hatcher, Robert, et al. *Sexual Etiquette 101.* Atlanta, GA: Emory University School of Medicine.

✔ If you're at a loss for words, try these responses: "I like you a lot, but I'm not ready to have sex." "You're a great person, but sex isn't something I do to prove I like someone." "I'd like to wait until I'm married to have sex."

✔ If you're feeling pressured, let your date know that you're uncomfortable. Be simple and direct. Watch out for emotional blackmail. If your date says, "If you really liked me, you'd want to make love," point out that if he or she really liked you, he or she wouldn't try to force you to do something you don't want to do.

✔ If you're a woman, monitor your sexual signals. Men impute more sexual meaning to gestures (such as casual touching) that women perceive as friendly and innocent.[20]

✔ Communicate your feelings to your date sooner rather than later. It's far easier to say, "I don't want to go to your apartment," than to fight off unwelcome advances once you're there.

✔ Remember that if saying no to sex puts an end to a relationship, it wasn't much of a relationship in the first place.

Sexual Behavior

From birth to death, we are sexual beings. Our sexual identities, needs, likes, and dislikes emerge in adolescence and become clearer as we enter adulthood, but we continue to change and evolve throughout our lives. In men sexual interest is most intense at age 18; in women, it reaches a peak in the 30s. Although age brings changes in sexual responsiveness, we never outgrow our sexuality.

Sexuality in Childhood

For infants, the mouth is the principal source of sensual pleasure, but they are also sensitive to genital and general body contact. By the age of 3 or 4, children recognize the genital differences between males and females, and may develop childhood romances. Curiosity about adults' and other children's genitals, about where babies come from, and about breasts on women and beards on men continues until age 8 or 9. At that time, interest in sex play becomes less common; but curiosity about sex and where babies come from remains high.

"Unless they don't watch TV, don't go to movies and don't talk with friends, children will be curious about sex," says Nancy Adler, Ph.D., professor of medical psychology at the University of California, San Francisco. "Even if they didn't, they'd probably still want to know about sex." It is crucially important for today's parents to answer children's questions about sex as honestly as they can. The primary message to convey, Adler suggests, is simple: Sex is a normal part of life that's done responsibly by two people in a loving relationship.[21] While some awkwardness may be inevitable, parents can master the art of honest, open, and comfortable conversation.

Strategies for Change

Talking to Children About Sex

✔ Start early. Even with very young children, look for "teachable" moments, such as the birth of a litter of puppies, to talk about reproduction.

✔ Keep talks short and simple. Talk at the level a child is capable of understanding. Rather than delivering a long lecture, spread out the information in many small talks, repeating what you've already said several times.

✔ Stress the context of sexual activity. Go beyond the physical aspects of sex and convey your family's values. When watching television, for instance, comment on concepts such as sexual decision making and responsibility.

✔ Never laugh at a child's questions or comments or dismiss them as silly or trite. Children who learn early that they can bring up sex without fear of ridicule, rebuke, or embarrassment develop a trust that pays great dividends in adolescence.

✔ If you feel nervous, admit it. You might say, "I know this feels kind of awkward for both of us. But when I was growing up, I wished I could have talked to my parents about sex. Even though it may be a little embarrassing at first, I want you to know that in our house it's okay to talk about sex, and I'll try to be as open as I can."

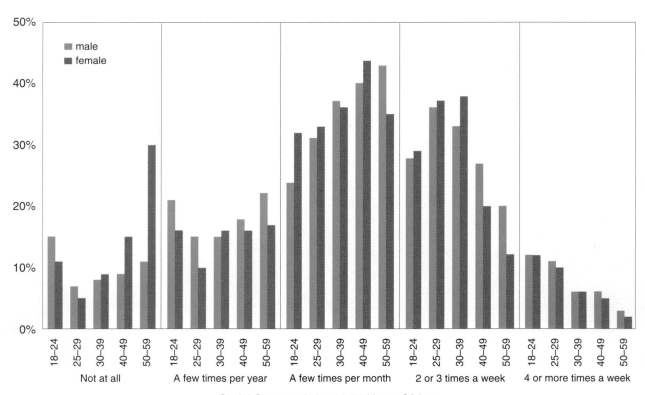

Source: Michael, Robert et al. *Sex in America: A Definitive Survey.* Boston: Little Brown, 1994.

Figure 9-5

How often do Americans have sex?

Adolescent Sexuality

Early in adolescence, sexual curiosity explodes, and sexual exploration—both alone and with a partner—takes on new meaning and intensity. Sexual education programs can make a difference by helping young people become sexually responsible, enable them to form satisfying relationships, help them assess their own attitudes toward sex, and give them information on sexuality. Good programs can clarify values and enhance communication.[22]

It's not unusual for teenage boys to experience frequent erections during the day and night, including **nocturnal emissions**, or wet dreams, during which ejaculation occurs. **Masturbation** (discussed later in this chapter) is the primary form of sexual expression for many teenagers, especially boys. Self-stimulation helps teens learn about their bodies and their sexual potential and serves as an outlet for sexual tension. By the end of adolescence, the majority of teens have masturbated to orgasm.

Other common sexual activities during adolescence include kissing and petting—erotic physical contact that may include holding, touching, manual stimulation of the genitals, and oral sex. As many as 25% of teens experience some same-sex attractions. Although many experiment with heterosexual and homosexual sexual experiences, adolescent sexual behavior does not always foretell sexual orientation. Young people, who often feel confused about their sexual identity, may engage in sexual activity with members of the same or the other sex as a way of testing how they really feel.[23]

Over the last several decades, the number of teenage boys and, even more dramatically, girls engaging in sexual intercourse has increased significantly. However, in 1997, the percentage of teenagers who have had sexual intercourse declined for the first time after increasing steadily for more than two decades. According to the National Center for Health Statistics, 50% of girls 15 to 19 years of age have had sexual intercourse—down from 55% in 1990. A similar trend is occurring with teenage boys ages 15 to 19. The percentage who have had intercourse declined from 60% in 1988 to 55%. There also has been an increase in the use of contraceptives at the time of first intercourse.[24]

Approximately 16% of girls whose first intercourse was before age 16 reported that their initial sexual experience had not been voluntary. Among these girls, 66% reported that their partner was under 18, 21% said their partner was 18 or 19, 7% said their partner was 20 to 22, and 7% had partners older than age 23.[25]

Even though American teens are not more sexually active than those in other countries, the United States continues to have the highest rate of teen pregnancy in the Western world. Of the 11 million unmarried adolescent females who are sexually active, about 1 million

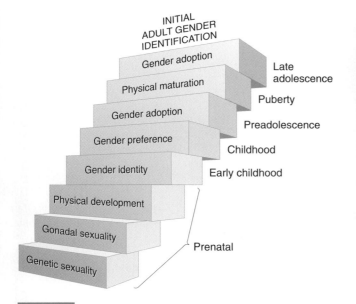

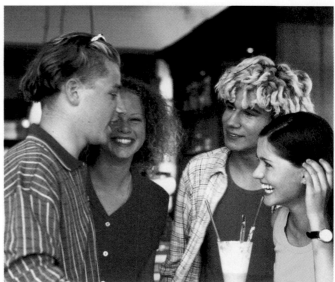

Figure 9-6

Sexuality has biological and psychological components. During adolescence sexuality develops rapidly: teens explore different social and intimate relationships as they begin to develop a sexual identity.

become pregnant each year. An estimated 40% of these pregnancies end in abortion; 50%, in live births; the others, in miscarriage.[26] (See the discussion of teen pregnancy in Chapter 10.)

Early sex education does have an impact. The more teenagers know about sex, sexually transmitted diseases, and how to say no to sex, the less likely they are to engage in risky sexual behaviors. In a study funded by the National Institute of Child Health and Human Development, researchers found that inner-city African-American teenage boys who participated in a sex education program were less likely to become sexually active than those who had not participated. Also, those who were already sexually active chose safer forms of sexual behavior.[27] Other studies have found that teens who come from a two-parent family, receive sex education, and have positive sexual attitudes are less likely to engage in premarital intercourse.

Sex on Campus

As seen in Campus Focus: "College Students and Sexuality," most college students—87.8% of women and 84%

of men—have had sexual intercourse. A much smaller but significant percentage—31.8% of women and 37.8% of men—had six or more sex partners during their lifetime.[28]

Yet most students, as indicated by a report on 272 students at a Midwestern university, don't believe it's embarrassing to be a virgin. Of those who are sexually active, many college students worry about STDs, yet they don't always take precautions to reduce the risk of disease, often because they believe that HIV and other infections simply couldn't happen to them. But concern about STDs has had some impact on the sexual habits of college students. In a study of 132 women students, 41% said that they used condoms during intercourse, an increase over reported use in previous decades.[29] As the women became seriously involved with men, however, they tended to use less, rather than more, protection. This is a potentially dangerous practice, since just knowing someone better doesn't make sex safer. Today's students also seem just as willing as their counterparts of two decades ago to engage in oral or anal sex and to have multiple partners.[30]

A study of 61 homosexual college men at a large mid-Atlantic state university found considerable concern

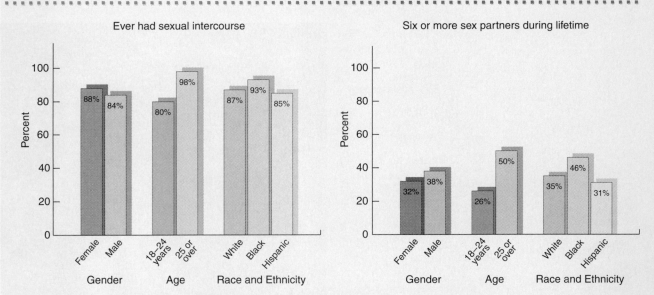

CAMPUS FOCUS: COLLEGE STUDENTS AND SEXUALITY

Ever had sexual intercourse

Six or more sex partners during lifetime

SOURCE: Douglas, Kathy, et al. "Results from the 1995 National College Health Risk Behavior Survey." American Journal of College Health, Vol. 46, September 1997.

about HIV infection. More than a quarter of the men had not engaged in homosexual activity. Of the 72% who had had sex with a man, some had made dramatic changes in their sexual behavior because of their fear of HIV: 7% had become celibate, and 14% no longer engaged in anal intercourse. About half had limited the number of people with whom they had sex and reported being more selective in choosing partners; 36% refused to have sex without a condom.[31]

The Sex Life of American Adults

The scientific study of Americans' sexual behavior began in 1938, when Alfred Kinsey, Ph.D., a professor of biology at the University of Indiana, and his colleagues asked some 5300 white men and 5940 white women about their sexual practices. In his landmark studies—*Sexual Behavior in the Human Male*, published in 1948, and *Sexual Behavior in the Human Female*, published in 1953—Kinsey reported that 73% of men and 20% of women had premarital intercourse by age 20 and 37% of men and 17% of women had some homosexual experience in their lifetime.

Even though Kinsey's research sample was not representative of the population as a whole, for decades his work remained the most definitive and revealing account of the sex lives of ordinary people. In the 1980s, after the emergence and recognition of the HIV epidemic, researchers and public health officials felt an urgent need for contemporary population-based studies that might help develop strategies to prevent HIV transmission. The last decade has seen several national surveys of sexual behavior.

The Janus Report on Sexual Behavior, published in 1993, was based on a survey of 2765 individuals across the United States. A larger survey, conducted by researchers at the University of Chicago, was based on face-to-face interviews with 3432 Americans, aged 18 to 59. It became the basis for two books published in 1994: *Sex in America*, aimed at a lay audience, and *The Social Organization of Sexuality*, a more scholarly work. Since then, the researcher's General Social Survey (GSS) database on sexual activity has grown to nearly 10,000 respondents, about three times larger than the 1992 study.

The GSS data indicate that overall sexual activity in America is relatively infrequent, with an average of 58 episodes per year, or slightly more than one a week. Yet there was a 5% increase in sexual activity in 1996, compared with earlier years—even though the population is aging, works longer hours, and can choose among a growing number of distractions. According to this analysis, about 15% of adults engage in half of all sexual activity; 42% of adults engage in 85% of all sex.[32]

The average adult reports having sex about once a week. However, one in five Americans has been celibate for at least a year, and one in twenty engages in sex at least every other day. Men report more sexual frequency than women—not because men are more boastful about their prowess, the researchers contend, but because the sample of women includes many widows and older women without partners. Among married people, the frequency reports of husbands and wives (not in the same couples) are within one episode per year—58.6 for married men and 57.9 for married women. And if other differences between men and women are statistically controlled (such as sexual preference, age, and educational attainment), married women actually report a slightly higher frequency than men.

People who are married, have children at home, and work long hours report having more sex. Those who work more than 60 hours a week are about 10% more sexually active than other workers, and even those who have preschool-aged children report having more sex than average. Even after their answers are controlled for differences in age, gender, and other factors, Americans with the longest work hours report higher sexual frequency.

The main reason why married people have sex more often is that they have easy access to a partner. Affluent, well-educated people, those in the top one-tenth of the income distribution, also report above-average sexual frequency. Even then, the rich only report about 5% more sex. In fact, adjustment for age and marital status reveals that Americans at the lower rungs of the income ladder may have slightly higher sexual frequency.

Sexual frequency peaks among those with some college education, then decreases among four-year college graduates, and declines even further among those with professional degrees. Americans who have attended graduate school are the least sexually active educational group in the population. These respondents may be more honest than others in reporting sexual activity, or they may be more precise in their definition of what counts as sex.

Sexual frequency increases among those who engage in other pleasurable pursuits, such as attending concerts, sporting events, and active forms of leisure. Yet it also increases along with television viewing. The more TV individuals watch, the more often they have sex. "It is not clear," the researchers observe, "whether the sexual response is stimulated by what is on the screen, or by boredom. And for some reason, watching PBS seems more positively related with increased sexual behavior than watching regular prime-time drama."

Sexual activity is higher among self-defined political liberals than among moderates or conservatives, and it is highest among those who describe themselves as "extreme liberals" and among "extreme conservatives." Catholics are slightly more sexually active than Protestants. But both Christian groups are about 20% less active than are Jews or agnostics. Among Protestant groups, Baptists are slightly above average and Presbyterians and Lutherans are slightly below average. Those who attend religious services of any sort at least once a week are less sexually active.

The most sexually active Americans are far more likely than average to approve of premarital or extramarital sex, to see positive benefits in pornography, to watch X-rated movies, and to favor giving birth control pills to teenagers. But those with liberal attitudes aren't the only sexually active individuals. People who own guns also have higher-than-average sexual frequency.

Does sex make people happier or healthier? Based on their analysis, the researchers concluded that the more sex a person has, the more likely he or she is to report having a happy life and a happy marriage. This connection is stronger among women than men. A second and more important predictor of sexual frequency is the feeling that one's life is exciting rather than routine or dull. "Being excited by life is most strongly associated with being happier," the researchers noted. "It seems that increased sexual activity is one of the many benefits of having a positive attitude."

Sex and Aging

According to *American Demographics,* the average frequency of sex remains steady throughout the 20s and mid-30s, but it falls nearly 20% among those aged 35 to 44. It drops another 25% for those aged 45 to 54, and another 25% for those aged 55 to 64. But the steepest declines happen after age 65. Sexual activity among those aged 65 to 74 is more than 60% lower than it is among 55- to 64-year-olds, and there is another drop of 50% for those aged 75 and older.[33]

Age-related declines in sexual activity are more drastic for women than for men. The rate for women drops 50% after age 55, then 90%, to near-complete inactivity, after age 75. In other words, women aged 65 to 74 average about ten episodes of sex a year, but that drops to two a year for those aged 75 and older. Also, sex among the oldest old is restricted to a fortunate few. Eighty-five percent of sexual activity among men and women aged 75 and older happens among 8% of this population.[34]

Sexual Diversity

Human beings are diverse in all ways—including sexual preferences and practices. Physiological, psychological, and social factors attract us to members of a certain sex; this attraction is our **sexual orientation**. Sigmund Freud argued that we all start off **bisexual**, or attracted to both sexes. But by the time they reach adulthood, most males prefer female sexual partners, and most females prefer male partners. **Heterosexual** is the term used for individuals whose primary orientation is toward members of the other sex. In virtually all cultures, some men and women are **homosexuals**, preferring partners of their own sex.

In our society, we tend to view heterosexuality and homosexuality as very different. In reality, these orientations are opposite ends of a spectrum of sexual preferences. Sex researcher Alfred Kinsey devised a seven-point continuum representing sexual orientation in American society. At one end of the continuum are those exclusively attracted to members of the opposite sex; at the other end are people exclusively attracted to members of the same sex. In between are varying degrees of homosexual and heterosexual orientation.

According to Kinsey's original data, 4% of men and 2% of women are exclusively homosexual. More recent studies have found lower numbers. For instance, in the University of Chicago's national survey, 2.8% of the men and 1.4% of the women defined themselves as homosexual. However, when asked if they'd had sex with a person of the same gender since age 18, about 5% of men and 4% of women said yes. If asked if they found members of the same sex sexually attractive, 6% of men and 5.5% of women said yes.

Bisexuality

Bisexuality—sexual attraction to both males and females—can develop at any point in one's life. In some cultures, bisexual activity is considered part of normal sexual experimentation. Among the Sabmia Highlanders in Papua New Guinea, for instance, boys perform oral sex on one another as part of the rites of passage into manhood.[35]

Some people identify themselves as bisexual even if they don't behave bisexually. Some are "serial" bisexuals—that is, they are sexually involved with same-sex partners for a while and then with partners of the other sex, or vice versa. An estimated 7 to 9 million men, about twice the number thought to be exclusively homosexual, could be described as bisexual during some extended period of their lives. The largest group are married, rarely have sexual relations with women other than their wives, and have secret sexual involvements with men.

Fear of HIV infection has sparked great concern about bisexuality, particularly among heterosexual women who worry about becoming involved with a bisexual man. About 20% to 30% of women with AIDS were infected by bisexual partners, and health officials fear that bisexual men who hide their homosexual affairs could transmit HIV to many more women. (See Chapter 11.)

Homosexuality

Homosexuality—social, emotional, and sexual attraction to members of the same sex—exists in almost all cultures. Men and women homosexuals are commonly referred to as *gay*; women homosexuals are also called *lesbians*.

Homosexuality threatens and upsets many people, perhaps because homosexuals are viewed as different, or perhaps because no one understands why some people are heterosexual and others homosexual. Homophobia has led to an increase in "gay bashing" (attacking homosexuals) in many communities, including college campuses. Some blame the emergence of AIDS as a societal danger. However, researchers have found that fear of AIDS has not created new hostility but has simply given bigots an excuse to act out their hatred.

Violations of basic human rights for gays and lesbians remain common around the globe. Amnesty International has documented abuses, ranging from exile to

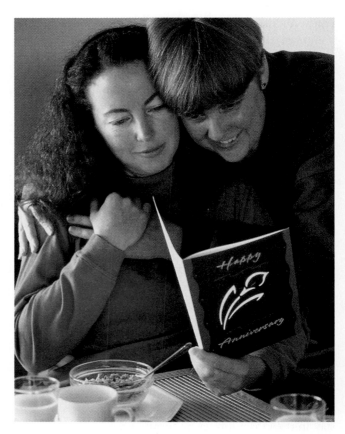

Happy together. Close-couple homosexual relationships are similar to stable heterosexual relationships.

labor camps in China to "social cleansing" death squads in Colombia to the death penalty for homosexual acts in Iran.

The Roots of Homosexuality

For decades, behavioral and medical specialists have debated whether homosexuality is biologically or socially determined. Some say that sexual orientation is genetically determined. Others contend that prenatal hormones influence sexual preference. Some psychotherapists have argued that mothers foster homosexuality by loving their sons too much and their daughters too little. Others have traced homosexuality to broken homes, seductive friends, and failure at "dating and mating."

Researchers have found structural differences in the brains of heterosexual and homosexual men that might indicate a biological basis for sexual orientation. In gay men, one segment of the hypothalamus, part of the forebrain, is typically about one-quarter to one-half the size of the same region in heterosexual men. Also, a cord of nerve fibers that allows the two halves of the brain to communicate with one another is larger in homosexual men than in either heterosexual men or in women. Such findings have raised many questions and controversies about the roots and nature of sexual orientation.[36]

Homosexual Lifestyles

Extensive studies of male and female homosexuals have shown that only a minority have problems coping with their homosexuality. The happiest and best adjusted tend to be those in close-couple relationships, the equivalent of stable heterosexual partnerships. An estimated 3 to 5 million gays and lesbians have conceived children in heterosexual relationships; others have become parents through adoption or artificial insemination. These men and women describe their families as much like any other; and studies of lesbian mothers have found that their children are essentially no different from average in self-esteem, gender-related issues and roles, sexual orientation, and general development.

Different ethnic groups respond to homosexuality in different ways. To a greater extent than white homosexuals, gays and lesbians from ethnic groups tend to stay in the closet longer rather than risk alienation from their families and communities. Often they feel forced to choose between their gay and ethnic identities.

In general, the African-American community has stronger negative views of homosexuals than whites, possibly because of the influence of strong fundamentalist Christian beliefs. Hispanic culture, with its emphasis on machismo, also has a very negative view of male homosexuality. Asian cultures, which tend to view an individual as a representative of his or her family, tend to view open declarations of sexual orientation as shaming the family and challenging their reputation and future.[37]

Sexual Activity

Part of learning about your own sexuality is having a clear understanding of human sexual behaviors. Understanding frees us from fear and anxiety, so that we may accept ourselves and others as the natural sexual beings we all are.

Celibacy

A celibate person practices sexual abstinence and does not engage in sexual activity. Complete **celibacy** means that the person doesn't masturbate (stimulate himself or herself sexually) or engage in sexual activity with a partner. In partial celibacy, the person masturbates but doesn't have sexual contact with others. Many people decide to be celibate at certain times of their lives. Some don't have sex because of concerns about pregnancy or STDs; others haven't found a partner for a permanent, monogamous relationship. Many simply have other priorities, such as finishing school or starting a career and realize that sex outside of a committed relationship is a threat to their physical and psychological well-being.

Fantasy

The mind is the most powerful sex organ in the body, and erotic mental images can be sexually stimulating. Sexual fantasies can accompany sexual activity or be pleasurable in themselves. Fantasies generally enhance sexual arousal, reduce anxiety, and boost sexual desire. They're also a way to anticipate and rehearse new sexual experiences, as well as to bolster a person's self-image and feelings of desirability. Part of what makes fantasies exciting is that they provide an opportunity for expressing forbidden desires, such as sex with a different partner or with a past lover.

In the University of Chicago survey, more than half the men (54%)—but only 19% of the women—said they thought about sex every day or several times a day. Men and women also have different types of sexy thoughts, with men's fantasies containing more explicit genital images and culminating in sexual acts more quickly than women's. In women's fantasies, emotional feelings play a greater role, and there is more kissing and caressing rather than genital contact. For many women, fantasy helps in reaching orgasm during intercourse; a loss of fantasy often is a sign of low sexual desire.[38]

Sex in Cyberspace

The Internet, designed for communication of very different sorts, has become a new medium for relationships, including those that might be described as sexual. In certain chat rooms, individuals can share explicit sexual fantasies or engage in the cyberspace equivalent of mutual fantasizing. In some ways, the Internet is the perfect venue for a safe form of sexual risk-taking. Individuals can assume any name, gender, race, or personality and can pretend to lead lives entirely different from their actual existences.

In one survey, 12% of college men and 10% of college women reported that they had tried cyberspace sexual contact. Many see it as a harmless way of adding an extra erotic charge to their daily lives. In some cases, individuals who meet in cybersex chat rooms develop what they come to think of as a meaningful relationship and arrange to meet in person. Sometimes these meetings are awkward; sometimes they do lead to a real-life romance. However, they rarely survive the intrusive reality of everyday existence and sometimes they end disastrously in disappointment and danger.[39]

For some individuals, particularly gays and lesbians, the Internet provides the opportunity to join a virtual community. In addition to sexual exchanges, they can find access to information and resources that may not be available elsewhere. For adolescents struggling with gender identity or for closeted homosexuals, going online can be their only opportunity to be open about their sexuality.

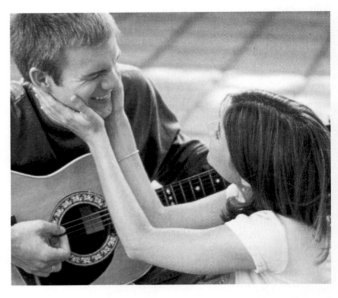

The magic of touch. Thrilling, soothing, stimulating—touch is a powerful nonverbal communication.

Masturbation

Not everybody masturbates, but most people do. Kinsey estimated that seven out of ten women and nineteen out of twenty men masturbate (and admit they do). Their reason is simple: It feels good. Masturbation produces the same physical responses as sexual activity with a partner and can be an enjoyable form of sexual release.

Masturbation has been described as immature; unsocial; tiring; frustrating; and a cause of hairy palms, warts, blemishes, and blindness. None of these myths is true. Even Freud felt that masturbation was normal for children. Sex educators recommend masturbation to adolescents as a means of releasing tension and becoming familiar with their sexual organs. Throughout adulthood, masturbation often is the primary sexual activity of individuals not involved in a sexual relationship and can be particularly useful when illness, absence, divorce, or death deprives a person of a partner. In the University of Chicago survey, about 25% of men and 9% of women said they masturbate at least once a week.

White men and women have a higher incidence of masturbation than African-American men and women. Latino women have the lowest rate of masturbation, compared with Latino men, white men and women, and black men and women. Individuals with a higher level of education are more likely to masturbate than those with less schooling, and people living with sexual partners masturbate more than those who live alone.[40]

Masturbation helps some people make better decisions about getting sexually involved with others. Self-stimulation also can aid women learning to experience orgasms or men experimenting with ways of delaying ejaculation. Some people find that masturbation enables them to relax and fall asleep more easily at night.

Kissing and Touching

A kiss is a universal sign of affection. A kiss can be just a kiss—a quick press of the lips—or it can lead to much more. Usually kissing is the first sexual activity that couples engage in, and even after years of sexual experimentation and sharing, it remains an enduring pleasure for partners (see Table 9-1).

Touching is a silent form of communication between friends and lovers. Although a touch to any part of the body can be thrilling, some areas, such as the breasts and genitals, are especially sensitive. Stimulating these **erogenous** regions can lead to orgasm in both men and women. Though such forms of stimulation often accompany intercourse, more couples are gaining an appreciation of these activities as primary sources of sexual fulfillment—and as safer alternatives to intercourse.

Intercourse

Vaginal **intercourse**, or coitus, refers to the penetration of the vagina by the penis (see Figure 9-7). This is the preferred form of sexual intimacy for most heterosexual couples, who may use a wide variety of positions. The most familiar position for intercourse in our society is the so-called missionary position, with the man on top, facing the woman. An alternative is the woman on top,

TABLE 9-1 SEXUAL PLEASURES: WHAT MEN AND WOMEN LIKE

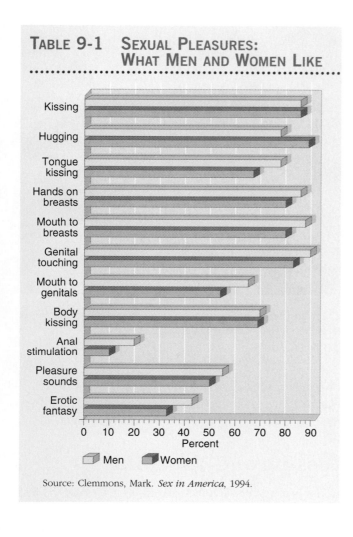

Source: Clemmons, Mark. *Sex in America*, 1994.

either lying down or sitting upright. Other positions include lying side by side (either face to face or with the man behind the woman, his penis entering her vagina from the rear); lying with the man on top of the woman in a rear-entry position; and kneeling or standing (again, in either a face-to-face or rear-entry position). Many couples move into several different positions for intercourse during a single episode of lovemaking; others may have a personal favorite, or may choose different positions at different times. (See Spotlight on Diversity: "Cultural Variations in Sexual Arousal.")

Sexual activity, including intercourse, is possible throughout a woman's menstrual cycle. However, some women prefer to avoid sex while menstruating because of uncomfortable physical symptoms, such as cramps, or concern about bleeding or messiness. Others use a diaphragm or cervical cap (see Chapter 10) to hold back menstrual flow. Since different cultures have different views on intercourse during a woman's period, partners should discuss their own feelings and try to respect each other's views. If they choose not to have intercourse, there are other gratifying forms of sexual activity.

Vaginal intercourse, like other forms of sexual activity involving an exchange of bodily fluids, carries a risk of sexually transmitted diseases, including HIV infection. In many other parts of the world, in fact, heterosexual intercourse is the most common means of HIV transmission. (See Chapter 11.)

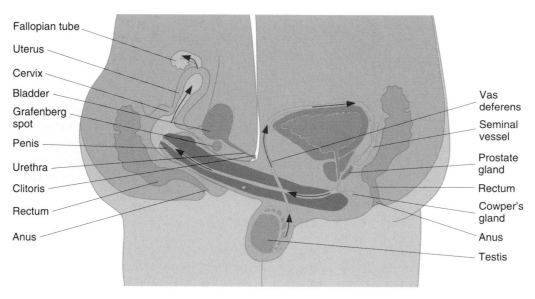

Figure 9-7

A cross-sectional view of sexual intercourse. Sperm are formed in each of the testes and stored in the epididymis. When a man ejaculates, sperm, in semen, travel up the vas deferens. (The prostate gland and seminal vesicles contribute components of the semen.) The semen is expelled from the penis through the urethra and deposited in the vagina, near the cervix. During sexual excitement and orgasm in a women, the upper end of the vagina enlarges and the uterus elevates. After orgasm, these organs return to their normal states, and the cervix descends into the pool of semen.

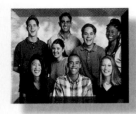

Spotlight on Diversity
Cultural Variations in Sexual Arousal

While the biological mechanisms underlying human sexual arousal and response are essentially universal, the particular sexual stimuli or behaviors that people find arousing are greatly influenced by cultural conditioning. For example, in Western societies, where the emphasis during sexual activity tends to be heavily weighted toward achieving orgasm, genitally focused activities are frequently defined as optimally arousing. In contrast, devotees to Eastern Tantric traditions (where spirituality is interwoven with sexuality) often achieve optimal pleasure by emphasizing the sensual and spiritual aspects of shared intimacy rather than orgasmic release (Devi, 1977). In the following paragraphs, we will provide brief examples of some other facets of cultural diversity in human sexual arousal.

Kissing on the mouth, a universal source of sexual arousal in Western society, may be rare or absent in many other parts of the world. Certain North American Eskimo people and inhabitants of the Trobriand Islands would rather rub noses than lips, and among the Thonga of South Africa, kissing is viewed as odious behavior. The Hindu people of India are also disinclined to kiss because they believe such contact symbolically contaminates the act of sexual intercourse. In their survey of 190 societies, Clellan Ford and Frank Beach (1951) found that mouth kissing was acknowledged in only 21 societies and practiced as a prelude or accompaniment to coitus in only 13.

Oral sex (both cunnilingus and fellatio) is a common source of sexual arousal among island societies of the South Pacific, in industrialized nations of Asia, and in much of the Western world. In contrast, in Africa (with the exception of northern regions), such practices are likely to be viewed as unnatural or disgusting behavior.

Foreplay in general, whether it be oral sex, sensual touching, or passionate kissing, is subject to wide cultural variation. In some societies, most notably those with Eastern traditions, couples may strive to prolong intense states of sexual arousal for several hours (Devi, 1977). While varied patterns of foreplay are common in Western cultures, these activities often are of short duration as lovers move rapidly toward the "main event" of coitus. In still other societies, foreplay is either sharply curtailed or absent altogether. For example, the Lepcha farmers of the southeastern Himalayas limit foreplay to men briefly caressing their partners' breasts, and among the Irish inhabitants of Inis Beag, precoital sexual activity is reported to be limited to mouth kissing and rough fondling of the woman's lower body by her partner (Messenger, 1971).

Another indicator of cultural diversity is the wide variety in standards of attractiveness. Although physical qualities exert a profound influence on human sexual arousal in virtually every culture, standards of attractiveness vary widely, as can be seen in the accompanying photos of women and men from around the world who are considered to be attractive in their own cultures. What may be attractive or a source of erotic arousal in one culture may seem strange or unattractive in others. For instance, while some island societies attach erotic significance to the shape and textures of female genitals, most Western societies do not. To cite a final example, in many societies bare female breasts are not generally viewed as erotic stimuli, as they are in America. In fact, aside from general indicators of good health (healthy skin, hair, teeth, etc.), there is little agreement among the world's diverse cultures about what makes a potential sexual partner attractive.

From Crooks, Robert, and Baur, Karla. *Our Sexuality*, 7th ed. Pacific Grove, CA: Brooks/Cole, 1999.

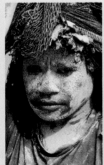
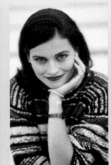
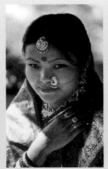
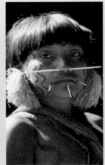
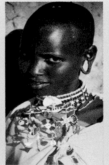
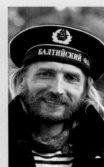

Our Standards of physical attractiveness vary widely, as can be seen in these six photos of women and men from around the world who are considered in their cultures to be attractive.

Oral-Genital Sex

Our mouths and genitals give us some of our most intense pleasures. Though it might seem logical to combine the two, some people are very uncomfortable with it. Some people consider oral-genital sex a perversion; it is against the law in many states, and a sin in some religions. However, others find it normal and acceptable. (The same comments apply to anal sex as well—see the next section.)

The formal terms for oral sex are **cunnilingus**, which refers to oral stimulation of the woman's genitals, and **fellatio**, oral stimulation of the man's genitals. For many couples, oral-genital sex is a regular part of their lovemaking. For others, it's an occasional experiment. Oral sex with a partner carrying a sexually transmitted disease, such as herpes or HIV infection, can lead to infection, so a condom should be used (with cunnilingus, a condom cut in half to lay flat can be used).

Different groups of the population have diverse views of oral sex. In one survey, more African-Amercian than white men reported never having performed or received oral sex.[41] Among American women, career women are more likely than homemakers to consider oral sex a normal act.[42]

Anal Stimulation and Intercourse

Because the anus has many nerve endings, it can produce intense erotic responses. Stimulation of the anus by the fingers or mouth can be a source of sexual arousal; anal intercourse involves penile penetration of the anus. An estimated 25% of adults have experienced anal intercourse at least once.[43] However, anal sex involves important health risks, such as damage to sensitive rectal tissues, and the transmission of various intestinal infections, hepatitis, and STDs, including HIV.

Sexual Response

Sexuality involves every part of you: mind and body, muscles and skin, glands and genitals. The pioneers in finding out exactly how human beings respond to sex were William Masters and Virginia Johnson, who first studied more than 800 individuals in their laboratory in the 1950s. They discovered that sexual response is a well-ordered sequence of events, so predictable it could be divided into four phases: excitement, plateau, orgasm, and resolution (see Figure 9-8). In real life, indi-

viduals don't necessarily follow this well-ordered pattern. But the responses for both sexes are remarkably similar. And sexual response always follows the same sequence, whatever the means of stimulation.

Excitement

Stimulation is the first step: a touch, a look, a fantasy. In men, sexual stimuli set off a rush of blood to the genitals, filling the blood vessels in the penis. Because these vessels are wrapped in a thick sheath of tissue, the penis becomes erect. The testes lift.

Women respond to stimulation with vaginal lubrication within 10 to 20 seconds of exposure to sexual stimuli. The clitoris becomes larger, as do the vaginal lips (the labia), the nipples, and later the breasts. The vagina lengthens, and its inner two-thirds increase in size. The uterus lifts, further increasing the free space in the vagina.

Plateau

During this stage, the changes begun in the excitement stage continue and intensify. The penis further increases in both length and diameter. The outer one-third of the vagina swells. During intercourse, the vaginal muscles grasp the penis to increase stimulation for both partners. The upper two-thirds of the vagina become wider as the uterus moves up; eventually its diameter is $2\frac{1}{2}$ to 3 inches.

Orgasm

Men and women have remarkably similar **orgasm** experiences. Both men and women typically have 3 to 12 pelvic muscle contractions approximately four-fifths of a second apart and lasting up to 60 seconds. Both undergo contractions and spasms of other muscles, as well as increases in breathing and pulse rates, and blood pressure. Both can sometimes have orgasms simply from kisses, stimulation of the breasts or other parts of the body, or fantasy alone.

The process of **ejaculation** (the discharge of semen by a male) requires two separate events. First, the vas deferens, the seminal vesicles, the prostate, and the upper portion of the urethra contract. The man perceives these subtle contractions deep in his pelvis just before the point of no return—which therapists refer to as the point of "ejaculatory inevitability." Then, seconds later, muscle contractions force semen out of the penis via the urethra.

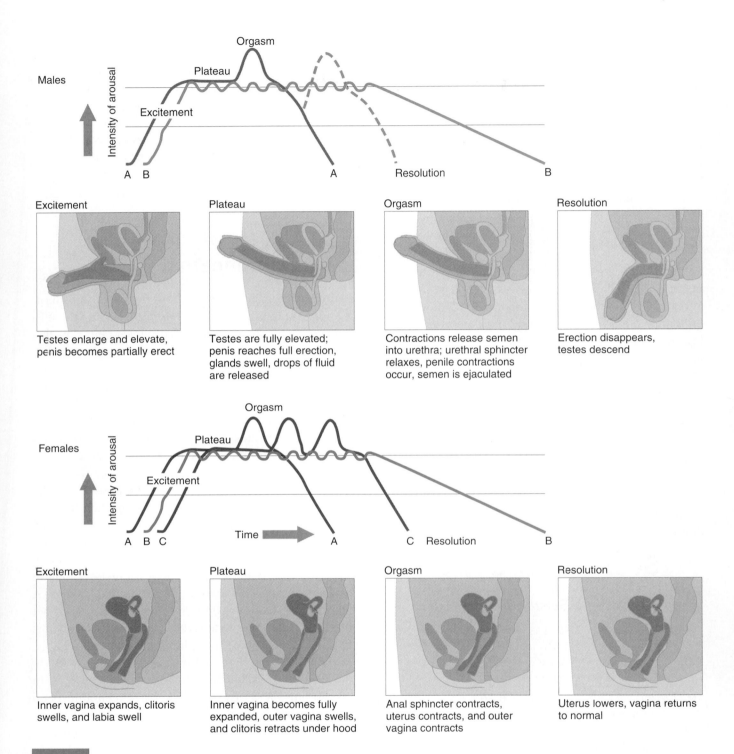

Figure 9-8

Human sexual response is a well-ordered sequence: excitement, plateau, orgasm, and resolution.

Female orgasms follow several patterns. Some women experience a series of mini-orgasms—a response sometimes described as "skimming." Another pattern consists of rapid excitement and plateau stages, followed by a prolonged orgasm. This is the most frequent response to stimulation by a vibrator.

Female orgasms are primarily triggered by stimulat-

ing the clitoris. When stimulation reaches an adequate level, the vagina responds by contracting. Although it sometimes seems that vaginal stimulation alone can set off an orgasm, the clitoris is usually involved—at least indirectly during full penile penetration.

Some researchers have identified what they call the *Grafenberg (or G) spot* (or area) just behind the front wall of the vagina, between the cervix and the back of the pubic bone (see Figure 9-7). When this region is stimulated, women report various sensations, including slight discomfort, a brief feeling that they need to urinate, and increasing pleasure. Continued stimulation may result in an orgasm of great intensity, accompanied by ejaculation of fluid from the urethra. However, other researchers have failed to confirm the existence and importance of the G spot, and sex therapists disagree about its significance for a woman's sexual satisfaction.

Resolution

The sexual organs of men and women return to their normal, nonexcited state during this final phase of sexual response. Heightened skin color quickly fades after orgasm, and the heart rate, blood pressure, and breathing rate soon return to normal. The clitoris also resumes its normal position and appearance very shortly thereafter, whereas the penis may remain somewhat erect for up to 30 minutes.

After orgasm, men typically enter a **refractory period**, during which they are incapable of another orgasm. The duration of this period varies from minutes to days, depending on age and the frequency of previous sexual activity. If either partner doesn't have an orgasm after becoming highly aroused, resolution may be much slower and may be accompanied by a sense of discomfort.

Strategies for Change
Improving a Sexual Relationship

✔ Use "I" statements, such as "I really enjoy making love, but I'm so tired right now that I won't be a responsive partner. Why don't we get the kids to bed early tomorrow so we can enjoy ourselves a little earlier?"

✔ When your partner is talking, do not dismiss what he or she is saying as crazy, irrational, or selfish.

✔ If your partner has temporarily lost interest in sex, express concern and ask what the two of you might do to make things better. Don't blame yourself.

✔ Speak up if something hurts during sex. Be specific.

✔ If you would like to try something different, say so. Practice saying the words first if they embarrass you. If your partner feels uncomfortable, don't force the issue, but do try talking it through.

✔ Set aside time for a regular sex talk. Take turns bringing up topics. Mention special pleasures or particular problems.

✔ If you want to request changes or tackle a touchy topic, start with positive statements. Let your partner know how much you enjoy having sex, and then express your desire to enjoy lovemaking more often or in different ways.

✔ Encourage small changes. If you want your partner to be less inhibited, start slowly, perhaps by suggesting sex in a different room or place.

Sexual Concerns

Many sexual concerns stem from myths and misinformation. There is no truth, for instance, behind the misconception that men are always capable of erection, that sex always involves intercourse, that partners should experience simultaneous orgasms, or that people who truly love each other always have satisfying sex lives.

Cultural and childhood influences can affect our attitudes toward sex. Even though America's traditionally Puritanical values have eased, our society continues to convey mixed messages about sex. Some children, repeatedly warned of the evils of sex, never accept the sexual dimensions of their identity. Others—especially young boys—may be exposed to macho attitudes toward sex and feel a need to prove their virility. Young girls may feel confused by media messages that encourage them to look and act provocatively and a double-standard that blames them for leading boys on. In addition, virtually everyone has individual worries. A woman may feel self-conscious about the shape of her breasts; a man may worry about the size of his penis; both partners may fear not pleasing the other.

The concept of sexual normalcy differs greatly in different times, cultures, or racial and ethnic groups. In certain times and places, only sex between a husband and wife has been deemed normal. In other circumstances, "normal" has been applied to any sexual behavior—alone or with others—that does not harm others or produce great anxiety and guilt. The following are some of the most common contemporary sexual concerns.

Safer Sex

Having sex is never completely safe; the only 100% risk-free sexual choice is abstinence. If you choose to be sexually active, you can greatly reduce your risk by restricting sexual activity to the context of a mutually

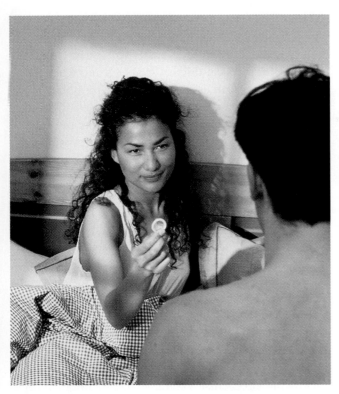

Don't forget. Be sexually responsible—for your own and your partner's sake. Using condoms is one way you can lower your risks of contracting STDs.

exclusive, monogamous relationship in which both partners know, on the basis of laboratory testing, that neither has an STD or HIV antibodies.

For centuries, sexually transmitted diseases, such as gonorrhea and syphilis, caused great suffering and many deaths. Modern medicine has developed effective treatments for these health threats, but other STDs, such as herpes and chlamydia, have become serious health problems. However, no STD in recent history has had as terrifying an impact as infection with HIV, which causes AIDS, a disease that has taken the lives of thousands of people in their prime. (Chapter 11 provides a complete discussion of the symptoms, diagnosis, and treatment of sexually transmitted diseases, including HIV infection and AIDS.)

Sex with a person who has never been exposed to HIV or to other STDs is safe (for you), regardless of what type of sexual activity you engage in. The only way of knowing for certain that a prospective partner doesn't have an STD or is not infected with HIV is through laboratory testing (see Chapter 11). Sex educators and health professionals strongly encourage couples to abstain from any sexual activity that puts them at risk for STDs until they both undergo medical examina-

tions and testing for STDs. This process greatly reduces the danger of disease transmission and can also help foster a deep sense of mutual trust and commitment. Many campus and public health clinics provide exams or laboratory testing either free of charge or on a sliding scale determined by your income.

Sexual Difficulties

A sexual difficulty may occur anywhere in the sexual response sequence. A man's penis may not become erect; a woman's vagina may not become moist. A man may lose his erection while attempting intercourse; the woman's vagina may become dry after penetration. Some men and women become excited, enjoy the plateau stage, but then don't achieve an orgasm; or their sexual cycle may be too long or too short for one of the partners. Sometimes the cause of the problem is alcohol or drugs (see Table 9-2), disease, injury, stress, or chronic pain. Often, however, it's fear, anxiety, or ignorance.

Sexual Anxiety

One of the most common feelings associated with sex—along with curiosity, desire, and love—is anxiety. No one is born knowing about sex. Most of us learn from our experiences, and—as with most activities, from ski-

TABLE 9-2	SEXUAL EFFECTS OF SOME DRUGS
Alcohol:	Chronic alcohol abuse causes hormonal alterations (reduces size of testes and suppresses hormonal function) and permanent damage to the circulatory and nervous systems.
Marijuana:	Reduces testosterone levels in men and decreases sexual desire.
Tobacco:	Adversely affects small blood vessels in the penis and decreases the frequency and duration of erections (Mannino et al., 1994).
Cocaine	Causes erectile disorder and inhibited orgasm.
Amphetamines:	In high doses and with chronic use, inhibits orgasm, decreases erection and lubrication.
Barbiturates	Causes decreased desire, erectile disorders, delayed orgasm.

SOURCE: Finger et al., 1997.

ing to speaking French—our first attempts tend to be awkward. A caring, loving relationship can make all the difference.

Problems with Arousal

The most frequent problem sex therapists and marriage counselors see is lack of sexual desire. Perfectly healthy couples, with no physical impairment, simply become bored with sex, even though they love each other and find each other attractive and enjoyable. Men and women are equally likely to lose interest in sex, and often neither partner has had previous arousal or orgasm problems.

Often stress—perhaps caused by a recent move, a new baby, or a high-pressure job—is the real culprit. Severe stress can short-circuit normal sexual response. Couples who try to unwind by drinking or using tranquilizers usually make the problem worse by further dampening their sexual responses.

Erectile Disorders

Erectile disorders, or **impotence**, affect many men as they age (see Figure 9-9). Virtually all men are occasionally unable to achieve or maintain an erection because of fatigue, stress, alcohol, or drug use. As clinically defined, impotence means that a man cannot get an

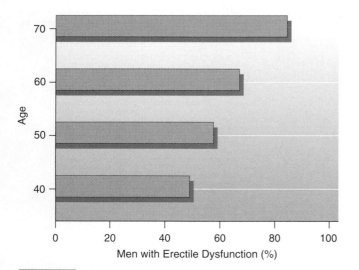

The Incidence of Erectile Disorder and Age

Men with Erectile Dysfunction (%)

Figure 9-9

Age itself does not cause erectile disorder, but the increased incidence of diseases such as diabetes, high blood pressure, and cardiovascular problems that accompany aging take their toll.

SOURCE: Kerin and Lipshultz, 1997.

erection more often than once in four attempts. Psychological factors, such as anxiety about performance, may cause impotence. But in as many as 80% of cases, the problem has physical origins. Diabetes and reactions to drugs—including an estimated 200 prescription medications—are the most frequent organic causes. Even cigarettes can create erection problems for men sensitive to nicotine. According to the Impotence Information Center, smoking ten or more cigarettes a day increases the likelihood of impotence.

New treatments for physiologic impotence include medications such as Viagra, which was released in 1998, or vacuum devices that increase blood flow to the penis to induce erection; injectable drugs (such as Caverject) that produces an erection within 20 minutes of injection into the base of the penis; vascular reconstruction (grafts of arteries from the lower abdomen are placed around narrowed branches of the main artery leading to the penis to restore blood flow); and penile implants (some inflatable, some permanently rigid) that enable impotent men to have sexual intercourse. The first oral medicine for erectile problems, Viagra, relaxes smooth muscle cells. Other experimental medications include Spontane, which affects the part of the brain that triggers erection, and Vasomax, which blocks adrenaline and dilates arteries.[44]

Failure to Respond

Women probably fail to become aroused at least as often as men, but it doesn't seem to be as upsetting to them as the inability to become erect is to men partly because it isn't as noticeable. Our culture is also more accepting of women who say they simply "don't feel like sex." The myth that a man should become aroused at every opportunity urges many men to have sex—or try to—regardless of how they feel.

Orgasm Problems in Men

For men, a common concern is **premature ejaculation**, which is defined as ejaculating within 30 to 90 seconds of inserting the penis into the vagina, or after 10 to 15 thrusts. Another definition is that a premature ejaculator cannot control or delay his ejaculation long enough to satisfy a responsive partner at least half the time. By this definition, a man may be premature with some women but not with others.

To delay orgasm, men may try to think of baseball or other sports, but this just makes sex boring. Others may masturbate before intercourse, hoping to take advantage of the refractory period, during which they cannot ejaculate again. Others may bite their lips or dig their nails into their palms—although usually this just results in premature ejaculators with bloody lips and scarred palms. Some physicians prescribe drugs, including antidepressants, and androgens (male sex hormones), to cure premature ejaculation. Topical anesthetics used to prevent climax dull pleasurable sensations for the woman as well as for the man.

Men can learn to control their ejaculation by concentrating on their sexual responses, rather than by trying to distract themselves or ignore their reactions. Some men find that they have greater control by lying on their backs with their partner on top, by relaxing during intercourse, and by communicating with their partner about when to stop or slow down movements.

Other techniques for delaying ejaculation include *stop-start,* in which a man learns to sense the feelings that precede ejaculation and stop his movements before the point of ejaculatory inevitability, allowing his arousal to subside slightly before restarting sexual activity. In the *squeeze technique,* a man's partner applies strong pressure with her thumb on the frenum and her second and third fingers on the top side of the penis, one above and one below the corona, until the man loses the urge to ejaculate.

Intercourse and Orgasm Problems in Women

Some women experience **dyspareunia**, or pain during intercourse. An extreme form of painful intercourse is **vaginismus**, in which involuntary contractions of the muscles of the outer third of the vagina are so intense that they totally or partially close the vaginal opening. This problem often derives from a fear of being penetrated. Relaxation techniques, such as *Kegel exercises* (alternately tightening and relaxing the muscles of the pelvic floor), or the use of fingers or dilators to gradually open the vagina, can make penetration easier.

The female orgasm has long been a controversial sexual topic. According to recent estimates, about 90% of sexually active women have experienced orgasm, but only a much smaller percentage achieve orgasm through intercourse alone. Even fewer reach orgasm if intercourse isn't accompanied by direct stimulation of the clitoris. Is intercourse without orgasm a sexual problem? The best answer is that it is a problem if a woman wants to experience orgasm during intercourse but doesn't.

Many counseling programs urge women who have never had orgasms to masturbate. They are then encouraged to share with their partners what they've learned, communicating with words or gestures what is most pleasing to them. Some women regularly want or need more than a single orgasm during intercourse. Partners can help by varying positions and experimenting with sexual techniques. However, in sexual response, more is not necessarily better, and the couple should keep in mind that no one else is counting.

Sex Therapy

Modern sex therapy, pioneered by Masters and Johnson in the 1960s, views sex as a natural, healthy behavior that enhances a couple's relationship. Their approach emphasizes education, communication, reduction of performance anxiety, and sexual exercises that enhance sexual intimacy.

Today most sex therapists, working either alone or with a partner, have modified Masters and Johnson's approach. Most see couples once a week for eight to ten weeks; the focus of therapy is on correcting dysfunctional behavior, not exploring underlying psychodynamics.

Contrary to common misconceptions, sex therapy does not involve conducting sexual activity in front of therapists. The therapist may review psychological and physiological aspects of sexual functioning and evaluate the couple's sexual attitudes and ability to communicate. The core of the program is the couple's "homework"—a series of exercises, carried out in private, that enhances their sensory awareness and improve nonverbal communication. These techniques have proven effective for couples regardless of their age or general health.[45]

Strategies for Change
....
When to Seek Help

You and your partner should consider consulting a sex therapist if any of the following is true for you:

✔   Sex is painful or physically uncomfortable.

✔   You're having sex less and less frequently.

✔   You have a general fear of, or revulsion toward, sex.

✔   Your sexual pleasure is declining.

✔   Your sexual desire is diminishing.

✔   Your sexual problems are increasing in frequency or persisting for longer periods.

Drugs and Sex

Many recreational drugs, such as alcohol and marijuana, are believed to enhance sexual performance. However, none of the popular drugs touted as *aphrodisiac*—including amphetamines, barbiturates, cantharides ("Spanish fly"), cocaine, LSD and other psychedelics, marijuana, amyl nitrite ("poppers") and L-dopa (a medication used to treat Parkinson's disease)—is truly a sexual stimulant. In fact, these drugs often interfere with normal sexual response. Researchers are studying one drug that may truly enhance sexual performance: yohimbine hydrochloride, which is derived from the sap of the tropical yohimbe tree that grows in West Africa.

Because many psychiatric problems can lower sexual desire and affect sexual functioning, medications appropriate to the specific disorders can help. In addition, psychiatric drugs may be used as part of therapy. Drugs such as certain antidepressants may be used to prolong sexual response in conditions such as premature ejaculation.

Medications can also cause sexual difficulty. In men, drugs that are used to treat high blood pressure, anxiety, allergies, depression, muscle spasms, obesity, ulcers, irritable colon, and prostate cancer can cause impotence, breast enlargement, testicular swelling, priapism (persistent erection), loss of sexual desire, inability to ejaculate, and reduced sperm count. In women, they can diminish sexual desire, inhibit or delay orgasm, and cause breast swelling or secretions.

Atypical Behavior

Although sexual desire and response are universal, some individuals develop sexual appetites or engage in activities that are not typical sexual behaviors.

Sexual Addiction

Some men and women can get relief from their feelings of restlessness and worthlessness only through sex (either masturbation or with a partner). Once the sexual high ends, however, they're overwhelmed by the same negative feelings and driven, once more, to have sex.

Some therapists describe this problem as **sexual addiction**; others, as **sexual compulsion**. Professionals continue to debate exactly what this controversial condition is, how to diagnose it, and how to overcome it. However, most agree that for some people, sex is more than a normal pleasure: It is an overwhelming need that must be met, even at the cost of their careers and marriages.

Sex addicts can be heterosexual or homosexual, male or female. Their behaviors include masturbation, phone sex, reading or viewing pornography, attending strip shows, having affairs, engaging in anonymous sex with strangers or prostitutes, exhibitionism, voyeurism, child molestation, incest, and rape. Many were physically and emotionally abused as children or have family members who abuse drugs or alcohol. They typically feel a loss of control and a compulsion for sexual activity, and they continue their unhealthy sexual behavior despite the dangers, including the risk of contracting STDs. Characteristics exhibited by sex addicts include:

- A preoccupation with sex so intense and chronic that it interferes with a normal sexual relationship with a spouse or lover.

- A compulsion to have sex again and again within a short period of time, and to engage in sexual behavior that results in feelings of anxiety, depression, guilt, or shame.

- A great deal of time spent away from family or work, in order to look for sex partners or engage in sex.

- Use of sex to hide from troubles.

With help, sex addicts can deal with the shame that both triggers and follows sexual activity. Professional therapy may begin with a month of complete sexual abstinence, to break the cycle of compulsive sexual behavior. Several organizations, such as Sexaholics Anonymous and Sexual Addicts Anonymous, offer support from people who share the same problem.

Sexual Deviations

Sexual deviations listed by the American Psychiatric Association include the following:

- *Fetishism:* Obtaining sexual pleasure from an inanimate object or an asexual part of the body, such as the foot.
- *Pedophilia:* Sex between an adult and a child.
- *Transvestitism:* Becoming sexually aroused by wearing the clothing of the opposite sex.
- *Exhibitionism:* Exposing one's genitals to an unwilling observer.
- *Voyeurism:* Obtaining sexual gratification by observing people undressing or involved in sexual activity.

- *Sadism:* Becoming sexually aroused by inflicting physical or psychological pain.
- *Masochism:* Obtaining sexual gratification by suffering physical or psychological pain.

Psychiatrists distinguish between passive sexual deviancy, which doesn't involve actual contact with another, and aggressive deviancy. Most voyeurs and obscene phone callers don't seek physical contact with the objects of their sexual desire. These behaviors are performed predominantly, but not exclusively, by males. Psychiatric medications used to treat obsessive-compulsive disorder (discussed in Chapter 4) may provide help.[46]

Transgenderism

Transgendered individuals, formerly called *transsexuals,* have gender identities opposite their biological sex. Most are males who feel deeply that they are more truly females. More than 3000 Americans have undergone complex medical procedures to change their genital and secondary sex characteristics. Those who desire *sex-change operations* should be carefully screened and counseled to determine whether such extreme measures would be appropriate and beneficial.

The Business of Sex

Sex, without affection and individuality, becomes a product to be packaged, marketed, traded, bought, and sold. Two of the billion-dollar industries that treat sex as a commodity are prostitution and pornography.

Prostitution, described as the world's oldest profession, is a nationwide industry grossing more than $1 billion annually. In every state except Nevada (and in all but a few counties there), prostitution is illegal. Besides the threat of jail and fines, prostitutes and their clients face another danger: sexually transmitted diseases, including HIV infection and hepatitis B.

Pornography is a multimedia industry—books, magazines, movies, the Internet, phone lines, and computer games are available to those who find sexually explicit material entertaining or exciting. Most laws against pornography are based on the assumption that such materials can set off uncontrollable, dangerous sexual urges, ranging from promiscuity to sexual violence. Research indicates that exposure to scenes of rape or other forms of sexual violence against women, or to scenes of degradation of women, does lead to tolerance of these hostile and brutal acts.

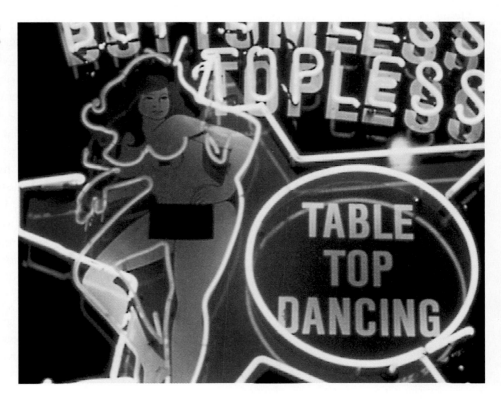

Sex sells. Topless bars and strip clubs are among the businesses that cater to those who enjoy sexual stimulation outside a loving relationship.

Making This Chapter Work for You
Responsible Sexuality

- A person's gender is determined not only by his or her physiological sex, but also by psychological and sociological factors.

- Our sexual hormones—in the female, estrogen and progesterone; in the male, testosterone—play a key role in sexual development. At puberty, estrogen causes a girl to develop female secondary sex characteristics—including enlarged external genitals and full breasts and hips and prepares her body for conception and pregnancy. Testosterone stimulates the development of male secondary sex characteristics, which include a deeper voice, facial and body hair growth, and enlarged genitals.

- Men and women think, act and react in such different ways, and the debate over whether nature and nurture causes gender differences continues. However, the real issue may not be what makes the genders different, but what difference—if any—the differences make.

- More women and men are shattering sexual stereotypes by choosing roles and occupations that have traditionally been closed to them. Individuals who allow themselves to express both their masculine and feminine traits are called androgynous.

- Women and men have different sexual organs, hormones, and different health problems. Awareness of these differences can help individuals take better care of their own sexual health and be more sensitive to the needs of their partners.

- A woman's menstrual cycle is a monthly process involving all her reproductive organs. Once a month, her ovary releases an egg cell, or ovum, that travels through the fallopian tube to the uterus. If the egg isn't fertilized, the uterine lining is shed during menstruation.

- Menstrual cycle problems include premenstrual syndrome, premenstrual dysphoric disorder, dysmenorrhea, and amenorrhea. Between the approximate ages of 45 and 54, menopause occurs when a woman's menstrual cycles stop.

- Sexual health issues for males include circumcision, which has some health advantages as well as some potential complications, such as increased risk of urinary tract infection. As men grow older, they are at risk for prostatitis, prostate enlargement, and prostate cancer. At midlife, men often experience a period of change and possible crisis.

- Making responsible sexual decisions—especially important in an age of sexual risks—requires accurate information, honest communication, consideration of all your options (including abstinence), determining whether you and your partner are ready for sex, and recognition of every individual's right to say no.

- Sexual behavior, which begins with the sexual curiosity of childhood, changes over the lifespan. Adolescents are initiating sexual activity at earlier ages than in the past but generally do not engage in frequent sex with many partners. Most college students are sexually active. Although concerned about HIV, many have not changed their sexual practices.

- Several national surveys have shown that most Americans have had several sex partners, have intercourse more often if they're married or under age 39, and engage in a range of sexual practices.

- Sexual orientation may be predominantly heterosexual, bisexual, or homosexual. Regardless of sexual orientation, healthy sexuality involves an understanding of your own body, your partner's needs and desires, and responsible sexual behavior.

- Sexual behaviors include celibacy, erotic fantasizing, kissing and touching, masturbation, intercourse, and oral sex.

- Whatever the type of sexual stimulation, the body's response always follows the same sequence: excitement, plateau, orgasm, and resolution.

- The safest sex practices are abstinence or sexual relations with only one partner who has never been exposed to HIV or other STDs.

- Sexual concerns include sexual anxiety, lack of sexual interest, sexual unresponsiveness, and sexual impairment due to the use of recreational drugs or medications. In men, common sexual problems include erectile disorders and premature ejaculation; women are more likely to have orgasm difficulties.

- Sexual addiction, transgenderism, and sexual deviations are considered atypical sexual behaviors. Prostitution and pornography strip sex of its emotional, deeply human meaning and transform it into a business.

By caring for your sexual health and treating your partner with respect, you prepare yourself to become a responsible, responsive sexual partner. By avoiding the dangers of sexually transmitted diseases, you assume responsibility for your safety and health. By dealing with any sexual problems that arise, you take charge of a key aspect of your health and behavior.

Health Online

Online Sexual Disorders Screening

http://www.med.nyu.edu/Psych/screens/sdsf.html (women)
http://www.med.nyu.edu/Psych/screens/sdsm.html (men)

These pages from the New York University School of Medicine present separate questionnaires for men and women that screen for the possible presence of sexual disorders. There are also links to referrals for counseling and medical treatment, and more information on sexual disorders.

Think about it ...

- Many of these symptoms are experienced by most people at one time or another. At what point do you think sexual problems become "disorders"?

- According to this screening test, do you have symptoms of a sexual disorder? If so, what do you think might be the causes of this problem?

▶ Key Terms

The terms listed here are used within the chapter. Page numbers are included for each term.
A definition of each term is given in the green Glossary pages at the end of this book.

Review Questions

1. What factors influence sexual identity in our society? Are they the same influences that affect gender identity? What are some differences between the two?

2. Name the different parts of the male reproductive system, and briefly explain the function of each part. Name the different parts of the female reproductive system, and briefly explain the function of each part.

3. What are some conditions that are unique to women's sexual health? men's sexual health? Are there any conditions that affect both men and women's sexual health?

4. What is the human sexual response cycle? List and briefly describe each step. Are there any differences in the sexual response cycles of males and females?

5. What are some preventive behaviors that can reduce an individual's chances of becoming HIV infected?

6. What are some common concerns among men and women regarding sexual performance difficulties? How might these problems be overcome?

 ## Critical Thinking Questions

1. Anita insists that her boyfriend, Bill, has never taken any sexual risks. But when she suggested that they get tested for STDs, he was furious and refused. Now Anita says she doesn't know what to believe. Is he telling the truth, or is he hiding something? She doesn't want to take any risks, but she doesn't want to lose him either. What would you advise her to say or do?

2. Tommy has always been fascinated with pornography. While his friends were discussing the latest sports stories, he hung out alone with his stash of porn magazines—the raunchier, the better. When asked if this habit has become an addiction, Tommy gets very defensive. He says he's just exercising his First Amendment rights. Do you think he needs help? Do you think it's okay to read or look at pornographic books, magazines, and videos? Why or why not?

3. Some people support the legalization of homosexual marriages. Some gay people feel that they will never be fully accepted in society unless they can legally marry. Other gay people oppose the idea as too imitative of straight couples. Some heterosexuals think that gay marriages would violate the sanctity of marriage. Do you think homosexual marriages should be accepted? Why or why not?

 ## Connections to Personal Health Interactive

To enhance your understanding of the material covered in this chapter, check out the following study aids on the **Personal Health Interactive CD-ROM**. *Each numbered icon within the chapter corresponds to an appropriate activity listed here.*

9.1 The Double Standard
9.2 Study Page: Female Sexual Anatomy
9.3 Study Page: Male Sexual Anatomy

9.4 Personal Insights: How Sexual Are You?
9.5 Survey of Sexual Knowledge
9.6 Chapter 9 Review

 ## References

1. Hess, Rex, et al. "Estrogen Linked to Sperm Count, Male Fertility." *Nature*, December 4, 1997.
2. McClintock, Martha, and Gilbert Herdt. "Rethinking Puberty: The Development of Sexual Attraction." *Current Directions in Psychological Science*, Vol. 9, No. 6, December 1996.
3. Herman-Giddens, Marcia, et al. "Second Sexual Charac-teristics and Menses in Young Girls Seen in Office Practice: A Study from the Pediatric Research in Office Settings Network." *Pediatrics*, Vol. 80, No. 4, April 1997.
4. Kimura, Doris. Personal interview.
5. Halpern, Diane. Personal interview.
6. Wiederman, Michael, et al. "The Attractiveness of Gender-typed Traits at Different Relationship Levels: Androgynous

Characteristics May Be Desirable After All." *Personality & Social Psychology Bulletin*, Vol. 20, No. 3, June 1994.

7. Blumenthal, Susan. "Improving Women's Mental and Physical Health: Federal Initiative and Programs." *American Psychiatric Press Review of Psychiatry*, Vol. 14. Washington, DC: American Psychiatric Press, 1995. Pinn, Vivian. "Women's Health Research." *Journal of the American Medical Association,* October 14, 1992. Clancy, Carolyn, and Charlea Massion. "American Women's Health Care." *Journal of the American Medical Association,* October 14, 1992.

8. "PMS: 66 Years of Research." *University of California, Berkeley Wellness Letter*, Vol. 14, No. 1, October 1997.

9. Yonkers, Kimberly A.; Halbreich, Uriel; Freeman, Ellen; Brown, Candace; and others. " Symptomatic Improvement of Premenstrual Dysphoric Disorder with Sertraline Treatment: A Randomized Controlled Trial." *Journal of the American Medical Association*, Vol. 278, No. 12, September 24, 1997.

10. Ozio, Ron. "Fewer Parents Choosing Circumcision." *Baylor College of Medicine News*, October 31, 1997.

11. Crooks, Robert, and Karla Baur. *Our Sexuality,* 7th ed. Pacific Grove, CA: Brooks/Cole, 1999.

12. Wiswell, Thomas. "Circumcision Circumspection." *New England Journal of Medicine*, Vol. 336, No. 17, April 24, 1997.

13. Laumann, Edward, et al. "Circumcision in the United States: Prevalence, Prophylactic Effects, and Sexual Practice." *Journal of the American Medical Association*, Vol. 277, No. 13, April 2, 1997.

14. "Prostate Problems: Medical and Nonmedical Treatments for Benign Prostate Hypertrophy." *Geriatrics,* June 1991. Carlson, Robert. "The Other Prostate Problem." *American Health,* October 1992.

15. Hatcher, Robert, et al. *Sexual Etiquette 101*. Atlanta, GA: Emory University School of Medicine.

16. Crooks and Baur, *Our Sexuality*.

17. Morrow, Lance. "Fifteen Cheers for Abstinence." *Time*, October 2, 1995.

18. Laumann, Edward, et al. *The Social Organization of Sexuality*. Chicago: University of Chicago, 1994.

19. Ibid.

20. Kowalski, Robin M. "Inferring Sexual Interest from Behavioral Cues: Effects of Gender and Sexually Relevant Attitudes." *Sex Roles: A Journal of Research,* Vol. 29, No. 2, July 1993.

21. Adler, Nancy. Personal interview.

22. Haffner, Debra W., and Goldfarb, Eva. "But Does It Work? Improving Evaluations of Sexuality Education." *SIECUS Report*, Vol. 25, No. 6, August–September 1997.

23. Campbell, Lisa. "Adolescent Sexual Behavior Does Not Always Foretell Sexual Orientation." *The Brown University Child and Adolescent Behavior Letter*, Vol. 10, No. 12, December 1994.

24. Crooks and Baur, *Our Sexuality*, 1999.

25. Ibid.

26. Alan Guttmacher Institute, 1994.

27. Ku, Leighton, et al. "The Association of AIDS Education and Sex Education with Sexual Behavior and Condom Use Among Teenage Men." *Family Planning Perspectives,* May–June 1992. Folkenberg, Judy. "AIDS Education Lowers Risky Sexual Behavior Among Black Male Adolescents." *NIH Healthline,* April–May 1992.

28. Douglas, Kathy, et al. "Results from the 1995 National College Health Risk Behavior Survey." *Journal of American College Health*, Vol. 46, September 1997.

29. DeBuono, Barbara, et al. "Sexual Behavior of College Women in 1975, 1986 and 1989." *New England Journal of Medicine*, March 22, 1990.

30. Reinisch, June, et al. "High-Risk Sexual Behavior Among Heterosexual Undergraduates at a Midwestern University." *Family Planning Perspectives*, May–June 1992.

31. D'Augelli, Anthony. "Sexual Behavior Patterns of Gay University Men: Implications for Preventing HIV Infection." *College Health*, July 1992.

32. Robinson, John, and Geoffrey Godbey. "No Sex, Please…We're College Graduates." *American Demographics*, February 1998.

33. Ibid.

34. Ibid.

35. Crooks, and Baur. *Our Sexuality*.

36. Risch, Neil, et al. "Male Sexual Orientation and Genetic Evidence." *Science*, Vol. 262, December 24, 1993. LeVay, S. "A Difference in Hypothalamic Structure Between Heterosexual and Homosexual Men." *Science,* Vol. 253, 1991, pp. 1034–1037.

37. Crooks and Baur, *Our Sexuality*, 1999.

38. Maltz, Wendy, and Boss, Suzie. *In the Garden of Desire: The Intimate World of Women's Sexual Fantasies*. New York: Broadway Books, 1997. Luker, Kristin. *Dubious Conceptions: The Politics of Teenage Pregnancy*. Cambridge, MA: Harvard University Press, 1996.

39. Crooks and Baur, *Our Sexuality*.

40. Laumann, et al. *The Social Organization of Sexuality*.

41. Billy, J. O., et al. "The Sexual Behavior of Men in the United States." *Family Planning Perspectives*, Vol. 25, 1993.

42. Janus, Samuel, and Cynthia Janus. *The Janus Report on Sexual Behavior*. New York: Wiley, 1993.

43. Seidman, Stuart, and Ronald Rieder. "Sexual Behavior Through the Life Cycle: An Empirical Approach." *American Psychiatric Press Review of Psychiatry*, Vol. 14. Washington, DC: American Psychiatric Press, 1995.

44. Horvitz, Leslie Alan. "Can Better Sex Come with a Pill? The Nineties' Impotence Cure." *Insight on the News*, Vol. 13, No. 46, December 15, 1997.

45. Bronner, Gila. "Helping Health Care Professionals on Issues of Intimacy and Sexuality Among the Aging." *SIECUS Report*, Vol. 25, No. 5, June–July 1997.

46. Schmidt, Chester. "Sexual Psychopathology and DSM-IV." *American Psychiatric Press Review of Psychiatry*, Vol. 14. Washington, DC: American Psychiatric Press, 1995. Bradford, J. M. W., et al. "Pharmacological Treatment of the Paraphilias." *American Psychiatric Press Review of Psychiatry*, Vol. 14. Washington, DC: American Psychiatric Press, 1995.

CHAPTER 10

REPRODUCTIVE CHOICES

After studying the material in this chapter, you should be able to:

Explain the process of conception in humans.

List the major options available for contraception, and **explain** the advantages and risks of each.

Define *abortion,* and **list** the commonly used abortion methods.

Define and **give examples** of *preconception care*.

Describe the physiological effects of pregnancy on a woman, including the most frequent complications of pregnancy.

Briefly **describe** the growth and development of a fetus from embryo to birth.

Describe the three stages of labor and birth.

Explain the options available to infertile couples wishing to have children.

As human beings, we have a unique power: the ability to choose to conceive or not to conceive. No other species on earth can separate sexual activity and pleasure from reproduction. However, simply not wanting to get pregnant is never enough to prevent conception, nor is wanting to have a child always enough to get pregnant. Both desires require individual decisions and actions.

Anyone who engages in vaginal intercourse must be willing to accept the consequences of that activity—the possibility of pregnancy and responsibility for the child who might be conceived—or take action to avoid those consequences. A heterosexual woman in Western countries spends 90% of her reproductive years trying to prevent pregnancy and 10% of these years trying to become or being pregnant.[1] This chapter provides information on conception, birth control, and the processes by which a new human life develops and enters the world.

Conception

The equation for making a baby is quite simple: one sperm plus one egg equals one fertilized egg, which can develop into an infant. But the processes that affect or permit **conception** are quite complicated. The creation of sperm, or **spermatogenesis**, starts in the male at puberty. As discussed in Chapter 9, the production of sperm is regulated by hormones. Sperm cells form in the seminiferous tubules of the testes and are passed into the epididymis, where they are stored until ejaculation (see Figure 10-1); a single male ejaculation may contain 500 million sperm. Each of the sperm released into the vagina during intercourse moves on its own, propelling itself toward its target, an ovum.

To reach its goal, the sperm must move through the acidic secretions of the vagina, enter the uterus, travel up the fallopian tube containing the ovum, then fuse with the nucleus of the egg **(fertilization)**. Just about every sperm produced by a man in his lifetime fails to accomplish its mission.

There are far fewer human egg cells than there are sperm cells. Each woman is born with her lifetime supply of ova, and between 300 and 500 eggs eventually mature and leave her ovaries during ovulation. As discussed in Chapter 9, every month, one or the other of the woman's ovaries releases an ovum to the nearby fallopian tube. It travels through the fallopian tube until it reaches the uterus, a journey that takes three to four days. An unfertilized egg lives for about 24 to 36 hours, disintegrates, and, during menstruation, is expelled along with the uterine lining.

Even if a sperm, which can survive in the female reproductive tract for two to five days, meets a ripe egg in a fallopian tube, its success is not assured. It must penetrate the layer of cells and a jellylike substance that surrounds each egg. Every sperm that touches the egg deposits an enzyme that dissolves part of this barrier. When a sperm bumps into a bare spot, it can penetrate the egg membrane and merge with the egg. (See Figure 10-2.) The fertilized egg travels down the fallopian tube, dividing to form a tiny clump of cells called a **zygote**. When it reaches the uterus, about a week after fertiliza-

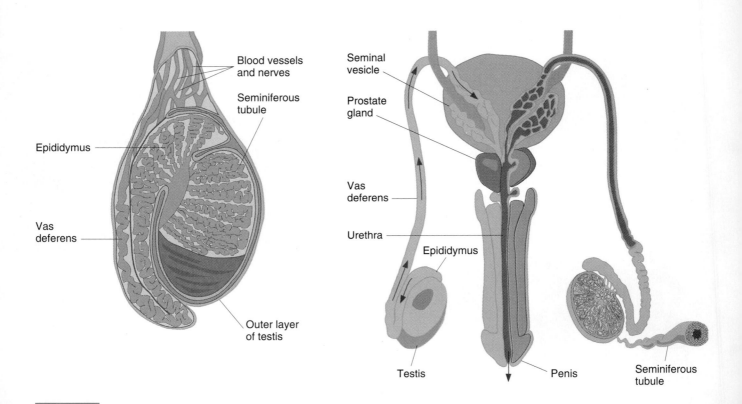

Figure 10-1

The testes. Spermatogenesis takes place in the testes. Sperm cells form in the seminiferous tubules and are stored in the coils of the epididymis. Eventually, the sperm drain into the vasa deferentia ready for ejaculation.

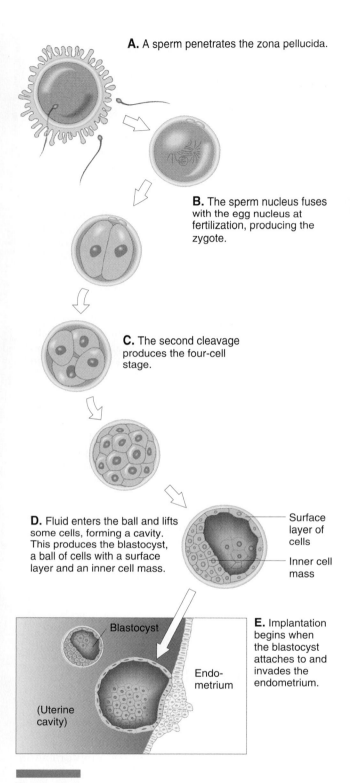

A. A sperm penetrates the zona pellucida.

B. The sperm nucleus fuses with the egg nucleus at fertilization, producing the zygote.

C. The second cleavage produces the four-cell stage.

D. Fluid enters the ball and lifts some cells, forming a cavity. This produces the blastocyst, a ball of cells with a surface layer and an inner cell mass.

Surface layer of cells

Inner cell mass

Blastocyst

Endo-metrium

(Uterine cavity)

E. Implantation begins when the blastocyst attaches to and invades the endometrium.

Figure 10-2

Fertilization. (A) The efforts of hundreds of sperm may allow one to penetrate the ovum's corona radiata, and outer layer of cells, and then the zona pellucida, a thick inner membrane. (B) The nuclei of the sperm and the egg cells approach. The nuclei merge, and the male and female chromosomes in the nuclei come together, forming a zygote. (C) The zygote divides into two cells, then four cells, and so on. (D) As fluid enters the ball, cells form a ball of cells called a blastocyst. (E) The blastocyst implants itself in the endometrium.

tion, it burrows into the endometrium, the lining of the uterus. This process is called **implantation**.

Conception can be prevented by **contraception**. Some contraceptive methods prevent ovulation or implantation, and others block the sperm from reaching the egg. Some methods are temporary; others permanently alter one's fertility.

The Basics of Birth Control

Since ancient times, men and women have tried to lower the odds of conceiving. In different cultures, women have used camel or alligator dung to absorb semen, or they have consumed gunpowder, foam from a camel's mouth, or water that had been used to wash a corpse. Roots, rags, grass, feathers, balls, honey, and opium have served as vaginal plugs. Men have worn condoms made of tortoise shell, horn, leather, linen, or goat's bladders. The ancient Greeks and Romans are believed to have used a plant called silphion as the first oral contraceptive.[2]

Today's sexually active couples have more appealing, though far-from-perfect choices (see Pulsepoints: "Ten Ways to Avoid Getting Pregnant"). According to the National Center for Health Statistics, the leading method of contraception in the United States is female sterilization, followed by oral contraceptives, the male condom, and male sterilization.[3]

Although many people are concerned about the risks associated with contraception, using birth control is safer and healthier than not using it. According to the Population Reference Bureau, the use of contraceptives, including oral contraceptives, saves millions of lives each year.[4] Some forms of contraception also reduce the risk of sexually transmitted diseases (STDs).

Ideally, two partners should decide together which form of birth control to use. However, according to a national 1995 Harris poll, more than 70% of men and women said men were "not responsible enough" to choose a birth control method. Both sexes believed that men were uninvolved because they "don't care" and because they consider birth control the "female's responsibility." Among those surveyed, 57% of the women using birth control said they were the ones who made sure contraception was used; 35% shared the decision with their male partners; the male took responsibility in the remaining instances.[5] The general lack of male involvement may account for 40% of each year's unwanted pregnancies.

Pulsepoints

Ten Ways to Avoid Getting Pregnant

1. Abstain. The only 100% safe and effective way to avoid unwanted pregnancy is not to engage in heterosexual intercourse.

2. Limit sexual activity to "outercourse." You can engage in many sexual activities—kissing, hugging, touching, massage, oral-genital sex—without risking pregnancy.

3. Talk about birth control with any potential sex partner. If you are considering sexual intimacy with a person, you should feel comfortable enough to talk about contraception.

4. Know what doesn't work—and don't rely on it. There are lots of misconceptions about ways to avoid getting pregnant, such as having sex in a standing position or during menstruation. Only the methods described in

this chapter are reliable forms of birth control.

5. Talk with a health care professional. A great deal of information and advice is available—in writing, from family planning counselors, from physicians on the Internet. Check it out.

6. Choose a contraceptive method that matches your personal habits and preferences. If you can't remember to take a pill every day, oral contraceptives aren't for you. If you're constantly forgetting where you put things, a diaphragm might not be a good choice.

7. Consider long-term implications. Since you may well wish to have children in the future, find out about the reversibility of various methods and possible effects on future fertility.

8. Resist having sex without contraceptive protection "just this once." It only takes once—even the very first time—to get pregnant. Be wary of drugs and alcohol. They can impair your judgement and make you less conscientious about using birth control—or using it properly.

9. Use backup methods. If there's a possibility that a contraceptive method might not offer adequate protection (for instance, if it's been almost three months since your last injection of Depo-Provera), use an additional form of birth control.

10. Inform yourself about emergency contraception. Just in case a condom breaks or a diaphragm slips, find out about the availability of forms of after-intercourse contraception.

Another barrier to birth control is cost. Many health insurers do not cover the cost of reversible methods of birth control—despite evidence that contraception, when used properly, is far more cost-effective than an unplanned pregnancy.[6] Even when birth control is affordable and available, many college students do not use it consistently. As Campus Focus: "College Students and Contraception" shows about 20% of students did not use contraceptives during their last sexual intercourse.[7]

If you are engaging in sexual activity that could lead to conception, you have to be realistic about your situation. This may mean assuming full responsibility for your reproductive ability, whether you're a man or a woman. You also have to recognize the risks associated with various methods of contraception. If you're a woman, the risks are chiefly yours. Although most women never experience any serious complications, it's

important to be aware of the potential for long-term risks. Risks that are acceptable to others may not be acceptable to you.

Choosing a Method

When it comes to deciding which form of birth control to use, there's no one "right" decision. (See Self-Survey: "Which Contraceptive Method Is Best for You?") However, good decisions are based on sound information. You should consult a physician or family-planning counselor if you have questions or want to know how certain methods might affect existing or familial medical conditions, such as high blood pressure or diabetes.

As Table 10-1 indicates, contraception doesn't always work. As you evaluate any contraceptive, always consider its **effectiveness** (the likelihood that it will

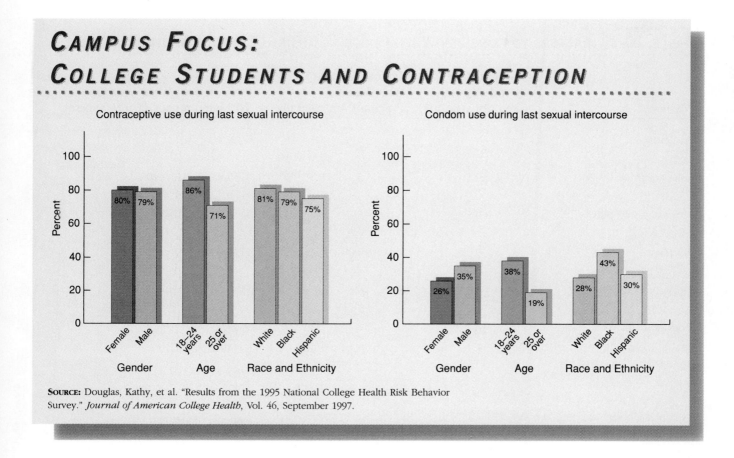

CAMPUS FOCUS:
COLLEGE STUDENTS AND CONTRACEPTION

Contraceptive use during last sexual intercourse

- Gender: Female 80%, Male 79%
- Age: 18–24 years 86%, 25 or over 71%
- Race and Ethnicity: White 81%, Black 79%, Hispanic 75%

Condom use during last sexual intercourse

- Gender: Female 26%, Male 35%
- Age: 18–24 years 38%, 25 or over 19%
- Race and Ethnicity: White 28%, Black 43%, Hispanic 30%

SOURCE: Douglas, Kathy, et al. "Results from the 1995 National College Health Risk Behavior Survey." *Journal of American College Health*, Vol. 46, September 1997.

indeed prevent pregnancy). Inevitably, theoretical effectiveness, based on statistical estimates, is greater than actual effectiveness. The **failure rate** for a contraceptive refers to the number of pregnancies that occur per year for every 100 women using a particular method of birth control.[8]

Some couples use withdrawal or **coitus interruptus**, removal of the penis from the vagina before ejaculation, to prevent pregnancy, even though it is not a reliable form of birth control. About half the men who have tried coitus interruptus find it unsatisfactory, either because they don't know when they're going to ejaculate or because they can't withdraw quickly enough. Also, the Cowper's glands, two pea-sized structures located on each side of the urethra, often produce a fluid that appears as drops at the tip of the penis any time from arousal and erection to orgasm. This fluid can contain active sperm and, in infected men, HIV.

As many as 3 million unintentional pregnancies each year in the United States are the result of contra-

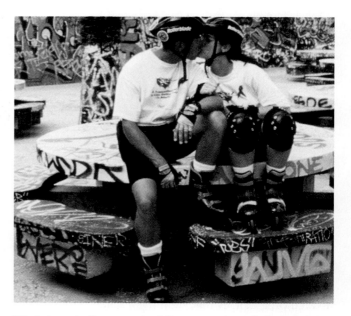

What does abstinence mean? Some couples refrain from intercourse but engage in "outercourse," or intimacy that includes kissing, hugging, and sensual touching.

TABLE 10-1 FACTORS TO CONSIDER WHEN CHOOSING A BIRTH CONTROL METHOD

Method	Failure Rate* If Used Correctly and Consistently	Typical Number* Who Become Pregnant Accidentally	Cost (in dollars per year for 100 occurrences of intercourse)
Abstinence	0	0	0
Estogen-progestin pills	0.1	3	$130–$260 ($10–$20 per cycle)
Progestin-only pills	0.5	3	$130–$260 ($10–$20 per cycle)
Norplant	0.09	0.09	$130–$170 if kept 5 years
Depo-Provera	0.3	0.3	$140 ($35 per injection)
Condoms (male)	3	12	$50 (50¢ each)
Condoms (female)	5	21	$250 ($2.50 each)
Diaphragm with spermicide	6	18	$155–$255 ($20 diaphragm, $50–$150 for fitting, $85 for spermicide)
Cervical cap			Same as diaphragm
Woman has become pregnant	26	36	
Woman never pregnant	9	18	
Spermicides	6	21	$85 (85¢ per application)
Progestasert T IUD	1.5	2	$160
Copper-T IUD	0.6	0.8	$160 1st year; less if kept more years
Tubal sterilization	0.4	0.4	$1,200–$2,500
Vasectomy	0.1	0.15	$250–$1,000
Fertility awareness: "rhythm"calendar, basal temperature, cervical mucus	1–9	20	0
Withdrawal	4	19	0
No method	85	85	0

* Number of women who become pregnant by the end of the first year of using a particular method.

SOURCE: Hatcher, et al., *Contraceptive Technology*. New York: Irvington, 1994.

ceptive failure, either from problems with the drug or device itself or from improper use. Half of the 1.5 million abortions performed in this country each year involve pregnancies that stem from failed birth control. Partners can lower the risk of unwanted pregnancy by using backup methods—that is, more than one form of contraception simultaneously. Emergency or post-inter- course contraception (discussed later in this chapter) could prevent as many as 2.3 million unwanted pregnancies each year.[9]

Always discuss contraception with your partner. Men shouldn't automatically shift this responsibility to women simply because women are the ones who get pregnant. And women shouldn't assume that men don't want to be

TABLE 10-1   CONTINUED...

Advantages	Disadvantages
No medical side effects. Helps develop nonintercourse sexual intimacy	Risk of unplanned intercourse
Very effective; no interruption of sexual experience; reduced menstrual cramps and flow	Possible side effects; increased risk of pregnancy if forgotten
Very effective; no interruption of sexual experience; no estrogen-related side effects	Breakthrough bleeding
Very effective; no interruption of sexual esperience; don't have to remember to take it; no estrogen-related side effects	Breakthrough bleeding; difficult removal
Very effective; no interruption of sexual experience; don't have to remember on daily basis; no estrogen-related side effects	Breakthrough bleeding side effects; clinic visit and injection every 3 months
Some protection from STDs; available without a prescription	Interruption of sexual experience; reduces sensation
Same as male condoms	Same as male condoms
No side effects; can be put in prior to sexual experience	Needs practice to use correctly
Same as diaphragm	Same as diaphragm
No prescription necessary; some protection from STDs	Interruption of sexual experience, skin irritation for some
Very effective; no interruption of sexual activity; don't have to remember to use	Side effects; increased menstrual flow and cramps; may be expelled
Highly effective; permanent	Not easy to reverse for fertility
Easier procedure than tubal sterilization	Not easy to reverse for fertility
Acceptable to Catholic Church; no medical side effects	Uncertainty of "safe times"; periods of abstinence from intercourse or use of other methods
No medical side effects	Interruption of intercourse
Acceptable only if pregnancy desired	

consulted or participate, nor should they hesitate to discuss sharing the costs with their partners. It takes two people to conceive a baby, and two people should be involved in deciding *not* to conceive a baby. In the process, they can also enhance their skills in communication, critical thinking, and negotiating. (See Personal Voices: "What Students Say About Birth Control.")

Abstinence and "Outercourse"

The contraceptive methods discussed in this chapter are designed to prevent pregnancy as a consequence of vaginal intercourse. Couples who choose abstinence make a very different decision—to abstain from vaginal intercourse and other forms of sexual activity (any in

Self-Survey

Which Contraceptive Method Is Best for You?

Answer Yes or No to each statement as it applies to you and, if appropriate, your partner.

1. You have high blood pressure or cardiovascular disease. _____

2. You smoke cigarettes. _____

3. You have a new sexual partner. _____

4. An unwanted pregnancy would be devastating to you. _____

5. You have a good memory. _____

6. You or your partner have multiple sexual partners. _____

7. You prefer a method with little or no bother. _____

8. You have heavy, crampy periods. _____

9. You need protection against STDs. _____

10. You are concerned about endometrial and ovarian cancer. _____

11. You are forgetful. _____

12. You need a method right away. _____

13. You're comfortable touching your own and your partner's genitals. _____

14. You have a cooperative partner. _____

15. You like a little extra vaginal lubrication. _____

16. You have sex at unpredictable times and places. _____

17. You are in a monogamous relationship and have at least one child. _____

Scoring:

Recommendations are based on Yes answers to the following numbered statements:

The combination pill: 4, 5, 6, 8, 9, 16

The progestin-only pill: 1, 2, 5, 7, 16

Condoms: 1, 2, 3, 6, 9, 12, 13, 14

Norplant and Depo-Provera: 1, 2, 4, 7, 11, 16

Diaphragm or cervical cap: 1, 2, 13, 14

The IUD: 1, 2, 7, 11, 13, 16, 17

Spermicides: 1, 2, 12, 13, 14, 15

Making Changes ....
Choosing a Contraceptive

Your responses may indicate that there's more than one appropriate method of birth control for you. Remember that you may choose different types of birth control at different stages of your life, or switch contraceptives for various reasons. Here are some factors you and your partner should always consider and discuss:

- **Effectiveness.** Keep in mind that your own conscientiousness will play an important role. If you forget to take your daily pill, or if you decide not to use a condom "just this once," you'll increase the odds of pregnancy by interfering with effective birth control.

- **Suitability.** If you don't have sex very often, a contraceptive with many risks and side effects, such as the pill, may be wrong for you. If you have many sexual partners and are at risk of contracting a sexually transmitted disease, a condom may provide protection against pregnancy and infection, especially if used with a diaphragm or cervical cap.

- **Side effects.** Some complications related to contraceptives are serious health threats. Be sure to ask questions and gather as much information as possible about what side effects to expect.

- **Safety.** The risks of certain contraceptives, such as the pill, may be too great to allow their use, if, for example, you have high blood pressure. Be honest in describing your medical history to your physician.

- **Future fertility.** Some women don't return to regular menstrual cycles for six months to a year after discontinuing oral contraceptives. This possibility may or may not be important to you now, but you should try to look ahead.

- **Cost.** The only free contraceptive methods are abstinence and rhythm methods. If you're on a tight budget, you might consider the relative costs of a year's prescription of oral contraceptives compared to a year's supply of condoms or spermicidal foam or jelly. However, you should also think about the long-term costs and consequences.

- **Reduced risk of sexually transmitted diseases.** Some forms of contraception, in particular barrier contraceptives and spermicides, help reduce the risk of transmission of some STDs. However, none provides complete protection.

SOURCE: Hales, 1994.

which ejaculation occurs near the vaginal opening) that could result in conception. Abstinence is the only form of birth control that is 100% effective and risk-free. It is also an important, increasingly valued lifestyle choice. A growing number of individuals, including some who have been sexually active in the past, are choosing abstinence until they establish a relationship with a long-term partner.

Individuals who choose abstinence from vaginal intercourse often engage in activities sometimes called "outercourse," such as kissing, hugging, sensual touching, and mutual masturbation. Outercourse can prevent pregnancy, but couples must be careful to avoid any penis-vagina contact. If the man ejaculates near the vaginal opening, sperm can swim up into the vagina and fallopian tubes to fertilize an egg. Except for oral-genital and anal sex, outercourse also may lower the risk of contracting sexually transmitted diseases. Some couples routinely restrict themselves to outercourse; others

choose such sexual activities temporarily when it is inadvisable for them to have vaginal intercourse—for example, after childbirth.

Hormone-Based Contraceptives

These reversible forms of birth control for women use forms of estrogen and progesterone to inhibit ovulation, alter the mucus lining of the cervix so that it blocks the passage of sperm, or prevent successful implantation of the fertilized egg in the uterus.

The Birth Control Pill

"The pill"—the popular term for **oral contraceptives**—is the method of birth control preferred by unmarried women and by those under age 30, including college students. Women 18 to 24 years old are most likely to

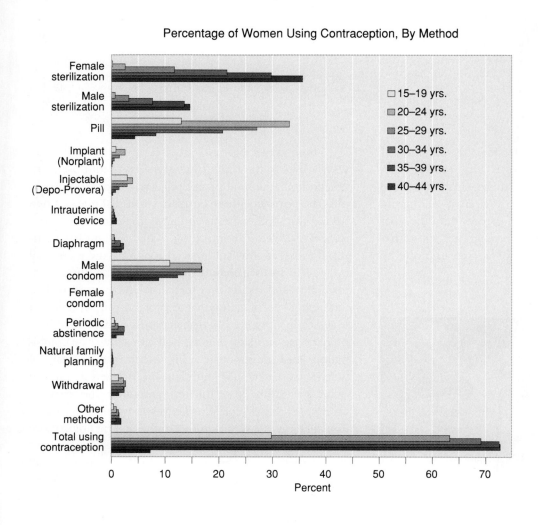

Figure 10-3

Percentage of women using contraception, by method.

SOURCE: Abma, J. C., et al. Fertility Planning and Women's Health, new data from the 1995 National Survey of Family Growth. National Center For Health Statistics. *Vital Health Statistics*, Vol. 23, No. 19, 1997.

Personal Voices   What Students Say About Birth Control

A Couple's Dialogue on the Condom:

He: "I love you. Would I give you an infection?"

She: "Not intentionally. But many people don't know they're infected. That's why condoms are best for both of us."

He: "Just this once?"

She: "Once is all it takes."

He: "But using condoms is like wearing a raincoat in a shower."

She: "We can work together to make it romantic and pleasurable. Besides, you won't feel anything if you don't use a condom."

"The first time I used a rubber, I relaxed inside her after I came, holding her for a while. Then I withdrew, leaving the rubber behind. My first thought was, 'Oh no, it's dissolved!' I reached inside her vagina and found the rubber. We used some foam right away, but were nervous until her next period."

"I really like the pill I'm taking. My periods are light, and the bad cramps I used to have are gone. I hadn't been using anything before taking the pill. It's a tremendous relief to make love and not be afraid of getting pregnant."

A pregnant university student insisted that she had never had intercourse without her diaphragm in place, and she had always used jelly. Discussion of how she maintained her diaphragm before use revealed that after each use and after washing her diaphragm carefully, she would tack it to the back of the headboard of her bed with a thumbtack.

"Since I've been using the diaphragm, I've moved more slowly into sexual relations. I want to discuss my method with a new partner before we have intercourse. When I'm feeling like I'm not comfortable enough to talk about birth control, I'm not ready to have intercourse."

"My husband heard of the possible problems women had taking pills. So

after two years, he said I had accepted the responsibility of contraception for a long while, and now it was his turn."

"At the age of 17, I unexpectedly got pregnant. I was devastated because I had planned to go to college, and I had so many things I wanted to do before settling down to have a family. My partner gave me so much support and encouragement, thus I was able to go through with an abortion. Now I am on the pill, and I am still going out with the same guy. Unfortunately, I learned my lesson the hard way, but it worked out fine. I am seriously taking precautions now and using contraception so I don't get pregnant."

"Five good reasons to use a condom: AIDS, herpes, gonorrhea, chlamydia, and 'Honey, I'm pregnant.'"

SOURCES: Hatcher, Robert, et al. *Sexual Etiquette 101.* Atlanta, GA: Emory University School of Medicine (no year cited); "Authors' Files," Crooks, Robert, and Karla Baur. *Our Sexuality,* 7th ed. Pacific Grove, CA: Brooks/Cole, 1999.

---

choose oral contraceptives. In use for 30 years, the pill is one of the most researched, tested, and carefully followed medications in medical history—and one of the most controversial. Although many women incorrectly think that the risks of the pill are greater than those of pregnancy and childbirth, long-term studies show that oral contraceptive use does not increase mortality rates.[10]

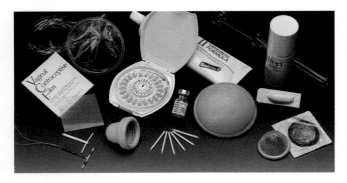

There is a wide variety of contraceptives available to couples.

Three types of oral contraceptives are currently widely used in the United States: the constant-dose combination pill, the multiphasic pill, and the progestin-only pill. The **constant-dose combination pill** releases two hormones, synthetic estrogen and progestin, which play important roles in controlling ovulation and the menstrual cycle, at constant levels throughout the menstrual cycle. The **multiphasic pill** mimics normal hormonal fluctuations of the natural menstrual cycle by providing different levels of estrogen and progesterone at different times of the month. Multiphasic pills reduce total hormonal dose and side effects. Both constant-dose combination and multiphasic pills block the release of hormones that would stimulate the process leading to ovulation. They also thicken and alter the cervical mucus, making it more hostile to sperm, and they make implantation of a fertilized egg in the uterine lining more difficult.

The **progestin-only**, or **minipill**, contains a small amount of progestin and no estrogen. Unlike women who take constant-dose combination pills, those using minipills probably ovulate at least occasionally. The minipills make the mucus in the cervix so thick and tacky, however, that sperm can't enter the uterus. Minipills also may interfere with implantation by altering the uterine lining.

Advantages   Birth control pills have several advantages: They are reversible, so a woman may easily stop using them. They do not interrupt sexual activity. Women on the pill have more regular periods, less cramping, and fewer tubal, or ectopic, pregnancies (discussed later in this chapter). The pill reduces the likelihood of benign breast lumps, ovarian cysts, and cancer of the lining of the uterus (endometrial cancer). In addition, the pill is one of the most effective forms of contraception. In actual use, the failure rate is 1% to 5% for estrogen/progesterone pills and 3% to 10% for minipills.

Disadvantages   The pill does not protect against HIV infection and other sexually transmitted diseases, so condoms and spermicide should also be used. In addition, the hormones in oral contraceptives may cause various side-effects, including spotting between periods, weight gain or loss, nausea and vomiting, breast tenderness, and decreased sex drive. Some women using the pill report emotional changes, such as mood swings and depression. Oral contraceptives can interact with other medications and diminish their effectiveness; women should inform any physician providing medical treatment that they are taking the pill.

Current birth control pills contain much lower levels of estrogen than early pills. As a result, the risk of heart disease and stroke among users is much lower than it once was; the danger may be lowest with the minipill. Yet there still is a risk of cardiovascular problems associated with use of the pill, primarily for women over 35 who smoke and those with other health problems, such as high blood pressure. Heart attacks strike an estimated 1 in 14,000 pill users between the ages of 30 and 39, and 1 in 1500 between the ages of 40 and 44. Strokes occur five times more frequently among women taking oral contraceptives, and clots in the veins develop in 1 out of every 500 previously healthy women.

Women generally worry more about the association of the newer pills with cancer than with cardiovascular disease. On the one hand, oral contraceptives may lower the risk of endometrial and ovarian cancer. On the other, some studies have found an increased risk of breast cancer, especially in women who take the pill when they're in their teens or early twenties.

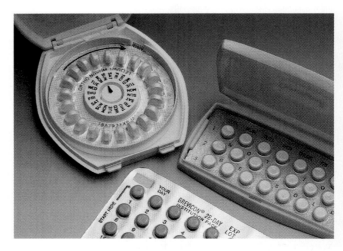

Oral Contraceptives. The birth control pill.

Strategies for Prevention

Before You Take the Pill

Before starting on the pill, you should undergo a thorough physical examination that includes the following tests:

✔   Routine blood pressure test.

✔   Pelvic exam, including a Pap smear.

✔   Breast exam.

✔   Blood test.

✔   Urine sample.

You should also let your doctor know about any personal or family incidence of high blood pressure or heart disease, diabetes, liver dysfunction, hepatitis, unusual menstrual history, severe depression, sickle-cell anemia, cancer of the breast, ovaries, or uterus, high cholesterol levels, or migraine headaches.

How to Use Oral Contraceptives   The pill usually comes in 28 day packets: 21 of the pills contain the hormones, and 7 are "blanks," included so that the woman can take a pill every day, even during her menstrual period. If a woman forgets to take one pill, she should take it as soon as she remembers. However, if she forgets during the first week of her cycle or misses more than one pill, she should rely on another form of birth control until her next menstrual period.

Even if you experience no discomfort or side effects while on the pill, see a physician at least once a year for an examination, which should include a blood pressure test and a pelvic and breast exam. Notify your doctor at once if you develop severe abdominal pain, chest pain, coughing, shortness of breath, pain or tenderness in the calf or thigh, severe headaches, dizziness, faintness, muscle weakness or numbness, speech disturbance, blurred vision, a sensation of flashing lights, a breast lump, severe depression, or yellowing of your skin. The acronym ACHES summarizes the most serious of these side effects. (See Table 10-2.)

Generally, when a woman stops taking the pill, her menstrual cycle resumes the next month, but it may be irregular for the next couple of months. However, 2% to 4% of pill users experience prolonged delays. Women who become pregnant during the first or second cycle after discontinuing use of the pill may be at greater risk of miscarriage; they also are more likely to conceive twins. Most physicians advise women who want to conceive to change to another method of contraception for three months after they stop taking the pill.

Contraceptive Implants (Norplant)

About 1% of women use hormonal implants, such as Norplant, which prevent pregnancy for up to five years (see Figure 10-4).[11] Six thin silicone rubber capsules release a low, continuous dose of a synthetic form of progestin called levonorgestrel. Other implants are currently being developed.

Norplant works primarily by suppressing ovulation, but it also thickens the cervical mucus (which inhibits sperm migration), inhibits the development and growth of the uterine lining, and limits secretion of progesterone during the second or luteal half of the menstrual cycle. The best candidates for Norplant are women who desire reversible long-term contraception, those who don't want to have to insert or ingest a contraceptive regularly, those who cannot take estrogen-containing oral contraceptives, those who would face high medical risks if they did become pregnant, and those who are undecided about sterilization. Adolescents using Norplant are considerably less likely than pill users to become pregnant unintentionally.[12] An estimated 1.8 million women have used Norplant worldwide.

Advantages   Norplant has proven to be ten times more effective than the pill in preventing pregnancy, with a pregnancy rate of only four or five pregnancies per 1000 users per year, compared with 20 to 50 pregnancies per 1000 users of oral contraceptives. Norplant is most effective in women who weigh less than 110 pounds and somewhat less effective in those weighing more than 154 pounds. However, even in heavier women, Norplant is more effective than oral contraceptives.

For sexually active adolescents and young adults, who often do not use birth control pills and other forms of contraception consistently, Norplant's primary advantage is its long duration of action and the fact that they do not need to remember to use it. In clinical studies, teenagers reported more side effects with Norplant than

TABLE 10-2 SYMPTOMS AND PROBLEMS ASSOCIATED WITH THE PILL

Symptoms of possible serious problems with the birth control pill, represented by their initials.

Initial	Symptom	Possible Problem
A	Abdominal pain (severe)	Gallbladder disease, liver tumor, or blood clot
C	Chest pain (severe) or shortness of breath	Blood clot in lungs or heart attack
H	Headaches (severe)	Stroke, high blood pressure, or migraine headache
E	Eye problems: blurred vision, flashing lights, or blindness	Stroke, high blood pressure, or temporary vascular problems at many possible sites
S	Severe leg pain (calf or thigh)	Blood clot in legs

Source: Adapted from Hatcher et al., 1994.

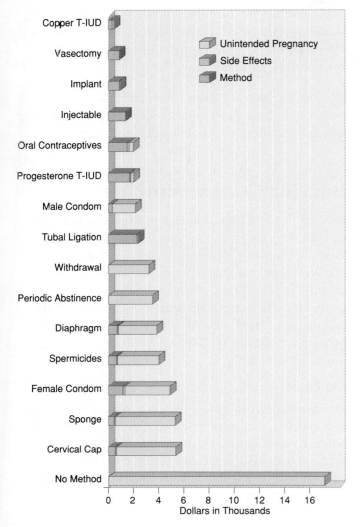

**Five-Year Costs of Family
Planning Methods**
(Managed Payment Model)

Legend:
- Unintended Pregnancy
- Side Effects
- Method

Methods (top to bottom): Copper T-IUD, Vasectomy, Implant, Injectable, Oral Contraceptives, Progesterone T-IUD, Male Condom, Tubal Ligation, Withdrawal, Periodic Abstinence, Diaphragm, Spermicides, Female Condom, Sponge, Cervical Cap, No Method

X-axis: 0 2 4 6 8 10 12 14 16
Dollars in Thousands

Source: Trussell, J., et al. "The Economic Value of Contraception: A Comparison of 15 Methods." *American Journal of Public Health*, Vol. 85, No. 4, 1995.

Figure 10-4

with oral contraceptives. Nevertheless, 93% of adolescents who had used Norplant for six months in one study expressed satisfaction.[13]

Disadvantages Common side effects of Norplant include menstrual irregularities, spotting, and amenorrhea; these are most likely to occur in the first year of use. Other possible complications include ovarian cysts, headaches, acne, weight changes, breast discharge, and hair growth. Because Norplant doesn't include estrogen

(as birth control pills do), there is no risk of clotting or high blood pressure. However, the FDA advises women with acute liver disease, unexplained vaginal bleeding, breast cancer, or blood clots in the lungs, legs, or eyes to avoid Norplant.

After Norplant became available in the United States in 1991, initial user satisfaction was high. However, satisfaction has declined, primarily because of side effects (cramps, headache, weight gain, and nausea are most common) and difficulties with removal of the implants. In one study, more than one in ten women had implants removed within one year because of side effects. Because of scarring and permanent nerve damage caused during implant removal, a class-action lawsuit was filed against Norplant's manufacturer. Physicians and nurse practitioners have subsequently developed removal techniques that they believe can lessen the risk of such complications.[14]

Controversy also arose over the suggestion that women on welfare or convicted of child abuse be ordered or given incentives to use Norplant. The American Medical Association's board of trustees has stated its opposition to the involuntary use of long-acting contraceptives because such a policy inhibits a person's fundamental rights to refuse medical treatment, not to receive cruel and unusual punishment, and to procreate.[15]

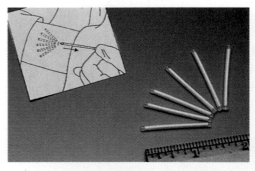

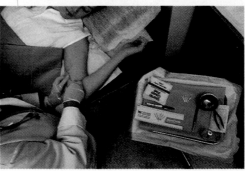

How Norplant works.

How to Use Norplant A qualified health-care professional, using a local anesthetic, implants the Norplant capsules with a needle under the skin of a woman's upper arms. The simple surgical procedure generally takes about five to ten minutes. Once in place, the capsules can be felt and may be visible, particularly in slender women. Removal of the capsules again requires minor surgery, lasting 15 to 20 minutes, with a local anesthetic. Complications can occur during removal; the most common are bruising, slight bleeding, and pain at the removal site. After removal, fertility generally returns with the next menstrual cycle. According to various studies, most former users of Norplant began ovulating again within seven weeks of implant removal, and most of those who wished to conceive did so within one year.

Depo-Provera

One injection of Depo-Provera, a synthetic version of the natural hormone progesterone, provides three months of contraceptive protection. This long-acting hormonal contraceptive, approved for use in the United States in 1992, raises levels of progesterone, thereby simulating pregnancy. The pituitary gland doesn't produce FSH and LH, which normally cause egg ripening and release. The endometrial lining of the uterus thins, preventing implantation of a fertilized egg.

Advantages Because Depo-Provera contains only progestin, it can be used by women who cannot take oral contraceptives containing estrogen (such as those who've had breast cancer). Its main advantage is that women do not need to take a daily pill or use a barrier method during sexual activity. It also may have some protective action against endometrial and ovarian cancer.

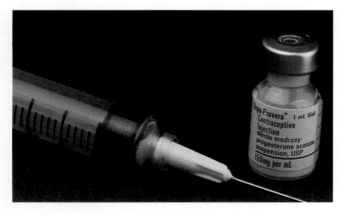

Depo-Provera, which is given by injection every 12 weeks.

Disadvantages Depo-Provera provides no protection against HIV and other STDs. It causes menstrual irregularities in most users; a delayed return of fertility; excessive endometrial bleeding; and other side effects, including decreased libido, depression, headaches, dizziness, weight gain, frequent urination, and allergic reactions in a small percentage of users.

How to Use Depo-Provera Women must receive an injection of Depo-Provera once every 12 weeks, ideally within five days of the beginning of menstruation.

Barrier Contraceptives

As their name implies, **barrier contraceptives** block the meeting of egg and sperm by means of a physical barrier (a condom, diaphragm, or a cervical cap), or a chemical one (vaginal spermicide in jellies, foams, creams, suppositories, or film). These forms of birth control have become increasingly popular because they can do more than prevent conception; they can also help reduce the risk of STDs.

Condoms

The male **condom** covers the erect penis and catches the ejaculate, thus preventing sperm from entering the woman's reproductive tract (see Figure 10-5). Most are made of thin surgical latex or sheep membrane; a new type is made of polyurethane, which is thinner, stronger, more heat-sensitive, and more comfortable than latex. Condoms with a spermicidal lubricant (nonoxynol-9) kill most sperm on contact and are thus more effective than other brands.

Although the theoretical effectiveness rate for condoms is 97%, the actual rate is only 80% to 85%. The condom can be torn during the manufacturing process or during its use; testing by the manufacturer may not be as strenuous as it could or should be. Careless removal can also decrease the effectiveness of condoms. However, the major reason that condoms have such a low actual effectiveness rate is that couples don't use them each and every time they have sex.

Condoms are second only to the pill in popularity among college-age adults.[16] Men purchase about half of the traditional male condoms sold in the United States, but condom use among never-married females tripled between 1982 and 1995, from 4 to 14%.[17] In one survey 88% of women said they are likely to insist on condom use with their next sex partner. Refusing to have sex unless a partner uses a condom is the most common approach followed by women to encourage condom use.[18]

Advantages Condoms made of latex or polyurethane, especially when used with spermicides containing nonoxynol-9, can help reduce the risk of certain STDs, including syphilis, gonorrhea, chlamydia, and herpes. They appear to lower a woman's risk of pelvic inflammatory disease (PID) and may protect against some parasites that cause urinary tract and genital infections. Public health officials view condoms as the best available defense against HIV infection.[19] They are available without a prescription or medical appointment, and their use does not cause harmful side effects. Some men appreciate the slight blunting of sensation they experi-

ence when using a condom because it helps prolong the duration of intercourse before ejaculation.

Disadvantages Condoms are not 100% effective in preventing pregnancy or STDs, including infection with HIV or HPV (human papilloma virus, discussed in Chapter 11). For anyone not in a monogamous relationship with a mutually exclusive, healthy partner—heterosexual or homosexual—condoms can reduce the risks of sexual involvement, but they cannot eliminate them. Condoms may have manufacturing defects, such as pin-size holes, or they may break or slip off during intercourse.[20] Some couples feel that putting on a condom interferes with sexual spontaneity; others incorporate it into their sex play. Some men dislike the reduced penile sensitivity or will not use them because they believe they interfere with sexual pleasure. Others cannot sustain an erection while putting on a condom. A small number are allergic to latex condoms.

How to Use a Condom Most physicians recommend prelubricated, spermicide-treated American-made latex or polyurethane condoms, not membrane condoms ("natural" or "sheepskin"). Before using a condom, check the expiration date, and make sure it's soft and pliable. If it's yellow or sticky, throw it out. Don't check for leaks by blowing up a condom before using it; you may weaken or tear it.

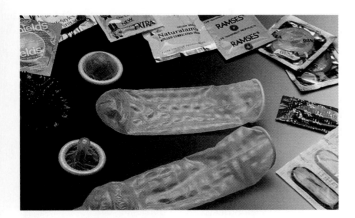

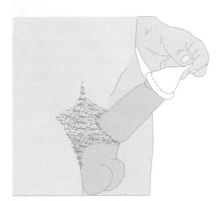

Pinch or twist the tip of the condom, leaving one-half inch at the tip to catch the semen.

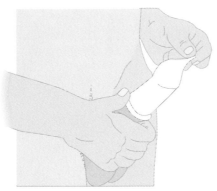

Holding the tip, unroll the condom.

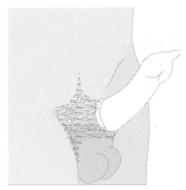

Unroll the condom until it reaches the pubic hairs.

Figure 10-5

The male condom. Condoms effectively reduce the risk of pregnancy as well as STDs. Using them consistently and correctly are important factors.

The condom should be put on at the beginning of sexual activity, before genital contact occurs (Figure 10-5). There should be a little space at the top of the condom to catch the semen. Wait until just before intercourse to apply spermicide. Any vaginal lubricant should be water-based. Petroleum based creams or jellies (such as Vaseline, baby oil, massage oil, vegetable oils, or oil-based hand lotions) can deteriorate the latex. After ejaculation, the condom should be held firmly against the penis so that it doesn't slip off or leak during withdrawal. Couples engaging in anal intercourse should use a water-based lubricant as well as a condom, but should never assume the condom will protect them from HIV infection or other STDS.

Strategies for Prevention

Insisting on Condoms

Increasingly, health advocates are urging women to say no to intercourse with any man who says no to condoms for several reasons, including the following:

✔ If sexual intercourse does lead to conception, the woman is the one who will have to face abortion or pregnancy.

✔ Women are at least three times more likely than men to contract a sexually transmitted disease, including HIV infection, from a single act of intercourse.

✔ Some STDs can cause extensive damage to a woman's reproductive system and lead to permanent infertility.

The Female Condom

The female condom, made of polyurethane, consists of two rings and a polyurethane sheath, and is inserted into the vagina with a tampon-like applicator (see Figure 10-6). Once in place, the device loosely lines the walls of the vagina. Internally, a thickened rubber ring keeps it anchored near the cervix. Externally, another rubber ring, two inches in diameter, rests on the labia and resists slippage. The female condom should be used with a spermicide and water-based lubricant.

Advantages The female condom gives women more control in reducing their risk of pregnancy and STDS. It does not require a prescription or medical appointment. One size fits all.

Disadvantages The failure rate for the female condom is higher than for other contraceptives. The statistical failure rate is 12.2%, which means that 12 of every 100 women using the device could expect to get pregnant

Figure 10-6

The female condom. This method is less effective than the male condom for preventing pregnancy and STDs (since no spermicide is used). Women may prefer the female condom as a way to control their risk of pregnancy and STDs. Like the male condom, this method does not require a prescription.

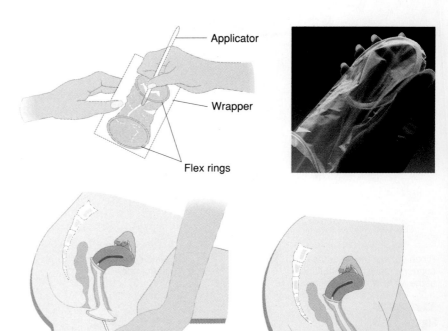

Applicator

Wrapper

Flex rings

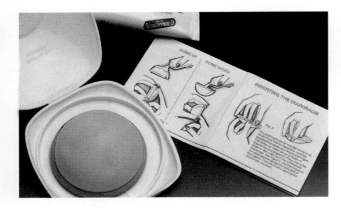

Figure 10-7

The diaphragm. When used correctly and consistently and with a spermicide, the diaphragm is effective in preventing pregnancy and STDs. It must be fitted by a health-care professional.

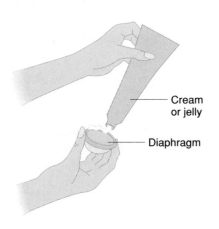

Cream or jelly

Diaphragm

Squeeze spermicide into dome of diaphragm and around the rim.

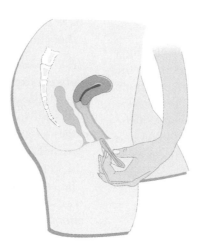

Squeeze rim together; insert jelly-side up.

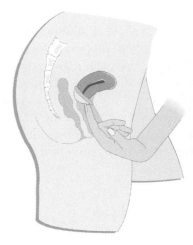

Check placement to make certain cervix is covered.

during a six-month period. In clinical trials, the actual failure rate was even higher—20.6%. Since it does not have spermicide on it, the female condom does not provide as much risk-reduction against STDs as male condoms with spermicide.

How to Use the Female Condom   As illustrated in Figure 10-6), a woman removes the condom and applicator and inserts the condom slowly by gently pushing the applicator toward the small of the back. When properly inserted, the outer ring should rest on the folds of skin around the vaginal opening, and the inner ring (the closed end) should fit against the cervix.

The Diaphragm

The **diaphragm** is a bowl-like rubber cup with a flexible rim that is inserted into the vagina to cover the cervix and prevent the passage of sperm into the uterus during sexual intercourse (see Figure 10-7). When used

with spermicide, the diaphragm is both a physical and a chemical barrier to sperm. The effectiveness of the diaphragm in preventing pregnancy depends on strong motivation (to use it faithfully) and a precise understanding of its use. If diaphragms with spermicide are used consistently and carefully, they can be 95% to 98% effective. Without a spermicide, the diaphragm is not effective.

Advantages   Diaphragms have become increasingly popular, most likely because of concern about the side effects of hormonal contraceptives. Many women feel that using a diaphragm makes them more knowledgeable and comfortable about their bodies.

Disadvantages   Some people find that the diaphragm is inconvenient and interferes with sexual spontaneity or that the spermicidal cream or jelly is messy, detracts from oral-genital sex, and may cause irritation. A poorly fitted diaphragm can cause discomfort during sex; some women report bladder discomfort, urethral irritation, or recurrent cystitis as a result of diaphragm use.

How to Use a Diaphragm Diaphragms are fitted and prescribed by a qualified health-care professional in sizes ranging from 2 to 4 inches (50–105 millimeters) in diameter. The diaphragm's main function is to serve as a container for a spermicidal (sperm-killing) foam or jelly, which is available at pharmacies without a prescription. Do not use oil-based lubricants because they will deteriorate the latex. A diaphragm should remain in the vagina for at least six hours after intercourse to assure that all sperm are killed. If intercourse occurs again during this period, additional spermicide cream or jelly must be inserted with an applicator tube.

The key to proper use of the diaphragm is having it available. A sexually active woman should keep it in the most accessible place—her purse, bedroom, bathroom. Before every use, a diaphragm should be checked for tiny leaks (hold up to the light or place water in the dome). A health-care provider should check its fit and condition every year when the woman has her annual Pap smear.

The Cervical Cap

Like the diaphragm, the **cervical cap**, combined with spermicide, serves as both a chemical and physical barrier blocking the path of the sperm to the uterus. The rubber or plastic cap is smaller and thicker than a diaphragm and resembles a large thimble that fits snugly around the cervix (see Figure 10-8). It is about as effective as a diaphragm.

Advantages Women who cannot use a diaphragm because of pelvic-structure problems or loss of vaginal muscle tone can often use the cap. Also, the cervical cap does not require additional applications of spermicide if intercourse occurs more than once within several hours.

Disadvantages Cervical caps are more difficult to insert and remove and may damage the cervix. Some women have difficulty getting a cervical cap that fits properly; others find it uncomfortable to wear.

How to Use a Cervical Cap Like the diaphragm, the cervical cap is fitted by a qualified health-care professional. For use, the woman fills it one-third to two-thirds full with spermicide and inserts it by holding its edges together and sliding it into the vagina. The cup is then pressed onto the cervix. (Most women find it easiest to do so while squatting or in an upright sitting position.) The cap can be inserted up to six hours prior to intercourse and should not be removed for at least six hours afterward. It can be left in place up to 24 hours. Pulling on one side of the rim breaks the suction and allows easy removal. Oil-based lubricants should not be used with the cap because they can deteriorate the latex.

Figure 10-8

The cervical cap. This method is very similar to the diaphragm and may work better for some women. It is smaller than the diaphragm and covers only the cervix.

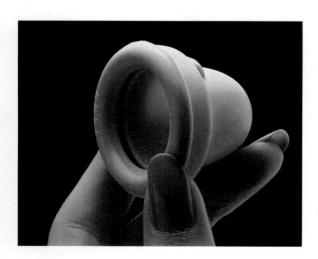

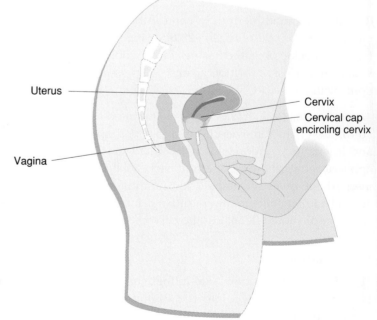

Uterus

Vagina

Cervix

Cervical cap encircling cervix

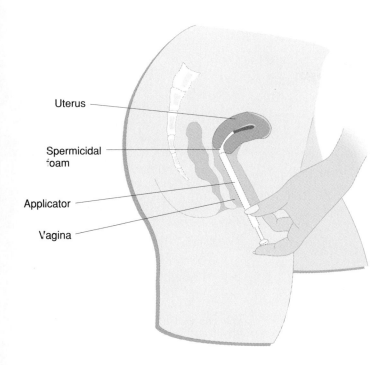

- Uterus
- Spermicidal foam
- Applicator
- Vagina

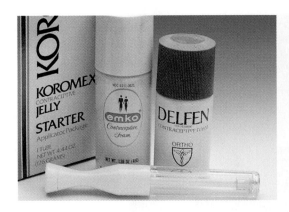

Figure 10-9

Vaginal spermicides. These various creams and jellies are available without a prescription and have minimal side effects. They are most effective in preventing pregnancy and STDs when used together with a condom.

Vaginal Spermicides

The various forms of **vaginal spermicides** include chemical foams, creams, jellies, vaginal suppositories, and gels (see Figure 10-9). Some creams and jellies are made for use with a diaphragm; others can be used alone. Several vaginal suppositories claim high effectiveness, but no American studies have confirmed these claims. In general, failure rates for vaginal suppositories are as high as 10% to 25%.

Advantages   Conscientious use of a spermicide together with another method of contraception, such as a condom, can provide safe and effective birth control and reduce the risk of some vaginal infections, pelvic inflammatory disease, and STDs. The side effects of vaginal spermicides are minimal.

Disadvantages   Even though spermicides can be applied in less than a minute, couples may feel that they interfere with sexual spontaneity. Some people are irritated by the chemicals in spermicides, but often a change of brand solves this problem. Others find foam spermicides messy or feel they interfere with oral-genital contact. Spermicidal suppositories that do not dissolve completely can feel gritty.

How to Use Vaginal Spermicides   The various types of spermicide come with instructions that should be followed carefully for maximum protection. Contraceptive

vaginal suppositories take about 20 minutes to dissolve and cover the vaginal walls. Foam, inserted with an applicator, goes into place much more rapidly. You must apply additional spermicide before each additional intercourse. After sex, women should shower rather than bathe to prevent the spermicide from being rinsed out of the vagina and should not douche for at least six hours.

Vaginal Contraceptive Film (VCF)

Available from pharmacies without a prescription, the 2-inch-by-2-inch thin film known as the **vaginal contraceptive film (VCF)** is laced with spermicide (Figure 10-10). Once folded and inserted into the vagina, it dissolves into a stay-in-place gel. Its theoretical effectiveness is similar to that of other forms of spermicide; paired with a condom, it is almost 100% effective.

Advantages   VCF film can be used by people allergic to foams and jellies. Unlike foams and jellies, it dissolves gradually and almost unnoticeably.

Disadvantages   Some people feel that insertion, even though it takes only seconds, interrupts sexual spontaneity.

How to Use VCF   A woman inserts the film by folding it and guiding it in with a finger so that it covers her cervix. VCF can be inserted from a minimum of 5 min-

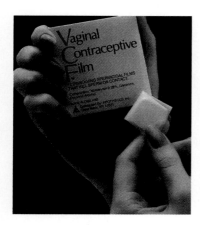

Figure 10-10

Vaginal contraceptive film (VCF). This thin film is laced with spermicide. Its effectiveness is similar to other vaginal spermicides, and it is most effective paired with a condom.

**How to Use
Vaginal Contraceptive Film**

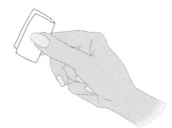

Remove the square of film from the convenient sealed envelope and fold it in half.

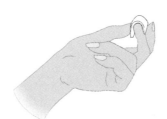

Make sure your fingers are dry, place on your second or third finger.

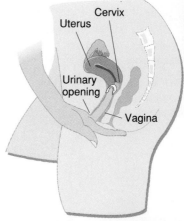

With one swift movement, place it high in your vagina against the cervix. VCF is effective for one hour. One film should be used for each act of intercourse. Follow the instructions in the product leaflet.

utes to a maximum of 90 minutes before intercourse. It is effective for up to two hours and need not be removed. A new VCF must be inserted if intercourse occurs again after two hours.

The Intrauterine Device

The **intrauterine device** (IUD) is a small piece of molded plastic, with a nylon string attached, that is inserted into the uterus through the cervix. It prevents pregnancy by interfering with implantation. Once widely used, IUDs became less popular after most brands were removed from the market because of serious complications such as pelvic infection and infertility. However, the currently available IUDs have not been shown to increase the risk of such problems for women in mutually monogamous relationships. (See Figure 10-11.)

According to manufacturers' estimates, about 2% of American women using contraception currently rely on IUDs. Throughout the world more than 25 million IUDs have been distributed in 70 countries.[21] Progestaser System is a T-shaped device containing progesterone, which prevents implantation; it must be replaced every year. The Copper T (Paragard) contains copper, which interferes with the growth of a fertilized egg by causing biochemical reactions with the uterine lining. The Copper T remains effective for ten years,

making it the longest-acting reversible contraceptive available to women in the United States. Its cumulative failure rate is 2.6.[22]

Advantages The IUD is highly effective and easy to reverse. According to recent analyses, the Copper T is the cheapest and most cost-effective form of birth control. Current models cause fewer complications than the pill. The IUD does not interrupt sexual activity, and 98% of IUD users in one survey said they are happy with this method.[23]

Disadvantages The most serious disadvantage is the possibility of increased risk of PID, which can lead to scarring and infertility. Many gynecologists recommend other forms of birth control for childless women who someday may want to start a family. In addition, women with many sexual partners, who are at highest risk of PID, are not good candidates for this method. During insertion of an IUD, women may experience discomfort, cramping, bleeding, or pain, which may continue for a few days or longer. The hormonal IUD causes less excess bleeding and cramping than the Copper-T. An estimated 2 to 20% of users expel an IUD within a year of insertion.

If a woman using an IUD does become pregnant, the IUD is removed to reduce the risk of miscarriage (which can be as high as 50%). Physicians generally

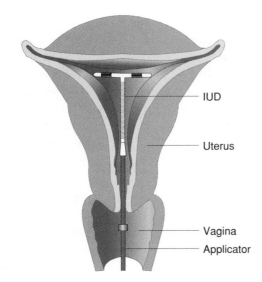

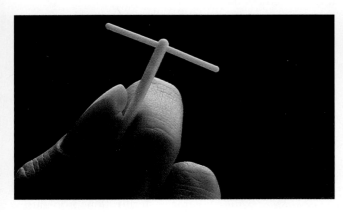

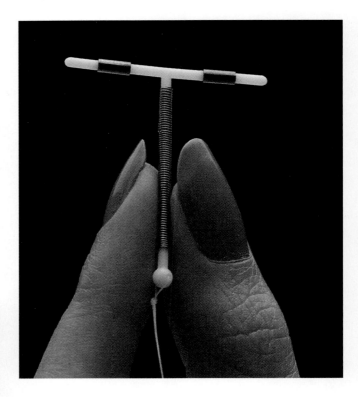

Figure 10-11

The IUD. The intrauterine device is effective and cost-efficient for preventing pregnancy, although some women may expel the device. The IUD does not offer protection against STDs, and there is increased risk of pelvic inflammatory disease (PID).

offer therapeutic abortion to the woman because of the serious risks (including infection, premature delivery, and possibly a higher rate of birth defects) of continuing the pregnancy.

How to Use an IUD A physician inserts an IUD during the woman's period, when the cervix is slightly softened and dilated. Antibiotics may be prescribed to lower any risk of infection. An IUD can be removed at any time during her cycle. A woman should check regularly, particularly after each menstrual period, for the nylon string attached to the IUD, because she may not otherwise notice if an IUD has been expelled.

Sterilization

The most popular method of birth control among married couples in the United States is **sterilization** (surgery to end a person's reproductive capability). Each

year an estimated 1 million men and women in the United States undergo sterilization procedures.

Advantages Sterilization has no effect on sex drive in either men or women. Many couples report that their sexual activity increases after sterilization, because they're free from the fear of pregnancy or the need to deal with contraceptives.

Disadvantages Sterilization should be considered permanent and should be used only if both individuals are sure they want no more children. Although sterilization doesn't usually create psychological or sexual problems, it can worsen existing problems, particularly marital ones. Couples should discuss sterilization, together and with a physician, to understand fully the possible physical and emotional consequences. Although a link between vasectomy and an increased risk of prostate cancer was reported, the most recent research—including a study of almost 74,000 men in Denmark—did not find a correlation.[24]

Male Sterilization   An estimated 13% of married couples rely on male sterilization.[25] In men, the cutting of the *vas deferens,* the tube that carries sperm from one of the testes into the urethra for ejaculation, is called **vasectomy**. During the 15- or 20-minute office procedure, done under a local anesthetic, the doctor makes small incisions in the scrotum, lifts up each vas deferens, cuts them, and ties off the ends to block the flow of sperm (see Figure 10-12). Sperm continue to form, but they are broken down and absorbed by the body.

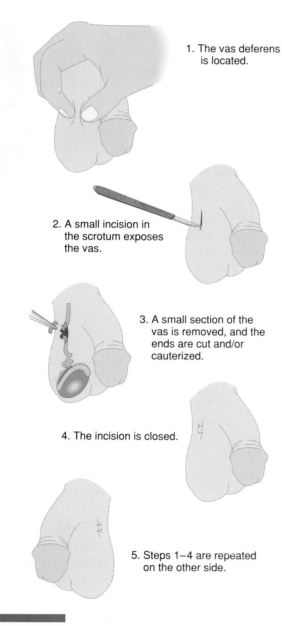

1. The vas deferens is located.

2. A small incision in the scrotum exposes the vas.

3. A small section of the vas is removed, and the ends are cut and/or cauterized.

4. The incision is closed.

5. Steps 1–4 are repeated on the other side.

Figure 10-12

Male sterilization, or vasectomy.

The man usually experiences some local pain, swelling, and discoloration for about a week after the procedure. More serious complications, including the formation of a blood clot in the scrotum (which usually disappears without treatment), infection, and an inflammatory reaction, occur in a small percentage of cases. The National Institute of Child Health and Human Development, in a 15-year followup study of nearly 5000 men, found that sterilization poses no increased danger of heart disease, even decades after the procedure. The pregnancy rate among the wives of men who've had vasectomies is about 15 in 10,000 women per year. Most result from a couple's failure to wait several weeks after the operation, until all sperm stored in each vas deferens have been ejaculated, before having unprotected coitus.

Sometimes men want to reverse their vasectomies, usually because they want to have children with a new spouse. Although anyone who chooses to have a vasectomy should consider it permanent, surgical reversal *(vasovasostomy)* is sometimes successful. New microsurgical techniques have led to annual pregnancy rates for the wives of men undergoing vasovasostomies of about 50%, depending on such factors as the doctor's expertise and the time elapsed since the vasectomy.

Female Sterilization   Female sterilization procedures modify the fallopian tubes, which each month normally carry an egg from the ovaries to the uterus. These operations may soon surpass the pill as the first contraceptive choice among women under, as well as over, age 30. The two terms used to describe female sterilization are **tubal ligation** (the cutting or tying of the fallopian tubes) and **tubal occlusion** (the blocking of the tubes). The tubes may be cut or sealed with thread, a clamp, or a clip, or by coagulation (burning) to prevent the passage of eggs from the ovaries (see Figure 10-13). They can also be blocked with bands of silicone.

The procedures used for sterilization are laparotomy, laparoscopy, and colpotomy. **Laparotomy** involves making an abdominal incision about 2 inches long and cutting the tubes. A laparotomy usually requires a hospital stay and up to several weeks of recovery. It leaves a scar and carries the same risks as all major surgical procedures: the side effects of anesthesia, potential infection, and internal scars. In a **minilaparotomy**, an incision about an inch long is made just above the pubic hairline. Most often the tubes are tied and cut. They can

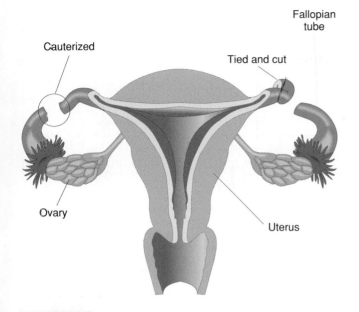

Fallopian
tube

Cauterized

Tied and cut

Ovary

Uterus

Figure 10-13
Female sterilization, or tubal ligation.

Methods Based on the Menstrual Cycle (Fertility Awareness Methods)

Awareness of a woman's cyclic fertility can help in both conception and contraception. The different methods of birth control based on a woman's menstrual cycle are sometimes referred to as natural family planning or fertility awareness methods. They include the cervical mucus method, the calendar method, and the basal-body-temperature method (all described below).

Advantages   Birth control methods based on the menstrual cycle involve no expense, no side effects, and no need for prescriptions or fittings. On the days when the couple can have intercourse, there is nothing to insert, swallow, or check. In addition, abstinence during fertile periods complies with the teachings of the Roman Catholic Church.

Disadvantages   During times of possible fertility (usually eight or nine days a month), couples must abstain from vaginal intercourse—which some may find difficult—or use some form of contraception. Conscientious planning and scheduling are essential. Women with irregular cycles may not be able to rely on the calendar method. Others may find the mucus or temperature methods difficult to use. For all these reasons, this approach to birth control is less reliable than many others. In theory, the overall effectiveness rate for the various fertility awareness methods is 80%. In practice, of every 100 women using one of these methods for a year, 24 become pregnant. However, using a combination of the basal-body-temperature method *and* the cervical mucus method may be 90% to 95% effective in preventing pregnancy (see Figure 10-14).

Cervical Mucus Method   This method, also called the **ovulation method**, is based on the observation of changes in the consistency of the mucus in the vagina. In the first days after menstruation, the vagina feels dry because of a decline in hormone production, indicating a safe period for unprotected intercourse. Within a few days, estrogen levels rise, and the mucus begins to thin out and becomes less cloudy: The fertile period begins. At peak estrogen levels, the mucus is smooth, stretchable, and slippery (like raw egg white), and very clear. Mucus with these characteristics is usually observed within 24 hours of ovulation and lasts one to two days, signaling maximum fertility. The mucus becomes sticky

also be sealed by electrical coagulation, which causes extensive damage to the tubes; there is also the risk of burns to nearby organs. The operation can be performed by a skilled physician in 10 to 30 minutes, usually under local anesthesia, and the woman can generally go home the same day. The failure (pregnancy) rate is only 1 in 1000.

Tubal ligation or occlusion can also be performed with the use of **laparoscopy**, commonly called "belly-button" or "band-aid" surgery. This procedure is done on an outpatient basis and takes 15 to 30 minutes. A lighted tube called a laparoscope is inserted through a half-inch incision made right below the navel, giving the doctor a view of the fallopian tubes. Using surgical instruments that may be inserted through the laparoscope or through other tiny incisions, the doctor then cuts or seals the tubes, most commonly by electrical coagulation. The possible complications are similar to those of minilaparotomy, as is the failure rate.

In a **colpotomy**, the fallopian tubes are reached through the vagina and cervix. This procedure leaves no external scar, but is somewhat more hazardous and less effective. A **hysterectomy** (removal of the uterus) is a major surgical procedure that is too dangerous to be used as a method of sterilization, unless there are other medically urgent reasons for removing the uterus.

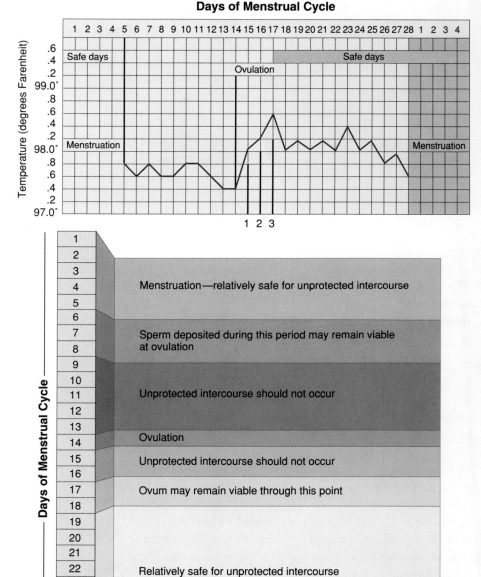

Figure 10-14

Fertility awareness methods. These methods are based on a woman's menstrual cycle and involve charting basal body temperature (top), careful calculation of the menstrual cycle (bottom), or careful observation of cervical mucus. Periods of abstinence are a necessary part of these methods.

and cloudy again three days thereafter, and the second safe period begins. Most women using this method have to refrain from unprotected intercourse for about 9 days of each 28-day menstrual cycle.

Calendar Method This approach, often called the **rhythm method**, involves counting the days after menstruation begins to calculate the estimated day of ovula-

tion. Ideally, a woman first keeps a chart of her monthly cycles for about a year so she knows the average length of her cycle. The first day of menstruation is day one. She counts the number of days until the last day of her cycle, which is the day before menstrual flow begins. To determine the starting point of the period during which she should avoid unprotected intercourse, she subtracts 18 from the number of days in her shortest cycle. For instance, if her shortest cycle was 28 days, day 10 would be her first high-risk day. To calculate when she can again have unprotected intercourse, she subtracts 10 from the number of days in her longest cycle. If her longest cycle is 31 days, she could resume intercourse on day 21. Other forms of sexual activity can continue from day 10 to day 21. This method requires careful timing to avoid the possible meeting of a ripe egg and active sperm in the woman's Fallopian tube.

Basal-Body-Temperature Method In this method the woman measures her **basal body temperature**, the body temperature upon waking in the morning, using a specially calibrated rectal thermometer, which is more precise than an oral one. She records her temperature on a chart (see Figure 10-14). The basal body temperature remains relatively constant from the beginning of the menstrual cycle to ovulation. After ovulation, however, basal body temperature rises by more than 0.5 degrees F. The woman knows that her safe period has begun when her temperature has been elevated for three consecutive days. After eight to ten months, she should have a sense of her ovulatory pattern, in addition to knowing her daily readings.

Emergency, or After-Intercourse, Contraception

In cases where unprotected intercourse has occurred, a condom has broken or slipped off, or another form of contraception has failed, there are options for preventing implantation of a fertilized egg and possible pregnancy. **After-intercourse methods** of birth control include higher doses of standard oral contraceptives; the so-called *morning-after pill*, which prevents implantation of a fertilized egg; insertion of an IUD; *menstrual extraction*, in which the uterine lining is suctioned out; and *dilation and curettage (D and C)*, in which the uterine contents are scraped out. Many individuals are not aware that options for post-intercourse contraception exist. Yet some methods have been used in rape crisis centers for more than 20 years and are available from physicians, family planning clinics, and more than 80% of college health centers.[26]

Some oral contraceptives, taken within 72 hours after intercourse, safely prevent pregnancy and bring on menstruation. Physicians often prescribe two standard pills (Ovral) or four low-dose pills (Lo/Ovral, Nordette, Levlen, Triphasil, or TriLevlen) to be taken as soon after intercourse as possible, followed 12 hours later by two more. Such *emergency contraceptive pills (or ECP)* are 70% to 80% effective—far less than other forms of contraception. Moreover, ECP does not work if taken more than 72 hours after intercourse.[27]

Morning-after pills do not prevent conception but rather interfere with the implantation of a fertilized egg. The pill currently used contains ethinyl estradiol or conjugated equine estrogens. It is not recommended except in cases of rape, incest, or complicated high-risk pregnancy factors. If menstruation doesn't follow use of the morning-after pill, a dilation and curettage (D and C) procedure or an aspiration (suctioning) is performed to remove the contents of the uterus. An alternative for women who cannot take hormonal agents because of medical reasons is insertion of an intrauterine device (IUD) within five to seven days following unprotected intercourse in the middle of the menstrual cycle to prevent implantation of a fertilized egg. This approach should never be used, however, if there is a high risk of exposure to a sexually transmitted disease.

Another option for emergency contraception is the copper IUD, which may be inserted up to seven days following unprotected intercourse and left in place to provide ongoing contraception. Its failure rate is less than 1%, which makes the copper IUD the most effective form of emergency contraception, and, if left in place, the most cost effective.[28]

Menstrual extraction—considered a form of abortion by some—involves removing the contents of the uterus by suction with a device that doesn't require cervical dilation or anesthesia. Some women perform this procedure at home if their menstrual periods are a few days late. However, because the risk of infection is high, such home treatment is not recommended.

Future Contraceptives

There has not been a new male method of birth control in almost 200 years, when the vulcanization of rubber made possible the mass production of condoms. However, researchers are actively searching for a safe, effective, reliable form of contraception for men. Among the possibilities: weekly injections or implants of *testosterone enanthate,* a synthetic version of the male sex hormone, to lower and eventually stop sperm production; vaccines that impair sperm production; and progestin-related drugs to reduce sperm counts.

A Brazilian pharmaceutical company is testing a contraceptive pill for men, called NoFertil, that destroys male sperm without affecting potency. Its primary ingredient is gossypol, a substance derived from the cotton plant that, in prior tests in China, had caused permanent infertility in 10 to 15% of the men who used it. Chinese scientists also are testing another plant, tripergium, which can produce a significant reduction in sperm density and motility.[29]

Some medical professionals worry about the effects any hormones might have on a man's higher vulnerability to heart disease. Others fear that men, who never face the prospect of pregnancy in their bodies, would not be willing to accept potential dangers or side effects. However, the high number of men opting for vasectomies indicates that men want to take on the responsibilities and risks associated with birth control.

Future birth control options for women may include implants, based on the same principle as Norplant, but that dissolve harmlessly in the body and do not require removal. Researchers are experimenting with different types of disposable diaphragms, a new cervical cap, and IUDs of varying shapes and hormonal compounds. They also are studying agents, such as the so-called abortion pill (discussed later in this chapter), that might be taken late in the menstrual cycle to prevent or interfere with implantation of a fertilized egg.

Abortion

The purposeful termination of a pregnancy—**elective abortion**—should not be considered a form of contraception, but an alternative to giving birth to an unplanned child. Abortion is too risky, too expensive, and too complex a procedure to be viewed as anything other than an emergency backup if contraception fails.

More than 1.5 million abortions are performed in the United States every year; about 25% of all pregnancies in the United States end in abortion.[30] Three of every 100 American women between the ages of 15 and 44 have chosen to terminate a pregnancy. About half of all abortions are performed because of failed contraception; the others occur in the 9% of sexually active women who don't use birth control. In this country, 90% of abortions are performed within 12 weeks of fertilization; only 2 of every 1000 are performed more than 20 weeks after fertilization.[31]

Thinking Through the Options

A woman faced with an unwanted pregnancy—often alone, unwed, and desperate—can find it extremely difficult to decide what to do. The political debate over the right to life almost always is secondary to practical and emotional matters, such as the quality of her relationship to the baby's father, their capacity to provide for the child, the impact on any children she already has, and other important life issues.

Giving up her child for adoption, discussed later in this chapter, is an option for women who do not feel abortion is right for them. Because the number of would-be adoptive parents greatly exceeds the number of available newborns, some women considering adoption may feel pressured by offers of money from couples eager to adopt. Others, particularly minority women, may feel cultural pressures to keep a child—regardless of their age, economic situation, or ability to care for an infant. Advocates of adoption reform are pressing for mandatory counseling for all pregnant women considering adoption (available now in agency-arranged, but not private, adoptions) and for extending the period of time during which a new mother can change her mind about giving her child up for adoption.

In deciding whether or not to have an abortion, women report asking themselves many questions, including the following[32] :

- How do I feel about the man with whom I conceived this baby? Do I love him? Does he love me? Is this man committed to staying with me?

- What sort of relationship, if any, have we had or might we have in the future?

- If I continue the pregnancy and give birth, could I love the baby?

- Who can help me gain perspective on this problem?

- Have I thought about adoption? Do I think I could surrender custody of my baby? Would it make a difference if the adoption process were open and I could know the adoptive parents?

- If I keep my child, can I care for him or her properly? How would the birth of another baby affect my other children?

- Do I have marketable skills, an education, an adequate income? Would I be able to go to school or keep my job if I have a child? Who would help me?

- Would this child be born with serious abnormalities? Would it suffer or thrive?

- How does each option fit with what I believe is morally correct? Could I handle each of the options emotionally?

Answering these questions honestly and objectively may help women as they think through the realities of their situation.

Medical Abortion

A hormonal compound called RU-486 (mifepristone), which is not yet available in the United States, can end a pregnancy if taken within nine weeks of a woman's last menstrual period. RU-486, which is 96% effective in inducing abortion, blocks progesterone, the hormone that prepares the uterine lining for pregnancy. Two days after taking this compound, a woman takes a prostaglandin to increase uterine contractions. The uterine lining is expelled along with the fertilized egg (see Figure 10-15). Women have compared the discomfort of this experience to severe menstrual cramps. Common side effects include excessive bleeding, nausea, fatigue, abdominal pain, and dizziness. About 1 woman in 100 requires a blood transfusion following her use of RU-486.

Scientists also are testing other chemicals that could induce early abortions. These include methotrexate (a drug in use as a treatment for cancer, rheumatoid arthritis, psoriasis, and ectopic pregnancies) and misoprostol (an ulcer treatment that causes uterine contractions). Reported side effects of these agents include mild diarrhea, nausea, vomiting, and severe cramping.

Other Abortion Methods

Medically, first-trimester abortion is less risky than childbirth. However, the likelihood of complications increases when abortions are performed in the second trimester (that is, the second three-month period) of pregnancy.

Suction curettage, usually done from seven to thirteen weeks after the last menstrual period, involves the gradual dilation (opening) of the cervix, often by inserting into the cervix one or more sticks of *laminaria* (a sterilized seaweed that absorbs moisture and expands, thus gradually stretching the cervix). Some women feel pressure or cramping with the laminaria in place. Occasionally, the laminaria itself starts to bring on a miscarriage.

At the time of abortion, the laminaria is removed, and dilators are used to enlarge the cervical opening further, if needed. The physician inserts a suction tip into the cervix, and the uterine contents are drawn out via a vacuum system (see Figure 10-16). A curette (a spoon-shaped surgical instrument used for scraping) is used to check for complete removal of the contents of the uterus. With suction curettage, the risks of complication are low. Major complications, such as perforation of the

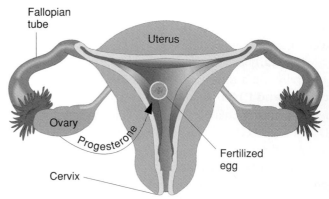

Progesterone, a hormone produced by the ovaries, is necessary for the implantation and development of a fertilized egg.

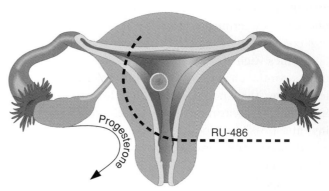

Taken early in pregnancy RU-486 blocks the action of progesterone and makes the body react as if it isn't pregnant.

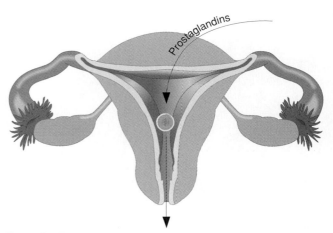

Prostaglandins, taken two days later, cause the uterus to contract and the cervix to soften and dilate. As a result, the fertilized egg is expelled in 97% of the cases.

Figure 10-15

How RU-486, known as the abortion pill, works.

uterus, occur in fewer than 1 in 100 cases. About 90% of the abortions performed in this country are done by this technique.

For early-second-trimester abortions, physicians generally use a technique called **dilation and evacuation (D and E)**, in which they open the cervix and use medical instruments to remove the fetus from the uterus. D and E procedures are performed under local or general anesthesia.

To induce abortion from week 16 to week 20, prostaglandins (natural substances found in most body tissues) are administered as vaginal suppositories or injected into the amniotic sac by inserting a needle through the abdominal wall. They induce uterine contractions, and the fetus and placenta are expelled within 24 hours. Other methods for second-trimester abortions include injecting saline or urea solutions into the amniotic sac; they terminate the pregnancy by fetus-triggering contractions that expel the fetus and placenta. Sometimes vaginal suppositories or drugs that help the uterus contract are used. Complications from abortion techniques that induce labor include nausea, vomiting, diarrhea, tearing of the cervix, excessive bleeding, and possible shock and death.

Hysterotomy involves surgically opening the uterus and removing the fetus. It is generally done from week 16 to week 24 of the pregnancy, primarily

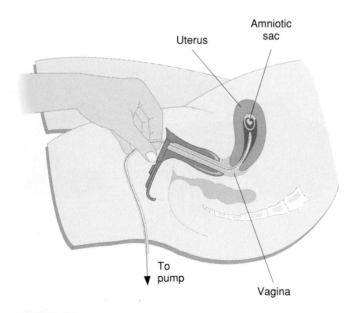

Uterus

Amniotic sac

To pump

Vagina

Figure 10-16

Suction curettage. The contents of the uterus are extracted through the cervix with a vacuum apparatus.

in emergency situations when the woman's life is in danger, or when other methods of abortion are considered too risky. However, late pregnancy abortions increase the risk of spontaneous abortion or premature labor in subsequent pregnancies and should be avoided if possible.

Psychological Responses After Abortion

The most common response of women who have just gotten an abortion is relief. While they may feel regret, sadness, or guilt following abortion, those with an unplanned pregnancy who obtain a legal abortion early in pregnancy typically report positive emotional effects. Moreover, emotional health and satisfaction typically continue to improve for one to two years following abortion. Researchers have found no evidence of so-called abortion trauma syndrome. The incidence of psychiatric illness and hospitalization is higher after childbirth than after abortion. Indeed, many women have reported that the decision to terminate a pregnancy was a "maturational point in their lives, one at which they experienced taking charge of their futures for the first time."[33]

Fewer than 10% of women who have abortions have long-term negative emotional reactions. The women most vulnerable to emotional stress after abortion are those terminating pregnancies that are wanted and personally meaningful, those who lack support from their partners or parents for the abortion, and those who aren't sure of their decision to have an abortion. The incidence of depression and other psychiatric problems is higher in women who have a second-trimester abortion for genetic or medical reasons. Often these women experience the same grief reactions that accompany a miscarriage. Counseling can help overcome feelings of guilt or decreased self-worth.[34]

The Politics of Abortion

Abortion is one of the most controversial political, religious, and ethical issues of our time. The issues of when life begins, a woman's right to choose, and an unborn child's right to survival are among the most divisive Americans have ever faced. Abortions were legal in the United States until the 1860s. For decades after that, women who decided to terminate unwanted pregnancies did so by attempting to abort themselves or by

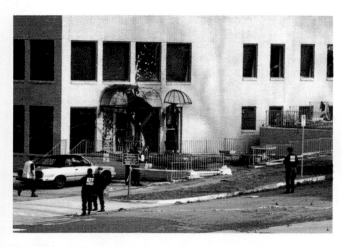

Opposition to legal abortions has often become violent. A security guard was killed and a nurse severely injured when a Birmingham, Alabama abortion clinic was bombed in January 1998.

obtaining illegal abortions—often performed by untrained individuals using unsanitary and unsafe procedures. In the late 1960s, some states began to change their laws to make abortions legal. In 1973, the U.S. Supreme Court, following a 1970 ruling on the case of *Roe v. Wade* by the New York Supreme Court, said that an abortion in the first trimester of pregnancy was a decision between a woman and her physician and was protected by privacy laws. The Court further ruled that abortion during the second trimester could be performed on the basis of health risks and that abortion during the final trimester could be performed only for the sake of the mother's health.

Since then, several laws have restricted the availability of legal abortions for low-income women. In 1989, the U.S. Supreme Court narrowed the interpretation of *Roe v. Wade* by upholding a law that sharply restricted publicly funded abortions and required doctors to test if a fetus could survive if they suspected a woman was more than 20 weeks pregnant. In 1992, in *Planned Parenthood v. Casey,* the Court upheld the right to legalized abortion but gave states the right to restrict abortion as long as they did not place an "undue burden" on a woman. This has limited the availability of abortion to young, rural, or low-income women.[35]

More than 25 years after *Roe v. Wade*, the debate over abortion continues to stir passionate emotion, with pro-life supporters arguing that life begins at conception and that abortion is therefore immoral, and pro-choice advocates countering that an individual woman should have the right to make decisions about her body

and health. The controversy over abortion has at times become violent: Physicians who performed abortions have been shot and killed; abortion clinics have been bombed, wounding and killing patients and staff members.

From 1990 to 1998, the number of abortions performed in the United States declined (see Figure 10-17), and the death rate from abortions has plummeted. More than half of all abortions (54%) are performed within the first eight weeks of pregnancy. Only about 1% of abortions occur after 20 weeks, but in the late 1990s Congress considered a ban on late abortions—or, as some labeled them, "partial birth abortions." In this procedure, the woman is sedated and her cervix dilated; the fetus is removed from her vagina. It is most often performed in cases when the fetus has life-threatening defects or if carrying the baby to term would seriously endanger the health of the mother.

Since *Roe v. Wade*, technology has had a major impact on abortion procedures as well as politics. Because of home pregnancy tests, women can detect pregnancy sooner. A new surgical procedure, called early manual vacuum aspiration, enables women to have an abortion as early as eight days after conception. And the new medicines available for abortion, described previously, also offer new options for early termination of a pregnancy. RU-486, the so-called French abortion pill, has gained a tentative approval for marketing in the United States. In nations where RU-486 is available, 60% of the women who choose abortion choose the pill, which must be used in the first seven weeks of pregnancy.

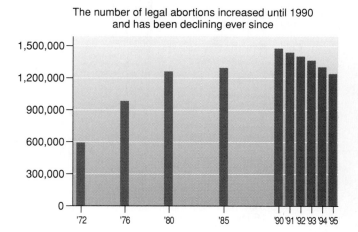

Figure 10-17

Although the majority of Americans continue to support abortion, many feel that it should be more restricted and difficult to obtain. While 61% of Americans say abortion should be permitted during the first three months of pregnancy, only 15% support second-trimester abortions and 7% feel that abortions in the last trimester should be legal.[36]

A Cross-Cultural Perspective

Throughout the world an estimated 10 to 20 million illegal abortions are performed each year. About 1 in 100 women dies as a result. Women who survive illegal abortions may suffer chronic health problems related to the lack of adequate medical care.

In other countries, abortion laws vary greatly. (See Figure 10-18). In Eastern Europe, where abortions were once legal and common, the collapse of communism has led to new restrictions on abortion. By contrast, Spain's supreme court has relaxed legal restrictions on abortions performed on social grounds. In Pakistan, new, more liberal rules on abortion state that abortion is no longer a crime if carried out to provide "necessary treatment." In Latin America, where anti-abortion laws are very strict, Cuba is the only country in which abortion on request is legal in early pregnancy. In other nations of Central and South America, women obtaining abortions and those performing them face criminal penalties, including imprisonment.

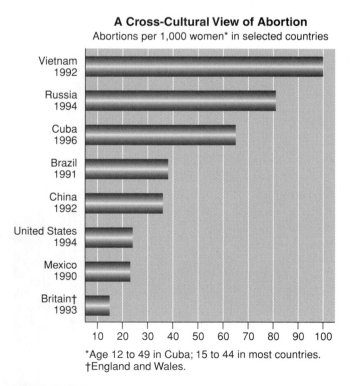

A Cross-Cultural View of Abortion
Abortions per 1,000 women* in selected countries

*Age 12 to 49 in Cuba; 15 to 44 in most countries.
†England and Wales.

Figure 10-18

SOURCE: Alan Guttmacher Institute

Pregnancy

After an upswing in the 1980s, the U.S. birth rate has declined, a trend that the Census Bureau expects to continue throughout the 1990s. The average age of mothers has risen, but about 70% of babies are still born to women in their twenties. Mothers are now averaging slightly fewer than two children each. Not every married couple is opting for parenthood. One-third of all married couples say that they plan *not* to have children; a generation ago, only one-fifth of all married couples were childless—and often not by choice. Childless couples are at least as likely—if not more likely—to be content with their marriages as couples with children.

Of course, you don't have to be part of a couple to want or to conceive a child. The number of never-married college-educated and career women who are becoming single parents has risen dramatically. They want children—with or without an ongoing relationship with a man—and may feel that, because of their age, they can't delay getting pregnant any longer.

Preconception Care: A Preventive Approach

The time *before* a child is conceived can be crucial in assuring that an infant is born healthy, full-size, and full-term. Women who smoke, drink alcohol, take drugs, eat poorly, are too thin or too heavy, suffer from unrecognized infections or illnesses, or are exposed to toxins at work or home may start pregnancy with one or more strikes against them and their unborn babies. The best chance for lowering the infant mortality rate and preventing birth defects is before pregnancy. **Preconception care**—the enhancement of a woman's health and well-being prior to conception in order to ensure a healthy pregnancy and baby— includes risk assessment (including evaluation of medical, genetic, and lifestyle risks), health promotion (such as teaching good nutrition guidelines), and interventions to reduce risk (such as treatment of infections and other diseases or assistance in quitting smoking or drug use.

Strategies for Prevention

Do You Need Preconception Counseling?

To determine whether you might benefit from preconception counseling, ask yourself the following questions:

✔ Do you have a major medical problem, such as diabetes, asthma, anemia, or high blood pressure?

✔ Do you know of any family members who have had a child with a birth defect or mental retardation?

✔ Have you had a child with a birth defect or mental retardation?

✔ Are you concerned about inherited diseases, such as Tay-Sachs disease, sickle-cell anemia, hemophilia, or thalassemia?

✔ Are you 35 years of age or older?

✔ Do you smoke, drink alcohol, or take illegal drugs?

✔ Do you take prescription or over-the-counter medications regularly?

✔ Do you use birth control pills?

✔ Do you have a cat?

✔ Are you a strict vegetarian?

✔ Are you dieting or fasting for any reason?

✔ Do you run long distances or exercise strenuously?

✔ Do you work with chemicals, toxic substances, radiation, or anesthesia?

✔ Do you suspect that you or your partner may have a sexually transmitted disease?

✔ Have you had German measles (rubella) or a German measles vaccination?

✔ Have you ever had a miscarriage, ectopic pregnancy, stillbirth, or complicated pregnancy?

✔ Have you recently traveled outside the United States?

If your answer to any of these questions is yes, you definitely should seek counseling from an obstetrician, nurse-midwife, or family practitioner three to six months before you hope to conceive a child.

How a Woman's Body Changes During Pregnancy

The 40 weeks of pregnancy transform a woman's body. At the beginning of pregnancy, the woman's uterus becomes slightly larger, and the cervix, softer and bluish due to increased blood flow. Progesterone and estrogen trigger changes in the milk glands and ducts in the breasts, which increase in size and feel somewhat tender. The pressure of the growing uterus against the bladder causes a more frequent need to urinate. As the pregnancy progresses, the woman's skin stretches as her body shape changes, her center of gravity changes as her abdomen protrudes, and her internal organs shift as the baby grows (see Figure 10-19). Pregnancy is typically divided into three-month periods called trimesters.

How a Baby Grows

Silently and invisibly, over a nine-month period , a fertilized egg develops into a human being. When the zygote reaches the uterus, it's still smaller than the head of a pin. Once nestled into the spongy uterine lining, it becomes an **embryo**. The embryo takes on an elongated shape, rounded at one end. A sac called the **amnion** envelopes it (see Figure 10-20). As water and other small molecules cross the amniotic membrane, the embryo floats freely in the absorbed fluid, cushioned from shocks and bumps. At nine weeks the embryo is called a **fetus**.

A special organ, the **placenta**, forms. Attached to the embryo by the umbilical cord, it supplies the growing baby with fluid and nutrients from the maternal bloodstream and carries waste back to the mother's body for disposal (see Figure 10-21).

Emotional Aspects of Pregnancy

Almost all prospective parents worry about their ability to care for a helpless newborn. By talking openly about their feelings and fears, however, they can strengthen the bonds between them, so that they can work together as parents as well as partners. Psychological problems, such as depression, can occur during pregnancy. The availability of social support and other resources for coping with stress can make a great difference in the potential impact of emotional difficulties.[37]

The physiological changes of pregnancy can affect a woman's mood. In early pregnancy, she may feel weepy, irritable, or emotional. As the pregnancy continues, she may become calmer and more energetic. Men, too, feel a range of intense emotions about the prospect of having a child: pride, anxiety, hope, fears for their unseen child and for the woman they love. Although many men want to be as supportive as possible, they may think that they have to be strong and calm—and may therefore pull away from their wives. The more involved fathers become in preparing for birth, the closer they feel to their partners and babies afterward.

Figure 10-19

Physiological changes of pregnancy.

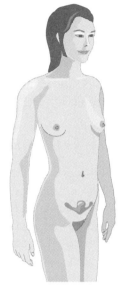

Before conception

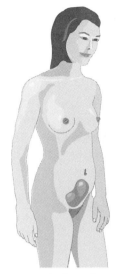

At 4 months

First Trimester

Increased urination because of hormonal changes and the pressure of the enlarging uterus on the bladder.

Enlarged breasts as milk glands develop.

Darkening of the nipples and the area around them.

Nausea or vomiting, particularly in the morning.

Fatigue.

Increased vaginal secretions.

Pinching of the sciatic nerve, which runs from the buttocks down through the back of the legs, as the pelvic bones widen and begin to separate.

Irregular bowel movements.

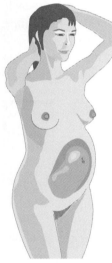

Second Trimester

Thickening of the waist as the uterus grows.

Weight gain.

Increase in total blood volume.

Slight increase in size and change in position of the heart.

Darkening of the pigment around the nipple and from the navel to the pubic region.

Darkening of the face.

Increased salivation and perspiration.

Secretion of colostrum from the breasts.

Indigestion, constipation, and hemorrhoids.

Varicose veins.

At 7 months

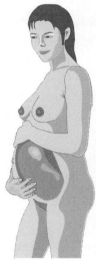

At 9 months

Third Trimester

Increased urination because of pressure from the uterus.

Tightening of the uterine muscles (called Braxton-Hicks contractions).

Shortness of breath because of increased pressure by the uterus on the lungs and diaphragm.

Heartburn and indigestion.

Trouble sleeping because of the baby's movements or the need to urinate.

Descending ("dropping") of the baby's head into the pelvis about two to four weeks before birth.

Navel pushed out.

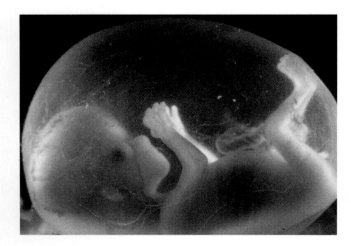

Figure 10-20

The amnion, or amniotic sac, surrounds and cushions the fetus.

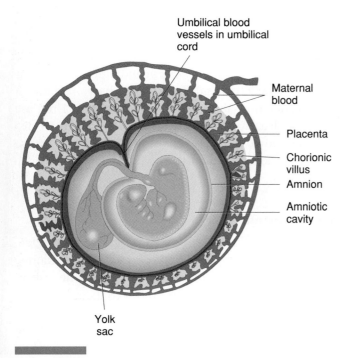

Figure 10-21

The placenta. The placenta supplies the growing embryo with fluid and nutrients from the maternal bloodstream and carries waste back for disposal.

Prenatal Care: Taking Care of Yourself and Your Baby

A pregnant woman has to take good care of herself to provide good care for her unborn child. This means regular medical and dental checkups. A woman should have her first prenatal visit as soon as she discovers that she's pregnant. A study group of the American College of Obstetricians and Gynecologists (ACOG) has recommended seven or eight prenatal visits for women with low-risk pregnancies; women at higher risk require more frequent checkups. Many teenage and unmarried pregnant women don't get adequate prenatal care, and some don't see a health-care professional until late in their pregnancy, because they can't afford or don't have access to medical services.

Age

The risk of a poor pregnancy outcome increases with age. Women 30 or older face a 40% greater risk of late fetal death, compared with women ages 20 to 24. Women over 35 also face an increased risk of very low birth weight, preterm delivery, and small-for-gestational-age (SGA) infants. Preconception and prenatal care, including good nutrition and careful monitoring, increase the chances of a healthy baby for older mothers.

Nutrition

A well-balanced diet throughout pregnancy is critical for a mother and her fetus both before and at birth. If a woman—regardless of her prepregnancy weight—gains too little weight, the risk to the growing fetus is high.[38] ACOG recommends a weight gain of 22 to 27 pounds during pregnancy. The National Academy of Sciences' Food and Nutrition Board advises a maximum weight gain of 35 pounds, based on findings that weight gain aids fetal growth and lowers the risk of infant mortality and mental retardation.

No vitamin supplement can replace a well-balanced diet, but a multivitamin can help reduce or avoid deficiencies. According to the CDC, women who take a simple daily multivitamin containing a B vitamin called folate (or folic acid) before conception can cut in half the risk that their children will suffer neural tube defects, which stem from faulty development of the spinal column. These conditions include spina bifida, a defect in which the bones of the spine, the vertebrae, are incompletely formed.

Activity and Rest

Almost all pregnant women can benefit from exercise throughout pregnancy—as long as they don't push too hard or too far. Regular exercise (three times a week) is better, safer, and more effective than occasional workouts. While women who were athletic prior to pregnancy generally can continue their physical activity, they should be aware of warning signs that could indicate a

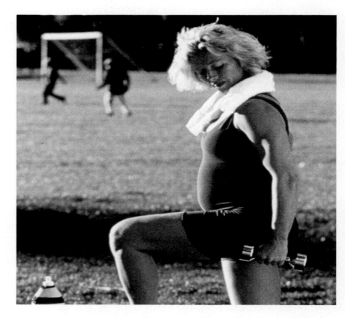

How much exercise? Most pregnant women benefit from regular, moderate exercise. For women who were very active before their pregnancies, a higher level of activity is probably fine.

potential problem, such as faintness, dizziness, pain, or vaginal bleeding.[39]

Rest is as important as exercise; the pregnant woman who's not used to taking naps may have to make time in her schedule for rest periods. If insomnia or the frequent need to urinate during the night becomes a problem, she may have to rely on catnaps during the day. She should *not* take sleeping pills.

Substance Use

Smoking endangers two lives: the mother's and the fetus's. The sooner a mother-to-be stops smoking, the better the chances that the fetus will develop normally. Smoking increases the risk of miscarriage, stillbirth, low birth weight, heart defects, and premature birth, and also impairs growth.[40] The fetus's oxygen supply is impaired by the increased levels of carbon monoxide in the smoking mother's bloodstream. Passive smoking (inhaling other people's smoke) can be hazardous for the mother and fetus as well.[41] (See Chapter 16.) Mothers who quit smoking in the first trimester have fewer preterm deliveries and low-birth-weight infants than those who continue smoking.[42]

Approximately 16% of pregnant women report drinking in the previous month.[43] According to the CDC, more than 8000 alcohol-damaged babies are born every year. One out of every 750 newborns has a cluster of physical and mental defects called **fetal alcohol syndrome (FAS)**: low birth weight, smaller-than-normal head circumference, smaller and shorter size, irritability as newborns, and permanent mental impairment as a result of their mothers' alcohol consumption. The milder forms of these problems, particularly impaired intellectual ability and school performance, are called fetal alcohol effects (FAE). (See Chapter 15.)

The risk of fetal alcohol syndrome is greatest if a mother drinks 3 ounces or more of pure alcohol (the equivalent of six or seven cocktails) a day. However, moderate drinking—one or two cocktails daily—may also have an effect. Even one drink a day has been associated with birth defects; binge drinking (five or more drinks on one occasion) is most toxic. The National Institute on Alcohol Abuse and Alcoholism and the Surgeon General advise pregnant women—and those trying to become pregnant—to abstain from drinking alcohol.

Moderate to heavy caffeine users are at greater risk of miscarriage than women who use little or no caffeine. Even more than one cup of coffee a day is linked with low birth weight. The FDA's advice is for pregnant women to "avoid caffeine containing products or use them sparingly."

At least one out of every ten newborns is exposed to illegal drugs before birth. The consequences of drug use during pregnancy include severe damage to the child's brain and nervous system and birth defects. Marijuana smokers have smaller, sicker babies and a higher risk of stillbirths, according to some research. Drug use also may lead to "neurochemical" birth defects by disrupting normal development of the brain. Cocaine use increases the risk of premature birth, stillbirths, and malformations.

Environmental Risks

According to a study of over 23,000 pregnant women, exposure to heat from a hot tub, sauna, or fever during the first trimester of pregnancy increases the risk of neural tube defects. Hot tubs presented the greatest single danger, while exposure to heat from multiple sources led to even greater risk. Electric blankets were not associated with increased risk.[44]

High levels of radiation of the type used for cancer therapy have been associated with birth defects. Diagnostic X rays should be avoided during pregnancy if possible, but they're not a significant threat, particularly after the first trimester. At least in theory, the rapidly developing fetus is especially vulnerable to pollutants, toxic wastes, heavy metals, pesticides, gases, and other hazardous compounds in the environment.

Strategies for Prevention

A Mother-to-Be's Guide to a Healthy Pregnancy

✔ ACOG recommends consuming about 300 more calories a day than before pregnancy and concentrating on eating the right foods, not on watching your weight. *Never* diet during pregnancy. Don't restrict salt intake either, unless specifically directed to by your doctor.

✔ Drink six to eight glasses of liquids each day, including water, fruit and vegetable juices, and milk.

✔ Don't exercise strenuously for more than 15 minutes, ACOG advises. Avoid vigorous exercise in hot, humid weather. Never let your body temperature rise above 100°F or your heart rate climb above 140 beats per minute.

✔ Stretch and flex carefully because the joints and connective tissue soften and loosen during pregnancy. After the fourth month of pregnancy, don't do any exer cises while lying on your back, as this could impair blood flow to the placenta.

✔ Walk, swim, and jog in moderation; and play tennis only if you played before pregnancy. Ski only if you're experienced, and stick to low altitudes and safe slopes. Do not water-ski, surf, or ride a horse.

Prenatal Testing

All parents worry that their unborn baby might not be normal and healthy. Sophisticated new tests can answer some, but not all, of their questions and can identify more than 250 diseases and defects. Prenatal tests are being performed earlier and with less risk to a fetus than ever before. The most common prenatal tests include the following:

- *Ultrasonography* uses high-frequency sound waves to produce an image of the fetus on a video screen and as a photographic picture. Ultrasound can check fetal age and spot certain birth defects.

- *Alpha-fetoprotein (AFP) screening,* performed from the 13th to 20th week of pregnancy, measures a substance produced by the baby's kidneys in the mother's blood. Levels that are too high could indicate a neural tube defect; levels that are too low may signal Down syndrome.

- *Amniocentesis,* performed from the 14th to 16th week of pregnancy, consists of removing a small amount of the amniotic fluid surrounding the fetus. This fluid contains cells shed by the fetus, which can be grown in tissue culture and then checked for any chromosomal or genetic defects (see Figure 10-22a).

- *Chorionic villi sampling (CVS),* performed from the eighth to tenth week of pregnancy, involves suctioning a small sample of the chorionic villi, the tissue surrounding the fetus, for laboratory analysis (see Figure 10-20b). Results are generally available within a week.

There are no known risks for ultrasonography and AFP screening. For both amniocentesis and CVS, there is about a 1% risk of miscarriage. Some testing centers have reported a higher incidence of both limb defects and miscarriage following CVS than others using this technique. Before choosing a facility for testing, pregnant women should inquire about that facility's experience and complication rate. Prenatal tests are usually recommended only if the mother is over age 35, has had a child with a genetic disorder, or is a known carrier of a detectable genetic disorder.

Complications of Pregnancy

In about 10% to 15% of all pregnancies, there is increased risk of some problem, such as a baby's failure to grow normally. **Perinatology**, or maternal-fetal medicine, focuses on the special needs of high-risk mothers and their unborn babies. Perinatal centers, with state-of-the-art equipment and 24-hour staffs of specialists in this field, have been set up around the country. Several of the most frequent potential complications of pregnancy are discussed below.

Ectopic Pregnancy

Any woman who is of childbearing age, has had intercourse, and feels abdominal pain with no reasonable cause may have an **ectopic pregnancy**. In this type of pregnancy, the fertilized egg remains in the fallopian tube instead of traveling to the uterus. Ectopic, or tubal, pregnancies have increased dramatically in recent years, now accounting for 2% of all reported pregnancies. STDs, particularly chlamydia infections (discussed in Chapter 11), have become a major cause of ectopic pregnancy.[45] Other risk factors include previous pelvic surgery, particularly involving the fallopian tubes; pelvic inflammatory disease; infertility; and use of an IUD.

In an ectopic pregnancy, a misplaced egg develops normally, producing the usual signs of pregnancy, until the cramped amniotic sac bursts, damaging the fallopian tube. The woman will bleed internally and feel lower abdominal pains; or she may feel an aching in her shoulders, as the blood flows upward toward the diaphragm. If the bleeding is substantial, the woman can go into shock, with low blood pressure and a high pulse rate. Symptoms are hot and cold flashes, nausea, dizziness, fainting, pelvic pain, and irregular bleeding.

Treatment for the damaged fallopian tube is usually removal, but microsurgery can often repair the damage. About 50% of the women who have had an ectopic pregnancy conceive again; 10% have another ectopic pregnancy. Ectopic pregnancies can lead to permanent infertility.

Miscarriage

About 10% to 20% of pregnancies end in **miscarriage**, or spontaneous abortion, before the 20th week of gestation. Major genetic disorders may be responsible for 33% to 50% of pregnancy losses. About 0.5% to 1% of women suffer three or more miscarriages, possibly because of genetic, anatomic, hormonal, infectious, or autoimmune

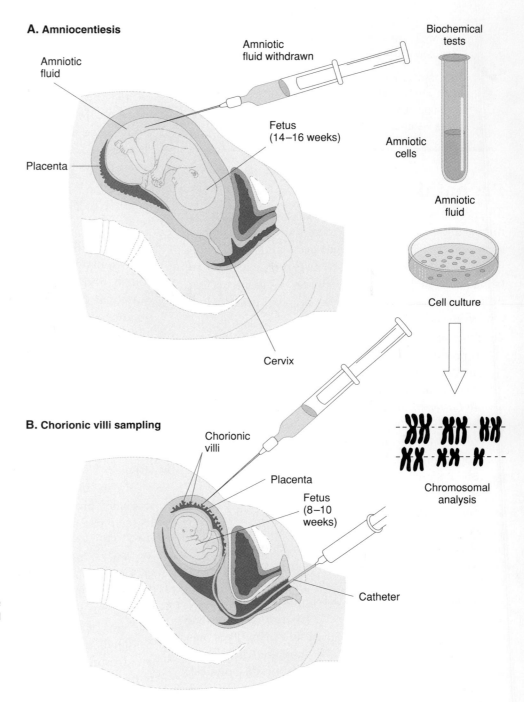

A. Amniocentesis

Amniotic fluid

Amniotic fluid withdrawn

Biochemical tests

Placenta

Fetus (14–16 weeks)

Amniotic cells

Amniotic fluid

Cell culture

Cervix

B. Chorionic villi sampling

Chorionic villi

Placenta

Fetus (8–10 weeks)

Chromosomal analysis

Catheter

Figure 10-22

Prenatal testing. (A) In amniocentesis, a sample of the amniotic fluid is withdrawn; fetal cells found in that fluid can then be grown in tissue culture and checked for chromosomal defects. (B) In chorionic villi sampling (CVS), a tissue sample of the villi is removed from the uterus and analyzed for chromosomal defects.

factors.[46] An estimated 70% to 90% of women who miscarry eventually become pregnant again.

Physicians typically recommend bed rest if a woman begins bleeding or cramping early in pregnancy. In some cases, the cramping stops, and the pregnancy continues normally. In others, the bleeding becomes intense, the cervix widens, and the embryo is expelled. If the miscarriage is complete, the bleeding stops; and the uterus returns to its normal state and shape. If it is incomplete, a physician has to remove any bits of tissue remaining in the uterus by performing a D and C.

Few medical events are more emotionally devastating than a pregnancy loss. Women often feel the loss in an extremely intense, almost physical way. Many who miscarry had not reached the point in pregnancy where the fetus seems separate from them. Typically, women feel both vulnerable and responsible, as if they did something to cause the loss or should have, could have, done something to prevent it. They try to identify what they did wrong: exercising or not exercising, working or not working; eating too much or not enough. Some women interpret a loss as a punishment for past sins, imagined or real. Such self-inflicted guilt, allowed to fester, can lead to major depression.[47]

Fathers, of course, also grieve but in different ways and at different times. At first, their greatest pain is their helplessness. They see their partners hurting so badly that they cannot find the words to console them. Not knowing what to do or say, some men pull away, burying themselves in work or drowning their sorrow in alcohol. Some strive to put the loss behind them and get on with their lives.[48]

Infections

The infectious disease most clearly linked to birth defects is **rubella** (German measles). All women should be vaccinated against this disease at least three months prior to conception, to protect themselves and any children they may bear. (See Chapter 11 for more on immunization.) The most common prenatal infection today is *cytomegalovirus*. This infection produces mild flulike symptoms in adults but can cause brain damage, retardation, liver disease, cerebral palsy, hearing problems, and other malformations in unborn babies.

STDs, such as syphilis, gonorrhea, and genital herpes, can be particularly dangerous during pregnancy if not recognized and treated. If a woman has a herpes outbreak around the date her baby is due, her physician will deliver the baby by caesarean section to prevent infecting the baby. HIV infection endangers both a pregnant woman and her unborn baby, and all pregnant women and new mothers should be aware of the HIV epidemic, the risks to them and their babies, and the availability of anonymous testing.

Premature Labor

Approximately 10% of all babies are born too soon (before the 37th week of pregnancy). According to a 1995 study, prematurity is the main underlying cause of stillbirth and infant deaths within the first few weeks after birth.[49] Bed rest, close monitoring, and, if necessary, medications for at-risk women can buy more time in the womb for their babies. But women must recognize the warning signs of **premature labor**—dull, low backache; a feeling of tightness or pressure on the low-

er abdomen; and intestinal cramps, sometimes with diarrhea—early enough. Low-birthweight premature babies face the highest risks, but comprehensive, enriched programs can reduce developmental and health problems.

Pregnancy and Age

Teen pregnancy and birth rates have dropped throughout the 1990s. Every year approximately 1 million American girls become pregnant. Most had not been using contraceptives consistently or correctly. Of those who carry to term, 90% keep their babies.

Most teen pregnancies (85 to 95%, compared with 55% for older women) are unplanned. And a sexually active teenager is actually less likely to get pregnant today than in the 1950s (when teen pregnancy rates reached an all-time high). Largely because of increased use of contraceptives, the odds of a sexually active girl getting pregnant have fallen to one in five, down from the one-in-four odds faced by teens in the 1970s. Throughout the 1990s, the pregnancy rate among American teenagers has also declined—yet it remains two to eight times higher than rates in other Western countries such as The Netherlands, Great Britain, and Scandinavia.[50]

In the past, most teenage mothers married the fathers of their unborn children. Today most do not. Many teenage girls who become pregnant have partners who are aged 20 or older. However, according to a government analysis, the role of older men may have been overestimated. Many of the teen mothers involved with men over age 20 are themselves aged 18 or 19. Nearly one-quarter of minors who have had a child with an older partner are married at the time of the infant's birth; only 21% of births to unmarried teens are fathered by substantially older men.[51]

Why do so many teens in the United States become pregnant? When surveyed, girls themselves cite various reasons, including lack of attention and love from their parents and lack of access to contraceptives. Many, as one girl poignantly put it, "are looking for someone to love them back."

As teen births have begun to decline, the number of women deciding to have children later in life has increased. One of every five women in the United States now has her first baby after age 35; first births among women older than 40 have increased 50% in the last 15 years.[52]

There are greater risks to the fetus when mothers are older than 35, primarily an increase in fetal birth defects due to chromosomal abnormalities, such as Down syndrome. At age 30, the estimated risk is 2.6 per thousand; the incidence rises to 5.6 per thousand at age 35; 15.8 at age 40; and 53.7 at age 45.[53] However, pregnancy itself for healthy women over age 35 is safe. As discussed later in this chapter, assisted reproductive technologies have enabled women in their forties, fifties, and even sixties to have successful pregnancies.

Childbirth

A generation ago, delivering a baby was something a doctor did in a hospital. Today parents can choose from an almost bewildering array of birthing options. The first decision parents-to-be face is choosing a birth attendant, who can be a physician or a nurse-midwife. Certified nurse-midwives in the United States deliver more than 90,000 babies a year, mostly in hospitals and birth centers. Their approach is based on the belief that the typical pregnant woman can deliver her baby naturally without technological intervention. Lay midwives have a similar orientation but less formal training; only a handful of states permit lay midwives to deliver babies.

When interviewing physicians or midwives, look for the following:

- Experience in handling various complications.
- Extensive prenatal care.
- A commitment to be at the mother's side for the entire labor in order to spot complications quickly and provide assistance.
- A compatible philosophy toward childbirth and medical interventions.

Where to Have Your Baby

A hospital with trained specialists and a nursery for newborns is recommended for high-risk women. However, if their pregnancies are normal and uncomplicated, mothers-to-be have alternatives almost unheard of a generation ago. A woman at low risk for complications may consider having her baby in an independent birth center, which offers a homelike setting. If a couple chooses to have their baby in a hospital, they may do so in a birthing room decorated to look like a comfortable bedroom. In many facilities, specially shaped birthing chairs are available, so a woman can stay in an upright position to push her baby into the world.

Only about 1% of American babies are born at home. ACOG opposes home births because of potential hazards to mother and child. But the safety of a home birth can be maximized if the pregnant woman has been carefully screened and a skilled doctor or nurse-midwife is attending.

Preparing for Childbirth

The most widespread method of childbirth preparation is **psychoprophylaxis**, or the **Lamaze method**. Fernand Lamaze, a French doctor, instructed women to respond to labor contractions with prelearned, controlled breathing techniques. As the intensity of each contraction increases, the laboring woman concentrates on increasing her breathing rate in a prescribed way. Her partner coaches her during each contraction and helps her cope with discomfort.

Women who have had childbirth preparation training tend to have fewer complications and require fewer medications. However, painkillers or anesthesia are always an option if labor is longer or more painful than expected. The lower body can be numbed with an **epidural block**, which involves injecting an anesthetic into the membrane around the spinal cord, or a **spinal block**, in which the injection goes directly into the spinal canal. General anesthesia is usually used only for emergency caesarean births.

Labor and Birth

There are three stages of **labor**. The first starts with *effacement* (thinning) and *dilation* (opening up) of the cervix. Effacement is measured in percentages, and dilation in centimeters (cm) or finger-widths. Around this time, the amniotic sac of fluids usually breaks, a sign that the woman should call her doctor or midwife.

The first contractions of the early, or *latent*, phase of labor are usually not uncomfortable; they last 15 to 30 seconds, occur every 15 to 30 minutes, and gradually increase in intensity and frequency. The most difficult contractions come after the cervix is dilated to about 8 cm, as the woman feels greater pressure from the fetus. The first stage ends when the cervix is completely dilated to a diameter of 10 cm (or five finger-widths) and the baby is ready to come down the birth canal (see Figure 10-23). For women having their first baby, this first stage of labor averages 12 to 13 hours. Women having another child often experience shorter first-stage labor.

When the cervix is completely dilated, the second stage of labor occurs, during which the baby moves into the vagina, or birth canal, and out of the mother's body. As this stage begins, women who have gone through

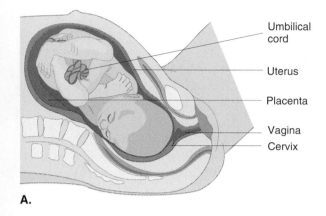

Umbilical cord

Uterus

Placenta

Vagina

Cervix

A.

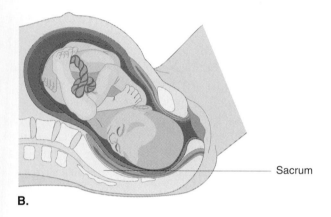

Sacrum

B.

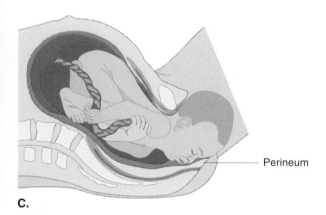

Perineum

C.

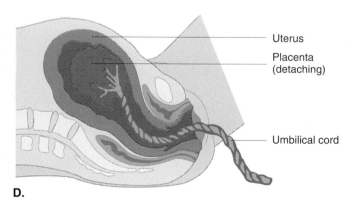

Uterus

Placenta (detaching)

Umbilical cord

D.

Figure 10-23

Birth. (A) The cervix is partially dilated, and the baby's head has entered the birth canal. (B) The cervix is nearly completely dilated. The baby's head rotates so that it can move through the birth canal. (C) The baby's head extends as it reaches the vaginal opening, and the head and the rest of the body pass through the birth canal. (D) After the baby is born, the placenta detaches from the uterus and is expelled from the woman's body.

childbirth preparation training often feel a sense of relief from the acute pain of the transition phase and at the prospect of giving birth.

This second stage can take up to an hour or more. Strong contractions may last 60 to 90 seconds and occur every two to three minutes. As the baby's head descends, the mother feels an urge to push. By bearing down, she helps the baby complete its passage to the outside.

As the baby's head appears, or *crowns,* the doctor may perform an *episiotomy*—an incision from the lower end of the vagina toward the anus to enlarge the vaginal opening. The purpose of the episiotomy is to prevent the baby's head from causing an irregular tear in the vagina, but routine episiotomies have been criticized as unnecessary. Women may be able to avoid this procedure by trying different birthing positions or having an attendant massage the perineal tissue.

Usually the baby's head emerges first, then its shoulders, then its body. With each contraction, a new part is born. However, the baby can be in a more difficult position, facing up rather than down, or with the feet or buttocks first (a **breech birth**), and a caesarean birth may then be necessary.

In the third stage of labor, the uterus contracts firmly after the birth of the baby; and, usually within five minutes, the placenta separates from the uterine wall. The woman may bear down to help expel the placenta, or the doctor may exert gentle external pressure. If an episiotomy has been performed, the doctor sews up the incision. To help the uterus contract and return to its normal size, it may be massaged manually, or the baby may be put to the mother's breast to stimulate contraction of the uterus.

Caesarean Birth

In a **caesarean delivery** (also referred to as a caesarean section), the doctor lifts the baby out of the woman's body through an incision made in the lower abdomen

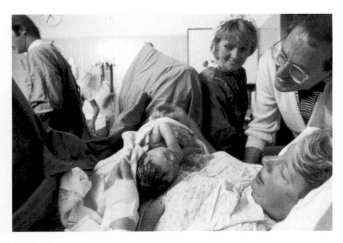

Family time. Fathers are routinely present at the birth of their children and often act as breathing coaches after both parents train in Lamaze techniques.

and uterus. The most common reason for caesarean birth is "failure to progress," a vague term indicating that labor has gone on too long and may put the baby or mother at risk. Other reasons include the baby's position (if feet or buttocks are first) and signs that the fetus is in danger. Thirty years ago, only 5% of babies born in America were delivered by caesarean birth; the current rate is 22.6%—substantially higher than in most other industrialized countries.

About 36% of caesarean sections are performed because the woman has had a previous caesarean birth. Yet research indicates that more than two-thirds of women who undergo caesarean births because of failure to progress in labor, and approximately four of every five women who have had caesarean births for other reasons, can have successful vaginal deliveries in subsequent pregnancies.

Caesarean birth involves abdominal surgery, so many women feel more physical discomforts after a caesarean than a vaginal birth. These discomforts include nausea, pain, and abdominal gas. Women who have had a caesarean section must refrain from strenuous activity, such as heavy lifting, for several weeks.

Following Birth

Hospital stays for new mothers have gotten shorter. The average length of stay is now only 2.6 days for a vaginal delivery and 4.1 days after a caesarean birth. A primary reason has been pressure to reduce medical costs. Obstetricians have voiced concern that the rush to release new mothers may jeopardize their well-

being and the health of their babies, who are more likely to require emergency care for problems such as jaundice. The American College of Obstetricians and Gynecologists and the American Academy of Pediatrics recommend that women remain in the hospital two days after a vaginal delivery and four days after a caesarean birth.

For the new mother, the high of delivery may be followed by a low known as **postpartum depression**. This time of fatigue, anxiety, and fluctuating moods is so common that it is listed in obstetrics texts as a normal consequence of delivery. For most women, it is a temporary feeling. For others, the depression, combined with fatigue and the new demands of the newborn, can persist and deepen. If postpartum depression lasts more than three or four weeks, the woman should seek help from a qualified psychotherapist.

It takes a while for the mother's body to return to normal after having given birth. The woman usually loses about 11 pounds at delivery and an additional 4 to 5 pounds in the following weeks. Usually four to eight weeks are required for the woman's reproductive organs, especially the uterus, to return to normal. Breast-feeding hastens this process, and exercises help restore the abdomen's size, shape, and tone. For three to six weeks after birth, there is a vaginal discharge called **lochia**, a mixture of blood from the site in the uterus where the placenta was attached, and tissue from the uterine lining. If the mother doesn't breast-feed her infant, menstruation typically resumes about four to ten weeks after giving birth.

Breast-Feeding Versus Bottle-Feeding

A generation ago, most middle- and upper-class women bottle-fed their babies. Today, an increasing number of mothers and medical professionals feel that breast milk is best. Breast-fed babies have fewer illnesses and a much lower hospitalization rate. Their mortality rate is also lower. Breast milk seems not only to prevent disease, but also to help bring infection under control. When breast-fed babies do get sick, they recover more quickly.

Despite the benefits of breast-feeding, there are valid reasons to choose bottle-feeding. According to the American Council on Science and Health, at least 20% of women are unable to breast-feed after their first deliveries, and 50% of new mothers encounter significant difficulties nursing. Sometimes the woman's breasts become inflamed, or she must take medications that would endanger her infant; sometimes the infant is unable to suckle vigorously enough to get an adequate milk supply. Another problem is that in certain areas of the country, the levels of pesticides and other chemical contaminants in mother's milk can be high.

Babies at Risk

According to the National Center for Health Statistics, a record percentage of U.S. newborns are surviving to their first birthday. The infant mortality rate, as reported in 1995, is a record low of 7.9 deaths per 1000 live births—a continued decline that puts the nation on track to reach its goal of no more than 7 infant deaths per 1000 births by the year 2000. However, African-American babies are not faring as well. Their mortality rate was 16.5 in 1992—making them 2.4 times more likely to die, primarily because of prematurity and dangerously low birth weight, before their first birthday. This gap has widened from just a 60% greater risk in 1950. Babies of Chinese and Japanese descent have the lowest mortality rates.[55]

In all, more than 1.3 million newborns each year require special care after birth because of prematurity, low birth weight, birth defects, jaundice, respiratory difficulties, or other problems. About 6% of newborns—more than 200,000 babies a year—require immediate intensive care for potentially life-threatening problems that developed before, during, or after birth.

Genetic Disorders

Two to 4% of babies are born with a genetic abnormality. The most common include the following:

- *Cystic fibrosis.* The most common genetic problem among white Americans, this is a disabling abnormality of the respiratory system and sweat and mucous glands.

- *Down syndrome.* This disorder is caused by an extra number 21 chromosome and occurs in one out of every 600 to 1000 births. Infants are born with varying degrees of physical and mental retardation. The chances of a woman delivering an infant with Down syndrome increase with her age. At age 25, the chances are 1 in 1200; at age 35, they rise to 1 in 365; and at age 40, they are 1 in 100.

- *Sickle-cell anemia.* About 8% to 10% of North America's 25 million African Americans carry a gene for sickle-cell anemia, a blood disorder that occurs when hemoglobin, the oxygen-carrying protein of red blood cells, is abnormal and causes red blood cells to assume a crescent (sickle) shape. Unable to provide adequate oxygen to vital organs of the body, sickled cells cause fatigue, loss of interest and appetite, pain, and a host of other symptoms. Blood transfusions can prolong a victim's life, but there's no cure for sickle-cell anemia. About half the victims die before age 20.

- *Phenylketonuria (PKU).* This disease occurs when the liver enzyme needed by the body for the metabolism of the amino acid phenylalanine is absent. If both parents are carriers, there's a one-in-four chance that the child will develop phenylketonuria (PKU). In most states, the law requires testing newborns for PKU. If PKU is detected, an immediate, long-term phenylalanine-free diet can reduce the effects of the disorder. If untreated, the victim becomes severely mentally retarded.

- *Tay-Sachs disease.* Occurring almost exclusively among young children of Eastern European Jewish ancestry, Tay-Sachs disease is caused by an enzyme deficiency. Infants with this disorder appear normal for perhaps nine months, but then gradually deteriorate physically and mentally. Death usually occurs before the fifth birthday. Carriers can be identified by a blood test.

The Littlest Addicts

Cocaine and crack babies suffer major complications, including withdrawal and permanent disabilities. (See Chapter 14 for a discussion of these drugs.) They have higher-than-normal incidences of respiratory and kidney troubles, premature birth, and low birth weight, and may be at greater risk of sudden infant death syndrome. Visual problems, lack of coordination, and developmental retardation are also common.

Crib Death: Sudden Infant Death Syndrome (SIDS)

SIDS, or **crib death**—the unexplained death of an apparently healthy baby under one year of age—is the second-leading cause of infant mortality in the United States. Typically, a seemingly healthy infant, usually 1 to 7 months old, is put to bed according to the daily routine. The baby may have some signs of a cold or cough. When the parents return to the crib, they find the child dead. There is no sign of a struggle, nor does the baby suffocate in the blankets. Determining the cause of death often proves impossible. Premature and very small babies are the most vulnerable. A newly recognized risk factor, based on studies of 20,000 infants during the first week of life, is the "resonance frequency" of each cry—an acoustic measure of a child's cry that cannot be easily determined by listening. Computer analysis found that infants with a high-resonance frequency were more likly to die of SIDS. A screening test based on this factor may be developed to detect newborns at risk.

Based on a review of studies on SIDS from around the world, health professionals have found that sleeping on its stomach increases a baby's risk of SIDS. As a result, many pediatricians now recommend that normal, full-term infants be placed on their backs for the first six months—a simple step that might cut the number of SIDS deaths in half and save the lives of 2000 infants in the United States every year. According to a 1995 report, more parents are indeed changing the position in which they lay their babies down to sleep.[56]

Infertility

The World Health Organization defines infertility as the failure to conceive after one year of unprotected intercourse. About 85% of couples will conceive during one year, rising to almost 90% by two years. The main causes of infertility are ovulation problems, tubal damage, or sperm dysfunction. Less common causes are endometriosis, cervical factors, or coital difficulties. Even after intensive investigation, 10 to 20% of couples have "unexplained infertility" in which no cause can be demonstrated.[57]

Of the couples who marry this year, 1 in 12 won't be able to conceive a child, and 10% of couples already married won't be able to have additional children. About 6.1 million women reported impaired fertility in 1995, compared with 4.9 million in 1988. **Infertility** is a problem of the couple, not of the individual man or woman. In 40% of cases, infertility is caused by female problems; in 40% by male problems; in 10% by a combination of male and female problems; and in 10% by unexplained causes. A thorough diagnostic workup can reveal a cause for infertility in 90% of cases. Almost two-thirds of the couples who seek medical help for infertility eventually succeed in having a child.[58]

In women, the most common causes of subfertility or infertility are age, abnormal menstrual patterns, suppression of ovulation, and blocked fallopian tubes. (See Figure 10-24.) Other gynecologic disorders that can lead to infertility include endometriosis, in which cells from the endometrium (the lining of the uterus) migrate to other locations within the pelvic cavity; fibroids, benign growths of tissue within the uterus that can interfere with conception; uterine defects; problems with the cer-

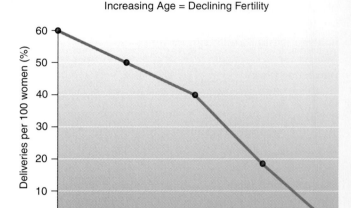

Increasing Age = Declining Fertility

SOURCE: Cohen, B. The Reproductive Cycle. *Management of Infertility: A Clinician's Manual.* 2nd ed. Durant, OK: Essential Information Systems, 1991, pp. 15–38.

Figure 10-24

Impact of age on fertility outcome in women.

vical mucus; and an immunological reaction to a man's sperm. The prevention of STDs can help prevent some cases of infertiltiy in women.[59]

Male subfertility or infertility is usually linked to either the quantity or the quality of sperm, which may be inactive, misshapen, or insufficient (less than 20 million sperm per milliliter of semen in an ejaculation of 3 to 5 ml). Sometimes the problem is hormonal or a blockage of a sperm duct. Some men suffer from the inability to ejaculate normally, or from retrograde ejaculation—in which some of the semen travels in the wrong direction, back into the body of the male. Another problem is a *varicocele,* an enlarged vein that carries too much blood and makes the testicle too warm. An undergarment that uses a small amount of water to cool the testicles may help overcome this problem; some men require surgery to eliminate the varicocele. The use of drugs such as cocaine and marijuana can also interfere with the creation of sperm.[60]

Medical treatment can identify the cause of infertility in about 90% of affected couples. The odds of successful pregnancy range from 30% to 70%, depending on the specific cause of infertility. One result of successful infertility treatments has been a boom in twins, triplets, and quadruplets. Some obstetricians have urged less aggressive treatment for infertility to avoid such high-risk multiple births.

Infertility can have an enormous emotional impact. Often, the wife begins to worry first because infertility touches on a core aspect of femininity. Many women long to experience pregnancy and childbirth and feel great loss if they cannot conceive. Their self-esteem may be diminished, and they may become obsessed with success and outcome. Women in their thirties and forties fear that their "biological clock" is running out of time. Men may be confused and surprised by the intensity of their partners' emotions. Most are more concerned about their wives than about having a baby, but they feel helpless and frustrated in their husbandly role of fixing matters for the wife. Although they both need each other's support more than ever, they may pull away because of their sadness and a sense of losing control over their lives.[61]

Artificial Insemination

Since the 1960s, **artificial insemination**—the introduction of viable sperm into the vagina by artificial means—has led to an estimated 250,000 births in the United States, primarily in couples in which the husband was infertile. However, some states do not recognize such children as legitimate; others do, but only if the woman's husband gave his consent for the insemination.

There have been complaints about unethical treatment in infertility centers. Fertility specialists and government licensing agencies have been working together to set uniform standards for licensing. Infertile couples should carefully obtain as much information as possible, including the credentials of any fertility specialists, who should be board-certified in obstetrics and gynecology, with additional training in reproductive endocrinology and infertility. Those performing surgery should be members of the Society of Reproductive Surgeons; centers offering in vitro fertilization or alternative techniques should be staffed by members of the Society of Assisted Reproductive Technology.

Assisted Reproductive Technology

New approaches to infertility include microsurgery, sometimes with lasers, to open destroyed or blocked egg and sperm ducts; new hormone preparations to induce ovulation; and the use of balloons, inserted through the cervix and inflated, to open blocked fallop-

ian tubes (a procedure called *balloon tuboplasty*). However, less than 2% of infertile women undergo assisted reproductive technologies in order to conceive.

Among the most promising techniques that can help couples overcome fertility problems is *in vitro fertilization,* which involves removing the ova, often with a long needle, from a woman's ovary just before normal ovulation would occur. The woman's egg and her mate's sperm are placed in a special fertilization medium (a substance that encourages fertilization) for a specific period of time, and are then transferred to another medium to continue developing. If the fertilized egg cell shows signs of development, within several days it is returned to the woman's uterus by means of a hollow tube placed through the vagina and cervix. The egg cell implants itself in the lining of the uterus, and the pregnancy continues as normal. The success rate varies from center to center but is generally less than 20%; and the costs are high. In a 1994 study, in vitro fertilization costs per successful delivery ranged from $66,667 for the first cycle of IVF to $114,286 by the sixth attempt.[62]

Less time-consuming and less expensive than in vitro fertilization, *gamete intrafallopian transfer (GIFT)* involves placing sperm and eggs into the fallopian tubes. GIFT mimics nature by allowing fertilized eggs to develop in the fallopian tubes according to a normal timetable. The success rate is about 20%. In *zygote intrafallopian transfer (ZIFT),* eggs are collected from the mother-to-be and combined with the father's sperm in a laboratory dish. One day after fertilization occurs, the single-celled zygote that forms is placed in the fallopian tube. In a variation called *intracytoplasmic sperm injection (ICSI),* several eggs are harvested, and each is injected with a single sperm by means of a fine hollow needle. (This overcomes problems related to the inability of sperm to penetrate the egg.) The fertilized eggs are then placed in the fallopian tube.[63]

Fertilization rates are comparable to in vitro fertilization with sperm from normal ejaculation.[64] There is also a new technique called *gestational surrogacy,* in which an embryo is conceived in a laboratory dish using a woman's egg and her partner's sperm and then implanted into another woman's (the surrogate's) uterus. Alternatively, the fertilized donor egg can later be transferred to the uterus of the infertile woman, who carries and delivers the developing embryo. Embryos may be frozen for later implantation in a process (called *cryopreservation)* that is highly controversial because of legal issues concerning the "ownership" of the unborn.

Older women are just as likely as younger women to have a successful pregnancy after implantation of a donor embryo. In some experimental and controversial cases, donor eggs and embryos have been implanted in women in their forties, fifties, and (in at least two cases) sixties. The use of a donor egg from a younger woman eliminates the risk of increased genetic problems. There are ethical questions about using expensive assisted reproductive technologies for the sake of enabling older women to become mothers or of allowing creation of "designer" babies of a certain racial or ethnic identity or with certain attributes, such as sex, height, or intelligence.

Fertility drugs and assisted reproduction techniques have extended the limits of motherhood. In 1996 Arceli Keh, a 63-year-old bank teller in southern California, became the oldest mother on record when she gave birth to a baby girl. She had lied about her age to qualify for infertility treatments. In 1997 Bobbi McCaughey in Des Moines, Iowa, after treatment with fertility drugs, gave birth to seven babies—and earned her own place in the annals of reproduction as the mother of the only surviving set of septuplets.

These births set off both a media frenzy and a firestorm of controversy. Many questioned the ethics of a woman becoming a mother at over age 60. In Bobbi McCaughey's case, doctors pointed out that the chance of miscarrying and losing all the babies was greater than 50%.[65] Assisted reproductive techniques involve some problems, including high costs and a low success rate. One attempt at in vitro fertilization ranges from $6,000 to $10,000 and insurance rarely covers these expenses. The overall success rate for any form of assisted pregnancy is about 25%.

Of the pregnancies achieved by fertility treatments, 20 to 30% result in multiple births. As a result of hormonal stimulation, the woman's ovaries usually release several eggs; often more than one is fertilized. To increase the chances of conception, fertility specialists usually implant more than one embryo. The more that survive, the greater the risk of prematurity, low birth weight, birth defects, and death in the womb or after birth. In some cases, one or more fetuses are aborted to increase the likelihood that at least one other will survive.

There also has been controversy over whether the hormones used to stimulate the ovaries in infertility treatment may increase the risk of ovarian cancer. However, an analysis of all the research on this topic concluded that, as currently used, ovarian-stimulating drugs do not increase this risk.[66]

Adoption

Men and women who cannot conceive children biologically can still become parents. **Adoption** matches would-be parents yearning for youngsters to love with infants or children who need loving. Couples interested in adoption can work with either public agencies or private counselors who contact obstetricians directly. Or they can contact organizations that arrange adoptions of children in need from other countries.

Each year some 50,000 U.S. children become available for adoption—far fewer than the number of would-be parents looking for youngsters to love. By some estimates, only 1 in 30 couples receive the child they want—and they spend an average of two years and as much as $100,000 on the adoption process.

Not only are the stakes high, but adoption arrangements often are chaotic. As psychologist David Brodzinsky, Ph.D., of Rutgers University, coauthor of *Being Adopted*, puts it, "in adoption in the 1990s, anything goes."[67] Private adoptions are legal in some states, banned in others. In some places, birth mothers sign over all claims to a child within seventy-two hours of giving birth; in others they have up to a year to change their minds. Sometimes foster parents are encouraged to adopt—particularly if they're African Americans caring for an African-American child. In others, they face a daunting series of bureaucratic barriers. What's needed most, say experts on every side of the issue, are uniform adoption laws in all fifty states.

An increasing number of people support *open adoptions*, which allow for visiting and communication

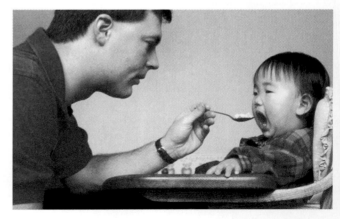

Adoption gives people the option to become parents when they would not otherwise be able to have children.

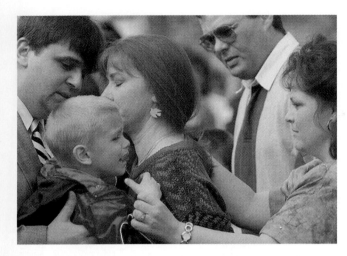

Adoption controversies. The rights of adoptive and biological parents come into conflict in cases such as those of Baby Richard and Baby Jessica. In both of these cases courts ordered the adoptive parents to relinquish custody to the biological parents.

with the biological parents even though the adoptive parents retain legal custody. Even after a *closed adoption,* the biological (or birth) parents may at some point search for their children, if only to explain why they chose to give them up for adoption.

Although fewer than 2% of each year's 50,000 adoptions of American children are contested, adoptive parents are nervous and confused.

"Adoptive or foster parents have no rights whatsoever until the rights of the biological parents are legally terminated," says Mary Beth Style, Vice President for policy and practice for the National Council on Adoption[68]—even when they have nurtured a child for months or years, as often happens in foster care. Although mental health professionals contend that the courts should recognize the rights of a child's "psychological" parents, most rulings have placed little importance on such bonds. Political pressure for reform has increased, which makes birthparent support groups earful. "There's a rush to sever quickly and permanently the biological bonds between parents and their children," says Janet Fenton, President of Concerned United Birthparents. "The focus in adoption is shifting from finding homes for children who need them to finding babies for couples who can't have them."[69]

The best advice for prospective adoptive parents is to learn as much as they can about their state's adoption laws and to prepare for the reality that their plans might not work out.

Making This Chapter Work for You
Responsible Reproductive Choices

- Simply not wanting to conceive is never enough to prevent conception. Before you become sexually active, you have to decide about birth control. The fact that women bear children does not mean that men aren't equally responsible for birth control.

- A sexually active couple that doesn't use contraception has an 80% chance of conceiving a child within a year. If you decide to take that gamble, the stakes are your future, your partner's future, and the future of the child you may conceive.

- To prevent conception, you can make the survival of sperm in the vagina more difficult, or you can block the sperm's path into the vagina, uterus, and fallopian tubes. By preventing ovulation, you can make sure that the sperm doesn't find a ready, ripe egg; or you can prevent the fertilized egg from implanting itself in the uterine wall.

- Abstinence and sexual activities that do not involve vaginal intercourse ("outercourse") are completely safe and 100% effective—as long as couples are committed to this practice and make sure that sperm is never ejaculated near the vaginal opening.

- Hormonally based birth control methods include oral contraceptives (the pill); hormone implants (Norplant), which inhibit ovulation and alter the cervical mucus so that sperm are prevented from entering the uterus; and Depo-Provera, an injectable hormone that provides three months of contraceptive protection.

- The barrier contraceptives provide a physical or chemical barrier that prevents sperm from reaching an egg. They include the condom, diaphragm, cervical cap, and spermicidal foam, jelly, suppositories, and film. Use of condoms with spermicides containing nonoxynol-9 can also reduce the risk of pregnancy and some sexually transmitted diseases.

- Intrauterine devices (IUDs), made with a hormonal compound or copper, prevent implantation of a fertilized egg. They are highly effective and long-acting but are recommended only for women in monogamous relationships.

- Couples using natural family planning or fertility awareness methods refrain from unprotected vaginal

Health Online

Successful Contraception   http://www.arhp.org/success/index.html

Sponsored by the Association of Reproductive Health Professionals, this site includes an interactive program to help you choose the best birth control method for you. It takes into consideration your health history, lifestyle factors, and personal preferences. There is also information on assessing your birth control choices and details on each method.

Think about it ...

- Does this program recommend any birth control methods for you that you haven't considered before? What would be the advantages and disadvantages of these methods compared to the one you are currently using?

- What are the most important considerations for you in choosing a method of birth control? Cost, effectiveness, accessibility, convenience, or other factors?

- If you are not currently sexually active, have you thought about what method of contraception you might use if you do start having sex?

intercourse during the days just preceding and just following ovulation. They may use cervical mucus, a monthly calendar, or body temperature changes to determine a woman's period of greatest fertility.

- The most popular and effective, but permanent, birth control method among married couples is sterilization: vasectomy in a man and tubal ligation or occlusion in a woman.

- After-intercourse methods of birth control include higher doses of oral contraceptives; the so-called morning-after pill, which prevents implantation of a fertilized egg; insertion of an IUD; and menstrual extraction, in which the uterine lining is auctioned out.

- One of the most controversial and divisive issues today is legalized induced abortion, the termination of pregnancy by the removal of the uterine contents. A hormonal compound, RU-486, often called the abortion pill, available only at research centers, can terminate a pregnancy in its first weeks. Commonly used abortion methods in the United States are suction curettage, dilation and evacuation (D and E), prostaglandin injection, and hysterotomy.

- Good prenatal care includes good nutrition; adequate rest and exercise; and avoiding risks, such as smoking, alcohol, caffeine, harmful drugs, and exposure to radiation. Among the serious complications of pregnancy are ectopic pregnancy, in which the fertilized egg implants itself at sites other than in the uterus; miscarriages, which usually occur before the sixteenth week of pregnancy; infections, which may cause disease, brain damage, and malformations of the fetus; and premature labor, which occurs after week 20 and before week 37 of the pregnancy.

- Labor and delivery consists of three stages. During the first stage, the cervix thins and dilates to a diameter of 10 centimeters. In the next stage, the baby passes through the birth canal. The placenta is expelled during the third stage. A caesarean, or surgical, birth may be necessary to overcome certain risks. After birth, the woman's body begins to return to its prepregnant state. The woman may choose to breast-feed, which can help protect the newborn from various illnesses, or bottle-feed her baby.

- Infertile couples may decide to attempt to have a child by such medical procedures as in vitro fertilization or other assisted forms of birth technology.

Another alternative is adoption, although the number of available babies is far fewer than the number of would-be parents hoping to adopt.

Choices about sexual behavior invariably lead to choices about reproduction. Sexual responsibility means recognizing that fact and acting with full awareness of the consequences of sexual activity. You must think not just of yourself, but also of your partner, because your decisions and actions may affect both of you, now and in the future. You must also consider the baby you might conceive if you don't use contraception. If you should decide to have a child, your responsibilities extend to the new life you helped to create.

▶ Key Terms

The terms listed here are used within the chapter. Page numbers are included for each term.
A definition of each term is given in the green Glossary pages at the end of this book.

adoption *322*
after-intercourse methods *303*
amnion *309*
artificial insemination *321*
barrier contraceptives *292*
basal body temperature *303*
breech birth *317*
caesarean delivery *317*
cervical cap *000*
coitus interruptus *283*
colpotomy *301*
conception *280*
condom *292*
constant-dose combination pill *288*
contraception *281*
crib death *319*
diaphragm *295*
dilation and evacuation (D and E) *306*
ectopic pregnancy *313*
elective abortion *304*
effectiveness *282*

embryo *309*
epidural block *316*
failure rate *283*
fertilization *280*
fetal alcohol syndrome (FAS) *312*
fetus *309*
hysterectomy *301*
hysterotomy *306*
implantation *281*
infertility *320*
intrauterine device (IUD) *298*
labor *316*
Lamaze method *316*
laparoscopy *301*
laparotomy *300*
lochia *318*
minilaparotomy *300*
minipill *288*
miscarriage *313*
multiphasic pill *288*
oral contraceptives *287*
ovulation method *301*

perinatology *313*
placenta *309*
postpartum depression *318*
preconception care *308*
premature labor *314*
progestin-only pill *288*
psychoprophylaxis *316*
rhythm method *302*
rubella *315*
spermatogeneis *280*
spinal block *316*
sterilization *299*
suction curettage *305*
sudden infant death syndrome (SIDS) *319*
tubal ligation *300*
tubal occlusion *300*
vaginal contraceptive film (VCF) *297*
vaginal spermicides *297*
vasectomy *300*
zygote *280*

▶ Review Questions

1. What is conception? What is preconception care? Who should practice it? How? When does it occur?

2. What are some common methods of contraception? List an advantage and disadvantage for each method.

3. If an infertile couple wishes to have children, what are their options? What are the benefits or risks of those options?

4. What is abortion? List and describe the various methods of abortion.

5. What happens to a woman when she becomes pregnant? Describe the physiological changes that occur during pregnancy.

6. What are some of the most frequent complications of pregnancy? How can the risk of complications be minimized or avoided?

Personal Health 10.3 *INTERACTIVE*

Critical Thinking Questions

1. After reading about the various methods of contraception, which do you feel would be most effective for you? What factors enter into your decision (convenience, risks, effectiveness, etc.)?

2. In Wyoming, a pregnant woman went to the police station to report that her husband had beaten her. Instead of charges being brought against him, she was arrested for intoxication and charged with abusing her fetus by drinking. Across the country, other women who use hard drugs or alcohol while pregnant or whose newborns test positive for drugs have been arrested and put on trial for abusing their unborn children. Prosecutors argue that they are defending the innocent victims of substance abuse. Some health officials, on the other hand, argue that addicted women need help, not punishment. What do you think? Why?

3. When Bobby McCaughey gave birth to septuplets in 1997, some people felt that the power of fertility drugs had gone too far. If you or your partner took fertility drugs and then became pregnant with seven fetuses, would you carry them all to term? What if you knew that the chances of them all surviving were very slim and that eliminating some of them would improve the odds for the others? What ethical issues do cases like these raise?

 ## Connections to Personal Health Interactive

To enhance your understanding of the material covered in this chapter, check out the following study aids on the **Personal Health Interactive CD-ROM**. *Each numbered icon within the chapter corresponds to an appropriate activity listed here.*

10.1 Do You Want to Be a Parent?
10.2 Fetal Brain Development
10.3 Chapter 10 Review

References

1. Mahoney, from Robert Crooks and Karla Baur, *Our Sexuality*, 7th ed. Pacific Grove, CA: Brooks/Cole, 1999.
2. Riddle, John, and J. Worth Estes. "Oral Contraceptives in Ancient and Medieval Times." *American Scientist*, May–June 1992.
3. Lancashire, Jeff. "New Report Documents Trends in Childbearing, Reproductive Health." National Center for Health Statistics, June 5, 1997.
4. "Family Planning Saves Millions of Women and Children's Lives." *WIN News*, Vol. 23, No. 2, Spring 1997.
5. Steinhauer, Jennifer. "Men Avoiding Obligation for Birth Control." *New York Times*, May 25, 1995.
6. Trussell, James, et al. "The Economic Value of Contraception." *American Journal of Public Health*, Vol. 2, No. 9, May 4, 1995. Tamkins, Theresa. "Many Insurers Do Not Pay for Birth Control." *Medical Tribune*, Vol. 2, No. 9, May 4, 1995.
7. Douglas, Kathy, et al. "Results from the 1995 National College Health Risk Behavior Survey." *Journal of American College Health*, Vol. 46, September 1997.
8. Walling, Anne. "Overview of the Failure Rate of Contraceptive Methods." *American Family Physician*, Vol. 55, No. 1, January 1997.
9. Hanson, Vivien. "How to Provide Postcoital Contraception." *Patient Care*, April 15, 1997.
10. Hatcher, Robert, et al. *Contraceptive Technology*. New York: Irvington, 1994. Colditz, G. "Oral Contraceptive Use and Mortality During 12 Years of Follow-Up: The Nurses' Health Study." *Annals of Internal Medicine*, Vol. 120, 1994.
11. Lancashire, "New Report Documents Trends in Childbearing, Reproductive Health."
12. Berenson, Abbey, and Constance Wiemann. "Use of Levonorgestrel Implants versus Oral Contraceptives in Adolescents: A Case-Control Study." *American Journal of Obstetrics & Gynecology*, Vol. 171, No. 4, April 1995.
13. Berenson, Abbey, and Constance Wiemann. "Use of Levonorgestrel Implants versus Oral Contraceptives in Adolescents: A Case-Control Study." *American Journal of Obstetrics & Gynecology*, Vol. 171, No. 4, April 1995.
14. Dunson, Thomas, et al. "Complications and Risk Factors Associated with the Removal of Norplant Implants." *Obstetrics & Gynecology*, Vol. 85, No. 4, April 1995. Klaisle, Cynthia, and Philip Darney. "A Guide to Removing Contraceptive Implants." *Contemporary Nurse Practitioner*, Vol. 1, No. 2, March–April 1995. Darney, Philip.

"Contraceptive Implants: Proper Technique for Rapid, Problem-Free Removal." *Women's Health Reports*, Vol. 1, No. 2, May 1, 1995.

15. Board of Trustees, American Medical Association. "Requirements or Incentives by Government for the Use of Long-Acting Contraceptives." *Journal of the American Medical Association,* April 1, 1992.

16. Hatcher et al., *Contraceptive Technology.*

17. Lancashire, "New Report Documents Trends in Childbearing, Reproductive Health."

18. De Bro, S., et al. "Influencing a Partner to Use a Condom." *Psychology of Women Quarterly,* Vol. 18, 1994.

19. Pinkerton, Steven, and Paul Abrahamson. "Condoms and the Prevention of AIDS." *American Scientist,* Vol. 85, No. 4, July–August 1997.

20. Lindberg, Laura Duberstein, et al. "Young Men's Experience with Condom Breakage." *Family Planning Perspectives,* Vol. 29, No. 3, May–June 1997.

21. "A New Look at an Old Device: Can IUDs Make a Comeback?" *Contraceptive Technology Update,* Vol. 16, No. 5, May 1995. Klitsch, Michael. "IUD Use and Tubal Infertility." *Family Planning Perspectives,* August 1992.

22. Volm, from Crooks, Robert, and Karla Baur, *Our Sexuality.*

23. Hatcher et al., *Contraceptive Technology.*

24. Giovannucci, E., et al. "A Long-Term Study of Mortality in Men Who Have Undergone Vasectomy." New *England Journal of Medicine,* May 21, 1992.

25. Lancashire, "New Report Documents Trends."

26. Grimes, David. "Emergency Contraception—Expanding Opportunities for Primary Prevention." *New England Journal of Medicine*, Vol. 337, No. 15, October 9, 1997.

27. Cates, Willard, and Elizabeth Raymond. "Annotation: Emergency Contraception—Parsimony and Prevention in the Medicine Cabinet." *American Journal of Public Health*, Vol. 87, No. 6, June 1997.

28. Trussell, James, et al. "Preventing Unintended Pregnancy: The Cost-Effectiveness of Three Methods of Emergency Contraception." *American Journal of Public Health*, Vol. 87, No. 6, June 1997.

29. Crooks and Baur.

30. Gober, Patricia. "The Role of Access in Explaining State Abortion Rates." *Social Science & Medicine*, Vol. 44, No. 7, April 1997.

31. Hatcher et al., *Contraceptive Technology.*

32. Maloy, Katie, and Maggie Patterson. *Birth or Abortion? Private Struggles in a Political World.* New York: Plenum Press, 1992.

33. Stotland, Nada. "The Myth of the Abortion Trauma Syndrome." *Journal of the American Medical Association,* October 21, 1992.

34. Rosenfeld, Jo Ann. "Emotional Responses to Therapeutic Abortion." *American Family Physician,* January 1992.

35. Gober, "The Role of Access."

36. Golberg, Carey, with Janet Elder. "Public Still Backs Abortion, But Wants Limits, Poll Says." *New York Times,* January 16, 1998.

37. Seguin, Louise, et al. "Chronic Stressors, Social Support and Depression During Pregnancy." *Obstetrics & Gynecology*, Vol. 85, No. 4, April 1995.

38. Copper, Rachel, et al. "The Relationship of Maternal Attitude Toward Weight Gain During Pregnancy and Low Birth Weight." *Obstetrics & Gynecology*, Vol. 85, No. 4, April 1995.

39. Artal, Raul, and Philip Buckenmeyer. "Exercise During Pregnancy and Postpartum." *Contemporary Ob/Gyn*, May 1995. Stressguth, Ann, et al. "Prenatal Alcohol and Offspring Development: The First Fourteen Years." *Drug & Alcohol Dependence*, Vol. 36, No. 2, October 1994.

40. "Medical-Care Expenditures Attributable to Cigarette Smoking During Pregnancy—United States, 1995." *Journal of the American Medical Association*, Vol. 278, No. 23, December 17, 1997.

41. Centers for Disease Control and Prevention. *Morbidity and Mortality Weekly Review*, May 13, 1994.

42. Milunsky, Aubrey, et al. "Maternal Heat Exposure and Neural Tube Defects." *Journal of the American Medical Association,* August 19, 1992.

43. "Drinking in Pregnancy." *Morbidity and Mortality Weekly Report*, U.S. Centers for Disease Control, April 1997 .

44. Hillard, Paula. "Increase in Ectopic Pregnancies." *Contemporary Ob/Gyn*, May 1995.

45. Coste, J., et al. "Sexually Transmitted Diseases as Major Causes of Ectopic Pregnancy." *Fertility and Sterility*, Vol. 62, 1994.

46. Moore, Peter."Tackling Autoantibody-linked Pregnancy Loss." *Lancet*, Vol. 350, No. 9073, July 26, 1997. Cowchock, Susan. "Autoantibodies and Pregnancy Loss." *New England Journal of Medicine*, Vol. 337, No. 3, July 17, 1997.

47. Lynch, Denis, et al. "Major Depressive Disorder Following Miscarriage." *Journal of the American Medical Association*, Vol. 277, No. 19, May 21, 1997.

48. Puddifoot, John, and Martin Johnson. "The Legitimacy of Grieving: The Partner's Experience at Miscarriage." *Social Science & Medicine*, Vol. 45, No. 6, Sept 15, 1997.

49. Wilcox, Allen, et al. "Birthweight and Perinatal Mortality." *Journal of the American Medical Association*, Vol. 273, No. 9, March 1, 1995.

50. National Center for Health Statistics. "Fact Sheet on Adolescent Pregnancy." Public Information Office, 1997.

51. Lindberg, Laura, et al. "Age Differences Between Minors Who Give Birth and Their Adult Partners." *Family Planning Perspectives*, Vol. 29, No. 2, March–April 1997.

52. Muldoon, from Crooks, and Baur, *Our Sexuality.*

53. Crooks and Bauer. *Our Sexuality.*

54. Quilligan, Edward. "Obstetrics and Gynecology." *Journal of the American Medical Association*, Vol. 273, No. 21, June 7, 1995.

55. Singh, Gopal, and Stella Yu. "Infant Mortality in the United States." *American Journal of Public Health*, Vol. 85, No. 7, July 1995.

56. Gibson, E., et al. "Infant Sleep Positions Following New

AAP Guidelines." *Pediatrics*, Vol. 88, No. 1, July 1995. Guntheroth, Warren, and Philip Spiers. "Sleeping Prone and the Risk of Sudden Infant Death Syndrome." *Journal of the American Medical Association*, May 6, 1992.

57. "Infertility: Its Investigation and Treatment." *WIN News*, Vol. 23, No. 2, Spring 1997.

58. "Infertility Statistics." *Focus on Fertility*, Vol. 1, No. 2, Spring 1995.

59. DeLisle, Susan. "Preserving Reproductive Choice: Preventing STD-Related Infertility in Women." *SIECUS Report*, Vol. 25, No. 3, February–March 1997.

60. de Kretser, D. M. "Male Infertility." *Lancet*, Vol. 349, No. 9054, March 15, 1997.

61. Schreiber, Pamela. "From Your Patient's Perspective: The Emotional Impact of Infertility." *Focus on Fertility*, Vol. 1, No. 2, Spring 1995.

62. Neuman, P.J., et al. "The Cost of a Successful Delivery with In-Vitro Fertilization." *New England Journal of Medicine*, Vol. 331, 1994.

63. Huffman, Grace Brooke. "Intracytoplasmic Sperm Injection and Genetic Risk." *American Family Physician*, Vol. 55, No. 5, April 1997.

64. Crooks and Baur, *Our Sexuality*.

65. Kolata, Gina. "Many Specialists Are Left in No Mood for Celebration." *New York Times*, November 21, 1997.

66. Mosgaard, Berit Jul. "Infertility, Fertility Drugs, and Invasive Ovarian Cancer: A Case-Control Study." *Journal of the American Medical Association*, Vol. 278, No. 12, September 24, 1997.

67. Brodzinsky, David, Marshall Schechter, and Robin Marantz Henig. *Being Adopted*. New York: Doubleday, 1992.

68. Style, Mary Beth. Personal interview.

69. Fenton, Janet. Personal interview.

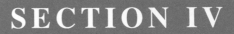

PERSONAL HEALTH RISKS

*E*very day you make choices that affect both the quantity and the quality of your life. The right choices aren't always easy to make or to sustain. The chapters in this section can help by providing information you can use in making and implementing healthful decisions. By understanding the risks to your health, you can prepare to overcome them—and not simply live life, but celebrate it every day.

CHAPTER 11

DEFENDING YOURSELF FROM INFECTIOUS DISEASES

After studying the material in this chapter, you should be able to:

Explain how the different agents of infection spread disease.

Describe how your body protects itself from infectious disease.

List and **describe** some common infectious diseases.

List the sexually transmitted diseases and the symptoms and treatment for each.

Define HIV infection, and **describe** its symptoms.

List the methods of HIV transmission.

Explain some practical methods for preventing HIV infection and other sexually transmitted diseases.

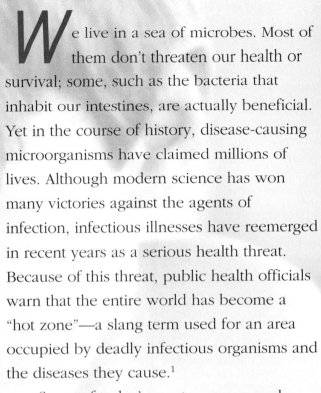

We live in a sea of microbes. Most of them don't threaten our health or survival; some, such as the bacteria that inhabit our intestines, are actually beneficial. Yet in the course of history, disease-causing microorganisms have claimed millions of lives. Although modern science has won many victories against the agents of infection, infectious illnesses have reemerged in recent years as a serious health threat. Because of this threat, public health officials warn that the entire world has become a "hot zone"—a slang term used for an area occupied by deadly infectious organisms and the diseases they cause.[1]

Some of today's most common and dangerous infectious illnesses spread primarily through sexual contact, and their incidence has skyrocketed. Sexually transmitted diseases (STDs) cannot be prevented in the laboratory. Only you, by your behavior, can prevent and control them.

This chapter is a lesson in self-defense against all forms of infection. The information it provides can help you boost your defenses, recognize and avoid enemies, protect yourself from STDs, and realize when to seek help.

Understanding Infection

Infection is a complex process, triggered by various **pathogens** (disease-causing organisms) and countered by the body's own defenders. Physicians explain infection in terms of a **host** (either a person or a population) that contacts one or more agents in an environment. A **vector**—a biological or physical vehicle that carries the agent to the host— provides the means of transmission.

Agents of Infection

The types of microbes that can cause infection are viruses, bacteria, fungi, protozoa, and helminths (parasitic worms) (see Figure 11-1).

Viruses

The tiniest pathogens—**viruses**—are also the toughest; they consist of a bit of nucleic acid (DNA or RNA, but never both) within a protein coat. Unable to reproduce on its own, a virus takes over a body cell's reproductive machinery and instructs it to produce new viral particles, which are then released to enter other cells.

Among the most common viruses are the following:

- *Rhinoviruses and adenoviruses,* which get into the mucous membranes and cause upper-respiratory tract infections and colds.

- *Influenza viruses,* which can change their outer protein coats so dramatically that individuals resistant to one strain cannot fight off a new one.

- *Herpes viruses,* which take up permanent residence in the cells and flare up periodically.

- *Papilloma viruses,* which cause few symptoms in women and almost none in men, but may be responsible, at least in part, for a rise in the incidence of cervical cancer among younger women.

- *Hepatitis viruses,* which cause several forms of liver infection, ranging from mild to potentially life threatening.

- *Slow viruses,* which give no early indication of their

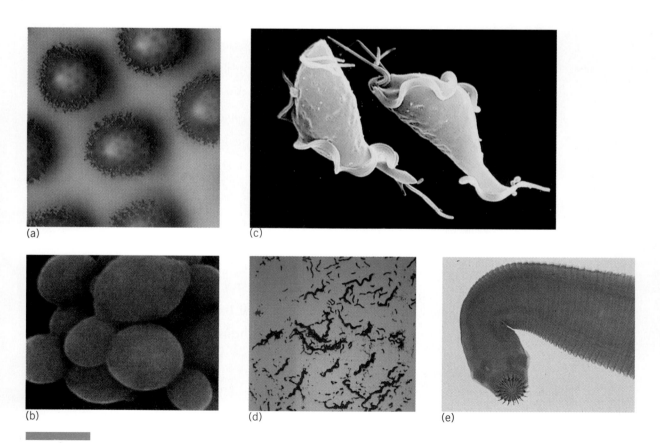

(a)

(b)

(c)

(d)

(e)

Figure 11-1

Examples of the major categories of organisms that cause disease in humans. Except for the helminths (parasitic worms), pathogens are microorganisms that can be seen only with the aid of a microscope. (a) Viruses: common cold, (b) Fungi: yeast, (c) Protozoa: trichomonas, (d) Bacteria: syphilis, (e) Helminths: tapeworm.

presence but can produce fatal illnesses within a few years.

- *Retroviruses,* which are named for their backward ("retro") sequence of genetic replication compared to other viruses. One retrovirus, human immunodeficiency virus (HIV), causes acquired immune deficiency syndrome (AIDS). Scientists have identified different retroviruses that have been linked to several diseases, including some forms of leukemia and lymphoma (cancers of the blood and lymph glands, respectively).

- *Filoviruses,* which are newly identified viruses that resemble threads and are extremely lethal. Most of those infected with the two known filoviruses, Marburg and Ebola, develop *viral hemorrhagic fever,* which causes uncontrollable bleeding and usually proves fatal.[2]

The problem in fighting viruses is that it's difficult to find drugs that harm the virus and not the cell it has commandeered. **Antibiotics** (drugs that inhibit or kill bacteria) have no effect on viruses. **Antiviral drugs** (such as amantadine for influenza and acyclovir for herpes simplex) don't completely eradicate a viral infection, although they can decrease its severity and duration. Because viruses multiply very quickly, antiviral drugs are most effective when taken before an infection develops or in its early stages.

Bacteria

Simple one-celled organisms, **bacteria** are the most plentiful microorganisms as well as the most pathogenic. Most kinds of bacteria don't cause disease; some, like the *Escherichia coli* that aid in digestion, play important roles within our bodies. Even friendly bacteria, however, can get out of hand and cause acne, urinary tract infections, vaginal infections, and other problems.

Bacteria harm the body by releasing enzymes that digest body cells or toxins that produce the specific effects of such diseases as diphtheria or toxic shock. In self-defense the body produces specific proteins (called *antibodies*) that attack and inactivate the invaders. Tuberculosis, tetanus, gonorrhea, scarlet fever, and diphtheria are examples of bacterial diseases.

Because bacteria are sufficiently different from the cells that make up our bodies, antibiotics can kill them without harming our cells. Some of these drugs are produced by microorganisms; others are synthetic agents. Antibiotics work only against specific types of bacteria. If your doctor thinks you have a bacterial infection, tests of your blood, pus, sputum, urine, or stool can identify the particular bacterial strain. Antibiotic medication is prescribed after determination of the bacteria.

Antibiotics may cause undesirable and sometimes serious side effects, including allergic reactions. Furthermore, frequent exposure of bacteria to a particular antibiotic may cause the bacteria to become resistant to that drug so that the antibiotic loses its effectiveness. As a result, in recent years, more virulent treatment-resistant forms of bacterial infections (discussed later in this chapter) have developed.

Fungi

Single-celled or multicelled organisms, **fungi** consist of threadlike fibers and reproductive spores. These plants, lacking chlorophyll, must obtain their food from organic material, which may include human tissue. Fungi release enzymes that digest cells, and are most likely to attack hair-covered areas of the body, including the scalp, beard, groin, and external ear canals. They also cause athlete's foot. Treatment consists of antifungal drugs.

Protozoa

These single-celled, microscopic animals release enzymes and toxins that destroy cells or interfere with their function. Diseases caused by **protozoa** are not a major health problem in this country, primarily because of public health measures. Around the world, however, some 2.24 billion people (more than 40% of the world's population) are at risk for acquiring one protozoa-caused disease—malaria—every year. Up to 3 million die of this disease annually.[3] Many more come down with amoebic dysentery. Treatment for protozoa-caused diseases consists of general medical care to relieve the symptoms, replacement of lost blood or fluids, and drugs that kill the specific protozoa.

The most common disease caused by protozoa in the United States is *giardiasis*, an intestinal infection caused by microorganisms in human and animal feces. It has become a threat at day-care centers, as well as among campers and hikers who drink contaminated water. Once ingested, giardia organisms use an adhesive sucker to stick to the intestinal walls, where they multiply and absorb nutrients from their host. Symptoms include nausea, lack of appetite, gas, diarrhea, fatigue, abdominal cramps, and bloating. Many people recover in a month or two even without treatment. However, in some cases, the microbe causes recurring attacks over many years. Giardiasis can be life-threatening in small children and the elderly, who are especially prone to severe dehydration from diarrhea. Treatment usually consists of antibiotics.

Helminths (Parasitic Worms)

Small parasitic worms that attack specific tissues or organs and compete with the host for nutrients are called **helminths**. One major worldwide health problem is *shistosomiasis,* a disease caused by a parasitic worm, the fluke, that burrows through the skin and enters the circulatory system. Infection with another helminth, the tapeworm, may be contracted from eating undercooked beef, pork, or fish containing larval forms of the tapeworm. Helminthic diseases are treated with appropriate medications.

Transmission of Infectious Diseases

The major vectors, or means of transmission, for infectious disease are animals/insects, person-to-person, food, water, and airborne.

Animals/Insects

Disease may be transmitted by house pets, livestock, or wild animals. Insects also spread a variety of diseases. The housefly may spread dysentery, diarrhea, typhoid fever, or trachoma (an eye disease rare in the United States but common in other parts of the world). Other insects, including mosquitoes, ticks, mites, fleas, and lice, can transmit such diseases as malaria, yellow fever, encephalitis, dengue fever (a growing threat in Mexico), and Lyme disease (discussed later in this chapter). In 1998, 1.4 million hens in Hong Kong were killed to prevent the spread of avian flu.[4]

Person-to-Person

The people you're closest to can transmit pathogens by coughing, sneezing, kissing, or sharing food or dishes with you. To avoid infection, stay out of range of anyone who's coughing, sniffling, or sneezing. Carefully wash your dishes, utensils, and hands, and abstain from sex or make self-protective decisions about sexual partners. (See the sections on STDs later in this chapter.)

Food

Every year foodborne illnesses strike millions of Americans, sometimes with fatal consequences. Bacteria account for two-thirds of foodborne infections, and thousands of suspected cases of infection with *Escherichia coli* bacteria in undercooked or inadequately washed food have been reported. (See Chapter 6 for a discussion of food safety.)

Every year as many as 4 million Americans have a bout with *salmonella* bacteria, which have been found in about a third of all poultry sold in the United States. These infections can be serious enough to require hospitalization, and can lead to arthritis, neurological problems, and even death. Consumers can greatly reduce the number of salmonella infections by following proper handling, cooking, and refrigeration.

A deadly food disease, *botulism,* is caused by certain bacteria that grow in improperly canned foods. Although its occurrence is rare in commercial products, botulism is a danger in home canning. Another uncommon threat is *trichinosis,* caused by the larvae of a parasitic roundworm in uncooked meat. This infection, which causes nausea, vomiting, diarrhea, fever, thirst, profuse sweating, weakness, and pain, can be avoided by thoroughly cooking meat.

Water

Waterborne diseases, such as typhoid fever and cholera, are still widespread in less developed areas of the world. They have been rare in the United States, although outbreaks caused by inadequate water purification have occurred. In 1993, for instance, water contaminated with the parasite *Cryptosporidium* sickened thousands in Milwaukee and caused severe, long-lasting bouts with diarrhea.

The Process of Infection

If someone infected with the flu sits next to you on a bus and coughs or sneezes, tiny viral particles may travel into your nose and mouth. Immediately the virus finds or creates an opening in the wall of a cell, and the process of infection begins. During the **incubation period**, the time between invasion and the first symptom, you're unaware of the pathogen multiplying inside you. In some diseases, incubation may go on for months, even years; for most, it lasts several days or weeks.

The early stage of the battle between your body and the invaders is called the *prodromal* period. As infected cells die, they release chemicals that help block the invasion. Other chemicals, such as *histamines,* cause blood vessels to dilate, thus allowing more blood to reach the battleground. During all of this, you feel mild, generalized symptoms, such as headache, irritability, and discomfort. You're also highly contagious. At the height of the battle—the typical illness period—you cough, sneeze, sniffle, ache, feel feverish, and lose your appetite.

Recovery begins when the body's forces gain the advantage. With time, the body destroys the last of the invaders and heals itself. However, the body is not able to develop long-lasting immunity to certain viruses, such as colds, flu, or HIV.

How Your Body Protects Itself

Various parts of your body safeguard you against infectious diseases and provide **immunity**, or protection, from these health threats. Your skin, when unbroken, keeps out most potential invaders. Your tears, sweat, skin oils, saliva, and mucus contain chemicals that can kill bacteria. Cilia, the tiny hairs lining your respiratory passages, move mucus, which traps inhaled bacteria, viruses, dust, and foreign matter, to the back of the throat, where it is swallowed; the digestive system then destroys the invaders.

When these protective mechanisms can't keep you infection-free, your body's immune system, which is on constant alert for foreign substances that might threaten the body, swings into action. The immune system includes structures of the lymphatic system, which includes the spleen, thymus gland, lymph nodes, and vessels called lymphatics that help filter impurities from the body (see Figure 11-2). More than a dozen different types of white blood cells are concentrated in the organs of the lymphatic system or, by way of the blood and lymph vessels, patrol the entire body. The two basic types of immune mechanisms are humoral and cell-mediated.

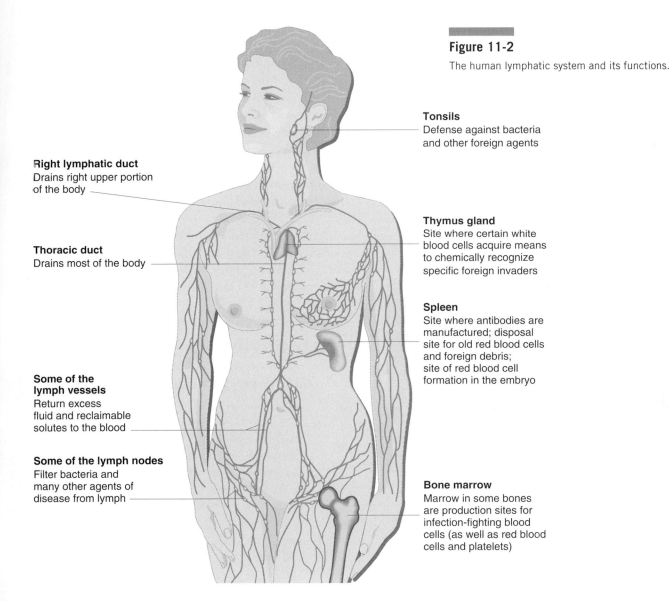

Figure 11-2
The human lymphatic system and its functions.

Tonsils
Defense against bacteria and other foreign agents

Right lymphatic duct
Drains right upper portion of the body

Thoracic duct
Drains most of the body

Thymus gland
Site where certain white blood cells acquire means to chemically recognize specific foreign invaders

Spleen
Site where antibodies are manufactured; disposal site for old red blood cells and foreign debris; site of red blood cell formation in the embryo

Some of the lymph vessels
Return excess fluid and reclaimable solutes to the blood

Some of the lymph nodes
Filter bacteria and many other agents of disease from lymph

Bone marrow
Marrow in some bones are production sites for infection-fighting blood cells (as well as red blood cells and platelets)

Humoral immunity refers to the protection provided by antibodies, proteins derived from white blood cells called B lymphocytes or B cells (see Figure 11-3). Humoral immunity is most effective during bacterial or viral infections. An *antigen* is any substance that enters the body and triggers production of an antibody. Once the body produces antibodies against a specific antigen—the mumps virus, for instance—you're protected against that antigen for life. If you're again exposed to mumps, the antibodies previously produced prevent another episode of the disease.

But you don't have to suffer through an illness to acquire immunity. Inoculation with a vaccine containing synthetic or weakened antigens can give you the same protection. The type of long-lasting immunity in which the body makes its own antibodies to a pathogen is called *active* immunity. Immunity produced by the injection of **gamma globulin**, the antibody-containing part of the blood, from another person or animal that has developed antibodies to a disease, is called *passive* immunity.

The various types of T cells are responsible for cellular, or **cell-mediated**, immunity. These lymphocytes are manufactured in the bone marrow and carried to the thymus for maturation. Cell-mediated immunity mainly protects against parasites, fungi, cancer cells, and foreign tissue (see Figure 11-3b). Thousands of different T cells work together to ward off disease. Some T cells activate other immune cells; others help in antibody-mediated responses; and still others suppress lymphocyte activity while others carry out different functions.

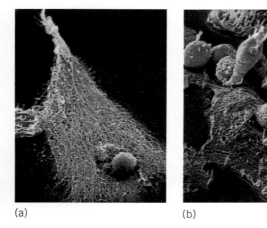

(a)   (b)

Figure 11-3

Types of lymphocytes. (a) B cell covered with bacteria. The B cells function in humoral immunity by producing antibodies. (b) T cells attack a caner cell. The T cells function in cell-mediated immunity.

Immune Response

Attacked by pathogens, the body musters its forces and fights. Sometimes the invasion is handled like a minor border skirmish; other times a full-scale battle is waged throughout the body. Together, the immune cells work like an internal police force. When an antigen enters the body, the T cells aided by *macrophages* (large scavenger cells with insatiable appetites for foreign cells, diseased and run-down red blood cells, and other biological debris), engage in combat with the invader. Meanwhile, the B cells churn out antibodies, which rush to the scene and join in the fray. Also busy at surveillance are natural killer cells that, like the elite forces of a SWAT team, seek out and destroy viruses and cancer cells.

The **lymph nodes**, or glands, are small tissue masses in which some protective cells are stored. If pathogens invade your body, many of them are carried to the lymph nodes, where they are then destroyed. This is why the lymph nodes often feel swollen when you have a cold or the flu.

If the microbes establish a foothold, the blood supply to the area increases, bringing oxygen and nutrients to the fighting cells. Tissue fluids, as well as antibacterial and antitoxic proteins, accumulate. You may develop redness, swelling, local warmth, and pain—the signs of **inflammation**. As more tissue is destroyed, a cavity, or **abscess**, forms, and fills with fluid, battling cells, and dead white blood cells (pus). If the invaders aren't killed or inactivated, the pathogens are able to spread into the bloodstream and cause what is known as **systemic disease**. The toxins released by the pathogens cause fever, and the infection becomes more dangerous.

Strategies for Prevention

Natural Ways to Bolster Immunity

✔ *Eat a balanced diet* to be sure you get essential vitamins and minerals. Severe deficiencies in vitamins B-6, B-12, and folic acid impair immunity. Keep up your iron and zinc intake. Iron influences the number and vigor of certain immune cells, whereas zinc is crucial for cell repair. Too little vitamin C may also increase susceptibility to infectious diseases.

✔ *Avoid fatty foods.* A low-fat diet can increase the activity of immune cells that hunt down and knock out cells infected with viruses.

✔ *Get enough sleep.* Without adequate rest, your immune system cannot maintain and renew itself.

✔ *Exercise regularly.* Aerobic exercise stimulates the production of an immune-system booster called interleukin-2.

✔ *Don't smoke.* Smoking decreases the levels of some immune cells.

✔ *Control your alcohol intake.* Heavy drinking interferes with normal immune responses and lowers the number of defender cells.

Immunity and Stress

Whenever we confront a crisis, large or small, our bodies produce powerful hormones that provide extra energy. However, this stress response dampens immunity, reducing the number of some key immune cells and the responsiveness of others. (See Chapter 2 for more on how our bodies respond to stress.)

As research into the field of psychoneuroimmunology (discussed in Chapter 4) has shown, psychological factors can affect immunity. When people are grieving for a loved one or lose their jobs, for instance, their immune systems show measurable impairment. People living with daily stress (caring for a parent with Alzheimer's disease, for example) or with episodic stress (such as final examinations in college) also have weakened immune responses. On the other hand, social contacts, through friendships, intimate relationships, or marriage, may bolster immunity.

Immune Disorders

Sometimes our immune system overreacts to certain substances, or mistakes the body's own tissues for enemies, or doesn't react adequately. The result is an immune disorder. The most common are **allergies**, which essentially represent a hypersensitivity to a substance in one's environment or diet.

One of the most costly of chronic conditions, allergies run up annual tabs of $1.8 to $2 billion in doctor visits, diagnostic tests, prescriptions, and decreased productivity. Every year they account for more than 10 million workdays missed; every day they keep 10,000 children out of school.

"Allergies may seem trivial to people who don't have them, but they have an enormous effect on a person's quality of life," says Robert Miles, M.D., of Lynchburg, VA, president-elect of the American College of Allergy, Asthma and Immunology.[5] Their symptoms are many and miserable: itching, nasal congestion, eye irritation, coughing, wheezing, hives, vomiting, and diarrhea (from food allergies), even sudden, life-threatening collapse (from anaphylaxis, the most extreme allergic reaction). While victims seldom die of allergies, they just as rarely recover. And when individuals try to outrun allergies by moving away from one region's irritants, they often end up acquiring new sensitivities on their new home ground.

A list of allergic triggers, or allergens, reads like an inventory of creation, including life's pleasures (such as foods and flowers), perils (insect stings and poison ivy), and inescapable realities (like mold and dust). The very air we breathe can be a danger. The symptoms of allergy and of its more sinister sister-disease, asthma, increase along with pollutants, such as diesel fumes, and the number of small particles in the environment.

But breakthroughs in treatments are helping many allergy sufferers breathe more easily. "In the past, allergy symptoms and medications both made people so drowsy that they often couldn't concentrate or function at their best," says Miles, who notes that today's allergy sufferers no longer have to choose between feeling better or feeling alert. Treatment options include oral medications, nasal sprays, and immunotherapy, which consists of a series of injections of small but increasing doses of an allergen. In its newest form, "rush" immunotherapy speeds up the normal schedule for allergy shots—sometimes from once a day to three to eight shots in a day. On this accelerated schedule, immunization can be completed in three to five days. Whatever the timetable, about 85% of allergy sufferers feel better after completing immunotherapy.[6]

Autoimmune disorders result when the immune system fails to recognize body tissue as self and attacks it. Many of these severely disabling diseases, such as myasthenia gravis, rheumatoid arthritis, and systemic lupus erythematosus, primarily strike women systematically in their childbearing years. These diseases, which often worsen with time, may be treated with drugs that suppress the immune system.

Some people have an **immune deficiency**—either inborn or acquired. A very few children are born without an effective immune system; their lives can be endangered by any infection. Although still experimental, genetic therapy to implant a missing or healthy gene may offer new hope for a normal life.

Immunization: The Key to Prevention

One of the great success stories of American medicine has been the development of vaccines that provide protection against many infectious diseases. Unfortunately, many Americans, including large numbers of children in urban centers, haven't been properly immunized. As a result, some diseases that had been considered under control, such as measles, mumps, and whooping cough (pertussis), have been occurring more often. At particular risk are children in poorer sections of large American cities, who often aren't immunized against measles and other so-called childhood diseases because of the cost.[7]

As shown in Table 11-1, the American Academy of Pediatrics recommends that all children be immunized against measles, mumps, German measles (rubella), diphtheria, tetanus, chickenpox, and hepatitis B. Although some vaccines confer lifelong protection, others do not. The protection provided by diphtheria and tetanus vaccinations, for example, diminishes over time, so booster vaccinations are required every ten years. Health officials also recommend measles booster shots for students entering college, and suggest that people born after 1956 be revaccinated for polio,

measles, and other infectious diseases before visiting developing countries.

If you're uncertain about your past immunizations, check with family members or your doctor. If you can't find answers, a blood test can show whether you carry antibodies to specific illnesses.

If you're pregnant or planning to get pregnant within the next three months, do not get a measles, mumps, rubella, or oral polio vaccination. If you're allergic to neomycin, consult your doctor before getting a measles, mumps, rubella, or intramuscular polio vaccination. Those with egg allergies should also check with a doctor before getting a measles, mumps, or flu vaccination. Also, never get a vaccination when you have a high fever.

Poliomyelitis

Immunization has greatly reduced the incidence of polio in the United States. A basic series of three oral-vaccine doses is recommended for infants at 2, 4, and 6 months of age. Boosters are recommended at 18 months of age and when entering school. These may be given along with the diphtheria, tetanus, and pertussis (DPT) vaccination, but many physicians prefer to separate the two. Additional boosters for polio aren't necessary, except when traveling to an area where the disease is common.

TABLE 11-1 RECOMMENDED CHILDHOOD IMMUNIZATION SCHEDULE

Vaccines are listed under the routinely recommended ages. Bars indicate range of acceptable ages for immunization. Catch-up immunization should be done during any visit when feasible. Shaded ovals indicate vaccines to be assessed and given if necessary during the early adolescent visit.

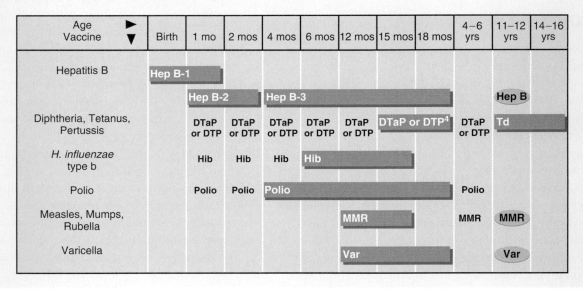

Age ▶ / Vaccine ▼	Birth	1 mo	2 mos	4 mos	6 mos	12 mos	15 mos	18 mos	4–6 yrs	11–12 yrs	14–16 yrs
Hepatitis B	Hep B-1	Hep B-2		Hep B-3						Hep B	
Diphtheria, Tetanus, Pertussis		DTaP or DTP	DTaP or DTP	DTaP or DTP	DTaP or DTP	DTaP or DTP	DTaP or DTP[4]		DTaP or DTP	Td	
H. influenzae type b		Hib	Hib	Hib	Hib						
Polio		Polio	Polio	Polio					Polio		
Measles, Mumps, Rubella						MMR			MMR	MMR	
Varicella						Var				Var	

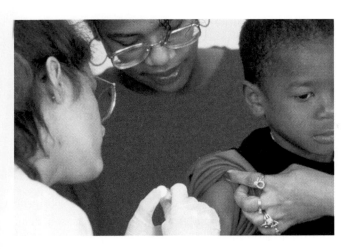

Immunizations are an important protection against childhood diseases. Neighborhood clinics in urban centers offer immunizations to those children at particular risk.

Tetanus (Lockjaw)

Tetanus is an uncommon disease transmitted via a variety of injuries. Since the tetanus germ cannot grow in the presence of air, puncture wounds, such as those caused by stepping on a nail or gardening rake, pose the greatest danger. Tetanus is often called "lockjaw," because the characteristic symptom is a stiffening of the jaws so severe that the patient is unable to open his or her mouth. Everyone should get booster inoculations for tetanus at least once every ten years.

Diphtheria

Diphtheria, a dangerous disease, is rare because of immunization. An average of fewer than three cases per year have been reported in the last decade.[8] Diphtheria and tetanus vaccinations (toxoids) are usually given in combination with the pertussis (whooping cough) vaccine-part of the DTP shot. The schedule for these consists of a basic series and two boosters prior to entering school. Older children and adults receive only diphtheria and tetanus toxoid (DT) in a more dilute form. Adults as well as children should get booster shots every ten years.

Pertussis

Pertussis (whooping cough), a bacterial infection that can develop into pneumonia, is potentially fatal. Until recently, the pertussis vaccine was made with killed whole pertussis cells and mixed with diphtheria and tetanus vaccines to make the whole cell DTP shot. For years parents have been concerned about its safety because of reports of permanent brain damage and even death. Careful analysis by many investigators found that any increased risk of permanent neurological damage was so small as to be virtually unmeasurable. However, new *acellular* pertussis vaccines, made of only a few parts of the pertussis cell, have proven effective against pertussis and produce fewer side effects.[9]

Measles

Measles, a potentially deadly infection, remains a serious health threat among high school and college students and inner-city preschool children. Although measles can be a mild disease in healthy children, the risk of severe complications, including permanent brain damage and death, increases with age. Measles occurs predominantly in unvaccinated preschoolers, particularly in urban areas and among African-American and Latino populations.

Symptoms include a rash on the face and body, runny nose, high fever, cough, eye inflammation, and fatigue. Ten to 15% of measles patients develop serious complications, such as ear infections, diarrhea, or pneumonia. One out of every 1000 develops encephalomyelitis, an inflammation of the brain that can be fatal or lead to mental retardation, or to movement, behavioral, or neurological disorders.

Centers for Disease Control (CDC) officials estimate that 5% to 15% of college students are susceptible to measles because they were vaccinated at 12 months of age rather than the currently recommended 15 months, or did not receive a second dose of the vaccine between ages 4 and 12. Others were given immune globulin, which was intended to lower the risk of reaction but which also reduced the vaccine's effectiveness. Many colleges are requiring students to submit proof of measles immunization before allowing them to enroll. In all, some 3 million Americans, aged 20 to 37, are at risk.

Rubella (German Measles)

About 85% of adults are immune to rubella, even if they have no history of the disease. The most serious result of this mild disease is the destructive effect it has on an unborn baby if the mother is infected in early pregnancy. All children should be immunized against rubella at 1 year of age or later.

Adults who are not immune may be immunized at any age, but women should not receive the vaccine during pregnancy or during the two to three months immediately preceding pregnancy. All unimmunized children in a pregnant woman's household should be immunized against rubella, for they are the most likely potential carriers. Recent outbreaks of rubella among newborns have been blamed on the lack of routine rubella screening and followup vaccination of susceptible women of childbearing age.

Varicella (Chickenpox)

A vaccine against chicken pox, a common childhood disease that causes itchy red pustules, was approved by the FDA and became available in 1995. The American Academy of Pediatrics recommends universal vaccination at the same time as first MMR vaccinations (see Table 11-1), as well as immunization for susceptible older children. After age 13, adolescents who have not been immunized previously and have not had chickenpox should receive two doses of the vaccine four to eight weeks apart.[10]

Hepatitis B

The U.S. Public Health Service recommends that children and adolescents be immunized against hepatitis B along with vaccinations for other illnesses. Vaccination also is recommended for all sexually active individuals.

HIB Infection

In the United States, *Hemophilus* influenza type B, or HIB, is the leading cause of bacterial *meningitis*, a life-threatening infection of the lining of the brain and spinal cord that afflicts 12,000 to 15,000 children each year and kills 5% to 10% of them. A vaccine protects children from this potentially deadly infection of the central nervous system. Sometimes found in children attending day-care programs, HIB often goes undiagnosed before irreparable damage is done; therefore, vaccination is particularly crucial and beneficial. The frequency of HIB infection has dropped by 95% in the 1990s.

Infectious Diseases

An estimated 500 microorganisms cause disease; no effective treatment exists for about 200 of these illnesses.[11] Although infections can be unavoidable at times, the more you know about their causes, the more you can do to protect yourself.

Who's at Highest Risk?

Like human bullies, the viruses responsible for the most common infectious illnesses tend to pick on those least capable of fighting back. Among the most vulnerable are the following groups:

- *Children and their families.* Youngsters get up to a dozen colds annually; adults average two a year. When a flu epidemic hits a community, about 40% of school-age boys and girls get sick, compared with only 5% to 10% of adults. But their parents get up to six times as many colds as other adults.[12]

- *The elderly.* Statistically, fewer older men and women are likely to catch a cold or flu, yet when they do, they face greater danger than the rest of the population. People over 65 who get the flu have a one in ten chance of being hospitalized for pneumonia or other respiratory problems, and a one in fifty chance of dying from the disease.[13]

- *The chronically ill.* Lifelong diseases, such as diabetes, kidney disease, or sickle cell anemia, decrease an individual's ability to fend off infections. Individuals taking medications that suppress the immune system, such as steroids, are more vulnerable to infections, as are those with medical conditions that impair immunity, such as infection with HIV, the virus that causes AIDS.

- *Smokers and those with respiratory problems.* Smokers are a high-risk group for respiratory infections and serious complications, such as pneumonia. Chronic breathing disorders, such as asthma and emphysema, also greatly increase the risk of respiratory infections.

- *Those who live or work in close contact with someone sick.* Health-care workers who treat high-risk patients, nursing home residents, and others living in close quarters—such as students in dormitories—face greater odds of catching others' colds and flus.

- *Residents or workers in poorly ventilated buildings.* The technology of the twentieth century has helped spread certain airborne illnesses, such as tuberculosis, via recirculated air. Indoor air quality may be closely linked with disease transmission in winter, when people spend a great deal of time in tightly sealed rooms.

The Common Cold

There are more than 200 distinct cold viruses, or rhinoviruses. Although in a single season you may develop a temporary immunity to one or two, you may then be hit by a third. Colds can strike in any season, but different cold viruses are more common at different times of years. Rhinoviruses cause most spring, summer, and early fall colds, and tend to cause more symptoms above the neck (stuffy nose, headache, runny eyes). Adenoviruses, parainfluenza viruses, corona viruses, influenza viruses, and others that strike in the winter are more likely to get into the bronchi and trachea (the breathing passages) and cause more fever and bronchitis. Cold viruses spread by coughs, sneezes, and touch. Cold-sufferers who sneeze and then touch a doorknob or countertop leave a trail of highly contagious viruses behind them.[14]

When cold symptoms do develop, what should you do? According to the latest word from health experts, less treatment may be more effective. Aspirin and acetaminophen (Tylenol) may suppress the antibodies the body produces to fight cold viruses and may actually increase some symptoms, such as nasal stuffiness. If you want an alternative to relieve achiness, try ibuprofen (brand names include Motrin, Advil, and Nuprin), which doesn't seem to affect immune responses. Moreover, children, teenagers, and young adults should never take aspirin for a cold or flu, because of the danger of Reye's syndrome, a potentially deadly disorder that can cause convulsions, coma, swelling of the brain, and kidney damage.

Not too long ago millions of Americans gulped Vitamin C to ward off colds, but large-scale research studies found no proof to back up this premise. Now many cold sufferers are thinking zinc, but the research remains inconclusive. In one study at the Cleveland Clinic Foundation, 100 adults who'd had cold symptoms for less than 24 hours sucked either on zinc gluconate lozenges or placebos every two hours during the day. The zinc users felt better in a median of 4.4 days, compared with 7.6 days for the others, and reported less coughing, hoarseness, nasal congestion, sore throat, and headache.[15]

The major complaints of the zinc-licking volunteers were a bad metallic taste, nausea, and mouth ulcers. Other studies have had conflicting results. Researchers caution that some zinc lozenges, particularly those sweetened with mannitol or sorbitol or containing citric acid, may not release as much zinc as the pure zinc compounds that have been tested.[16]

Echinacea, a flower derivative used in many herbal remedies, also is being touted as a cold cure. But there have been no scientific studies to prove it works—and some scientists fear that it may actually interfere with a healthy immune response. "Echinacea has never been tested properly to see if it works," says Jack Gwaltney, M.D., head of the Division of Epidemiology and Virology at the University of Virginia and one of the nation's premier cold experts. "Why waste your money and maybe even risk your health by trying something that hasn't been tested when effective symptom-relievers are available?"[17]

Although pharmacy shelves are brimming with an estimated 800 different cold remedies, most contain the same basic ingredients. Physicians advise against multi-symptom remedies, which usually provide medication (and side effects) for symptoms you don't have as well as those you do. Choose medications tailored to relieve specific symptoms, says Gwaltney, whose personal recommendation for a head cold is a 12-hour antihistamine and a nonsteroidal anti-inflammatory drug (such as ibuprofen), taken from first symptom for two or three days. "The more we study the first-generation antihistamines in scientific double-blind trials, the better they look," he says. "Combined with a painkiller, they work like gangbusters in relieving runny nose, sneezing, coughing, and malaise."

The main drawback of antihistamines is drowsiness, which can impair a person's ability to drive or operate machinery safely. Another ingredient, pseudoephedrine, can open and drain sinus passages without drowsiness but can speed up heart rate and cause complications for individuals with high blood pressure, diabetes, heart disease, or thyroid disorders. Nasal sprays can clear a stuffy nose, but they invariably cause a rebound effect. "The nose goes from stuffy to clear, stuffy to clear, and after three days a lot of people develop a sore throat. They blame the cold, but it's really from the spray dripping back through the sinuses," says Gwaltney.

For a cough, the ingredient to look for in any suppressant is dextromethrophan, which turns down the brain's cough reflex. In expectorants, the only medicine the FDA has deemed effective is guaifenesin, which helps liquefy secretions so you can bring up mucus from the chest. Unless you're coughing up green or foul yellow mucus—signs of a "secondary" bacterial infection—antibiotics won't help. They have no effect against viruses and may make your body more resistant to such medications when you develop a bacterial infection in the future.

Your own immune system can do something modern science cannot: cure a cold. All that it needs is time, rest, and plenty of fluids. Warmth also is important, because the aptly named "cold" viruses replicate at lower temperatures. Hot soups and drinks (particularly those with a touch of something pungent, like lemon or ginger) both raise body temperature and help clear the nose. Even more important is getting off your feet. Taking it easy reduces demands on the body, which helps speed recovery.

Strategies for Prevention

Taking Care of Your Cold

✔ Drink plenty of liquids (except alcohol) to liquify mucus, replace lost fluids, and prevent complications such as ear infections and bronchitis.

✔ If you have a sore throat, gargle with warm, salty water. While sprays or lozenges can relieve the pain of a sore throat, none cures the inflammation causing the discomfort.

✔ If you have a cough, a cold-mist humidifier or steam vaporizer will liquefy secretions and help more than expectorants (drugs that bring up the mucus in your chest). If you do use an expectorant, make sure it contains guaifenesin, the only ingredient the FDA has found effective. The primary benefit of cough suppressants is that they allow a person with a dry, hacking cough to sleep through the night.

✔ Symptoms requiring medical attention include: fever lasting more than four or five days, or rising over 104°F; yellow-green or rust-colored discharge from the nose or throat; significant pain in the throat, sinuses, eyes, or chest; or a cough that persists.

Influenza

Although similar to a cold, **influenza**—or the flu—causes more severe symptoms that last longer (see Table 11-

2). Some 25 to 50 million Americans come down with the flu every year. According to CDC estimates, influenza and pneumonia have accounted for 10,000 to 45,000 deaths in the last 20 years.

Flu viruses, transmitted by coughs, sneezes, laughs, and even normal conversation, are extraordinarily contagious, particularly in the first three days of the disease. The usual incubation period is two days, but symptoms can hit hard and fast. Two varieties of viruses—influenza A and influenza B—cause most flus. In recent years, the deadliest flu epidemics have been caused by various forms of influenza A viruses.

A vaccine against the flu is available, but it is not foolproof. "Because the flu virus is constantly changing, you need a new shot every year," explains Edwin Kilbourne, M.D., of New York Medical College, who has decided the components of each year's flu shots for 22 years. "And because it takes the body time to manufacture antibodies to the new viruses, you should get a vaccination at least 10 to 14 days before an outbreak hits your area."[18]

Long recommended for high-risk individuals, such as the elderly or chronically ill, flu shots now are advised for almost everyone. "The vaccine is so very safe, and the effects of the flu can be so serious that the only people we advise against it are those who are allergic to eggs. Doctors now recommend flu shots for pregnant women, particularly those who will be in the latter stages of pregnancy because flu could endanger an unborn child. "The vaccine is well proven to be safe and effective—providing 70 to 80 % protection against flu," says Kilbourne. The only individuals who should steer clear, as already noted, are those allergic to eggs, since the inactivated flu viruses are grown in chick embryos.

If you haven't had a flu shot and you develop symptoms of the flu, call your doctor. Two prescription medications—rimantadine and amantadine, taken as early as possible in the course of an infection—can reduce the severity and duration of symptoms. However, there is a risk of side effects, such as an increased risk of seizures in individuals with epilepsy, insomnia, loss of appetite, and jitteriness.

Scientists predict that better vaccines, flu drugs, cold remedies, and possibly even a cure are on the way. A new antiviral drug zanamivir can reduce the symptoms and lessen the duration of both types of flu viruses.[19] However, it can only be administered as an aerosol.[20]

TABLE 11-2   IS IT A COLD OR THE FLU?

	Cold	Flu
Symptoms		
Fever	Rare	Characteristic, high (102°F–104°F); lasts 3–4 days
Headache	Rare	Prominent
General aches, pains	Slight	Usual; often severe
Fatigue, weakness	Quite mild	Can last up to 2–3 weeks
Prostration (extreme exhaustion)	Never	Early and prominent
Stuffy nose	Common	Sometimes
Sneezing	Usual	Sometimes
Sore throat	Common	Sometimes
Chest discomfort, cough	Mild to moderate; hacking cough	Common; can become severe
Complications	Sinus congestion or earache	Bronchitis, pneumonia; can be life-threatening
Prevention	None	Annual vaccination; amantadine (an antiviral drug)
Treatment	Only temporary relief of symptoms	Amantadine within 24–48 hours after onset of symptoms

SOURCE: National Institutes of Health.

Strategies for Prevention

Protecting Yourself from Colds and Flus

✔ Wash your hands frequently with hot water and soap. In a public restroom, use a paper towel to turn off the faucet after you wash your hands, and avoid touching the doorknob. Wash objects used by someone contagious with a cold.

✔ Take good care of yourself: Make sure you're getting adequate sleep. Eat a balanced diet. Exercise regularly. Don't share food or drinks.

✔ Spend as little time as possible in crowds, especially in closed places, such as elevators and airplanes. When out, keep your distance from sneezers and coughers. Don't touch your eyes, mouth, and nose after being with someone who has cold symptoms.

✔ Use tissues rather than cloth handkerchiefs, which may harbor viruses for hours or days.

✔ Try to avoid irritating air pollutants. Don't smoke, which destroys protective cells in the airways and worsens any cough. Limit your intake of alcohol, which depresses white blood cells and increases the risk of bacterial pneumonia in flu sufferers.

Mononucleosis

You can get **mononucleosis** through kissing—or any other form of close contact. "Mono" is a viral disease that's most common among people 15 to 24 years old; its symptoms include a sore throat, headache, fever, nausea, and prolonged weakness. The spleen is swollen, and the lymph nodes are enlarged. You may also develop jaundice or a skin rash similar to German measles.

The major symptoms usually disappear within two to three weeks, but weakness, fatigue, and often depression may linger for at least two more weeks. The greatest danger is from physical activity that might rupture the spleen, resulting in internal bleeding. The liver may also become inflamed. A blood test can determine whether you have mono. However, there's no specific treatment for it, other than rest.

Chronic Fatigue Syndrome (CFS)

More than 3 million Americans have the array of symptoms known as **chronic fatigue syndrome (CFS)**.[21] According to the CDC, symptoms of chronic fatigue syndrome include chills or low grade fever, sore throat, tender lymph nodes, muscle pain, muscle weakness, extreme fatigue that doesn't improve with rest, headaches, joint pain (without swelling), neurological problems (confusion, memory loss, visual disturbances), and sleep disorders. Symptoms may begin suddenly and persist for six months to several years. Depression and anxiety attacks generally develop after ten months of illness.

Once dismissed as the yuppie flu, CFS has long baffled scientists. For several years, the number-one suspect was Epstein-Barr Virus (EBV), which causes mononucleosis and is a permanent resident in more than 90% of American adults, usually in latent form. However, the cause of CFS remains unknown. Some researchers contend that a single agent, perhaps a retrovirus, triggers the collapse of the immune system. Others think that repeated, undetected infections by bacteria, viruses, fungi, and parasites may lead to a gradual decline, while another theory blames symptoms on chronic low blood pressure.

Diagnosis of CFS remains difficult, although numerous studies have found significant immune abnormalities, such as high levels of certain immune cells (B lymphocytes and cytokines) that act as if they were constantly battling a viral infection. Researchers are working to develop a blood test that will definitively diagnose CFS. No specific treatments have proven effective for all patients, although some have responded to experimental drugs used to treat HIV infection and AIDS.

Hepatitis

At least five different viruses, referred to as **hepatitis** A, B, C, Delta, and E, can cause this inflammation of the liver. Newly identified viruses also may be responsible for some causes of what is called "non-A, non-B" hepatitis. An estimated 500,000 Americans contract hepatitis each year; about 6000 people die as a result.

All forms of hepatitis target the liver, the body's largest internal organ. Symptoms include headaches, fever, fatigue, stiff or aching joints, nausea, vomiting, and diarrhea. The liver becomes enlarged and tender to the touch; sometimes the yellowish tinge of jaundice develops. Treatment consists of rest, a high-protein diet, and the avoidance of alcohol and drugs that may stress the liver until the disease runs its course. Alpha interferon, a protein that boosts immunity and prevents viruses from replicating, may be used for some forms.

Most people begin to feel better after two or three weeks of rest, although fatigue and other symptoms can linger. As many as 10% of those infected with hepatitis B and up to two-thirds of those with hepatitis C become carriers of the virus for several years or even life. Some have persistent inflammation of the liver, which may cause mild or severe symptoms and increase the risk of liver cancer.

Hepatitis A, a less serious form, is generally transmitted by poor sanitation, primarily fecal contamination of food or water, and is less common in industrialized nations than in developing countries. Among those at highest risk in the United States are children and staff at day-care centers, residents of institutions for the mentally handicapped, sanitation workers, and workers who handle primates, such as monkeys. Gamma globulin can provide short-term immunity; vaccines against hepatitis A have been approved by the FDA.[22]

Hepatitis B, a potentially fatal disease transmitted through the blood and other bodily fluids, infects an estimated 350,000 people around the world each year. Once spread mainly by contaminated tattoo needles, needles shared by drug addicts, or transfusions of contaminated blood, hepatitis B is now transmitted mostly through sexual contact. It can cause chronic liver infection, cirrhosis, and liver cancer. At highest risk are male homosexuals, heterosexuals with multiple sex partners, health-care workers with frequent contact with blood, IV-drug abusers, and infants born to infected mothers. Vaccination can prevent hepatitis B and is recommended for children, teens, and adults at high risk.[23]

Hepatitis C, spread in the same way as hepatitis B, is the most common serious complication of blood transfusions. However, more effective screening tests have greatly reduced the risk of getting blood contaminated by hepatitis C virus. Hepatitis D, sometimes called the delta virus, can only infect individuals already suffering from hepatitis B. Because it is incomplete, this virus needs to borrow some proteins from the B virus in order to replicate. Like hepatitis B and C, it is spread by blood and bodily fluids. In the United States, it is most common among individuals who are in frequent contact with blood and among users of IV drugs. Hepatitis E is transmitted primarily through water contaminated by sewage. Although rare in the United States, this potentially deadly virus has caused epidemics in Africa and Asia.

Strategies for Prevention

Preventing Hepatitis

✔ Practice good personal hygiene, especially careful handwashing.

✔ If exposed to hepatitis A, get an injection of immune globulin serum, a solution containing antibodies against the virus.

✔ Obtain a vaccination against hepatitis B, if you're not already immunized.

✔ Do not use illegal drugs. If you must inject drugs (such as insulin), never share hypodermic needles.

✔ Avoid risky sexual behaviors. The safest sexual practices are abstinence or a monogamous relationship with an uninfected partner.

Pneumonia

An inflammation of the lungs, **pneumonia** fills the fine, spongy networks of the lungs' tiny air chambers with fluid. It can be caused by bacteria, viruses (including flu), or foreign material in the lungs (such as smoke). The symptoms of classic bacterial pneumonia are fever, shortness of breath, and general weakness. Along with influenza, pneumonia is the fifth-leading killer of Americans and the most common infectious cause of death.

The typical signs of pneumonia include cough, a fever of more than 101°F, difficulty breathing, chills, and excessive yellow green phlegm. Symptoms of pneumonia can develop either gradually or else so quickly that a person's life is in danger within hours. Antibiotics can control bacterial pneumonia, but they must be given before microbes erode local tissues and spread through the blood elsewhere in the body, causing a condition known as septicemia, or blood poisoning. Because of the dangers of pneumonia, you should see a doctor if there's any chance you have it. Severe cases may require hospitalization and high doses of antibiotics.

Vaccination against pneumonia is recommended for those who've had pneumonia in the past, those with impaired immune function, and those over age 50. The pneumonia vaccine greatly reduces the risk of this disease, especially for women and those with impaired immunity.

Tuberculosis

A bacterial infection of the lungs that was once the nation's leading killer, **tuberculosis (TB)** claims the lives of more people than any acute infectious disease other than pneumonia (Figure 11-4). One-third of the world's population is infected with the TB organism, although not all develop active disease. Each year the infection spreads to another 8 million people. In the United States, TB cases, after declining for decades, increased from the mid-1980s to the early 1990s. The reasons include immigration from countries where TB is common, poverty, homelessness, alcoholism and drug abuse, the HIV/AIDS epidemic, and the emergence of resistant strains of TB. By the mid-1990s, some cities reported a decline in TB, thanks to better infection control and greater monitoring to ensure completion of treatment.[24]

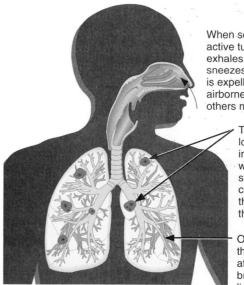

When someone with active tuberculosis exhales, coughs, or sneezes, tuberculosis is expelled in tiny airborne droplets that others may inhale.

The TB bacteria lodge mainly in the lungs, where they slowly multiply, creating patches, then cavities, in the lungs.

Other parts of the lung are affected, including bronchi and the lining of the lung.

If untreated, TB can eventually spread to and damage the brain, bone, eyes, liver and kidneys, spine, and skin.

Figure 11- 4

How tuberculosis spreads.

Although TB is most prevalent among high-risk groups, the overall danger increases as more people develop active disease because TB is highly contagious. TB outbreaks have occurred throughout the country in hospitals, nursing homes, prisons, and office buildings, where inadequate ventilation increases the risk of infection.

Most TB patients recover completely after six months of taking a combination of three different medicines. Drug-resistant forms of the tuberculosis microorganism strike mostly patients who start drug treatment but don't follow through with it. Because they don't take enough of the medication to kill all the TB bacteria in their system, those that survive become resistant. Even with full treatment, the risk of dying from drug-resistant tuberculosis is 50%. HIV infection greatly increases susceptibility to infection with TB and the risk of dying if infected with treatment-resistant forms.[25]

If you think you may have been exposed to TB or if you develop suspicious symptoms (loss of appetite and weight, low-grade fever, fatigue, chills, night sweats, coughing), see your doctor for a TB test. This consists of an injection just under the skin. The area of the arm where the test was administered should be checked by a health-care professional. The test results help to determine the presence of the TB bacteria; further tests confirm the diagnosis. If the skin test is positive, indicating that TB is present, you'll be monitored with yearly chest X rays. You may also require treatment with a drug such as refampin or isoniazid (also called INH).

Group A and Group B Strep Infection

Sore throats are common winter complaints, but those caused by group A streptococcus bacteria—"strep throats"—are more than a trivial threat. If not treated promptly with antibiotics, strep bacteria can travel to the kidneys, the liver, or the heart, where they can cause rheumatic fever—an inflammation of the heart that can cause weakness, shortness of breath, joint pain, and an abnormal heartbeat. In recent years clusters of rheumatic fever have sprung up in several major cities. Pediatricians are urging parents to consult their doctors if a youngster complains of a sore throat or if strep is widespread in the community. Rapid new diagnostic tests can identify strep within minutes. If the test is positive, treatment with penicillin or a similar antibiotic is indicated.

A new danger linked with group A strep is toxic streptococcal shock syndrome, or toxic strep. This is an invasive form of the disease in which strep gains access to the blood and causes a drop in blood pressure, a very high fever, and the production of exotoxins (substances that can attack various organs, such as the kidneys, heart or, in rare cases, flesh). Toxic strep is rather rare and usually doesn't occur with strep throats. Prompt treatment is critical.[26]

Group B streptococcus (GBS), the leading cause of life-threatening perinatal infections in the United States, is primarily a threat to newborns. Because some 15% to 40% of pregnant women carry GBS but have no symptoms, the American Academy of Pediatrics has called for universal screening of expectant mothers. Each year 12,000 newborns are infected, most of them during childbirth; more than 1600 die, and another 1600 suffer permanent brain damage from meningitis. Women at high risk of infecting their newborns with GBS are those who have premature labor, early rupture of their amniotic membranes, fever, and a high group B strep count before or during pregnancy, or who have previously borne an infant infected with GBS. Also at risk are diabetics, poor women, and those under age 20. Treating all high-risk pregnant women could prevent most GBS infections in newborns.

Toxic Shock Syndrome

As discussed in Chapter 9, **toxic shock syndrome (TSS)** is a potentially deadly disease associated with the use of tampons, particularly high-absorbency types. It is caused by *Staphylococcus aureus* and group A *Streptococcus pyogenes* bacteria that release toxins (poisonous waste products) into the bloodstream. Symptoms include a high fever; a rash that leads to peeling of the skin on the fingers, toes, palms, and soles; dizziness; dangerously low blood pressure; and abnormalities in several organ systems (the digestive tract and the kidneys) and in the muscles and blood.

In addition to women who use high-absorbency tampons, or leave their tampons in too long, those who have given birth within the preceding six to eight weeks are at greater risk.[27] Children (including newborns), men, and postmenopausal women also have developed TSS, which usually has been traced to bacteria in skin abscesses, boils, cuts, or postsurgical wounds.

Without prompt treatment, TSS can cause severe and permanent damage, including muscle weakness, partial paralysis, amnesia, disorientation, an inability to concentrate, and impaired lung and kidney function. Sometimes toxic shock weakens the blood vessels, increasing the risk of heart problems. Victims can enter the state of life-threatening crisis called shock, in which blood flow throughout the body is inadequate to sustain life. Treatment usually consists of immediate hospitalization, intravenous administration of fluids, medications to raise blood pressure, and powerful antibiotics; intravenous administration of immunoglobins that attack the toxins produced by these bacteria may also be beneficial.

Lyme Disease

Lyme disease, a bacterial infection, is spread by ticks carrying a kind of bacterium, the spirochete *Borrelia burgdorferi*. An infected person may have various symptoms, including joint inflammation, heart arrhythmias, blinding headaches, and memory lapses. The disease can also cause miscarriages and birth defects. Lyme disease is by far the most commonly reported vector-borne infectious disease in the United States.[28]

The vast majority of all reported cases have occurred in just ten states; those leading the list are New York, New Jersey, Connecticut, Pennsylvania, and Wisconsin.[29] Nationwide cases of Lyme disease dropped 36% in 1997, compared with 1991.[30]

The primary culprit in most cases of Lyme disease is the deer tick, although other ticks, including the Western black-legged tick, the dog tick, and the Lone Star tick, also may transmit the bacterium that causes Lyme disease as well as organisms that transmit other diseases, such as Rocky Mountain spotted fever and babesiosis.

Hunters and campers are more likely to test positive for Lyme disease. Pet owners are not at additional risk. The most important preventive step is to check yourself for ticks whenever you come in from the outdoors. However, detecting some types of ticks can be difficult. In their nymphal stage, when they're most likely to bite, ticks are about the size of a poppyseed. Even as adults, some ticks are no bigger than a sesame seed.

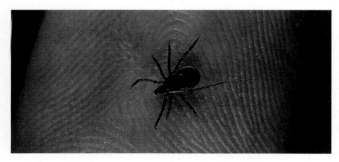

Ticks are responsible for the spread of Lyme disease. If you spot a tick, remove it as soon as possible with tweezers or small forceps. Put it in a plastic bag or sealed bottle and save it. If you develop a rash or other symptoms, take it with you to the doctor.

Regardless of whether or not they've spotted a tick, residents of infested areas should check regularly for signs of a bite. About two-thirds of those bitten develop some skin changes from two days to four weeks afterward. The classic skin lesion is a small, clear-centered red doughnut that expands, but most people simply have a red blotch or two blotches. However, the rash always expands, usually to about 2 inches in diameter. In some cases, it may cover a person's entire chest or thigh; others develop rashes far from the bite, caused by spirochetes that travel through the bloodstream. More sensitive diagnostic tests allow detection of extremely low numbers of spirochetes and make earlier diagnosis possible.

Strategies for Prevention

Protecting Yourself

✔ If you live in the North Atlantic states, the north central Midwest, or along the Pacific coast, wear long pants rather than shorts, and tuck your pants into your socks when walking through woods or fields of high grass.

✔ Stick to the center of trails when hiking, and avoid piles of leaves and branches.

✔ In tick-infested areas, use insect repellents. People who use insect repellents are half as likely to get Lyme disease as those who don't.

✔ After spending time outdoors, examine yourself for ticks or bites every day. Check less obvious places, such as the scalp and behind the ears.

✔ If you do spot a tick, remove it right away. Using tweezers or forceps, grasp the tick firmly as close to its head and as near to your skin as possible. Gently pull backward, without squeezing the tick's body, until its hold is released. Wash your hands thoroughly. Treat the wound with rubbing alcohol.

The Threat of Emerging and Re-Emerging Infectious Diseases

As defined by the National Institute of Allergy and Infectious Diseases (NIAID), emerging infections are those that have been recently recognized, are increasing in humans, or threaten to spread to new areas in the near future. The most widespread is HIV, which is believed to have emerged from Central Africa less than 20 years ago.

Other emerging viruses, such as Hantavirus, Ebola, dengue, Lassa, and Marburg, have been responsible for deadly outbreaks around the globe (see Spotlight on Diversity: "A World of Viruses"). The most well-known may be Ebola, a particularly virulent virus that is transmitted by direct contact with blood or bodily fluids. In several outbreaks in Africa, this filovirus has resisted all medication and killed up to 90% of its victims.[31]

Another threat comes from mutated, or changed, forms of familiar microbes (such as those that cause tuberculosis) that have become resistant to standard medications. Why, despite enormous scientific progress, do emerging and resistant microbes remain such a formidable foe? "Viruses and bacteria have the capacity to reinvent themselves rapidly," says John La Montagne, Ph.D, of NIAID. "Because they have few genes compared to people, one mutation can change an organism's ability to infect, spread, or cause disease."[32] There are other reasons why deadly infections are becoming a greater threat. As civilization spreads into previously undeveloped areas, such as the rainforests of Central Africa, and goods and animals are imported from distant lands, more human beings are encountering microbes that were once confined to very remote regions.

Reproductive and Urinary Tract Infections

Reproductive and urinary tract infections are very common. Many are not spread exclusively by sexual contact, and so they are not classified as sexually transmitted diseases (STDs), discussed later in this chapter.

Vaginal Infections

The most common vaginal infections are **trichomoniasis**, **candidiasis**, and **bacterial vaginosis**.

Protozoa (*Trichomonas vaginalis*) that live in the vagina can multiply rapidly, causing itching, burning, and discharge—all symptoms of trichomoniasis. Male carriers usually have no symptoms, although some may develop urethritis or an inflammation of the prostate and seminal vesicles. All patients with this infection should be screened for syphilis, gonorrhea, chlamydia, and HIV. Sexual partners must be treated with oral medication (metronidazol; trade name Flagyl), even if they have no symptoms, to prevent reinfection.

Populations of a yeast called *Candida albicans*—normal inhabitants of the mouth, digestive tract, and

vagina—are usually held in check. Under certain conditions, however (such as poor nutrition, stress, or antibiotic use), the microbes multiply, causing burning, itching, and a whitish discharge. Common sites for candidiasis, which is also called moniliasis, are the vagina, vulva, penis, and mouth. Vaginal medications, such as GyneLotrimin and Monistat, available as OTC drugs for women with recurrent infections, provide effective treatment. Male sexual partners may be advised to wear condoms during outbreaks of candidiasis. Women should keep the genital area dry and wear cotton underwear.

Bacterial vaginosis is characterized by alterations in the microorganisms that live in the vagina, including depletion of certain bacteria and overgrowth of others. It typically causes a white or gray vaginal discharge with a distinctive fishy odor similar to that of trichomoniasis. Its underlying cause is unknown, although it occurs most frequently in women with multiple sex partners. Long-term dangers include pelvic inflammatory disease (PID), (discussed later in this chapter) and pregnancy complications. Metronidazole, either in the form of a pill or a vaginal gel, is the primary treatment. According to CDC guidelines, treatment for male sex partners appears to be of little benefit, but some health practitioners recommend treatment for both partners in cases of recurrent infections.[33]

Urinary Tract Infections (UTIs)

A urinary tract infection (UTI) can be present in any of the three parts of the urinary tract: the urethra, bladder, or kidney. An infection involving the urethra is known as **urethritis**. If the bladder is also infected, it's called **cystitis**. If it reaches the kidneys, it's called **pyelonephritis**.

Three times as many women as men develop UTIs, probably for anatomical reasons. A woman's urethra is only 1.5 inches long; a man's is 6 inches. Therefore bacteria, the major cause of UTIs, have a shorter distance to travel to infect a woman's bladder and kidneys. About one-fourth to one-third of all women between ages 20 and 40 develop UTIs, and 80% of those who experience one infection develop recurrences.

Conditions that can set the stage for UTIs include irritation and swelling of the urethra or bladder as a result of pregnancy, bike riding, irritants (such as bubble bath, douches, or a diaphragm), urinary stones, enlargement in men of the prostate gland, vaginitis, and stress. Early diagnosis is critical, because infection can spread

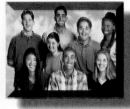

Spotlight on Diversity
A World of Viruses

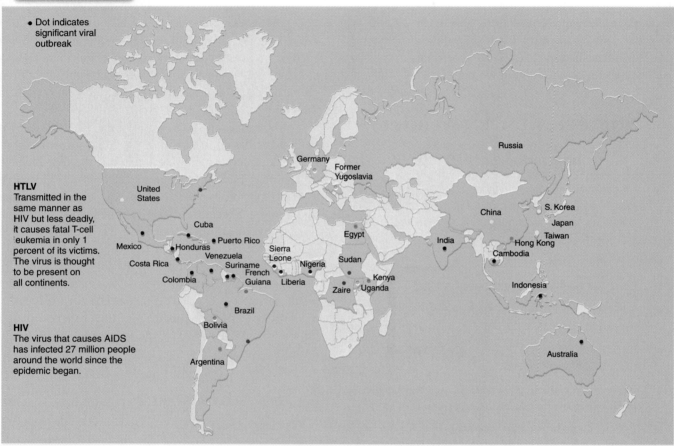

• Dot indicates
  significant viral
  outbreak

HTLV
Transmitted in the
same manner as
HIV but less deadly,
it causes fatal T-cell
leukemia in only 1
percent of its victims.
The virus is thought
to be present on
all continents.

HIV
The virus that causes AIDS
has infected 27 million people
around the world since the
epidemic began.

Russia

Germany
Former
Yugoslavia

S. Korea
Japan
China
Taiwan
Hong Kong
Cambodia
Indonesia
India

United
States
Cuba
Puerto Rico
Mexico
Honduras
Venezuela
Costa Rica
Suriname
French
Colombia
Guiana
Sierra
Leone
Nigeria
Egypt
Sudan
Liberia
Zaire
Uganda
Kenya
Brazil
Bolivia
Argentina
Australia

Key

In the past decades, more than a dozen threatening viruses have emerged. Whether they are due to people encroaching on untouched land, faster travel, or reasons still unknown, these infections are taxing an already depleted global health network. Some better-known cases:

• **"Bird Flu"** — Hong Kong. A new flu strain that emerged in the winter of 1997–1998.

• **Dengue** — Severe strains of this mosquito-borne tropical virus have emerged in Asia and Latin America since the mid-70s. There were 116,000 infections in Latin America alone in 1990.

• **Ebola** — (*filovirus*) With a fatality rate of up to 90 percent, it killed hundreds in Zaire and western Sudan in 1976 and 1979. A new outbreak in Kikwit, Zaire, has killed scores.

• **Hanta Virus** — A new form of this East Asian, rodent-borne virus appeared in the southwestern U.S. in May 1993, taking 12 lives; 106 cases, more than half fatal, have since been reported in 23 states.

• **Junín** — (*arenavirus*) First identified in 1953 near the Junín River in northern Argentina. Spread by field mice, it kills 20 percent of its victims.

• **Lassa** — (*arenavirus*) The virus that causes African hemorrhagic fever infects 200,000 to 400,000 annually in West Africa, killing approximately 5,000.

• **Machupo** — (*arenavirus*) This rodent-borne virus re-emerged last year in northern Bolivia when 7 family members were infected in Magdalena; 6 died.

• **Marburg** — (*filovirus*) Closely related to Ebola, this virus was identified in 1967 when 31 people were infected in West Germany and Yugoslavia by Ugandan green monkeys. 7 died.

• **Oropouche** — (*arbovirus*) Identified in 1961 after causing flulike symptoms in 11,000 residents of Belém, Brazil. Transmitted by the biting midge, or sandfly.

• **Rift Valley Fever** — (*arbovirus*) In the 1950s, this mosquito-borne virus was recognized in northern Kenya. An epidemic occurred in Egypt's Nile River delta in 1977, with more than 10,000 infected.

• **Sabiá** — (*arenavirus*) This new virus was identified in 1990 in Sao Paulo, Brazil. Last year a Yale scientist accidentally infected himself and survived.

SOURCES: World Health Organization, Pan American Health Organization; *Newsweek*.

to the kidneys and, if unchecked, result in kidney failure. Symptoms include frequent burning, painful urination, chills, fever, fatigue, and blood in the urine.

Recurrent UTIs, a frequent problem among young women, have been linked with a genetic predisposition, sexual intercourse, and the use of diaphragms. Postintercourse treatment with antibiotics can lower the risk. Frequent recurrence of symptoms may not be caused by infection but by interstitial cystitis, a little-understood bladder inflammation that affects an estimated 450,000 Americans, almost all of them women.[34]

Strategies for Prevention

How to Prevent UTIs

✔ Be conscientious about general cleanliness. Since a major cause of UTIs is the bacteria normally found in stools, be sure to wipe from front to back after bowel movements.

✔ Drink five to six glasses of water a day.

✔ Don't wait when you feel the urge to urinate.

✔ Don't use chemical irritants, such as perfumed hygiene sprays or bubble bath.

✔ If you use a diaphragm, have the fit checked regularly, especially after giving birth.

✔ If UTIs seem to follow sex, ask about prophylactic medication. Urinate immediately after intercourse.

✔ If you have a relapse after treatment or have recurrent infections, ask your partner to get a checkup too.

Sexually Transmitted Diseases (STDs)

Venereal diseases (from the Latin *venus*, meaning "love" or "lust") are more accurately called **sexually transmitted diseases (STDs)**. Around the world, more than 250 million cases of STDs are diagnosed each year (more than a million are of HIV).[35] Almost 700,000 people are infected every day with one of the over 20 STDs tracked by world health officials. STDs are much more widespread (or "prevalent") in developing nations because of lack of adequate health standards, prevention practices, and access to treatment.

More Americans are infected with STDs now than at any other time in history. They are among the top ten most frequently reported diseases in the United States,

and their annual economic cost is $17 billion.[36] The major cause of preventable sterility in America, STDs have tripled the rate of ectopic (tubal) pregnancies, which can be fatal if not detected early. STD complications, including miscarriage, premature delivery, and uterine infections after delivery, affect more than 100,000 women annually. Moreover, infection with an STD greatly increases the risk of HIV transmission (discussed later in this chapter). The incidence of STDs is highest in young adults and homosexual men. Others affected by STDs include unborn and newborn children who can "catch" potentially life-threatening infections in the womb or during birth.

Although each STD is a distinct disease, all STD pathogens like dark, warm, moist body surfaces, particularly the mucous membranes that line the reproductive organs; they hate light, cold, and dryness. It is possible to catch or have more than one STD at a time. Curing one doesn't necessarily cure another, and treatments don't prevent another bout with the same STD. (See Table 11-3.)

Many STDs, including early HIV infection and gonorrhea in women, may not cause any symptoms. As a result, infected individuals can continue their usual sexual activity without realizing that they're jeopardizing others' well-being. (See the Self-Survey: "STD Attitude Scale.")

STDs, Adolescents, and Young Adults

STDs strike both sexes, all classes, and all ages. However, the young are at greatest risk. According to the CDC, 86% of all STDs in the United States occur among 15- to 29-year-olds; as many as half of all young people may develop an STD by age 30.[37]

Recently, the rate of HIV infection among American teenagers has begun to skyrocket. No one knows precisely how many teens are HIV-positive. However, many more girls than boys are infected through heterosexual intercourse. According to the CDC, in the category of those under age 25, 39% of females and 5% of males were exposed to HIV infection through heterosexual contact.[38]

Various behaviors put teenagers at risk of STDs, including:

• *Feelings of invulnerability*, which lead to risk-taking behavior. Even when they are well-informed of the risks, adolescents may remain unconvinced that anything bad can or will happen to them.

• *Multiple partners.* In a survey of 11,631 high school

TABLE 11-3   COMMON SEXUALLY TRANSMITTED DISEASES (STDS): MODE OF TRANSMISSION, SYMPTOMS, AND TREATMENT

STD	TRANSMISSION	SYMPTOMS	TREATMENT
Chlamydial infection	The *Chlamydia trachomatis* bacterium is transmitted primarily through sexual contact. It may also be spread by fingers from one body site to another.	In women, PID (pelvic inflammatory disease) caused by *Chlamydia* may include disrupted menstrual periods, pelvic pain, elevated temperature, nausea, vomiting, headache, infertility, and ectopic pregnancy. In men, chlamydial infection of the urethra may cause a discharge and burning during urination. *Chlamydia*-caused epididymitis may produce a sense of heaviness in the affected testicle(s), inflammation of the scrotal skin, and painful swelling at the bottom of the testicle.	Doxycycline, azithromycin, or ofloxacin
Gonorrhea ("clap")	The *Neisseria gonorrhoeae* bacterium ("gonococcus") is spread through genital, oral–genital, or genital–anal contact.	The most common symptoms in men are a cloudy discharge from the penis and burning sensations during urination. If disease is untreated, complications may include inflammation of scrotal skin and swelling at base of the testicle. In women, some green or yellowish discharge is produced but commonly remains undetected. Later, PID (pelvic inflammatory disease) may develop.	Dual therapy of a single dose of ceftriaxone, cefixime, ciprofloxacin, or ofloxacin plus doxycycline for seven days
Non-gonococcal urethritis (NGU)	Primary causes are believed to be the bacteria *Chlamydia trachomatis* and *Ureaplasma urealyticum*, most commonly transmitted through coitus. Some NGU may result from allergic reactions or from *Trichomonas* infection.	Inflammation of the urethral tube. A man has a discharge from the penis and irritation during urination. A woman may have a mild discharge of pus from the vagina but often shows no symptoms.	Doxycycline or erythromycin
Syphilis	The *Treponema pallidum* bacterium ("spirochete") is transmitted from open lesions during genital, oral–genital, or genital–anal contact.	*Primary stage:* A painless chancre appears at the site where the spirochetes entered the body. *Secondary stage:* The chancre disappears and a generalized skin rash develops. *Latent stage:* There may be no visible symptoms. *Tertiary stage:* Heart failure, blindness, mental disturbance, and many other symptoms occur. Death may result.	Benzathine penicillin G, doxycycline, tetracycline, or erythromycin
Chancroid	The *Haemophilus ducreyi* bacterium is usually transmitted by sexual interaction.	Small bumps (papules) in genital regions eventually rupture and form painful, soft, craterlike ulcers that emit a foul-smelling discharge.	Single doses of either ceftriaxone or azithromycin or seven days of erythromycin
Herpes	The genital herpes virus (HSV-2) seems to be transmitted primarily by vaginal, anal, or oral–genital intercourse. The oral herpes virus (HSV-1) is transmitted primarily by kissing.	Small, painful red bumps (papules) appear in the genital region (genital herpes) or mouth (oral herpes). The papules become painful blisters that eventually rupture to form wet, open sores.	No known cure; a variety of treatments may reduce symptoms; oral or intravenous acyclovir (Zovirax) promotes healing and suppresses recurrent outbreaks.

continued

TABLE 11-3   CONTINUED...

STD	TRANSMISSION	SYMPTOMS	TREATMENT
Genital warts (condylomata acuminata)	The virus is spread primarily through vaginal, anal, or oral-genital sexual interaction.	Hard and yellow-gray on dry skin areas; soft, pinkish-red, and cauliflowerlike on moist areas.	Freezing, application of topical agents like trichloroacetic acid or podofilox, cauterization, surgical removal, or vaporization by carbon dioxide laser
Viral hepatitis	The hepatitis B virus may be transmitted by blood, semen, vaginal secretions, and saliva. Manual, oral, or penile stimulation of the anus are strongly associated with the spread of this virus. Hepatitis A seems to be primarily spread via the fecal–oral route. Oral–anal sexual contact is a common mode for sexual transmission of hepatitis A.	Vary from nonexistent to mild, flulike symptoms to an incapacitating illness characterized by high fever, vomiting, and severe abdominal pain.	No specific therapy; treatment generally consists of bed rest and adequate fluid intake.
Bacterial vaginosis	The most common causative agent, the *Gardnerella vaginalis* bacterium, is sometimes transmitted through coitus.	In women, a fishy- or musty-smelling, thin discharge, like flour paste in consistency and usually gray. Most men are asymptomatic.	Metronidazole (Flagyl) by mouth or intravaginal applications of topical metronidazole gel or clindamycin cream
Candidiasis (yeast infection)	The *Candida albicans* fungus may accelerate growth when the chemical balance of the vagina is disturbed; it may also be transmitted through sexual interaction.	White, "cheesy" discharge; irritation of vaginal and vulval tissues.	Vaginal suppositories or topical cream, such as clotrimazole and miconazole, or oral fluconazole
Trichomoniasis	The protozoan parasite *Trichomonas vaginalis* is usually passed through genital sexual contact.	White or yellow vaginal discharge with an unpleasant odor; vulva is sore and irritated.	Metronidazole (Flagyl) for both women and men
Pubic lice ("crabs")	*Phthirus pubis*, the pubic louse, is spread easily through body contact or through shared clothing or bedding.	Persistent itching. Lice are visible and may often be located in pubic hair or other body hair.	Preparations such as A-200 pyrinate or Kwell (gamma benzene hexachloride)
Scabies	*Sarcoptes scabiei* is highly contagious and may be transmitted by close physical contact, sexual and nonsexual.	Small bumps and a red rash that itch intensely, especially at night.	5% permethrin lotion or cream
Acquired immuno-deficiency syndrome (AIDS)	Blood and semen are the major vehicles for transmitting HIV, which attacks the immune system. It appears to be passed primarily through sexual contact, or needle sharing among injecting drug users.	Vary with the type of cancer or opportunistic infections that afflict an infected person. Common symptoms include fevers, night sweats, weight loss, chronic fatigue, swollen lymph nodes, diarrhea and/or bloody stools, atypical bruising or bleeding, skin rashes, headache, chronic cough, and a whitish coating on the tongue or throat.	Commence treatment early after seroconversion with a combination of three antiviral drugs ("triple drug therapy") plus other specific treatment(s), if necessary, of opportunistic infections and tumors.

Source: Crooks, Robert, and Baur, Karla. *Our Sexuality*, 7th ed. Pacific Grove, CA: Brooks Cole, 1999.

Self-Survey

STD Attitude Scale

Directions: Please read each statement carefully: STD means sexually transmitted diseases, once called venereal diseases. Record your first reaction by marking an "X" through the letter that best describes how much you agree or disagree with the idea.

Use This Key: SA = Strongly agree; A = Agree; U = Undecided; D = Disagree; SD = Strongly disagree.

Remember: STD means sexually transmitted disease, such as gonorrhea, syphilis, genital herpes, and AIDS.

1. How one uses his/her sexuality has nothing to do with STDs.

    SA   A   U   D   SD

2. It is easy to use the prevention methods that reduce one's chances of getting an STD.

    SA   A   U   D   SD

3. Responsible sex is one of the best ways of reducing the risk of STDs.

    SA   A   U   D   SD

4. Getting early medical care is the main key to preventing harmful effects of STDs.

    SA   A   U   D   SD

5. Choosing the right partner is important in reducing the risk of getting an STD.

    SA   A   U   D   SD

6. A high rate of STDs should be a concern for all people.

    SA   A   U   D   SD

7. People with an STD have a duty to get their sex partners to seek medical care.

    SA   A   U   D   SD

8. The best way to get a sex partner to STD treatment is to take him/her to the doctor with you.

    SA   A   U   D   SD

9. Changing one's sex habits is necessary once the presence of an STD is known.

    SA   A   U   D   SD

10. I would dislike having to follow the medical steps for treating an STD.

    SA   A   U   D   SD

11. If I were sexually active, I would feel uneasy doing things before and after sex to prevent getting an STD.

    SA   A   U   D   SD

12. If I were sexually active, it would be insulting if a sex partner suggested we use a condom to avoid STDs.

    SA   A   U   D   SD

13. I dislike talking about STDs with my peers.

    SA   A   U   D   SD

14. I would be uncertain about going to the doctor unless I was sure I really had an STD.

    SA   A   U   D   SD

15. I would feel that I should take my sex partner with me to a clinic if I thought I had an STD.

    SA   A   U   D   SD

16. It would be embarrassing to discuss STDs with one's partner if one were sexually active.

    SA   A   U   D   SD

17. If I were to have sex, the chance of getting an STD makes me uneasy about having sex with more than one person.

    SA   A   U   D   SD

18. I like the idea of sexual abstinence (not having sex) as the best way to avoid STDs.

    SA   A   U   D   SD

19. If I had an STD, I would cooperate with public health persons to find the sources of the STD.

    SA   A   U   D   SD

20. If I had an STD, I would avoid exposing others while I was being treated.

    SA   A   U   D   SD

21. I would have regular STD checkups if I were having sex with more than one partner.

    SA   A   U   D   SD

22. I intend to look for STD signs before deciding to have sex with anyone.

    SA   A   U   D   SD

23. I will limit my sex activity to just one partner because of the chances I might get an STD.

    SA   A   U   D   SD

24. I will avoid sex contact anytime I think there is even a slight chance of getting an STD.

    SA   A   U   D   SD

25. The chance of getting an STD would not stop me from having sex.

    SA   A   U   D   SD

26. If I had a chance, I would support community efforts toward controlling STDs.

    SA   A   U   D   SD

27. I would be willing to work with others to make people aware of STD problems in my town.

    SA   A   U   D   SD

Self-Survey   Continued...

Scoring: Calculate total points for each subscale and total scale, using the point values below.

For items 1, 10–14, 16, 25:

Strongly agree = 5 points;   Disagree = 2 points; and
Agree = 4 points;   Strongly disagree = 1 point.
Undecided = 3 points;

For items 2–9, 15, 17–24, 26, 27:

Strongly agree = 1 point;   Disagree = 4 points; and
Agree = 2 points;   Strongly disagree = 5 points.
Undecided = 3 points;

Total scale: items 1–27
Belief Subscale: items 1–9
Feeling Subscale: items 10–18
Intention to Act Subscale: items 19–27

Interpretation ....

High score predisposes one toward high-risk STD behavior. Low score predisposes one toward low-risk STD behavior.

Yarber, Torabi, and Veenker (1989) developed the STD Attitudes Scale by administering three experimental forms of 45 items each. Respondents were 2980 students in six secondary school districts in the Midwest and East. Based on statistical analysis, the scale was reduced to the final 27 items. Reliability coefficients for the entire scale and the three subscales ranged from .48 to .73. The developers reported evidence of construct validity in that the scale was sensitive to positive attitude changes resulting from STD education.

Reference: Yarber, W. L., Torabi, M. R., and Veneer, C. H. Development of a Three-Component STD Attitude Scale. *Journal of Sex Education and Therapy*, Vol. 15, 1989, pp. 36–39. Used by permission.

students, 26.7% of the boys and 11.8% of the girls reported having had four or more sex partners during their lifetime.[39]

- *Failure to use condoms.* Among those who reported having had sexual intercourse in the previous three months, fewer than half reported condom use. Students who'd had four or more sex partners were significantly *less* likely to use condoms than those who'd had fewer partners.

- *Widespread substance abuse.* Teenagers who drink or use drugs are more likely to engage in sexually risky behaviors, including sex with partners whose health status and history they do not know and unprotected intercourse.[40]

The college years are a prime time for contracting sexually transmitted diseases. According to the American College Health Association, chlamydia and human papilloma virus (HPV) have reached epidemic levels at many schools—although many of those infected aren't even aware of it. Among college women who tested positive for chlamydia in a screening study, 79% had no symptoms.[41]

An estimated 1 to 2 per 100 college students are HIV-positive. While students are at lower risk of HIV infection than other groups, such as gay men or injecting drug users, they engage in many behaviors, such as alcohol and drug use and unsafe sexual practices, that place them at increased risk. Even though the current rates of HIV infection are relatively low, health officials feel that the potential exists for rapid spread of HIV on college campuses. Although studies show that many college students are well-informed about STDs, this knowledge often does not translate into behavioral change. Even students targeted as "opinion leaders"—individuals who serve as sources of information for a wide range of individuals and shape the opinions of many—are no better informed and no more likely to practice safer sex.[42]

Educators and health officials have struggled to find ways to bridge the gap between what college students know about the threat of STDs and what they do to protect themselves. Some universities are experimenting with alternatives to workshops or traditional informational materials, such as peer counseling. Others have invited individuals who are HIV-positive or who have AIDS to meet with students and talk about their experiences. In a study of psychology students, those who listened to a lecturer with HIV had significantly higher scores in terms of knowledge and behavioral intent to practice safer sex, compared with their scores before the lecture and with students who had no AIDS education. Many health professionals believe that education must begin much earlier and so are endeavoring to introduce HIV/AIDS education programs at the elementary school level.

Prevention and Protection

Abstinence is the only guarantee of sexual safety—and one that more and more young people are choosing. As discussed in Chapter 9, the choice of an abstinent (or

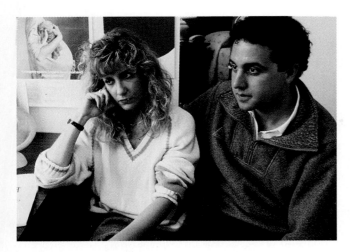

Talking openly about STDs and being tested with your partner protects your health and can foster a sense of trust and commitment.

celibate) lifestyle offers many advantages, both in the present and the future. By choosing not to be sexually active with a partner, individuals can safeguard their physical health, their fertility, and their future.

For men and women who are sexually active, a mutually faithful sexual relationship with just one healthy partner is the safest option. For those not in such relationships, safer-sex practices are essential for reducing risks (see Pulsepoints: "Ten Ways to Prevent Sexually Transmitted Diseases"). Some experts believe that condom use may be a more effective tactic than any drug or vaccine in preventing STDs.[43]

How can you tell if someone you're dating or hope to date has been exposed to an STD? The bad news is, you can't. But the good news is, it doesn't matter—as long as you avoid sexual activity that could put you at risk of infection. Ideally, before engaging in any such behavior, both of you should talk about your prior sexual history (including number of partners and sexually transmitted diseases) and other high-risk behavior, such as the use of injection drugs. If you know someone well enough to consider having sex with that person, you should be able to talk about STDs. If the person is unwilling to talk, you shouldn't have sex.

Even if you do talk openly, you can't be sure a potential partner is telling you the truth. In various surveys of college students, a significant proportion of the men and women said they would lie to a potential partner about having an STD or testing positive for HIV. The only way of knowing for certain that a prospective partner is safe is through laboratory testing. Sex educators and health professionals strongly encourage couples to abstain from any sexual activity that puts them at risk for

STDs until they both undergo medical examinations and laboratory testing to rule out STDs. This process greatly reduces the danger of disease transmission and can also help foster a deep sense of mutual trust and commitment. Many campus and public health clinics provide exams or laboratory testing either free of charge or on a sliding scale determined by your income.

Strategies for Prevention

Telling a Partner That You Have an STD

✔ *Talk before sex.* If you have a chronic STD, such as herpes, discuss it before you have sex. Emphasize that herpes is preventable and that you are committed to using proper precautions.

✔ *Be honest.* If you know or suspect you might have an STD, tell anyone with whom you have had sex exactly what it is.

✔ *Don't accuse.* If you suspect that your partner gave you an STD, you may well be angry. However, there is little to be gained by blaming. Inform your partner of your condition and suggest that he or she seek medical attention.

✔ *Try to be calm and clear.* If you respond with guilt, fear or disgust, your partner is more likely to react in the same emotional way.

✔ *Be sensitive.* Rather than becoming defensive if your partner is angry or resentful, show that you're willing to listen and that you genuinely care.

✔ *Do not engage in sexual activities.* Wait until you both get a thorough medical evaluation, appropriate treatment, and reassurance that you are no longer contagious.

Chlamydia

The most widespread sexually transmitted bacterium in the United States is *Chlamydia trachomatis*, which causes 3 to 5 million **chlamydial infections** each year.[44] *Chlamydia trachomatis* infections are more common in younger than in older women, in African-American than in white women, and in unmarried than in married pregnant women. They also occur more often in both men and women with gonorrhea.

Those at greatest risk of chlamydial infection are individuals 25 years old or younger who engage in sex with more than one new partner within a two-month period and women who use birth control pills or other

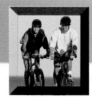

Pulsepoints

Ten Ways to Prevent Sexually Transmitted Diseases (STDs)

1. Abstain from sexual intercourse. You don't have to abstain from all sexual activity. Fantasizing, masturbating, touching, hugging, and petting are all safe and pleasurable.

2. Don't rush into a sexual relationship. Get to know a potential partner well over a period of several months or more. Share your sexual histories, and build an honest, mutually caring, and trusting relationship.

3. Get checked out. The only accurate way to assess the risks of STDs is a thorough medical examination, including laboratory testing.

4. Maintain a mutually faithful sexual relationship with just one uninfected partner. An exclusive sexual relationship with a person who has never been exposed to any STD is safe, regardless of what type of sexual activity you engage in.

5. Always use condoms and spermicides. Although their use reduces your risk, keep in mind that doing so does not guarantee protection.

6. Don't have sex with multiple partners. The risk of STDs increases along with the number of sexual partners. Also avoid sexual contact with individuals who've had multiple or anonymous sexual partners.

7. Inspect your partner's genitals before sex. Although some STDs produce no visible signs, it is possible to see herpes blisters, chancres, rashes, genital warts, and the like.

8. Wash your own—and your partner's—genitals before and after sex. Although it's not clear how effective soap and water are, washing—especially of the penis—is generally believed to have some benefits.

9. Don't have sexual contact with individuals who use injection drugs. Regardless of the type of drug—anabolic steroids, cocaine, heroin, and so on—users are at higher risk for several STDs, including hepatitis and HIV infection.

10. Keep a clear head. Don't make decisions about sexual activity while under the influence of alcohol or drugs that could affect your judgment.

nonbarrier contraceptive methods. Many physicians recommend testing for any woman who has more than one sexual partner in a year; for anyone who seeks medical treatment for an STD; for those seeking health care at adolescent or family planning clinics where chlamydia is seen often; and for young individuals, particularly in urban settings, with multiple sexual partners.

There are two general types of genital chlamydial infections in women: infection of the mucosa of the lower reproductive tract (urethritis or cervicitis, infection of the cervix), in which women may experience few if any symptoms. They may include a mild irritation or itching, burning during urination, and a slight vaginal discharge. The second type involves infection of the upper reproductive tract, or pelvic inflammatory disease (PID) (discussed later in this chapter). Women with lower reproductive tract infections are generally unaware that they have the disease until informed that their sexual partners have it, because most experience no symptoms. New tests have been developed that may be able to detect many cases of chlamydia in women that had been missed in the past.

In men, *Chlamydia trachomatis* causes an estimated half of all cases of epididymitis (infection of the tube that leads out of the testicle) and nongonococcal urethritis (NGU) (inflammation of the urethra not caused by gonorrhea). About 30% of men with NGU develop no or few symptoms. Others experience symptoms similar to those of gonorrhea, including discharge from the penis and mild burning during urination. About 60% to 70% of infected mothers pass the organism to their babies during birth, resulting in eye infections or chlamydial pneumonia, which affects 30,000 newborns every year. Chlamydia has been linked to various problems in pregnancy, including premature rupture of the membranes and early delivery, small-for-gestational-age babies, low-birthweight infants, and perinatal death. Unless treated, many infants remain infected for months or even years. However, treatment significantly improves the odds for a healthy pregnancy and baby.

According to CDC guidelines, the treatment of choice for uncomplicated chlamydia infections is a seven-day regimen of doxycycline or a single, 1-gram dose of azithromycin. Because chlamydia often occurs along with gonorrhea, some health practitioners prescribe seven days of ofloxacin, a drug effective against both chlamydial and gonorrheal infections. The use of condoms with spermicide can reduce, but not eliminate, the risk of chlamydial infection. Sexual partners should be examined and treated if necessary.

Pelvic Inflammatory Disease (PID)

Infection of a woman's fallopian tubes or uterus, called **pelvic inflammatory disease (PID)**, is not actually an STD, but rather a complication of STDs. About one in every seven women of reproductive age has PID; by the year 2000, half of all adult women may have had it. Each year, about 1 million new cases are reported.

Ten to 20% of initial episodes of PID lead to scarring and obstruction of the fallopian tubes severe enough to cause infertility. Other long-term complications are ectopic pregnancy and chronic pelvic pain. The risk of these complications rises with subsequent PID episodes, bacterial vaginosis (discussed earlier in this chapter), and use of IUDs. Smoking also may increase the likelihood of PID. Two bacteria—gonococcus (the culprit in gonorrhea) and chlamydia—are responsible for one-half to one-third of all cases of PID. Other organisms are responsible for the remaining cases.

Most cases of PID occur among women under age 25 who are sexually active. Gonococcus-caused cases tend to affect poor women; those caused by chlamydia range across all income levels. One-half to one-third of all cases are transmitted sexually, and others have been traced to some IUDs that are no longer on the market. Several studies have shown that women with PID are more likely to have used douches than those without the disease.[45]

PID is a silent disease that, in half of all cases, often produces no noticeable symptoms as it progresses and causes scarring of the fallopian tubes. Experts are encouraging women with mild symptoms, such as abdominal pain or tenderness, to seek medical evaluation and physicians to test these patients for infections.[46] Women may learn that they have PID only after discovering that they cannot conceive, or after they develop an ectopic pregnancy (see Chapter 10). PID causes an estimated 15% to 30% of all cases of infertility every year, and about half of all cases of ectopic pregnancy. Most women do not experience any symptoms, but some may develop abdominal pain, tenderness in certain sites

during pelvic exams, or vaginal discharge. Treatment may require hospitalization and intensive antibiotics therapy.

Gonorrhea

Gonorrhea (sometimes called the "clap" in street language) is one of the most common STDs in the United States and is increasing in occurrence. By some estimates, there may be approximately 1 million new cases every year. The incidence is highest among teenagers and young adults. Sexual contact, including oral-genital sex, is the primary means of transmission.

Most men who have gonorrhea know it. Thick, yellow-white pus oozes from the penis, and urination causes a burning sensation. These symptoms usually develop two to nine days after the sexual contact that infected them. Men have a good reason to seek help: It hurts too much not to. Women also may experience discharge and burning on urination. However, as many as eight out of ten infected women have no symptoms.[47]

Gonococcus, the bacterium that causes gonorrhea, can live in the vagina, cervix, and fallopian tubes for months, even years, and continue to infect the woman's sexual partners. Approximately 5% of sexually active American women have positive gonorrhea cultures but are unaware that they are silent carriers.

If left untreated in men or women, gonorrhea spreads through the urinary-genital tract. In women, the inflammation travels from the vagina and cervix, through the uterus, to the fallopian tubes and ovaries. The pain and fever are similar to those caused by stomach upset, so a woman may dismiss the symptoms.

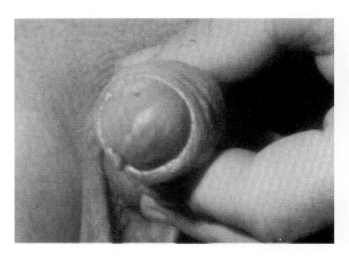

A cloudy discharge is symptomatic of gonorrhea.

Eventually these symptoms diminish, even though the disease spreads to the entire pelvis. Pus may ooze from the fallopian tubes or ovaries into the peritoneum (the lining of the abdominal cavity), sometimes causing serious inflammation. However, this, too, can subside in a few weeks. Gonorrhea, the leading cause of sterility in women, can cause PID. In pregnant women, gonorrhea becomes a threat to the newborn. It can infect the infant's external genitals and cause a serious form of conjunctivitis, an inflammation of the eye that may lead to blindness. As a preventive step, newborns may have penicillin dropped into their eyes at birth.

In men, untreated gonorrhea can spread to the prostate gland, testicles, bladder, and kidneys. Among the serious complications are urinary obstruction and sterility caused by blockage of the vas deferens (the excretory duct of the testis). In both sexes, gonorrhea can develop into a serious, even fatal, bloodborne infection that can cause arthritis in the joints, attack the heart muscle and lining, cause meningitis, and attack the skin and other organs.

Although a blood test has been developed for detecting gonorrhea, the tried-and-true method of diagnosis is still a microscopic study and analysis of cultures from the male's urethra, the female's cervix, and the throat and anus of both sexes.

In the last decade, antibiotic-resistant strains of gonorrhea have emerged, and the current CDC treatment guidelines suggest the use of drugs effective against both resistant and nonresistant strains of *Neisseria gonorrhoeae*. Because gonorrhea often occurs along with chlamydia, practitioners often use an agent effective against both, such as ofloxacin. Antibiotics taken for other reasons may not affect or cure the gonorrhea because of their dosage or type. And you can't develop immunity to gonorrhea; within days of recovering from one case, you can catch another.

Nongonococcal Urethritis (NGU)

The term ***nongonococcal urethritis*** (NGU) refers to any inflammation of the urethra that is not caused by gonorrhea. NGU is the most common STD in men, accounting for 4 million to 6 million visits to a physician every year.[48] Two separate microorganisms, *Chlamydia trachomatis* and *Ureaplasma urealyticum*, are the primary causes; the usual means of transmission is sexual intercourse. Other infectious agents, such as fungi or

bacteria, allergic reactions to vaginal secretions, or irritation by soaps or contraceptive foams or gels may also lead to NGU.

In the United States, NGU is more common in men than gonoccocal urethritis. The symptoms in men are similar to those of gonorrhea, including discharge from the penis (usually less than with gonorrhea) and mild burning during urination. Women frequently develop no symptoms or very mild itching, burning during urination, or discharge. Symptoms usually disappear after two or three weeks, but the infection may persist and causes cervicitis or PID in women and, in men, may spread to the prostate, epididymis, or both. Treatment usually consists of doxycline or erythromycin and should be given to both sexual partners after testing. For men, a single oral dose of azithromycin has proven as effective as a standard seven-day course of doxycycline.[49]

Syphilis

A corkscrew-shaped, spiral bacterium called *Treponema pallidum* causes **syphilis**. This frail germ dies in seconds if dried or chilled, but grows quickly in the warm, moist tissues of the body, particularly in the mucous membranes of the genital tract. Entering the body through any tiny break in the skin, the germ burrows its way into the bloodstream. Sexual contact, including oral sex or intercourse, is a primary means of transmission. Genital ulcers caused by syphilis may increase the risk of HIV infection, while individuals with HIV may be more likely to develop syphilis.

The incidence of syphilis has increased and decreased several times over recent decades, rising in the 1970s and early 1980s, declining in the mid-1980s and rising again in the closing years of the 1980s, mostly among the urban poor. Several studies have shown a link between increases in syphilis, gonorrhea, AIDS, and other STDs and the use of crack cocaine, along with the exchange of sex for drugs or money.[50] Other influences include unemployment, poverty, poor education, and inadequate health care, which in turn can lead to crime, prostitution, substance abuse, family disruption, and despair. Public education programs, expanded screening and surveillance, increased tracing of contacts, and condom promotion have helped to control the spread of syphilis in some areas.

There are clearly identifiable stages of syphilis:

- *Primary syphilis.* The first sign of syphilis is a lesion, or chancre (pronounced "shanker"), an open lump or crater the size of a dime or smaller, teeming with bacteria. The incubation period before its appearance ranges from 10 to 90 days; three to four weeks is average. The chancre appears exactly where the bacteria entered the body: in the mouth, throat, vagina, rectum, or penis. Any contact with the chancre is likely to result in infection.

- *Secondary syphilis.* Anywhere from one to twelve months after the chancre's appearance, secondary-stage symptoms may appear. Some people have no symptoms. Others develop a skin rash or a small, flat rash in moist regions on the skin; whitish patches on the mucous membranes of the mouth or throat; temporary baldness; low-grade fever; headache; swollen glands; or large, moist sores around the mouth and genitals. These are loaded with bacteria; contact with them, through kissing or intercourse, may transmit the infection. Symptoms may last for several days or several months. Even without treatment, they eventually disappear as the syphilis microbes go into hiding.

- *Latent syphilis.* Although there are no signs or symptoms, no sores or rashes at this stage, the bacteria are invading various organs inside the body, including the heart and brain. For two to four years, there may be recurring infectious and highly contagious lesions of the skin or mucous membranes. However, syphilis loses its infectiousness as it progresses: After the first two years, a person rarely transmits syphilis through intercourse.

After four years, even congenital syphilis is rarely transmitted. Until this stage of the disease, however, a pregnant woman can pass syphilis to her unborn child. If the fetus is infected in its fourth month or earlier, it may be disfigured or may even die. If infected late in pregnancy, the child may show no signs of infection for months or years after birth, but may then become disabled with the symptoms of tertiary syphilis.

- *Tertiary syphilis.* Ten to twenty years after the beginning of the latent stage, the most serious symptoms of syphilis emerge, generally in the organs in which the bacteria settled during latency. Syphilis that has progressed to this stage has become increasingly rare. Victims of tertiary syphilis may die of a ruptured aorta or of other heart damage, or may have progressive brain or spinal cord damage, eventually leading to blindness, insanity, or paralysis. About a third of those who are not treated during the first three stages of syphilis enter the tertiary stage later in life.

Health experts are urging screening for syphilis for everyone who seeks treatment for an STD, especially adolescents; for everyone using illegal drugs; and for the partners of these two groups. They also recommend that anyone diagnosed with syphilis be screened for other STDs and be counseled about voluntary testing for HIV.

Early diagnosis of syphilis can lead to a complete cure. The most widely used diagnostic techniques are the Venereal Disease Research Laboratory (VDRL) test or the rapid-plasma-reagin (RPR) test. However, these may be positive only during the secondary stage of the disease, when the bacteria have reached the bloodstream. A positive finding always requires additional information, including a physical exam and other laboratory tests, to confirm the diagnosis and help in planning treatment.

Penicillin is the drug of choice for treating primary, secondary, or latent syphilis. The earlier treatment begins, the more effective it is. Those allergic to penicillin may be treated with doxycycline, tetracycline, or erythromycin. An added danger of not getting treatment for syphilis is an increased risk of HIV transmission.

Herpes

Herpes (from the Greek word that means "to creep") collectively describes some of the most common viral infections in humans. Characteristically, **herpes simplex** causes blisters on the skin or mucous membranes. Herpes simplex exists in several varieties. Herpes simplex virus 1 (HSV-1) generally causes cold sores and fever blisters around the mouth. Herpes simplex virus 2 (HSV-2) may cause blisters on the penis, inside the vagina, on the cervix, in the pubic area, on the buttocks, or on the

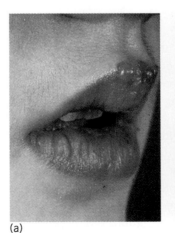
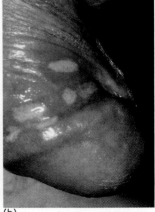

(a)   (b)

Herpes. (a) Herpes simplex virus 1, or HSV-1, as a mouth sore. (b) Herpes simplex virus 2, or HSV-2, usually causes genital sores.

thighs. With the increase of oral-genital sex, some doctors report finding Type 2 herpes lesions in the mouth and throat.

The incidence of herpes infection has soared. Since the late 1970s, the proportion of Americans with herpes simplex type 2 virus has increased by almost one-third. One in five women and one in seven men over age 12—some 45 million people—carry this virus. Two out of three people with the virus do not know they are infected and potentially contagious. Recent research with a new, more sensitive test reveals that individuals without any obvious symtoms shed the virus "subclinically" whether or not they have lesions. Most people with herpes contract it from partners who were not aware of any symptoms or of their own contagiousness.[51] Standard methods of diagnosing genital herpes in women, which rely primarily on physical examination and viral cultures, may miss as many as two-thirds of all cases. Newly developed blood tests are more effective in detecting unrecognized and subclinical infections with HSV-2.

HSV transmission occurs through close contact with mucous membranes or abraded skin. Condoms help prevent infection but aren't foolproof. When herpes sores are present, the infected person is highly contagious and should avoid bringing the lesions into contact with someone else's body through touching, sexual interaction, or kissing. However, HSV also can be transmitted when there are no signs or symptoms of the disease.

A newborn can be infected with genital herpes while passing through the birth canal, and the frequency of mother-to-infant transmission seems to be increasing. Most infected infants develop typical skin sores, which should be cultured to confirm a herpes diagnosis. Some physicians recommend treatment with acyclovir. Because there is a risk of severe damage and possible death, caesarean delivery may be advised for a woman with active herpes lesions.[52]

The virus that causes herpes never entirely goes away; it retreats to nerves near the lower spinal cord, where it remains for the life of the host. Herpes sores can return without warning weeks, months, or even years after their first occurrence, often during menstruation or times of stress, or with sudden changes in body temperature. Of those who experience HSV recurrence, 10% to 35% do so frequently— that is, about six or more times a year. In most people, attacks diminish in frequency and severity over time. Herpes, like other STDS, can trigger feelings of shame, guilt, and depression.

Acyclovir (Zovirax), a prescription drug, has proven effective in treating and controlling herpes. Available as an ointment, in capsules, and in injection form, it relieves the symptoms but doesn't kill the virus. Whereas the ointment works only for the initial bout with herpes, acyclovir in injectable and pill form dramatically reduces the length and severity of herpes outbreaks. Continuing daily oral acylcovir can reduce recurrences by about 80%. However, its safety in pregnant women has not been established. Infection with herpes viruses resistant to acyclovir is a growing problem, especially in individuals with immune-suppressing disorders.[53]

Various treatments—compresses made with cold water, skim milk, or warm salt water, ice packs, or a mild anesthetic cream—can relieve discomfort. Herpes sufferers should avoid heat, hot baths, or nylon underwear. In recent years physicians have tried a host of therapies, including topical ointments, various vaccines, exposure to light, and ultrasonic waves—all with little success. Some physicians have used laser therapy to vaporize the lesions. Clinical trials of an experimental vaccine to protect people from herpes infections are underway.

Human Papilloma Virus Infection (Genital Warts)

Infection with **human papilloma virus (HPV)**, a pathogen that can cause genital warts, is the most common viral STD. By some estimates, 20 million or more women in the United States are infected with HPV, as are three out of four of their male sexual partners.

HPV is transmitted primarily through vaginal, anal, or oral-genital sex. More than half of HPV-infected individuals do not develop any symptoms. Genital warts may appear from three weeks to eighteen months after contact, with an average period of about three months after contact with an infected individual. These are treated by freezing, cauterization, chemicals, or surgical removal. Recurrences are common, for the virus remains in the body.

HPV infection may invade the urethra and cause urinary obstruction and bleeding. It greatly increases a woman's risk of developing a precancerous condition called cervical intraepithelial neoplasia, which can lead to cervical cancer. There also is a strong association between HPV infections and cancer of the vagina, vulva, urethra, penis, and anus.[54] Adolescent girls

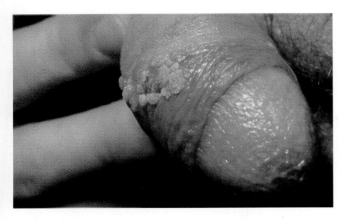

Human papilloma virus, which causes genital warts, is the most common viral STD.

infected with HPV appear to be particularly vulnerable to developing cervical cancer. It is not known if HPV itself causes cancer or acts in conjunction with cofactors (such as other infections, smoking, or suppressed immunity). HPV transmission may be the reason women are five to eleven times as likely to get cervical cancer if their steady sexual partner has had 20 or more previous partners.

Women who have had an HPV infection should get an annual Pap smear. However, this standard diagnostic test for cervical cancer doesn't identify HPV infection. A newer, more specific test can recognize HPV soon after it enters the body. Women who test positive should undergo checkups for cervical changes every six to twelve months. If precancerous cells develop, surgery or laser treatment can prevent further growth. Smoking may interact with HPV to increase the risk of cancer.

HPV may also cause genital warts in men and increase the risk of cancer of the penis. HPV-infected men, who may not develop any symptoms, can spread the infection to their partners. People with visible genital warts also may have asymptomatic or subclinical HPV infections that are extremely difficult to treat.

No form of therapy has been shown to eradicate HPV completely, nor has any single treatment been uniformly effective in removing warts or preventing their recurrence. CDC guidelines suggest treatments that focus on the removal of visible warts—cryotherapy (freezing) and topical applications of podofilox, pdophyllin, or trichloroacetic acid—and then eradication of the virus. At least 20% to 30% of treated individuals experience recurrence. In experimental studies, interfer-

on—a biologic substance produced by virus-infected cells that inhibits viral replication—has proven helpful.[55]

Chancroid

A **chancroid** is a soft, painful sore or localized infection caused by the bacterium *Haemophilus ducrevi* and usually acquired through sexual contact. Half of the cases heal by themselves. In other cases, the infection may spread to the lymph glands near the chancroid, where large amounts of pus can accumulate and destroy much of the local tissue. The incidence of this STD, widely prevalent in Africa and tropical and semitropical regions, is rapidly increasing in the United States, with outbreaks in several states, including Louisiana, Texas, and New York. Chancroids, which may increase susceptibility to HIV infection, are believed to be a major factor in the heterosexual spread of HIV. This infection is treated with antibiotics (ceftriaxone, azithromycin, or erythromycin) and can be prevented by keeping the genitals clean and washing them with soap and water in case of possible exposure.

Strategies for Change

What to Do If You Have an STD

✔ If you suspect that you have an STD, don't feel too embarrassed to get help through a physician's office or a clinic. Treatment relieves discomfort, prevents complications, and halts the spread of the disease.

✔ Following diagnosis, take oral medication (which may be given instead of or in addition to shots) exactly as prescribed.

✔ Try to figure out from whom you got the STD. Be sure to inform that person, who may not be aware of the problem.

✔ If you have an STD, never deceive a prospective partner about it. Tell the truth—simply and clearly. Be sure your partner understands exactly what you have and what the risks are.

Pubic Lice and Scabies

These infections are sometimes, but not always, transmitted sexually. Pubic lice (or "crabs") are usually found in the pubic hairs, although they may migrate to any

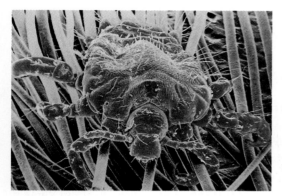

Actual
size

A pubic louse, or "crab."

hairy areas of the body. Lice lay eggs called nits that attach to the base of the hair shaft. Irritation from the lice may produce intense itching. Scratching to relieve the itching can produce sores. Scabies is caused by a mite that burrows under the skin and lays eggs that hatch and undergo many changes in the course of their life cycle, producing great discomfort, including intense itching.

Lice and scabies are treated with applications of Kwell or A-200 pyrinate shampoo (which kills the adult lice but not always the nits) to all the areas of the body where there are concentrations of body hair (genitals, armpits, scalp). You must repeat treatment in seven days to kill any newly developed adults. Wash or dry-clean clothing, and bedding.

HIV/AIDS

Thirty years ago, no one knew what the **human immunodeficiency virus (HIV)** was. No one had ever heard of **acquired immunodeficiency syndrome (AIDS)**. Today HIV/AIDS has been recognized as the most serious epidemic of our time. In the United States, the number of AIDS cases has been declining since 1995, with a 5% drop from 1995 to 1996 and a 12% decrease from 1996 to 1997. However, HIV infection and AIDS remain a grave health threat. Between 35,000 and 40,000 people are newly infected with HIV every year. According to the Centers for Disease Control and Prevention (CDC), an estimated 400,000 and 600,000 Americans are HIV-positive.[56]

Globally, HIV, once seen as an epidemic affecting primarily gay men and injecting drug users, has taken on a very different form. Today, heterosexuals in developing countries have the highest rates of infection and mortality.

As indicated by the chart on page 363, the incidence of HIV varies greatly from country to country and continent to continent. More than 60% of the world's HIV-infected adults live in sub-Saharan Africa, which is home to less than 10% of the world's population. In Botswana, Zimbabwe, Zambia, Uganda, and Malawi, more than 30% of adults between the ages of 15 and 49 are infected. In contrast, China, one of the world's most populous countries, has less than 0.2% of all cases of adults infected with HIV.

The Spread of HIV

HIV came to the United States in the late 1970s. Several factors—including frequent sexual activity with multiple, anonymous partners and high-risk sexual practices, such as anal intercourse—may have caused its quick spread through gay communities in the 1980s. As more became known about HIV transmission, many homosexual men adopted safer ways of sexual expression, reduced their number of sexual partners, or entered into monogamous relationships. As a result, the spread of HIV among gay men—especially older men in metropolitan areas—slowed. However, the incidence of AIDS in young gay men and homosexual men in rural or suburban areas increased steadily in the early 1990s.[57]

In the 1980s, HIV also spread among injecting drug users, who, by sharing contaminated needles, injected the virus directly into their bloodstream. Injection drug use has been the number-one source of HIV infection in heterosexual men and women in this country. Sex with an infected injecting drug user is also a major cause of HIV infection. (See Chapter 14 for further discussion of drug use.) Almost one-third of reported cases of AIDS have been directly or indirectly related to injection drug use. CDC-sponsored studies indicate that needle exchange programs that provide drug users with sterile needles could significantly reduce HIV transmission.[58]

HIV also spread through blood transfusions, blood products, and organ transplants from HIV-positive individuals during the period between 1978 and 1985, before testing to identify contaminated blood became routine. Today's blood and organ supply is much safer, primarily because of more sophisticated testing of donated blood, blood products used for hemophiliacs, and donated organs, tissues, and sperm. There have been several documented cases of HIV infection through artifical insemination performed prior to 1986. Even today, women who use semen from men who have not been tested for HIV are at risk of infection.[59]

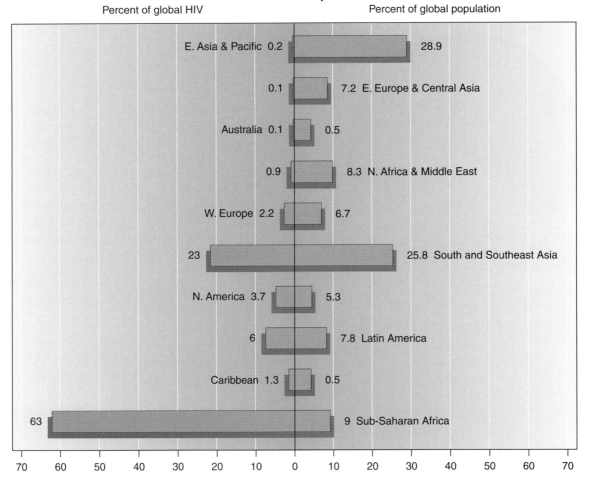

HIV and World Population

Percent of global HIV | Percent of global population

E. Asia & Pacific 0.2 | 28.9
0.1 | 7.2 E. Europe & Central Asia
Australia 0.1 | 0.5
0.9 | 8.3 N. Africa & Middle East
W. Europe 2.2 | 6.7
23 | 25.8 South and Southeast Asia
N. America 3.7 | 5.3
6 | 7.8 Latin America
Caribbean 1.3 | 0.5
63 | 9 Sub-Saharan Africa

SOURCE: World Health Organization, 1998.

Figure 11-5   While AIDS has taken a heavy toll worldwide, the vast number of HIV infections in Sub-Saharan Africa is cataclysmic.

Increasingly, HIV is being transmitted via heterosexual contact. More than 10% of known AIDS cases have occurred among heterosexuals. Although both men and women are at risk if they engage in unprotected sex, women are far more likely to contract HIV from an infected male partner than men are from an infected female partner. The reason may be that semen contains a much higher concentration of HIV than is found in vaginal fluids, and a greater area of mucosal tissue is exposed in the female genital tract than in the male.

HIV is transmitted to infants by HIV-positive mothers in three possible ways: before birth via circulation; during labor and birth; or after birth, through infected breast milk. Every year about 7000 HIV-infected women give birth. Treatment of both mothers and newborns with zidovudine (AZT) can reduce the risk of HIV transmission from mother to child from one in four to less than one in ten—a 67.5% reduction.[60]

Accidental contact with HIV-contaminated blood or bodily fluids has led to some cases of HIV infection and AIDS. According to the CDC, HIV is transmitted among health-care workers in about 1 per 250 instances of their accidental injection with needles containing HIV-positive blood.

The threat of transmission from infected health-care professionals to patients has proven to be very low. To protect both health-care workers and their patients, the CDC requires all professionals to follow basic precautions, such as wearing protective gloves while performing medical procedures. The CDC has also issued guidelines urging health-care workers to inform patients if they are infected with HIV and to stop performing surgery or any procedure in which bleeding might occur.

A small number of cases of HIV infection in heterosexual men in the United States have been traced to prostitutes. However, in big cities, as many as half the prosti-

Adult and adolescent exposure to AIDS, July 1996–June 1997

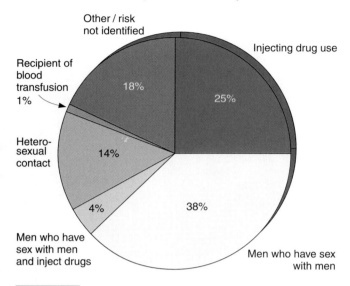

Figure 11-6

Percent of adult and adolesent exposure to AIDS, from July 1996–June 1997

SOURCE: Centers for Disease Control, 1998.

tutes tested have been exposed to HIV, almost all through injection drug use or sex with injecting drug users.

Reducing the Risk of HIV Transmission

HIV/AIDS can be so frightening that some people have exaggerated its dangers, whereas others understate them. The fact is that although no one is immune to HIV, you can reduce the risk if you abstain from sexual activity, remain in a monogamous relationship with an uninfected partner, and do not inject drugs. If you're not in a long-term monogamous relationship with a partner you're sure is safe, and you're not willing to abstain from sex, there are things you can do to lower your risk of HIV infection. Remember that the risk of HIV transmission depends on sexual behavior, not sexual orientation. Homosexual, heterosexual, and bisexual individuals all need to know about the kinds of sexual activity that increase their risk.

Here's what you should know about HIV transmission (see Figure 11-7):

- Casual contact does *not* spread HIV infection. Compared to other viruses, HIV is extremely difficult to get. HIV can live in blood, semen, vaginal fluids, and breast milk. Many chemicals, including household bleach, alcohol, and hydrogen peroxide, can inactivate it. In studies of family members sharing dishes, food, clothing, and frequent hugs with people with HIV infection or AIDS, those who have contracted the virus have shared razor blades, toothbrushes, or had other means of blood contact.

- You cannot tell visually whether a potential sexual partner has HIV. A blood test is needed to detect the antibodies that the body produces to fight HIV, thus indicating infection.

- HIV can be spread in semen and vaginal fluids during a single instance of anal, vaginal, or oral sexual contact between heterosexuals, bisexuals, or homosexuals. The risk increases with the number of sexual encounters with an infected partner.

- Teenage girls may be particularly vulnerable to HIV infection because the immature cervix is easily infected.

- Anal intercourse is an extremely high-risk behavior because HIV may enter the bloodstream through tiny breaks in the lining of the rectum. HIV transmission is much more likely to occur during unprotected anal intercourse than vaginal intercourse.[61]

- Other behaviors that increase the risk of HIV infection include having multiple sex partners, engaging in sex without condoms or virus-killing spermicides, sexual contact with persons known to be at high risk (e.g., prostitutes or injecting drug users), and sharing injection equipment for drugs.

- Individuals are at greater risk if they have an active sexual infection. Sexually transmitted diseases, such as herpes, gonorrhea, and syphilis, facilitate transmission of HIV during vaginal or rectal intercourse.

- No cases of HIV transmission by deep kissing have been reported, but it could happen. Studies have found blood in the saliva of healthy people after kissing; other lab studies have found HIV in saliva. Social (dry) kissing is safe.

- Oral sex can lead to HIV transmission. The virus in any semen that enters the mouth could make its way into the bloodstream through tiny nicks or sores in the mouth. A man's risk in performing oral sex on a woman is smaller because an infected woman's genital fluids have much lower concentrations of HIV than does semen.

- HIV infection is not widespread among lesbians, although there have been documented cases of pos-

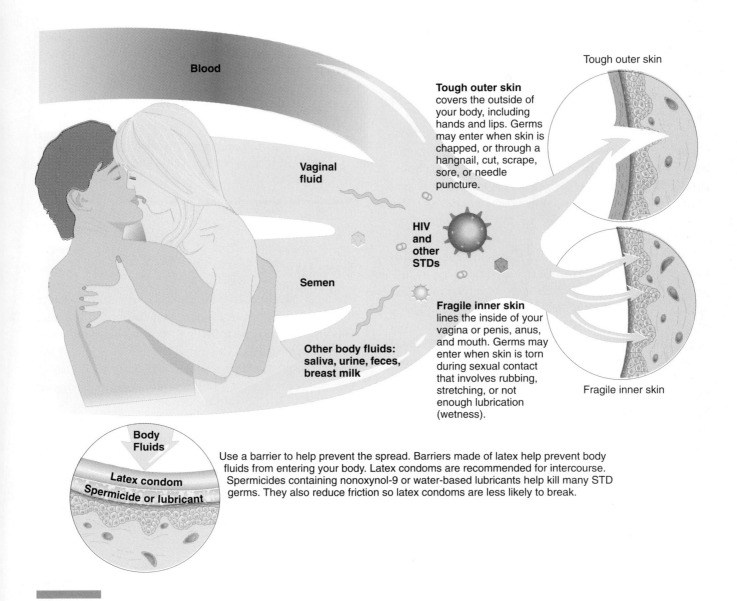

Figure 11-7

How HIV infection and other STDs are spread. Most STDs are spread by viruses, such as HIV, or bacteria carried in certain body fluids.

sible female-to-female HIV transmission. In each instance, one partner had had sex with a bisexual man or male injecting drug user or had injected drugs herself.[62]

HIV Infection

HIV infection refers to a spectrum of health problems that result from immunologic abnormalities caused by the virus when it enters the bloodstream. In theory, the body may be able to resist infection by HIV. In reality, in

almost all cases, HIV destroys the cell-mediated immune system, particularly the CD4+ T-lymphocytes (also called T4 helper cells). The result is greatly increased susceptibility to various cancers and opportunistic infections (infections that take hold because of the reduced effectiveness of the immune system).

According to new insights into the pathogenesis of HIV—the way in which HIV attacks the immune system—researchers now know that HIV triggers a state of all-out war within the immune system. Almost immediately following infection with HIV, the immune system responds aggressively by manufacturing enormous numbers of CD4 cells. However, it eventually is overwhelmed as the viral particles continue to replicate, or multiply. The intense war between HIV and the immune system indicates that the virus itself, not a breakdown in the immune system, is responsible for disease progression.[63]

Shortly after becoming infected with HIV, individuals may experience a few days of flulike symptoms, which most ignore or attribute to other viruses. Some people develop a more severe mononucleosis-type syndrome. After this stage, individuals may not develop any signs or symptoms of disease for a period ranging from weeks to more than 12 years.

HIV infection can itself be a serious illness and is associated with a variety of HIV-related diseases, including different cancers and dangerous infections. HIV-infected individuals may develop persistent generalized lymphadenopathy, enlargement of the lymph nodes at two or more different sites in the body. This condition typically persists for more than three months without any other illness to explain its occurrence. Diminished mental function may appear before other symptoms. Tests conducted on infected, but apparently healthy, men have revealed impaired coordination, problems in thinking, or abnormal brain scans.

Strategies for Prevention

Lowering Your Risk of Exposure to HIV

✔ Abstain from sexual contact with anyone who is infected with HIV, whether or not he or she has symptoms, or with anyone who is at high risk of HIV infection because of his or her behavior.

✔ Avoid sexual contact with anyone who has had sex with people at risk of HIV infection. Avoid multiple or anonymous sex partners. Avoid sex with anyone who has had multiple or anonymous sex partners, or with anyone who has had a sex partner infected with HIV.

✔ Use a condom during every sexual act, including oral sex, from start to finish. Also use a spermicide that provides extra protection against STDS.

✔ Don't have sexual contact with individuals who use injection drugs.

✔ Avoid receptive anal intercourse, as well as the insertion of fingers or objects into your anus, because these acts could tear your rectal tissues, allowing direct access to your bloodstream. Avoid contact with your partner's blood, semen, urine, and feces.

✔ Don't use amyl nitrite (poppers), a sexual stimulant that may be associated with the development of a cancer characteristic of AIDS.

✔ Don't have sex with prostitutes.

✔ Don't share needles (or other injection drug equipment), razor blades, or toothbrushes.

✔ In addition to their partner's use of a condom, women should use a diaphragm with a spermicide for extra protection.

Testing for HIV

The most widely used HIV antibody tests do not detect the virus itself but antibodies that the body forms in response to exposure to HIV. A negative result indicates no exposure to HIV. But since it can take three to six months for the body to produce the telltale antibodies, a negative result may not be accurate, depending on the timing of the test.

There are means of isolating HIV, but they are expensive and not widely available. Tests that measure HIV antigens (substances that stimulate the production of antibodies) are considered relatively insensitive; doctors use them mainly to determine a patient's prognosis and to measure the effects of antiviral drugs. The standard laboratory blood tests used to detect infection by the HIV virus are the following:

- *Enzyme-linked immunosorbent assay (ELISA)*. A test that detects protein antibodies produced by an infected individual's immune system to fight against particles of HIV.

- *Western blot*. A more accurate and expensive test that's done to confirm the results of a positive ELISA test.

When perfectly performed, both tests can detect antibodies in 99.6% of infected people and can correctly give negative results in uninfected people at least 99% of the time. However, actual percentages of false reading are higher than the 99% implies. Most testing centers repeat the test if the initial results are positive. Experienced counselors can refer men and women with two positive readings to physicians who specialize in HIV-related problems.

Home HIV testing kits are available at health centers and pharmacies. By means of a finger prick, users produce a few drops of blood that they apply to a special card and mail to a laboratory. Usually within seven days, thay can call a toll-free number, identify themselves by a number, and get results anonymously. According to preliminary reports from one manufacturer of HIV tests, 99% of those who use the home tests are HIV-negative. For those who do get positive results, it is important to undergo more precise laboratory testing and to take advantage of counseling services.

Health officials, who estimate that at least 110,000 HIV-positive individuals are unaware of their status, recommend HIV testing for the following individuals:

- Men who have had sex with other men, regardless of whether they consider themselves homosexual.

- Anyone who uses injection drugs and has shared needles, or has had sex with someone who has done so.

- Women who have had sex with bisexual men.

- Anyone who has had sex with someone from an area with a high incidence of HIV infection.

- Individuals who have had sex with people they do not know well.

- Anyone who received blood transfusions or blood products between 1978 and 1985. (Their sexual partners or, if they are new mothers, their infants may also be at risk.)

AIDS

Until recently, a diagnosis of AIDS was made only when an HIV-positive person developed one of more than 23 severe, debilitating illnesses, such as pneumonia or cancer. Since 1993, the definition of AIDS has been expanded to include anyone with HIV whose immune system is severely impaired, as indicated by a CD4 count of less than 200 cells per cubic millimeter of blood, compared to normal CD4 cell counts in healthy people not infected with HIV of 800 to 1200 per cubic millimeter of blood. In addition, the expanded definition included those persons with HIV infection who experience recurrent pneumonia, invasive cervical cancer, or pulmonary tuberculosis.

People with AIDS also may experience persistent fever, diarrhea that persists for more than one month, or involuntary weight loss of more than 10% of normal body weight. Generalized lymphadenopathy may persist. Neurological disease—including dementia (confu-

sion and impaired thinking) and other problems with thinking, speaking, movement, or sensation—may occur. Secondary infectious diseases that may develop in people with AIDS include *Pneumocystis carinii* pneumonia, tuberculosis, or oral candidiasis (thrush). Secondary cancers associated with HIV infection include Kaposi's sarcoma and cancer of the cervix.

The number of AIDS deaths in the United States has been declining. According to the Centers for Disease Control and Prevention, the number of deaths caused by AIDS declined by 44% in the first half of 1997, compared with the same period in 1996. The declines were greatest in New York City and Los Angeles.[64]

Treatments

The improvements in severe illness and death are due primarily to new forms of therapy, particularly protease inhibitor drugs, which have been remarkably effective in boosting levels of protective T cells and reducing "viral load"—the amount of HIV virus in the bloodstream. Administering these medications in combination with AZT early after infection preserves the body's store of T helper cells, which otherwise are depleted by the HIV virus. In most patients who can tolerate this combination therapy, concentrations of the HIV virus drop to undetectable levels.[65, 66]

This drug regimen is expensive and can run more than $10,000 to $12,000 a year. Only 20% of Americans who carry the HIV virus have insurance that pays this cost.[67] While this "cocktail therapy," as some call it, has had a dramatic effect, the benefits seem to decline in about half of those treated. After being knocked into temporary submission, levels of the HIV virus rise, even though patients often continue to feel well.[68]

The search for a true cure for AIDS continues. Researchers are studying the small number of HIV-infected individuals who remain healthy and do not suffer loss of immune function. Learning more about the genetics of individuals who manage to survive with HIV may lead to therapies that can help others do the same.[69]

Researchers also are working on new *microbicides*, agents that kill pathogens that might be especially helpful in protecting women from infection without the aid or consent of their partners.[70] Another potentially promising approach is *gene therapy*, in which the immune system might be reconstituted with genetically altered cells that could resist infection by HIV. Scientists also are testing a vaccine against HIV.

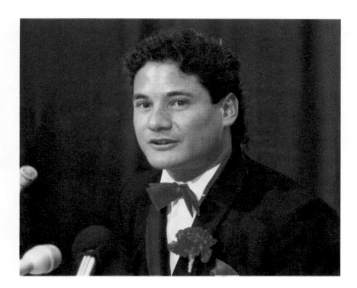

The Americans with Disabilities Act prohibits discrimination against people with HIV/AIDS.

The Personal Impact of HIV

In recent years, the announcements that celebrities such as basketball star Earvin (Magic) Johnson, Jr., are HIV positive have made many Americans far more aware of these problems. Because of greater awareness and medical advances, infection with HIV is viewed less as a death sentence than as a life sentence and more individuals are living with AIDS (see Figure 11-8).

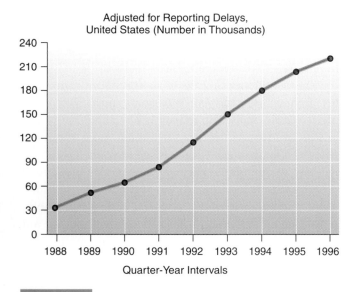

Figure 11-8 Adults and adolescents living with AIDS, from January 1988 to September 1996.

SOURCE: CDC/National AIDS Case Surveillance Data.

In addition to medical dangers, many Americans infected with HIV, including children, have had to deal with physical or verbal abuse because of their disease. Individuals with HIV/AIDS have become more outspoken in defending their rights, in part because of a federal law, the Americans with Disabilities Act, which prohibits discrimination against all people with illnesses or disabilities. The courts have upheld the right of children with HIV infection to public education and the right of HIV-positive employees to remain on the job. However, in some cases, conflicts between personal rights and public health goals remain.

Strategies for Change
....
When a Friend Has HIV or AIDS

HIV has become so widespread among people in the prime of life that almost everyone knows someone either at risk or infected with the virus. While you may feel helpless or inadequate when a friend becomes seriously ill, you can offer comfort:

✔ Touch your friend. A simple squeeze of the hand or a hug can let him or her know that you care.

✔ Respond to your friend's emotions. Weep with your friend when he or she weeps. Laugh when your friend laughs. It's healthy to share these intimate experiences.

✔ Check in with your friend's partner or roommate and offer to take over any caregiving that is needed to provide him or her with a break.

✔ It's okay to ask about the illness, but be sensitive to whether your friend wants to discuss it. You can find out by asking, "Would you like to talk about how you're feeling?" But don't pressure your friend if the response is no.

Making This Chapter Work for You
Guarding Against Infectious Diseases

■ Infectious illnesses remain a serious health threat. Disease-causing organisms called pathogens, carried by various vectors, can infect a host (either a person or a population) in various ways.

■ The types of microbes that can cause infection are viruses, which invade a body cell and take over its reproductive processes; bacteria, one-celled organisms that release disease-causing toxins; fungi, microscopic plants that feed on human tissue; protozoa, one-celled organisms that release substances that destroy or damage cells; and helminths, parasitic worms that invade body tissue.

■ During the incubation period, a pathogen is multiplying; in the prodromal period, symptoms appear; during active infection, symptoms are most intense; during recovery, symptoms subside.

■ Antibacterial drugs, sulfa drugs, and antibiotics treat diseases caused by bacteria, but they have no effect on viruses or other pathogens. Antiviral drugs can damage cells invaded by viruses.

■ The body's natural defenses against pathogens include the skin; antibacterial substances in tears, sweat, saliva, and mucus; and the immune system, which includes many different types of defenders. Humoral immunity involves an antigen-antibody response. Cell-mediated immunity refers to the activity of various types of protective cells. Once a person has produced antibodies to a pathogen, he or she has developed active immunity and is usually protected from that disease for life.

■ Immune system disorders include allergies, autoimmune disorders, and acquired immunodeficiency syndrome (AIDS).

■ Immunizations are the best method of prevention against infectious diseases such as polio, tetanus, diphtheria, rubella, measles, chickenpox, hepatitis B, and HIB. College-age men and women may be especially vulnerable to measles and may require revaccination.

■ Infectious diseases caused by viruses include the common cold, influenza, viral pneumonia, mononucleosis, and hepatitis. Bacterial infections include bacterial pneumonia, tuberculosis, group A and group B strep, toxic shock syndrome, and Lyme disease.

■ Emerging infections are those recently recognized, increasing in humans, or threatening to spread to new areas in the near future. They include HIV, Hantavirus, Ebola, dengue, Lassa, and Marburg, which have been responsible for deadly outbreaks around the globe.

■ Reproductive and urinary tract infections are very common and include trichomoniasis, candidiasis, and bacterial vaginosis, as well as infections of the urethra, bladder, or kidney.

■ The incidence of sexually transmitted diseases (STDs) is increasing. Because many STDs do not cause any

symptoms in their initial stages, infected individuals may continue their usual sexual activity without realizing that they're jeopardizing others' well-being.

■ While STDs strike both sexes, all classes, and all ages, young Americans are at greatest risk. According to the CDC, as many as half of all young people may develop an STD by age 30.

■ The most widespread sexually transmitted bacterium in the United States is *Chlamydia trachomatis*, which causes 3 to 5 million infections each year, most in individuals 25 years old or younger.

■ Infection of a woman's fallopian tubes or uterus, called pelvic inflammatory disease (PID), is the second-most serious STD affecting women (after HIV infection). About one in every seven women of reproductive age has PID.

■ One of the most common and dangerous STDs in the United States is gonorrhea, which is caused by the gonococcus bacterium and is diagnosed with a blood test or a culture. The incidence is highest among teenagers and young adults.

■ Nongonoccal urethritis (NGU) refers to any inflammation of the urethra that is not caused by gonorrhea. Two separate microorganisms, *Chlamydia trachomatis* and *Ureaplasma urealyticum*, are the primary causes.

■ Syphilis, caused by a bacterium, is easily treated in its stages but can progress and, over time, invade various organs inside the body, including the heart and brain.

■ Herpes simplex virus causes painful blisters during flareups and never entirely leaves the body. Human papilloma virus (HPV) and chancroid infections are other STDs that are spreading rapidly.

■ Human immunodeficiency virus (HIV) is a retrovirus that attacks the body's immune system and causes various problems, ranging from symptomatic infection to generalized swelling of the lymph glands. It is spread through anal, vaginal, and oral sexual contact; contaminated needles of drug abusers; blood transfusions, blood products, and organ transpants from HIV-positive individuals; from HIV-positive mothers to their babies before, during, or after birth; and accidental contact with HIV-contaminated blood or bodily fluids.

■ Acquired immunodeficiency syndrome (AIDS) is diagnosed when HIV severely impairs a person's immune system, as indicated by a CD4 count of less than 200 cells per cubic millimeter of blood. People

Health Online

Cells Alive! http://www.cellsalive.com/

This site features interactive animations and other illustrations plus clear written descriptions to help explain how pathogens and the immune system work in the human body. Topics include HIV infection, making antibodies, penicillin, parasites, and streptococcus.

Think about it ...

- How does the HIV virus go about damaging the immune system? Where might researchers developing drugs to treat people with HIV try to interrupt this process?

- What are some recurring themes in the descriptions of infections and immunity? What could you do to make your immune system stronger?

- Do animated illustrations like these help you understand the process of infection better than still printed illustrations like those in this text?

---

with AIDS also may experience persistent fever, diarrhea, involuntary weight loss, neurological disease, and secondary infectious diseases and cancers.

■ HIV/AIDS has been recognized as the most serious epidemic of our time although the death rate for AIDS has dropped in recent years. HIV is transmitted through sexual contact, blood transfusions, organ transplants, and sharing contaminated needles.

Infectious diseases threaten everyone's health, but—as with many other illnesses—you can do a great deal to reduce your odds of becoming a victim. Prevention is always the wisest course. Cleanliness is an important first step. The liberal use of soap and hot water kills many pathogens. Colds and flus are, in the long run, inevitable; but preventive measures, such as avoiding obvious carriers, can help reduce your risk.

Sexually transmitted diseases are a particularly personal responsibility. You owe it to yourself, to those you love, and to the children you might conceive to be aware of the signs, symptoms, and stages of STDs and to avoid exposure and take the protective steps described in Pulsepoints: "Ten Ways to Prevent Sexually Transmitted Diseases." You can do more than anyone else to prevent sexual infections. If you fear that you've been exposed, don't wait for serious symptoms to develop. Self-treatment doesn't work for STDS; you need a doctor's help.

 Key Terms

The terms listed here are used within the chapter. Page numbers are included for each term.
A definition of each term is given in the green Glossary pages at the end of this book.

abscess *336*
acquired immunodeficiency syndrome (AIDS) *362*
allergy *337*
antibiotics *333*
antiviral drug *333*

autoimmune *337*
bacteria *333*
bacterial vaginosis *348*
candidiasis *348*
cell-mediated *336*
chanchroid *361*

chlamydial infections *355*
chronic fatigue syndrome (CFS) *344*
cystitis *348*
fungi *333*
gamma globulin *336*

Review Questions

1. How does an agent of infection spread disease? Explain the process of transmission and infection using a common agent of infection as an example.

2. What factors bolster or weaken the immune system? Name some different types of immunity.

3. What is an infectious disease? Name some of the common ones and effective methods of prevention.

4. What are HIV infection and AIDS? How is HIV transmitted? Who is most at risk for contracting HIV?

5. How does a person contract a sexually transmitted disease? List and describe some different kinds of STDS, their symptoms, and treatment.

6. How can a person avoid HIV and other sexually transmitted diseases? What are the best methods of preventing STDS?

 ## Critical Thinking Questions

1. What are several practices that you know of or use to avoid contracting infectious diseases? Briefly explain the convenience, advantages, and disadvantages of each practice.

2. The U.S. military and some employers routinely screen personnel for HIV. Some hospitals test patients and note their HIV status on their charts. Some insurance companies test for HIV before selling a policy. Do you believe that an individual has the right to refuse to be tested for HIV? Should a physician be able to order an HIV test without a patient's consent? Can a surgeon refuse to operate on an HIV-infected patient or one who refuses HIV testing? Do patients have the right to know if their doctors, dentists, or nurses are HIV-positive?

3. A man who developed herpes sued his former girlfriend. A woman who became sterile as a result of pelvic inflammatory disease (PID) took her ex-husband to court. A woman who contracted HIV infection from her dentist, who had died of AIDS, filed suit against his estate. Do you think that anyone who knowingly transmits a sexually transmitted disease should be held legally responsible? Do you think such an act should be a criminal offense?

 ## Connections to Personal Health Interactive

*To enhance your understanding of the material covered in this chapter, check out the following study aids on the **Personal Health Interactive CD-ROM**. Each numbered icon within the chapter corresponds to an appropriate activity listed here.*

11.1 Personal Insights: Do You Prevent Disease?
11.2 Chapter 11 Review

▶ References

1. National Institute of Allergy and Infectious Diseases (NIAID). "The World As A Hot Zone: New and Re-Emerging Diseases." Bethesda, MD: National Institutes of Health, 1995.
2. Garret, Laurie. *The Coming Plague.* New York: Ballantine, 1994.
3. Miller, Louis. "Malaria." *NIAID Tips Sheet for Science Writers,* February 21, 1995. Angier, Natalie. "Malaria's Genetic Game of Cloak and Dagger." *New York Times,* August 22, 1995.
4. Marwick, Charles. "Could Virulent Virus Be Harbinger of 'New Flu?'" *Journal of the American Medical Association,* Vol. 279, No. 4, January 28, 1998. Altman, Lawrence. "Hunt in Sealed Lab Seeks Deadly Secrets of 'Bird Flu.'" *New York Times,* January 11, 1998. Lee, William. "Hepatitis B Virus Infection." *New England Journal of Medicine,* Vol. 337, No. 24, December 11, 1997. Ulene, Art. *How to Outsmart Your Allergies.* Asthma and Allergy Foundation of America.
5. Miles, Robert. Personal interview.
6. "New Treatment Options Bring Relief to Allergy Sufferers." American College of Allergy and Asthma, Annual Meeting, November 1997.
7. American Academy of Pediatrics. "Implementation of the Immunization Policy." *Pediatrics,* August 1995. Bowman, Marjorie, and Thomas Schwenk. "Family Medicine." *Journal of the American Medical Association,* Vol. 273, No. 21, June 7, 1995.
8. Unti, Lisa, et al. "Incentives and Motivators in School-based Hepatitis B Vaccination Programs." *Journal of School Health,* Vol. 67, No. 7, September 1997.
9. Folkers, Greg. "Acellular Pertussis Vaccines Effective, Safe in NIAID-Sponsored Trials." *NIAID News,* July 13, 1995.
10. American Academy of Pediatrics. "Chicken Pox Vaccine Recommendations." *Pediatrics,* May 1995.
11. Centers for Disease Control and Prevention.
12. Sniadack, David. Medical epidemiologist, National Center for Infectious Diseases, Centers for Disease Control and Prevention, Atlanta. Personal interview.
13. Centers for Disease Control and Prevention.
14. Gwaltney, Jack M., Jr., and Scott B. Halstead. "Contagiousness of the Common Cold." *Journal of the American Medical Association,* Vol. 278, No. 3, July 16, 1997.
15. "Zinc Lozenges Reduce the Duration of Common Cold Symptoms." *Nutrition Reviews,* Vol. 55, No. 3, March 1997.
16. Apgar, Barbara. "Effectiveness of Zinc in the Treatment of the Common Cold." *American Family Physician,* Vol. 56, No. 3, September 1, 1997.
17. Gwaltney, Jack. Personal interview.
18. Kilbourne, Edwin. Personal interview.
19. Hayden, Frederick, et al. "Efficacy and Safety of the Neuraminidase Inhibitor Zanamivir in the Treatment of Influenza Virus Infection." *New England Journal of Medicine,* Vol. 337, No. 13, September 25, 1997.
20. Couch, Robert. "A New Antiviral Agent for Influenza—Is There a Clinical Niche?" *New England Journal of Medicine,* Vol. 337, No. 13, September 25, 1997.
21. Wessely, Simon, et al. "The Prevalence and Morbidity of Chronic Fatigue and Chronic Fatigue Syndrome." *American Journal of Public Health,* Vol. 87, No. 9, September 1997.
22. "The FDA Has Approved the First Vaccine in the United States to Prevent Hepatitis A." *American Health,* May 1995.
23. Lee, William. "Hepatitis B Virus Infection." *New England Journal of Medicine,* Vol. 337, No. 24, December 25, 1997.
24. Stoeckle and Douglas. "Infectious Diseases."
25. Miller, Jeff. "TB: Too Tough to Kill?" *UCSF Magazine,* October 1995.
26. Unti. "Incentives and Motivators in School-based Hepatitis B."
27. "Tampons: Reducing Toxic Shock Risk." *University of California, Berkeley Wellness Letter,* Vol. 14, No. 3, December 1997.
28. Fix, Alan, et al. "Tick Bite and Lyme Disease in an Endemic Setting." *Journal of the American Medical Association,* Vol. 279, No. 3, January 21, 1998.
29. Ostfeled, Richard. "The Oncology of Lyme Disease Risk." *American Scientist,* Vol. 85, No. 4, July–August 1997.
30. Health Report. *Time,* Vol. 150, No. 17, October 27, 1997.
31. Strausbaugh, Larry. "Emerging Infectious Diseases: A Challenge to All." *Journal of the American Medical Association,* Vol. 278, No. 5, August 6, 1997.
32. "Malicious Microbes Warrant Basic Biomedical Research." *NIAID News,* February 20, 1995.
33. Braverman, P., and V. Strasburger. "Adolescent Sexual Activity." *Clinical Pediatrics,* Vol. 32, 1994.
34. Dranov, Paula. "Urinary Tract Infections." *American Health,* May 1995.
35. Quinn, T. "Recent Advances in Diagnosis of Sexually Transmitted Disease." Vol. 21, 1994.
36. "Sexually Transmitted Diseases in the United States." *SIECUS Report,* Vol. 25, No. 3, February–March 1997.
37. Braverman and Strasburger. "Adolescent Sexual Activity."
38. Centers for Disease Control and Prevention. HIV/AIDS Surveillance Report, Vol. 7, No. 1, 1995.
39. Braverman and Strasburger. "Adolescent Sexual Activity."
40. Centers for Disease Control and Prevention.
41. DePunzio, C., et al. "Epidemiology and Therapy of Chlamydia Trachomatis Genital Infection in Women." *Journal of Chemotherapy,* June 1992.
42. Schneider, Dona, et al. "Evaluating HIV/AIDS Education in the University Setting." *Journal of American College Health,* Vol. 43, July 1994. O'Leary, A., et al. "Predictors of Safer Sex on the College Campus: A Social Cognitive Theory Analysis." *Journal of American College Health,* May 1992. Jaccard, James, et al. "Student Opinion Leaders and HIV/AIDS Knowledge and Risk Behavior." *Journal of American College Health,* Vol. 43, March 1995.
43. Pinkerton, Steven, and Paul Abramsom. "Condoms and the Prevention of AIDS." *American Scientist,* Vol. 85, No. 4, July–August 1997.
44. Biro, F., et al. "A Comparison of Diagnostic Methods in Adolescent Girls With and Without Symptoms of Chlamy-

dia Urogenital Infection." *Pediatrics*, Vol. 93, 1994. "*Chlamydia trachomatis* Antibody Testing Is More Accurate Than Hysterosalpingography in Predicting Tubal Factor Infertility." *Fertility and Sterility*, Vol. 61, 1994.

45. Zhang, Jun, et al. "Vaginal Douching and Adverse Health Effects." *American Journal of Public Health*, Vol. 87, No. 7, July 1997.

46. MacKay, Trent, et al. "PID: Suspect More, Treat More, Hospitalize Less." *Patient Care*, Vol. 31, No. 12, July 15, 1997.

47. Newland, Jamesetta. "Gonorrhea in Women." *American Journal of Nursing*, Vol. 97, No. 8, August 1997.

48. Schmid, George, and Phil Fontanarosa. "Evolving Strategies for Management of the Nongonococcal Urethritis Syndrome." *Journal of the American Medical Association*, Vol. 274, No. 7, August 16, 1995.

49. Stamm, Walter, et al. "Azithromydin for Empirical Treatment of the Nongonococcal Urethritis Syndrome in Men." *Journal of the American Medical Association*, Vol. 274, No. 7, August 16, 1995.

50. Crooks, Robert, and Karla Baur. *Your Sexuality*, 6th ed. Pacific Grove, CA: Brooks Cole, 1996.

51. Arvin, Ann, and Charles Prober. "Herpes Simplex Virus Type 2—A Persistent Problem." *New England Journal of Medicine*, Vol. 337, No. 16, October 16, 1997.

52. Overall, J. "Herpes Simplex Virus Infection of the Fetus and Newborn." *Pediatric Annals*, Vol. 23, 1994.

53. NAIAD. "Scientists Tackle Resistant Herpes."

54. Braverman and Strasburger. "Adolescent Sexual Activity."

55. Ferenczy, Alex, et al. "Current Treatment Strategies in the Management of Human Papillomavirus Infection." *American Journal of Obstetrics and Gynecology*, Vol. 172, No.4, April 1995.

56. Centers for Disease Control and Prevention, February 1998.

57. Saag, Michael. "HIV Pathogenesis: The Evolving Understanding of HIV Disease." *HIV/AIDS Reporter*, Vol. 1, April 1995.

58. Marwick, Charles. "Released Report Says Needle Exchanges Work." *Journal of the American Medical Association*, Vol. 273, No. 13, April 5, 1995.

59. "HIV Threat for Women Artificially Inseminated before '86." *American Medical News*, March 20, 1995.

60. Wilbanks, George. "Protecting the Unborn Against AIDS." *ACOG Women's Health*, July 24, 1995.

61. Billy, J., et al. "The Sexual Behavor of Men in the United States." *Family Planning Perspectives*, 1993.

62. Seidman, S., and R. Rieder. "A Review of Sexual Behavior in the United States." *American Journal of Psychiatry*, Vol. 151, 1994.

63. Centers for Disease Control.

64. CDC.

65. Balter, Michael. "How Does HIV Overcome the Body's T Cell Bodyguards?" *Science*, Vol. 278, No. 5342, November 21, 1997.

66. Landay, Alan. "Immune Restoration Following Treatment." *Journal of the American Medical Association*, Vol. 278, No. 18, November 12, 1997.

67. Lacayo, Richard."Hope with an Asterisk." *Time*, Vol. 148, No. 29, December 30, 1996.

68. "Setbacks for Many on Drugs for AIDS." *New York Times*, September 30, 1997.

69. Dean, Michael, and Stephen O'Brien. "In Search of AIDS-Resistance Genes." *Scientific American*, Vol. 277, No. 3, September 1997. Pinkerton, Steven, and Paul Abramson. "Condoms and the Prevention of AIDS." *American Scientist*, Vol. 85, No. 4, July–August 1997.

70. Voelker, Rebecca. "Scientists Zero in on New HIV Microbicides." *Journal of the American Medical Association*, Vol. 273, No. 13, April 5, 1995.

CHAPTER 12

KEEPING YOUR HEART HEALTHY

After studying the material in this chapter, you should be able to:

Describe how the heart functions.

List and **explain** the controllable and uncontrollable risk factors for cardiovascular disease.

Explain the relationship of cholesterol to the risk of heart attack.

Define hypertension, and **list** its common risk factors.

Define atherosclerosis, and **list** effective treatments for it.

Explain what happens during a myocardial infarction (MI) (heart attack) and what can be done to prevent and treat such attacks.

Define stroke and transient ischemic attacks (TIAs), and **explain** their cause, prevention, and treatment.

The news about cardiovascular disease—disorders of the heart and blood vessels—is heartwarming. Although still the nation's top killer, the annual mortality rate from heart disease has been declining.[1] The medical advances described in this chapter have helped, but much of the credit goes to lifestyle changes, such as quitting smoking and making dietary changes that lower blood pressure and cholesterol levels.

Yet we still have a long way to go to keep the hearts of all Americans healthy. One out of every four men and women in the United States has some form of cardiovascular illness. Heart-related disorders account for almost as many deaths as the *combined* total for cancer, accidents, influenza, pneumonia, AIDS, and all other causes.

The time to start protecting your heart is now. Many people mistakenly think of cardiovascular disorders as illnesses of middle and old age. However, the events leading up to heart disease often begin in childhood, develop more rapidly throughout adolescence, and become a serious health threat to men in their thirties and forties and to women in their forties and fifties. It's never too soon to start being heart smart. This chapter provides the information you need about risk factors: silent dangers, such as high blood pressure; and medical advances that can help your chances to have a healthier heart and a longer life.

How Your Heart Works

The heart is a hollow, muscular organ with four chambers that serve as two pumps (see Figure 12-1). It is about the size of a clenched fist. Each pump consists of a pair of chambers formed of muscles. The upper two—each called an **atrium**—receive blood, which then flows through valves into the lower two chambers, the **ventricles**, which contract to pump blood out into the arteries through a second set of valves. A thick wall divides the right side of the heart from the left side; but even though the two sides are separated, they contract at almost the same time. Contraction of the ventricles is called **systole**; the period of relaxation between contractions is called **diastole**. The heart valves, located at the entrance and exit of the ventricular chambers, have flaps that open and close to allow blood to flow through the chambers of the heart.

The myocardium (heart muscle) consists of branching fibers that enable the heart to contract or beat between 60 and 80 times per minute, or about 100,000 times a day. With each beat, it pumps about 2 ounces of blood. This may not sound like much, but it adds up to nearly 5 quarts of blood pumped by the heart in one minute, or about 75 gallons per hour.

The heart is surrounded by the pericardium, which consists of two layers of a tough membrane. The space between the two contains a lubricating fluid that allows the heart muscle to move freely. The endocardium is a smooth membrane lining the inside of the heart and its valves.

Blood circulates through the body by means of the pumping action of the heart, as shown in Figure 12-2. The right ventricle (on your own right side) pumps blood, via the *pulmonary arteries*, to the lungs, where it picks up oxygen (a gas essential to the body's cells) and gives off carbon dioxide (a waste product of metabolism). The blood returns from the lungs via the *pulmonary veins* to the left side of the heart, which pumps it, via the **aorta**, to the arteries in the rest of the body.

The arteries divide into smaller and smaller branches, and finally into **capillaries**, the smallest blood vessels of all (only slightly larger in diameter than a single red blood cell). The blood within the capillaries supplies oxygen and nutrients to the cells of the tissues, and takes up various waste products. Blood returns to the heart via the veins: The blood from the upper body (except the lungs) drains into the heart through the *superior vena cava*, while blood from lower body returns via the *inferior vena cava*.

The workings of this remarkable pump affect your entire body. If the flow of blood to or through the heart or to the rest of the body is reduced, or if a disturbance occurs in the small bundle of highly specialized cells in the heart that generate electrical impulses to control

Figure 12-1

The healthy heart. The heart muscle is nourished by blood from the coronary arteries, which arise from the aorta. The pericardium is the outer covering of the heart.

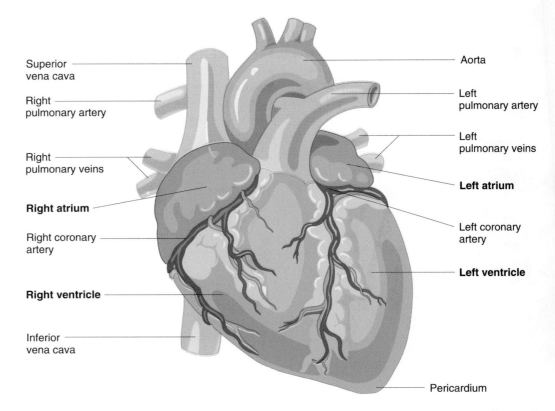

Superior vena cava

Right pulmonary artery

Right pulmonary veins

Right atrium

Right coronary artery

Right ventricle

Inferior vena cava

Aorta

Left pulmonary artery

Left pulmonary veins

Left atrium

Left coronary artery

Left ventricle

Pericardium

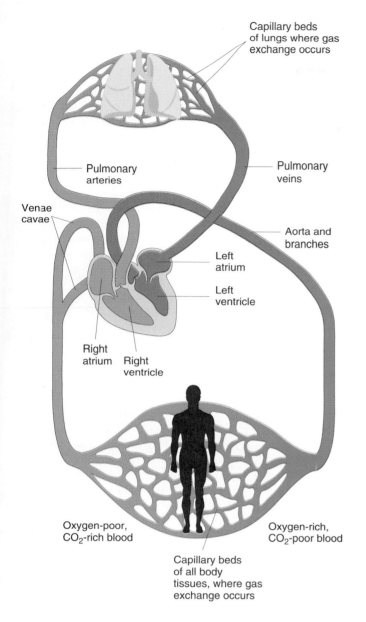

Capillary beds of lungs where gas exchange occurs

Pulmonary arteries

Pulmonary veins

Venae cavae

Aorta and branches

Left atrium

Left ventricle

Right atrium

Right ventricle

Oxygen-poor, CO_2-rich blood

Oxygen-rich, CO_2-poor blood

Capillary beds of all body tissues, where gas exchange occurs

Figure 12-2

The path of blood flow. Blood is pumped from the right ventricle into the pulmonary arteries, which lead to the lungs, where gas exchange (oxygen for carbon dioxide) occurs. Oxygenated blood returning from the lungs drains into the left atrium and is then pumped into the left ventricle, which sends the blood into the aorta and its branches. The oxygenated blood flows through the arteries, which extend to all parts of the body. Again, gas exchange occurs in the body tissues; this time oxygen is "dropped off" and carbon dioxide "picked up." Photo depicts a computer-enhanced image of a healthy heart.

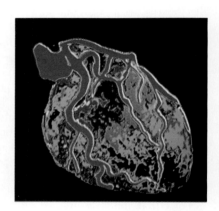

heartbeats, the result may at first be too subtle to notice. However, without diagnosis and treatment, these changes could develop into a life-threatening problem.

Preventing Heart Problems

Heart disease starts slowly and silently. Autopsy studies, in which researchers have examined the hearts of youngsters killed in accidents, have found fatty streaks in the arteries of children as young as age 3. Doctors are paying more attention to childhood risk factors, but medical experts disagree as to whether all children should be routinely screened for risk factors for coronary heart disease. Most physicians regularly check children's blood pressure but do not take routine cholesterol measurements.

According to a survey of 1503 college students, young adults are aware of the risk factors for heart disease, including high blood pressure, elevated cholesterol, smoking, and lack of exercise. However, only a third of those surveyed exercised or had their cholesterol levels checked regularly. As with other health-related behaviors, there is a gap between what students know about the risks of heart disease and what they do to protect themselves.[2] (See Personal Voices: "Dave's Heart.")

At any age, lifestyle changes can make a difference. Physical activity is particularly beneficial. Regular exercise reduces the risk of heart attack, helps maintain a desirable body weight, lowers blood pressure, and improves metabolism. If rigorous and frequent enough, it also may increase longevity.[3] Dietary changes (such as limiting total fat and cholesterol intake) also help pre-

Personal Voices Dave's Heart

Dave and his Dad used to spend hours watching baseball on TV. Smoking one cigarette after another as he always did, his Dad would explain the plays and tell Dave stories about the players he'd seen in his day. He'd been a pretty fair player when he was young. Of course, he didn't play anymore. Even playing catch with Dave would leave him breathless.

Dave's Mom called him and his father her "big guys" and produced lavish home-cooked meals for them. His Dad loved bacon and eggs, thick steaks, and Mom's pies. "The Millers are big people," Dave's Mom used to say. "They have good appetites."

Dave's father had his first heart attack when Dave was 10. Dave never forgot the terror he felt watching this big, strong man lying on the floor, his face twisted in pain, his fist pressed against his chest. Dave's father seemed different when he came home from the hospital, as if something had gone out of him. But his face would still light up with an impish grin, especially when he'd sneak a cigarette and wink at Dave so he wouldn't tell his Mom.

The second heart attack came four years later. This time Dave's Dad didn't come home. At the funeral, neighbors and relatives murmured, "What a pity," "Such a young man. How sad." Dave's own heart ached as he struggled to hold back his tears.

When Dave went off to college, he was so busy that he didn't think much about his Dad. He missed his Mom's cooking, though. He lived on double cheeseburg-ers, french fries, pizza, and beer. Not that there was an ounce of fat on him. He lifted weights three times a week, played softball with his friends, and swam whenever he got a chance. Even when he hardly got any sleep, he felt strong as a horse.

After his father's death, Dave had sworn he'd never smoke. But working late on term papers and hanging out at sports bars, he got in the habit of lighting up. He didn't know when one or two cigarettes a day became a dozen or when a dozen became a pack. Still, he never felt winded, not even after a workout.

After graduation, Dave, whose mother always said he had a way with people, discovered that he was a born salesman. He moved from company to company, always for a better commission, a bigger territory, a greater opportunity. Taking clients to dinner was part of his job—one that Dave enjoyed. But the long hours meant he had little or no time to exercise. Some nights he'd go back to the office and work until midnight, smoking cigarettes and sipping coffee to stay awake.

When he was 30, Dave got married. His wife nagged him about smoking, so he cut out cigarettes at home. She also lectured him about the fatty foods he loved. Every time he reached for an extra pat of butter, she'd glare at him. Dave would laugh it off. "Hey, I'm a big guy. I've got a big appetite," he'd say. The truth was that Dave was bigger than ever—well over 240 pounds, 50 pounds more than he weighed in college. Sometimes playing tag with Brian, his little boy, he'd find himself gasping for breath—just like his own Dad.

When Dave was in his late thirties, his wife insisted that he get a physical. He was sure there would be nothing wrong. The physician took Dave's family history, noted his weight and blood pressure, tested his blood cholesterol, and asked, "Do you know what I see? A heart attack waiting to happen." At first Dave couldn't even believe her words. He felt too good. He was too young. He'd cut down on his smoking. Maybe in another ten years or so, he'd have to watch it a little more. But not now, not yet.

One night, as Dave was tucking his son into bed, the little boy asked, "Are you going to die, Daddy?" "Not as long as you need me," he replied. "But, Daddy," Brian sobbed. "I'll always need you." Dave felt his eyes fill with tears as he thought back to his Dad and all the times he'd needed him and he hadn't been there.

The very next day Dave made another appointment with his physician. This time he listened carefully. With his physician's supervision, he began a regular exercise program. He got information on heart healthy meals and nutrition. He threw out his last pack of cigarettes and, even though he craved them, never bought another. When he went back for a checkup a year later, he asked his physician if she still thought she was looking at a heart attack waiting to happen. "No," she replied. "Now I'm looking at a heart attack that doesn't have to happen."

—D.H.

vent heart disease. Foods rich in cell-protecting **antioxidants** (discussed in Chapter 6), as well as folic acid and supplements of Vitamin E, have been linked with a lower risk of heart disease.[4]

Strategies for Prevention
. . . .
What You Can Do to Avoid Heart Disease

✔ *Eat a low-fat diet.* Get no more than 30% of your daily calories from fat in any form and no more than 10% from saturated fat. (See Chapter 6 for a discussion of types of fat.)

✔ *Limit your cholesterol intake to 300 milligrams a day.* (See Chapter 6.)

✔ *Exercise.* Regular aerobic exercise—walking, cycling, swimming, or jogging—is best.

✔ *Watch your weight.* Extra pounds can mean extra risk for high blood pressure and other forms of cardiovascular disease.

✔ *Don't smoke.* Smokers have twice the risk of heart attack and two to four times the risk of sudden cardiac death that nonsmokers have.

✔ *Limit your intake of alcohol.* Alcohol can increase blood pressure and directly affect the heart; drink no more than

3 ounces, or the equivalent of two alcoholic drinks, a day.

✔ *Hold the salt.* Along with losing weight, significantly cutting down on your intake of sodium can reduce blood pressure. (See Chapter 6.)

Risk Factors for Cardiovascular Disease

Several major risk factors contribute to disorders of the heart and blood vessels. The greater the number or severity of these risk factors, the greater your overall risk. (See Self-Survey: "Are You Headed for a Heart Attack?")

Risks You Can Control

The choices individuals make and the habits they follow can have a significant impact on whether or not their hearts remain healthy. The following are potential risks that you can avoid for the sake of your heart's health.

Physical Inactivity

According to the Centers for Disease Control and Prevention (CDC), the leading culprit in deaths from heart attack is sedentary living. People who are not even somewhat physically active face a much greater risk of fatal heart attack than those who engage in some form of exercise or activity. Individuals who work out rigorously and regularly have the healthiest hearts and the lowest risks of heart disease. (See Chapter 5 for a discussion of the benefits of minimal, moderate, and vigorous exercise.)

Cigarette Smoking

Each year smoking causes more than 250,000 deaths from cardiovascular disease—far more than it causes from cancer and lung disease. Smokers who have heart attacks are more likely to die from them than are non-smokers. Smoking is the major risk factor for *peripheral vascular disease,* in which the blood vessels that carry blood to the leg and arm muscles get hardened and clogged. Both active and passive smoking accelerate the process by which arteries become clogged and increase the risk of heart attacks and strokes.[5] Passive smoking also reduces beneficial blood fats and increases harmful ones in children.[6]

Cigarette smoking may damage the heart in several ways:

- The nicotine may repeatedly overstimulate the heart.

- Carbon monoxide may take the place of some of the oxygen in the blood, which reduces the oxygen supply to the heart muscle.

- The tars and other smoke residues may damage the lining of the coronary arteries, making it easier for cholesterol to build up and narrow the passageways.

- Smoking also increases blood clotting, leading to a higher incidence of clotting in the coronary arteries and subsequent heart attack. Clotting in the peripheral arteries is also increased, which can cause leg pain with walking and, ultimately, stroke.

- New research indicates that ex-smokers may have irreversible damage to their arteries.[7]

High Blood Pressure (Hypertension)

Blood pressure is a result of the contractions of the heart muscle, which pumps blood through your body, and the resistance of the walls of the vessels through which the blood flows. Each time your heart beats, your blood pressure goes up and down within a certain range. It's highest when the heart contracts; this is called *systolic blood pressure.* It's lowest between contractions; this is called *diastolic blood pressure.* A blood pressure reading consists of the systolic measurement "over" the diastolic measurement, recorded in millimeters of mercury (mmHg) by a sphygmomanometer (see Figure 12-3).

High blood pressure, or **hypertension**, occurs when the artery walls become constricted so that the force exerted as the blood flows through them is greater than it should be. Physicians see blood pressure as a continuum: the higher the reading, the greater the risk of stroke and heart disease. (See also the further discussion of high blood pressure later in this chapter.)

As a result of the increased work in pumping blood, the heart muscle of a person with hypertension can become stronger and also stiffer. This stiffness increases resistance to filling up with blood between beats, which can cause shortness of breath with exertion. Hypertension can also act on the kidney arteries, which can lead to kidney failure in some cases. In addition, hypertension accelerates the development of plaque buildup within the arteries. Especially when combined with obesity, smoking, high cholesterol levels, or diabetes, hypertension increases the risks of cardiovascular problems several times. However, you can control high blood pressure through diet, exercise, and medication (if necessary).

Self-Survey

Are You Headed for a Heart Attack?

If you're like most people, you don't think about your heart until something goes wrong. But consider this: having any one of the risk factors more than doubles your chance of developing coronary heart disease. Take a minute to assess your risk factors by placing a check in the appropriate column for each statement below.

	Yes	No
High Blood Cholesterol		
You often eat high-fat foods or foods high in cholesterol, such as butter and eggs.	____	____
Your blood cholesterol level of fatty substances in your blood is over 200 mg/dL.	____	____
You're unaware of your total blood cholesterol level.	____	____
Smoking		
You are a cigarette, pipe, or cigar smoker.	____	____
You smoke four or more cigarettes a day.	____	____
You have little motivation to quit smoking.	____	____
High Blood Pressure		
You're overweight and eat lots of salty foods.	____	____
Your blood pressure is above 140/90.	____	____
You're unaware of your blood pressure level.	____	____
Other Risk Factors		
You have diabetes or a family history of diabetes.	____	____
You don't have a regular exercise or stress management program.	____	____

	Yes	No
You're a woman on birth control pills and also have high blood cholesterol or high blood pressure.	____	____
You're a man whose father or other male relative had a heart attack at an early age.	____	____

The More Times You Answered Yes

The higher your score, the greater your risk of developing coronary heart disease. But take heart. Once you understand more about your heart and your risk factors, you'll know what changes you can make to keep your heart healthy.

SOURCE: Adapted from Daly City, CA: Krames Communications, 1988.

Making Changes
Reducing Your Risk

- Try to quit smoking permanently.
- Have your blood pressure checked regularly. If your blood pressure is high, see your physician. Remember, blood pressure medicine is effective only if taken regularly.
- Try to fit a half hour of brisk walking, swimming, or other enjoyable aerobic activity into your day.
- If you're overweight or eat a lot of foods high in saturated fat or cholesterol (whole milk, cheese, eggs, butter, fatty foods, fried foods), you need to change your diet (see Chapter 6 for details).

SOURCE: Adapted from the American Heart Association.

Blood Fats

Cholesterol is a fatty substance found in certain foods and also manufactured by the body (see Chapter 6). The measurement of cholesterol in the blood is one of the most reliable indicators of the formation of plaque, the sludgelike substance that builds up on the inner walls of arteries. You can lower blood cholesterol levels by cutting back on high-fat foods and exercising more, thereby reducing the risk of a heart attack. According to the National Heart, Lung, and Blood Institute (NHLBI), for every 1% drop in blood cholesterol, studies show a 2% decrease in the likelihood of a heart attack. (See the Cholesterol Connection, later in this chapter.)

Triglycerides

These fats, which flow through the blood after meals, have been linked to increased risk of coronary artery disease, especially in women. **Triglyceride** levels tend to be highest in those whose diets are high in calories, sugar, alcohol, and refined starches. High levels of these fats may increase the risk of obesity, but cutting back on these foods can reduce high triglyceride levels.

According to the NHLBI, triglyceride levels should be between 30 and 150 milligrams per decaliter (mg/dL) of blood. Triglyceride levels in the range of 250–500 mg/dL are a danger sign of an increased risk of heart disease. Higher levels, especially over 1000 mg/dL, also

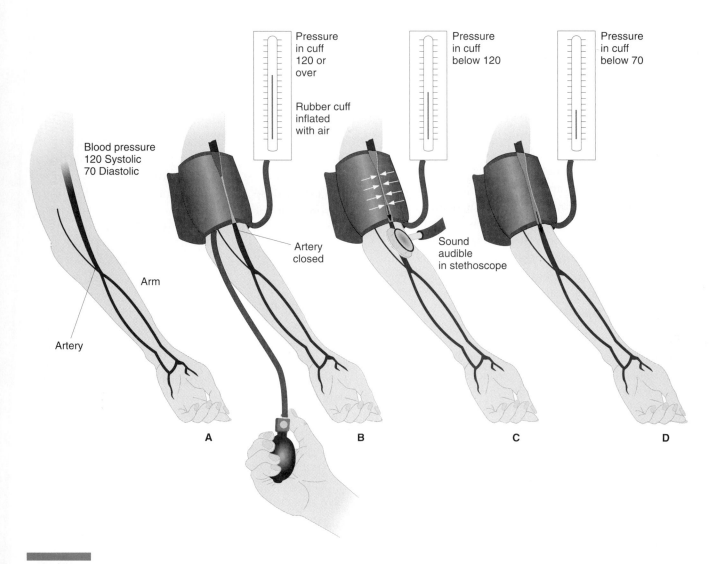

Figure 12-3

Measurement of blood pressure. Assume a blood pressure of 120/70 in a young, healthy individual. (A) The brachial artery of the arm is used to measure blood pressure. (B) The cuff of the sphygmomanometer (blood pressure cuff) is wrapped snugly around the arm just above the elbow and inflated until the blood flow into the brachial artery is stopped. This stoppage is detected with a stethoscope. (C) The cuff is gradually loosened, while the examiner listens carefully for pulse sounds with the stethoscope. The pressure reading as the first soft tapping sounds are heard (as a small amount of blood spurts through the constricted artery) is the systolic pressure. (D) As the cuff is loosened still further, the sounds become louder and more distinct. When the artery is no longer constricted and blood flows freely, however, the pulse sounds can no longer be heard. The reading at which the sounds disappear is recorded as the diastolic pressure.

increase the risk of pancreatitis, an inflammation of the pancreas requiring immediate medical attention.

Lipoproteins

Lipoproteins are compounds in the blood that are made up of proteins and fat. The different types are classified by their size or density. The heaviest are *high-density lipoproteins*, or HDLs, which have the highest portion of protein. These "good guys," as some cardiologists refer to them, pick up excess cholesterol in the blood and carry it back to the liver for removal from the body. *Low-density lipoproteins*, or LDLs, carry more cholesterol than HDLs and deposit it on the walls of arteries—they're the bad guys.

HDLs are most plentiful in the people least likely to get cardiovascular disease, such as young women and athletes. The higher the level of HDL and the higher the ratio of HDL to total cholesterol (HDL plus other blood fats), the lower the likelihood of heart disease. An HDL level of less than 45 mg/dL and an HDL-cholesterol ratio of less than 1 to 5 increase a man's risk of coronary artery disease. Women should have an HDL level above

55 mg/dL and an HDL-cholesterol ratio of more than 1 to 4.10. (See the Cholesterol Connection for ways to lower elevated levels.)

Diabetes Mellitus

Diabetes mellitus, a disorder of the endocrine system, increases the likelihood of hypertension and atherosclerosis, thereby increasing the risk of heart attack and stroke. A physician can detect diabetes and prescribe a diet, exercise program, and, if necessary, medication to keep it in check. Even before developing diabetes, individuals at high risk for this disease—those who are overweight, have a family history of the disease, have mildly elevated blood pressure and blood sugar levels, and above-ideal levels of harmful blood fats—may already be at increased risk of heart disease. (See Chapter 13 for more information on diabetes.)

Weight

According to the National Heart, Lung, and Blood Institute, losing weight at any age can help reduce the risk of heart problems. For women, obesity is as great a cause of excess death and disability from heart disease as smoking and heavy drinking. Even mild to moderately obese women are more likely to suffer chest pain or a heart attack than thinner women.[8] (See Chapter 7 for a discussion of weight control.)

Psychological Factors

As discussed in Chapter 2, the way we respond to everyday sources of stress can affect our hearts as well as our overall health. While we may not be able to control the sources of stress, we can change how we habitually respond to it. The significance of Type-A behavior (see Chapter 2) has been debated for more than 30 years. Initial studies showed a clearly increased risk of coronary artery disease; more recent ones have not. Of all Type-A traits, anger and hostility have been most closely linked to heart disease. These negative emotions may send adrenaline and other stress hormones into the bloodstream, where they cause fat to be dumped into the blood, driving up cholesterol levels. Recent studies indicate that depression may increase the risk of heart disease as well.

Risks You Can't Control

Heredity

Anyone whose parents, siblings, or other close relatives suffered heart attacks before age 50 is at increased risk of developing heart disease. Certain risk factors, such as abnormally high blood levels of lipids, can be passed down from generation to generation. Although you can't rewrite your family history, individuals with an inherited vulnerability to cardiovascular disease can lower the danger by changing the risk factors within their control. Your heart's health depends to a great extent on your behavior, including the decisions you make about the foods you eat, or the decision not to smoke. As an added preventive step, cardiologists may prescribe a small daily dose of aspirin to individuals with a history of coronary artery disease who are at risk of forming clots that could block blood supplies to the heart, brain, and other organs. (*Note*: Daily aspirin is not advised for individuals who are not at risk because of their age or health history.)

Race and Ethnicity

African Americans are twice as likely to develop high blood pressure as are whites. African Americans also suffer strokes at an earlier age and of greater severity. Poverty may be an unrecognized risk factor for members of this minority group, who are less likely to receive medical treatments or undergo corrective surgery. Family history, lifestyle, diet, and stress may also play a role, starting early in life. However, researchers have found no single explanation for why African-American youngsters, like their parents, tend to have higher blood pressure than white children.[9]

Age

Almost four out of five people who die of heart attacks are over age 65. Heart disease accounts for more than 40% of deaths among people between 65 and 74 and almost 60% at age 85 and above. However, the risk factors that are likely to cause heart disease later in life, including high blood pressure and cholesterol levels, may begin to develop in childhood. Nevertheless, although cardiovascular function declines with age, heart disease is not an inevitable consequence of aging. Many 80- and 90-year-olds have strong, healthy hearts.[10]

Gender

Men have a higher incidence of cardiovascular problems than women, particularly before age 40. Coronary artery disease tends to develop about a decade later in women than in men, possibly because younger women have high blood levels of heart-healthy HDLs. The female sex hormone estrogen may also have a protective effect by increasing HDL levels and decreasing harmful LDL levels. After menopause or surgical removal of the ovaries, women's estrogen levels drop and their LDL levels tend to go up. Postmenopausal hormone replacement therapy (HRT) can protect women against heart disease by keeping their HDL levels up and their LDL levels down. However, the question of which women should take estrogen remains controversial (see Chapter 9).[11]

Because heart disease has been perceived as a man's problem, research on women's hearts has lagged behind. The current recommendations for blood pressure, cholesterol levels, and prevention are based almost entirely on research on men. However, heart disease is the fourth-leading cause of death among women aged 30 to 34, third among women aged 35 to 39, second among women aged 40 to 64, and first among women over age 65. Although heart disease causes greater disability in women, it is routinely treated less aggressively than in men.

Heart disease takes different forms in men and women. Middle-aged men are more likely to have a heart attack or sudden heart stoppage, while women in their middle years are more likely to suffer angina or chest pain (discussed later in this chapter). However, the rate of heart attacks increases in women in their sixties or older. And a woman's risk of dying within a month of a heart attack is 75% higher than for a man, possibly because she generally is older and has other health problems, such as hypertension and diabetes.

Male Pattern Baldness

Male pattern baldness (the loss of hair at the vertex, or top, of the head) is associated with increased risk of heart attack in men under age 55. A study of 1437 men showed a "modest" increased risk for those men who'd lost hair at the top of their heads but not for those with receding hairlines. The speed at which men lose their hair also may be an indicator of risk. Scientists speculate that men with male pattern baldness who lose their hair quickly may metabolize male sex hormones differently than others, thereby increasing the likelihood of heart disease.

Although it's premature to say that baldness is definitely "bad news for the heart," health experts advise bald men to follow basic guidelines, such as not smoking and controlling their cholesterol levels, to lower any possible risk.[12]

The Cholesterol Connection

Cholesterol levels have dropped steadily among Americans since 1980; this change alone may account for an 8 to 17% decline in the incidence of heart disease.[13] For the sake of a healthy heart, all adults should know what their cholesterol level is, whether it's too high and if it is, what they can do to lower cholesterol.

What's Normal?

When it comes to cholesterol, "normal" isn't good enough. The average cholesterol level for middle-aged men and women in the United States is about 215 mg/dL of blood—more than the recommended desirable limit set by the NHLBI. Adults with a cholesterol level of 220 mg/dL may be more than twice as likely to get heart disease as those with a level of 180 mg/dL; for those with levels of 300 mg/dL or higher, the risk is four times greater.

According to the NHLBI:

- Total cholesterol should be below 200 mg/dL of blood for men and below 210 mg/dL for women.

- A total cholesterol reading of 201–239 mg/dL is considered borderline and presents a moderate to high risk for heart disease. Americans with cholesterol levels below 240 mg/dL account for more than 60% of the cases of coronary heart disease in this country.

- Total cholesterol levels of 240 or more mg/dL are dangerously high.

- LDL levels should be less than 130 mg/dL: a level of 160 mg/dL or more is high.

- HDL levels should be at least 35 mg/dL.

Persons in the moderate- to high-risk categories (as many as half of all adults, according to some estimates) should undergo a test of the concentrations of the different types of lipoproteins (HDLs and LDLs), the protein-fat complexes that carry cholesterol in the blood.

Cholesterol and Children

Watching cholesterol levels isn't just for grownups anymore. In its guidelines for children, the National Cholesterol Education Program recommends cholesterol testing for youngsters at possible risk of heart disease, including those who have any of the following risk factors:

- A parent or grandparent who developed atherosclerosis (narrowing of the arteries due to plaque buildup) at or before age 55.

- A parent or grandparent who suffered a heart attack at or before age 55.

- A parent whose blood cholesterol level is over 240 mg/dL.

Federal health officials aren't advising cholesterol screening for all youngsters, in part because children with high cholesterol levels don't necessarily end up with high blood cholesterol as adults. About 25% of American children may have cholesterol levels higher than the ideal of 170 mg/dL. Most of these are in the range of 190 to 200, although a small percentage are 300 or higher. For those with moderately elevated cholesterol levels, the suggested treatment is a low-fat, high-fiber diet, identical to the one most beneficial for adults' hearts. For children whose blood cholesterol is within normal ranges, doctors advise a balanced diet, with moderate amounts of a full range of nutrients.[14]

Cholesterol and the Elderly

After age 70, elevated cholesterol levels seem less of a threat—at least in men. In a study of nearly 1000 people at Yale University, high cholesterol did not increase the risk of heart disease in those over age 70. This study suggests that the 2 million elderly people taking cholesterol-lowering drugs may be receiving little, if any benefit and may even be risking some harm. However, another 1995 report concluded that, in older women, elevated cholesterol may indeed predict a greater risk of potentially fatal heart disease.[15]

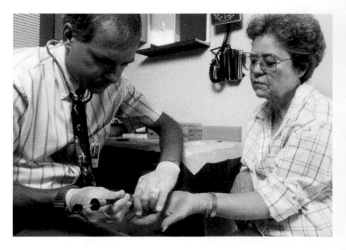

Getting a cholesterol test is a quick, simple, and relatively painless procedure.

Strategies for Prevention
···

What You Need to Know About Cholesterol Testing

✔ Go to your usual primary health-care provider to have your cholesterol level checked. Although cholesterol tests at shopping malls or health fairs can help identify people at risk, the analyzers are often not certified technicians, and the readings may occasionally be inaccurate. In addition, without a health expert to counsel them, some people may be unnecessarily frightened by a high reading—or falsely reassured by a low one.

✔ Ask about accuracy. Even at first-rate laboratories, cholesterol readings are often inaccurate. Find out if the lab is using the National Institutes of Health (NIH) standards, and ask about the lab's margin for error (which should be less than 5%).

✔ Think about timing. A cholesterol test is most accurate after a 12- to 14-hour fast. Schedule the test before breakfast if you can, or at least two hours after eating. Women may not want to get tested at the end of their menstrual cycles, when minor elevations in cholesterol levels occur because of lower estrogen levels. Choles-

terol levels can also rise 5% to 10% during periods of stress. Reschedule the test if you come down with an intestinal flu, because the viral infection could interfere with the absorption of food and thus with cholesterol levels. Let your doctor know if you're taking any drugs. Common medications, including birth control pills and hypertension drugs, can affect cholesterol levels.

✔ Sit down before allowing blood to be drawn or your finger to be pricked, because fluids pool differently in the body when you're standing than when you're sitting. Don't let a technician squeeze blood from your finger, because that forces fluid from cells, diluting the blood sample and possibly leading to a falsely low reading.

✔ Get real numbers. Don't settle for "normal" or "high," because laboratories can label results inaccurately. Find out exactly what your reading is. Find out your HDL/LDL ratio. If your cholesterol level is high, have it retested; ask to find out HDL and LDL levels as well.

✔ Some physicians advise getting two or three tests in the same month and averaging the result. A person's cholesterol levels vary so much from day to day that a single measurement may be meaningless.

Lowering Cholesterol Levels

There are various ways to reduce cholesterol levels—and the risk of heart disease. The best way to begin is by reducing cholesterol and fat in your diet (see Chapter 6). Your goal should be to limit all fats to no more than 30% of the calories you consume every day and saturated fats to no more than 10%. Controlling your weight and increasing physical activity also can help.

If cholesterol levels are dangerously high and exercise and diet therapy fail, medications to lower cholesterol can be highly effective. Researchers at the University of California's Lawrence Berkeley Laboratory found that, over several years, the combination of a low-fat diet and cholesterol-lowering drugs can reduce and even reverse clogging of the arteries.[16] The American College of Cardiology has reported that at least two cholesterol-lowering drugs, simvastatin and provastatin, can halt or delay the progression of heart disease and prolong life.[17] However, preventive treatment of individuals who have high cholesterol readings but no evidence of coronary artery disease with cholesterol-lowering drugs remains controversial.[18]

There also is some question about whether too-low cholesterol levels might cause different health problems over time. Numerous reports have linked total blood cholesterol levels of 160 or lower with greater mortality from liver cancer, lung disease, hemorrhagic stroke, suicide, and alcoholism. There are many reasons why a person's cholesterol levels may be low—genetics, an extremely rigorous diet and exercise regimen, or illness, including anemia and diseases of the lungs or liver.

The Silent Killers

The two most common forms of cardiovascular disease in this country are high blood pressure (hypertension) and coronary artery disease, the gradual narrowing of the blood vessels of the heart. Often these two problems go together.

High Blood Pressure

Hypertension forces the heart to pump harder than is healthy. Because the heart must force blood into arteries that are offering increased resistance to blood flow, the left side of the heart often becomes enlarged (see Figure 12-4). The term *essential hypertension* indicates that the cause is unknown, as is usually the case. Occasionally, abnormalities of the kidneys or the blood vessels feeding

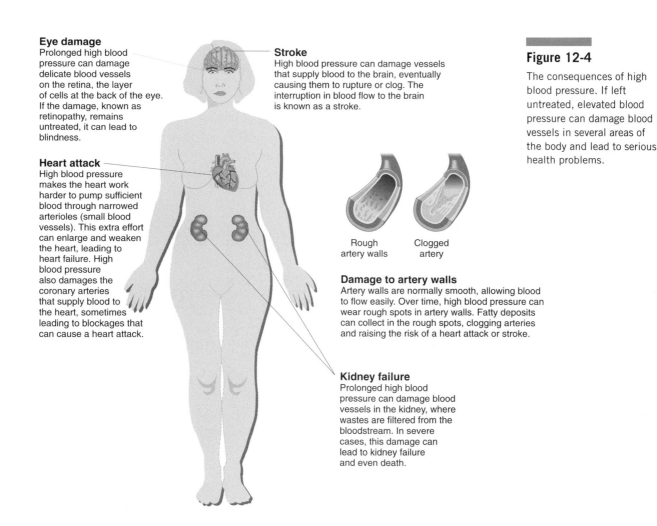

Eye damage
Prolonged high blood pressure can damage delicate blood vessels on the retina, the layer of cells at the back of the eye. If the damage, known as retinopathy, remains untreated, it can lead to blindness.

Stroke
High blood pressure can damage vessels that supply blood to the brain, eventually causing them to rupture or clog. The interruption in blood flow to the brain is known as a stroke.

Heart attack
High blood pressure makes the heart work harder to pump sufficient blood through narrowed arterioles (small blood vessels). This extra effort can enlarge and weaken the heart, leading to heart failure. High blood pressure also damages the coronary arteries that supply blood to the heart, sometimes leading to blockages that can cause a heart attack.

Rough artery walls

Clogged artery

Damage to artery walls
Artery walls are normally smooth, allowing blood to flow easily. Over time, high blood pressure can wear rough spots in artery walls. Fatty deposits can collect in the rough spots, clogging arteries and raising the risk of a heart attack or stroke.

Kidney failure
Prolonged high blood pressure can damage blood vessels in the kidney, where wastes are filtered from the bloodstream. In severe cases, this damage can lead to kidney failure and even death.

Figure 12-4

The consequences of high blood pressure. If left untreated, elevated blood pressure can damage blood vessels in several areas of the body and lead to serious health problems.

them, or certain substances in the bloodstream, are identified as the culprits. Whatever its cause, hypertension is dangerous because excessive pressure can wear out arteries, leading to serious cardiovascular diseases, vision problems, and kidney disease.

More than 40 million Americans have high blood pressure that requires monitoring or treatment. While most are under age 65, hypertension has become increasingly common among people in their twenties and thirties. Physicians urge all adults to have their blood pressure checked at least once a year.

A blood pressure reading that's slightly above normal isn't necessarily proof of a blood pressure problem. Due to nervousness, blood pressure may shoot up when anxious individuals enter a medical office, causing what's known as *white coat hypertension*. Other factors, such as warm weather or variations in how health-care practitioners do the test, also can cause elevated readings.[19] It can help to take blood pressure readings at home and compare them with your physician's readings. (Equipment for measuring blood pressure is sold at most pharmacies.)

Normal blood pressure in most young adults is 120/80 mmHg (120 systolic pressure, 80 diastolic pressure) under relaxed conditions. Borderline hypertension is 140/90 to 160/95; definite hypertension is 160/95 and above. The lower, or diastolic, number has increasingly been used in categorizing high blood pressure, with 90 to 104 indicating mild hypertension; 105 to 114, moderate; and 115 and over, severe. A high diastolic reading indicates an increased risk of heart disease, even if the systolic pressure is normal (see Table 12-1). According to a 1995 report, people whose systolic blood pressure is slightly above normal also face increased health risks of heart disease and stroke, compared with those whose blood pressure is under 140.[20]

Experts disagree on the definitions of hypertension, particularly mild forms of it. Only the United States has set the lower limit for high diastolic blood pressure at 90 mmHg; other countries start at 95 or 100. The World Health Organization (WHO) calls diastolic blood pressures from 90 to 94 borderline and recommends that patients with a diastolic reading below 95 be monitored for six months.

In evaluating individual patients, most health-care professionals look not just at the numbers but also at other risk factors, such as cholesterol levels and family history. Physicians have warned that people with borderline hypertension may sustain damage to their heart and blood vessels and should seek more aggressive treatment for their high blood pressure. Even people with blood pressure of 130/93 may show early signs of cardiovascular problems, such as changes in the heart muscle such that it cannot relax completely between contractions.

Prevention pays off when it comes to high blood pressure. The most effective preventive measures involve lifestyle changes. Losing weight has been demonstrated to be the best approach for individuals with high normal values. Exercise may be effective in lowering mildly elevated blood pressure. Restriction of sodium intake also helps. There are no data showing an association between individuals with normal blood pressure, salt intake, and the risk of heart attack.[21] However,

TABLE 12-1 Classification of High Blood Pressure

Category	Systolic Reading	Diastolic Reading	Followup Recommended
Normal	Less than 130	Less than 85	Check again in two years.
High normal	130–139	85–89	Check in one year. Many physicians recommend lifestyle modifications at this stage.
Hypertension			
Stage 1	140–159	90–99	Modify lifestyle. Begin drug treatment if lifestyle modifications are not effective within six months.
Stage 2	160–179	100–109	Begin drug treatment and modify lifestyle.
Stage 3	180–209	110–119	Begin drug treatment and modify lifestyle.
Stage 4	More than 210	More than 120	Immediate medical evaluation and treatment with drugs. Modify lifestyle.

Source: Joint National Committee on Detection, Evaluation, Treatment of High Blood Pressure.

individuals with hypertension who are sensitive to sodium are at about twice the risk of heart attack and stroke as others.[22] Among the approaches that have not proven effective are dietary supplements, such as calcium, magnesium, potassium, and fish oil.

The same lifestyle changes that work as preventive measures are the best forms of nondrug (or nonpharmacologic) treatment for hypertension (see Pulsepoints: "Ten Keys to a Healthy Heart"). However, there is no single ideal prescription for reducing high blood pressure in all patients. The most current recommendations are:

- Achieve and maintain appropriate body weight.
- Limit alcohol to one ounce a day.
- Get some exercise daily.
- Keep sodium intake below 2.4 grams a day.
- Consume adequate dietary amounts of potassium, calcium, and potassium.
- Don't smoke.
- Cut down on saturated fats, cholesterol, and "trans-fats."

If exercise, dietary changes, and restriction of salt intake fail to bring down blood pressure, some health experts argue that even those with mild hypertension should take drugs to prevent damage to the heart and blood vessels. There is controversy about the best medications for treating hypertension. The Fifth Joint National Committee on the Detection, Evaluation, and Treatment of High Blood Pressure recommended hydrochlorthiazide, a diuretic agent that increases fluid elimination, and cardiac drugs known as betablockers as the initial treatment for most patients. However, a 1997 review of all antihypertensive prescriptions at approximately 35,000 pharmacies in the United States found that the use of these medications had decreased, and more physicians are prescribing other drugs, such as calcium antagonists and ACE inhibitors, for their patients. [23]

Coronary Artery Disease

The general term for any impairment of blood flow through the blood vessels, often referred to as "hardening of the arteries," is **arteriosclerosis**. The most common form is **atherosclerosis**, a disease of the lining of the arteries in which plaque—deposits of fat, fibrin (a clotting material), cholesterol, other cell parts, and calcium—narrows the artery channels.

Clogging the Arteries

Atherosclerosis, which may begin in childhood, worsens with the continued buildup of plaque on the arterial lining (see Figure 12-5). The arteries lose their ability to expand and contract. Blood moves with increasing difficulty through the narrowed channels, making it easier for a clot (thrombus) to form, perhaps blocking the channel and depriving vital organs of blood. When such a blockage is in a coronary artery, the result is coronary

---

Pulsepoints

Ten Keys to a Healthy Heart

1. Don't smoke. There's no bigger favor you can do your heart—and lungs!

2. Watch your weight. Even relatively modest gains can have a big effect on your risk of heart disease.

3. Cut down on saturated fats and cholesterol. This could help prevent high blood cholesterol levels, obesity, and heart disease.

4. Get moving. Engage in regular physical activity. A little is better than none; more is even better.

5. Lower your stress levels. If too much stress is a problem in your life, try the relaxation techniques described in Chapter 2.

6. Know your family history. Inheriting a predispositon to high blood pressure or heart disease means that your heart needs extra preventive care.

7. Get your blood pressure checked regularly. Knowing your numbers can alert you to a potential problem long before you develop any symptoms.

8. Tame your temper. Hostility can be hazardous to the heart. Look for other ways of releasing anger and frustration.

9. Find out your cholesterol levels. You can't know if your heart is in danger unless you know if your cholesterol is too high. Get a blood test at your next physical, and discuss the results with your physician.

10. Take appropriate medications. Those with high cholesterol or high blood pressure should seek their physicians' advice.

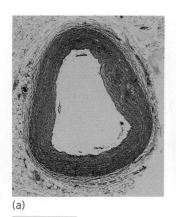 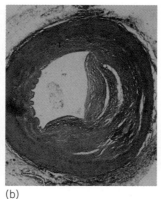

(a)   (b)

Figure 12-5

(A) A healthy coronary artery. (B) An artery partially blocked by the buildup of atherosclerotic plaque.

thrombosis, one form of heart attack. When the clot occurs in the brain, the result is cerebral thrombosis, one form of stroke (discussed later in this chapter).

Unclogging the Arteries

For years, heart specialists said that, once clogged, arteries couldn't be unclogged. However, recent research has shown that it is possible to reverse the buildup of plaque inside the arteries by means of cholesterol-lowering drugs and a low-fat diet. A strict program of dietary and lifestyle change without any medication, developed by Dean Ornish, M.D., of the University of California, San Francisco, also has proven effective in reversing coronary artery disease. The following are the key elements of this approach:

- A very low-fat, vegetarian diet, including nonfat dairy products and egg whites, keeping fat intake to below 8% of total calories consumed. Ornish's recommended diet allows no meat, poultry, fish, butter, cheese, ice cream, or any form of oil.

- Moderate exercise, consisting of an hour of aerobic activity three times a week. Walking is recommended because more rigorous exercise might be dangerous for heart patients, who may develop increased risk of blood clots, irregular heartbeats, or coronary artery spasms during exertion.

- Stress counseling. Ornish's patients learn how the body's stress response can cause a rapid heartbeat and narrowing of the arteries, and how stress reduction can reduce cholesterol levels.

- An hour a day of yoga, meditation, breathing, and progressive relaxation. Some patients use visualiza-

tion, for instance, imagining their arteries being cleared by a tunneling machine.

Ornish believes that a less strict version of his treatment program might help prevent arteries from becoming blocked in the first place.[24]

Crises of the Heart

For many people, the first sign of heart disease is pain, ranging from mild to excruciating. They may be experiencing angina pectoris, spasms of the coronary artery, or myocardial infarction (heart attack). According to the American Heart Association (AHA), as many as 1.5 million men and women have heart attacks each year; almost 5 million Americans alive today have had a heart attack, chest pain, or both.

Angina Pectoris

A temporary drop in the supply of oxygen to the heart tissue causes feelings of pain or discomfort in the chest known as **angina pectoris**. Some people suffer angina only when the demands on their hearts increase, such as during exercise or when under stress. Many people have angina for years and yet never suffer a heart attack; in some, the angina even disappears. However, angina should be considered a warning of danger if it becomes more severe or more frequent, occurs with less activity or exertion, begins to waken a person from a sound sleep at night, persists for more than ten to fifteen minutes, or causes unusual perspiration.

Angina is most commonly treated with beta blockers, calcium channel blockers, or nitrates.

Coronary Artery Spasms

Sometimes the arteries tighten suddenly or go into a spasm, cutting off or reducing blood flow. Spasms can produce heart attacks, as well as angina, and can be fatal. Several factors may trigger spasms in the heart, including the following:

- *Clumping of platelets.* When *platelets* (a type of blood cell) clump together, they produce a substance called thromboxane A-2, which causes the narrowing of a blood vessel.

- *Smoking.* When some angina victims stop smoking, their chest pain declines or disappears.

- *Stress.* No one knows exactly how stress may lead to

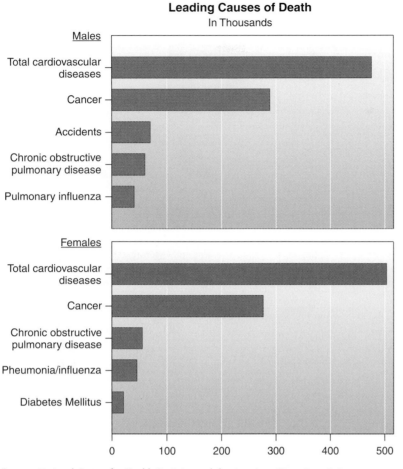

Leading Causes of Death
In Thousands

Males
- Total cardiovascular diseases
- Cancer
- Accidents
- Chronic obstructive pulmonary disease
- Pulmonary influenza

Females
- Total cardiovascular diseases
- Cancer
- Chronic obstructive pulmonary disease
- Pheumonia/influenza
- Diabetes Mellitus

0   100   200   300   400   500

Source: National Center for Health Statistics and the American Heart Association.

Figure 12-6

Cardiovascular diseases are the leading causes of death among men and women in the United States.

spasms, but many heart specialists believe that it's a culprit.

- *Increased calcium flow.* Calcium regularly flows into smooth muscle cells; too much calcium, however, may lead to a spasm. (This calcium flow is not regulated by the amount of calcium in your diet.)

Myocardial Infarction (Heart Attack)

The medical name for a heart attack, or coronary, is **myocardial infarction (MI)**. The *myocardium* is the cardiac muscle layer of the wall of the heart. It receives its blood supply, and thus its oxygen and other nutrients, from the coronary arteries. If an artery is blocked by a clot or plaque, or by a spasm, the myocardial cells do not get sufficient oxygen, and the portion of the myocardium deprived of its blood supply begins to die (see Figure 12-7). Although such an attack may seem sudden, usually it has been building up for years, par-

ticularly if the person has ignored risk factors and early warning signs.

Individuals should seek immediate medical care if they experience the following symptoms:

- A heavy, squeezing pain or discomfort in the center of the chest, which may last for several minutes.
- A pain that may radiate to the shoulder, arm, neck, back, or jaw.
- Anxiety.
- Sweating.
- Nausea and vomiting.
- Shortness of breath.
- Dizziness or fainting.

The two hours immediately following the onset of such symptoms is the most crucial period. About 40% of those who suffer an MI die within this time. According to the American Heart Association, most patients wait three hours after the initial symptoms begin before seeking help. By that time, half of the affected heart

Figure 12-7

The making of a heart attack. (A) The bulk of the heart is composed mainly of the myocardium, the muscle layer that contracts. (B) A clot in one of the arteries that feeds into the myocardium can cut off the blood supply to part of the myocardium, causing cells in that area to die. This is called a myocardial infarction, or heart attack.

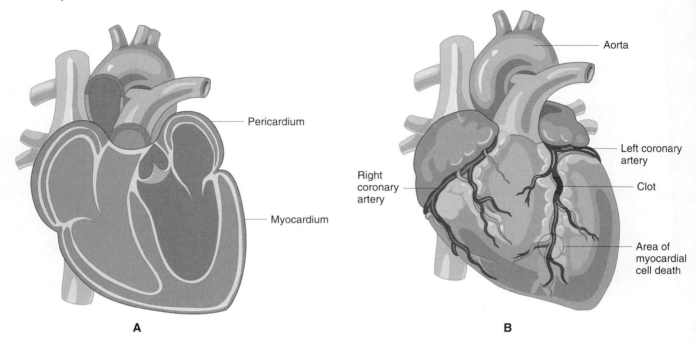

A

B

muscle may already be lost. Public health officials have launched a nationwide campaign urging Americans to "call fast, call 911."[25] In addition, more doctors' offices, airlines, and public meeting places, such as casinos, are purchasing heart defibrillators. This life-saving equipment may seem expensive, at an estimated $3500, but according to one recent study at a medical school, the cost of defibrillators and training teams of nurses in their use came to only about a nickel per paying patient.[26] State-of the-art treatments for heart attacks include clot-dissolving drugs, early administration of medications to thin the blood, intravenous nitroglycerin, and, in some cases, a beta blocker (which blocks many of the effects of adrenaline in the body, particularly its stimulating impact on the heart).

Clot-dissolving drugs called thrombolytic agents are the treatment of choice for acute myocardial infarction in most clinical settings. Administered through a *catheter* (flexible tube) threaded through the arteries to the site of the blockage (the more effective method of delivery) or injected intravenously (the faster, cheaper method of delivery), these agents can save lives and dissolve clots, but don't remove the underlying atherosclerotic plaque. Patients receiving such therapy may require further procedures, such as bypass surgery or **angioplasty**, which can reduce their risk of another heart attack or death.

Emergency balloon angioplasty has shown greater effectiveness than clot-dissolving medication in restoring blood flow in arteries immediately after an attack. With this approach, arteries are less likely to close down again and patients have shorter hospital stays and fewer hospital readmissions. Angioplasty patients also are less likely to die of the heart attack or to experience repeat attacks. However, only 20% of American hospitals perform angioplasty, and not all can do it on an emergency basis.[27]

Strategies for Prevention

What to Do If a Heart Attack Strikes

✔ If you develop chest discomfort that lasts for two minutes or more, call the local emergency rescue service immediately.

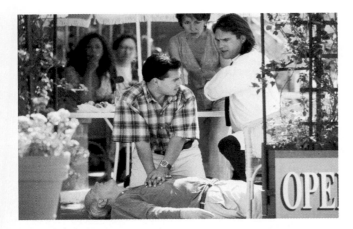

If you witness someone who appears to be experiencing a heart attack, the best thing you can do is call for emergency help immediately. Only after medical emergency personnel are called should you begin any CPR efforts.

✔ If you're with someone who's exhibiting the classic signs of heart attack, and if they last for two minutes or more, act at once. Expect the person to deny the possibility of anything as serious as a heart attack, but insist on taking prompt action.

✔ Call for help. Bystanders should call the emergency medical system (available by dialing 911 in many places) immediately. The odds of survival are greatest if emergency teams get to a heart attack victim quickly and administer advanced cardiac life support. Individuals trained in **cardiopulmonary resuscitation (CPR)**, a combination of mouth-to-mouth breathing and chest compression for victims of cardiac arrest, should use this technique only after calling or having someone else call for emergency help.[28]

Heart Rate Abnormalities

The heart has its own electrical system, which produces an evenly timed, regular beat. When relaxed, most adults have a heart rate of between 60 and 80 beats per minute—slower if they're in good physical condition. During strenuous activity or stress, the heart beats faster. Sometimes the heart seems to skip a beat or experience premature (or early) heartbeats. In many cases, these irregularities are no cause for alarm; but they can be dangerous in an MI victim. Caffeine, long suspected of triggering irregular heartbeats, doesn't seem to be a culprit.

A very fast heart rate (over 100 beats per minute) is known as **tachycardia**; a very slow one (under 60 beats

per minute) is **bradycardia**. Resting heart rates of under 60 beats per minute aren't necessarily signs of illness, even though they meet the definition of bradycardia; in fact, they may reflect excellent physical condition. In **atrial fibrillation**, electrical impulses spread in all directions through the heart, while the ventricle continues to beat. Various drugs are effective in correcting such irregularity, or **arrhythmia**.

Patients with very slow or irregular heartbeats who don't respond to drugs may need an implanted electrical pacemaker that stimulates contractions of the heart at a normal rate. Such pacemakers, compact battery-powered systems, deliver a series of small electrical impulses to the heart muscle. A new, still experimental alternative involves cauterization of tiny portions of the heart by means of a thin wire threaded through a vein. This removes unwanted paths of conductivity that give rise to rapid-fire heartbeats.

Congestive Heart Failure

When the heart's pumping power is well below normal capacity, fluid begins to collect in the lungs, hands, and feet. The heart is then said to be in failure. As blood fluids accumulate in the lungs, pulmonary congestion occurs, causing shortness of breath. In other parts of the body, fluid seeps through the thin capillary walls and causes swelling (edema), especially in the ankles and legs. **Congestive heart failure** usually results from myocardial infarction, but can also be the result of rheumatic fever, birth defects, hypertension, or atherosclerosis. It is treated by reducing the workload on the heart, modifying salt intake, administering drugs that rid the body of excess fluid, and using medications (such as digitalis) to improve the heart's pumping efficiency.

Rheumatic Fever

Rheumatic fever, which strikes most often between the ages of 5 and 15, is a disease that causes painful, swollen joints; skin rashes; and heart damage in half its victims. It is always preceded by a streptococcal infection (see Chapter 11 on infectious diseases). A new strain of streptococcal bacteria has caused a resurfacing of rheumatic fever, which had been considered a disease of the past. The first step to prevention is early identification of the streptococcal infection; the second is treatment with antibiotics to avoid permanent scarring of the heart valves.

Congenital Defects

Approximately 8 out of every 1000 children born in the United States have congenital heart disease. The most common defects are holes in the ventricular septum, the wall dividing the lower chambers of the heart. Holes may also occur in the atrial septum, the wall between the upper chambers. Sometimes the arteries delivering blood to the body and lungs are transposed and thus attached to the wrong ventricles. Such babies have a bluish color because their blood isn't carrying sufficient oxygen.

Heart Savers

A generation ago physicians had no way of detecting problems before the symptoms of heart disease began and could offer little more than bed rest as a therapy after they struck. The last decade, however, has brought tremendous progress in the diagnosis and treatment of heart problems. Today men and women with heart problems can learn of possible dangers much earlier than in the past and undergo treatments that may add years to their lives.

Diagnostic Tests

The **electrocardiogram (ECG, EKG)**, a recording of the electrical activity of the heart, is the traditional method of evaluating the heart's health (see Figure 12-8). An exercise ECG—or *stress test*—is one method of finding out whether an area of the heart begins to run out of blood during the stress of an athletic workout. The subject walks or jogs on a treadmill while the ECG monitors the heart's response.

Thallium scintigraphy uses radioactive isotopes that are injected into the bloodstream. A special imaging device called a *scintillation*, or gamma camera, picks up the rays emitted by the isotopes; a computer translates these signals into images of the heart as it pumps. The test can be performed while the patient is either resting or exercising on a treadmill or bicycle. Adding a thallium scan to an exercise ECG increases the probability of detecting existing heart disease by 70% to 90%.

In **coronary angiography**, the most complete and accurate diagnostic test for heart problems, a thin tube is threaded through the blood vessels of the heart, a radiopaque dye is injected, and X rays are taken to detect any blockage of the arteries. Angiography is extremely precise, but it's also costly and risky: About one out of every 1500 patients dies as a result of the test.

Treatments

Most people with heart disease can be treated successfully with medications. Other alternatives are bypass surgery, balloon angioplasty, heart transplants, and external and implanted mechanical devices.

Medications

The main types of drugs used to treat high blood pressure and heart disease include diuretics; beta blockers; calcium channel blockers; and angiotensin converting enzyme (ACE) inhibitors, which block a hormone known as angiotensin that strongly influences blood

Figure 12-8

ECG readings. (A) A recording of normal electrical activity in the heart. (B) Grossly irregular activity seen in an acute heart attack.

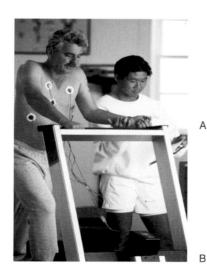

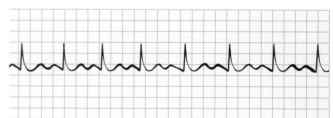

A

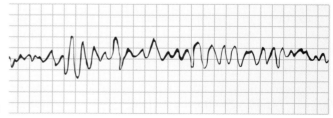

B

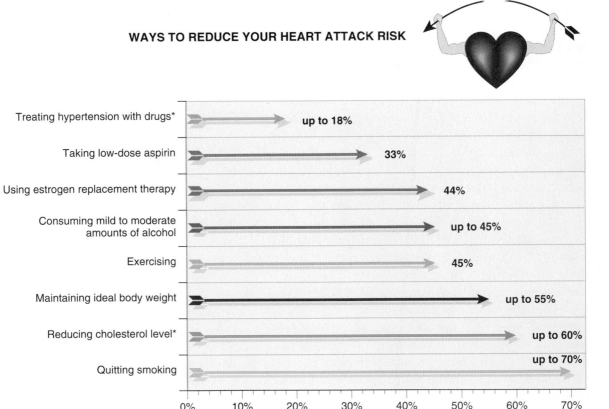

WAYS TO REDUCE YOUR HEART ATTACK RISK

Treating hypertension with drugs*   — up to 18%

Taking low-dose aspirin   — 33%

Using estrogen replacement therapy   — 44%

Consuming mild to moderate amounts of alcohol   — up to 45%

Exercising   — 45%

Maintaining ideal body weight   — up to 55%

Reducing cholesterol level*   — up to 60%

Quitting smoking   — up to 70%

0%   10%   20%   30%   40%   50%   60%   70%

*Because studies of these lifestyle changes have mostly involved men, the benefits are less clear for women.

SOURCE: *American Health*, March 1993, p. 14.

Figure 12-9

pressure. Side effects range from lethargy and fatigue to an increased risk of chest pain and heart attack if certain drugs are discontinued abruptly. The newer, more expensive agents—calcium channel blockers and ACE inhibitors—have become more popular, even though they have not proved more effective than older medications such as diuretics and beta blockers. Unlike the older drugs, the new ones are less likely to cause side effects such as impotence, insomnia, lethargy, and depression. The newer drugs can be taken in lower doses with negligible side effects.

Recent reports have found dangers associated with several widely used heart medications, including a modestly increased risk of heart attack in patients taking some calcium channel blockers, which are used to lower blood pressure, raise cardiac output in heart failure, relieve various forms of angina, and control arrhythmias.[29] They work by countering the flow of calcium ions into the heart muscle cells; calcium is believed to stimulate and contract heart muscle, occasionally causing a sudden spasm that can completely close an artery.

Beta blockers lower the heart's demand for blood by producing changes in the autonomic (involuntary) nervous system. A variety of beta blockers are widely used for medical problems, including migraine headaches and glaucoma (a serious eye disease), as well as heart disease. Other cardiac medications include thrombolytic drugs and antiarrythmics. These drugs are not risk-free, and there have been recent reports that some may actually increase the likelihood of a heart attack.

Surgical Procedures and Mechanical Aids

A **coronary bypass** is a procedure in which an artery from the patient's leg or chest wall is grafted onto a coronary artery to detour blood around the blocked area. Each year hundreds of thousands of coronary bypasses are performed in the United States; about 1% to 5% of these patients die as a result of surgical complications.

For many patients, the results of bypass surgery are positive. But about one out of five patients suffers subtle, long-lasting impairment of mental performance, including problems concentrating and learning, remembering new information, and performing mental tasks as quickly as before the surgery. About 20% remain depressed a year after their operations; their mood changes may stem from damage sustained in the surgery.

Coronary bypasses do not extend life for individuals with mild to moderate angina unless the left main coronary artery was the one that was blocked. If drugs fail to control angina, a coronary bypass can eliminate pain. But surgery is not a cure for the atherosclerotic process that caused the blockage; indeed, in as many as 80% of bypass patients, the grafts themselves develop blockages within ten years.

Percutaneous transluminal coronary angioplasty (PTCA), also called balloon angioplasty, is now the most often performed heart operation. Less costly and less risky than bypass surgery, PTCA opens blood vessels in the heart that are narrowed but not completely blocked. PTCA involves a precise, time-consuming technique called *cardiac catheterization*—the threading of a narrow tube or catheter through an artery to the heart. An X ray taken with a special dye injected into the arteries reveals the location and extent of a blockage. By inflating a tiny balloon at the tip of the catheter, physicians can break up the clog and widen the narrowed artery. When they deflate the balloon, circulation is restored. Balloon angioplasties are not without risks, however; and balloon-opened arteries can clog up again.

In the near future, heart specialists may be able to sand plaque off artery walls with a tiny rotating sander, although this method has risks similar to those of balloon angioplasty. The most promising and commonly used nonballoon method is coronary stents, which can reduce complications and the risk of later renarrowing.

For a variety of heart disorders in which the heart muscle has become so damaged that it can no longer effectively pump blood throughout the body, the only hope is a heart transplant. In recent years the survival rates for transplant recipients have improved dramatically. *Left-ventricular-assist devices (LVADs)* enhance the pumping action of the heart. Used as external, temporary measures until a donor heart becomes available, fully implantable models may someday serve as permanent blood-pumping devices.

Artificial hearts also have been used to keep desperately ill patients alive while waiting for a donor heart. One man lived 620 days with an experimental artificial heart. However, he suffered serious complications, including strokes, infections, high fevers, and seizures. Other recipients of artificial hearts also developed serious complications and died within briefer periods.

Stroke: From No Hope to New Hope

When the blood supply to a portion of the brain is blocked, a cerebrovascular accident, or **stroke**, occurs. About 500,000 people suffer strokes each year, and strokes rank third, after heart disease and cancer, as a cause of death in this country. After decades of steady decline, the number of strokes per year has begun to rise. The main reasons seem to be that more Americans are living longer, advanced medical care is allowing more people to survive heart disease, and doctors are better able to diagnose and detect strokes. Yet 80% of strokes are preventable, and key risk factors can be modified through either lifestyle changes or drugs.[30]

Strategies for Prevention
. . . .
How to Prevent a Stroke

✔ Quit smoking. Smokers have twice the risk of stroke that nonsmokers have. When they quit, their risk drops 50% in two years. Within five years after quitting, their risk is nearly the same as nonsmokers.

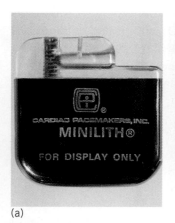
(a)

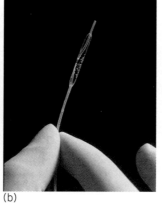
(b)

Medical technology has more options now for treating heart disorders. (a) The pacemaker can be surgically implanted in the chest to deliver electrical impulses that normalize a weak or irregular heartbeat. (b) A catheter with a tiny balloon is used in balloon angioplasty to widen a clogged artery.

✔ Keep blood pressure under control. Treating hypertension with medication can lead to a 40% reduction in fatal and nonfatal strokes.

✔ Eat a low-fat, low-cholesterol diet, which reduces your risk of fatty buildup in blood vessels.

✔ Avoid obesity, which burdens the blood vessels as well as the heart.

✔ Exercise. Moderate amounts of exercise improve circulation and may help dissolve deposits in the blood vessels that can lead to stroke.

Causes of Strokes

One of the most common causes of stroke is the blockage of a brain artery by a thrombus, or blood clot—a *cerebral thrombosis*. Clots generally form around deposits sticking out from the arterial wall. Sometimes a wandering blood clot (embolus), carried in the bloodstream, becomes wedged in one of the cerebral arteries. This is called a *cerebral embolism*, and it can completely plug up a cerebral artery (see Figure 12-10a).

A stroke can also be caused by the bursting of a diseased artery in the brain, which floods the surrounding

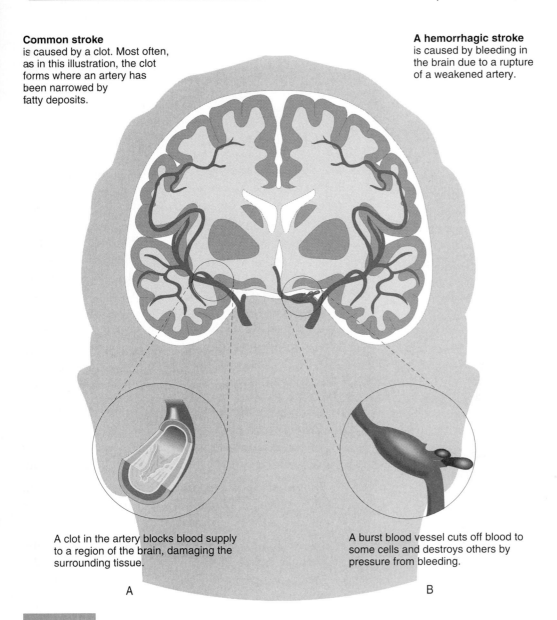

Common stroke is caused by a clot. Most often, as in this illustration, the clot forms where an artery has been narrowed by fatty deposits.

A hemorrhagic stroke is caused by bleeding in the brain due to a rupture of a weakened artery.

A clot in the artery blocks blood supply to a region of the brain, damaging the surrounding tissue.

A

A burst blood vessel cuts off blood to some cells and destroys others by pressure from bleeding.

B

Figure 12-10

Two types of strokes. Blockage of an artery by a blood clot can cause what is termed a common stroke. The bursting of an artery in the brain is called a hemorrhagic stroke, or cerebral hemorrhage.

tissue with blood. This is called a *cerebral hemorrhage*. The cells nourished by the artery are deprived of blood and can't function, and the blood from the artery forms a clot that may interfere with brain function. This is most likely to occur if the patient suffers from a combination of hypertension and atherosclerosis. Hemorrhage (bleeding) may also be caused by a head injury or by the bursting of an aneurysm, a blood-filled pouch that balloons out from a weak spot in the wall of an artery (see Figure 12-10b).

Brain tissue, like heart muscle, begins to die if deprived of oxygen, which may then cause difficulty speaking and walking, and loss of memory. These effects may be slight or severe, temporary or permanent, depending on how widespread the damage is and whether other areas of the brain can take over the function of the damaged area. About 30% of stroke survivors develop dementia, a disorder that robs a person of memory and other intellectual abilities.[31]

The following symptoms should alert you to the possibility that you or someone with you has suffered a stroke:

- Sudden weakness, loss of strength, or numbness of face, arm, or leg.
- Loss of speech, or difficulty speaking or understanding speech.
- Dimness or loss of vision, particularly double vision in one eye.
- Unexplained dizziness.
- Change in personality.
- Change in pattern of headaches.

Transient Ischemic Attacks (TIAs)

Sometimes a person will suffer **transient ischemic attacks (TIAs)**, "little strokes" that cause minimal damage but serve as warning signs of a potentially more severe stroke. One out of three people who suffer TIAs will have a stroke during the following five years if they don't get treatment. The two major types of TIAs are:

- *Transient monocular blindness.* Blurring, a blackout or whiteout of vision, a sense of a shade coming down, or another visual disturbance in one eye.
- *Transient hemispheral attack.* Diminished blood flow to one side of the brain, causing numbness or

weakness of one arm, leg, or side of the face, or problems speaking or thinking.

Many TIAs are caused by a narrowing of blood vessels in the neck (carotid arteries) because of a buildup of plaque. Specialists can diagnose this problem by feeling and listening to the arteries, by ultrasound, by measuring the pressure or circulation rate from the carotid arteries to the eyes, or by arterial angiography (injection of a dye into the arteries as X rays are taken), a procedure that can be dangerous, even deadly, or lifesaving.

Surgery to widen the carotid arteries may be recommended for individuals under age 60 with significant narrowing (50% to 80% or more). However, this is a risky procedure, and often physicians advise it only when clearly necessary. For other patients, aspirin and other drugs that make platelets less sticky and interfere with clotting may be effective.

Risk Factors for Strokes

People who've experienced TIAs are at the highest risk for stroke. Other risk factors, like those for heart disease, include some that can't be changed (such as gender and race) and some that can be controlled:

- *Gender.* Men have a greater risk of stroke than women do. Past studies have shown an association between oral contraceptive use and stroke, particularly in women over age 35 who smoke. The newer low-dose oral contraceptives have not shown an increased stroke risk among women ages 18 to 44.[32]
- *Race.* African Americans have a much greater risk of stroke than whites do. Hispanics also are more likely to develop hemorrhagic strokes than whites.[33]
- *Age.* A person's risk of stroke more than doubles every decade after age 55.
- *Hypertension.* Detection and treatment of high blood pressure are the best means of stroke prevention.
- *High red blood cell count.* A moderate to marked increase in the number of a person's red blood cells increases the risk of stroke.
- *Heart disease.* Heart problems can interfere with the flow of blood to the brain; clots that form in the heart can travel to the brain, where they may clog an artery.
- *Blood fats.* Although the standard advice from cardiologists is to lower harmful LDL levels, what may be

more important for stroke risk is a drop in the levels of protective HDL. In one study of 200 men in their 50s, 60s, and 70s—all of whom had desirably LDL levels—nearly 90% of those who had unhealthfully low amounts of HDL (under 35 milligrams per liter of blood) had thickening of the walls of the arteries that carry blood from neck to the brain—a potentially ominous sign.[34]

- *Diabetes mellitus.* Diabetics have a higher incidence of stroke than nondiabetics.

Treatments for Strokes

A small ("baby") aspirin a day cuts in half the risk of strokes caused by abnormal heartbeats, which strike 75,000 Americans each year. Extremely rapid beating of the heart's upper chambers causes blood clots to form; they may enter the bloodstream and travel to the brain, where they can get stuck and choke off the blood supply. In the past, the only way to prevent such strokes was regular use of a medication called warfarin, which inhibits blood clotting and therefore increases the risk of severe bleeding. However, aspirin proved as effective as warfarin—without that dangerous side effect.

Increasingly, surgeons are operating on carotid arteries that may have been narrowed by a buildup of atherosclerotic plaque—a condition that contributes to 20% to 30% of strokes, some in individuals with no symptoms—by cleaning them out in a procedure called *carotid endarterectomy.* This procedure has been shown to be effective in preventing stroke in patients with and without early symptoms of stroke.[35]

It now seems possible to save brain cells for a brief time after a thrombotic stroke occurs. Thrombolytic drugs, used for heart attack victims, can restore brain blood flow after a thrombotic stroke; other medications called heparinoids can reduce the blood's tendency to clot. In order for thrombolytic drugs to be effective, they must be administered within 90 minutes after the stroke; heparinoids must be given within 24 hours. However, many stroke victims do not seek help for 24 hours or longer.

In addition, drugs such as nimodipine and other agents undergoing clinical testing at major medical centers, are being used to protect brain cells from damage. Clinicians also are experimenting with ways to tie off tiny, bleeding, cranial arteries with tiny clothespins or to suction off blood that is exerting pressure on the brain.

Using stereotactic radioimagery, which relies on a three-dimensional imaging system, surgeons can focus an X-ray beam on a clot or hemorrhage and destroy it.

Making This Chapter Work for You
Becoming Heart Smart

- Heart disease develops over time; the processes leading to heart disease often begin in childhood. Early recognition of risks and lifestyle changes to reduce them can have a dramatic impact in lowering the likelihood of heart-related problems in middle and old age.

- Factors predisposing an individual to heart disease or stroke include risks you can control, such as lack of exercise, cigarette smoking, obesity, high blood pressure, and high cholesterol levels. Other predisposing factors include diabetes mellitus, a family history of heart disease, age, race, and, to a certain degree, gender.

- Men tend to develop heart disease about a decade earlier in life than women, but women are less likely to respond as well to various treatments and are more likely to die as the result of a heart attack.

- Individuals with high cholesterol levels are at risk of developing atherosclerosis and having a heart attack. Federal health officials, supported by dozens of medical organizations, have called upon all Americans to lower their cholesterol levels by reducing their intake of saturated fats and cholesterol-rich foods. All adults should undergo cholesterol testing every five years. Dietary changes and exercise can lower cholesterol readings. Treatment with cholesterol-lowering drugs has proven effective in reducing and reversing coronary artery disease.

- Hypertension, or high blood pressure, occurs when the arterial walls offer too much resistance to blood flow. Health officials have recently learned that even borderline or mildly elevated blood pressure can be dangerous. Treatment of mild hypertension includes diet modification, exercise, and restriction of salt intake. For more severe hypertension, medication to widen the blood vessels or to decrease cardiac output may be necessary.

- The most common form of coronary artery disease is atherosclerosis, in which blood flow is impaired as the arteries narrow and lose their ability to dilate and

Health Online

contract because of plaque deposits inside the arteries. Thrombosis, or blockage of an artery by a thrombus, is the major danger of atherosclerosis, because a blocked artery can cause a heart attack or stroke.

- Some people suffer from chest pains, or angina pectoris, caused by periodic and temporary inadequate blood flow to the heart. Chest pain may also be a result of coronary artery spasms caused by the clumping of platelets, which results in a narrowing of the blood vessel.

- Myocardial infarction, or heart attack, occurs when heart muscle tissue in the myocardium begins to die because its supply of oxygen and other nutrients has been cut off by a blocked artery. The damage caused by a heart attack can be reduced with early treatment, including the use of clot-dissolving drugs or tiny balloons to unclog arteries (a procedure called angioplasty).

- Other heart problems include heartbeat irregularities, or arrhythmias; congestive heart failure, which occurs when the heart is unable to pump at its normal capacity; heart damage from rheumatic fever; and congenital heart defects.

- Doctors can evaluate the heart's condition through such procedures as electrocardiography, angiography, and nuclear scanning, and through various types of imaging procedures. Hypertension, heart failure, angina, and arrhythmias can be treated with drugs. Surgical treatments for heart disease include the coronary bypass operation, balloon angioplasty, pacemaker implantation, heart transplants, and external and implanted mechanical devices.

- A stroke, or cerebrovascular accident, occurs when the blood supply to the brain is restricted or blocked, and can be caused by a cerebral thrombosis, cerebral embolism, or cerebral hemorrhage. Transient ischemic attacks (TIAs) may precede a serious stroke.

- Surgery to unclog the carotid arteries carrying blood to the brain can reduce the risk of stroke.

- In the past, physicians believed that little could be done once a stroke occurred. However, speedy treatment with clot-dissolving drugs can limit braincell damage and prevent death.

Cardiovascular disease claims fewer lives than in the past, largely because of lifestyle changes, including smoking less, exercising more, and avoiding fatty foods. More Americans are helping to protect their own hearts and save their own lives. You can join in this heart-warming, health-enhancing campaign by following the guidelines in Pulsepoints.

Key Terms

The terms listed here are used within the chapter. Page numbers are included for each term.
A definition of each term is given in the green Glossary pages at the end of this book.

angina pectoris *388*
angioplasty *390*
antioxidants *378*
aorta *376*
arrhythmia *391*
arteriosclerosis *387*
atherosclerosis *387*
atrial fibrillation *391*
atrium *376*
bradycardia *391*
capillary *376*
cardiopulmonary

resuscitation (CPR) *391*
cholesterol *380*
congestive heart failure *391*
coronary angiography *392*
coronary bypass *393*
diastole *376*
electrocardiogram (ECG, EKG) *392*
hypertension *379*
lipoprotein *381*
male pattern baldness *383*
myocardial infarction (MI) *389*

percutaneous transluminal coronary angioplasty (PTCA) *394*
stroke *394*
systole *376*
tachycardia *391*
thallium scintigraphy *392*
transient ischemic attacks (TIAs) *396*
triglyceride *380*
ventricle *376*

Review Questions

1. Name the different parts of the heart, and explain how they function.
2. Explain the difference between the systolic and diastolic blood pressure readings.
3. What are the uncontrollable risk factors for cardiovascular disease? Which risk factors are controllable? What preventive steps can you take to minimize these risks?
4. What is the relationship between cholesterol and the development of heart disease or incidence of heart attacks? How can cholesterol intake be modified to decrease the risk of adverse health effects?
5. What are some health effects associated with hypertension? Atherosclerosis? List the risk factors and any effective treatments for each.
6. What is a stroke? What are TIAs? What are the causes of each and common treatments? What can be done to prevent their occurrence?

Critical Thinking Questions

1. Have you had your blood pressure checked lately? If your reading was high, what steps are you now taking to help reduce your blood pressure?
2. Have you had a cholesterol reading lately? Do you think it's necessary for you to obtain one? If your reading was/is borderline or high, what lifestyle changes can you make to help control your cholesterol level?
3. The costs for a heart transplant are over $100,000. The annual price tag for a year's worth of cyclosporine, the drug that prevents rejection and must be taken for the rest of a transplant recipient's life, is about $5000. The total medical bill can come to hundreds of thousands of dollars—enough to fund programs to improve the nutrition of poor pregnant women, to treat alcoholism, or to provide regular preventive care. Does treatment of any single individual justify such huge costs? Should our society try to balance the costs versus the benefits of such heroic measures as heart transplants? How would you go about making such decisions?

Connections to Personal Health Interactive

To enhance your understanding of the material covered in this chapter, check out the following study aids on the **Personal Health Interactive CD-ROM**. *Each numbered icon within the chapter corresponds to an appropriate activity listed here.*

12.1 Personal Insights: Is Your Heart Happy?   **12.2** Chapter 12 Review

References

1. National Center for Health Statistics, 1995.
2. Frost, R. "Cardiovascular Risk Modification in the College Student: Knowledge, Attitude, and Behaviors." *Journal of General Internal Medicine*, May–June 1992.
3. Blair, Steven, et al. "Changes in Physical Fitness and All-Cause Mortality: A Prospective Study of Healthy and Unhealthy Men." *Journal of the American Medical Association*, Vol. 273, No. 14, April 12, 1995. Lee, I-Min, et al. "Exercise Intensity and Longevity in Men: The Harvard Alumni Health Study." *Journal of the American Medical Association*, Vol. 273, No. 14, April 19, 1995.
4. Hodis, Harold, et al. "Serial Coronary Angiographic Evidence that Antioxidant Vitamin Intake Reduces Progression of Coronary Artery Atherosclerosis." *Journal of the American Medical Association*, Vol. 273, No. 23, June 21, 1995.
5. Werner, Rachel, and Thomas Pearson. "What's So Passive About Passive Smoking?" *Journal of the American Medical Association*, Vol. 278, No. 2 , January 14, 1998.
6. Moore, Peter. "Passive Smoking Changes Lipid Profiles in At-Risk Children." *Lancet*, Vol. 350, No. 9070, September 6, 1997.
7. Howard, George, et al. "Cigarette Smoking and Progression of Atherosclerosis." *Journal of the American Medical Association*, Vol. 278, No. 2, January 14, 1998.
8. Manson, JoAnn, et al. "A Prospective Study of Obesity and Risk of Coronary Heart Disease in Women." *New England Journal of Medicine*, March 29, 1990.
9. Murray, Robert. "Skin Color and Blood Pressure." *Journal of the American Medical Association*, February 6, 1991.
10. National Institute on Aging. Hearts and Arteries. *What Scientists Are Learning About Age and the Cardiovascular System*. Gaithersburg, MD: NIA Information Center, 1995.
11. Quilligan, Edward. "Obstetrics and Gynecology." *Journal of the American Medical Association*, Vol. 273, No. 21, June 7, 1995.
12. Lesko, Samuel, et al. "A Case-Control Study of Baldness in Relation to Myocardial Infarction in Men." *Journal of the American Medical Association*, February 24, 1993. Wilson, Peter, and William Kannel. "Is Baldness Bad for the Heart?" *Journal of the American Medical Association*, February 24, 1993.
13. Katzenstein, Larry. "Good News About Heart Disease." *American Health*, December 1994. Hoffman, Carolyn, and Theresa Turner. "Strategies for Using University Health Services for Cholesterol Screening." *Journal of American College Health*, Vol. 43, No. 2, September 1994.
14. Bao, Weihang, et al. "Longitudinal Changes in Cardiovascular Risk from Childhood to Young Adulthood in Offspring of Parents with Coronary Artery Disease." *Journal of the American Medical Association*, Vol. 278, No. 21, December 3, 1997.
15. Krumholz, H. M., et al. "Lack of Association Between Cholesterol and Coronary Heart Disease Mortality and Morbidity and All-Cause Mortality in Persons Older Than 70 Years." *Journal of the American Medical Association*, Vol. 272, November 19, 1994. Corti, Maria-Chiara, et al. "HDL Cholesterol Predicts Coronary Heart Disease Mortality in Older Persons." *Journal of the American Medical Association*, Vol. 274, No. 7, August 16, 1995.
16. Katzenstein, Larry. "Reversing Heart Disease." *American Health*, November 1994.
17. "People with Heart Disease." *American Health*, June 1995.
18. Gore, Joel, and James Dalen. "Cardiovascular Disease." *Journal of the American Medical Association*, Vol. 274, No. 7, August 16, 1995.
19. Reeves, Richard. "Does This Patient Have Hypertension?" *Journal of the American Medical Association*, Vol. 273, No. 15, April 19, 1995.
20. "Systolic Blood Pressure." *American Health*, June 1995.
21. Whalley, Helen. "Salt and Hypertension: Consensus or Controversy?" *Lancet*, Vol. 350, No. 9092, December 6, 1997.
22. Morimoto, Atsushi, et al. "Sodium Sensitivity and Cardiovascular Events in Patients with Essential Hypertension." *Lancet*, Vol. 350. No. 9093, December 13, 1997.
23. Siegel, David, and Julio Lopez. "Trends in Antihypertensive Drug Use in the United States: Do the JNC-V Recommendations Affect Prescribing." *Journal of the American Medical Association*, Vol. 278, No. 21, December 3, 1997.
24. Dienstrey, Harris. "What Makes the Heart Healthy? A Talk with Dean Ornish." *Advances: The Journal of Mind Body Health*, Spring 1992.
25. Meischke, Hendrika, et al. "'Call Fast, Call 911: A Direct Mail Campaign to Reduce Patient Delay in Acute Myocardial Infarction." *American Journal of Public Health*, Vol. 87, No. 10, October 1997.
26. Peberdy, Mary Ann. Presentation, American Heart

Association annual meeting, November 1997. Weaver, W., et al. "Comparison of Primary Coronary Angioplasty and Intravenous Thrombolytic Therapy for Acute Myocardial Infarction." *Journal of the American Medical Association*, Vol. 278, No. 23, December 17, 1997. Yusuf, Salim, and Janice Pogue. "Primary Angioplasty Compared with Thrombolyic Therapy for Acute Myocardial Infarction." *Journal of the American Medical Association*, Vol. 278, No. 23, December 17, 1997.

27. Katzenstein, Larry. "A Better Treatment for Heart Attacks." *American Health*, July–August 1995.

28. American Heart Association.

29. Cutler, Jeffrey, et al. *Archives of Internal Medicine,* April 25, 1995. Chrebet, Jennifer. "A Report That a Widely Prescribed Class of Blood Pressure Drugs Increases Heart Attack Risk." *American Health*, May 1995.

30. McBride, Gail. "Stroke: A Prevention and Survival Kit." *American Health*, January–February 1995.

31. Henry, Brian. "Memory-Robbing Disorder Detected in One in Three Stroke Survivors." American Heart Association, December 1997.

32. Schwartz, Stephen. "Use of Low-Dose Oral Contraceptives and Stroke in Young Women." *Journal of the American Medical Association*, Vol. 278, No. 23, December 17, 1997.

33. Henry, Brian. "Hispanics Face Higher Risk for Bleeding Strokes Than Whites, Native Americans." American Heart Association, December 1997.

34. "Low HDL-Cholesterol Raises Stroke Risk." *Tufts University Health & Nutrition Letter*, Vol. 15, No. 10, December 1997.

35. Brody, Jane. "To Prevent Strokes, Surgeons Turn to a Direct Attack on Clogged Arteries." *New York Times*, July 12, 1995.

CHAPTER 13

LOWERING YOUR RISK OF CANCER AND OTHER MAJOR DISEASES

After studying the material in this chapter, you should be able to:

Define cancer, and **list** the seven warning signs.

List and **explain** the risk factors for cancer.

Describe practical behaviors to reduce the risk.

Describe appropriate treatment for cancer.

Define *diabetes mellitus,* and **describe** the early symptoms and treatment for this disease.

List and **explain** other major noninfectious illnesses.

Whether or not you will get a serious disease at some time in your life may seem to be a matter of odds. Genetic tendencies, environmental factors, and luck affect your chances of having to face many health threats. However, you do have some control over such risks, and even if a major illness may be inevitable, you can often prevent or delay it for years, even decades. Cancer is an excellent example. For the first time since 1900, the overall cancer death rates in the United States are coming down. According to the American Cancer Society, the number of cancer deaths has fallen from a peak of 135 per 100,000 in 1990 to 130 per 100,000—and this trend may accelerate in the next century. Some experts predict that within 20 years, cancer deaths could be cut an additional 25%.[1]

Prevention and health promotion hold great promise for the other noninfectious illnesses discussed in this chapter: diabetes mellitus; epilepsy; respiratory diseases; anemias; liver disorders; kidney problems; digestive diseases; disorders of the muscles, joints, and bones; and skin disorders. This chapter also explains the causes, risk factors, development, diagnosis, and treatment of these disorders and discusses special needs related to differences in physical and mental abilities.

Understanding Cancer

The declining rate of cancer deaths does not stem from research breakthroughs or development of a "magic bullet" to cure cancer. Most of the gains that have been made are the result of changes in lifestyle—most importantly, a reduction in smoking. Among white males, who have reduced smoking more than other groups in recent years, lung cancer death rates have dropped by more than 6%. Among white women, who have increased smoking, death rates from lung cancer have risen 6%.

Early detection also is helping to save lives. Thanks to refinements in diagnostic tests for breast cancer, for instance, tumors as small as 2 centimeters in size can now be detected; just a few years ago, only 3-centimeter tumors could be spotted on mammograms. This may be one reason why mortality rates from breast cancer also have dropped in the 1990s.[2]

The National Cancer Institute (NCI) estimates that approximately 7.4 million Americans alive today have a history of cancer. About 1,382,400 new cancers of various types (excepting basal and squamous cell skin cancers) will be diagnosed this year. In the course of a lifetime, men in the United States have a one in two lifetime risk of developing cancer; for women, the risk is one in three.[3]

The uncontrolled growth and spread of abnormal cells causes cancer. Normal cells follow the code of instructions embedded in DNA (the body's genetic material); cancer cells do not. Think of the DNA within the nucleus of a cell as a computer program that controls the cell's functioning, including its ability to grow and reproduce itself. If this program or its operation is altered, the cell goes out of control. The nucleus no longer regulates growth. The abnormal cell divides to create other abnormal cells, which again divide, eventually forming **neoplasms** (new formations), or tumors.

Tumors can be either *benign* (slightly abnormal, not considered life-threatening) or *malignant* (cancerous). The only way to determine whether a tumor is benign is by microscopic examination of its cells. Cancer cells have larger nuclei than the cells in benign tumors, they vary more in shape and size, and they divide more often.

Without treatment, cancer cells continue to grow, crowding out and replacing healthy cells. This process is called **infiltration**, or invasion. They may also **metastasize**, or spread to other parts of the body via the bloodstream or lymphatic system (see Figure 13-1). For many cancers, as many as 60% of patients may have metastases (which may be too small to be felt or seen without a microscope) at the time of diagnosis.

Although all cancers have similar characteristics, each is distinct. Some cancers are relatively simple to cure, whereas others are more threatening and mysterious. The earlier any cancer is found, the easier it is to treat and the better the patient's chances of survival. Cancers are classified according to the type of cell and the organ in which they originate, such as the following:

- *Carcinoma,* the most common kind, which starts in the epithelium, the layers of cells that cover the body's surface or line internal organs and glands.

- *Sarcomas,* which form in the supporting, or connective, tissues of the body: bones, muscles, blood vessels.

- *Leukemias,* which begin in the blood-forming tissues (bone marrow, lymph nodes, and the spleen).

- *Lymphomas,* which arise in the cells of the lymph system, the network that filters out impurities.

Figure 13-1

Metastasis, or spread of cancer. Cancer cells can travel through the blood vessels to spread to other organs, or through the lymphatic system to form secondary tumors.

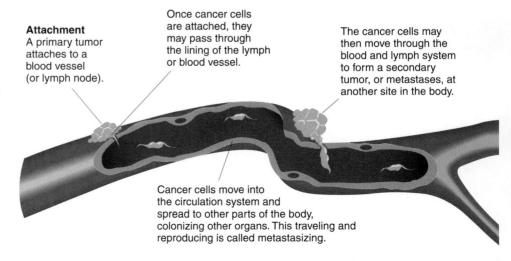

Attachment
A primary tumor attaches to a blood vessel (or lymph node).

Once cancer cells are attached, they may pass through the lining of the lymph or blood vessel.

The cancer cells may then move through the blood and lymph system to form a secondary tumor, or metastases, at another site in the body.

Cancer cells move into the circulation system and spread to other parts of the body, colonizing other organs. This traveling and reproducing is called metastasizing.

Leading Sites of New Cancer Cases and Deaths — U.S. 1998 Estimates

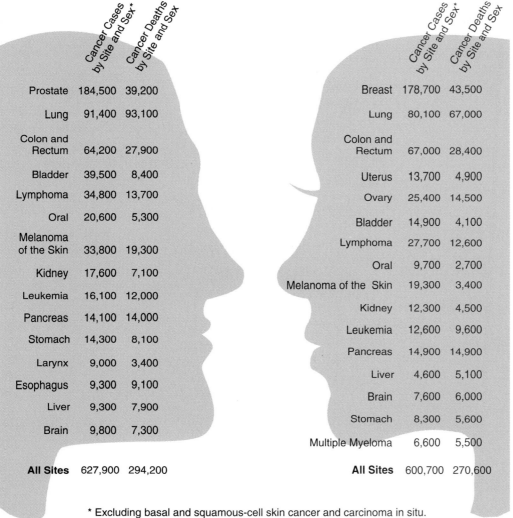

	Cancer Cases by Site and Sex*	Cancer Deaths by Site and Sex			Cancer Cases by Site and Sex*	Cancer Deaths by Site and Sex
Prostate	184,500	39,200		Breast	178,700	43,500
Lung	91,400	93,100		Lung	80,100	67,000
Colon and Rectum	64,200	27,900		Colon and Rectum	67,000	28,400
Bladder	39,500	8,400		Uterus	13,700	4,900
Lymphoma	34,800	13,700		Ovary	25,400	14,500
Oral	20,600	5,300		Bladder	14,900	4,100
Melanoma of the Skin	33,800	19,300		Lymphoma	27,700	12,600
Kidney	17,600	7,100		Oral	9,700	2,700
Leukemia	16,100	12,000		Melanoma of the Skin	19,300	3,400
Pancreas	14,100	14,000		Kidney	12,300	4,500
Stomach	14,300	8,100		Leukemia	12,600	9,600
Larynx	9,000	3,400		Pancreas	14,900	14,900
Esophagus	9,300	9,100		Liver	4,600	5,100
Liver	9,300	7,900		Brain	7,600	6,000
Brain	9,800	7,300		Stomach	8,300	5,600
				Multiple Myeloma	6,600	5,500
All Sites	627,900	294,200		**All Sites**	600,700	270,600

* Excluding basal and squamous-cell skin cancer and carcinoma in situ.

Figure 13-2

Cancer appears to be on the rise, possibly because of environmental factors—and possibly because we now have the tests and the general awareness to be able to detect more cancers.

SOURCE: American Cancer Society, *Cancer Facts and Figures*, 1998.

Bad News, Good News

Millions of Americans, regardless of their family histories or other risk factors, worry about cancer—and with reason. Cancer rates have risen steadily in recent decades. A middle-aged American man is now twice as likely to develop cancer as his grandfather was. A woman's cancer risk has increased 30% to 50% over her grandmother's.[4]

"We don't know the reasons for the increase," says oncologist Charles Loprinzi, M.D., of the Mayo Clinic. "The American lifestyle, the environment, the Western diet—all could be risk factors. But it also could be that we're detecting a lot more cancers than we did in the past because we have more sophisticated tests."[5] (See Figure 13-2.) Whatever the cause, the scary statistics—and the equally alarming headlines about dangers in

dyes, cellular phones, electric blankets—have convinced some people that everything causes cancer and little, if anything, can be done about it. That's definitely not the case.

"It's not all doom and gloom," says epidemiologist Margaret Spitz, M.D., of the University of Texas M.D. Anderson Cancer Center in Houston.[6] Two out of three Americans *never* get cancer. And thanks to dramatic advances in diagnosing and treating cancer, more people with cancer are being cured every year, and the quality of their life has improved dramatically.[7]

The greatest surge for any cancer at any age has been in malignant melanoma, a deadly form of skin cancer (discussed later in this chapter) that has increased by 600% in the last 60 years. Some scientists believe that its incidence will continue to skyrocket as the earth's protective layer of ozone, which blocks harmful ultraviolet rays, diminishes. (See Chapter 21 for a discussion of the shrinking ozone layer.) Among the other cancers that are increasing in incidence are lung and breast cancer in women, prostate cancer in men, and brain cancer. However, cancers vary greatly in their severity and lethality. Screening tests can detect some—but not all—cancers at early stages, when the chance for a cure is best.

There also is good news about cancer "cures." In the 1930s, only about one in four patients survived for five years after treatment. Today about four in ten—40%—of those diagnosed with cancer this year are expected to be alive five years after diagnosis. This is the so-called observed cancer survival rate. When adjusted for normal life expectancy, the "relative" five-year survival rate for all cancer is 56%.[8]

Strategies for Prevention

The Seven Warning Signs of Cancer

If you note any of the following seven warning signs, immediately schedule an appointment with your doctor:

✔ **C**hange in bowel or bladder habits.

✔ **A** sore that doesn't heal.

✔ **U**nusual bleeding or discharge.

✔ **T**hickening or lump in the breast, testis, or elsewhere.

✔ **I**ndigestion or difficulty swallowing.

✔ **O**bvious change in a wart or mole.

✔ **N**agging cough or hoarseness.

How Cancer Develops

For decades researchers have tried to figure out exactly how a normal cell turns into a cancer cell. In the last few years, they've made dramatic progress in unraveling this mystery by studying **oncogenes**, normal genes that control growth but have gone awry. For reasons that scientists don't yet understand, the DNA in these genes changes. In addition, other genes, called *tumor suppressor* genes, which normally control cell growth, fail to stop cells from dividing before they become cancerous. More than half of all known types of cancer, including those of the colon, brain, lung, breast, bone, and blood, have been linked to defects in one particular tumor suppressor gene: *p53*.[9]

The normal function of the *p53* gene is to help cells respond when their DNA has been damaged.[10] When this gene is mutated or missing, however, it allows injured cells to reproduce damaged DNA. People born with a mutation in one copy of the *p53* gene are at extremely high risk for cancer. If the second copy is damaged, clusters of precancerous cells grow. If additional genetic mutations occur, the cell growth can develop into full-blown cancer.

Often genetic and environmental risk factors interact. In colon cancer, for instance, an individual may inherent a gene that has been linked to colon cancer and develop hundreds to thousands of benign adenomatous polyps, which can progress to cancer if not treated. However, the trigger for polyp growth may be in a gene involved in fat metabolism; therefore, eating a high-fat diet greatly increases any inherited vulnerability.[11]

Most cancers develop over a period of many years. Once detected, cancers are classified in terms of how far they've spread and to which organs. An *in situ* cancer is contained in the place where it originated. An invasive cancer has spread to surrounding tissues. A metastasized cancer has traveled to distant sites in the body.

Cancer Risk Factors That You Cannot Control

No one is immune from cancer, but many factors can influence an individual's risk. (See Table 13-1 and the Self-Survey: "Are You at Risk of Cancer?")

TABLE 13-1 THE MOST SURVIVABLE CANCERS

Five-year survival rates for many types of cancer:

Thyroid	100%	Kidney	88%
Testis	99%	Larynx	84%
Prostate	99%	Oral (mouth)	81%
Breast (female)	97%	Stomach	61%
Melanoma (skin)	95%	Lung	48%
Uterus	95%	Brain	34%
Urinary bladder	93%	Esophagus	22%
Ovary	92%	Liver	13%
Cervix	91%	Pancreas	13%
Colon & rectum	91%		

SOURCE: *Cancer Facts & Figures 1997.*

Self-Survey

Are You at Risk of Cancer?

Answer the following questions:

1. Do you protect your skin from overexposure to the sun? _____
2. Do you abstain from smoking or using tobacco in any form? _____
3. If you're over 40 or if family members have had colon cancer, do you get routine digital rectal exams? _____
4. Do you eat a balanced diet that includes the RDA for vitamins A, B, and C? _____
5. If you're a woman, do you have regular Pap tests and pelvic exams? _____
6. If you're a man over 40, do you get regular prostate exams? _____
7. If you have burn scars or a history of chronic skin infections, do you get regular checkups? _____
8. Do you avoid smoked, salted, pickled, and high-nitrite foods? _____
9. If your job exposes you to asbestos, radiation, cadmium, or other environmental hazards, do you get regular checkups?
10. Do you limit your consumption of alcohol? _____
11. Do you avoid using tanning salons or home sunlamps? _____
12. If you're a woman, do you examine your breasts every month for lumps? _____
13. Do you eat plenty of vegetables and other sources of fiber? _____
14. If you're a man, do you perform regular testicular self-exams? _____
15. Do you wear protective sunglasses in sunlight?
16. Do you follow a low-fat diet? _____
17. Do you know the cancer warning signs? _____

Scoring:

If you answered no to any of the questions, your risk for developing various kinds of cancer may be increased.

Making Changes ....
Cutting Your Cancer Risk

You may not be able to control every risk factor in your life or environment, but you can protect yourself from the obvious ones.

- *Avoid excessive exposure to ultraviolet light.* If you spend a lot of time outside, you can protect your skin by using sunscreen and wearing long-sleeve shirts and a hat. Also, wear sunglasses to protect your eyes. Don't purposely put yourself at risk by binge-sunbathing or by using sunlamps.
- *Avoid obvious cancer risks.* Besides ultraviolet light, other environmental factors that have been linked with cancer include tobacco, asbestos, and radiation.
- *Keep yourself as healthy as possible.* The healthier you are, the better able your body is to ward off diseases that can predispose you to cancer. Get regular exercise; eat a balanced, high-fiber, low-fat diet; and avoid excessive alcohol use.
- *Be alert to changes in your body.* You know your body's rhythms and appearance better than anyone else, and only you will know if certain things aren't right. Changes in bowel habits, skin changes, unusual lumps or discharges—anything out of the ordinary may be clues that require further medical investigation.
- *Don't put off seeing your doctor if you detect any changes.* Procrastination can't hurt anyone but you.

Heredity

Heredity may account for about 10% of all cancers, and an estimated 13 to 14 million Americans may be at risk. Yet most people—and many physicians who haven't kept up with the dramatic breakthroughs in cancer genetics in recent years—don't realize that a person's genetic legacy can be a significant risk factor.[12] (See Personal Voices: "Living with a Lethal Legacy.")

In hereditary cancers, such as retinoblastoma (an eye cancer that strikes young children) or certain colon cancers, a specific cancer-causing gene is passed down from generation to generation. The odds of any child with one affected parent inheriting this gene and developing the cancer are fifty-fifty. In familial cancers, close relatives develop the same types of cancer, but no one knows exactly how the disease is transmitted. In the future, genetic tests may be able to identify individuals who are born with an increased susceptibility. Tracing cancers through a family tree is one simple way of checking your own risk.

The most likely sites for inherited cancers to develop are the breast, brain, blood, muscles, bones, and adrenal gland. The telltale signs of inherited cancers include the following:

Personal Voices Living with a Lethal Legacy

Susan inherited her mother's brown eyes, bouyant sense of humor, and "the bad gene"—the cancer-causing one that had killed her grandmother and great-grandmother. Susan's mother was 42 years old when she learned that she, too, had breast and ovarian cancer. She died two years later, leaving behind eight sisters. Within the next decade, six of them had developed breast or ovarian cancer.

Growing up in Minneapolis, Susan—one of five girls—swore that she'd outsmart the disease that had devastated her family. She became a nurse, married her college sweetheart, and had four children—three of them girls—while still in her twenties. "I decided to have my breasts removed when I turned 30," recalls Susan, "I didn't want my children to have to go through what I did when I lost my mother." But Susan, a marathon runner, was fit and healthy, and four mammograms showed only some cystic growths.

"The doctors told me I had perfect breasts and acted as if I was crazy to want them cut off," she recalls. Her husband, who had been urging her to have prophylactic mastectomies, insisted she see a cancer specialist, who also saw no immediate need for surgery. Still Susan worried, especially after she felt a pea-sized growth in her left breast. Night after night she'd lie in bed, nervously fingering the lump and wondering if it had grown.

Reassured by her doctors that there was no need to rush, Susan, then 32, postponed a biopsy for several months until after her family got settled into a new home. The results shocked every-one: the lump was malignant, and the cancer had spread to three lymph nodes. After removal of both breasts and seven months of chemotherapy, Susan underwent a prophylactic total hysterectomy to reduce her risk of ovarian cancer.

Since her diagnosis, Susan has identified almost 40 cases of breast or ovarian cancer among her relatives, and researchers estimate that every girl in the family faces fifty-fifty odds of developing cancer. All four of her sisters—including the youngest, who is 26—have had mastectomies; two have had prophylactic hysterectomies. "The biggest mistake I made in my life was not having preventive surgery," says Susan.

Not everyone with hereditary cancers needs to take such drastic steps. Marian, a nurse in San Francisco, has worried about cancer ever since she was a child. "My mother was diagnosed with breast cancer when I was 3 and died when I was 10," she recalls. "When I was 17, I learned that my grandmother had also died of breast cancer, and I became paranoid as hell."

Ever since Marian has done everything she can to lower her risk of breast cancer. She had her two children in her twenties and nursed both of them for more than a year. She doesn't smoke or drink. She's always eaten a low-fat diet and watched her weight. By "keeping in touch with" her breasts, she's discovered two breast lumps—both of which turned out to be benign. And she started having annual mammograms when she was 35.

Two years ago, when she turned 49—the age at which her mother died—Marian took a new and unusual step toward lowering her cancer risk: She volunteered for a nationwide clinical trial of tamoxifen, an estrogen-like drug that may prevent breast tumors. "One of my life goals is to die of something other than breast cancer," she says. "I don't know if tamoxifen will help, but the study provides ten years of very close monitoring, and that could save my life."

Like breast and ovarian cancer, colon cancer can run in a family. Gary's father, who died at age 55, was the thirty-ninth person in his extended family to die of this disease. Gary, a Chevrolet dealer in Iowa, didn't want to become the forti-eth. "I feel fortunate that I knew I was at risk and could do something about it," he says, "Ever since my dad's death, I tried to get regular cancer checkups." Several years ago, when he was 45, a colonoscopy revealed a growth in Gary's colon. Initial tests indicated it was benign, but because of Gary's family history, his doctor performed another biopsy. This time the test revealed malignant cells.

"My surgeon says it was the earliest they'd ever found a tumor, and I didn't have to go through chemotherapy or radiation," says Gary, who underwent a colonectomy that removed about 18 inches of his lower intestine. "To me, the operation was no big deal. It was like going to the dentist. I'd been told that I had a fifty-fifty chance of getting colon cancer by the time I was 50, so I kind of expected it. I'm just fortunate that I knew the odds and my doctors were on top of the situation."

- *Early development.* Genetic forms of certain diseases strike earlier than noninherited cancers. For example, the average age of women diagnosed with breast cancer is 62. But if breast cancer is inherited, the average age at diagnosis is 44, an 18-year difference.

- *Family history.* Anyone with a close relative (mother, father, sibling, child) with cancer has about three times the usual chance of getting the same type of cancer.

- *Multiple targets.* The same type of hereditary cancer often strikes more than once—in both breasts or both kidneys, for instance, or in two separate parts of the same organ.

- *Unusual gender pattern.* Genes may be responsible for cancers that generally don't strike a certain gender—for example, breast cancer in a man.

- *Cancer family syndrome.* Some families, with unusually large numbers of relatives affected by cancer, seem clearly cancer-prone. For instance, in Lynch syndrome (a form of colon cancer), more than 20% of the family members in at least two generations develop cancer of both the colon and endometrium.

Race and Culture

Cancer rates vary greatly among different ethnic and racial groups and in different cultures. In the United States, the cancer rate among African Americans is higher than that among whites, and a higher proportion of African Americans who get cancer die from the disease. The American Cancer Society (ACS) estimates that at least half of the differences in survival rates between African Americans and whites is due to poor access to medical care and late diagnosis of cancer among people who are economically disadvantaged.

An ACS study found that fewer public information materials are available in Spanish and that Latinos are less aware of symptoms and signs of cancer than are whites or African Americans. In addition, Latinos express greater fear of cancer and view it as a death sentence that they can do little, if anything, to change. This "fatalismo" may explain why, in three studies of women with cancer, the Latinos delayed seeking care for cancer-related symptoms or didn't go to the doctor until their symptoms were more advanced. Vietnamese-American women, whose cervical cancer rate is three times higher than it is for Caucasian Americans, also are less likely to undergo regular checkups and Pap smears.[13]

Viruses

Researchers have long known that viruses can cause tumors in animals, but only recently have they shown a connection between several different viruses and cancer in humans. Viruses have been implicated in certain leukemias (cancers of the blood system) and lymphomas (cancers of the lymphatic system), cancers of the nose and pharynx, liver cancer, and cervical cancer. Human immunodeficiency virus (HIV) can lead to certain lymphomas and leukemias and to a type of cancer called Kaposi's sarcoma. Human papilloma virus (HPV) has been linked to an increased risk of cervical cancer and cancer of the penis.[14] (See Chapter 11 on infectious diseases.)

Environmental Risks

Many chemicals used in industry today are carcinogens, and employees as well as people living near a factory that creates smoke, dust, or gases are at risk. Among the known dangers are nickel, chromate, asbestos, and vinyl chloride. (See Chapter 21 for more information on environmental risks.)

Three to 5% of all cancers might be caused by radiation, including medical, occupational, and environmental exposures. Large doses clearly cause cancer; the effects of lower doses are not as clear. Among those at greater risk are workers at and residents near nuclear facilities, pregnant women and their fetuses, and children exposed to nuclear fallout. Clinical studies have revealed a long latent period before a radiation-induced cancer appears (usually a minimum of five years). Electromagnetic radiation, such as that produced by electric blankets, may increase the risk of brain cancer and leukemia in children whose mothers used them during pregnancy.

Personality

Are certain types of people, particularly meek, unassuming "nice guys," more prone to cancer than others? Yes, says psychologist Lydia Temoshok. In her studies of patients with malignant melanoma, she observed that 75% had characteristics of what she calls the Type-C personality: always patient and cooperative, bottling up feelings, rarely expressing anger, constantly putting others' needs first, trying to please everyone. However, other researchers have challenged this theory, noting that personality may be one of many factors that can contribute to or protect against cancer. The personality traits most often associated with a good outcome when cancer strikes include a fighting spirit, emotional expressiveness, and optimism. However, no long-range studies of large groups have confirmed a relationship between personality and cancer development or recovery.[15]

Reducing Your Cancer Risk

Environmental factors may cause between 80 and 90% of cancers and, at least in theory, can be prevented by avoiding cancer-causing substances (such as tobacco and sunlight) or using substances that protect against cancer-causing factors (such as antioxidants and vitamin D).[16] How do you start protecting yourself? Simple changes in lifestyle—not smoking, protecting yourself from the sun, exercising regularly—are essential (see Pulsepoints: "Ten Ways to Protect Yourself from Cancer" for practical guidelines).

Cancer-Smart Nutrition

"Eating more fruits and vegetables is the number-one dietary guideline you need to know and follow to lower your cancer risk," says Marion Nestle, Ph.D., chair of nutrition at New York University, "There are huge arguments about whether specific nutrients—beta carotene, Vitamin C, Vitamin E—can prevent cancer, but there is absolutely no argument that the best diet for reducing cancer risk is one containing a large proportion of its calories from fruits, vegetables and whole grains."[17]

In a review of 156 studies linking diet to cancer, researchers found "extraordinarily consistent scientific evidence" that fruits and vegetables protect against a variety of cancers, including tumors of the breast, cervix, ovary, endometrium, lung, stomach, colon, bladder, pancreas, esophagus, mouth and larynx.[18] Which fruits and veggies are best? Researchers have identified beneficial antioxidants in many fresh fruits and vegetables, as well as specific cancer-blocking compounds in broccoli and other *crucifers*, such as brussels sprouts, cauliflower and cabbage, and other potentially protective phytochemicals in carrots, greens (spinach, chicory, kale), tomatoes and citrus fruits. (See Chapter 6 on nutrition.) However, your best bet is eating as many different types of fruits and vegetables as possible—for a total of five to nine servings a day.[19]

"The key to good nutrition is always variety," says Nestle. "If you eat different fruits and vegetables, you'll get vitamins and minerals, you'll get plenty of fiber, you'll lower the fat in your diet—all of which are known to lower cancer risks. Besides, there are hundreds of nutrients—known and unknown—in real food. That's why you shouldn't rely on supplements."

Another way to lower your cancer risk is to reduce the fat in your diet. There is solid evidence that cutting back on fat can lower the risks of colon, ovarian, and pancreatic cancer.[20] A low-fat diet may reduce the risk of actinic keratosis, a warty skin condition caused by sunlight exposure that can be an indication of sun-induced skin damage leading to cancer.[21] In a Harvard study of 47,855 men between ages 40 and 75, those men who ate a high-fat diet, especially those in which the fat came from red meat, had a significantly greater chance of developing advanced cases of prostate cancer, although there was no correlation with overall prostate cancer rates and dietary fat.[22]

Pay attention to food processing and preparation as well. Whenever possible, select foods close to their natural state, grown locally and without pesticides. Avoid cured, pickled, or smoked meats. When cooking, try not to fry or barbecue often; these cooking methods can produce mutagens that induce cancer in animals. The process of smoking or charcoal-grilling releases carcinogenic tar that may increase the risk of cancer of the stomach and esophagus.

Strategies for Prevention

Eating to Reduce Your Cancer Risk

✔ Eat at least five servings of fruits and vegetables a day: at least one rich in vitamin A (e.g., cantaloupe, carrots, spinach, or sweet potatoes), at least one high in vitamin C (e.g., grapefruit, oranges, cauliflower, or green peppers), at least one high-fiber selection (e.g., winter squash, corn, figs, or apples).

✔ Have cabbage family (cruciferous) vegetables several times a week.

✔ Don't fry or barbecue often. Safer cooking methods are baking, boiling, steaming, microwaving, poaching, and roasting.

✔ Choose foods without added chemicals or pesticides. Whenever possible, select foods that are close to their natural state, grown locally, and freshly picked.

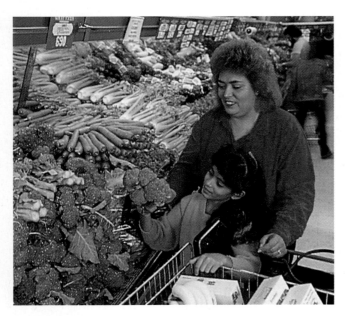

Eating cruciferous vegetables, including broccoli, brussels sprouts, and cabbage, can help reduce your cancer risk.

Cigarette Smoke and Environmental Tobacco Smoke

Cigarette smoking is the single most devastating and preventable cause of cancer deaths in the United States. People who smoke two or more packs of cigarettes a

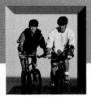

Pulsepoints   Ten Ways to Protect Yourself from Cancer

1. Don't smoke. Cigarette smoke is the number-one carcinogen in this country, responsible for one in every three cancers.

2. Stay out of the sun. Wearing sunscreen (with a Sun Protection Factor of at least 15) is better than not using any, but protective clothing is better—and staying in the shade is best.

3. Limit your intake of alcohol. Heavy drinkers are more likely to develop oral cancer and cancers of the larynx, throat, esophagus, liver, and breast.

4. Watch your weight. Obesity increases the risks of several cancers, including endometrial cancer and, particularly among postmenopausal women, breast cancer.

5. Get moving. Exercise—the heart strengthener and stamina builder—also can reduce the risk of colon can-

cer. Women who exercised early in life are less likely to develop breast cancer as adults.

6. Be sexually cautious. Cervical cancer has been linked with intercourse at an early age, multiple sex partners, and infection with the human papilloma virus (HPV), the virus that causes genital warts. The incidence of prostate cancer in men increases with multiple sexual partners and a history of frequent sexually transmitted diseases.

7. Check yourself out. Scan your skin for suspicious moles every month. If you're a woman, examine your breasts. If you're a man, check your testicles. Follow ACS recommendations for other cancer checkups.

8. Protect yourself from possible environmental carcinogens. Many chemicals used in industry can increase

the risk to employees and people living near a factory that creates smoke, dust, or gases. Follow safety precautions at work, and check with local environmental protection officials about possible hazards in your community.

9. Watch what you eat. Cut down on fat; eat more fruits, vegetables and whole grains. High-fat foods have been linked to several cancers, including breast, prostate, colon. Fruits, vegetables, and grains are rich in potentially protective antioxidants.

10. Inform yourself. Know the warning signs of cancer (see page 406), and see a physician if you develop any of them. Find out about any history of cancer in your family. Even though heredity accounts for a relatively small percentage of cancer cases, the more you know about potential risks, the more you can do to protect yours.

day are 15 to 25 times more likely to die of cancer than are nonsmokers. Cigarettes cause most cases of lung cancer and increase the risk of cancer of the mouth, pharynx, larynx, esophagus, pancreas, and bladder. Pipes, cigars, and smokeless tobacco also increase the danger of cancers of the mouth and throat.

Environmental tobacco smoke can increase the risk of cancer even among those who've never smoked. For example, researchers have found that exposure to others' tobacco smoke for as little as three hours a day can increase the risk of developing cancer threefold.[23] (See the discussion of passive smoking in Chapter 16.)

Possible Carcinogens

Although it may not be possible to avoid all possible **carcinogens** (cancer-causing chemicals), you can take steps to minimize your danger. Many chemicals used in industry, including nickel, chromate, asbestos, and vinyl chloride, are carcinogens, and employees as well as people living near a factory that creates smoke, dust, or gases are at risk. If your job involves their use, follow safety precautions at work. If you are concerned about

possible hazards in your community, check with local environmental protection officials (see Chapter 21 on environmental health).

Women and men who dye their hair frequently, particularly with very dark shades of permanent coloring, may be at increased risk for leukemia (cancer of blood-forming cells), non-Hodgkin's lymphoma (cancer of the lymph system), multiple myeloma (cancer of the bone marrow) and, in women, ovarian cancer. Lighter shades and less permanent tints do not seem to be a danger.[24]

Chemoprevention

In recent years scientists have focused on what has long seemed revolutionary: **chemoprevention**, the use of natural or laboratory-made substances to reduce the risk of developing cancer. Many of these substances resemble or are isolated from compounds found in foods. They are believed to work by halting or reversing the process by which a cell becomes cancerous.

To identify possible chemopreventive agents, scientists analyze data from studies of selected groups of

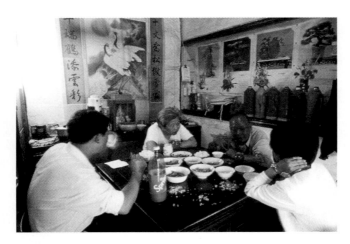

Chemoprevention is a growing area of study. Researchers seek to understand how dietary supplements lowered cancer risk in China but may have slightly increased certain cancer risks in Finland.

people—for example, those with a lower than average rate of cancer—to determine whether they eat large amounts of certain types of foods. They then isolate compounds from these foods and test them in animals/or human cancer cells grown in the laboratory to see whether the compounds might halt or reverse the process of cancer development. If a substance shows promise, researchers may then evaluate it in clinical trials.

Studies of chemoprevention with dietary supplements have produced contradictory—and confusing—results. In research sponsored by the National Cancer Institute (NCI) in China, daily vitamin and mineral supplements reduced the risk of dying of cancer in a population whose diet is very low in fresh fruits and vegetables. But another study of Finnish men, all smokers over age 50, found that beta carotene and Vitamin E supplements provided no benefit and may have somewhat increased their risk of dying of lung cancer. Ongoing NCI studies are investigating possible benefits from vitamin-A related compounds, folic acid, selenium, and calcium.[25]

NCI also is sponsoring studies of two drugs that might prevent breast or prostate cancer. One is tamoxifen, which blocks the hormone estrogen from binding with receptors in cancer-prone body tissues. Earlier studies have shown that it can protect some women from a recurrence of breast cancer after surgery. Current clinical trials are studying its use in healthy women at high risk of breast cancer because of their family histo-

ry. This form of prevention may carry a price however: a small but significant increase in uterine cancer.[26]

A similar chemoprevention trial is looking at the possible preventive benefits of finasteride (Proscar), a drug used to treat benign swelling of the prostate, a common problem in aging men. Unlike tamoxifen, it is not known to increase other cancer risks, but it does have side effects. Five percent of the men taking it report impotence; another 5% notice a decrease in ejaculate.[27]

Will agents like tamoxifen and Proscar someday become part of an anti-cancer program for many, if not most, Americans? "We won't have the answers for years, because a lot more research needs to be done," says Otis Brawley, M.D., a senior investigator in the Division of Cancer Prevention and Control of the NCI. "Chemoprevention is a very young science. Right now these agents should be studied, not advocated."[28]

What to Do If You're High Risk

The only way of knowing if you are at risk for hereditary cancers is by learning your family history. Ask parents, aunts, uncles, and cousins whether close relatives developed cancer, which types, and at what age. If you discover several cases, talk with your physician, who may recommend genetic counseling, which is available at university medical centers throughout the country, or DNA tests to reveal whether family members have inherited specific genes that greatly increase their likelihood of developing cancer. (These tests are not recommended for the general population.)

Although cancer surveillance should be part of everyone's routine health care, those at increased risk should take extra precautions. Young women with two or more relatives with ovarian cancer, for instance, might consider taking oral contraceptives. Studies by the Centers for Disease Control have shown that the longer a woman uses birth control pills, the lower her risk of ovarian and endometrial cancer—a benefit that persists for at least 15 years after discontinuing use of the pill. (See Table 13-2 for a list of screening guidelines for high-risk individuals.)

Types of Cancer

Cancer refers to a group of more than a hundred diseases characterized by abnormal cell growth. The most common are discussed in the following sections.

TABLE 13-2 WHAT TO LOOK FOR

Cancer	On your own	At the doctor's Test	What the test reveals
Breast	Lumps, swelling, or other changes found in manual self-exam	Mammogram yearly for women over 40; clinical manual exam	Lumps, swelling, or other abnormalities
Cervical	Unusual vaginal bleeding or discharge	Pap smear yearly	Precancerous or cancerous cells
Colorectal	Blood in the stool, change in bowel habits such as persistent and unexplainable diarrhea or constipation	Starting at age 50: Digital rectal exam every 5 years	Lumps or lesions or other rectal abnormalities
		Fecal occult blood test yearly	Blood in the stool
		Sigmoidoscopy every 5 years	Unusual growths or lesions
Oral	Persistent sores or other lesions in the mouth or on the lips	Visual exam by a doctor or dentist yearly	Oral lesions
Prostate	Change in urinary habits, such as difficulty urinating (The cause is usually benign prostate enlargement, but the symptoms could indicate prostate cancer.)	Starting by age 50: Digital rectal exam	Swelling of the prostate gland, lumps, or other abnormalities
		Prostate-specific antigen (PSA) test	Elevated levels of prostate-specific antigen (a protein produced by prostate cells), which may indicate prostate cancer
Skin	Changes or irregularities in the size of moles; unusual growths	Visual exam by a doctor every year for those over 40; every 3 years for ages 20–40.	Changes or irregularities in moles; precancerous lesions

SOURCE: *American Health*, September 1995.

Skin Cancer

Sunlight is the primary culprit in the 600,000 new cases of skin cancer that develop every year. Most damage is caused by exposure to the B range of ultraviolet light (UVB); the longer wavelength of light known as UVA also may be damaging to the skin. Tanning salons or sunlamps also increase the risk of skin cancer because they produce ultraviolet radiation. A half-hour dose of radiation from a sunlamp can be equivalent to the amount you'd get from an entire day in the sun. (See Figure 13-3.)

The most common skin cancers are basal-cell (involving the base of the epidermis, the top level of the skin) and squamous-cell (involving cells in the epidermis). Smoking and exposure to certain hydrocarbons in asphalt, coal tar, and pitch may increase the risk

Figure 13-3

Three types of skin cancer. Squamous-cell cancer; malignant melanoma, the deadliest form of cancer; and basal-cell cancer.

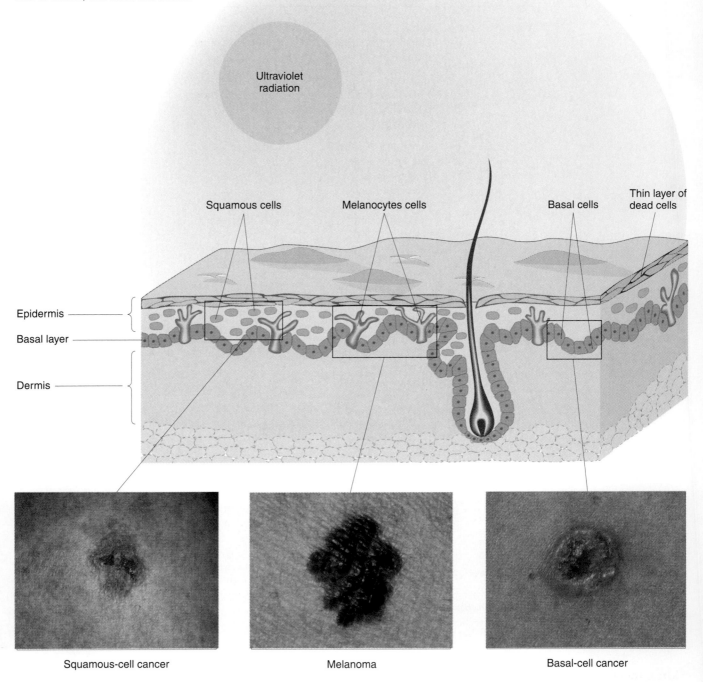

Ultraviolet radiation

Squamous cells   Melanocytes cells   Basal cells   Thin layer of dead cells

Epidermis

Basal layer

Dermis

Squamous-cell cancer   Melanoma   Basal-cell cancer

of squamous-cell skin cancer. Both types can usually be treated with surgery. However, individuals who develop such cancers are at higher risk for developing subsequent tumors of the same type.

The incidence of the deadliest type, malignant melanoma, is rising by 4% to 5% per year. The overall risk of getting melanoma for Americans is about 1 in 120, but increases for individuals with any of the following characteristics:

- Blond or red hair.

- Marked freckling of the upper back.
- Rough red bumps on the skin called actinic keratoses.
- A family history of melanoma.
- Three or more blistering sunburns in the teenage years.
- Three or more years at an outdoor summer job as a teenager.

Any one or two of these factors increases a person's risk of melanoma three or four times. A combination of three or more factors increases the risk 20 to 25 times. Other risk factors include occupational exposure to carcinogens and inherited skin disorders, such as xeroderma pigmentosum and familial atypical multiple-mole melanoma.

If detected early, melanoma is highly curable. However, once a tumor is thicker than an eighth of an inch—about the thickness of a dime—it probably has metastasized. Treatment may consist of surgery, radiation, electrodesiccation (tissue destruction by heat), cryosurgery (tissue destruction by cold), or a combination of these therapies. Individuals who've had melanoma may be at high risk for developing this cancer again.[29]

Strategies for Prevention

Scanning Your Skin

Here's how to screen yourself for possible changes that may indicate skin cancer:

✔ Once a month, stand in front of a full-length mirror to examine your front and back, and your left and right sides with your arms raised. Check the backs of your legs, the tops and soles of your feet, and the surfaces between your toes. Use a hand mirror to check the back of your neck, behind your ears, and your scalp.

✔ Watch for changes in the size, color, number, and thickness of moles. Suspicious moles are likely to be asymmetrical (one half doesn't match the other), with ragged, notched, or blurred edges. Also look for any signs of darkly pigmented growth, oozing, scaliness, bleeding, or a change in sensation, itchiness, tenderness, or pain.

✔ Don't put too much faith in sunscreens. Wearing sunscreen (with a Sun Protection Factor, or SPF, of at least 15) is good, but protective clothing is better—and staying in the shade is best.[30]

✔ Check your shadow. One simple guideline for reducing the risk of skin cancer risk is avoiding the sun anytime your shadow is shorter than you are. According to NCI, this shadow method—based on the principle that the closer the sun comes to being directly overhead, the stronger its ultraviolet rays—works for any location and at any time of year.

✔ Check for photosensitivity. If you are taking any drugs, ask your doctor or pharmacist to see if the medication could make you more sensitive to sun damage. Be especially cautious about sun exposure if you have been using a synthetic preparation derived from vitamin A (Retin A) as an acne or anti-wrinkle treatment; it can increase your susceptibility.

Breast Cancer

The disease American women fear most, according to a survey commissioned by the National Council on the Aging, is breast cancer. Yet, the number-one killer of American women is heart disease, which claims the lives of one in every two women in the United States. By comparison, breast cancer accounts for 4% of annual deaths.[31]

One reason for women's concern is the oft-quoted statistic that one in nine American women will develop breast cancer. However, age is a crucial factor. The NCI estimates the risk for women under age 35 as only 1 in 622, rising to 1 in 93 by age 45, 1 in 33 by age 55, 1 in 17 by age 65, and 1 in 9 by age 85.

Although the incidence of breast cancer has been increasing, mortality rates have been declining in recent years. Most researchers credit the statistics on improved survival to the increased use of mammography and improvements in treatments. The risk factors for breast cancer include being over age 50, having a personal or family history of the disease, having no children, having had a first child after age 30, early onset of puberty, late menopause, exposure to radiation, obesity (for postmenopausal women), and, in premenopausal women with a family history of breast cancer, certain types of benign breast disease.

Causes Researchers have identified specific "breast cancer genes," including those known as BRCA1 and BRCA2. Women with defects in these genes have a greater risk of cancer than others. On average, women with at least one genetic mutation have a 56% chance of getting breast cancer by age 70 (compares with 13% for women in the general population) and a 16% chance of ovarian cancer (compared with 1.6%). However, genes aren't the only determinant of cancer risk, and a woman with one or more breast cancer genes will not inevitably develop cancer. At this time, most physicians do not recommend testing except for women in families at high risk of breast or ovarian cancer.[32]

Estimates of the number of women with a family history of breast cancer range from 5% to 20%. A small subset of such women come from families with a striking incidence of breast and other cancers often associated with family history. Currently, physicians recommend that women at high risk undergo breast examinations and mammography every 6 to 12 months beginning between ages 25 and 35. Although there is no conclusive evidence that *prophylactic* (preventive) surgery reduces risk, some women opt for this choice.[33]

African-American women are more than twice as likely to die of breast cancer than white women, largely because their disease more often reaches an advanced stage before it is diagnosed.[34] The delay in seeking treatment accounted for 40% of the higher death rate, while 15% was attributed to the tumor being more aggressive in black women (a factor that may be related to diet and environment). According to a 1995

Looking

Stand in front of a mirror with your upper body unclothed. Look for changes in the shape and size of the breast, and for dimpling of the skin or "pulling in" of the nipples. Any changes in the breast may be made more noticeable by a change in position of the body or arms. Look for any of the above signs or for changes in shape from one breast to the other.

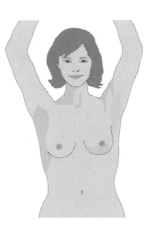 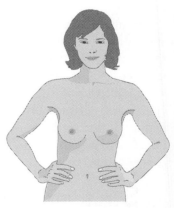

1. Stand with your arms down.

2. Raise your arms overhead.

3. Place your hands on your hips and tighten your chest and arm muscles by pressing firmly.

Feeling

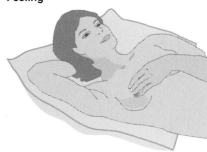 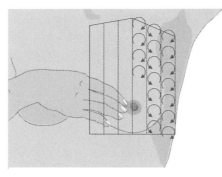 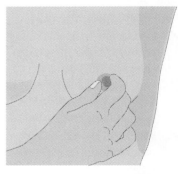

1. Lie flat on your back. Place a pillow or towel under one shoulder, and raise that arm over your head. With the opposite hand, you'll feel with the pads, not the fingertips, of the three middle fingers, for lumps or any change in the texture of the breast or skin.

2. The area you'll examine is from your collarbone to your bra line and from your breastbone to the center of your armpit. Imagine the area divided into vertical strips. Using small circular motions (the size of a dime), move your fingers up and down the strips. Apply light, medium, and deep pressure to examine each spot. Repeat this same process for your other breast.

3. Gently squeeze the nipple of each breast between your thumb and index finger. Any discharge, clear or bloody, should be reported to your doctor immediately.

Figure 13-4

Breast self-exam. The best time to examine your breasts is after your menstrual periods, every month.

report in the *Journal of the National Cancer Institute*, the chances of dying of breast cancer may be influenced more by where a woman lives as an adult than by where she was born and grew up.[35]

The question of risk related to diet and alcohol use remains unresolved, with different studies suggesting different degrees of risk. There also is continuing controversy over the role of postmenopausal hormone replacement therapy (HRT) and an increased risk of breast cancer. Some studies have found an increased risk as high as 30% to 70%, whereas others have found no increased risk of breast cancer.[36] (For a complete discussion of the pros and cons of HRT, see Chapter 18 on aging.)

Detection To detect lumps or changes that could signal breast cancer, all women should perform monthly breast self-exams seven to ten days after their periods (see Figure 13-4) and have a professional breast exam yearly if over 40 and every three years if between ages 20 and 40.

The best tool for early detection is the diagnostic X-ray exam called **mammography**. Overall, screening mammograms could reduce breast cancer deaths by 25%. Mammograms can detect a tumor two to three years before it can be detected by manual exam (see Figure 13-5).

Although annual mammograms have long been routinely recommended for women over 50, there's been considerable controversy over screening recommendations for women in their forties. At an NIH consensus conference, an international panel of experts—after reading more than 100 reports and listening to 32 presentations by invited speakers—decided not to decide. Rather then advising for or against routine mammography in this age group, the panel recommended that each woman make her own choice in consultation with her physician. This proclamation stirred intense controversy. Ultimately, in March 1997, the ACS and National Cancer Society recommended that all women begin routine mammographic screening by age 40.[37]

Subsequent studies have shown that annual mam-

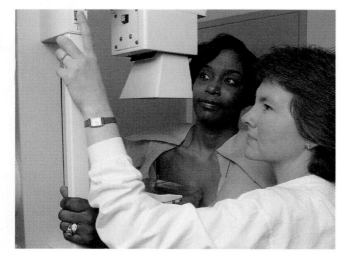

Figure 13-5

This comparison of cancer sizes found by various breast-cancer detection methods shows the difference between mammography and other methods. Mammography, a diagnostic X ray technique, is able to detect a lump that is much smaller than what a woman can find with regular breast self-exams.

Cancer calcifications of this size and smaller can be seen on mammograms.	Average-size lump found by mammogram.	Average-size lump found by women practicing frequent breast self-exam.	Smallest-size cancer that can be felt by physician's palpation exam.	Average-size lump found by women practicing occasional breast self-exam.
0.1 cm	0.4 cm (5/32 in.)	0.8 cm (5/16 in.)	1 cm (4/10 in.)	1.7 cm (11/16 in.)

mograms in a woman's forties are not only safe but highly effective in reducing breast cancer risks. According to scientists' estimates, annual mammography screening would reduce deaths due to breast cancer by at least 35% in women aged 40 to 49, compared to 24% when mammograms are given every other year. Any possible risks associated with radiation exposure are considered negligible, if present at all.[38]

Mammography techniques have improved markedly in recent years, and more refinements should enhance accurate and early detection of breast cancer in the future. For example, digital mammography projects an image onto a television screen, allowing magnification of suspicious areas. Computers also are being used to interpret mammograms with greater precision, and new biopsy techniques, such as sentinel node biopsy, can rule out noncancerous tumors.

Treatment If a mammogram detects a lump or suspicious area, a tissue biopsy is performed to confirm the diagnosis of cancer. Depending on the size and site of the tumor, surgeons may recommend **lumpectomy** (local removal of a tumor and surrounding tissue) or more extensive surgery, such as a **quadrantectomy** (which removes a larger area of the breast and lymph glands). These "breast-conserving" procedures lead to survival rates that are equal to those following **mastectomy** (removal of the entire breast). Followup chemotherapy with a drug such as tamoxifen (previously discussed as a form of chemoprevention) blocks estrogens (female sex hormones) that can stimulate tumor growth, and can decrease the risk of recurrences and increase survival times.[39]

Cervical Cancer

The risk factors for cervical cancer include early age of first intercourse, multiple sex partners, genital herpes, human papilloma virus (HPV) infection, and significant exposure to passive smoking. The standard screening test for cervical cancer is the Pap smear (described in Chapter 20). Each year this test detects about 1.2 million cases of abnormal cell growth. Since Pap tests were introduced, the death rate from cervical cancer has decreased by 70%. However, they can fail to detect cancerous cells in as many as 20%–40% of the women tested.

Warning signs for cervical cancer include irregular bleeding or unusual vaginal discharge. In precancerous stages, cervical cells may be destroyed by laser surgery or freezing in a doctor's office. More advanced cancer may require more extensive surgery, sometimes in combination with chemotherapy or radiation.[40]

Ovarian Cancer

Ovarian cancer is the leading cause of death from gynecological cancers, with 24,000 new cases diagnosed and 13,600 deaths each year. Risk factors include a family history of ovarian cancer; personal history of breast cancer; obesity; infertility (because the abnormality that interferes with conception may also play a role in cancer development); and low levels of transferase, an enzyme involved in the metabolism of dairy foods. Often women develop no obvious symptoms until the advanced stages, although they may experience painless swelling of the abdomen; irregular bleeding; lower abdominal pain; digestive and urinary abnormalities; fatigue; backache; bloating; and weight gain.

The lifetime risk of ovarian cancer in a woman with no affected relatives is 1 in 70. The risk for a woman with one first-degree relative with ovarian cancer is 1 in 20, and the risk increases with additional affected relatives. For women who may have a hereditary ovarian cancer syndrome, the lifetime risk may be as high as one in two. Routine screening is not recommended for women who are not at known risk. For those at increased risk, an NIH consensus panel has recommended annual pelvic and rectal exams, and ultrasound imaging of the pelvic region and a blood test for a substance called CA125 every six months.[41] In cases of very high risk, some oncologists (cancer specialists) recommend prophylactic removal of the ovaries when childbearing is completed or by no later than age 35. "Every case is different, of course, based on an individual's risk," says M. Steven Piver, M.D., an oncologist at Roswell Park Cancer Institute in Buffalo, New York.[42]

Colon and Rectal Cancer

Colon and rectal cancer claims about 60,000 lives a year. Most cases occur after age 50 and slightly more often among women than men. Risk factors include a personal or family history of colon and rectal cancer, polyps (growths) in the colon or rectum, and ulcerative colitis (described later in this chapter). Early signs of colorectal cancer are bleeding from the rectum, blood in the stool, or a change in bowel habits.

The simplest test for this common cancer detects blood in a person's stool. According to the Congressional Office of Technology Assessment, such tests, which cost only about $4, could prevent 23,000 cancers a year among those aged 65 or older. The other standard screening tests for colon cancer are a digital rectal exam, which should be performed annually after age 40, a stool blood slide test that detects blood in feces (recommended every year after age 50), and proctosigmoidoscopy, which involves inserting a fiber-optic tube for visual inspection of the colon and rectum (recommended every three to five years after age 50). Scientists have also developed a gene test for colon cancer that could identify those at highest genetic risk.[43]

Treatment may involve surgery, radiation therapy, or chemotherapy. Regular exercise can lower the risk of colon and rectal cancer in both men and women. Hormone replacement after menopause may significantly reduce women's risk of colon cancer.[44]

Prostate Cancer

Prostate cancer is the most frequently diagnosed non-skin cancer among American men, with an estimated 200,000 new cases each year (ACS).[45] African-American men have the highest rate of prostate cancer in the world; their death rate from this cancer is twice that of white men ("Action").[46]

The risk of prostate cancer increases with age, family history, exposure to the heavy metal cadmium, high number of sexual partners, and history of frequent sexually transmitted diseases. (Researchers have found no evidence that vasectomies might increase prostate cancer risk, as had once been thought.) Saturated fats, those in animal products like butter and meat, do greatly increase the risk of prostate cancer.

The development of a simple screening test that measures levels of a protein called prostate-specific antigen (PSA) in the blood has revolutionized the diagnosis of prostate cancer. Although PSA testing has proven more accurate than previous methods in detecting prostate cancers at early stages, it has created an ethical dilemma for physicians. Because PSA also can be elevated in men with a benign condition called prostatic hyperplasia, the test can indicate cancer where none exists.[47]

In addition, there seem to be different forms of the cancer—some aggressive and deadly, some "low grade" and slow moving. Among men older than age 70, life expectancy without treatment is nearly identical to survival following definitive treatments. Many older men with low-grade prostate cancer may expect a normal life span without undergoing potentially debilitating surgery or radiation.

Men whose brothers or fathers had the disease should begin getting tested at age 40. All men over age 50 should also undergo an annual rectal examination, in which a doctor inserts a gloved finger into the rectum and feels the prostate for abnormal growths that may indicate cancer. As noted above, a chemoprevention trial is looking at the possible preventive benefits of Proscar (finasteride), a drug used to treat benign swelling of the prostate, a common problem in aging men.

Early warning signs of prostate cancer are frequent or difficult urination, blood in the urine, painful ejaculation, or constant lower-back pain. Treatments include surgical removal of the prostate, conventional radiation, implanting "seeds" of radioactive iodine in the prostate, and hormone therapy.

Testicular Cancer

This cancer is not common, accounting for only 3% of cancers of the male genitals and urinary tract. What is more, it occurs mostly among young men between the ages of 18 and 35, who are not normally at risk of cancer. At highest risk are men with an undescended testicle (a condition that is almost always corrected in childhood to prevent this danger). To detect possibly cancerous growths, men should perform monthly testicular self-exams, as shown in Figure 13-6. Often the first sign of this cancer is a slight enlargement of one testicle. There also may be a change in the way it feels when touched. Sometimes men with testicular cancer report a dull ache in the lower abdomen or groin, along with a sense of heaviness or sluggishness. Lumps on the testicles also may indicate cancer.

A man who notices any abnormality should consult a physician. If a lump is indeed present, a surgical biopsy is necessary to find out if it is cancerous. If the biopsy is positive, a series of tests generally is needed to determine whether the disease has spread. Treatment for testicular cancer generally involves surgical removal of the diseased testis, sometimes along with radiation therapy, chemotherapy, and the removal of nearby

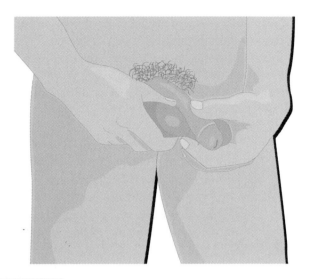

Figure 13-6

Testicular self-exam. The best time to examine your testicles is after a hot bath or shower, when the scrotum is most relaxed. Place your index and middle fingers under each testicle and the thumb on top, and roll the testicle between the thumb and fingers. If you feel a small, hard, usually painless lump or swelling, or anything unusual, consult a urologist.

lymph nodes. The remaining testicle is capable of maintaining a man's sexual potency and fertility. Only in rare cases is removal of both testicles necessary. Testosterone injections following such surgery can maintain potency. The chance for a cure is very high if testicular cancer is spotted early.

Leukemia

Risk factors for this cancer of the blood include Down syndrome and other inherited abnormalities and excessive exposure to radiation or certain chemicals, such as benzene. Leukemia can be difficult to detect early because its symptoms are often similar to those of less serious conditions, such as influenza. Diagnosis is based on blood tests and a bone-marrow biopsy. Treatment may involve chemotherapy, drugs, blood transfusions, and bone-marrow transplants.

Lung Cancer

Cigarettes cause most cases of lung cancer, which is the leading cause of cancer deaths in women and the second leading cause in men. Risk factors include smoking for twenty or more years; exposure to certain

industrial substances, particularly asbestos; passive smoking; radiation exposure; and radon exposure. A smoker's risk of developing lung cancer drops almost to that of a nonsmoker within ten years after his or her last cigarette, although the lungs may still be damaged. (See Figure 13-7.)

Lung cancer is very difficult to detect early. Warning signs include a persistent cough, sputum streaked with blood, chest pain, recurring bronchitis, or pneumonia. Diagnosis is based on a chest X-ray, sputum cytology (cell) testing, and fiber-optic bronchoscopy (direct examination of the lungs by means of a specially lighted tube). Treatment generally involves surgery, chemotherapy, and/radiation.

Oral Cancer

Heavy smoking of cigarettes, cigars, or pipes; excessive drinking; and the use of chewing tobacco increase the risk of oral cancer. Those who drink as well as smoke are particularly vulnerable. Early signs include a mouth sore that bleeds easily and doesn't heal; a lump or thickening; a reddish or whitish patch; and difficulty chewing, swallowing, or moving the tongue or jaws. Regular exams by your dentist or primary care physician can detect oral cancers. Surgery and radiation are the standard treatments.

New Hope Against Cancer

Because of advances in diagnosis and treatment, cancer is no longer a death sentence. Cancer survivors make up one of the fastest growing groups in the United States. Many have had no evidence of cancer for five years. Others survive in remission, a state in which patients have no symptoms, and the spread of cancerous cells is assumed to be temporarily stopped. ACS officials believe that by applying today's state-of-the-art treatments, survival rates for both men and women could increase by another 10% to 15% by the end of the 1990s. So many people now survive that specialists debate whether long-term followup for certain cancers, such as cancer of the colon or rectum, is necessary—or just creates unwarranted anxiety.[48]

Cancer Therapy

The following are the primary forms of treatment for cancer:

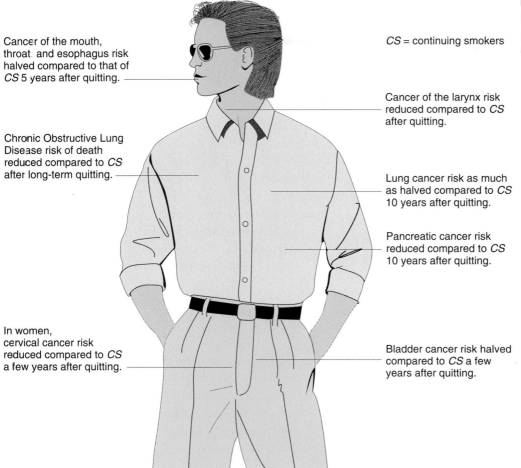

Figure 13-7
Lowered health risks from quitting smoking.

Cancer of the mouth, throat. and esophagus risk halved compared to that of *CS* 5 years after quitting.

Chronic Obstructive Lung Disease risk of death reduced compared to *CS* after long-term quitting.

In women, cervical cancer risk reduced compared to *CS* a few years after quitting.

CS = continuing smokers

Cancer of the larynx risk reduced compared to *CS* after quitting.

Lung cancer risk as much as halved compared to *CS* 10 years after quitting.

Pancreatic cancer risk reduced compared to *CS* 10 years after quitting.

Bladder cancer risk halved compared to *CS* a few years after quitting.

- *Surgery* to remove a tumor and surrounding cells. The oldest and most widely used approach, surgery is most effective for small, localized cancers.

- *Radiation therapy*, which exposes the involved area of the body to powerful radiation, which destroys cancer cells. Radiation therapy is sometimes used as an adjuvant, or supplementary, treatment along with surgery or chemotherapy.

- *Chemotherapy*, which uses powerful drugs or hormones, taken orally or through injection, to interfere with the reproduction of fast-multiplying cancer cells.

- *Immunotherapy*, which stimulates the body's own immune system to attack cancer cells. One approach uses biological response modifiers (BRMs), substances normally produced by the immune system in small amounts to fight infection. The most commonly used BRMs include interferons (proteins produced by cells to resist viruses) and interleukins (proteins released by certain white blood cells to support the growth of others). A related approach uses monoclonal antibodies (made by combining a cancer cell with an antibody forming cell) that can target and kill cancer cells without damaging healthy cells.

Another treatment, **bone-marrow transplantation**, involves extremely high doses of radiation or, increasingly, chemotherapy to kill cancer cells; however, the marrow in the patient's body is also destroyed. The patient then receives healthy bone-marrow cells, either his or her own (which may have undergone treatment in a laboratory) or a carefully matched donor's. *Autologous* transplants (those using the person's own blood) have produced long-term survival rates of more than 50% for certain leukemias and lymphomas (cancer of the immune system). They're also being used experimentally in treating other cancers, including breast and ovarian tumors.

Most cancer treatments affect normal, healthy cells as well as cancerous ones. Most vulnerable to radiation and chemotherapy are the fastest-growing body cells: hair cells, cells of the gastrointestinal tract, cells in the reproductive organs, and cells of the blood-producing tissue, the bone marrow.

Promising advances in cancer treatment that may save lives in the future include new and more powerful forms of chemotherapy and adding immunotherapy agents to standard anticancer drugs to make chemotherapy more effective. Researchers at the NCI are also experimenting with **gene therapy**, the insertion of genes into a patient, as a possible cancer treatment, and with the development of cancer vaccines.[49]

Using the Mind to Help the Body

The powers of the mind can be a powerful resource for cancer patients. In fact, knowledge itself can be powerful. According to recent studies, cancer patients who participate in educational programs that explain their disease and treatment have significantly higher survival rates. Support groups also affect both the quality and quantity of life. Patients with melanoma who attended support groups did much better both on psychological tests and on measures of tumor-fighting immune cells.[50]

In another landmark study, women with metastatic breast cancer who participated in weekly support groups reported less depression, anxiety, fatigue, and pain and greater self-esteem than women who received standard medical care. Participation in the groups, which focused on the psychological impact of cancer, doctor-patient issues, and pain control, also doubled their survival times. Average survival time for group members was 36.6 months from diagnosis, compared to 18.9 months for those in the control group.[51]

Diabetes Mellitus

About 100 million people around the world—including an estimated 14 million people in the United States—have **diabetes mellitus**, a disease in which the body doesn't produce or respond properly to insulin, a hormone essential for daily life. In those who have diabetes, the pancreas, which produces insulin (the hormone that regulates carbohydrate and fat metabolism) doesn't function as it should. When the pancreas either stops producing insulin or doesn't produce sufficient insulin to meet the body's needs, almost every body system can be damaged.

Diabetes may be caused by an autoimmune reaction in which the insulin-producing areas of the pancreas are attacked by immune cells. Scientists also have found that a virus may play a role in triggering the onset of Type 1 diabetes. According to recent studies, some people who have a certain genetic profile may develop a viral infection that causes the immune system to overreact and attack the pancreas. The viruses that have been implicated are Coxsackie viruses, polio-related viruses that cause upper respiratory infections. This discovery could lead to development of a vaccine for people with a family history of diabetes.[52]

What Is Diabetes?

Glucose is the primary form of sugar that the body cells use for energy. When a healthy person eats a meal, the level of glucose in the blood rises, triggering the production and release of insulin by special cell clusters in the pancreas called the islets of Langerhans. Insulin enhances the movement of glucose into various body cells, bringing down the level of glucose in the blood. In those who have diabetes, however, insulin secretion is either nonexistent (referred to as Type 1 or *insulin-dependent diabetes*) or deficient (referred to as Type 2 or *non insulin-dependent diabetes*). Without sufficient insulin, the glucose in the blood is unable to enter most body cells, so the cells' energy needs aren't met. The levels of glucose in the blood rise higher and higher after each meal. This unused glucose eventually passes through the kidneys, which are unable to process the excessive glucose, and out of the body in urine.

Deprived of the fuel it needs, the body begins to break down stored fat as a source of energy. This process produces weak acids, called ketones. A buildup of ketones leads to ketoacidosis, an upheaval in the body's chemical balance that brings on nausea, vomiting, abdominal pain, lethargy, and drowsiness. Severe ketoacidosis can lead to coma and eventual death.

An estimated 5.4 million adults in the United States have undiagnosed diabetes. Type 2 diabetes, the most prevalent form of the disease, often causes no symptoms for many years. In order to identify individuals with this disease as early as possible, the American

TABLE 13-3 EARLY SIGNS OF DIABETES

Type 1
Insulin-dependent

Sudden appearance of these symptoms:
    Constant urination
    Abnormal thirst
    Unusual hunger
    Rapid weight loss
    Irritability
    Weakness or fatigue
    Nausea and vomiting
Symptoms may appear to be "flu"
Occurs in children or young adults
Requires administration of insulin for life

Type 2
Non insulin-dependent

Family history of diabetes
Gradual appearance of these symptoms:
    Drowsiness
    Itching
    Blurred vision
    Excessive weight
    Tingling and numbness in feet
    Easy fatigue
    Skin infections
    Slow healing of wounds
Symptoms may be confused with aging
Sedentary lifestyle, excess weight contribute
Occurs in those over age 30
Generally treated with diet and exercise
    programs, medication

SOURCE: American Diabetes Association.

Diabetes Association now recommends screening every three years for all men and women beginning at age 45.[53] Those at highest risk include relatives of diabetics (whose risk is two and a half times that of others); obese persons (85% of diabetics are or were obese); older persons (four out of five diabetics are over age 45); and mothers of large babies, because this is an indication of maternal prediabetes. A child of two parents with Type 2 diabetes faces an 80% likelihood of also becoming diabetic.

The early signs of diabetes are frequent urination, excessive thirst, a craving for sweets and starches, and weakness. (See Table 13-3.) Diagnosis is based on tests of the sugar level in the blood. Researchers are work-

ing to develop a test that would help identify telltale antibodies in the blood which could indicate that pancreas cells are being destroyed years before the first signs of diabetes.

The Dangers of Diabetes

Before the development of insulin injections, diabetes was a fatal illness. Today diabetics may have normal lifespans. However, both types of diabetes can lead to devastating complications, including increased risk of heart attack or stroke, kidney failure, blindness, and loss of circulation to the extremities. Although few people realize it, diabetes claims more than 100,000 women's lives a year—more than the number who succumb to breast cancer.[54]

Diabetic women who become pregnant face higher risks of miscarriage and serious birth defects; however, precise control of blood sugar levels before conception and in early pregnancy can lower the likelihood of these problems. The development of diabetes during pregnancy—called gestational diabetes—may pose potentially serious health threats to mother and child years later. Women who develop gestational diabetes are more than three times as likely to develop Type II diabetes if they have a second pregnancy; their infants may be at increased risk of caridovascular disease later in life.[55]

Strategies for Prevention

Lowering the Risk of Diabetes

✔ Eat a diet rich in complex carbohydrates (bread and other starches) and high-fiber foods, and low in sodium and fat.

✔ Eat fruits and vegetables that are rich in antioxidants, substances that prevent oxygen damage to cells.

✔ Avoid alcohol.

✔ Keep your weight down. Weight loss for those who are overweight can sometimes decrease or eliminate the need for insulin or oral drugs. For individuals at high risk of developing noninsulin-dependent diabetes, losing just half the pounds needed to reach their ideal weight can prevent the onset of the disease.

✔ Exercise regularly. Regular, vigorous aerobic activity reduces the risk of noninsulin-dependent diabetes in men and women.[56]

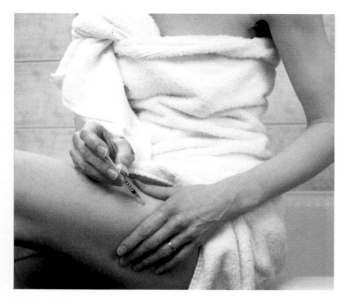

Many diabetics control their disease by injecting themselves with insulin.

Diabetes and Ethnic Minorities

Several minority groups, especially African Americans, Native Americans, and Latinos, are at high risk of developing diabetes. One in every ten African Americans and Latinos has this disease. And the members of some Native-American tribes are 300% more likely to develop diabetes than the general population. For many, obesity and unhealthy food choices increase the risk. Researchers now believe that the interaction of environmental factors and genes varies among different racial and ethnic groups.

Treatments for Diabetes

There's no cure for diabetes at this time. The best treatment option is to keep blood sugar levels as stable as possible to prevent complications, such as kidney damage. Home glucose monitoring allows diabetics to check their blood sugar levels as many times a day as necessary and to adjust their diet or insulin doses as appropriate.

Those with insulin-dependent diabetes require daily doses of insulin via injections, an insulin infusion pump, or oral medication. Those with noninsulin-dependent diabetes can control their disease through a well-balanced diet, exercise, and weight management. However insulin therapy may be needed to keep blood glucose levels near normal or normal, thereby reducing the risk of damage to the eyes, nerves, and kidneys.[57]

Medical advances hold out bright hopes for diabetics. Laser surgery, for instance, is saving eyesight. Bypass operations are helping restore blood flow to the heart and feet. Dialysis machines and kidney and pancreas transplants save many lives. Researchers are exploring various approaches to prevention, including early low-dose insulin therapy, oral insulin to correct immune intolerance, and immunosuppressive drugs. Still on the horizon is the promise of a true cure through transplanting insulin-producing cells from healthy pancreases. In very preliminary trials, this procedure has helped patients become insulin-independent, at least temporarily.

Other Major Illnesses

Other noninfectious diseases besides cancer and diabetes have a debilitating effect on many people. But most of the diseases discussed in this section can be controlled, if not cured.

Epilepsy and Seizure Disorders

About 10% of all Americans will have at least one seizure at some time. Between 0.5% and 1% of all Americans have recurrent seizures. Derived from the Greek word for seizure, **epilepsy** is the term used to refer to a variety of neurological disorders characterized by sudden attacks (seizures) of violent muscle contractions and unconsciousness. Epilepsy is rarely fatal; the primary danger to life is to suffer an attack while driving or swimming.

Seizures can be major, referred to as *grand mal*; minor, referred to as *petit mal*; or psychomotor. In a grand-mal seizure, the person loses consciousness, falls to the ground, and experiences convulsive body movements. Petit-mal seizures are brief, characterized by a loss of consciousness for 10 to 30 seconds, by eye or muscle flutterings, and occasionally by a loss of muscle tone. About 90% of all epileptics have grand-mal seizures; 40% suffer both petit-mal and grand-mal seizures. The frequency of attacks defines the severity of the epilepsy. Diagnosis is based on a history of recurring attacks and a study of the brain's electrical activity, called an electroencephalogram (EEG).

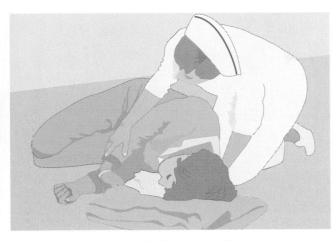

If someone is having an epileptic seizure, others should watch to be sure the person is not harmed, but should not restrict his or her movements.

About half of all cases of epilepsy have no known cause and are therefore classified as *idiopathic.* All others stem from conditions that affect the brain, such as trauma, tumors, congenital malformations, or inflammation of the membranes covering the brain. Idiopathic epilepsy usually begins between the ages of 2 and 14. Seizures before age 2 are usually related to developmental defects, birth injuries, or a metabolic disease affecting the brain. (Fever-induced convulsions are not related to epilepsy.) Seizures after age 14 are generally symptoms of brain disease or injury.

Seizure disorders don't reflect or affect intellectual or psychological soundness; people who suffer from them have normal intelligence. Therapy with anticonvulsant drugs can control seizures in most people, and once seizures are under control, epileptics can live full, normal lives by continuing to take their medications. However, about 10% to 20% of the 120,000 people who develop epilepsy every year continue to have seizures despite medical therapy. Technological advances have allowed doctors to identify more accurately where seizures originate in the brain; and surgery, though risky and expensive, is offering new hope to many epileptics.

If you're with a person who suffers a grand-mal seizure, make sure he or she isn't injured during the attack. Don't try to restrain the person or interfere with his or her movements, and don't try to force anything into the person's mouth. Medical treatment usually isn't needed unless the seizure lasts more than a couple of minutes or is almost immediately followed by another.

Respiratory Diseases

Noninfectious diseases of the respiratory system, including chronic bronchitis and emphysema, can also be causes of disability and death. (See Chapter 17 for the major infectious respiratory diseases, and Chapter 16 for smoking-induced problems.)

Asthma

Some 14 to 15 million Americans, including 4.8 million children, suffer from **asthma**, a disease characterized by constriction of the breathing passages.[58] As with allergy, asthma rates have skyrocketed in the last two decades. Since 1980 mortality rates have doubled, with asthma claiming the lives of 5000 Americans every year. The problem is especially severe in inner cities, where emergency room visits and asthma mortality rates run as high as eight times the national average.[59]

While asthma is not always linked to allergy, the two are related. Among people with asthma, 90% of the children, 70% of young adults, and 50% of older adults also have allergies. According to epidemiologic research, 23% of youngsters diagnosed with allergies by age 1 develop asthma by age 6. Of those diagnosed after age 1, 13% eventually become asthmatic. Symptoms include wheezing, coughing, shortness of breath, and chest tightness. If the symptoms are untreated or undertreated, they can worsen and damage the lungs.[60]

The two main approaches to asthma treatment are control of the underlying inflammation by means of anti-inflammatory drugs, such as corticosteroids, cromolyn sodium, and neodocromil, and short-term relief of symptoms with bronchodilators, such as albuterol, which expand the breathing passages. In its most recent official guidelines, the National Heart, Lung and Blood Institute encouraged more frequent use of inhaled steroids and less reliance on bronchodilators, which have little effect on the underlying inflammation. In one major study, the use of inhaled steroids decreased the risk of hospitalization by 50%.[61]

Some new asthma medications, such as Accolate and Zyflo, directly target leukotriene, one of the chemicals involved in an inflammatory response. These drugs seem useful in cases of mild to moderate asthma, but specialists are still uncertain of exactly how they'll fit into long-term asthma management. Experts also predict new options that will replace standard bronchodilator inhalers, which are being removed from the market because of the global ban on chlorofluorocarbons (CFCs). The first "environmentally friendly" inhaler, Proventil, which uses an alternative propellant, became available in 1997; more such drugs are expected in 1998.

Chronic Obstructive Lung Disease (COLD)

Chronic obstructive lung disease (COLD), also called chronic obstructive pulmonary disease (COPD), is characterized by progressively more limited flow of air into, and out of, the lungs. COLD consists of two separate but closely related conditions: chronic bronchitis and emphysema. Most COLD patients develop both forms. The major cause is cigarette smoking, although air pollution may also play a role. (See also Chapter 17.)

In chronic bronchitis, the bronchial passageways are constantly inflamed, and individuals develop a persistent, sputum-producing cough; shortness of breath; and wheezing. They must stop smoking, lose excess weight, exercise, and avoid or reduce contact with air pollutants.

Chronic bronchitis can lead to emphysema, a deterioration of the lungs that may begin in adolescence. Eventually, the alveoli, tiny air sacs in the lungs, tear, reducing the lungs' ability to exhale. This condition can lead to heart failure.

Anemias

The **anemias** are diseases affecting the oxygen-carrying capacity of the blood. Usually there's a reduced number of red blood cells or a reduced amount of hemoglobin, the oxygen-carrying component of red blood cells. Anemia can be caused by nutritional inadequacies; loss of blood, including heavy menstrual bleeding; deficiencies in red-cell production; or genetic disorders. Iron-deficiency anemia is a form of anemia caused by a lack of dietary iron, an essential component of the hemoglobin molecule that carries oxygen. It's the most common form of anemia and often goes undiagnosed in women.

- *Sickle-cell anemia* is a genetic blood disorder that occurs when the hemoglobin contained in the red blood cells is abnormal. The red blood cells become crescent-or sickle-shaped and unable to supply oxygen to body tissues (see Figure 13-8). This disease causes crippling, severe pain, and premature death. About 8% to 10% of African Americans carry the gene for sickle-cell anemia.

- *Pernicious anemia* results from a lack of vitamin B12 (cobalamine), which causes a deficiency in the formation of red blood cells. Although B-12 is usually present in the diet, some people lack a substance needed to absorb it into their blood. Injections of B12 can control this condition.

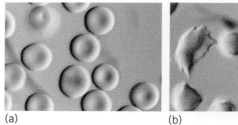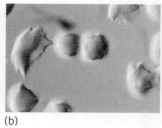

(a)   (b)

Figure 13-8

Sickle-cell anemia. (a) Normal mature red blood cells are disk-shaped and concave. (b) In sickle-cell anemia, the red blood cells are crescent-shaped and jagged, causing them to pile up and obstruct small blood vessels. Areas of the body are thus deprived of oxygen and nutrients.

- *Aplastic anemia*, most common in young adults and adolescents, interferes with the bone marrow's ability to form blood. Usually it results from ingesting a toxic agent, often a medication; symptoms include multiple internal hemorrhages. Whole-blood transfusions are the primary therapy, but the condition is usually fatal.

Liver Disorders

Cirrhosis is characterized by significant loss of liver cells and the formation of scar tissue that can interfere with circulation in the liver. The major cause of one of the most common forms of cirrhosis, Laennec's cirrhosis, is chronic alcoholism. Each year, about 30,000 Americans die of alcohol-related liver disorders. (See also Chapter 15.)

Early signs of liver damage include an enlarged liver (which your doctor can feel during a physical exam) and tiny, spiderlike blood vessels on the surface of the skin. Blood tests may show abnormal levels of certain enzymes, or enlarged red blood cells. Even people with advanced liver disease feel better and live longer once they've stopped drinking alcohol. Cirrhosis symptoms, which occur only in the advanced stages of the disease, include yellow discoloration of the skin and eyes (jaundice), accumulation of fluid in the abdomen, and mental confusion.

Liver transplants are the only hope for those with advanced liver disease. With improvements in surgical techniques and the use of antirejection drugs (including cyclosporin, a combination of cyclosporin and an antifungal medication, and a new drug called FK-506), 70%

or more of liver-transplant recipients—including some in their sixties and seventies—now live for at least a year. Some liver transplant recipients have lived longer than 20 years.

Kidney Diseases

A wide range of diseases can affect the kidneys and their ability to process fluids and waste. Some are acute, temporary problems; others are chronic, progressive illnesses that permanently impair kidney function. (See Chapter 12 for a description of kidney infections.)

Nephrosis refers to a cluster of symptoms indicating chronic damage to the kidneys, including chronic proteinuria (the loss of more than one gram of protein a day in the urine), hypercholesteremia (high levels of fats in the blood), and edema (fluid retention). The kidney damage can be the result of diabetes, heavy metal poisoning, allergic reactions to insect stings, or other disorders.

Kidney stones may form either from calcium salts or from minerals (the causes are unknown). Most stones eventually pass out of the body in urine, which can be extremely painful. They don't usually obstruct the flow of urine or interfere with kidney function. However, infection can develop behind a stone. Larger stones can be surgically removed or painlessly shattered into harmless fragments by high-frequency sound waves.

The various chronic and inflammatory diseases of the kidney can all lead to kidney failure. A mechanical process of clearing waste fluids from the body, called *dialysis*, can do the kidneys' job temporarily. Another alternative is a kidney transplant, either from a living, related donor or from a cadaver whose kidney has been carefully tissue-matched to the recipient to minimize the risk of rejection. New methods of controlling complications caused by rejection have led to great success. The longest-surviving recipients of transplanted kidneys have lived for more than 25 years with their donated organs. However, a lack of organ donors remains a critical obstacle to performing more of these lifesaving operations.

Digestive Diseases

Most disorders of the digestive tract affect only one section: either the esophagus, the stomach and duodenum, the small intestine, the large intestine, the liver, the pan-

creas, the gallbladder, or the rectum. The most dangerous are Crohn's disease and ulcerative colitis. According to the National Digestive Diseases Advisory Board, almost half of the U.S. population will suffer a digestive problem at some time in their lives.

Ulcers

Open sores, often more than an inch wide, that develop in the lining of the stomach or the duodenum (the first part of the small intestine) are called **ulcers**. They are caused by excessive acidic digestive juices. The major symptom is a burning pain felt throughout the upper abdomen. The pain may come and go, lasting up to three hours. It may begin either right after eating or several hours later.

One in five men and one in ten women get ulcers of the stomach or duodenum, but the number of ulcers is declining. Risk factors include heavy use of cigarettes, alcohol, or caffeine; the ingestion of large amounts of painkillers that contain aspirin or ibuprofen; and advanced age. Bleeding is not common but may be dangerous, even life-threatening. An untreated stomach ulcer can lead to serious weight loss and anemia.

Researchers have identified a bacterium, *Helicobacter pylori*, or *H. Pylori* (formerly named *Campylo bacter*), that may infect the digestive system and set the stage for ulcers. According to various studies, most ulcer patients carry this organism. One theory is that infection leads to an inflammation of the stomach lining called gastritis, which increases vulnerability to other stressors, such as smoking, alcohol, or anxiety.

H. Pylori can be detected in several ways. A blood test can reveal the presence of infection by detecting antibodies against *H. Pylori*. However, a blood test can be positive even if someone has long been free of the bacteria. The most definitive test requires endoscopy, a procedure in which a physician examines the lining of the stomach or duodenum by passing a thin flexible tube (an endoscope) down the patient's throat and snips a small bit of tissue for laboratory analysis to detect bacteria. Researchers are experimenting with a simpler diagnostic breath test in which patients drink a special liquid that triggers a response by *H. Pylori* bacteria in the stomach. Treatment with conventional antibiotics leads to improvement in most patients.

Conventional therapy for ulcers includes self-help measures, such as avoiding aspirin; eating small, frequent meals; taking antacids; and not smoking or drinking alcohol or caffeine. Drugs such as cimetidine, ranitidine, and sucralfate can reduce the amount of acid produced by the stomach and relieve ulcer symptoms. If a stomach ulcer doesn't heal after six to eight weeks of drug treatment, physicians may recommend surgery to remove the ulcer.

Inflammatory Bowel Disease (IBD)

As many as 2 million Americans—many in the prime of life—suffer from one of the two forms of **inflammatory bowel disease (IBD)**: *Crohn's disease*, which causes inflammation anywhere in the digestive tract, and *ulcerative colitis*, which creates severe ulcers in the inner lining of the colon and rectum. Both illnesses can trigger frequent and intense diarrhea, abdominal pain, gas, fever, and rectal bleeding.

The specific causes of IBD remain unknown, but scientists speculate that some irritating substance—perhaps a bacterium, virus, or chemical or environmental agent—somehow leaks through the intestine's thin lining into the bowel's deep inner wall. Inflammation develops, setting into motion a chain of harmful reactions by the body's protective immune system and causing swelling, pain, and damage to the intestinal wall. Ulcers (small perforations or holes) may form, exposing cells and tissues to destructive intestinal bacteria and enzymes. Blood and fluid from body tissues may leak into the intestines, showing up as diarrhea or blood in the stool. Twenty percent of cases involve a genetic or familial predisposition.

Treatment for IBD consists primarily of drugs, including powerful steroids, antibiotics, and medications that fight inflammation. Dietary changes can also help. Crohn's patients who don't improve on medication or who develop life-threatening complications, such as a severe intestinal blockage, may undergo surgery to remove or bypass the diseased part of the intestine and reconnect two healthy segments. However, the disease very often recurs in another part of the intestinal tract. For those with ulcerative colitis, removal of the entire colon brings an end to troubling symptoms—and to the increased risk of colon cancer that these individuals face. Most gastroenterologists advise patients with ulcerative colitis to undergo annual examinations of the colon (colonoscopies) to detect precancerous changes in cells.

Irritable Bowel Syndrome

Irritable bowel syndrome (also called irritable colon or spastic colon) is a common problem caused by intestinal spasms. The muscular contractions that move waste material through the intestines become irregular and uncoordinated, causing frequent feelings of a need to defecate, nausea, cramping, pain, gas, and a sensation that the rectum is never emptied.

Diagnostic tests, including X rays, stool samples, and examination of the colon with a sigmoidoscope, can rule out colon cancer and other problems. Travel, stress, changes in diet, and smoking often worsen these symptoms. Many people respond well to a high-fiber diet; others prefer a bland diet. There's no standard medical treatment for irritable bowel syndrome; some physicians prescribe stool softeners, laxatives, or drugs to reduce intestinal spasms.

Gallstones

An estimated 25 million Americans—about 10% of the population—have **gallstones**: clumps of solid material, usually cholesterol, that form in bile stored in the gallbladder. One-third to one-half of all gallstones produce no symptoms. However, some gallstones, carried out of the liver with bile, get stuck in the bile duct and cause intense pain that lasts for several hours. Ultrasound and special X rays called cholecystograms can detect gallstones.

During an attack of gallstone pain, a physician may recommend a painkiller. Some gallstones can be dissolved by long-term drug treatment. Another alternative to traditional gallbladder surgery is laparoscopic surgery, in which gallstones are removed without having to cut through the major abdominal muscles.

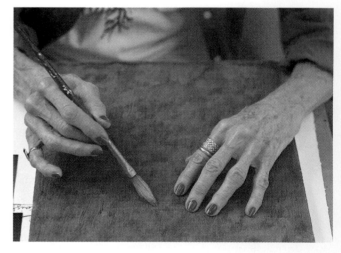

Those who suffer arthritis pain may tend to minimize movement in their joints, but moderate activity will help keep muscles functioning that stabilize the joints.

Disorders of the Muscles, Joints, and Bones

Because they're constantly being used, muscles, joints, and bones are more susceptible to damage from injury than are most other parts of the body.

Arthritis

More than 17 million people suffer from some form of **arthritis**, an inflammatory disease of the joints that takes over a hundred forms. Rheumatoid arthritis is an autoimmune disease in which the body attacks its own connective tissue; it's fairly common among younger people. Degenerative arthritis, or osteoarthritis, characterized by changes in bone tissue and cartilage, primarily at the joints, seems to be the result of normal wear and tear. Women are generally affected by arthritis three times more often than are men, until the seventh or eighth decade of life. Race and occupation don't seem to be factors; climate affects symptoms but not causes.

The goal of all treatments for arthritis is to maintain the patient's ability to function. Drugs can relieve pain and reduce inflammation; surgical treatments, including total joint replacement, and physical therapy are also used to maintain motion and strength, and to correct deformities.

Hernias

A **hernia** is a bulge of soft tissue that forces its way through or between strained or weakened muscles. Hernias can occur in many parts of the body, but they're most common in the abdominal wall. A surgeon can push the protruding tissue back into place and tighten or sew together the loose muscles.

Backaches

Back woes, which rank second only to headaches among modern miseries, eventually afflict seven of every ten adults. Anyone from a college athlete to a retired grandparent can suffer a back injury, but the risks increase with time as the deeper muscles and tendons surrounding the spine become less resilient. Yet age itself is rarely the only factor in a disabling back attack; almost always tense, injured, or weak muscles are to blame. Other risk factors include extra pounds, particularly if stuffed into a pot belly; lack of exercise; poor posture; and bending from the waist to hoist a heavy load.

Strain from use or abuse accounts for 80% of back ailments. Most vulnerable is the lower, or lumbar, part of the spine, which bears the greatest pressure when bending and lifting. Five to 10% of back problems involve the discs between the vertebrae. Most common is the protrusion (or herniation) of the soft center of a disc through the casing so that it presses on spinal nerves. Another 10% of back problems involve structural defects, which may be the result of injuries, tumors, arthritis, congenital malformations, osteoporosis (the weakening of the bones), or scoliosis (side-to-side curving of the spine). Sometimes a sore back is a symptom of diseases of other organs, such as the kidneys, gallbladder, or stomach. A physical exam and various tests, including electrodiagnostic studies, X rays, CT scans, and MRIs (magnetic resonance imaging), may be necessary to pinpoint the problem.

Bed rest, supplemented by moist heat or other muscle relaxants and anti-inflammatory drugs, eases most backaches. However, the days when doctors advised two weeks of bed rest for a bad back are gone. After two or three days, most back patients are urged to get up, start walking, and resume light activity.

Back specialists tailor treatment programs to an individual's needs. Different forms of physical therapy—including specific exercises, massage, heat, ultrasound, and electrical stimulation—often relieve pain and speed recovery. Some people successfully use chiropractic, acupuncture, hypnosis, biofeedback, or relaxation techniques to cope with back pain. Regardless of treatment, more than 85% of back-injury patients get well within two weeks. Fewer than 2% eventually require surgery to repair a herniated disc.

Strategies for Prevention

Preventing Back Problems

✔ When standing, shift your weight from one foot to the other. If possible, place one foot on a stool, step, or railing 4 to 6 inches off the ground. Hold in your stomach, tilt your pelvis toward your back, and tuck in your buttocks to provide crucial support for the lower back.

✔ Because sitting places more stress on the lower back than standing, try to get up from your seat at least once an hour to stretch or walk around. Whenever possible, sit in a straight chair with a firm back. Avoid slouching in overstuffed chairs or dangling your legs in midair. When driving, keep the seat forward so that your knees are raised to hip level; your right leg should not be fully extended. A small pillow or towel can help support your lower back.

✔ Sleep on a flat, firm mattress. The best sleep position is on your side, with one or both knees bent at right angles to your torso. The pillow should keep your head in line with your body so that your neck isn't bent forward or to the side.

✔ When lifting, bend at the knees, not from the waist. Get close to the load. Tighten your stomach muscles, but don't hold your breath. Let your leg muscles do the work.

✔ Always warm up and stretch before a workout. Exercise regularly, but don't push yourself too hard. The activities that are easiest on the back are swimming, cycling (in an upright position), walking, and jogging (preferably not on concrete). Activities that demand sudden stops and turns (such as tennis and other racket sports) or that involve a good chance of falling (such as downhill skiing) are most likely to spell trouble for your back—and you.

✔ Don't smoke. Smoking may interfere with circulation to the lower back; and a chronic smoker's cough can be so irritating that it provokes a back spasm.

Skin Disorders

Your skin is the largest organ of your body. Because of its visibility, none of its problems may seem trivial. The more serious skin diseases are discussed below. (See also the "A-to-Z Self-Care Guide" at the back of this book for a discussion of more common problems, such as acne and athlete's foot.)

Eczema and Dermatitis

Dermatitis is any inflammation of the skin. *Eczema*, a specific type of dermatitis usually caused by allergies, is a skin inflammation that results from internal processes. Symptoms of eczema include redness, flaking, blistering, and thickening of the skin. Self-help treatments include avoiding irritants, such as dishwater, and using steroid creams containing 0.5% hydrocortisone.

Psoriasis

In **psoriasis**, the rate of skin cell production is speeded up. As skin cells pile up faster than they can be shed, they produce scaly, deep-pink, raised patches on the skin. Triggers of psoriasis are stress, skin damage, and illness. Self-help measures include sunbathing or using

ultraviolet light to clear up the psoriasis. Physicians usually prescribe ointments, creams, or pastes, including some steroid preparations, or ultraviolet treatment.

Special Needs for Different Abilities

About 49 million Americans have physical or mental impairments, including blindness, deafness, disorders of the muscles or nerves, paralysis, loss of limbs, or mental retardation, that substantially limit one or more major life activities. Most are the result of illnesses, such as strokes, arthritis, or heart disease, and affect the ability to walk, speak, or live independently. Some congenital disorders, such as cerebral palsy, cause speech problems, muscular weakness, and mental retardation. Accidents are responsible for other disabilities, including paralysis (see Chapter 17).

Individuals with special needs and abilities can live full, happy, and productive lives. Famous people who've made major contributions to the world despite disabilities include the composer Ludwig van Beethoven, who wrote some of his most famous music after becoming deaf, the inventor Thomas A. Edison, who was deaf throughout much of his life, and President Franklin D. Roosevelt, who became paralyzed in both legs at the age of 39.

Few such problems can be cured, but a great deal can be done to overcome them. **Rehabilitation medicine**, the specialty dedicated to improving the condi-

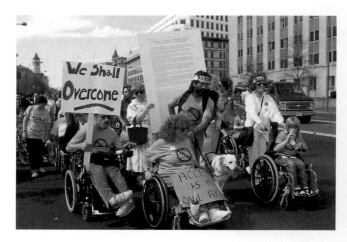

Disabled Americans have lobbied for changes in attitudes and for legislation that enables them to participate more fully in society.

tion of the disabled, can provide treatments such as surgery for certain types of blindness or deafness, medications to ease the crippling pain of arthritis, and physical therapy, including special exercises to build up endurance and muscle strength. Mechanical devices, such as electric wheelchairs, artificial limbs, and hearing aids, can open up wider worlds to the disabled. Occupational therapy teaches skills to help the disabled gain confidence. Vocational training prepares them to find employment.

Individuals with special needs face special challenges in their daily lives. Some are primarily physical, such as difficulty bathing, lifting groceries, opening cans and bottles, or going someplace. They also face many social and economic challenges. Because some people feel uncomfortable about disabilities, they may not treat individuals with special needs with the same acceptance and respect that they show to others. This can lead to discrimination from employers.

The U.S. Congress has taken action to affirm the rights of individuals of differing abilities, starting with equal educational opportunities. Until very recently, special education for children with physical, intellectual or behavioral disabilities meant separate education. These youngsters were taught in different classrooms, isolated from normally developing children, often in schools far from their homes. Most did poorly—in school and beyond—-and never graduated from high school, got jobs, or lived independently.

The federal Individuals with Disabilities Education Act mandates that children with disabilities be educated in "the least restrictive environment possible," a term that school districts around the country have been struggling to define. What has emerged is a hodge-podge of programs—usually called *inclusion* or *integration*—that have been opening up regular classrooms to youngsters many thought never could learn in such settings.

Heralded by some, criticized by others, inclusion has had its successes and its setbacks. In the best situations, teachers and students receive extra support and assistance. But in some schools, disabled children have simply been dumped into a classroom with little or no planning or teacher support. "The situation varies from state to state, county to country, school district to school district," says Jennifer York, Ph.D., an assistant professor of education at the University of Minnesota who has been studying the impact of inclusion.[62] In the limited number of studies that have been done—generally in communities that have made a major commitment to

inclusion—disabled youngsters in regular classrooms have shown solid gains, building much stronger communication skills and showing clear academic progress.

Since 1992 the Americans with Disabilities Act has protected disabled people from discrimination by private employers, required wheelchair access to public buildings and mass transportation, and ordered telephone companies to provide telephone relay services that allow people with impaired speech or hearing to make and receive calls. Many states now require insurers to provide coverage for high-risk individuals such as cancer survivors. The names of many of the organizations that help the disabled, such as the National Coalition for Cancer Survivorship and the National Council on Independent Living, are in "Your Health Directory" at the back of the book.

Strategies for Change
Helping Individuals with Special Needs

✔ *Be considerate, not condescending.* Treat others as you would like to be treated yourself. Any discomfort you feel about another's disability can appear to be a lack of understanding and respect.

✔ *Ask if the person needs help;* don't simply assume that he or she is helpless. Keep in mind that there are many ways to perform routine actions. If the person would like help, find out how you can be of assistance. Follow his or her instructions rather than doing things your way.

✔ *Stress abilities.* People with disabilities also have abilities. Recognizing these abilities shows respect for people with disabilities and allows them as much as possible to do things for themselves.

✔ *Don't deny the problem.* While it's important to recognize a disabled person's strengths, don't negate any prob-lems the person may be experiencing. Let them talk openly and express their feelings.

✔ *Don't be afraid to touch.* Everyone responds to a caring touch.

Making This Chapter Work for You
Staying Alive and Healthy

■ You can do a great deal to prevent or delay many serious illnesses, including the one we fear most: cancer. In all types of cancer, changes in the genetic

Health Online

An Introduction to Skin Cancer
http://www.maui.net/~southsky/introto.html

Did you know that it is estimated that one in seven Americans will get skin cancer at some point in their lives? This page is dedicated to skin cancer, its causes, determining personal risk, prevention, and treatment. There are many special features, like a daily UV forecast for 30 cities across the country.

Think about it ...

- What are your personal risk factors for skin cancer? What could you do to lower your chances of getting this disease?

- Check out today's UV forecast for the city nearest where you live. What does it mean? What precautions should you take, if any?

- Skin cancer cases are on the rise in the United States. Can you think of three possible reasons for this?

material in the cells cause normal cells to turn into abnormal cells and multiply to form malignant tumors, or neoplasms. Benign tumors are not normally life-threatening. Hereditary, viral, chemical, and physical factors can cause malignant, or cancerous, tumors.

■ Prevention is the best approach to cancer. Lifestyle changes—including not smoking; limiting sun exposure; restricting alcohol intake; eating a high-fiber, low-fat diet; and exercising—can reduce the risk of developing cancer. Scientists are experimenting with a new approach, called chemoprevention, which involves giving vitamins or drugs to healthy people at high risk of cancer, in order to prevent the development of tumors. Having regular cancer checkups, knowing the warning signs of cancer, and performing periodic self-exams can help identify potentially cancerous changes so that treatment can begin as early as possible.

■ Traditionally, cancer treatment includes some form or combination of chemotherapy (drug treatment), surgery, and radiation. Promising new developments in fighting cancer include more effective forms of treatment, such as powerful drug combinations, immunotherapy, and gene therapy. Psychological support can make a big difference in enhancing the quality and extending the quantity of life for cancer patients.

■ Diabetes mellitus is a serious medical problem in which the pancreas produces an insufficient amount of insulin, a hormone needed by the body's cells to metabolize glucose. Treatment for milder cases of diabetes is a carefully controlled diet; insulin is necessary in more severe cases.

■ Other major illnesses include epilepsy and seizure disorders, which can usually be controlled by medication or surgery.

■ A growing problem is asthma, which can be triggered by allergens, pollution, respiratory infections, and stress; complications and death rates for asthma are rising. The symptoms of chronic bronchitis, a common disorder among smokers, include a persistent cough, shortness of breath, and wheezing. In emphysema, the air sacs in the lungs lose their elasticity, and the lungs become enlarged.

■ Other major diseases include anemia, liver disease, kidney disorders, digestive diseases, and disorders of the muscles, joints, and bones.

■ Physical and mental impairments, whether caused by congenital disorders, illnesses, or accidents, affect millions of Americans; but a great deal can often be done to overcome their effects.

Serious disease may seem to be a matter of odds. Genetic tendencies, environmental factors, and luck do seem to affect your chances of having to face many of these health threats. However, you have more control over such risks than anyone or anything else in your life.

■ *Don't smoke*, and you all but eliminate the threat of lung cancer and many respiratory problems—and brighten your heart's future, too.

■ *Eat healthy foods*, and you not only look good but also keep your arteries free of fat, lower your blood pressure, reduce your cancer risk, and help prevent diabetes.

■ *Exercise regularly*, and you not only tone muscles but also strengthen your cardiovascular system.

■ *Have regular screening tests*, and you can cut off some life-threatening diseases before they get an edge on you.

 ## Key Terms

The terms listed here are used within the chapter. Page numbers are included for each term.
A definition of each term is given in the green Glossary pages at the end of this book.

anemia *426*
arthritis *429*
asthma *425*
**bone-marrow
  transplantation** *421*
carcinogen *410*
chemoprevention *410*
**chronic obstructive lung disease
  (COLD)** *426*
cirrhosis *426*
dermatitis *430*

diabetes mellitus *422*
epilepsy *424*
gallstones *428*
gene therapy *422*
hernia *429*
infiltration *404*
**inflammatory bowel disease
  (IBD)** *428*
irritable bowel syndrome *428*
kidney stones *427*
lumpectomy *418*

mammography *417*
mastectomy *418*
metastasize *404*
neoplasm *404*
nephrosis *427*
oncogene *406*
psoriasis *430*
quadrantectomy *418*
rehabilitation medicine *430*
ulcer *427*

 ## Review Questions

1. What is cancer? What warning signs should a person look for?

2. What factors put a person at greater risk of developing cancer? What cultural and racial groups are at greatest risk? What can be done to reduce the risk of developing some of the more common types of cancer?

3. What can be done to increase the likelihood of early detection of cancer?

4. List and describe the types of treatments available for cancer patients. What are some of the side effects of these treatments? Describe some of the new treatments being developed.

5. What is diabetes mellitus? Describe the early symptoms of the disease and methods of treatment.

6. Name some different types of noninfectious illnesses, and describe the symptoms and treatments for three of them.

 ## Critical Thinking Questions

1. A friend of yours, Karen, discovered a small lump in her breast during a routine self-examination. When she mentions it, you ask if she has seen a doctor. She tells you that she hasn't had time to schedule an appointment; besides, she says she's not sure it's really the kind of lump one has to worry about. It's clear to you that Karen is in denial and procrastinating about seeing a doctor. What advice would you give her?

2. Do you know someone who is disabled? How do their lifestyle practices differ from your own? What is the effect of their health-care practices and behaviors on your own behavior?

3. Because of advances in antirejection treatment, organ transplants have proven highly successful in helping many people who otherwise might have died. Even elderly patients have clearly benefited from donated kidneys and livers. However, because the demand for organs to transplant greatly exceeds the supply, health experts have debated setting priorities. Should a 30-year-old be placed higher on the waiting list for a particular organ than a 70-year-old? Should a nurse who needs a liver because she contracted hepatitis on the job get priority over an alcoholic whose liver has been destroyed by cirrhosis? Who, if anyone, should make such decisions? Would a lottery be more fair?

 ## Connections to Personal Health Interactive

To enhance your understanding of the material covered in this chapter, check out the following study aids on the **Personal Health Interactive CD-ROM** *. Each numbered icon within the chapter corresponds to an appropriate activity listed here.*

 ## References

13.1 Personal Insights: What Is Your Risk for Cancer?

13.2 Chapter 13 Review

1. American Cancer Society.

2. American Cancer Society.

3. National Cancer Institute.

4. Davis, Devra, et al. "Decreasing Cardiovascular Disease and Increasing Cancer Among Whites in the United States from 1973 Through 1987." *Journal of the American Medical Association*, Vol. 271, No. 6, February 9, 1994.

5. Loprinzi, Charles. Personal interview.

6. Spitz, Margaret. Personal interview.

7. DeVita, Elizabeth. "Conquering Cancer." *American Health*, November 1994.

8. American Cancer Society.

9. Levine, Arnold. "The Genetic Origins of Neoplasia." *Journal of the American Medical Association*, Vol. 273, No. 7, February 15, 1995.

10. Ward, Darrell. *Reporting on Cancer*. Columbus: Ohio State University, 1994.

11. Stephenson, Joan. "Fruits of Molecular Studies Include Gene Linking Diet and Cancer, Novel Markers for Malignancy." *Journal of the American Medical Association*, Vol. 274, No. 5, August 2, 1995.

12. Burtness, Barbara. "Oncology and Hematology." *Journal of the American Medical Association*, Vol. 273, No. 21, June 7, 1995.

13. Miller, Jeff. "Cancer Clues." *UCSF Magazine*, Vol. 15, No. 2, November 1994.

14. National Cancer Institute. "Human Papillomavirus." *Cancer Facts*. Bethesda, MD: National Institutes of Health.

15. Temoshok, Lydia, and Henry Dreher. *The Type C Connection*. New York: Random House, 1992. Barraclough, Jennifer. *Cancer and Emotion: A Practical Guide to Psycho-Oncology*. New York: John Wiley & Sons, 1994. Miller, Daniel. "Instincts, Feelings, and Homeostasis: A Psychophysiological Model of Cancer." *Advances: The Journal of Mind-Body Health*, Vol. 11, No. 2, Spring 1995.

16. Osborne, Michael, et al. "Cancer Prevention." *Lancet*, Vol. 349, No. 9063, May 17, 1997. Hong, Wan Ki an Michael Sporn. "Recent Advances in Chemoprevention of Cancer." *Science*, Vol. 278, No. 5340, November 7, 1997.

17. Nestle, Marion. Personal interview.

18. Miller, A. B., et al. "Diet in the Aetiology of Cancer: A Review." *European Journal of Cancer*, Vol. 30A, No. 2, 1994.

19. Harnack, Lisa, et al. "Association of Cancer Prevention-Related Nutrition Knowledge, Beliefs and Attitudes to Cancer Prevention Dietary Behavior." *Journal of the American Dietetic Association*, Vol. 97, No. 7, September 1997.

20. "Food Choices May Lower Risk for Ovarian Cancer." *Tufts University Diet & Nutrition Letter*, Vol. 12, No. 11, January 1995.

21. Black, Homer, et al. "Effect of a Low-Fat Diet on the Incidence of Actinic Keratosis." *New England Journal of Medicine*, Vol. 330, No. 18, May 5, 1994.

22. Roman, Mark. "Dietary Fat and Prostate Cancer." *American Health*, January–February 1994.

23. Robinson, John, and Tibbett Speer. "The Air We Breathe." *American Demographics*, Vol. 17, No. 6, June 1995.

24. Office of Cancer Communications. "Personal Use of Hair Coloring Products and the Risk of Cancer." National Institutes of Health, February 1, 1994. Thun, M. J., et al. "Hair Dye Use and Risk of Fatal Cancers in U.S. Women." *Journal of the National Cancer Institute*, February 2, 1994.

25. NCI. "Chemoprevention." *Cancer Facts*, November 11, 1994. NCI. "Alpha Tocopherol, Beta Carotene Cancer Prevention Study: Vitamin E and Beta Carotene Supplements Did not Prevent Lung Cancer in Male Smokers." *Cancer Facts*, April 4, 1994.

26. NCI. "Questions and Answers About the Breast Cancer Prevention Trial." *Cancer Facts*, February 1995.

27. "Questions and Answers About the Prostate Cancer Prevention Trial." *Cancer Facts*, October 1993.

28. Brawley, Otis. Personal interview.

29. NCI. Marwick, Charles. "New Light on Skin Cancer Mechanisms." *Journal of the American Medical Association*, Vol. 274, No. 6, August 9, 1995. *Melanoma Research Report*. Bethesda, MD: National Institutes of Health. NCI. *Skin Cancers: Basal Cell and Squamous Cell Carcinomas, Research Report*. Bethesda, MD: National Institutes of Health, 1994.

30. Naylor, Mark. "The Case for Sunscreens." *Journal of the American Medical Association*, Vol. 278, No. 21, December 3, 1997.

31. "Assessing the Odds." *Lancet*, Vol. 350, No. 9091, November 29, 1997.

32. Runowicz, Carolyn. "Breast Cancer Genes and What They Mean." *New England Journal of Medicine Health News*, June 18, 1997.

33. Hoskins, Kent, et al. "Assessment and Counseling for Women with a Family History of Breast Cancer." *Journal of the American Medical Association*, Vol. 273, No. 7, February 15, 1995.

34. American Cancer Society. *Cancer Facts & Figures—1995.*

35. Kliewer, Erich, and Ken Smith. "Breast Cancer and Location." *Journal of the National Cancer Institute*, August 3, 1995.

36. Colditz, G., et al. "The Use of Estrogens and Progestins and the Risk of Breast Cancer in Postmenopausal Women." *New England Journal of Medicine*, Vol. 332, May 15, 1995. Stanford, Janet, et al. "Combined Estrogen and Progestin Hormone Replacement Therapy in Relation to Risk of Breast Cancer in Middle-Aged Women." *Journal of the American Medical Association*, Vol. 274, No. 2, July 12, 1995. Adami, Hans-Olov, and Ingemar Persson. "Hormone Replacement and Breast Cancer: A Remaining Controversy?" *Journal of the American Medical Association*, Vol. 274, No. 2, July 12, 1995.

37. Woolf, Steven, and Robert Lawrence. "Lessons from the Consensus Panel on Mammography Screening." *Journal of the American Medical Association*, Vol. 278, No. 23, December 17, 1997.

38. Cady, Blake, et al. "Breast Cancer Update: Progress and Conflict." *Patient Care*, Vol. 31, No. 11, June 15, 1997.

39. NCI. *What You Need to Know About Breast Cancer*. Bethesda, MD: National Institutes of Health.

40. NCI. *What You Need to Know About Cervical Cancer*. Bethesda, MD: National Institutes of Health.

41. NIH Consensus Statement. *Ovarian Cancer: Screening, Treatment and Followup*. Bethesda, MD: National Institutes of Health, 1994.

42. Piver, Steven. Personal interview.

43. Leard, Lorriana. "Patient Preferences for Colorectal Cancer Screening." *Journal of the American Medical Association*, Vol. 278, No. 23, December 17, 1997.

44. Newcomb, Polly. *Journal of the National Cancer Institute*, July 19, 1995. NCI. *What You Need to Know About Cancer of the Colon and Rectum*. Bethesda, MD: National Institutes of Health.

45. American Cancer Society.

46. "Action Proposal on Prostate Cancer in African Americans Is Issued by the American Cancer Society." January 13, 1998.

47. Lange, Paul. "New Information About Prostate-Specific Antigen and the Paradoxes of Prostate Cancer." *Journal of the American Medical Association*, Vol. 273, No. 4, January 25, 1995.

48. Loprinzi, Charles. "Follow-Up Testing for Curatively Treated Cancer Survivors." *Journal of the American Medical Association*, Vol. 273, No. 23, June 21, 1995. Virgo, Katherine, et al. "Cost of Patient Follow-up After Potentially Curative Colorectal Cancer Treatment." *Journal of the American Medical Association*, Vol. 273, No. 23, June 21, 1995.

49. Skolnick, Andrew. "Essential Components Now in Place for Clinical Testing of Cancer Vaccine Strategies, Experts Say." *Journal of the American Medical Association*, Vol. 273, No. 7, February 15, 1995.

50. Chollar, Susan. "Mind over Cancer?" *American Health*, November 1994.

51. Spiegel, David. *Living Beyond Limits*. New York: Random House, 1995.

52. Collins, Clare. "Diabolical Diabetes." *American Health*, January–February 1993.

53. American Diabetes Association. "Screening for Type 2 Diabetes." *Diabetes Care*, Vol. 21, Supplement 1, Clinical Practice Recommendations, 1998.

54. Miller, Elizabeth. "Diabetes, a Greater Death Threat to Women than Breast Cancer." American Diabetes Association National Service Center, June 11, 1995.

55. Council on Pregnancy. "Symposium on Pathogenesis and Prevention of Diabetic Embryopathy." ADA annual meeting, June 1995. Miller, Elizabeth. "Threatening Risks of Gestational Diabetes Continue to Unfold." American Diabetes Association, National Service Center, June 11, 1995.

56. Bernstein, Gerald, and Suzanne LeVert. *Diabetes: Reducing Your Risk.* New York: Bantam Books, 1994.

57. Hayward, Rodney, et al. "Starting Insulin Therapy in Patients with Type 2 Diabetes." *Journal of the American Medical Association*, Vol. 278, No. 20, November 26, 1997.

58. Voelker, Rebecca. "Taking Asthma Seriously." *Journal of the American Medical Association*, Vol. 278, No. 1, July 2, 1997.

59. "Asthma Hospitalization and Readmissions Among Children and Young Adults." *Morbidity and Mortality Weekly Report*, Vol. 46, No. 1, August 8, 1997.

60. "NAEPP Guidelines: Progress in Asthma Management." *American Family Physician*, Vol. 56, No. 2, August 1997.

61. "NHLBI Issues Updated Guidelines for the Diagnosis and Management of Asthma." *American Family Physician*, Vol. 56, No. 2, August 1997.

62. York, Jennifer. Personal interview.

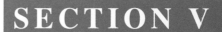

AVOIDING HARMFUL HABITS

We constantly hear messages encouraging us to take risks with our health, to try drugs, to have a drink, to smoke cigarettes. We also live with the consequences of others' drug abuse, alcoholism, and smoking. That's why it's important to know about potentially harmful habits— even if you never rely on drugs to pick you up or bring you down, never smoke, and never drink to excess. This section provides information you can use to avoid or overcome habits that could destroy your health, happiness, and life.

CHAPTER 14

DRUG USE, MISUSE, AND ABUSE

After studying the material in this chapter, you should be able to:

Explain factors affecting drug dependence.

Describe the methods of use, effects of, and treatments for cocaine and crack abuse.

Describe the common forms and effects of amphetamines, depressants, cannabis products, psychedelics and hallucinogens, and narcotic drugs.

Describe the issues affecting the treatment of drug dependence.

Define addiction, and **explain** the addictive process.

Explain codependency, and **list** and **explain** some ways that a codependent person can enable another person to continue an addictive behavior.

Describe the twelve-step plan for recovery from addiction.

*A*t a concert on campus, students pass around a marijuana joint while listening to the music. A bored teenager in an affluent suburb swallows a tab of LSD. At a party, a group of 20-something singles snort lines of cocaine. A middle-aged woman, troubled by worries and unable to relax, starts taking more and more of the medications she's gotten from various physicians to relieve her anxiety.

These people may not fit the image of a desperate addict that many conjure up when they think about drug users. Yet drugs are a fact of life for each of them, and each faces a risk of developing a substance abuse disorder. Although drug use has declined in the last two decades, the rates of drug abuse and drug-related problems remain high. About half of American adults surveyed report having used an illicit drug at some time in their lives; 15% say they did so in the preceding 12 months.[1]

No one who uses drugs expects to lose control. Even regular drug users believe they are smart enough, strong enough, or lucky enough not to get hooked. But after continued use, a person's need for a drug can outweigh everything else, including the values, people, and relationships he or she once held dearest.

This chapter provides information on the nature and effects of drugs, the impact of drugs on individuals and society, and the drugs Americans most commonly use, misuse, and abuse.

Understanding Drugs and Their Effects

A **drug** is a chemical substance that affects the way you feel and function. In some circumstances, taking a drug can help the body heal or relieve physical and mental distress. In other circumstances, taking a drug can distort reality, undermine well-being, and threaten survival. No drug is completely safe; all drugs have multiple effects that vary greatly in different people at different times. Knowing how drugs affect the brain, body, and behavior is crucial to understanding their impact and making responsible decisions about their use.

Drug misuse is the taking of a drug for a purpose or by a person other than that for which it was medically intended. Borrowing a friend's prescription for penicillin when your throat feels scratchy is an example of drug misuse. The World Health Organization defines **drug abuse** as excessive drug use that's inconsistent with accepted medical practice. Taking anabolic steroids, discussed later in this chapter, to look more muscular is an example of drug abuse.

There are risks involved with all forms of drug use. Even medications that help cure illnesses or soothe symptoms have side effects and can be misused. Some substances that millions of people use every day, such as caffeine, pose some health risks. Others—like the most commonly used drugs in our society, alcohol and tobacco—can lead to potentially life-threatening problems. With some illicit drugs, any form of use can be dangerous.

Many factors determine the effects a drug has on an individual. These include how the drug enters the body, the dosage, drug action, and presence of other drugs in the body—as well as the physical and psychological make-up of the person taking the drug and the setting in which the drug is used.

Routes of Administration

Drugs can enter the body in a number of ways (see Figure 14-1). The most common way of taking a drug is by swallowing a tablet, capsule, or liquid. However, drugs taken orally don't reach the bloodstream as quickly as drugs introduced into the body by other means. A drug taken orally may not have any effect for 30 minutes or more.

Drugs can enter the body through the lungs either by inhaling smoke, for example, from marijuana, or by inhaling gases, aerosol sprays, or fumes from solvents or other compounds that evaporate quickly. Young users

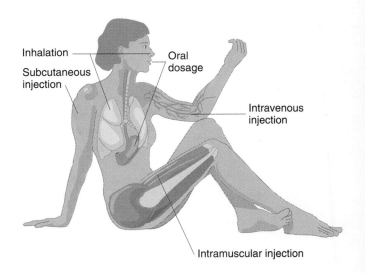

Figure 14-1

Routes of administration of drugs.

of such **inhalants**, discussed later in this chapter, often soak a rag with fluid and press it over their noses. Or they may place inhalants in a plastic bag, put the bag over their noses and mouths, and take deep breaths—a practice called *huffing* and one that can produce serious, even fatal consequences.

Drugs can also be injected with a syringe subcutaneously (beneath the skin), intramuscularly (into muscle tissue, which is richly supplied with blood vessels), or intravenously (directly into a vein). **Intravenous** (IV) injection gets the drug into the bloodstream immediately (within seconds in most cases); **intramuscular** injection, moderately fast (within a few minutes); and **subcutaneous** injection, more slowly (within ten minutes).

Approximately 1.5 million Americans use illegal IV drugs. This practice is extremely dangerous because many diseases, including hepatitis and infection with human immunodeficiency virus (HIV), can be transmitted by sharing contaminated needles. Indeed, an estimated 250,000 to 300,000 of the nation's IV-drug users are HIV-positive; they are the chief source of transmission of HIV among heterosexuals. About 70% of the AIDS cases in women and children are linked directly or indirectly to IV drug use. (See Chapter 11 for more on HIV infection and AIDS.)

Dosage

The effects of any drug depend on the amount an individual takes. Increasing the dose usually intensifies the effects produced by smaller doses. Also, there may be a change in the kind of effect at different dose levels. For example, low doses of barbiturates may relieve anxiety, while higher doses can induce sleep, loss of sensation, even coma and death.

Individual Differences

Each person responds differently to different drugs, depending on circumstances or setting. The enzymes in our bodies reduce the levels of drugs in our bloodstream; because there can be 80 variants of each enzyme, every person's body may react differently.

Often drugs intensify the emotional state a person is in. If you're feeling depressed, a drug may make you feel more depressed. A generalized physical problem, such as having the flu, may make your body more vulnerable to the effects of a drug. Genetic differences among individuals also may account for varying reactions.

Personality and psychological attitude also play a role in drug effects, so that one person may have a frighteningly bad trip on the same LSD dosage on which another person has a positive experience. To a certain extent, this depends on each user's **set** (or mind-set)—his or her expectations or preconceptions about using the drug. Someone who snorts cocaine to enhance sexual pleasure may feel more stimulated simply because that's what he or she expects.

Setting

The setting for drug use also influences its effects. Passing around a joint of marijuana at a friend's is not a healthy or safe behavior, but the experience of going to a crack house is very different—and entails greater dangers.

Toxicity

The dosage level at which a drug becomes poisonous to the body, causing either temporary or permanent damage, is called its **toxicity**. In most cases, drugs are eventually broken down in the liver by special body chemicals called *detoxification enzymes*.

Types of Action

A drug can act *locally,* as novocaine does to deaden pain in a tooth; *generally,* throughout a body system, as barbiturates do on the central nervous system; or *selectively,* as a drug does when it has a greater effect on one specific organ or system than on others, such as a spinal anesthetic. A drug that accumulates in the body because it's taken in faster than it can be metabolized and excreted is called *cumulative*; alcohol is such a drug.

Interaction with Other Drugs or Alcohol

A drug can interact with other drugs in four different ways:

- An **additive** interaction is one in which the resulting effect is equal to the sum of the effects of the different drugs used.

- A **synergistic** interaction is one in which the total effect of the two drugs taken together is greater than the sum of the effects the two drugs would have had if taken by themselves on separate occasions. Mixing barbiturates and alcohol, for example, has up to four times the depressant effect than either drug has alone.

- A drug can be **potentiating**—that is, one drug can increase the effect of another. Alcohol, for instance, can increase the drowsiness caused by antihistamines (antiallergy medications).

- Drugs can interact in an **antagonistic** fashion—that is, one drug can neutralize or block another drug with opposite effects. Tranquilizers, for example, may counter some of the nervousness and anxiety produced by cocaine.

The danger of mixing alcohol with other drugs cannot be emphasized too strongly. Alcohol and marijuana intensify each other's effects, making driving and many other activities extremely dangerous. Some people have mixed sedatives or tranquilizers with alcohol and never regained consciousness.

Medications

Many of the medications and pharmaceutical products available in this country do indeed relieve symptoms and help cure various illnesses. However, every year thousands of Americans are hospitalized because of complications caused by medications. Because drugs are powerful, it's important to know how to use them appropriately.

Over-the-Counter (OTC) Drugs

More than half a million health products—remedies for everything from bad breath to bunions—are readily available without a doctor's prescription. This doesn't mean, however, that they're necessarily safe or effective. Indeed, many widely used **over-the-counter (OTC) drugs** pose unsuspected hazards. Among the most

Self-Survey

Is It Drug Dependence or Abuse?

Individuals with a substance dependence or abuse disorder may

- Use more of an illegal drug or a prescription medication or use a drug for a longer period of time than they desire or intend. _____
- Try, repeatedly and unsuccessfully, to cut down or control their drug use. _____
- Spend a great deal of time doing whatever is necessary in order to get drugs, taking them, or recovering from their use._____
- Be so high or feel so bad after drug use that they often cannot do their job or fulfill other responsibilities. _____
- Give up or cut back on important social, work, or recreational activities because of drug use. _____
- Continue to use drugs even though they realize that they are causing or worsening physical or mental problems. _____
- Use a lot more of a drug in order to achieve a "high" or desired effect or feel fewer such effects than in the past. _____
- Use drugs in dangerous ways or situations. _____
- Have repeated drug-related legal problems, such as arrests for possession. _____
- Continue to use drugs, even though the drug causes or worsens social or personal problems, such as arguments with a spouse. _____
- Develop hand tremors or other withdrawal symptoms if they cut down or stop drug use. _____
- Take drugs to relieve or avoid withdrawal symptoms. _____

The more boxes that you or someone close to you checks, the more reason you have to be concerned about drug use. The most difficult step for anyone with a substance use disorder is to admit that he or she has a problem. Sometimes a drug-related crisis, such as being arrested or fired, forces individuals to acknowledge the impact of drugs. If not, those who care—family, friends, boss, physician—may have to confront them and insist that they do something about it. This confrontation, planned beforehand, is called an intervention and can be the turning point for drug users and their families.

This chapter provides information on drug dependence and abuse and specific drugs of abuse.

Making Changes ....
Alternatives to Drugs

If you are an addict, you must first admit that you have a problem before you can begin the process of recovery. Then you should seek help from health-care professionals. If your answers raised doubts about your drug use, try to stop using them. Consider these alternatives instead of drugs:

- If you need physical relaxation, try athletics, exercise, or outdoor hobbies. For adventure, sign up for a wilderness survival outing; or take up windsurfing or rock climbing.
- If you want to stimulate your senses, train yourself to be more sensitive to nature and beauty. Take time to appreciate the sensations you experience when you're walking in the woods or embracing a person you love.
- If you're anxious, depressed, or uptight and want relief from emotional pain, turn to people—either friends or professional counselors or support groups. If you want to find meaning in life or expand your personal awareness, explore various philosophical theories through classes, seminars, and discussion groups. Study yoga or meditation.
- If you want to enhance your creativity or appreciation of the arts, challenge your mind through reading, classes, creative games, discussion groups, memory training, or travel. Pursue training in music, art, singing, or writing. Attend more concerts, ballets, or museum shows.
- If you want to be accepted, volunteer in programs in which you can assist others and not focus solely on yourself. If you want to promote political or social change, volunteer in political campaigns, or join lobbying and political-action groups.

potentially dangerous is aspirin, the "wonder drug" in practically everyone's home pharmacy. When taken by someone who's been drinking (often to prevent or relieve hangover symptoms), for instance, aspirin increases blood-alcohol concentrations (see Chapter 15).[2] Along with other nonsteroidal anti-inflammatory drugs, such as ibuprofen (brand names include Advil and Nuprin), aspirin can damage the lining of the stomach and lead to ulcers in those who take large daily doses for arthritis or other problems (see Table 14-1). Kidney problems have also been traced to some pain relievers.

TABLE 14-1 COMPARING NONPRESCRIPTION PAIN RELIEVERS

Over-the-counter pain relievers all reduce pain, but they can cause different side effects and other reactions.

	Aspirin	Acetaminophen	Ibuprofen	Naproxen sodium
Some common brand names	Anacin, Ascriptin, Bayer, Bufferin, Ecotrin, Empirin	Excedrin Asprin-Free, Panadol, Tylenol	Advil, Ibuprin, Motrin IB, Nuprin	Aleve
Reduces pain and fever	Yes	Yes	Yes	Yes
Reduces inflammation	Yes	No	Not at maximum recommended dosage.	Not at maximum recommended dosage.
Inhibits blood clotting	Yes	No	Yes	Yes
Possible side effects	Gastrointestinal bleeding, stomach upset, and ulceration.	Unlikely when taken as directed.	Gastrointestinal bleeding, stomach upset, and ulceration.	Gastrointestinal bleeding, stomach upset.
Special concerns	Do not take if you have an allergy to aspirin or other over-the-counter pain relievers, asthma, bleeding in the digestive tract, or ulcers. Can cause Reye's syndrome in children with chickenpox.	Overdoses can be toxic to the liver. Alcohol may enhance the toxic effect of high doses.	Do not take if you have an allergy to other over-the-counter pain relievers, bleeding in the digestive tract, asthma, kidney problems, or ulcers.	Do not take if you have an allergy to other over-the-counter pain relievers, bleeding in the digestive tract, asthma, kidney problems, or ulcers.

SOURCE: Reprinted with permission from the Mayo Clinic Health Letter, April 1994. Reviewed by Daniel A. Hussar.

Some health products that aren't even considered true drugs can also cause problems. Many Americans take food supplements, even though the FDA has never approved their use for any medical disorder. OTC supplements of niacin, a vitamin that can help lower cholesterol levels, have produced liver damage in some people for reasons that doctors have not yet determined.

A growing number of drugs that once were available only with a doctor's prescription can now be bought over the counter. These include Gyne-Lotrimin and Monistat, which combat vaginal yeast infections, and famotidine (sold as Pepcid AC) and cimetidine (sold as Tagamet), which offer an alternative to antacids for people suffering from heartburn and acid indigestion. For consumers, the advantages of this greater availability include lower prices and fewer visits to the doctor. The disadvantages, however, are the risks of misdiagnosing a problem, and misusing or overusing medications.

Like other drugs, OTC medications can be used improperly, often simply because of a lack of education about proper use. Among those most often misused are the following:

• *Nasal sprays.* Nasal sprays relieve congestion by shrinking blood vessels in the nose. If they are used too often or for too many days in a row, however, the blood vessels widen instead of contracting, and the surrounding tissues become swollen, causing more congestion. To make the vessels shrink again, many people use more spray more often. The result can be permanent damage to nasal membranes, bleeding, infection, and partial or complete loss of smell.

• *Laxatives.* Believing that they must have one bowel movement a day (a common misconception), many people rely on laxatives. Brands that contain phenolphthalein imitate the lining of the intestines and cause muscles to contract or tighten, often making constipation worse rather than better. Bulk laxatives are less dangerous, but regular use is not advised. A high-fiber diet and more exercise are safer and more effective remedies for constipation.

- *Eye drops.* Eye drops make the blood vessels of the eye contract. However, as in the case of nasal sprays, with overuse (several times a day for several weeks), the blood vessels expand, making the eye look redder than before.
- *Sleep aids.* Although over-the-counter sleeping pills are widely used, there has been little research on their use and possible risks.[3]

Prescription Drugs

Medications are a big business in this country. However, the latest, most expensive drugs aren't necessarily the best. Each year the Food and Drug Administration (FDA) approves about 20 new drugs, yet no more than four are rated as truly meaningful advances. The others often are no better or worse than what's already on the market.

Both doctors and patients make mistakes when it comes to prescription drugs. The most frequent mistakes doctors make are over- or underdosing, omitting information from prescriptions, ordering the wrong dosage form (a pill instead of a liquid, for example), and not recognizing a patient's allergy to a drug.

Many prescribed medications aren't taken the way they should be; millions simply aren't taken at all. The dangers of **noncompliance** (not taking prescription drugs properly) include recurrent infections, serious medical complications, and emergency hospital treatment. The drugs most likely to be taken incorrectly are those that treat problems with no obvious symptoms (such as high blood pressure), that require complex dosage schedules, that treat psychiatric disorders, or that have unpleasant side effects.

Some people skip or stop taking medications because they fear that any drug can cause tolerance and eventual dependence. Others fail to let doctors know about side effects. For instance, patients may stop taking anti-inflammatory drugs because they irritate their stomachs. However, taking the drugs with food can eliminate this problem. The side effects of some other drugs may disappear as the person's body becomes accustomed to the drug.

Physical Side Effects

Most medications, taken correctly, cause only minor complications. However, no drug is entirely without side effects for all individuals taking it. Serious complications that may occur include heart failure, heart attack, seizures, kidney and liver failure, severe blood disorders, birth defects, blindness, memory problems, and allergic reactions.

Allergic reactions to drugs are common. The drugs that most often provoke allergic responses are penicillin and other antibiotics (drugs used to treat infection). Aspirin, sulfa drugs, barbiturates, anticonvulsants, insulin, and local anesthetics can also provoke allergic responses. Allergic reactions range from mild rashes to hives to anaphylaxis—a life-threatening constriction of the airways and sudden drop of blood pressure that causes rapid pulse, weakness, paleness, confusion, nausea, vomiting, unconsciousness, and collapse. This extreme response, which is rare, requires immediate treatment with an injection of epinephrine (adrenaline) to open the airways and blood vessels.

Psychological Side Effects

Dozens of drugs—both over-the-counter and prescription—can cause changes in the way people think, feel, and behave. Unfortunately, neither patients nor their physicians usually connect such symptoms with medications. Doctors may not even mention potential mental and emotional problems because they don't want to scare patients away from what otherwise may be a very effective treatment. But what you don't know about a drug's effects on your mind can hurt you.

Among the medications most likely to cause psychiatric side effects are drugs for high blood pressure, heart disease, asthma, epilepsy, arthritis, Parkinson's disease, anxiety, insomnia, and depression. Some drugs—such as the powerful hormones called corticosteroids, used for asthma, autoimmune diseases, and cancer—can cause different psychiatric symptoms, depending on dosage and other factors. Other drugs, such as ulcer medications, can cause delirium and disorientation, especially when given in high doses or to elderly patients. More subtle problems, such as forgetfulness or irritability, are common reactions to many drugs—but also are more likely to be ignored or dismissed.

The older you are, the sicker you are, and the more medications you're taking, the greater your risk of developing some psychiatric side effects. "Even medications that don't usually cause problems, such as antibiotics, can cause psychiatric side effects in some individuals," says Jack Gorman, M.D., a professor of clinical psychiatry at Columbia University School of Medicine. "Whenever you sense a change in yourself, always ask, 'Could a drug be causing this?'"[4]

Any medication that slows down bodily systems—as many high blood pressure and cardiac drugs do—

can cause depressive symptoms. Estrogen in birth control pills can cause mood changes. As many as 15% of women using oral contraceptives have reported feeling depressed or moody. For many people, switching to another medication quickly lifts a drug-induced depression.

All drugs that stimulate or speed up the central nervous system can cause agitation and anxiety—including the almost 200 allergy, cold, and congestion remedies containing pseudoephedrine hydrochloride (Sudafed). Other common culprits in inducing anxiety are caffeine and theophylline, a chemical relative of caffeine found in many medications for asthma and other respiratory problems. These drugs act like mild amphetamines in the body, making people feel hyper and restless.

Strategies for Prevention

Preventing Problems

✔ Always ask about possible side effects of a drug. Find out if any other medicines might be just as effective with fewer side effects.

✔ Inform your physician of any other medicines that you take regularly, including birth control pills and over-the-counter preparations, such as sleeping pills.

✔ Report exactly how much alcohol and caffeine you consume every day. Find out how these substances might interact with the medications you're taking. Don't hesitate to ask a pharmacist about drug interactions.

✔ Check on timing. For example, drugs with sedative effects shouldn't be taken during the day, while those with stimulant effects shouldn't be taken at bedtime. If

you're taking several medicines, take out one day's supply of pills at a time, make up a schedule for taking them, and check off each dose of each drug as you take it.

✔ If you've had a psychiatric problem, such as depression, in the past, or if you've ever experienced psychiatric side effects from drugs, tell your doctor.

✔ If you suspect that a medication is affecting your mind or behavior, tell your doctor exactly how you feel. Find out if you can switch to a lower dose or an alternative medication. If your physician says that there are no other options, consult a psychiatrist.

✔ Don't suddenly stop taking any medication on your own. You may endanger your physical well-being and end up feeling much greater anxiety, depression, or confusion.

Drug Interactions

OTC and prescription drugs can interact in a variety of ways. For example, mixing some cold medications with tranquilizers can cause drowsiness and coordination problems, thus making driving dangerous. Moreover, what you eat or drink can impair or completely wipe out the effectiveness of drugs or lead to unexpected effects on the body. For instance, aspirin takes five to ten times as long to be absorbed when taken with food or shortly after a meal than when taken on an empty stomach. Or if tetracyclines encounter calcium in the stomach, they bind together and cancel each other out.

To avoid potentially dangerous interactions, check the label(s) for any instructions on how or when to take a medication, such as "with a meal." If the directions say

Doug's Drugs
10 Crossway Blvd. Monterey, CA 52437
PHONE 782-4510
DR. GOLDSTEIN
Rx 74428   08/22/95
JOHNSON, RICHARD ALAN
 TAKE ONE TABLET EVERY 6 HRS.
AS NEEDED FOR SEVERE HEADACHE
(GEN TYLENOL #3)
CODEINE PHOSPHATE/APAP
#30   (PY)   30/300 TABLETS
POTENCY EXPIRES 1/99   #51

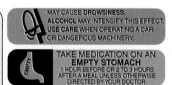
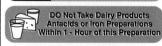
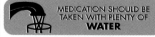
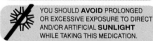
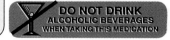

Drug interactions can alter the effectiveness of your medication. When you take a prescription medication, be sure to read warning labels about interactions, possible side effects, and whether the medication interacts with certain foods.

that you should take a drug on an empty stomach, do it at least one hour before eating or two or three hours after eating. Don't drink a hot beverage with a medication, because the temperature may interfere with the effectiveness of the drug. Don't open, crush, or dissolve tablets or capsules without checking first with your physician or pharmacist.

Whenever you take a drug, be especially careful of your intake of alcohol, which can change the rate of metabolism and the effects of many different drugs. Because it dilates the blood vessels, alcohol can add to the dizziness sometimes caused by drugs for high blood pressure, angina, or depression. Also, its irritating effects on the stomach can worsen stomach upset from aspirin, ibuprofen, and other anti-inflammatory drugs.

Generic Drugs

The **generic** name is the chemical name for a drug. A specific drug may appear on the pharmacist's shelf under a variety of brand names, which may cost more than twice the generic equivalent. About 75% of all prescriptions specify a brand name, but pharmacists may—and in some states must—switch to a generic drug unless the doctor specifically tells them not to. Prescriptions filled with generic drugs cost 20% to 85% less than their brand-name counterparts.

Generic drugs have the same active ingredients as brand-name prescriptions, but their fillers and binders, which can affect the absorption of a drug, may be different. For some serious illnesses, the generics may not be as effective; some experts recommend sticking with brand names for heart medications, psychiatric drugs, and anticonvulsant drugs (for epilepsy and other seizure disorders).

To determine whether you should buy the generic version of a drug, ask your physician whether it matters if you get a brand-name or generic drug. If it does, ask which brand name is best. Also, find out if switching to a generic or from one generic to another might harm your condition in any way.

Strategies for Prevention

Getting the Most Out of Medications

✔ Before you leave with a prescription, be sure to ask the following: What is the name of the drug? What's it supposed to do? How and when do I take it? For how long? What foods, drinks, other medications, or activities

should I avoid while taking this drug? Are there any side effects? What do I do if they occur? What written information is available on this drug? Are there other, possibly cheaper alternatives? Why do you recommend this particular drug? Are there nondrug alternatives, such as using a vaporizer, gargling with salt water, and drinking plenty of liquids for a viral infection; or losing weight and exercising to lower blood pressure?

✔ If you're taking a medication, tell your doctor if you plan to change your diet significantly—cutting calories or fat, stopping or starting vitamin supplements, or changing the amount of fiber you consume.

✔ Don't keep old medications around, and don't take drugs prescribed for someone else unless your doctor tells you to. Keep medications out of reach of small children.

✔ Ask your pharmacist how best to store your prescriptions. (A hot, damp bathroom medicine chest is often the worst place.) Have all prescriptions filled at the same pharmacy, and ask your pharmacist to keep a record of your medications to avoid hazardous interactions.

Caffeine Use and Misuse

Caffeine, which has been drunk, chewed, or swallowed since the stone age, is the most widely used **psychotropic** (mind-affecting) drug in the world. Eighty

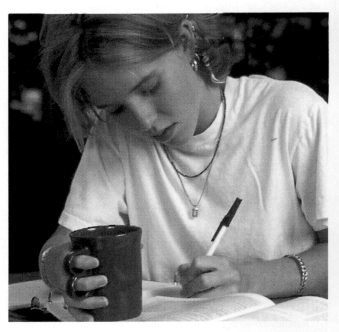

The coffee habit. Caffeine is one of the most widely used addictive substances.

percent of Americans drink coffee, our principal caffeine source—an average of 3.5 cups a day. Coffee contains 100 to 150 mg of caffeine per cup; tea, 40 to 100 mg; cola, about 45 mg. Most medications that contain caffeine are one-third to one-half the strength of a cup of coffee. However, some, such as Excedrin, are very high in caffeine (Table 14-2).

The effects of caffeine vary. Because it is a **stimulant**, it relieves drowsiness, helps in the performance of repetitive tasks, and improves capacity for work. Some athletes feel that caffeine gives them an extra boost that allows them to go farther and longer in endurance events. However, consumption of caffeine can also lead to dependence, anxiety, insomnia, faster breathing, upset stomach and bowels, and dizziness.[5]

Although there is no conclusive proof that caffeine causes birth defects, it does cross the placenta into the tissues of a growing fetus. Because of an increased risk of miscarriage, the U.S. surgeon general has recommended that pregnant women avoid or restrict their caffeine intake. Some fertility specialists also have urged couples trying to conceive to reduce caffeine to increase their chance of success.

It is possible to overdose on caffeine. The characteristic symptoms of caffeine intoxication are restlessness, nervousness, excitement, insomnia, flushed face, increased urination, digestive complaints, muscle twitching, rambling thoughts and speech, rapid heart rate or arrhythmias, periods of inexhaustibility, and physical restlessness. Some people develop these symptoms after as little as 250 mg of caffeine a day; others, only with much larger doses. Higher doses may produce ringing in the ears or flashes of light, grand mal seizures, and potentially fatal respiratory failure.

Caffeine withdrawal for those dependent on this substance can cause headaches. Those who must cut back should taper off gradually. One approach is to mix regular and decaffeinated coffee, gradually decreasing the quantity of the former.

Substance Use Disorders

People have been using mind-altering, or **psychoactive**, chemicals for centuries. Citizens of ancient Mesopotamia and Egypt used opium. More than 3000 years ago Hindus included cannabis products in religious ceremonies. For centuries the Inca Indians in South America have chewed the leaves of the coca bush. Yet while drugs existed in most societies, their use was usually limited to small groups. Today millions of Americans regularly turn to drugs to pick them up, bring them down, alter perceptions, or ease psychological pain.

The 1960s ushered in an explosive increase in drug use and in the number of drug users in our society. Marijuana use soared in the 1960s and 1970s; cocaine, in the 1980s. In 1986, crack—a cheap, smokeable form of cocaine—hit the streets and cities of America, and the number of regular cocaine users zoomed. In the years since, government officials, describing drugs as the number-one public health threat in our society, have declared war against them. Yet the abuse of both legal and illegal drugs continues to be an enormous problem. An estimated 5.5 million Americans are in need of treatment for drug abuse and dependence. Millions more are struggling to live drug-free lives.[6] (See Self-Survey: "Is it Drug Dependence or Abuse?")

Understanding Substance Use Disorders

In early Roman law, *addictus* referred to someone who, because he could not pay his debts, was sentenced into slavery. Indeed, one of the meanings of addiction given by the *Oxford Latin Dictionary* is "enslavement."[7] For much of the twentieth century, addiction to drugs was

TABLE 14-2 CAFFEINE COUNTS

Substance (typical serving)	Caffeine (milligrams)
No Doz (one pill)	200
Coffee (drip), one 5-ounce cup	130
Excedrin (two pills)	130
Espresso (2-ounce cup)	100
Instant coffee (5-ounce cup)	74
Coca-Cola (12 ounces)	46
Tea (5-ounce cup)	40
Dark chocolate (1 ounce)	20
Milk chocolate	6
Cocoa (5 ounces)	4
Decaffeinated coffee	3

viewed as a social or criminal problem, and the only people called addicts were "drug-crazed junkies" desperate for a fix. In the 1960s, however, when scientists switched to the *medical model* for understanding addictions, they began to view addictions to chemicals—such as alcohol and psychoactive drugs—as lifelong chronic diseases that affect a person's mind and body.

Today the word **addiction** has moved out of the realm of scientific terminology and into the mainstream of American life. Among laypeople, addiction refers to the habitual use of substances, such as alcohol, psychoactive drugs, and nicotine, and also to compulsive behaviors, such as overeating (discussed in Chapter 5). Like drugs, these activities can be used repeatedly to numb pain or enhance pleasure; some may alter a person's brain chemistry or create cravings; all can lead to a loss of internal control.

Today chemical addiction is viewed as a lifelong, chronic illness that affects mind, body, and spirit. Its key characteristics are repeated drug use, loss of control over how much or how often a person takes a drug, and continued use despite harmful consequences. Because addiction is considered too broad and judgmental a term for scientific use, mental health professionals describe drug-related problems in terms of dependence and abuse. However, they agree that there are four characteristic symptoms of addiction: compulsion to use the substance, loss of control, negative consequences, and denial.

Dependence

Individuals may develop **psychological dependence** and feel a strong craving for a drug because it produces pleasurable feelings or relieves stress or anxiety. **Physical dependence** occurs when a person develops *tolerance* to the effects of a drug and needs larger and larger doses to achieve intoxication or another desired effect. Individuals who are physically dependent and have a high tolerance to a drug may take amounts many times those that would produce intoxication or an overdose in someone who was not a regular user.

Men and women with a substance dependence disorder may use a drug to avoid or relieve withdrawal symptoms or consume larger amounts of a drug or use it over a longer period than they'd originally intended. They may try repeatedly to cut down or control drug use without success; spend a great deal of time obtaining or using drugs or recovering from their effects; give up or reduce important social, occupational, or recre-

ational activities because of their drug use; or continue to use a drug despite knowledge that the drug is likely to cause or worsen a persistent or recurring physical or psychological problem.

Specific symptoms of dependence vary with particular drugs. For instance, certain drugs, such as marijuana, hallucinogens, or phencyclidine, do not cause withdrawal symptoms. The degree of dependence also varies. In mild cases, a person may function normally most of the time. In severe cases, the person's entire life may revolve around obtaining, using, and recuperating from the effects of a drug.

Individuals with drug dependence become intoxicated or high on a regular basis—whether every day, every weekend, or several binges a year. They may try repeatedly to stop using a drug and yet fail—even though they realize that their drug use is interfering with their health, family life, relationships, and work.

Abuse

Some drug users do not develop the symptoms of tolerance and withdrawal that characterize dependence, yet they use drugs in ways that clearly have a harmful effect on them. These individuals are diagnosed as having a *psychoactive substance abuse disorder*. They continue to use drugs despite their awareness of persistent or repeated social, occupational, psychological, or physical problems related to drug use, or they use drugs in dangerous ways or situations (before driving, for instance). (See Pulsepoints: "Ten Ways to Tell If Someone Is Abusing Drugs.")

Intoxication and Withdrawal

Intoxication refers to maladaptive behavioral, psychological, and physiologic changes that occur as a result of substance use. **Withdrawal** is the development of symptoms that cause significant psychological and physical distress when an individual reduces or stops drug use. (Intoxication and withdrawal from specific drugs are discussed later in this chapter.)

Polyabuse

Most users prefer a certain type of drug but also use several others; this behavior is called **polyabuse**. The average user who enters treatment is on five different drugs. The more drugs anyone uses, the greater the chance of side effects, complications, and possibly life-threatening interactions (see Table 14-3).

Comorbidity

There is a great deal of overlap between mental disorders and substance abuse disorders. "A little more than

Pulsepoints

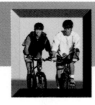

Ten Ways to Tell If Someone Is Abusing Drugs

1. An abrupt change in attitude. Individuals may lose interest in activities they once enjoyed or in being with friends they once valued.

2. Mood swings. Drug users may often seem withdrawn or "out of it," or they may display unusual temper flareups.

3. A decline in performance. Students may start skipping classes, stop studying, or not complete assignments; their grades may plummet.

4. Increased sensitivity. Individuals may react intensely to any criticism or become easily frustrated or angered.

5. Secrecy. Drug users may make furtive telephone calls or demand greater privacy concerning their personal possessions or their whereabouts.

6. Physical changes. Individuals using drugs may change their pattern of sleep, spending more time in bed or sleeping at odd hours. They also may change their eating habits and lose weight.

7. Money problems. Drug users may constantly borrow money, seem short of cash, or begin stealing.

8. Changes in appearance. As they

become more involved with drugs, users often lose regard for their personal appearance and look disheveled.

9. Defiance of restrictions. Individuals may ignore or deliberately refuse to comply with deadlines, curfews, or other regulations.

10. Changes in relationships. Drug users may quarrel more frequently with family members or old friends and develop new, strong allegiances with new acquaintances, including other drug users.

---

a third of those with a psychiatric disorder also have a chemical dependency problem, and a little more than a third of those with a chemical dependency problem have a psychiatric disorder," notes psychiatrist Richard Frances, M.D., the founding president of the American Association of Addiction Psychiatry.[8] Individuals with such "dual diagnoses" require careful evaluation and appropriate treatment for the complete range of complex and chronic difficulties that they face.

Strategies for Prevention

Saying No to Drugs

If people offer you a drug, here are some ways to say no:

✔ Let them know you're not interested. Change the subject. If the pressure seems threatening, just walk away.

TABLE 14-3   USE OF PSYCHOACTIVE DRUGS IN THE UNITED STATES

Drug	Number who used in the past month	Effects on dopamine
Heroin	200,000	Triggers release of dopamine; acts on other neurotransmitters
Amphetamines	800,000	Stimulate excess release of dopamine
Cocaine/Crack	1.5 million	Blocks dopamine absorption
Marijuana	10 million	Binds to areas of brain involved in mood and memory; triggers release of dopamine
Alcohol	11 million abusers	Triggers dopamine release; acts on other neurotransmitters
Nicotine	61 million	Triggers release of dopamine
Caffeine	130 million*	May trigger release of dopamine

*coffee drinkers

✔ Have something else to do: "No, I'm going for a walk now."

✔ Be prepared for different types of pressure. If your friends tease you, tease them back.

✔ Keep it simple. "No, thanks," "No," or "No way" all get the point across.

✔ Give them the cold shoulder: ignore them.

✔ Hang out with people who won't ask you questions you have to say no to.

What Causes Drug Dependence and Abuse?

No one fully understands why some people develop drug dependence or abuse disorders, while others, who may experiment briefly with drugs, do not. Inherited body chemistry, genetic factors, and sensitivity to drugs may make some individuals more susceptible. These disorders may stem from many complex causes.

The Biology of Addiction

A major breakthrough in understanding the roots of addiction has been the discovery that certain mood-altering substances and experiences—a puff of marijuana, a slug of whiskey, a snort of cocaine, a big win at black jack—trigger a rise in a brain chemical called dopamine associated with feelings of satisfaction and euphoria. This neurotransmitter, one of the crucial messengers that link neurons, or nerve cells, in the brain, rises during any pleasurable experience, whether it be a loving hug or a taste of chocolate.

Addictive drugs have such a powerful impact on dopamine and its receptors (its connecting cells) that they change the pathways within the brain's pleasure centers.[9] As Figure 14-2 indicates, in different ways, different substances create a craving for more of the same. According to this hypothesis—which remains incomplete and controversial—addicts do not specifically yearn for heroin, cocaine, or nicotine but for the rush of dopamine that these drugs produce.[10] Some individuals, born with low levels of dopamine, may be particularly susceptible to addiction.

Other Routes of Addiction

Although scientists do not believe there is an "addictive" personality, certain individuals are at greater risk of drug dependence because of psychological risk factors, including difficulty controlling impulses, a lack of values that might constrain drug use (whether based in reli-

NORMAL STATE

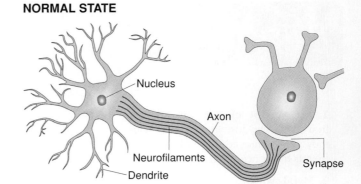

DRUG-ADDICTED STATE

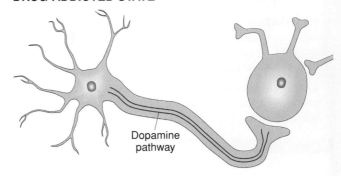

AFFECTED AREAS OF THE BRAIN

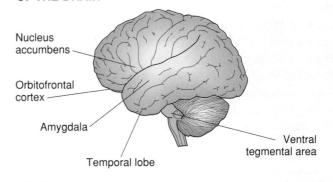

Figure 14-2

The normal vs. drug-addicted nervous system. Repeated drug doses overload normal neurotransmitter systems, and cells compensate by making dopamine less effective and becoming smaller. When doses stop, craving ensues.

SOURCE: *The Neuroscientist.*

gion, family, or society), low self-esteem, feelings of powerlessness, and depression. The one psychological trait most often linked with drug use is denial. Young people in particular are absolutely convinced that they will never lose control or suffer in any way as a result of drug use.

Many diagnosed drug users have at least one mental disorder, particularly depression or anxiety, and many people with psychiatric disorders abuse drugs. Individuals may self-administer drugs to treat psychiatric symptoms; for example, they may take sedating drugs to suppress a panic attack.

Individuals who are isolated from friends and family, or who live in communities, such as poor inner-city areas where drugs are widely used, have higher rates of drug abuse. Young people from lower socioeconomic backgrounds are more likely to use drugs than their more affluent peers, possibly because of economic disadvantage; family instability; a lack of realistic, rewarding alternatives and role models; and increased hopelessness.

Individuals whose companions are substance abusers are far more likely to use drugs. Peer pressure to use drugs can be a powerful factor for adolescents and young adults. Young people growing up in families in which parents or older sibling abuse drugs tend to develop drug problems themselves. The likelihood of drug abuse is also related to family instability, parental rejection, and divorce.

Drugs that produce an intense, brief high—like crack cocaine—lead to dependence more quickly than slower-acting agents, like cocaine powder. Drugs that cause uncomfortable withdrawal symptoms, such as barbiturates, may lead to continued use to avoid such discomfort.

Drug use involves certain behaviors, situations, and settings that users may, in time, associate with getting high. Even after long periods of abstinence, some former drug users find that they crave drugs when they return to a site of drug use or meet people with whom they used drugs. Former cocaine users report that the sight of white powder alone can serve as a cue that triggers a craving.

Most individuals who use drugs first try them as adolescents. Teens are likely to begin experimenting with tobacco, beer, wine, or hard liquor, then smoke marijuana or sniff inhalants. Some then go on to try sedative-hypnotics, stimulants (including cocaine), and hallucinogens such as LSD. A much smaller percentage of teens try the opioids. Over time some individuals give up certain drugs, such as hallucinogens, and return to old favorites, such as alcohol and marijuana. A smaller number continue using several drugs, a pattern called polysubstance abuse.

Mental health professionals have long debated whether experimentation with certain drugs, mainly marijuana, serves as a gateway to other substances of abuse. Recent research indicates that early use of illegal drugs, not cigarettes or alcohol, may predict drug and alcohol use at age 20, but neither appears to influence these habits by age 30.[11]

The Toll of Drugs

Drugs affect a person's physical, psychological, and social health; their effects can be *acute* (resulting from a single dose or series of doses) or *chronic* (resulting from long-term use). Acute effects vary with different drugs. Stimulants may trigger unpredictable rage; an overdose of heroin may lead to respiratory depression, a breathing impairment that can be fatal.

Over time, chronic drug users may feel fatigued, cough constantly, lose weight, become malnourished, and ache from head to toe. They may suffer blackouts, flashbacks, and episodes of increasingly bizarre behavior, often triggered by escalating paranoia. Their risk of overdose rises steadily, and they must live with constant stress: the fear of getting busted for possession or of losing a job if they test positive for drugs, the worry of getting enough money for their next fix, the dangers of associating with dealers and other users.

The toll of drug use can be especially great on teenagers. Teenage drug use disrupts many critical developmental tasks of adolescence and young adulthood. Use of drugs during the teen years can lead to drug-related crime (including stealing), poor achievement in high school or college, and job instability.

Strategies for Prevention

Spotting a Potential Drug Problem

In the early stages of drug use, before dependence develops, it is possible for individuals to recognize and change risky behavior. The following guidelines can help:

✔ Keep a diary for two weeks. You may want to use index cards or a small notebook that you can carry with you wherever you go. Write down everything you take into your body and everything you do. Don't edit or reread your diary for two weeks. Then underline or highlight the behaviors that appear again and again. Do they cause you any concern?

✔ Consider asking someone else to read your diary to spot any worrisome patterns. Also talk with family and friends about any differences they perceive in you. Ask if they feel you're spending less time with them. Have you disappointed them by breaking plans or promises? Have their feelings toward you changed?

✔ Consider your performance at school or work. Has the quality of your work declined? Have you missed deadlines or made errors in judgment? Has someone ever had to fill in or otherwise cover for you?

✔ If there is a potential problem, you might want to try

modifying your behavior for one month, to reduce or eliminate a substance or habit. During this time, record your feelings as well as what you take in and do. Note any symptoms or changes in energy, sleep, and so on.

✔ If you're able to modify your behavior over a full month, continue to reduce your substance use or behavior over time.

✔ If you can't make changes on your own or feel it's too hard to do so, get help. On campus, find out about counseling services, substance-abuse hotlines, and support groups. You could also contact one of the organizations dealing with specific addictive behaviors listed in "Your Health Directory" at the back of this book.

Drugs in America

Drug abuse has remained a major problem in the 1990s, even though by late 1997, drug use among teenagers seemed to be leveling off.[12] The estimated medical and social costs of drug abuse are believed to exceed $240 billion. Addiction to drugs, alcohol, or tobacco accounts for a third of all hospital admissions and a quarter of all deaths.[13]

According to the Survey Research Center at the University of Michigan at Ann Arbor, for the first time in more than five years, drug use among eighth graders stopped climbing in 1997: 29.4% said they had tried an illegal drug, compared with 31.2% in 1996. The eighth graders also expressed greater disapproval of drug users than in the past.

Older high school students, however, continue to smoke marijuana in increasing numbers. Nearly half of seniors reported smoking marijuana at least once. Nine in ten seniors, including many nonusers, said marijuana was easy to obtain. A much smaller percentage of high school seniors—8.7% in the 1997 survey—have experimented with cocaine; 2.1% said they had tried heroin.

As teenagers, in varying numbers, continue to experiment with drugs, experts debate the best approaches to prevention. The most popular antidrug program is DARE (for Drug Abuse Resistance Education), which is used by nearly 75% of the nation's schools. Critics charge that DARE, which focuses on knowledge and attitudes toward drugs, does not address the psychological and behavioral aspects of drug abuse. Increasingly, experts are urging more emphasis on "life skills training," a program that, in its initial evaluations, has significantly reduced alcohol and marijuana use among teens.[14]

Drugs in Society

There is no typical drug user. High school students, professional athletes, business executives, inner-city teenagers, rock musicians, doctors, truckers, teachers, and many others of different ages and ethnic groups use drugs regularly. However, we all pay a price for living in a drug-using society, including the costs of medical care, treatment, and imprisonment for addicts and drug traffickers. Other hidden costs include accidents caused by drug-using drivers and workers, drug-related violence and crime, and care for babies born to drug-dependent mothers.

In the last 20 years, the United States has spent nearly $70 billion fighting drugs. But victory is nowhere in sight. Criminal organizations in Latin America and Asia have increased production and become more sophisticated in distributing cocaine and heroin. Illicit drugs have become more available in more countries and at lower prices than ever before.

Critics of the nation's drug policy argue that the war is being fought on the wrong front. Currently, about two-thirds of federal spending for drug control goes toward law enforcement and only one-third toward prevention and treatment. Many contend that more should be spent on antidrug education for children, on treatment for addicts, and on researching drugs that could help in overcoming drug dependence.

There is evidence that prevention can and does work. According to the National Clearinghouse for Alcohol and Drug Information, each month prevention efforts keep approximately 3.5 million youngsters from drinking alcohol and 24 million young adults from using illicit drugs.[15] Experts have identified a set of principles that they see as essential for the success of prevention efforts, including the following realizations:

- Drug problems are too complex to be changed significantly through individual decision making alone. Programs must be developed to help young people build skills to resist pressures to take drugs.

- Shared responsibility is more appropriate than blaming the victim of drug abuse. Families, peers, and the community have to work together, because everyone benefits when an individual avoids drug abuse.

- Education is necessary but insufficient to produce needed change in societal attitudes and values related to drugs. Millions of Americans have banded together to support antidrunk-driving and nonsmoking laws; a similar approach could be effective in getting across the message that drug use will no longer be tolerated.

Strategies for Prevention

Preventing Temptation

You can take steps to protect yourself from the temptation to use drugs. Among them are the following:

✔ *Learn how to cope with stress.* Try some of the coping techniques, such as exercise, guided imagery, or meditation, described in Chapter 2.

✔ *Strengthen your self-esteem.* Take pride in your achievements, particularly when setbacks bruise your confidence.

✔ *Develop a range of interests.* Get into the habit of finding pleasure in swimming, dancing, playing an instrument, doing volunteer work, or taking long walks.

✔ *Practice assertiveness.* Cultivate the art of speaking up and voicing your opinion—regardless of the subject or circumstances.

Student Drug Use

On college campuses, alcohol (discussed in Chapter 15) is the number-one drug of abuse, while marijuana remains the most commonly used illegal drug. As indicated in the Campus Focus: "College Students and Illegal Drug Use," about half of college students have tried marijuana, although the percentage of current users is much lower: 11.6% of women and 17.1% of men. About 14% of college students have tried cocaine.

Various factors influence which students use drugs:

• *Gender.* Men are more likely to use drugs than are women, but the differences are not large. For instance, in one national survey, 30% of college men and 28% of college women reported using an illicit drug in the last year, while 28% of the men and 25% of the women said they had smoked marijuana. However, women who both drink alcohol and smoke marijuana may be more susceptible to addiction.[16]

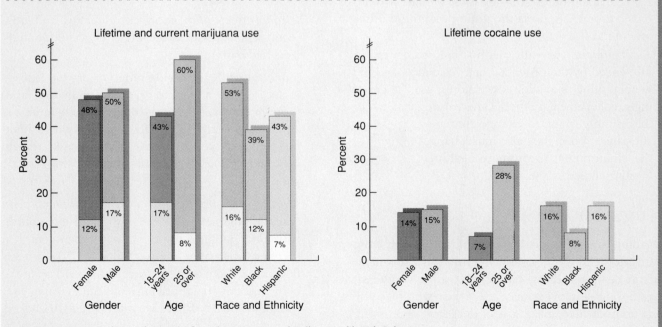

CAMPUS FOCUS:
COLLEGE STUDENTS AND ILLEGAL DRUG USE

SOURCE: Douglas, Kathy, et al. "Results from the 1995 National College Health Risk Behavior Survey." *Journal of American College Health*, Vol. 46, September 1997.

- *Race/ethnicity.* In general, white students have higher levels of alcohol and drug use than do African-American students. In a comparison of African-American students at predominantly white and predominantly black colleges, those at historically black colleges had lower rates of alcohol and drug use than did either white or African-American students at white schools. The reason, according to the researchers, may be that these colleges provide a greater sense of self-esteem, which helps prevent alcohol and drug use.

- *Perception of risk.* Students seem most likely to try substances they perceive as being "safe," or low-risk. Of these, the top three are caffeine, alcohol, and tobacco; marijuana is listed fourth in terms of perceived safety. Other agents—barbiturates, heroin, cocaine, PCP, speed, LSD, crack, and inhalants—are viewed as about equally risky and are used much less often. Why do today's students believe that using certain types of drugs is not harmful? Researchers have identified three possible explanations: In general, less public attention is being paid to the drug problem and to educating youngsters about drugs. Second, young people have less chance to learn about the dangers of drugs because fewer fellow students and celebrities have been abusers in recent year. Thus, they have not seen, either personally or in the media, the ravages drug use can cause. Third, an increased glorification of marijuana and other drugs by rock, grunge, and rap music groups supports the notion that these drugs are safe to use.[17]

- *Environment.* As with alcohol use, students are influenced by their friends, their residence, and the general public's attitude toward drug use.[18] Increasingly, college health officials are realizing that, rather than simply trying to change students' substance abuse, they also must change the environment to promote healthier lifestyle choices.

Drugs on the Job

According to the National Household Survey on Drug Abuse, workers of every variety—from truck drivers to stockbrokers—use drugs on the job. At the very least, drug-abusing employees may affect their workplace by being unproductive, making poor decisions, and having strained relationships with coworkers. Even more frightening, however, is the threat to themselves and others from accidents due to their drug use.

Along with alcohol and nicotine, cocaine and marijuana are the primary drugs of abuse on or off the job. As a result of widespread drug use, the military and a growing number of companies are requiring drug tests of job applicants and employees. However, drug testing is not 100% precise. For example, individuals who have recently eaten poppy seeds (as in a muffin or bagel) can test positive for opiates. Increasingly, employers are shifting from policing employees to setting up programs to help those with drug problems overcome their drug dependence.

Drug use is also common among the unemployed. According to a survey by the National Institute for Drug Abuse, of all adults between the ages of 18 and 34 who don't have jobs, 21.5% used illicit drugs in the prior month. Among those with full-time jobs, only 9.7% used drugs. In particular, unemployed young adults are much more likely to use cocaine and marijuana than those who are working full-time.[19]

Drugs and Driving

One important impact of drugs is their effect on driving ability (see Chapter 15). Alcohol and drug use are equally common in drivers injured in traffic accidents. Often drivers using alcohol also test positive for other drugs. Different drugs affect driving ability in different ways. Here are the facts from the National Institute on Drug Abuse:

- *Alcohol* affects perception, coordination, and judgment, and increases the sedative effects of tranquilizers and barbiturates.

- *Marijuana* affects a wide range of driving skills—including the ability to track (stay in the lane) through curves, brake quickly, and maintain speed and a safe distance between cars—and slows thinking and reflexes. Normal driving skills remain impaired for four to six hours after smoking a single joint.

- *Sedatives, hypnotics, and antianxiety agents* slow reaction time, and interfere with hand–eye coordination and judgment; the greatest impairment is in the first hour after taking the drug. The effects depend on the particular drug: some build up in the body and can impair driving skills the morning after use; others make drivers very sleepy and, therefore, incapable of driving safely.

- *Amphetamines*, after repeated use, impair coordination. They can also make a driver more edgy and less coordinated, and thus more likely to be involved in an accident.

- *Hallucinogens* distort judgment and reality, and cause confusion and panic, thus making driving extremely dangerous.

Common Drugs of Abuse

The psychoactive substances most often associated with both abuse and dependence include alcohol (discussed in Chapter 15); amphetamines; cocaine; cannabis (marijuana); hallucinogens; inhalants; opioids; phencyclidine (PCP); and sedative-hypnotic or anxiolytic (antianxiety) drugs. (See Table 14-4.)

Amphetamines

Amphetamines, stimulants that were once widely prescribed for weight control because they suppress appetite, have emerged as a global danger. In 1997, the United Nations reported a worldwide surge in amphetamine abuse and described this trend as "more dangerous than heroin and cocaine."[20] They trigger the release of epinephrine (adrenalin), which stimulates the central nervous system. Amphetamines are sold under a variety of names: amphetamine (brand name Benzedrine, street-name "bennies"), dextroamphetamine (Dexedrine, or "dex"), methamphetamine (Methedrine, or "meth" or "speed"), and Desoxyn ("copilots"). Related *uppers* include the prescription drugs methylphenidate (Ritalin), pemoline (Cylert), and phenmetrazine (Preludin).

Amphetamines are available in tablet or capsule form. Abusers may grind and sniff the capsules, or make a solution and inject the drug. "Ice" is a smokable form of methamphetamine that is highly addictive and produces an intense physical and psychological high that can last from four to fourteen hours. *Crank* is the street term for another central nervous system stimulant, propylexedrine, which is less potent than amphetamine. Abusers often extract the drug from the cotton plug of decongestant inhalants and inject it intravenously.

How Users Feel

Amphetamines produce a state of hyper-alertness and energy. Users feel confident in their ability to think clearly and to perform any task exceptionally well—although amphetamines do not, in fact, significantly boost performance or thinking. Higher doses make them feel "wired": talkative, excited, restless, irritable, anxious, moody.

If taken intravenously, amphetamines produce a characteristic "rush" of elation and confidence, as well as adverse effects, including confusion, rambling or incoherent speech, anxiety, headache, and palpitations. Individuals may become paranoid; be convinced they are having "profound" thoughts; feel increased sexual interest; and experience unusual perceptions, such as ringing in the ears, a sensation of insects crawling on their skin, or hearing their name called. Crank users may feel high and sleepy or may hallucinate and lose contact with reality.

Risks

Dependence on amphetamines can develop with episodic or daily use. Users typically take amphetamines in large doses to prevent crashing. "Bingeing"—taking high doses over a period of several days—can lead to an extremely intense and unpleasant crash—characterized by a craving for the drug, shakiness, irritablity, anxiety, and depression—that requires two or more days for recuperation.

Amphetamine intoxication may cause the following symptoms:

- Feelings of grandiosity, anxiety, tension, hypervigilance, anger, social hypersensitivity, fighting, jitteriness or agitation, paranoia, and impaired judgment in social or occupational functioning.
- Increased heart rate, dilated pupils, elevated blood pressure, perspiration or chills, and nausea or vomiting.
- Less frequent effects such as speeding up or slowing down of physical movement; muscular weakness, impaired breathing, chest pain, heart arrhythmia; confusion, seizures, impaired movements or muscle tone, or even coma.
- In high doses, a rapid or irregular heartbeat, tremors, loss of coordination, and collapse.

Smokeable methamphetamine, or "ice", also increases heart rate and blood pressure; high doses can cause permanent damage to blood vessels in the brain. Other physical effects of methamphetamine include dilated pupils, blurred vision, dry mouth, and increased breathing rate. Prolonged use can cause fatal lung and kidney disorders. Injecting propylexedrine can lead to convulsions, strokes, and respiratory and kidney failure. Abusers also may develop infected veins, and if they share needles, they risk infection with human immunodeficiency virus (HIV), which causes AIDS.

The long-term effects of amphetamine abuse include malnutrition; skin disorders; ulcers; insomnia;

TABLE 14-4   THE EFFECTS OF DRUGS

Drugs	What They Do	Health Effects	Major Risks
Amphetamines	Speed up physical and mental processes; create sense of heightened energy and confidence.	Loss of appetite, blurred vision, headache, dizziness, sweating, sleeplessness, trembling, anxiety, nausea or vomiting, suspiciousness, delusions, hallucinations, confusion, palpitations, jitteriness or agitation, unusual perceptions (such as a ringing in the ears or a sensation of insects crawling on the skin); increased heart rate; elevated blood pressure; muscular weakness; impaired breathing, movements, or muscle tone.	Dependence, chest pain, heart arrhythmias (disruption of heart rhythm); seizures; malnutrition; skin disorders; ulcers; lack of sleep; depression; paranoia; vitamin deficiencies; brain damage; sexual dysfunction; stroke; high fever; heart failure; violent behavior; coma; fatal overdose.
Cannabis (marijuana and hashish)	Relax the mind and body; alter mood; heighten perceptions.	Faster heartbeat and pulse, dry mouth and throat, impaired perception and reactions, lethargy, nausea, possible hallucinations, panic attacks, decreased motivation.	Psychological dependence; impaired thinking, perception, memory, and coordination; increased heart rate and blood pressure; impaired fertility; dampened immunity; bronchitis, emphysema, lung cancer.
Cocaine and crack	Speed up physical and mental processes; create sense of heightened energy and confidence.	Headaches, exhaustion, shaking, sweating, chills, blurred vision, nausea or vomiting, seizures, loss of appetite, impaired judgment, hyperactivity, babbling, speeding up or slowing down of physical activity, impaired breathing, chest pain, impaired movements or muscle tone.	Dependence; extreme suspiciousness; violence; damage to nose (if snorted), blood vessels, and heart; blood pressure irregularities; loss of sexual desire; impotence; seizures; chest pain; arrhythmias; heart attack; disruptions in heart rhythm; intracranial hemorrhage; damage to liver and lungs (if smoked); hepatitis, HIV infection, skin infections, inflammation of the arteries, and infection of the lining of the heart (if injected).
Hallucinogens (LSD, mescaline)	Alter perceptions and produce hallucinations, which may be frightening or pleasurable.	Increased heart rate, blood pressure, and body temperature; headache, nausea, sweating, trembling, heart palpitations, blurring of vision, tremors, poor coordination; "bad trips" and irrational acts on LSD.	With LSD, disturbing flashbacks, psychological dependence, delusional disorder.
Inhalants	Produce hallucinations and temporary feelings of well-being and giddiness.	Dizziness, involuntary eye movements, poor coordination, slurred speech, unsteady gait, lethargy, depressed reflexes, slowed-down movements, tremors, general muscle weakness, blurred vision, nausea, sneezing, coughing, nosebleeds, lack of	Hepatitis, liver failure, kidney failure, respiratory impairment, blood abnormalities, irregular heart beat, heart failure, destruction of bone marrow and skeletal muscles, stupor,

TABLE 14-4 CONTINUED

Drugs	What They Do	Health Effects	Major Risks
		coordination, loss of appetite, decreased heart and breathing rates, loss of consciousness, aggressiveness, impulsiveness, impaired judgment, increased risk of accidents or injuries.	or coma.
Opioids (opium, morphine, heroin, or synthetic narcotics)	Relax the central nervous system; relieve pain; produce temporary sense of well-being.	Restlessness, nausea, vomiting, slowed breathing, weight loss, lethargy, loss of sex drive, mood swings, slurred speech, sweating, impaired judgment, drowsiness, slurred speech, impaired attention or memory.	Dependence, malnutrition, lower immunity, infections of the heart lining and valves, skin abscesses, congested lungs, hepatitis, tetanus, liver disease; if injected, infections of the heart lining and valves, skin abscesses, hepatitis, tetanus, liver disease, and HIV transmission; depression of central nervous system; coma; fatal overdose.
Phencyclidine (PCP)	Produce changes in perceptions, including hallucinations, and distorted feelings, including delusions of great strength and invulnerability.	Increased heart rate and blood pressure, flushing, sweating, dizziness, painful sensitivity to sound, numbness, diminished sensitivity to pain, impaired coordination and speech, stupor.	Psychosis; increased danger of injury or harm to others because of impulsivity, aggressiveness, and violence; coma, convulsions, heart and lung failure, ruptured blood vessels in the brain, suicide, death.
Sedative-hypnotics and anxiolytic (antianxiety) drugs (including benzodiazepines and barbiturates)	Slow down the central nervous system; reduce or relieve tension; induce relaxation, drowsiness, or sleep; decrease alertness.	Drowsiness, impaired judgment, poor coordination, slowed breathing, weak and rapid heart beat, disrupted sleep, dangerously impaired vision, unsteady gait, sleepiness, confusion, irritability.	Dependence, stupor, coma, fatal overdose, or reaction to sudden withdrawal.

depression; vitamin deficiencies; and, in some cases, brain damage that results in speech and thought disturbances. Sexual dysfunction and impaired concentration or memory also may occur.

Withdrawal

When the immediate effects of amphephtamines wear off, users experience a "crash"—they crave the drug and become shaky, irritable, anxious, and depressed. Amphetamine withdrawal usually persists for more than 24 hours after cessation of prolonged, heavy use. Its characteristic features include fatigue, disturbing dreams, much more or less than usual sleep, increased appetite, and speeding up or slowing down of physical move-

ments. Those who are unable to sleep despite their exhaustion often take sedative-hypnotics (discussed later in this chaper) to help them rest and may become dependent on them as well as amphetamines. Symptoms usually reach a peak in two to four days, although depression and irritability may persist for months. Suicide is a major risk.[21]

Cannabis Products

Marijuana ("pot") and **hashish** —the most widely used illegal drugs—are derived from the *cannabis* plant. The major psychoactive ingredient in both is *THC (delta-9-tetrahydrocannabinol)*. Nearly one of every three Amer-

TABLE 14-5 ANNUAL PREVALENCE OF USE FOR VARIOUS TYPES OF DRUGS, 1995

Type of drug	Full-Time college students	Others
Any illicit drug	33.5%	34.0%
Marijuana	31.2	28.7
Inhalants	3.9	3.1
Hallucinogens	8.2	7.9
LSD	6.9	6.8
Cocaine	3.6	4.5
Crack	1.1	1.5
MDMA ("Ecstasy")	2.4	1.9
Heroin	0.3	0.7
Other Opiates	3.8	4.0
Stimulants	5.4	7.5
"Ice"	1.1	2.2
Barbiturates	2.0	4.0
Tranquilizers	2.9	4.4
Alcohol	83.2	80.8
Cigarettes	39.3	47.7

SOURCE: National Survey Results on Drug Abuse from the Monitoring the Future Study, National Institute on Drug Abuse, 1995.

and experienced smokers learn to hold the smoke for longer periods to increase the amount of drug diffused into the bloodstream. The circumstances in which marijuana is smoked, the communal aspects of its use, and the user's experience all can affect the way a pot-induced high feels.

How Users Feel

In low to moderate doses, marijuana typically creates a mild sense of euphoria, a sense of slowed time (five minutes may feel like an hour), a dreamy sort of self-absorption, and some impairment in thinking and communicating. Users report heightened sensations of color, sound, and other stimuli, relaxation, and increased confidence. The sense of being "stoned" peaks within half an hour and usually lasts about three hours. Even when alterations in perception seem slight, as noted earlier, it is not safe to drive a car for as long as four to six hours after smoking a single joint. Some users—particularly those smoking marijuana for the first time or taking a high dose in an unpleasant or unfamiliar setting—experience acute anxiety, which may be accompanied by a panicky fear of losing control. They may believe that their companions are ridiculing or threatening them and experience a panic attack, a state of intense terror.

The immediate physical effects of marijuana include increased pulse rate, bloodshot eyes, dry mouth and throat, slowed reaction times, impaired motor skills, increased appetite, and diminished short-term memory (see Figure 14-3). High doses reduce the ability to perceive and to react; all the reactions experienced with low doses are intensified, leading to sensory distortion and—in the case of hashish—vivid hallucinations and LSD-like psychedelic reactions. The drug remains in the body's fat cells 50 hours or more after use, so people may experience psychoactive effects for several days after use. Drug tests may produce positive results for days or weeks after last use.

Risks

Dependence or abuse usually develops with repeated use over a long period of time. Typically, individuals smoke more often rather than smoking a larger amount. With chronic heavy use, users may feel a lessening or loss of the pleasurable effect and may develop lethargy, a loss of pleasure in activities, and persistent attention and memory problems. Chronic marijuana use seems to impair thinking, reading comprehension, verbal and mathematical skills, coordination, and short-term memory. Teenagers who smoke pot regularly often lose

icans over age 12 has tried marijuana at least once. Some 12 million Americans use it; more than 1 million cannot control this use. Marijuana has been used therapeutically, primarily to ease the nausea of chemotherapy, and some researchers urge further study of its potential benefits.[22] However, "compassionate" use has been limited by law because some believe it undercuts government opposition to drug use.[23]

Different types of marijuana have different percentages of THC. Because of careful cultivation, the strength of today's marijuana is much greater than that of the pot used in the 1970s; the physical and mental effects are therefore greater. Usually, marijuana is smoked in a cigarette ("joint") or pipe; it may also be eaten as an ingredient in other foods (as when baked in brownies), though with a less predictable effect. The drug high is enhanced by holding the marijuana smoke in the lungs,

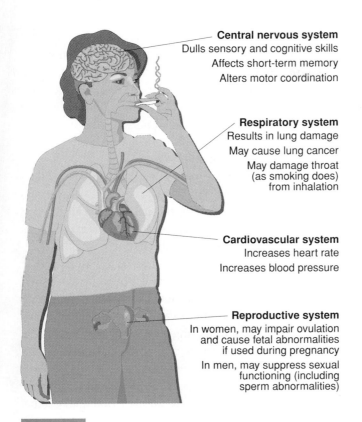

Central nervous system
Dulls sensory and cognitive skills
Affects short-term memory
Alters motor coordination

Respiratory system
Results in lung damage
May cause lung cancer
May damage throat
(as smoking does)
from inhalation

Cardiovascular system
Increases heart rate
Increases blood pressure

Reproductive system
In women, may impair ovulation
and cause fetal abnormalities
if used during pregnancy
In men, may suppress sexual
functioning (including
sperm abnormalities)

Figure 14-3
Some effects of long-term marijuana use on the body.

interest in school and do not remember what they learned when they were high. Some long-term regular users of marijuana may experience *burnout,* a dulling of their senses and responses termed *amotivational syndrome.*

A Harvard Medical School study that compared the cognitive functioning of college students who were heavy marijuana users (who'd smoked the drug 29 out of the previous 30 days), light users (who'd smoked marijuana once in the previous 30 days), and nonusers found significant impairments of thinking and specific cognitive abilities, such as sustained attention, in heavy users. These effects persisted even after a day of supervised abstinence from marijuana.[24] Over time, continued heavy marijuana use might interfere with students' ability to learn and perform well in school and in challenging careers.[25]

Chronic use can also lead to bronchitis, emphysema, and lung cancer. Smoking a single "joint," or marijuana cigarette, can be as damaging to the lungs as smoking five tobacco cigarettes. Marijuana may suppress ovulation and alter hormone levels in female users and may impair the fertility of male users. Frequent use of

marijuana during pregnancy can lower birth weight and cause abnormalities in the fetus similar to those of fetal alcohol syndrome.

Cocaine

Cocaine ("coke," "snow," "lady") is a white crystalline powder extracted from the leaves of the South American coca plant. Usually mixed with various sugars and local anesthetics like lidocaine and procaine, cocaine powder is generally inhaled. When sniffed or snorted, cocaine anesthetizes the nerve endings in the nose and relaxes the lung's bronchial muscles. Frequent snorting can irritate and damage the mucous membrane in the nose, cause sinusitis, destroy a user's sense of smell, and occasionally create a hole in the septum (the membrane between the nostrils).

Cocaine can be dissolved in water and injected intravenously. The drug is rapidly metabolized by the liver, so the high is relatively brief, typically lasting only about 20 minutes. This means that users will commonly inject the drug repeatedly, increasing the risk of infection and damage to their veins. Many intravenous cocaine users prefer the practice of *speedballing,* the intravenous administration of a combination of cocaine and heroin.

Cocaine alkaloid—or *freebase*—is obtained by removing the hydrocholoride salt from cocaine powder. "Freebasing" is smoking the fumes of the alkaloid form of cocaine. *Crack,* pharmacologically identical to freebase, is a cheap, easy-to-use, widely available, smokeable and potent form of cocaine named for the popping sound it makes when burned. Because it is absorbed rapidly into the bloodstream and large doses reach the brain very quickly, it is particularly dangerous. However, its low price and easy availability have made it a common drug of abuse in poor urban areas.[26]

How Users Feel

A powerful stimulant to the central nervous system, cocaine produces feelings of soaring well-being and boundless energy. Users feel that they have enormous physical and mental ability, yet are also restless and anxious. After a brief period of euphoria, users slump into a depression. They often go on cocaine binges, lasting from a few hours to several days, and consume large quantities of cocaine.

With crack, dependence develops quickly. As soon as crack users come down from one high, they want more crack. Whereas heroin addicts may shoot up several times a day, crack addicts need another hit within minutes. Thus, a crack habit can quickly become more expensive than heroin addiction. Some "crackheads" have $1000-a-day habits. Police in big cities have traced many brutal crimes and murders to young crack addicts, who often are extremely paranoid and dangerous. Smoking crack doused with liquid PCP, a practice known as *space-basing* has especially frightening effects on behavior.

With continuing use, cocaine users experience less pleasure and more unpleasant effects. Eventually they may reach a point at which they no longer experience euphoric effects and crave the drug simply to alleviate their persistent hunger for it. They think about it constantly, dream about it, spend all their money on it, and borrow, steal, or deal to pay for it. They cannot concentrate on work; they become increasingly irritable and confused. They may also become dependent on alcohol, sedatives, or opioids, which they use to calm down from cocaine's aftereffects.

Risks

Cocaine dependence is an easy habit to acquire. With repeated use, the brain becomes tolerant of the drug's stimulant effects, and users must take more of it to get high. Its grip is strong. Those who smoke or inject cocaine can develop dependence within weeks. Those who sniff cocaine may not become dependent on the drug for months or years. It is thought that 5% to 20% of all coke users—a group as large as the estimated total number of heroin addicts—are dependent on the drug.

The physical effects of acute cocaine intoxication include dilated pupils, elevated or lowered blood pressure, perspiration or chills, nausea or vomiting, speeding up or slowing down of physical activity, muscular weakness, impaired breathing, chest pain, and impaired movements or muscle tone.

Although some users initially try cocaine as a sexual stimulant, it does not enhance sexual performance. At low doses, it may delay ejaculation and orgasm and cause heightened sensory awareness, but men who use cocaine regularly have problems maintaining erections and ejaculating. They also tend to have low sperm counts, less active sperm, and more abnormal sperm than nonusers. Both male and female chronic cocaine users tend to lose interest in sex and have difficulty in reaching orgasm.

Cocaine use can cause blood vessels in the brain to clamp shut and can trigger a stroke, bleeding in the brain, and potentially fatal brain seizures. Cocaine users can also develop psychiatric or neurological complica-

tions (Figure 14-4). Repeated or high doses of cocaine can lead to impaired judgment, hyperactivity, nonstop babbling, feelings of suspicion and paranoia, and violent behavior. The brain never learns to tolerate cocaine's negative effects; users may become incoherent and paranoid and may experience unusual sensations, such as ringing in their ears, feeling insects crawling on the skin, or hearing their name called.

Cocaine can damage the liver and cause lung damage in freebasers. Smoking crack causes bronchitis as well as lung damage and may promote the transmission of HIV through burned and bleeding lips. Some smokers have died of respiratory complications, such as pulmonary edema (the buildup of fluid in the lungs).

Cocaine causes the heart rate to speed up and blood pressure to rise suddenly. Its use is associated with many cardiac complications, including arrhythmia (disruption of heart rhythm), angina (chest pain), and acute myocardial infarction (heart attack). These cardiac complications can lead to sudden death.

Cocaine users who inject the drug and share needles put themselves at risk for another potentially lethal problem: HIV infection. Other complications of injecting

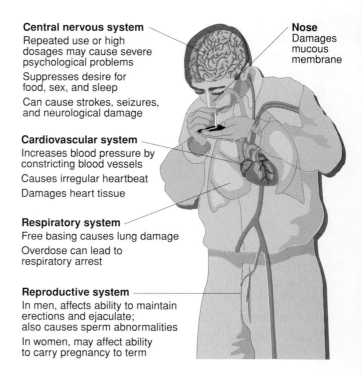

Central nervous system
Repeated use or high dosages may cause severe psychological problems
Suppresses desire for food, sex, and sleep
Can cause strokes, seizures, and neurological damage

Nose
Damages mucous membrane

Cardiovascular system
Increases blood pressure by constricting blood vessels
Causes irregular heartbeat
Damages heart tissue

Respiratory system
Free basing causes lung damage
Overdose can lead to respiratory arrest

Reproductive system
In men, affects ability to maintain erections and ejaculate; also causes sperm abnormalities
In women, may affect ability to carry pregnancy to term

Figure 14-4

Some effects of cocaine on the body.

cocaine include skin infections, hepatitis, inflammation of the arteries, and infection of the lining of the heart.

The most common ways of dying from cocaine use are persistent seizures that result in respiratory collapse, cardiac arrest from arrhythmias, myocardial infarction, and intracranial hemorrhage or stroke. The combination of alcohol and cocaine is particularly lethal. Alcohol and cocaine together are second only to the combination of heroin and alcohol in causing deaths related to substance abuse.

Cocaine is dangerous for pregnant women and their babies, causing miscarriages, developmental disorders, and life-threatening complications during birth. Women who use the drug while pregnant are more likely to miscarry in the first three months of pregnancy than women who do not use drugs or who use heroin and other opioids. When used early in pregnancy, cocaine can reduce the fetal oxygen supply, possibly interfering with the development of the fetus's nervous system. Infants born to cocaine and crack users can suffer withdrawal and may have major complications, or permanent disabilities. Cocaine babies have higher-than-normal rates of respiratory and kidney troubles, visual problems, and developmental retardation and may be at greater risk of sudden infant death syndrome.

Withdrawal

The symptoms of cocaine withdrawal include fatigue, vivid and disturbing dreams, excessive or too little sleep, irritability, increased appetite, and physical slowing down or speeding up. This initial crash may last one to three days after cutting down or stopping the heavy use of cocaine. Depression is common. Some individuals become violent, paranoid, and suicidal.

Symptoms usually reach a peak in two to four days, although depression, anxiety, irritability, lack of pleasure in usual activities, and low-level cravings may continue for weeks. As memories of the crash fade, the desire for cocaine intensifies. For many weeks after stopping, individuals may feel an intense craving for the drug. Experimental medical approaches for treating cocaine dependence include antidepressant drugs, anticonvulsant drugs, and the naturally occurring amino acids tryptophan and tryrosine. However, these have only limited benefit, and much more research into medical treatments is needed.[27]

Hallucinogens

The drugs known as **hallucinogens** produce vivid and unusual changes in thought, feeling, and perception.

The most widely used in the United States is *LSD (lysergic acid diethylamide*, or "acid"), which was initially developed as a tool to explore mental illness. It became popular in the 1960s and resurfaced among teenagers in the 1990s. LSD is taken orally, either blotted onto pieces of paper which are held in the mouth or chewed along with another substance, such as a sugar cube. Much less commonly used in this country is *peyote* (whose active ingredient is *mescaline*).

How Users Feel

LSD produces hallucinations, including bright colors and altered perceptions of reality. Effects from a single dose begin within 30 to 60 minutes and last 10 to 12 hours. During this time, there are slight increases in body temperature, heart rate, and blood pressure; sweating, chills and goose pimples appear. Some users develop headache and nausea. Mescaline produces vivid hallucinations—including brightly colored lights, animals, and geometric designs—within 30 to 90 minutes of consumption. These effects may persist for 12 hours.

The effects of hallucinogens depend greatly on the dose, the individual's expectations and personality, and the setting for drug use. Many users report religious or mystical imagery and thoughts; some feel they are experiencing profound insights. Usually the user realizes that perceptual changes are caused by the hallucinogen, but some become convinced that they have lost their minds. Drugs sold as hallucinogens are frequently mixed with other drugs, such as PCP and amphetamines, which can produce unexpected and frightening effects.

Hallucinogens do not produce dependence in the same way as cocaine or heroin. Individuals who have an unpleasant experience after trying a hallucinogen may stop using the drugs completely without suffering withdrawal symptoms. Others continue regular or occasional use because they enjoy the effects.

Risks

Physical symptoms include dilated pupils, rapid heart rate, sweating, heart palpitations, blurring of vision, tremors, and poor coordination. These effects may last eight to twelve hours. Hallucinogen intoxication also produces changes in emotions and mood, such as anxiety, depression, fear of losing one's mind, and impaired judgment.

LSD can trigger irrational acts. LSD users have injured or killed themselves by jumping out of windows, swimming out to sea, or throwing themselves in front of cars. Some individuals develop a delusional disorder, in which they become convinced that their distorted perceptions and thoughts are real. They may experience flashbacks (reexperiencing of symptoms felt while intoxicated), which include geometric hallucinations, flashes of color, halos around objects, and other perceptual changes.

Individuals having a "bad trip" may blame themselves and feel excessively guilty, tense, and so agitated that they cannot stop talking and they have trouble sleeping. They may fear that they have destroyed their brains and will never return to normal. Someone who already is depressed may take a hallucinogen to lift his or her spirits, only to become more depressed. Suicide is a real danger.

Inhalants

Inhalants or **deleriants** are chemicals that produce vapors with psychoactive effects. The most commonly abused inhalants are solvents, aerosols, model-airplane glue, cleaning fluids, and petroleum products like kerosene and butane. Some anesthetics and nitrous oxide (laughing gas) are also abused. Almost 20% of eighth graders surveyed have used household products, such as glue, solents, and aerosols, to get high.[28]

In order to inhale intoxicating vapors, individuals soak a rag in the substance, place it against the mouth and nose, and inhale; or inhale fumes from a substance placed in a paper or plastic bag; or inhale vapors directly from their containers. Young people, especially those who may not have money for or access to other drugs, are those most likely to try inhalants. Children between the ages of 9 to 13 tend to use inhalants with a group of peers who are likely to use alcohol and marijuana as well. Users are in all racial, socioeconomic, and gender groups, but the incidence of use is higher among poor minority youth than among others. Many users come from families that have separated or been affected by alcohol or drug problems; they often have school difficulties, such as truancy and poor grades, or problems adjusting to work.[29]

How Users Feel

Inhalants reach the lungs, bloodstream, and other parts of the body very rapidly. At low doses, users may feel slightly stimulated; at higher doses, they may feel less inhibited. Intoxication often occurs within five minutes and can last more than an hour. Inhalant users do not report the intense rush associated with other drugs, nor do they experience the perceptual changes associated with LSD. However, inhalants interfere with thinking and impulse control, so users may act in dangerous or destructive ways.

Often there are visible external signs of use: a rash around the nose and mouth, breath odors, residue on face, hands and clothing, redness, swelling, and tearing of the eyes, and irritation of throat, lungs and nose that leads to coughing and gagging. Nausea and headache also may occur.

Risks

Regular use of inhalants leads to tolerance, so that the sniffer needs more and more to attain the desired effects. Younger children who use inhalants several times a week may develop dependence. Older users who become dependent may use the drugs many times a day. Those who become dependent on inhalants are likely to have used many different substances as adolescents, and to have gradually turned to inhalants as their preferred substance.

Although some young people believe inhalants are safe to use, this is far from true. Inhalation of butane from cigarette lighters displaces oxygen in the lungs, causing suffocation. Users also can suffocate while covering their heads with a plastic bag to inhale the substance, or from inhaling vomit into their lungs while high. According to the International Institute on Inhalant Abuse, the effects of inhalants are unpredictable, and even a single episode could trigger asphyxiation or cardiac arrhythmia, leading to disability or death. Abusers also can develop difficulties with memory, with abstract reasoning, problems with coordination, and with uncontrollable movements of the extremities.

Opioids

The **opioids** include *opium* and its derivatives (i.e., *morphine, codeine,* and *heroin*) and nonopioid synthetic drugs that have similar sleep-inducing and pain-relieving properties. The opioids come from a resin taken from the seed pod of the Asian poppy. **Nonopioids**, such as *meperidine* (Demerol), *methadone*, and *propoxyphene* (Darvon), are chemically synthesized. These drugs are powerful narcotics, or painkillers.

Heroin, the most widely abused opioid, is illegal in this country. In other nations it is used as a potent painkiller for conditions such as terminal cancer. There are an estimated 400,000 to 600,000 heroin addicts in the United States, with men outnumbering women addicts

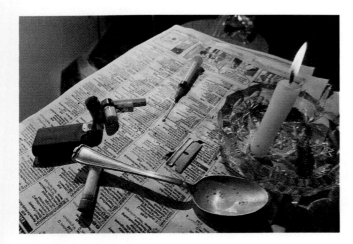

Opioid drugs, made from the Asian poppy, come in both legal and illegal forms. In any form, these substances can readily become addictive.

by three to one. Purer forms of heroin, available in many cities, can be snorted; this has led to a surge in the drug's popularity, especially among middle- and upper-class users.

Morphine, used as a painkiller and anesthetic, acts primarily on the central nervous system, eyes, and digestive tract and masks pain by producing mental clouding, drowsiness, and euphoria. It does not decrease the physical sensation of pain as much as it alters a person's awareness of the pain; in effect, he or she no longer cares about it.

Two semisynthetic derivatives of morphine are *hydromorphone* (trade name Dilaudid, or "little D"), with two to eight times the painkilling effect of morphine, and *oxycodone* (Percocet, Percodan, or "perkies"), similar to codeine but more potent. The synthetic narcotic *meperidine* (Demerol, or "demies") is now probably second only to morphine for use in relieving pain. It is also used by addicts as a substitute for morphine or heroin.

Codeine is a weaker painkiller and sedative than morphine. It is an ingredient in liquid products prescribed for relieving coughs, and in tablet and injectable form for relieving pain. The synthetic narcotic *propoxyphene* (Darvon) is a somewhat less potent painkiller than codeine; in fact, it is no more effective than aspirin in usual doses. It has been one of the most widely prescribed drugs for headaches, dental pain, and menstrual cramps. At higher doses, Darvon produces a euphoric high, which may lead to misuse.

Prescription opioids are taken orally in pill form but can also be injected intravenously. Heroin users typically inject the drug into their veins. However, individuals who experiment with whatever recreational drug is new and trendy often prefer *skin-popping* (subcutaneous injection) rather than *mainlining* (intravenous injection); they also may snort heroin as a powder, or dissolve it and inhale the vapors. To try to avoid addiction, some users begin by *chipping*, taking small or intermittent doses. Regardless of the method of administration, tolerance can develop rapidly.

Some individuals first take a medically prescribed opioid for pain relief or cough suppression, then gradually increase the dose and frequency of use on their own, often justifying this because of their symptoms rather than for the sensations the drug induces. They expend increasing efforts to obtain the drug, frequently seeking out several doctors to write prescriptions.

How Users Feel

All the opioids relax the user. When injected, they can produce an immediate "rush," or high, that lasts 10 to 30 minutes. For two to six hours thereafter, users may feel indifferent, lethargic, and drowsy; they may slur their speech and have problems paying attention, remembering and going about their normal routine. The primary attractions of heroin ("horse," "junk," "smack," or "downtown") are the euphoria and pain relief it produces. However, some people experience very unpleasant feelings, such as anxiety and fear. Other effects include a sensation of warmth or heaviness, dry mouth, facial flushing, and nausea and vomiting (particularly in first-time users).

Some addicts report a rush when heroin is injected directly into their veins. Since the effects of heroin do not last long—usually only two to four hours—addicts have to "shoot up" two to five times a day. With large doses, the pupils become smaller; and the skin becomes cold, moist, and bluish. Breathing slows down; the user cannot be awakened and may stop breathing completely.

Risks

Addiction is common. Almost all regular users of opioids rapidly develop drug dependence, which can lead to lethargy, weight loss, loss of sex drive, and the continual effort to avoid withdrawal symptoms through repeated drug administration. In addition, they experience anxiety; insomnia; restlessness; and craving for the drug. Users continue taking opioids as much to avoid the discomfort of withdrawal—a classic sign of addiction—as to experience pleasure.

Opioid intoxication is characterized by changes in mood and behavior, such as initial euphoria followed by apathy or discontent and impaired judgment. Physical symptoms include constricted pupils (although pupils may dilate from a severe overdose), drowsiness, slurred speech, and impaired attention or memory. Morphine affects blood pressure, heart rate, and blood circulation in the brain. Both morphine and heroin slow down—depress—the respiratory system; overdoses can cause fatal respiratory arrest.

Opioid poisoning or overdose causes shock, coma, and depressed respiration and can be fatal. Emergency medical treatment is critical, often with drugs called narcotic antagonists that rapidly reverse the effects of opioids when administered intravenously.

Over time, users who inject opioids may develop infections of the heart lining and valves, skin abscesses, and lung congestion. Infections from unsterile solutions, syringes, and shared needles can lead to hepatitis, tetanus, liver disease, and HIV transmission. The annual death rate among those dependent on opioids is 20 times higher than among other young people, primarily because of physical complications, overdose, suicide, and the violent lifestyle of many users.

Withdrawal

If a regular user stops taking an opioid, withdrawal begins within 6 to 12 hours. The intensity of the symptoms depends on the degree of the addiction; they may grow stronger for 24 to 72 hours and gradually subside over a period of 7 to 14 days, though some symptoms, such as insomnia, may persist for several months. Individuals may develop craving for an opioid, irritability, nausea or vomiting, muscle aches, runny nose or eyes, dilated pupils, sweating, diarrhea, yawning, fever, and insomnia. Desperately craving the drug, users may plead, demand, or manipulate others to obtain more. Opioid withdrawal usually is not life-threatening.

Methadone Maintenance

Opioid dependence is a very difficult addiction to overcome. Studies demonstrate that only 10% to 30% of heroin users are able to maintain abstinence. This fact contributed to the development of a unique, yet still controversial, treatment for opioid dependence: the use of methadone, a long-acting opioid that users can substitute for heroin or other opioids.

Methadone is used in two basic ways to treat opioid dependence: as an opioid substitute for detoxification, usually with a gradual tapering of methadone over a period of 21 to 180 days, and as a maintenance treatment. Methadone maintenance has been criticized by some as nothing more than the substitution of a legal opioid, methadone, for an illegal opioid, heroin. Critics charge that since methadone maintenance does not have abstinence as its goal, it contributes to continued use of other drugs, such as cocaine or alcohol. There also is concern, especially by those in law enforcement, that methadone recipients will engage in "diversion," the sale of take-home doses of methadone for profit. Despite these charges, methadone maintenance remains the mainstay of opioid dependence treatment and is the most successful treatment currently available.

Methadone maintenance may be the most thoroughly studied drug treatment. Research has clearly documented several important positive benefits, including decreased use of illicit opioids; decreased criminal behavior; decreased risk of contracting HIV infection (through sharing of infected needles); and improvements in physical health, employment, and other lifestyle factors. Individuals who have been on methadone maintenance for a long time (often years), have stable relationships and employment, have assimilated themselves into the nondrug culture, and are highly motivated to get off methadone have the best chance for successful detoxification from methadone.

A number of new drug therapies are emerging as useful agents in the treatment of opioid dependence. Naltrexone (Trexan) has been approved as medication for alcohol-dependence and opioid-dependence treatment. More recently, researchers have reported promising results with Temgesic (buprenorphine), a mild, nonaddicting opiate that, like heroin and methadone, bonds

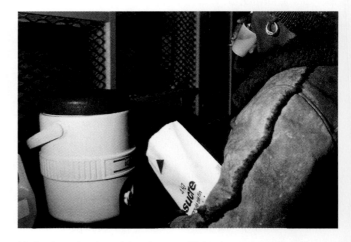

Methadone treatment has been criticized as a treatment for opioid addiction, but research clearly demonstrates positive benefits. Those who participate in long-term methadone maintenance programs usually move out of the drug culture and are candidates for eventually leaving methadone dependence behind them.

to certain receptors in the brain, blocking pain messages and persuading the brain that its cravings for heroin have been satisfied. As long as they take buprenorphine, even long-term junkies report they simply do not want heroin any more.[30]

Phencyclidine (PCP)

PCP (phencyclidine—brand name Sernyl; streetnames "angel dust," "peace pill," "lovely," and "green")—is an illicit drug manufactured as a tablet, capsule, liquid, flake, spray, or crystal-like white powder that can be swallowed, smoked, sniffed, or injected. Sometimes it is sprinkled on crack, marijuana, tobacco, or parsley, and smoked. A fine-powdered form of PCP can be snorted or injected. Once PCP was thought to have medicinal value as an anesthetic, but its side effects, including delirium and hallucinations, made it unacceptable for medical use.

PCP use peaked in the 1970s, but it remains a popular drug of abuse in both inner-city ghettos and suburban high schools. Often users think that it is the PCP that they take together with another illegal psychoactive substance, such as amphetamines, coke, or hallucinogens, that is responsible for the highs they feel, so they seek it out specifically.

How Users Feel

The effects of PCP are utterly unpredictable. It may trigger violent behavior or irreversible psychosis the first time it is used, or the twentieth time, or never. In low doses, PCP produces changes—from hallucinations to euphoria to feelings of emptiness or numbness—similar to those produced by other psychoactive drugs. Higher doses may produce a stupor that lasts several days, increased heart rate and blood pressure, flushing, sweating, dizziness, and numbness.

Risks

Some first-time users feel PCP is too unpredictable and do not try it again. Others quickly become heavy users. Many go on PCP binges or runs that can last several days. Some people use it daily, often along with alcohol and marijuana. It takes only a short period of occasional use for dependence or abuse to develop.

The behavioral changes associated with PCP intoxication, which can develop within minutes, include belligerence, aggressiveness, impulsiveness, unpredictability, agitation, poor judgment, and impaired functioning at work or in social situations. The physical symptoms of PCP intoxication include involuntary eye movements, increased blood pressure or heart rate, numbness or diminished responsiveness to pain, impaired coordination and speech, muscle rigidity, seizures, and a painful sensitivity to sound. Some people experience repetitive motor movements, such as facial grimacing, hallucinations, and paranoia. Suicide is a definite risk. Intoxication typically lasts four to six hours, but some effects can linger for several days. Delirium may occur within 24 hours of taking PCP or after recovery from an overdose and can last as much as a week.

PCP can trigger an episode of depression or anxiety that may persist for months. Some users reproach themselves constantly in the fear that they have destroyed their brains and will never return to normal. Some feel so restless that they cannot stop talking; some think they have superhuman strength. Large amounts can lead to convulsions, coma, heart and lung failure, ruptured blood vessels in the brain, and death.

Sedative-Hypnotics or Anxiolytic (Antianxiety) Drugs

These drugs depress the central nervous system, reduce activity, and induce relaxation, drowsiness, or sleep. They include the benzodiazepines and the barbiturates.

The **benzodiazepines**—the most widely used drugs in this category—are commonly prescribed for tension, muscular strain, sleep problems, anxiety, panic attacks, anesthesia, and in the treatment of alcohol withdrawal. They include such drugs as *chlordiazepoxide* (Librium), *diazepam* (Valium), *oxazepam* (Serax), *lorazepam* (Ativan), *flurazepam* (Dalmane), and *alprazolam* (Xanax). They differ widely in their mechanism of action, absorption rate, and metabolism, but all produce similar intoxication and withdrawal symptoms.

Benzodiazepine sleeping pills have largely replaced the **barbiturates**, which were used medically in the past for inducing relaxation and sleep, relieving tension, and treating epileptic seizures. These drugs are usually taken by mouth in tablet, capsule, or liquid form. When used as a general anesthetic, they are administered intravenously. Barbiturates such as *pentobarbital* (brand name Nembutal, or "yellow jackets"), *secobarbital* (Seconal, or "reds"), and *thiopental* (Pentothal) are short-acting and rapidly absorbed into the brain. The longer-acting barbiturates, such as *amobarbital* (brand name Amytal, or "blues" or "downers") and *phenobarbital* (Luminal, or "phennies"), which usually are taken orally and absorbed slowly into the

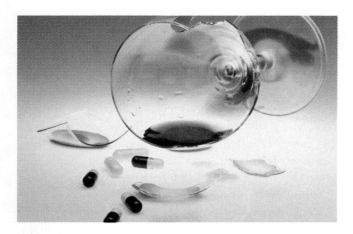

Antianxiety drugs react dangerously with alcohol.

bloodstream, take a while to reach the brain and have an effect for several days.

How Users Feel

The lower doses of these drugs may reduce or relieve tension, but increasing doses can cause a loosening of sexual or aggressive inhibitions. Individuals using this class of drugs may experience rapid mood changes, impaired judgment, and impaired social or occupational functioning. High doses produce slurred speech, drowsiness, and stupor.

Young people in their teens or early twenties who have used many illegal substances typically take sedative-hypnotic or anxiolytic drugs to obtain a high or a state of euphoria. Some use them in combination with other drugs. Less commonly, individuals may first obtain sedatives, hypnotics, or antianxiety medications by prescription from a physician for insomnia or anxiety and then gradually increase the dose or frequency of use on their own, often by seeking prescriptions from several physicians. While they justify this continued use because of their symptoms, the fact is that they reach a state in which they cannot function normally without the drug.

Risks

All the sedative-hypnotic and anxiolytic drugs can produce physical and psychological dependence within two to four weeks. A complication specific to sedatives is *cross-tolerance*—or cross-addiction—which occurs when users develop tolerance for one sedative or become dependent on it and develop tolerance for other sedatives as well. Individuals with a prior history of substance abuse are at greatly increased risk of abusing this class of drugs if they are prescribed by a physician. However, those who have not abused drugs or alcohol in the past rarely develop a substance-abuse problem

from these medications when they are prescribed for legitimate psychiatric disorders, such as panic disorder or generalized anxiety disorder.

Intoxication with these drugs can produce changes in mood or behavior, such as inappropriate sexual or aggressive acts, mood swings, and impaired judgment. Physical signs include slurred speech, poor coordination, unsteady gait, involuntary eye movements, impaired attention or memory, and stupor or coma.

Taken in combination with alcohol, these drugs have a synergistic effect that can be dangerous or even lethal. For example, an individual's driving ability, already impaired by alcohol, will be made even worse, increasing the risk of an accident. Alcohol in combination with sedative-hypnotics leads to respiratory depression and may result in respiratory arrest and death. Regular users of any of these drugs who become physically dependent should not try to cut down or quit on their own. If they try to quit suddenly, they run the risk of seizures, coma, and death.

Sedative-hypnotic and anxiolytic drugs can easily cross through the placenta, and cause birth defects and behavioral problems. Babies born to women who used these drugs during pregnancy may be physically dependent on the drugs and may develop breathing problems, feeding difficulties, disturbed sleep, sweating, irritability, and fever.

Withdrawal

Withdrawal from sedative-hypnotic and anxiolytic drugs may range from relatively mild discomfort to a severe syndrome with grand mal seizures, depending on the degree of dependence. Withdrawal symptoms include malaise or weakness, sweating, rapid pulse, coarse tremor of the hands, tongue, and eyelids, insomnia, nausea or vomiting, temporary hallucinations or illusions, physical restlessness, anxiety or irritability, and grand mal seizures. Withdrawal may begin within two to three days after stopping drug use, and symptoms may persist for many weeks.

Other Drugs of Abuse

Anabolic Steroids

Anabolic steroids, synthetic derivatives of the male hormone testosterone, are powerful compounds prescribed for the treatment of burns and injuries. An estimated 1 million Americans, half of them adolescents (many of whom started steroid use before age 16), use black-market steroids. Nonmedical distribution of steroids is a federal offense punishable by five years in prison. (See Chapter 5 for a discussion of steroid use as a means of building muscle strength and size.)

The potential side effects of anabolic steroids include an increased risk of heart disease, stroke, or obstructed blood vessels; liver tumors and jaundice; acne; transmission, through shared needles, of HIV; breast enlargement, atrophy of the testicles, and impotence in men; and deepened voice, breast reduction, and beard growth in women. Even a brief period of use in childhood or adolescence can have lasting effects on brain and body chemistry. Steroids may increase the risk of heart disease by lowering levels of high-density lipoproteins (HDL), the "good" blood fat believed to remove deposits from artery walls.[31] Steroids can also create the same problems with dependence and withdrawal as cocaine.

Adolescents who use anabolic steroids are more likely to engage in multiple drug use. In a survey of 12,267 students in grades 9 through 12, Harvard researchers found that adolescent steroid use was linked to the use of injected drugs, male gender, alcohol use, and strength training.[32] Higher levels of steroid use were reported in southern states.

Typical steroid users are male, middle-class, and white, who either want to boost their strength or look more muscular. They often take steroids in cycles of 4 to 18 weeks, followed by a break. Most "stack" the drugs, taking several pills or injectable drugs at once. Initially, they feel "juiced" or "pumped up," but they can also become irritable and aggressive. Some explode in unexpected violent outbursts, called "roid rages," or develop signs of mental illness, such as paranoia and delusions.

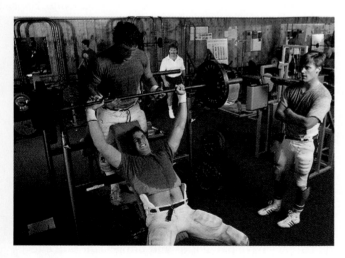

Pumping up. Steroids are an attractive—and highly dangerous— route to a muscular body. They are also illegal, and the side effects range from signs of mental illness to serious heart and liver damage.

A new alternative to steroids, the brain messenger chemical called *GHB (gammahydroxybutyrate)*, stimulates the release of human growth hormone but has no known effects on muscle growth. Although this substance is banned by the FDA, users obtain it illegally either for its high, which is similar to that caused by alcohol or marijuana, or for its alleged ability to trim fat and build muscles. However, GHB can act in unpredictable ways in the body, and the Centers for Disease Control (CDC) has reported at least 80 GHB-related hospitalizations, mostly for drug-induced comas or seizures.

New Drugs of Abuse

Designer Drugs

Designer drugs ("Adam," "Eve," "China White") are produced in chemical laboratories and sold illegally. Easy to manufacture from available raw materials, the drugs themselves were once technically legal because the law had to specify the exact chemical structure of an illicit drug. However, a law now bans all chemical "cousins" of illegal drugs.

Some of the drugs that emerged as dangers in the 1990s are legal and have legitimate medical uses (see Table 14-6). They include gamma hydroxybutyrate, or GHB or Liquid X (discussed above), a depressant with potential benefits for people with narcolepsy, and Rohypnol, a tranquilizer used overseas. Both are better known as date-rape or "easy-lay" drugs that are slipped into women's drinks to knock them out and cause short-term amnesia (see Chapter 17). Since the drugs are odorless and tasteless, a woman has no way of knowing whether her drink has been tampered with; the subsequent loss of memory leaves her with no explanation for where she's been or what's happened in the hours before she regains consciousness.[33]

Another new drug of abuse is "K," or ketamine, an anesthetic used by veterinarians. When cooked, dried, and ground into a powder for snorting, K blocks chemical messengers in the brain that carry sensory input. As a result, the brain fills the void with hallucinations. Too much K can cause such massive sensory deprivation that researchers compare the impact to a near-death experience. Ketamine is illegal in several states, but the federal government has not yet deemed it a controlled substance—a step that would substantially increase penalties for its use.[34]

Another synthetic, developed by college students in Pennsylvania in the early 1990s, is *methcathinone*, or "cat," a powerful synthetic stimulant that can produce a

TABLE 14-6   NEW DRUGS OF ABUSE

Drug	Street name	Medical use	Effect	Cost
Ketamine hydrochloride	K, Special K, Vitamin K	An anesthetic used in animals and frail humans	Hallucinations, sensory distortions	$40–$100 per gram of powder or 10-ml bottle of liquid
Gamma-hydroxybutyrate	Liquid X, Grievous bodily harm, G	A depressant that could possibly be used to treat narcolepsy	Relaxation and temporary euphoria	$5–$20 per dose
Flunitrazepam	Roofies, Roach	A strong sedative used overseas	Alcohol-like intoxication, drowsiness	$3–$5 per pill

high that lasts up to six days. Cat usually contains a mix of chemicals along with small doses of Drano or battery acid, which act as a catalyst.[35]

College and street chemists have also produced synthetic opiates that are particularly dangerous because they're far more potent than those derived from natural substances. Derivatives of *fentanyl*, an anesthetic widely used for surgery in the United States, are 20 to 2000 times as powerful as heroin, and the risk of a fatal overdose or brain damage is much greater.

MDMA (methylene dioxymethylamphetamine, commonly called "ecstasy") is somewhat related to mescaline and amphetamine. Psychiatrists once experimented with MDMA in patients because it alters a user's social and personal perceptions. However, the FDA has classified it, along with heroin and LSD, as a drug with "high potential for abuse and no medical usefulness." An estimated 500,000 to 4 million people—mostly college-age Americans—use the drug, which creates feelings of

warmth and openness. The use of ecstasy has increased greatly on campus, with almost one of every four students at some universities reporting its use.[36]

Users can develop insomnia, loss of appetite, muscle aches or stiffness, nausea, fatigue, and problems concentrating. MDMA destroys brain cells in animals; in humans it may damage the nerve cells that produce serotonin, a neurotransmitter involved in regulating responses to stress and pain, appetite, and sexual behavior. According to a 1995 report from Johns Hopkins University, the damage produced by ecstasy may do lasting harm by causing key nerve cells in the brain to grow back abnormally.[37]

In Great Britain, MDMA has killed at least 15 young persons and caused serious medical complications in many others. Almost all the victims took recreational doses at a club or party where crowds danced in all-night dance sessions called *raves*. Usually the stricken users collapse or develop seizures while dancing. Their body temperatures soar to as high as 110°F, while their pulses race and their blood pressures plummet. Some die, generally because of the effects of *hyperthermia* (elevated body temperature), within 2 to 60 hours. Prolonged vigorous dancing, particularly in hot, poorly ventilated rooms in which dancers can become dehydrated, may compound the dangers of this drug.

"Herbal" drugs also are being marketed as substitutes for standard street drugs. With names such as "herbal ecstasy," "nexus," and "ritual spirit," these tablets and capsules are advertised as safe and potent agents that can lead to "sacred visions," "tingly happy-happy buzz," and better sex. However, critics warn that the herbal pills have dangerous and unpleasant side effects, including stroke, heart attack, and a disfiguring skin condition. They are sold at head shops, night clubs, and raves. The FDA has been investigating these agents,

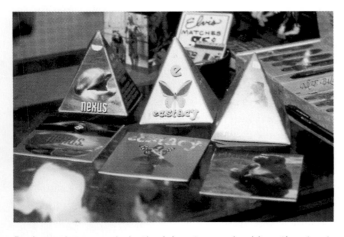

Designer drugs, made in the laboratory and sold on the street, aren't subject to quality controls and don't always contain what the buyer expects.

after receiving hundreds of complaints of strokes, seizures, and possibly even some deaths.

Treating Drug Dependence and Abuse

The most difficult step for a drug user is to admit that he or she *is* in fact an addict. If they are not forced to deal with their problem through some unexpected trauma, such as being fired or going bankrupt, those who care— family, friends, coworkers, doctors—may have to confront them and insist that they do something about their addiction. Often this intervention can be the turning point for addicts and their families.

Treatment may take place in an outpatient setting, a residential facility, or a hospital. Increasingly, treatment thereafter is tailored to address coexisting or dual diagnoses. A personal treatment plan may consist of individual psychotherapy, marital and family therapy, medication, and behavior therapy. Once an individual has made the decision to seek help for substance abuse, the first step usually is detoxification, which involves clearing the drug from the body. An exception is methadone maintenance, discussed earlier in this chapter, which does not rely on complete detoxification.

Controlled and supervised withdrawal within a medical or psychiatric hospital may be recommended if an individual has not been able to stop using drugs as an outpatient or in a residential treatment program. Detoxification is most likely to be complicated when a person is a polysubstance abuser and may require close monitoring and treatment of potentially fatal withdrawal symptoms. Other reasons for inpatient treatment include lack of psychosocial support for maintaining abstinence; the absence of a drug-free living environment; or a complicated drug history with addiction to multiple substances. However, restrictions on insurance coverage may limit the number of days of inpatient care. Increasingly, once individuals complete detoxification, they continue treatment in residential programs or as outpatients.

Medications are used in detoxification to alleviate withdrawal symptoms and prevent medical and psychiatric complications. Once withdrawal is complete, adjunctive medications are discontinued, so the individual is in a drug-free state. However, those with mental disorders may require appropriate psychiatric medication to manage their symptoms and reduce the risk of relapse. For example, a person suffering from major depression or panic disorder may require ongoing treatment with antidepressant medication.

The aim of chemical dependence treatment is to help individuals establish and maintain their recovery from alcohol and drugs of abuse. Recovery is a dynamic process of personal growth and healing that takes place as one makes the transition from a lifestyle of active substance use to drug-free recovery.

Whatever their setting, chemical dependence treatment programs initially involve some period of intensive treatment followed by one or two years of continuing aftercare. Most freestanding programs—those not affiliated with a hospital—follow what is known as the *Minnesota Model*, a treatment approach developed at Hazelden Recovery Center in Center City, Minnesota, more than 30 years ago. Its key principles include a focus on drug use as the primary problem, not as a symptom of underlying emotional problems; a multidisciplinary approach that addresses the physical, emotional, spiritual, family, and social aspects of the individual; a supportive community; and a goal of abstinence and health.

Outpatient programs for substance abuse, offered by freestanding centers, hospitals, and community mental health centers, often run four or five nights a week for four weeks to eight weeks, or in daily eight-hour sessions for seven to eight days, followed by weekly group therapy. These outpatient programs allow recovering drug users to go on with their daily lives and learn to deal with day-to-day work and family stresses. Mental health professionals in private practice also offer individually structured outpatient treatment.

Therapy groups provide an opportunity for individuals who have often been isolated by their drug use to participate in normal social settings. Small groups with other drug users can be especially valuable because they all share the experience of drug use; the members can confront one another with frankness and cut through lies and rationalizations. A professional therapist keeps members of the group from ganging up on one person.

Twelve-Step Programs

Since its founding in 1935, Alcoholics Anonymous (AA)—the oldest, largest, and most successful self-help program in the world—has spawned a movement (see Chapter 15). As many as 200 different recovery programs are based on the spiritual **twelve-step program** of AA Participation in twelve-step programs for drug abusers, such as Substance Anonymous, Narcotics Anonymous, and Cocaine Anonymous, is of fundamental importance in promoting and maintaining long-term abstinence.[38]

The basic precept of twelve-step programs is that members have been powerless when it comes to controlling their addictive behavior on their own. These programs don't recruit members. The desire to stop must come from the individual, who can call the number of a twelve-step program, listed in the telephone book, and find out when and where the next nearby meeting will be held. A representative may offer to send someone to the caller's house to talk about the problem and to escort him or her to the next meeting.

Meetings of various twelve-step programs are held daily in almost every city in the country. (Some chapters, whose members often include the disabled or those in remote areas, "meet" via electronic bulletin boards on their personal computers.) There are no dues or fees for membership. Many individuals belong to several programs because they have several problems, such as alcoholism, substance abuse, and pathological gambling. All have only one requirement for membership: a desire to stop an addictive behavior.

Strategies for Change

Getting the Most Out of a Twelve-Step Program

✔ Try out different groups until you find one you like and in which you feel comfortable.

✔ Once you find a group in which you feel comfortable, go back several times (some recommend a minimum of six meetings) before making a final decision on whether to continue.

✔ Keep an open mind. Listen to other people's stories and

ask yourself if you've had similar feelings or experiences.

✔ Accept whatever feels right to you, and ignore the rest. One common saying in twelve-step programs is, "Take what you like and leave the rest."

Relapse Prevention

The most common clinical course for substance abuse disorders involves a pattern of multiple relapses over the course of a lifespan. It is important for individuals with these problems and their families to recognize this fact. When relapses do occur, they should be viewed as neither a mark of defeat nor evidence of moral weakness. While painful, they do not erase the progress that has been achieved and ultimately may strengthen self-understanding. They can serve as reminders of potential pitfalls to avoid in the future.

One key to preventing relapse is learning to avoid obvious cues and associations that can set off intense cravings. This means staying away from the people and places linked with past drug use. Some therapists use conditioning techniques to give former users some sense of control over their urge to use the drug. The theory behind this approach, which is called *extinction* of conditioned behavior, is that with repeated exposure—for example, to videotapes of dealers selling crack cocaine—the arousal and craving will diminish. While this technique by itself cannot ward off relapses, it does seem to enhance the overall effectiveness of other therapies.

Another important lesson that therapists emphasize is that every "lapse" does not have to lead to a full-blown relapse. Users can turn to the skills acquired in treatment—calling people for support or going to meetings—to avoid a major relapse. Ultimately, users must learn much more than how to avoid temptation; they must examine their entire view of the world and learn new ways to live in it without turning to drugs. This is the underlying goal of the recovery process.

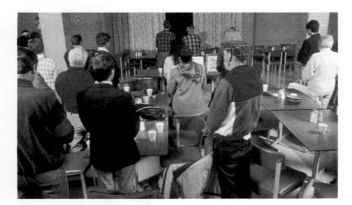

Twelve-step programs, based on the Alcoholics Anonymous model, have helped many people overcome behavioral addictions and addictions to alcohol, food, and drugs. The one requirement for membership is a desire to stop living out a pattern of addictive behavior.

Strategies for Prevention

Relapse-Prevention Planning

The following steps, from Terence Gorski and Merlene Miller's *Staying Sober* can lower the likelihood of relapses:

✔ *Stabilization and self-assessment.* Get control of yourself.

Find out what's going on in your head, heart, and life.

✔ *Education.* Learn about relapse and what to do to prevent it.

✔ *Warning-sign identification and management.* Make a list of your personal relapse warning signs. Learn how to interrupt them before you lose control.

✔ *Inventory training.* Learn how to become consciously aware of warning signs as they develop.

✔ *Review of the recovery program.* Make sure your recovery program is able to help you manage your warning signs of relapse.

✔ *Involvement of significant others.* Teach them how to help you avoid relapses.[39]

Outlook

Whatever the drug, recovery from dependence and abuse is a process of immense inner change that involves every aspect of a person's life. It does not follow a straight, even course, but moves back and forth between denial—of dependence, of loss of control, or of the severity of the problem—and awareness, ignorance and knowledge, craving and commitment. It often starts with a feeling of great relief, followed by a deep sense of emptiness. Individuals who have abused or become dependent on drugs must form a new identity, stop living in the past or future, give up their search for a quick fix, change the way they relate to family and old friends, find new things to do with the time they previously spent on their drug habit, learn new behaviors, and adopt new attitudes. Through treatment, education, and a reevaluation of what is meaningful in life, drug users can find a better way of living.

Valid statistics are difficult to obtain, but substance abuse counselors agree that eventually drug treatment works. But they emphasize that the high likelihood of relapse should not cause undue pessimism. Addiction, after all, is a chronic, progressive, often lifelong illness—not unlike many other medical problems.

"Would one ever place the expectation on a patient with diabetes or rheumatoid arthritis to be capable of overcoming their illness through some individual effort on their part?" asks Charles Connors, M.D., a psychiatrist at the Veterans Administration Medical Center in San Francisco. "The answer would certainly be no, but our inclination is to expect just this of patients with substance use disorders. We tend to conceptualize illnesses of addiction differently than medical illness and in so doing often place inordinate expectations on patients to

sustain 'abstinence' when, in fact, 'relapse' is the norm, just as 'progression of the illness' is the norm for medical illnesses such as diabetes or rheumatoid arthritis."[40]

Codependence

Codependence refers to the tendency of the spouses, partners, parents, and friends of individuals who use drugs or alcohol to allow, or *enable*, their loved ones to continue their drug use and self-destructive behavior. (Codependence is also discussed in Chapter 15.)

Codependents Anonymous, founded in 1986 for "men and women whose common problem is an inability to maintain functional relationships," sponsors support programs throughout the country. Nar-Anon provides groups for people affected by drug abuse. Both are listed in the resource directory at the back of this book; local chapters are in the white pages of the telephone directory.

Strategies for Change
. . . .
If Someone You Love Has a Drug Problem

✔ Get as much information as you can so that you understand what you—and your loved one—are up against. Also get some intervention training. Specially trained counselors work at most chemical-dependency units; some offer advice by phone.

✔ Confront the user. Along with other loved ones and, if possible, a professional counselor, detail incident after incident in which the drug abuse affected or hurt you, other members of your family, or the user.

✔ Don't expect a drug abuser to quit without help. Chemical dependence is a medical and psychological disorder that requires professional treatment. Offer your support, but make it clear that you expect your loved one to undergo therapy.

✔ If your loved one agrees to treatment, make sure that the program is based on a complete evaluation, checking for medical and emotional problems, as well as chemical dependency.

✔ Don't believe abusers who say they've learned to control their drug use. Abstinence is a cornerstone of any good rehabilitation program.

✔ Encourage a user to attend support groups, such as Cocaine Anonymous or Narcotics Anonymous, for at least one year after rehabilitation. Get help for yourself. Most hospitals and chemical-dependency programs offer educational programs for codependents.

Making This Chapter Work for You
Working Toward a Drug-Free Future

- Drugs—chemical substances that alter physiological or psychological processes—can be misused (used for a purpose—or person—other than that for which they were medically intended) or abused (used excessively or inappropriately). The misuse or abuse of psychoactive drugs can lead to physical and psychological dependence.

- Physical dependence occurs when physiological changes in the body caused by a drug result in an intense need for the drug. Psychological dependence occurs when users crave a drug for the emotional or mental changes it produces.

- Over-the-counter (OTC) drugs and prescription drugs can be misused or abused. The OTCs most often abused include painkillers and nasal inhalants. Prescription medications are often misused despite serious physical risks. The nonmedical, illegal use of anabolic steroids has become popular among young men who want to look muscular or build up their strength.

- Caffeine, though habit-forming and implicated in various health problems, doesn't seem to present any clear health threat if used in moderation.

- Amphetamine abusers may suffer from tremors, irregular heartbeat, loss of coordination, psychosis

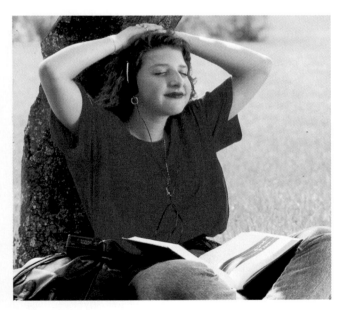

A quick fix? If drugs appear attractive as a "fix" for difficult times, try healthier remedies first, especially those that take you out-of-doors or get you active. Music is another nondrug aid to a change of mood, or even a "natural high."

and paranoia, malnutrition, skin disorders, ulcers, depression, brain damage, and heart failure. A form of smokeable methamphetamine, known as ice or glass, increases heart rate and blood pressure; high doses can cause permanent damage to blood vessels in the brain. Like ice, crank (propylhexedrine) produces effects similar to those of amphetamines.

- THC, the primary psychoactive ingredient in marijuana and hashish, can produce an increased heart rate, dry mouth and throat, and altered perception; high doses may result in distorted perception, hallucinations, and acute panic attacks. Long-term marijuana use may result in psychological dependence; lung damage; impairment of the central nervous system, reproductive system, and immune system; use of other drugs; mental and emotional dulling; loss of drive; and legal consequences.

- Cocaine, which produces feelings of high energy, may be snorted as a powder, smoked (or freebased) in a form called crack or rock, or dissolved in a solution that's then injected. The effects of cocaine use include impaired judgment, psychological disorders (including psychosis), headache, nausea, damaged nasal membranes in snorters, weight loss, liver damage, heart attack, stroke, brain seizure or hemorrhage, complications during pregnancy, and mental and physical damage to infants born to cocaine users.

- Sedative-hypnotics and antianxiety agents turn down the central nervous system. Barbiturate use can result in physical dependence, and because the addict needs increasingly larger doses, the risk of fatal overdose is high. Antianxiety medications, such as Valium and Xanax, can produce dependence, drowsiness, and slurred speech; withdrawal can produce coma, psychosis, and even death.

- Hallucinogens, including peyote and its active ingredient, mescaline; lysergic acid diethylamide (LSD); psilocybin; and phencyclidine (PCP) can produce hallucinations and, in some users, panic, paranoia, and psychotic episodes. PCP is a dangerous psychoactive drug because of its effects on behavior.

- The opiates, including opium, morphine, heroin, and codeine, may lead to infections of the heart, skin abscesses, and congested lungs, as well as tetanus, liver disease, hepatitis, and HIV infection from the use of unsterile syringes and needles. An addict who stops taking an opiate will experience withdrawal sickness—nausea, abdominal cramps, fever, sweating and chills, diarrhea, and severe aches

Health Online

Dapa-PC Drug Abuse Screening   http://www.danya.com/middle5.htm

Are you at risk for drug abuse? Take this online screening test and find out. The anonymous assessment looks at your drugtaking behavior, its effects on your life, and other physical, mental, emotional, and social risk factors for drug abuse.

Think about it ...

• According to this assessment, do you have any risk factors for drug abuse? What are they, and how might you avoid them?

• Have you ever misused a drug, even caffeine, or an over-the-counter medication? If so, why? What was the experience like?

• Do you think that there are situations in which it is okay to use an illegal psychoactive drug? Do you think using these drugs to enhance performance or as a recreational activity is legitimate? Why or why not?

and pains. The most abused synthetic opiates are Demerol and Darvon.

■ Inhalants, including amyl nitrite and butyl nitrite, can lead to serious complications. Designer drugs are illegally manufactured drugs that are far more potent than natural substances.

■ Treatment for drug dependence usually includes a combination of approaches, including detoxification in a hospital or as an outpatient; admission to a residential therapeutic community; or treatment in an outpatient drug-counseling program that may use behavioral, cognitive, and social-skills training techniques.

■ Codependence is an emotional and psychological behavioral pattern in which the spouses, partners, parents, and friends of individuals with addictive behaviors allow or enable their loved ones to continue their self-destructive habits. Codependents feel responsible for meeting others' needs, have low

self-esteem, and frequently have compulsions of their own.

Some therapists believe that addicts are never truly cured, but that like those with diabetes or arthritis, they can learn to live happy, fulfilling lives in spite of their illness. However, doing so demands self-esteem, self-confidence, and social and economic opportunities. "Drug addiction is a highly treatable disease when patients are motivated and have something to lose if they go back to drugs," says psychiatrist Richard Frances. "Individuals have to feel there's something better in the world than drugs."[41]

If drugs ever seem appealing as a quick fix to whatever is troubling you, consider alternative experiences that can help you solve your problems without creating new and bigger ones. Activities such as mountain biking or listening to music can produce a very real high, but there's a crucial difference between this sort of stimulation and drug dependence: With one, *you're* in control; with the other, drugs are.

▶ Key Terms

The terms listed here are used within the chapter. Page numbers are included for each term. A definition of each term is given in the green Glossary pages at the end of this book.

addiction *448*

additive *441*

amphetamine *455*

anabolic steroids *466*

antagonistic *441*

barbiturates *465*

benzodiazepines *465*

cocaine *459*

codependence *471*

Review Questions

1. What does it mean to be drug dependent? What are the contributing factors? How can you tell if someone is abusing drugs?

2. What are the differences between cocaine and crack? How can crack and cocaine addiction be treated?

3. What is an amphetamine? What are some common forms of amphetamines? Describe the uses of amphetamines and their effects on the user.

4. What are sedatives, hypnotics, and antianxiety drugs? What are some common forms of these drugs?

Describe their uses and the effects on the user.

5. List some methods of treatment for drug dependence. What are some of the issues affecting treatment? Can addiction be overcome?

6. Who is a codependent? What is enabling? What are some common modes of enabling?

7. How does a twelve-step program for recovery work? What are the basic rules or underlying beliefs? Why are such programs so successful?

Critical Thinking Questions

1. New testing procedures have been developed that allow one to detect the presence of drugs, such as marijuana, simply by using a sample of the drug user's hair. Parents could presumably use this test to determine if their children have been taking drugs. How do you feel about this? Is it fair? Would you use such a test on your children? What would you say if your parents used the test on you?

2. Alan has experimented with cocaine on a few occasions, and he talks about his experience in glowing terms. In fact, as your best friend, he'd like you to try it with him sometime. When you question him

about the dangers of addiction, he says, "Are you crazy? I don't do this more than once a month. I'm not addicted!" How would you respond to Alan?

3. Sheila was doing spring-cleaning when she came across a brown bag at the back of the linen closet. That evening she confronted her roommate about keeping an illegal substance in the apartment. Meg's response was: "Oh, I forgot that little bit of weed was even there. Besides, no one would *ever* find it. What are you so uptight about?" Sheila insisted, "I don't care if it's just a little—it's still illegal, and I don't want it here." How would you resolve their dispute?

 # Connections to Personal Health Interactive

To enhance your understanding of the material covered in this chapter, check out the following study aids on the **Personal Health Interactive CD-ROM**. *Each numbered icon within the chapter corresponds to an appropriate activity listed here.*

14.1 Study Page: Drug Effects
14.2 Personal Insights: How Do You Feel
About Drugs?

14.3 Chapter 14 Review

References

1. Warner, Lynn, et al. "Prevalence and Correlates of Drug Use and Dependence in the United States: Results from the National Comorbidity Survey." *Archives of General Psychiatry*, Vol. 52, March 1995.

2. "Aspirin." *Remedy*, Summer 1995.

3. Pilliteri, Janine, et al. "Over-the-Counter Sleep Aids: Widely Used But Rarely Studied." *Journal of Substance Abuse*, Vol. 6, No. 3, 1994.

4. Gorman, Jack. Personal interview.

5. "Caffeine's Hook." *Current Health*, Vol. 2, No. 24, January 1998.

6. Franklin, John. "Addiction Medicine." *Journal of the American Medical Association*, Vol. 273, No. 21, June 7, 1995.

7. Glare, P. G. W. *Oxford Latin Dictionary*. Oxford, England: Clarendon Press, 1985.

8. Frances, Richard. Personal interview.

9. Goleman, Daniel. "Brain Images Show the Neural Basis of Addiction As It Is Happening." *New York Times*, August 13, 1996.

10. Nash, J. Madeline. "Addicted." *Time*, May 5, 1997.

11. Labouvie, Erich, et al. "Age at First Use: Its Reliability and Predictive Utility." *Journal of Studies on Alcohol*, Vol. 58, No. 6, November 1997.

12. Wren, Christopher. "Survey Suggests Leveling Off in Use of Drugs by Students." *New York Times*, December 21, 1997.

13. Nash. "Addicted."

14. Kolata, Gina. "Experts Are at Odds on How Best to Tackle Rise in Teen-Agers Drug Use." *New York Times*, September 18, 1996.

15. Eigen, Lewis, and David Rowden. "The Success of Alcohol, Tobacco and Other Drug Prevention: A White Paper." National Clearinghouse for Alcohol and Drug Information, Rockville, MD, 1993.

16. Pacula, Rosalie. "Women and Substance Use: Are Women Less Susceptible to Addiction?" *American Economic Review*, Vol. 87, No. 2, May 1997.

17. Duitsman, Dalen, and Sheilia Lynds Colbry. "Perceived Risk and Use as Predictors of Substance Use among College Students." *Health Values*, Vol. 19, No. 2, March to April 1995.

18. Urberg, Kathryn, et al. "Close Friend and Group Influence on Adolescent Cigarette Smoking and Alcohol Use." *Developmental Psychology*, Vol. 130, No. 5, September 1997.

19. "Decrease in Drug Use by Adults Levels Off, Continues for Students." *Public Health Reports,* Vol. 107, No. 3, 1992.

20. Hoffman

21. Hales, Dianne, and Robert Hales. *Caring for the Mind*. New York: Bantam Books, 1995.

22. Lehrman, Sally. "Make Marijuana Research Easier, Panel Urges NIH." *Nature*, Vol. 388, No. 6643, August 14, 1997.

23. Grinspoon, Lester, and James Bakalar. "Marijuana as Medicine." *Journal of the American Medical Association,* Vol. 273, No. 23, June 21, 1995.

24. Pope, Harrison, and Deborah Yurgulen-Todd. "The Residual Cognitive Effects of Heavy Marijuana Use in College Students." *Journal of the American Medical Association*, Vol. 275, No. 7, February 21, 1996.

25. Concar, David. "A Dangerous Pathway." *New Scientist*, Vol. 155, No. 2089, July 5, 1997.

26. Brownsberger, William. "Prevalence of Frequent Cocaine Use in Urban Poverty Areas." *Contemporary Drug Problems*, Vol. 24, No. 2, Summer 1997.

27. Schmitz, Joy, et al. "Relapse Prevention Treatment for Cocaine Dependence." *Addictive Behaviors*, Vol. 22, No. 3, May–June 1997.

28. Chrebet, Jennifer. "Getting High on Household Products." *American Health*, November 1994.

29. International Institute on Inhalant Abuse, 450 West Jefferson Ave, Englewood, CO 80110.

30. Cloud, John. "A Way Out for Junkies?" *Time*, January 19, 1998.

31. Sachtleben, Thomas, et al. "Serum Lipoprotein Patterns in Long-term Anabolic Steroid Users." *Research Quarterly for Exercise and Sport*, Vol. 68, No. 1, March 1997.

32. DuRant, R. H., et al. "Anabolic-Steroid Use Among Adolescents in the United States," *Pediatrics*, Vol. 88, No. 1, July 1995.

33. Gorman, Christine. "Liquid X." *Time*, September 30, 1996.

34. Cloud, John. "Is Your Kid on K?" *Time*, October 20, 1997.

35. Monroe, Judy. "Designer Drugs: CAT & LSD." *Current Health*, Vol. 21, No. 1, September 1994.

36. Cuomo, Michael, et al. "Increasing Use of 'Ecstasy' (MDMA) and other Hallucinogens on a College Campus." *Journal of American College Health*, Vol. 42, No. 6, May 1994.

37. Ricaurte, George, et al. "Street Drug Ecstasy May Cause Lasting Brain Damage." *Journal of Neuroscience*, August 1995.

38. Lurtz, Linda. "Recovery, the 12-step Movement, and Politics." *Social Work*, Vol. 42, No. 14, July 1997.

39. Gorski, Terence J., and Marlene Miller. "Staying Sober: A Guide for Relapse Prevention." Independence, MO: Herald House, 1986.

40. Connors, Charles. Personal interview.

41. Frances, Richard. Personal interview.

CHAPTER 15

ALCOHOL USE, MISUSE, AND ABUSE

After studying the material in this chapter, you should be able to:

Describe the factors affecting a drinker's response to alcohol consumption.

List the effects of alcohol on the body systems.

Describe the impact of alcohol misuse among women and different ethnic groups.

Define alcoholism, and **list** common symptoms of this disease.

List the negative consequences to individuals, and to our society, from alcohol abuse.

Explain the common treatment methods for alcoholism.

Alcohol is the most widely used mind-altering substance in the world. In the United States, about half of all adults drink, at least occasionally. Ninety percent of college students use alcohol, and dangerous practices, such as drinking binges, are common on campuses across the country.[1]

The majority of people who use alcohol don't abuse it. The key to their responsible drinking isn't necessarily saying "No," but knowing when to say "No more." Even occasional drinkers need to learn their limits and recognize the point at which alcohol impairs their judgment or threatens their well-being. For some people in some circumstances, one drink may be too many.

When not used responsibly, alcohol can take an enormous toll. No medical conditions, other than heart disease, cause more disability and premature death than alcohol-related problems. No mental or medical disorders touch the lives of more families. No other form of disability costs individuals, employers, and the government more for treatment, injuries, reduced worker productivity, and property damage. The costs in emotional pain and in lost and shattered lives because of irresponsible drinking are beyond measure.

This chapter provides information about alcohol, its impact on the body, brain, behavior, and society, patterns of drinking, and the recognition, understanding, and treatment of drinking problems and of alcoholism.

Alcohol and Its Effects

Pure alcohol is a colorless liquid obtained through the fermentation of a liquid containing sugar. **Ethyl alcohol**, or *ethanol,* is the type of alcohol in alcoholic beverages. Another type—methyl, or wood, alcohol—is a poison that should never be drunk. Any liquid containing 0.5% to 80% ethyl alcohol by volume is an alcoholic beverage. However, different drinks contain different amounts of alcohol (see Figure 15-1).

One drink can be any of the following:

- One bottle or can (12 ounces) of beer, which is 5% alcohol.

- One glass (4 ounces) of table wine, such as burgundy, which is 12% alcohol.

- One small glass (2 1/2 ounces) of fortified wine, which is 20% alcohol.

- One shot (1 ounce) of distilled spirits (such as whiskey, vodka, or rum), which is 50% alcohol.

All of these drinks contain close to the same amount of alcohol—that is, if the number of ounces in each drink is multiplied by the percentage of alcohol, each drink contains the equivalent of approximately 1/2 ounce of 100% ethyl alcohol. With distilled spirits (such as bourbon, scotch, vodka, gin, and rum), alcohol content is expressed in terms of **proof**, a number that is *twice* the percentage of alcohol: 100-proof bourbon is 50% alcohol; 80-proof gin is 40% alcohol.

But the words "bottle" and "glass" can be deceiving in this context. Drinking a 16-ounce bottle of malt liquor, which is 6.4% alcohol, is *not* the same as drinking a 12-ounce glass of 3.2% beer. Two bottles of high-alcohol wines (such as Cisco), packaged to resemble much less powerful wine coolers, can lead to alcohol poisoning, especially in those who weigh less than 150 pounds. This is one reason why it is a serious danger for young people.

As with other substance use disorders, prevention is the best approach to alcohol problems. According to public health officials, if Americans drank less, the rates of alcohol dependence and abuse could be cut almost in half—from the current 15.5% of the population to 8.2%.[2]

How Much Can You Drink?

The best way to figure how much you can drink safely is to determine the amount of alcohol in your blood at any given time, or your **blood-alcohol concentration (BAC)**. BAC is expressed in terms of the percentage of alcohol in the blood and is often measured from breath or urine samples. Law enforcement officers use BAC to determine whether a driver is legally drunk. The Federal Department of Transportation has called on states to set 0.08%—the BAC that a 150-pound man would have after consuming about three mixed drinks within an hour—as the threshold at which a person can be cited for drunk driving. In the past, 0.1% was often the legal limit. (See Figure 15-2.)

A BAC of 0.05% indicates approximately 5 parts alcohol to 10,000 parts other blood components. Most people reach this level after consuming one or two drinks and experience all the positive sensations of drinking—relaxation, euphoria, and well-being—without feeling intoxicated. If they continue to drink past the 0.05% BAC level, they start feeling worse rather than better, gradually losing control of speech, balance, and emotions (see Table 15-1). At a BAC of 0.2%, they may pass out. At a BAC of 0.3%, they could lapse into a coma; at 0.4%, they could die.

For some people, even very low blood alcohol concentrations can cause a headache, upset stomach, or dizziness. These reactions often are inborn. People who have suffered brain damage—often as a result of head trauma or encephalitis—may lose all tolerance for alcohol, either temporarily or permanently, and behave abnormally after drinking small amounts. The

Figure 15-1

The alcohol content of different drinks.

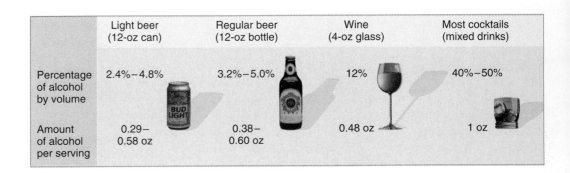

	Light beer (12-oz can)	Regular beer (12-oz bottle)	Wine (4-oz glass)	Most cocktails (mixed drinks)
Percentage of alcohol by volume	2.4%–4.8%	3.2%–5.0%	12%	40%–50%
Amount of alcohol per serving	0.29–0.58 oz	0.38–0.60 oz	0.48 oz	1 oz

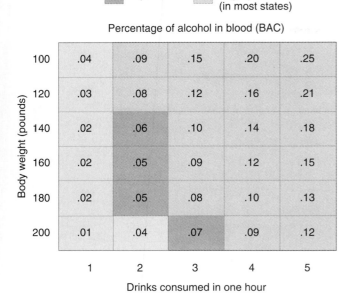

Figure 15-2

Blood-alcohol concentration and body weight. How fast one's BAC level rises depends on body weight and on how many drinks one has in a given amount of time. One drink is 12 oz of beer, 4 oz of wine, or $1\frac{1}{2}$ oz of 80-proof liquor.

elderly, as well as those who are unusually fatigued or have a debilitating physical illness, may also have a low tolerance to alcohol and respond inappropriately to a small amount.

How You Respond to Alcohol

Many factors affect an individual's BAC and response to alcohol, including the following:

- *How much and how quickly you drink.* The more alcohol you put into your body, the higher your

BAC. If you chug drink after drink, your liver, which metabolizes about 1/2 ounce of alcohol an hour, won't be able to keep up—and your BAC will soar.

- *What you're drinking.* The stronger the drink, the faster and harder the alcohol hits. Straight shots of liquor and cocktails such as martinis will get alcohol into your bloodstream faster than beer or table wine. Beer and wine not only contain lower concentrations of alcohol, but they also contain nonalcoholic substances that slow the rate of **absorption** (passage of the alcohol into your body tissues). If the drink contains water, juice, or milk, the rate of absorption will be slowed. However, carbon dioxide—whether in champagne, ginger ale, or a cola—whisks alcohol into your bloodstream. Also, the alcohol in warm drinks—such as a hot rum toddy or warmed sake—moves into your bloodstream more quickly than the alcohol in chilled wine or scotch on the rocks.

- *Your size.* If you're a large person (whether due to fat or to muscle), you'll get drunk more slowly than someone smaller who's drinking the same amount of alcohol at the same rate. Heavier individuals have a larger water volume, which dilutes the alcohol they drink.

- *Your gender.* Women have lower quantities of a stomach enzyme that neutralizes alcohol, so one drink for a woman has the impact that two drinks have for a man. Hormone levels also affect the impact of alcohol. Women are more sensitive to alcohol just before menstruation, and birth control pills and other forms of estrogen can intensify alcohol's impact. (See the section "Women and Alcohol" later in this chapter.)

- *Your age.* The same amount of alcohol produces higher BACs in older drinkers, who have lower vol-

TABLE 15-1 RECOGNIZING THE WARNING SIGNS OF ALCOHOLISM

- Experiencing the following symptoms after drinking: frequent head-aches, nausea, stomach pain, heartburn, gas, fatigue, weakness, muscle cramps, or irregular or rapid heartbeats.
- Needing a drink in the morning to start the day.

- Denying any problem with alcohol.
- Doing things while drinking that are regretted afterward.
- Dramatic mood swings, from anger to laughter to anxiety.
- Sleep problems.

- Depression and paranoia.
- Forgetting what happened during a drinking episode.
- Changing brands or going on the wagon to control drinking.
- Having five or more drinks a day.

Self-Survey

Do You Have a Drinking Problem?

This self-assessment, the Michigan Alcoholism Screening Test (MAST), is widely used to identify potential problems. This test screens for the major psychological, sociological, and physiological consequences of alcoholism. To complete it, simply answer Yes or No to the following questions, and add up the points shown in the right column for your answers.

	Yes	No	Points
1. Do you enjoy a drink now and then?	____	____	(0 for either)
2. Do you think that you're a normal drinker? (By normal, we mean that you drink less than or as much as most other people.)	____	____	(2 for no)
3. Have you ever awakened the morning after some drinking the night before and found that you couldn't remember part of the evening?	____	____	(2 for yes)
4. Does your wife, husband, a parent, or other near relative every worry or complain about your drinking?	____	____	(1 for yes)
5. Can you stop drinking without a struggle after one or two drinks?	____	____	(2 for no)
6. Do you ever feel guilty about your drinking?	____	____	(1 for yes)
7. Do friends or relatives think that you're a normal drinker?	____	____	(2 for no)
8. Do you ever try to limit your drinking to certain times of the day or to certain places?	____	____	(0 for either)
9. Have you ever attended a meeting of Alcoholics Anonymous?	____	____	(2 for yes)
10. Have you ever gotten into physical fights when drinking?	____	____	(1 for yes)
11. Has your drinking ever created problems for you and your wife, husband, a parent, or other relative?	____	____	(2 for yes)
12. Has your wife, husband, or other family members			

	Yes	No	Points
ever gone to anyone for help about your drinking?	____	____	(2 for yes)
13. Have you ever lost friends because of your drinking?	____	____	(2 for yes)
14. Have you ever gotten into trouble at work or school because of your drinking?	____	____	(2 for yes)
15. Have you ever lost a job because of your drinking?	____	____	(2 for yes)
16. Have you ever neglected your obligations, your family, or your work for two or more days in a row because of drinking?	____	____	(2 for yes)
17. Do you drink before noon fairly often?	____	____	(1 for yes)
18. Have you ever been told you have liver trouble? cirrhosis?	____	____	(2 for yes)
19. After heavy drinking, have you ever had delirium tremens (DTs) or severe shaking, or heard voices or seen things that weren't actually there?	____	____	(2 for yes*)
20. Have you ever gone to anyone for help about your drinking?	____	____	(5 for yes)
21. Have you ever been in a hospital because of your drinking?	____	____	(5 for yes)
22. Have you ever been a patient in a psychiatric hospital or on a psychiatric ward of a general hospital where drinking was part of the problem			

	Yes	No	Points

that resulted in hospitalization? _____ _____ (2 for yes)

23. Have you ever been seen
at a psychiatric or mental
health clinic or gone to
any doctor, social worker,
or clergyman for help
with any emotional prob-
lem where drinking was
part of the problem? _____ _____ (2 for yes)

24. Have you ever been
arrested for drunk driving,
driving while intoxicated,
or driving under the
influence of alcoholic
beverages? _____ _____ (2 for yes)

25. Have you ever been
arrested, or taken into
custody, even for a few
hours, because of
drunken behavior? _____ _____ (2 for yes)

(If Yes, How many times? _____**)

* Five points for delirium tremens
** Two points for *each* arrest

Scoring:

In general, five or more points places you in an alcoholic
category; four points suggests alcoholism; while three or
fewer points indicates that you're *not* alcoholic.

Making Changes
Spotting a Problem

Even if you don't show signs of alcoholism now, you should pay attention to your drinking pattern, and if it changes—if you find yourself drinking more than usual over an extended period—take this test again. If the test indicates that you show some symptoms of alcoholism, per-haps you hear yourself saying, "It may be a problem, but it's not that big a deal. I can quit any time." Maybe you've devised your own concept of alcoholism. You might think, for example, that you couldn't be alcoholic because you only drink on weekends, or because you don't start before 5:00 P.M., or because you drink only beer or wine.

Before you rule out the possibility of alcoholism, however, consider two things: First, the nature of the disease is to trick its victims into believing that they can control their drinking. Second, making an effort to control one's drinking is, by itself, a sign of alcoholism. People who don't have an alcohol problem don't think twice about how much they drink. They set a limit and stick to it. If your drinking causes problems in any area of your life—with your family, at work, in social settings, emotionally or physically, financial-ly, or with the law—it's worth finding out more about this disease.

If you've decided that you have a problem with alcohol, you deserve congratulations. You've made an important step toward recovery. Now you'll need to consider the treatment options described in this chapter.

SOURCE: Adapted from Barbara Yoder. *The Recovery Resource Book.* New York: Fireside Books, 1990.

umes of body water to dilute the alcohol than younger drinkers do.

- *Your race.* Many members of certain ethnic groups, including Asians and Native Americans, are unable to break down alcohol as quickly as Caucasians. This can result in higher BACs, as well as uncom-fortable reactions, such as flushing and nausea, when they drink. (See Spotlight on Diversity: "Drinking and Ethnic Groups.")

- *Other drugs.* Some common medications—including aspirin, acetaminophen (Tylenol), and ulcer medica-tions—can cause blood-alcohol levels to increase more rapidly. Individuals taking these drugs can be over the legal limit for blood-alcohol concentration after as little as a single drink. [3]

- *Family history of alcoholism.* Some children of alco-

holics don't develop any of the usual behavioral symptoms that indicate someone is drinking too much. It's not known whether this behavior is genetically caused or is a result of growing up with an alcoholic.

- *Eating.* Food slows the absorption of alcohol by diluting it, by covering some of the membranes through which alcohol would be absorbed, and by prolonging the time the stomach takes to empty.

- *Expectations.* In various experiments, volunteers who believed they were given alcoholic beverages but were actually given nonalcoholic drinks acted as if they were guzzling the real thing and became more talkative, relaxed, and sexually stimulated. [4]

- *Physical tolerance.* If you drink regularly, your brain becomes accustomed to a certain level of alcohol.

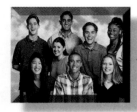

Spotlight on Diversity
Drinking and Ethnic Groups

Individuals in any racial and ethnic group can develop drinking problems, but certain groups suffer disproportionately high rates of alcohol dependence and abuse and related illnesses. These groups include African Americans, Latinos, and Native Americans. In addition, alcohol presents other concerns for Asians and Asian Americans. Increasingly, experts in alcohol treatment are recognizing racial and ethnic differences in risk factors for drinking problems, patterns of drinking, and most effective types of treatment. Increases in drinking have been traced to stresses related to immigration, acculturation, poverty, racial discrimination, and powerlessness. Environmental factors, such as aggressive marketing and advertising of alcoholic beverages in minority neighborhoods, also play a role.

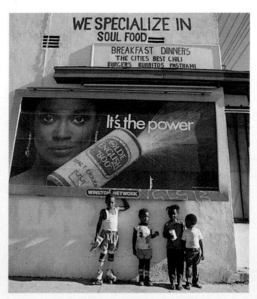

The makers of alcoholic beverages market their products aggressively in poor urban neighborhoods, where liquor stores and bars are common.

Few Latinos enter treatment, partly because of a lack of information, language barriers, and poor community-based services. Latino families generally try to resolve problems themselves, and their cultural values discourage the sharing of intimate personal stories, which characterizes Alcoholics Anonymous and other support groups. Churches often provide the most effective forms of help.

• **The Native-American Community** European settlers introduced alcohol to Native Americans. But because of the societal and physical problems resulting from excessive drinking, at the request of tribal leaders, the U.S. Congress in 1832 prohibited the use of alcohol by Native Americans. Many reservations still ban alcohol use, a policy that may force Native Americans who want to drink to travel long distances to obtain alcohol—and may contribute to the high death rate from hypothermia and pedestrian and motor-vehicle accidents among Native Americans. (Injuries are the leading cause of death among this group.)

Certainly, not all Native Americans drink, and not all who drink do so to excess. However, they have three times the general population's rate of alcohol-related injury and illness. Moreover, cirrhosis of the liver is the fourth-leading cause of death among this cultural group. While many Native-American women don't drink, those who do have high rates of alcohol-related problems, which affect both them and their children. Their rate of cirrhosis of the liver is 36 times that of white women. In some tribes, 10.5 out of every 1000 newborns have fetal alcohol syndrome, compared with 1–3 out of 1000 in the general population. (See the section on fetal alcohol syndrome in this chapter.)

Both a biological predisposition and socioeconomic conditions may contribute to alcohol abuse by Native Americans. In addition, according to their cultural beliefs, alcoholism is not a physical disease but a spiritual disorder—making it less likely that they'll seek appropriate treatment.

• **The African-American Community** Overall, African Americans consume less alcohol per person than whites, yet twice as many blacks die of cirrhosis of the liver each year. In some cities, the rate of cirrhosis is ten times higher among African-American than white men. Alcohol also contributes to high rates of hypertension, esophageal cancer, and homicide among African-American men.

The makers of alcoholic beverages market their products aggressively to African Americans, and there are many more liquor stores (per capita) in many African-American neighborhoods than in white communities. Peer pressure to drink, the easy accessibility of alcohol, and socioeconomic frustrations increase the likelihood of alcohol problems among African Americans. Moreover, recovery can be especially difficult because of the lack of treatment programs and role models in the African-American community, and the ongoing pressures to resume drinking.

• **The Latino Community** Latino societies discourage any drinking by women but encourage heavy drinking by men as part of their machismo, or feelings of manhood. According to the Department of Health and Human Services, Latino men have higher rates of alcohol use and abuse than the general population, and suffer a high rate of cirrhosis. Moreover, American-born Latino men drink more than those born in other countries.

• **The Asian-American Community** Asian Americans tend to drink very little or not at all, in part because of an inborn physiological reaction to alcohol that causes facial flushing, rapid heart rate, lowered blood pressure, nausea, vomiting, and other symptoms. A very high percentage of women of all Asian-American nationalities abstain completely. Some sociologists have expressed concern, however, that as Asian Americans become more assimilated into American culture, they'll drink more—and possibly suffer very adverse effects from alcohol.

SOURCES: Caetano, Raul. "Drinking and Alcohol-Related Problems Among Minority Women." *Alcohol Health & Research World*, Vol. 18, No. 3, Summer 1994. Atkinson, Donald, et al. "Mexican American and European American Ratings of Four Alcoholism Treatment Programs." *Hispanic Journal of Behavioral Sciences*, Vol. 16, No. 3, August 1994. Higuchi, Susumu, and Hiroaki KoNo. "Early Diagnosis and Treatment of Alcoholism: The Japanese Experience." *Alcohol & Alcoholism*, Vol. 29, No. 4, July 1994.

You may be able to look and behave in a seemingly normal fashion, even though you drink as much as would normally intoxicate someone your size. However, your driving ability and judgment will still be impaired.

Once you develop tolerance, you may drink more to get the desired effects from alcohol. In some people, this can lead to abuse and alcoholism. On the other hand, after years of drinking, some people become exquisitely sensitive to alcohol. Such reverse tolerance means that they can become intoxicated after drinking only a small amount of alcohol.

How Much Is Too Much?

Unlike many other drugs of abuse, including tobacco, any and all amounts of alcohol are not toxic. According to a 1997 study of nearly 500,000 people from ages 35 to 69, one drink a day can in fact be good for health. Those who had one serving (see Figure 15-1) of wine, beer, or hard liquor had a death rate 20% lower than nondrinkers over a nine-year period. Nearly all of the benefit came from a reduction in the risk of heart disease. However, the researchers cautioned that for women, a drink a day—while lowering the overall risk of deaths—increased by 30% the chance of dying from breast cancer.[5]

Federal health authorities at the National Institute of Alcohol and Alcohol Abuse (NIAAA) recommend that men have no more than two drinks a day and women, no more than one. The American Heart Association (AHA) advises that alcohol account for no more than 15% of the total calories consumed by an individual every day, up to an absolute maximum of 1.75 ounces of alcohol a day—the equivalent of three beers, two mixed drinks, or three and a half glasses of wine. Your own limit may well be less, depending on your sex, size, and weight. Some people—such as women who are pregnant or trying to conceive; individuals with prob-

lems, such as ulcers, that might be aggravated by alcohol; those taking medications such as sleeping pills or antidepressants; and those driving or operating any motorized equipment—shouldn't drink at all.

The dangers of alcohol increase along with the amount you drink. Heavy drinking destroys the liver, weakens the heart, elevates blood pressure, damages the brain, and increases the risk of cancer. Individuals who drink heavily have a higher mortality rate than those who have two or fewer drinks a day. However, the boundary between safe and dangerous drinking isn't the same for everyone. For some people, the upper limit of safety is zero: Once they start, they can't stop.

Intoxication

If you drink too much, the immediate consequence is that you get drunk—or, more precisely, intoxicated. According to the American Psychiatric Association's *Diagnostic and Statistical Manual of Mental Disorders*, 4th edition *(DSM-IV)*, **intoxication** consists of "clinically significant maladaptive behavioral or psychological changes," such as inappropriate sexual or aggressive behavior, mood changes, and impaired judgment and social and occupational functioning.[6] Alcohol intoxication, which can range from mild inebriation to loss of consciousness, is characterized by at least one of the following signs: slurred speech, poor coordination, unsteady gait, abnormal eye movements, impaired attention or memory, stupor, or coma. Medical risks of intoxication include falls, hypothermia in cold climates, and increased risk of infections because of suppressed immune function.

Time and a protective environment are the recommended treatments for alcohol intoxication. Anyone who passes out after drinking heavily should be monitored regularly to ensure that vomiting (the result of excess alcohol irritating the stomach) doesn't block the breathing airway. Always make sure that an unconscious drinker is lying on his or her side, with the head lower than the body. Intoxicated drinkers can slip into shock, a potentially life-threatening condition characterized by a weak pulse, irregular breathing, and skin-color changes. This is an emergency, and professional medical care should be sought immediately.

Strategies for Change
. . . .

How to Promote Responsible Drinking

✔ When preparing drinks for guests, measure the amount of alcohol you use, and figure out how many ounces your wine and beer glasses hold. Avoid pushing drinks on guests and refilling glasses quickly.

✔ Always serve food when serving drinks—but not the salty nuts, chips, and pretzels bars serve to increase thirst. Stop serving alcohol one hour before the evening is to end.

✔ Make sure nonalcoholic alternatives are available.

✔ Never serve alcohol to a guest who seems intoxicated.

✔ Never let an intoxicated person drive home. You could be legally, as well as morally, responsible in the event of an accident. Call a taxi, or have a friend who hasn't been drinking drive the person home. As a last resort, call the police. In many communities, they'll drive an intoxicated person home as a public service.

The Impact of Alcohol

Unlike drugs in tablet form or food, alcohol is directly and quickly absorbed into the bloodstream through the stomach walls and upper intestine. The alcohol in a typical drink reaches the bloodstream in 15 minutes and rises to its peak concentration in about an hour. The bloodstream carries the alcohol to the liver, heart, and brain. (See Figure 15-3.)

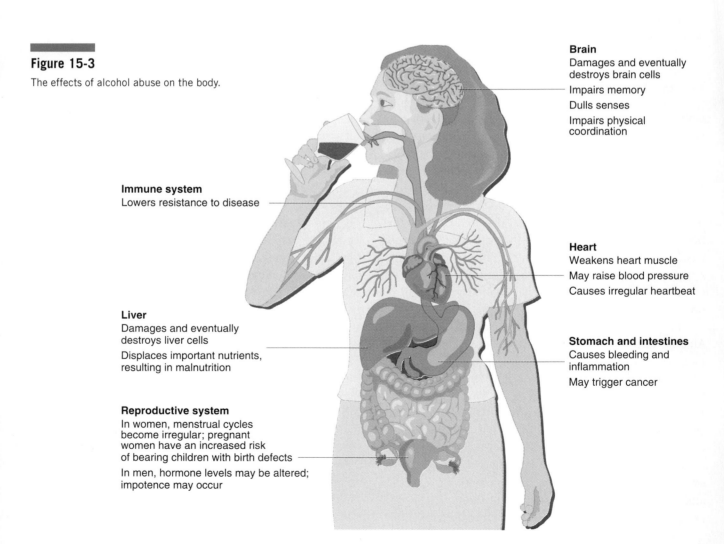

Figure 15-3
The effects of alcohol abuse on the body.

Brain
Damages and eventually destroys brain cells
Impairs memory
Dulls senses
Impairs physical coordination

Immune system
Lowers resistance to disease

Heart
Weakens heart muscle
May raise blood pressure
Causes irregular heartbeat

Liver
Damages and eventually destroys liver cells
Displaces important nutrients, resulting in malnutrition

Stomach and intestines
Causes bleeding and inflammation
May trigger cancer

Reproductive system
In women, menstrual cycles become irregular; pregnant women have an increased risk of bearing children with birth defects
In men, hormone levels may be altered; impotence may occur

Alcohol is a *diuretic*, a drug that speeds up the elimination of fluid from the body. Most of the alcohol you drink can leave your body only after metabolism by the liver, which converts about 95% of the alcohol to carbon dioxide and water. The other 5% is excreted unchanged, mainly through urination, respiration, and perspiration. Alcohol lowers body temperature, so you should never drink to get or stay warm.

Digestive System

Alcohol reaches the stomach first, where it is partially broken down. The remaining alcohol is absorbed easily through the stomach tissue into the bloodstream. When it's in the stomach, alcohol triggers the secretion of acids in the stomach, which irritate its lining. Excessive drinking at one sitting may result in nausea; chronic drinking may result in peptic ulcers (breaks in the stomach lining) and bleeding from the stomach lining.

The alcohol in the bloodstream eventually reaches the liver. The liver, which bears the major responsibility of fat metabolism in the body, converts this excess alcohol to fat. After a few weeks of four or five drinks a day, liver cells start to accumulate fat. Alcohol also stimulates liver cells to attract white blood cells, which normally travel throughout the bloodstream engulfing harmful substances and wastes. If white blood cells begin to invade body tissue, such as the liver, they can cause irreversible damage.

Cardiovascular System

Alcohol gets mixed reviews regarding its effects on the cardiovascular system. Moderate drinkers have healthier hearts, suffer fewer heart attacks, have less buildup of cholesterol in their arteries, and are less likely to die of heart disease than heavy drinkers or teetotalers.

Excessive drinking can clearly endanger the heart's health. Alcohol use can weaken the heart muscle directly, causing a disorder called cardiomyopathy.[7] The combined use of alcohol and other drugs, including tobacco and cocaine, greatly increases the likelihood of damage to the heart.

Immune System

Chronic alcohol use can inhibit the production of both white blood cells, which fight off infections, and red blood cells, which carry oxygen to all the organs and tissues of the body. Alcohol may increase the risk of infection with human immunodeficiency virus (HIV), by altering the judgment of users so that they more readily engage in activities, such as unsafe sexual practices, that put them in danger. If you drink when you have a cold or the flu, alcohol interferes with the body's ability to recover. It also increases the chance of bacterial pneumonia in flu-sufferers.

Brain and Behavior

At first, when you drink, you feel up. In low dosages, alcohol affects the regions of the brain that inhibit or control behavior, so you feel looser and act in ways you might not otherwise. However, you also experience losses of concentration, memory, judgment, and fine motor control; and you have mood swings and emotional outbursts. Moderate and heavy drinkers have shown signs of impaired intelligence, slowed-down reflexes, and difficulty remembering.[8]

Because alcohol is a central nervous system depressant, it slows down the activity of the neurons in the brain, gradually dulling the responses of the brain and nervous system. One or two drinks act as a tranquilizer or relaxant. Additional drinks result in a progressive reduction in central nervous system activity, leading to sleep, general anesthesia, coma, and even death. Moderate amounts of alcohol can have disturbing effects on perception and judgment, including the following:

- *Impaired perceptions.* You're less able to adjust your eyes to bright lights because glare bothers you more. Although you can still hear sounds, you can't distinguish between them or judge their direction well.

- *Dulled smell and taste.* Alcohol itself may cause some vitamin deficiencies, and the poor eating habits of heavy drinkers result in further nutrition problems.

- *Diminished sensation.* You may walk outside without a coat on a freezing winter night and not feel the cold.

- *Altered sense of space.* You may not realize, for instance, that you have been in one place for several hours.

- *Impaired motor skills.* Writing, typing, driving, and other abilities involving your muscles are impaired. This is why law enforcement officers sometimes ask suspected drunk drivers to touch their nose with a finger or to walk a straight line. Drinking large amounts of alcohol impairs reaction time, speed, accuracy, and consistency, as well as judgment.

- *Impaired sexual performance.* While drinking may increase your interest in sex, it may also impair sexual response, especially a man's ability to achieve or maintain an erection. As Shakespeare wrote, "It provokes the desire, but it takes away the performance."

Interaction with Other Drugs

Alcohol can interact with other drugs—prescription and nonprescription, legal and illegal. Of the 100 most frequently prescribed drugs, more than half contain at least one ingredient that interacts adversely with alcohol. Because alcohol and other psychoactive drugs may work on the same areas of the brain, their combination can produce an effect much greater than that expected of either drug by itself. The consequences of this synergistic interaction can be fatal (see Table 15-2). Alcohol is particularly dangerous when combined with depressants and antianxiety medications.

Aspirin—long used to prevent or counter alcohol's effects—may actually enhance its impact by significantly lowering the body's ability to break down alcohol in the stomach. In a study of healthy men between the ages of 30 and 45, volunteers who took two extra-strength aspirin tablets an hour before drinking a glass and a half of wine had a 30% higher BAC than when they drank alcohol alone. This increase could make a difference in impairment for individuals driving cars or operating machinery.

If you want to drink while taking medication, be sure you read the warnings on nonprescription-drug labels or prescription-drug containers; ask your doctor about possible alcohol–drug interactions; and check with your pharmacist if you have any questions about your medications, especially over-the-counter (OTC) products.

Increased Risk of Dying

Alcohol kills. The mortality rate for alcoholics is two and a half times higher that for nonalcoholics of the same age. The leading alcohol-related cause of death is injury, chiefly auto accidents involving a drunk driver. Alcohol is associated with at least half of all traffic fatalities, half of all homicides, and a quarter of all suicides.

The second leading cause of alcohol-related deaths is digestive disease, including *cirrhosis* of the liver, a chronic disease that causes extensive scarring and irreversible damage. In addition, as many as half of patients admitted to hospitals and 15% of those making office visits seek or need medical care because of the direct or indirect effects of alcohol.[9]

TABLE 15-2   INTERACTIONS OF ALCOHOL AND SOME COMMON DRUGS

Drug	Possible effects of interaction
Analgesics (painkillers)	
Narcotic (Codeine, Demerol, Percodan)	Increase in central nervous system depression, possibly leading to respiratory failure and death.
Nonnarcotic (aspirin, Tylenol)	Irritation of stomach, resulting in bleeding, and increased susceptibility to liver damage.
Antabuse	Nausea, vomiting, headache, high blood pressure, and erratic heartbeat.
Antianxiety drugs (Valium, Librium)	Increase in central nervous system depression; decreased alertness and impaired judgment.
Antidepressants	Increase in central nervous system depression; certain antidepressants in combination with red wine could cause a sudden increase in blood pressure.
Antihistamines (Actifed, Dimetap, and other cold medications)	Increase in drowsiness; driving more dangerous.
Antibiotics	Nausea, vomiting, headache; some medications rendered less effective.
Central nervous system stimulants (caffeine, Dexedrine, Ritalin)	Stimulant effects of these drugs may reverse depressant effect of alcohol but do not decrease intoxicating effects of alcohol.
Diuretics (Diuril, Lasix)	Reduction in blood pressure, resulting in dizziness upon rising.
Sedatives (Dalmane, Nembutal, Quaalude)	Increase in central nervous system depression, possibly leading to coma, respiratory failure, and death.

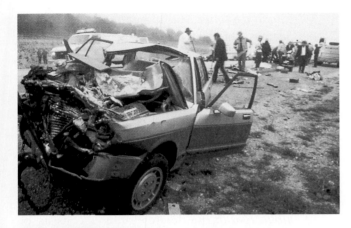

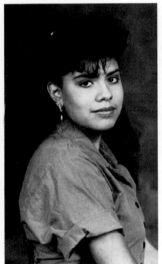

DRUNK DRIVING DOESN'T JUST KILL DRUNK DRIVERS.

Patricia Valencia, killed Nov. 10, 1991 at 2:10am on Hwy. 119, Dumas, TX.

Next time your friend insists on driving drunk, do whatever it takes to stop him.
Because if he kills innocent people, how will you live with yourself?

FRIENDS DON'T LET FRIENDS DRIVE DRUNK.

Driving and drinking don't mix! Alcohol is associated with at least half of all traffic fatalities—to the drunk driver and to others.

Young drinkers—teens and those in their early twenties—are at highest risk of dying from injuries, mostly car accidents. Older drinkers over age 50 face the greatest danger of premature death from cirrhosis of the liver, hepatitis, and other alcohol-linked illnesses.

Drinking in America

According to a survey of 47,485 households sponsored by the NIAAA, about half (52%) of American adults drink.[10] The survey showed little variation among the races with respect to quantity, frequency, and amount of alcohol consumed, although whites were more likely to be classified as daily or nearly daily drinkers than non-whites. A greater percentage of females than males reported a lifetime pattern of infrequent drinking (less than 12 drinks a year).[11] Men and women are most likely to drink between the ages of 21 and 34. Drinking typically declines with age.

The National Council on Alcoholism describes alcohol as the number-one drug problem among the nation's youth, with boys and girls experimenting with alcohol at younger ages than in previous decades. According to NIAAA statistics, the average age at which children take their first drink is now just under 13, and 40% have tasted alcohol by the age of 10. About 30% of teenagers experience negative consequences of alcohol abuse, including alcohol-related accidents, arrests, or impaired health or school performance.[12]

Why People Drink

The most common reason why people drink alcohol is to relax. Because it depresses the central nervous system, alcohol can make people feel less tense. Other motivations for drinking include the following:

- *Celebration.* Unless alcohol use violates family, ethnic, or religious values, people raise their glasses together on life's important occasions—births, graduations, weddings, promotions.

- *Friendship.* When friends visit, you may have a drink, or you may meet them somewhere "for a drink." Young people are much more likely to experiment with alcohol if their friends drink.[13]

- *Social ease.* When we use alcohol, we may seem bolder, wittier, sexier. At the same time, the people drinking with us become more relaxed and seem to enjoy our company more. Because alcohol lowers inhibitions, some people see it as a prelude to seduction.

- *Self-medication.* Like other drugs, alcohol may be the means some people use to treat—or escape from— painful feelings or bad moods.

- *Role models.* Athletes, some of the most admired celebrities in our country, have a long history of appearing in commercials for alcohol. Many advertisements feature glamorous women holding or sipping alcoholic beverages.

- *Advertising.* Brewers and beer distributors spend $15–$20 million a year promoting their products to college students. Their message: If you want to have fun, have a drink. Adolescents may be especially responsive to such sales pitches. In one survey, young men who recalled noticing more alcohol advertisements at age 15 drank more at 18.[14] Nearly two dozen national groups, including the American Medical Association, have petitioned the Federal Trade Commission to ban alcohol advertisements that link drinking to risky activities (such as driving, water skiing, and sky-diving) and that target youth.

Patterns of Alcohol Use

Because of concern about alcohol's health effects, increasing numbers of Americans are choosing not to drink at all. (See Pulsepoints: "Ten Steps to Responsible Drinking.") With alcohol consumption in the United States at its lowest level in 30 years, nonalcoholic beverages have grown in popularity. They appeal to drivers, boaters, pregnant women, individuals with health problems that could worsen with alcohol, those who are older and can't tolerate alcohol, anyone taking medicines that interact with alcohol (including antibiotics, antidepressants, and muscle relaxers), and everyone interested in limiting alcohol intake. Under federal law, these drinks can contain some alcohol, but a much smaller amount than regular beer or wine. Nonalcoholic beers and wines on the market also are lower in calories than alcoholic varieties.

Among the 52% of adults who drink, fewer than 10% ever develop drinking problems. They also vary greatly in how much and how often they drink. Although there are no standard definitions for drinking patterns, the following are generally recognized as most common:

- *Light drinking.* This is defined as having fewer than three alcoholic drinks a week. (As noted in Figure 15-1, a drink equals 1 ounce of spirits, a 4-ounce glass of table wine, or a 12-ounce can of beer, each of which contains approximately 12 grams of absolute alcohol.)

- *Infrequent drinking.* This term refers to frequency, not quantity. Infrequent drinkers have less than one drink a month but drink at least once a year. Some "low maximum" infrequent drinkers drink one to three times a month but never have five or more drinks at a sitting. "High maximum" infrequent drinkers do not drink more often, but they occasionally have five or more drinks at a sitting.

- *Moderate drinking.* Specialists in addiction research use different standards for defining moderation. According to a 1995 report in the *American Journal of Public Health*, moderate drinking consists of "drinking at levels that do not interfere with or threaten one's health, social relationships, daily obligations, or safety and the safety of others." According to the report, moderate drinking is defined as having an upper limit of four standard drinks on any day, on no more than three days a week. Women are advised to set their upper limit at three drinks a day, on no more than three days a week.[15]

- *Social drinking.* This term—used by laypeople rather than health-care professionals or researchers—refers to drinking patterns that are accepted by friends and peers. If your friends drink only on special occasions, you may think that having one glass of wine at a party is social drinking. On the other hand, if the people you socialize with drink regularly and heavily, you may mistakenly

Pulsepoints

Ten Steps to Responsible Drinking

1. Don't drink alone. Cultivate friendships with nondrinkers and responsible moderate drinkers.

2. Don't use alcohol as a medicine. Rather than reaching for a drink to put you to sleep, help you relax, or relieve tension, develop alternative means of unwinding, such as exercise, meditation, or listening to music.

3. Develop a party plan. Set a limit on how many drinks you'll have before you go out—and stick to it.

4. Alternate alcoholic and nonalcoholic drinks. At a social occasion, have a nonalcoholic beverage to quench your thirst.

5. Drink slowly. Never have more than one drink an hour.

6. Eat before and while drinking. Choose foods high in protein (cheese, meat, eggs, or milk) rather than salty foods, like peanuts or chips, that increase thirst.

7. Be wary of mixed drinks. Fizzy mixers, like club soda and ginger ale, speed alcohol to the blood and brain.

8. Don't make drinking the primary focus of any get-together. Cultivate other interests and activities that you can enjoy on your own or with friends.

9. Learn to say no. A simple "Thank you, but I've had enough" will do.

10. Stay safe. During or after drinking, avoid any tasks, including driving, that could be affected by alcohol.

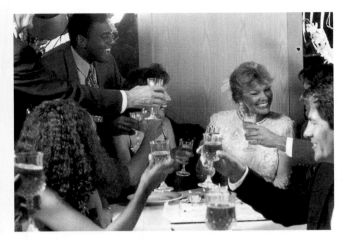

Alcohol can be part of many enjoyable social situations, as long as individuals know when to say "No more." Increasingly, many people are substituting nonalcoholic drinks.

think that having a six-pack of beer every night is social drinking.

- *Problem drinking.* Any kind of drinking that interferes with a major aspect of life, such as sleep, energy, family relationships, health, or safety, qualifies as problem drinking. Some of the problems associated with drinking—getting into fights, unwanted sexual activity, car accidents—are obvious. Others, such as alcohol-related damage to the digestive system, heart, liver or brain, may remain invisible for years.

- *Binge drinking.* When applied to alcohol, a binge consists of having five or more drinks at a single sitting for a man or four drinks at a single sitting for a woman. Binge drinking is most common among young men, especially those who are single, separated, or divorced, who drink beer, or who concentrate most of their drinking on weekends. Bingeing has been linked to a substantially increased risk of serious injury—especially from automobile accidents—as well as higher rates of unsafe sex, assault, and aggressive behavior. As discussed below, binge drinking is common in college.[16]

Drinking on Campus

Colleges today have been described as among the nation's "most alcohol-drenched institutions." Every year America's 12 million undergraduates drink 4 billion cans of beer, averaging 55 six-packs apiece, and spending $446 on alcoholic beverages—more than they spend on soft drinks and textbooks combined.[17]

Despite these figures, fewer students drink than in the past. In 1980, 9.5% of college students nationwide said they abstained from alcohol; by 1996, 17% did. According to the University of Michigan's Institute for Social Research, the percentage of students reported drinking daily also declined: from 6.5% in 1980 to 3.2%—as did those reporting binge drinking—from 44% to 38%. The National College Health Risk Behavior Survey, as shown in Campus Focus: "College Students and Alcohol Use" found that 6.6% of men and 2.2% of women reported "frequent" alcohol use, while a much higher percentage—43.8% of men and 27% of women—reported episodic heavy drinking.[18]

Why College Students Drink

Most college students drink for the same reasons undergraduates have always turned to alcohol. Away from home, often for the first time, many are both excited by and apprehensive about their newfound independence. When new pressures seem overwhelming, when they feel awkward or insecure, when they just want to let loose and have a good time, they reach for a drink.

Some students, however, seem especially vulnerable to problem drinking. In one new study, undergraduates who felt unable to cope with bad moods and had low expectations of their ability to handle emotional or other difficulties were more prone to having problems with alcohol. Rather than rely on coping strategies that would enable them to meet problems head on, they turned to alcohol.[19]

Students may be especially vulnerable to dangerous drinking in their freshman year as they struggle to adapt to an often bewildering new world. In a study of freshmen at a medium-sized state university and at a small, predominantly African-American university who were nondrinkers as high school seniors, almost half (46.5%) started to drink in college. They were less likely to do so if they had friends who discouraged them from drinking.

Other studies have also linked alcohol consumption with where students live on campus and what they perceive as the norm for acceptable drinking. Members of sororities and fraternities rated all drinking norms as more extreme and perceived fraternity drinking as particularly heavy—but these beliefs existed even before college.

According to a 1997 report, fraternity leaders are among the heaviest drinkers and most out-of-control partygoers. This survey found extensive drinking among all fraternity members, but the leaders showed the highest incidence of heavy drinking and bingeing.

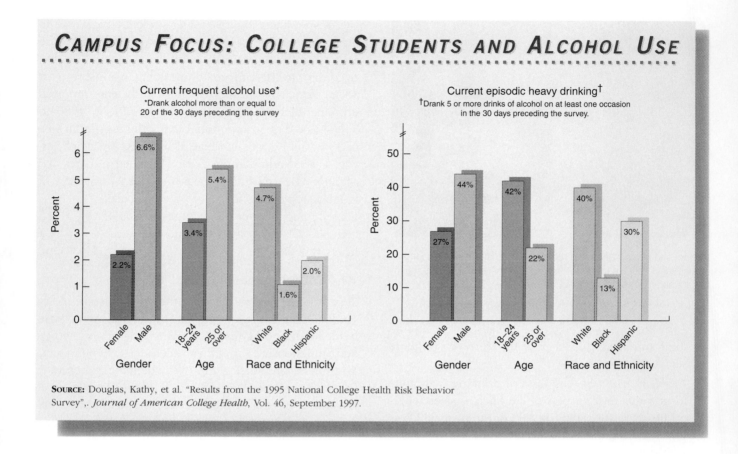

CAMPUS FOCUS: COLLEGE STUDENTS AND ALCOHOL USE

Current frequent alcohol use*
*Drank alcohol more than or equal to 20 of the 30 days preceding the survey

Current episodic heavy drinking†
†Drank 5 or more drinks of alcohol on at least one occasion in the 30 days preceding the survey.

SOURCE: Douglas, Kathy, et al. "Results from the 1995 National College Health Risk Behavior Survey",. *Journal of American College Health*, Vol. 46, September 1997.

Nearly 74% said they had engaged in binge drinking at some time in the past two weeks. The overall binge-drinking rate among fraternity brothers was 58%, compared with 42% among male students who did not belong to fraternities.[20] There was a similar trend in sororities: 54.6% of the leaders reported a binge-drinking episode in the last two weeks, compared with 45.5% of members and 25.9% of women not involved with sororities. Fraternity and sorority leaders also were more likely than those not in Greek houses to have had alcohol-related problems in the previous year, including blackouts and fights.

The most dramatic increases in college drinking have been among women: 86% of female undergraduates say they drink; 37%—compared with only 14% 1977—say they get drunk one to three times in a month. While men tend to drink as a way of partying, women on campus may drink for other reasons. Psychologists have theorized that college women may drink as a way of being with and relating to others, seeking acceptance from peers, and numbing the pain that comes from relationships that don't work.[21]

Yet women generally are not as casual about the risks of drinking as are men. In a 1994 survey of 177

men and 280 women, female students were more likely to assign a designated driver and to prevent someone from drinking and driving. They also were less likely to say it is socially acceptable to be intoxicated occasionally and to believe that most drinkers do not suffer health problems.[22]

Among both men and women, those with alcoholic parents and dysfunctional families are at greater risk of substance abuse. By some estimates, one of five college students comes from an alcoholic home and may be at increased risk of developing a drinking problem.[23]

Dangerous Drinking

Binge drinking has emerged as a serious threat to the health and lives of college students (see Personal Voices: "What Binge Drinking Can Do to You"). In a single month—November 1997—five college students died in alcohol-related accidents in the state of Virginia alone. At the University of Virginia, a survey found that 25% of students had participated in binge drinking three or more times in the previous two weeks.[24]

College students who binge on alcohol face other dangers: They are seven to ten times more likely to engage in unplanned or unprotected sex, to have problems with campus police, or to get hurt. Although female students drink less and less dangerously than men, female binge drinkers are more likely to engage in sexual activity, including intercourse, under the influence of alcohol than women who never binge. Binge-drinking women also report engaging in sexual behaviors when they would otherwise not have and not practicing safe sex, thereby putting themselves at greater risk. Binge drinkers create problems, not just for themselves, but for others (see Table 15-3). According to one survey, at schools where drinking was most popular, two-thirds of students reported having their sleep or studies interrupted by drunken students; more than half had been forced to care for a drunk friend; and at least a fourth had suffered an unwanted sexual advance.[25]

The American College Health Association estimates that drinking accounts for almost two-thirds of all violence on campus and about one-third of all emotional and academic problems among students. Alcohol may play a role in 90% of rapes and sexual assaults.[26] Drinking also claims the lives of many students each year, sometimes because of car accidents, and sometimes because of drinking games, in which individuals consume dangerously large quantities of alcohol.

Even though students report concern about alcohol, few seek counseling or other services.[27] Colleges are working to improve screening for alcohol problems

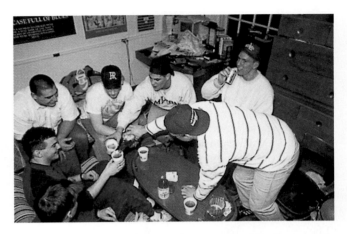

Binge drinkers can get into—and cause—trouble. Dangerously large amounts of alcohol can cause death, and heavy party drinking often results in violence.

among students and to educate students about responsible drinking.[28] At some schools, underage students caught drinking must attend a course that introduces the concepts of abstinence and controlled drinking.[29]

Students also are taking steps to ban drunkenness on campus. In addition, there's been an increase in on-campus chapters of national support groups such as AA, Al-Anon, Adult Children of Alcoholics, and a peer-education program called BACCHUS: Boost Alcohol Consciousness Concerning the Health of University Students.

TABLE 15-3 THE TROUBLES THAT "FREQUENT BINGE DRINKERS" CREATE FOR...

Themselves[1]	(% of those surveyed who admitted having had the problem)	And Others[2]	(% of those surveyed who had been affected)
Missed a class	61%	Had study or sleep interrupted	68%
Forgot where they were or what they did	54%	Had to care for drunken student	54%
Engaged in unplanned sex	41%	Been insulted or humiliated	34%
Got hurt	23%	Experienced unwanted sexual advances	26%
Had unprotected sex	22%	Had serious argument	20%
Damaged property	22%	Had property damaged	15%
Got into trouble withcampus or local police	11%	Been pushed or assaulted	13%
Had five or more alcohol-related problems in school year	47%	Had at least one of the above problems	87%

[1] "Frequent binge drinkers" were defined as those who had had at least four or five drinks at one time on at least three occasions in the previous two weeks.

[2] These figures are from colleges where at least 50% of students are binge drinkers.

SOURCE: Survey of 140 U.S. colleges by the Harvard School of Public Health.

Personal Voices What Binge Drinking Can Do to You

Here they were, the dead boy's family, parked in pretty much the same spot, doing some of the same things they did less than a month ago, only in reverse order. An enormous sadness created an automatic shield around them, too, as they carried the contents of his room down the steps and out the door of the old stone fraternity house on the Fenway in Boston.

All the clothes, books and pictures belonged to Scott Krueger. He arrived a few weeks ago in order to begin freshman year at MIT; arrived as bright and attractive as they come, ready and quite able to take his initial step away from home and right into a life that offered spectacular opportunity.

Too bad MIT and other institutions—academic, media, and corporate—do not view a six-pack or a pint of vodka as posing the same potentially lethal threat to life as a cigarette. The college is littered with no smoking signs, but they require an assembly before they can compose a sentence saying, "Get caught drinking and there will be no diploma."

Yet in the course of a normal day, alcohol absolutely ruins more American families and destroys more individual lives than a whole warehouse of filter-tips. However, because Jim Beam and Coors Lite employ better marketing experts and ad agencies, we read more editorials about lung cancer than about cirrhosis.

Now, on a pleasant fall weekend, we have an elite set of students, truly gifted people, using binge drinking as a badge of admission to some fraternity. What kind of "education" program do you concoct for people who scored 1,400 on their college boards and got into MIT? Is there a parent on this Earth tossing and turning because their son or daughter might smoke a cigarette on a Saturday night? But how many suffer from sleep deprivation hoping against hope that their child isn't behind the wheel, drunk, racing home to beat a curfew?

There aren't enough fingers to point at who caused the tragic events leading toward Scott Krueger's death: Who sold the booze? Who purchased it? Who moved his body? Who, if anyone, forced him to drink and drink and then drink some more?

Go to almost any city neighborhood, pause by nearly any corner, or park in the smallest of towns, and you will witness a huge national problem: Teenagers thinking they can act beyond their years by sneaking a couple of beers.

In the lineup of dark nightmares any parent thinks possible to befall a child—automobile crashes, robbery victim—death by drinking isn't even on the list. But as Scott Krueger's family packed his things for the long trip back out the Mass Pike to New York state, they drove off with the agonizing knowledge that their son was killed by alcohol and died within a culture that glibly assumes smoking is the only lethal social evil around.

N.Y. Times Service

Mike Barnicle is a Boston Globe columnist.
SOURCE: From *San Francisco Chronicle*, October 6, 1997.

Women and Alcohol

About half of women drink: of these, 45% are light drinkers; 3%, moderate drinkers; 2%, heavy drinkers; and 21%, binge drinkers.[30] According to the NIAAA, almost 4 million women suffer from alcohol abuse or dependence. But women who drink have different risk factors, potential dangers, and drinking patterns than men.

Why Women Drink

In the past, most people, including physicians and therapists, assumed that women who drank heavily did so primarily for social and psychological reasons—because they were lonely, isolated, broken-hearted. Many of these assumptions have proven to be false. The following are more likely to lead to drinking problems in women.

- *Inherited susceptibility.* In women, as in men, genetics account for 50% to 60% of a person's vulnerability to a serious drinking problem. But while heredity

increases the risk of alcoholism, life circumstances also play an important role in determining whether young women will have drinking problems. Female alcoholics are more likely than males to have a parent who abused drugs or alcohol, who had psychiatric problems, or who attempted suicide.[31]

- *Childhood traumas.* Female alcoholics often report that they were physically or sexually abused as children or suffered great distress because of poverty or a parent's death. In one 1997 study, 24% of women with alcohol problems reported abuse in childhood.

- *Depression.* "At all stages over the life span, female problem drinking is linked to depression," Edith Gomberg reports. Women are more likely than men to be depressed prior to drinking and to suffer from both depression and a drinking problem at the same time.

- *Relationship issues.* Single, separated, or divorced women drink both more and more often than married women; women with live-in male partners have

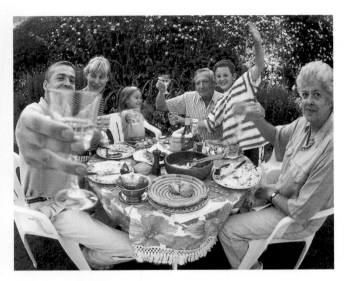

Genetics as well as life experience contribute to a woman's vulnerability to heavy drinking and alcohol dependence. Risk factors and drinking patterns are different for women and men.

the highest rates of drinking problems. "Functioning women alcoholics may be very successful in other areas of their lives but have problems in their relationships," says Sharon Wilsnack, Ph.D., a professor at the University of North Dakota School of Medicine who studied the drinking habits of more than 1,100 women over ten years.[32] Women involved with heavy drinkers are at risk of drinking heavily themselves, at least as long as the relationship continues.

- *Employment.* Women who work outside the home are less likely to become problem drinkers or alcoholics than those without paying jobs. The one exception: women in occupations still dominated by men, such as engineering, science, law enforcement and top corporate management. "Often women in these fields drink as a way of fitting in," observes Wilsnack. "Drinking takes on symbolic value. It's a way of signalling power, equality, status."

- *A lack or loss of roles.* Women of all ages, regardless of marital or employment status, tend to drink more and lean on alcohol when they lose a valued role, for example, when they're laid off from a job or their marriage ends in divorce.

- *Use of alcohol to self-medicate.* "In our society, women are permitted to use medication, so they feel it's permissible to use alcohol as if it were a medicine," observes Gomberg. "As long as they're taking it for a reason, it seems acceptable to them, even if they're drifting into a drinking problem."

Alcohol's Effects on Women

Problems directly related to a woman's alcohol use range from the consequences of risky sexual behavior after alcohol consumption (such as unwanted pregnancy or STDs) to severe physiological problems related to fertility and pregnancy.[33] Because they have far smaller quantities of a protective enzyme in the stomach to break down alcohol before it's absorbed into the bloodstream, women absorb about 30% more alcohol into their bloodstream than men do. The alcohol travels through the blood to the brain, so women become intoxicated much more quickly. And because there's more alcohol in the bloodstream to break down, the liver may also be adversely affected. In alcoholic women, the stomach seems to stop digesting alcohol completely, which may explain why women alcoholics are more likely to suffer liver damage than are men.

Among the other health dangers that alcohol holds for women are:

- *Gynecologic problems.* Moderate to heavy drinking may contribute to infertility, menstrual problems, sexual dysfunction, and premenstrual syndrome.[34]

- *Pregnancy and fetal alcohol syndrome (FAS).* When a woman drinks during pregnancy, her unborn child drinks, too. According to CDC estimates, more than 8000 alcohol-damaged babies are born every year. One out of every 750 newborns has a cluster of physical and mental defects called **fetal alcohol syndrome (FAS)**: small head, abnormal facial features (see Figure 15-4), jitters, poor muscle tone, sleep disorders, sluggish motor development, failure to thrive, short stature, delayed speech, mental retardation, or hyperactivity. Many more babies suffer **fetal alcohol effects (FAE)**—low birth weight, irritability as newborns, and permanent mental impairment—as a result of their mothers' alcohol consumption. (See Chapter 10 for further discussion of these conditions.)

  Labels on alcoholic beverages have had a proven but modest effect on reducing drinking in pregnancy, while community-based education efforts have been much more effective. Drug and alcohol abuse also can affect the quality of a woman's mothering.[35]

- *Breast cancer.* Numerous studies have suggested an increased risk of breast cancer among women who drink, and many physicians feel that those at high risk for breast cancer should stop, or at least reduce, their consumption of alcohol. (See Chapter 13 for more information on breast cancer risks.)

- *Osteoporosis.* As women become older, their risk of

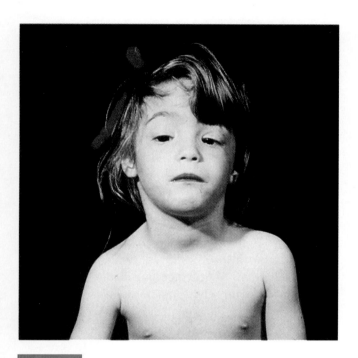

Figure 15-4

A child with fetal alcohol syndrome (FAS) has distinctive facial characteristics that vary with the severity of the disease, including droopy eyelids, a thin upper lip, and a wide space between the nose and upper lip.

osteoporosis, a condition characterized by calcium loss and bone thinning, increases. Alcohol can block the absorption of many nutrients, including calcium, and heavy drinking may worsen the deterioration of bone tissue (see Chapter 18).

- *Heart disease.* Women who are very heavy drinkers are more at risk of developing irreversible heart disease than are men who drink even more. In a study published in the *Journal of the American Medical Association* in 1995, a 121-pound woman who drank about 9 ounces of 86-proof liquor or about a liter of wine a day for 20 years put herself at risk for cardiomyopathy—a disease relatively uncommon among women in general.[36]

Alcohol Treatments for Women

Women who abuse alcohol also face a special burden: intense social disapproval. Many become cross-addicted to prescription medicines, or they develop eating disorders or sexual dysfunctions. Women often don't get the same care men do, frequently because of financial limitations and childcare responsibilities. Also, women are more likely to blame their symptoms on depression or anxiety, whereas men attribute them directly to alcohol.

As a result, women often obtain treatment later in the course of their illness, at a point when their problems are more severe. Increasingly, prevention programs are targeting high-risk women to recognize alcohol problems early and to tackle underlying problems, such as depression and low self-esteem.[37]

One of the most effective programs for women is Women for Sobriety, founded in 1975 by sociologist Jean Kirkpatrick, Ph.D. Its meetings focus on building self-esteem, self-confidence, and responsibility. "AA was started by men, and its message is very disempowering for women," says Kirkpatrick. "We view members as competent women who are struggling with issues that all women must face. Women don't need to recall the painful process of becoming alcoholics. They need to put the past behind them and move on, upward and onward." (See "Your Health Directory" at the back of this book.)[38]

Drinking and Driving

Drunk driving is the most frequently committed crime in the United States. In the last two decades, families of the victims of drunk drivers have organized to change the way America treats its drunk drivers. Because of the efforts of MADD (Mothers Against Drunk Driving), SADD (Students Against Driving Drunk), and other lobbying groups, cities, counties, and states are cracking down on drivers who drink. Since courts have held bars liable for the consequences of allowing drunk customers to drive, many bars and restaurants have joined the campaign against drunk driving. (There's even a group called Bartenders Against Drunk Driving, or BADD.) Many communities also provide free rides home on holidays and weekends for people who've had too much to drink.

To keep drunk drivers off the road, many cities have set up checkpoints, where they stop automobiles and inspect the drivers for intoxication. The U.S. Supreme Court has ruled that a driver's refusal to submit to a blood-alcohol concentration test at such checkpoints or at any other time can be used as evidence to prosecute him or her for drunk driving. An increasing number of states have toughened their enforcement of drunk-driving penalties. Some suspend a driver's license for several months for a first offense; repeat offenders can lose their licenses for a year or more.

These tougher policies seem to be working. Drunken-driving deaths have declined 31% since 1982.[39] However, they still account for more than 40% of automobile fatalities. According to studies by the National Highway Safety Administration, chronic drunk drivers continue to be a major safety threat. People with prior convictions for drunk driving represent fewer than 2% of all adults, yet they cause up to 60% of all alcohol-related deaths and injuries on U.S. roads.[40]

The National Commission Against Drunk Driving defines chronic drunk drivers as individuals who frequently drive with blood-alcohol levels of 0.15 or higher. These drivers tend to be single men between the ages of 25 and 45, with high school educations or less, blue-collar jobs, and a preference for beer rather than wine or hard liquor. They typically drive intoxicated four times a week, or 200 times a year.[41]

Strategies for Prevention

How to Prevent Drunk Driving

✔ When going out in a group, always designate one person who won't drink at all to serve as the driver.

✔ Never get behind the wheel if you've had more than two drinks within two hours, especially if you haven't eaten.

✔ Never let intoxicated friends drive home. Call a taxi, drive them yourself, or arrange for them to spend the night in a safe place.

Alcohol-Related Problems

The misuse and abuse of alcohol can lead to a range of problems, from intoxication to problem drinking to alcohol dependence or abuse. "For years, the United States lagged behind other countries in recognizing the spectrum of alcohol-related problems," says Frederick Bruhnsen, manager of DrinkWise at the University of Michigan, an innovative treatment program for problem drinkers. "Of all the people who drink, 20 to 25 percent develop some problem at some point. About four to five percent develop problems so severe as to be termed *alcoholic.*"[42]

By the simplest definition, problem drinking is the use of alcohol in any way that creates difficulties or potential difficulties or health risks for an individual. Like alcoholics, problem drinkers are individuals whose lives are in some way impaired by their drinking. The only difference is one of degree. Alcohol becomes a problem, and a person becomes an alcoholic, when the drinker can't "take it or leave it." He or she spends more and more time anticipating the next drink, planning when and where to get it, buying and hiding alcohol, and covering up secret drinking. Problem drinking affects more than the individual. In a study of eight nations, the higher the per-capita alcohol consumption, the higher the divorce rate.[43]

Alcohol abuse, as defined by the American Psychiatric Association's *Diagnostic and Statistical Manual of Mental Disorders,* 4th edition *(DSM-IV)*, involves continued use of alcohol despite awareness of social, occupational, psychological, or physical problems related to drinking, or drinking in dangerous ways or situations (before driving, for instance). A diagnosis of alcohol abuse is based on one or more of the following occurring at any time during a 12-month period:

- Recurrent alcohol abuse resulting in a failure to fulfill major role obligations at work, school, or home (such as missing work or school).

- Recurrent alcohol abuse in situations in which it is physically hazardous (such as before driving).

- Recurrent alcohol-related legal problems (such as drunk-driving arrests).

- Continued alcohol use despite persistent or recurring social or interpersonal problems caused or exacerbated by alcohol (such as fighting while drunk).[44]

Alcohol dependence is a separate disorder, in which individuals develop a strong craving for alcohol because it produces pleasurable feelings or relieves stress or anxiety. Over time they experience physiological changes that lead to *tolerance* of its effects; this means that they must consume larger and larger amounts to achieve intoxication. If they abruptly stop drinking, they suffer *withdrawal,* a state of acute physical and psychological discomfort. A diagnosis of alcohol dependence is based on three or more of the following symptoms occurring during any 12-month period:

- Tolerance, as defined by either a need for markedly increased amounts of alcohol to achieve intoxication or desired effect, or a markedly diminished effect with continued drinking of the same amount of alcohol as in the past.

- Withdrawal, as manifested by characteristic symptoms, including at least two of the following: sweating, rapid pulse, or other signs of autonomic hyperactivity; increased hand tremor; insomnia; nausea or vomiting; temporary hallucinations or illusions; physical agitation or restlessness; anxiety; or grand mal seizures; or

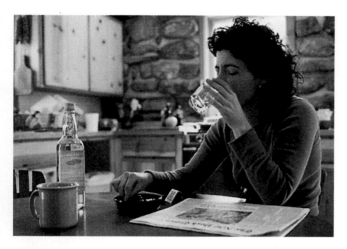

Alcohol dependence may spring from the perception that alcohol relieves stress and anxiety, or creates a pleasant feeling. Chronic drinking—especially daytime drinking and drinking alone—can be a sign of serious problems, even though the drinker may otherwise appear to be in control.

- Drinking to avoid or relieve these symptoms.
- Consuming larger amounts of alcohol, or over a longer period than was intended.
- Persistent desire or unsuccessful efforts to cut down or control drinking.
- A great deal of time spent in activities necessary to obtain alcohol, drink it, or recover from its effects.
- Important social, occupational, or recreational activities given up or reduced because of alcohol use.
- Continued alcohol use despite knowledge that alcohol is likely to cause or exacerbate a persistent or recurring physical or psychological problem.[45]

Alcoholism, as defined by the National Council on Alcoholism and Drug Dependence and the American Society of Addiction, is a primary, chronic disease in which genetic, psychosocial, and environmental factors influence its development and manifestations. The disease is often progressive and fatal. Its characteristics include impaired control of drinking, a preoccupation with alcohol, continued use of alcohol despite adverse consequences, and distorted thinking, most notably denial. Like other diseases, alcoholism is not simply a matter of insufficient willpower, but a complex problem that causes many symptoms, can have serious consequences, yet can improve with treatment.

A lack of obvious signs of alcoholism can be deceiving. If a person doesn't drink in the morning but feels that he or she must always have a drink at a certain time of the day, that may represent loss of control. If a person never drinks alone but always drinks socially with others,

that can camouflage loss of control. If a person is holding a job or taking care of the family, he or she may still spend every waking hour thinking about that first drink at the end of the day (preoccupation).

How Common Are Alcohol-Related Problems?

According to the NIAAA, 9% of adults meet the criteria for alcohol abuse or dependence. White males 18 to 29 years old have 2.4 times greater prevalence of abuse and dependence than nonwhites. Among those over age 64, nonwhites have a prevalence rate of abuse and dependence 28.4% higher than whites.[46]

Probably fewer than 5% of alcoholics and problem drinkers are "skid-row drunks." The other 95% are all around us, every day. (See Self-Survey: "Do You Have a Drinking Problem?") Alcoholism generally first appears between the ages of 20 and 40, although even children and young teenagers can become alcoholics. It takes 5 to 15 years of heavy drinking for an adult to become alcoholic, but just 6 to 18 months for an adolescent to develop the disease.

According to the National Comorbidity Survey, published in 1995, 23.5% of Americans may become dependent on or abuse alcohol in the course of a lifetime, while 9.7% experience these disorders in the course of a year. At all ages, men are two to five times more likely than women to abuse alcohol. In men, drinking usually starts in the late teens or twenties. Women tend to start drinking at a later age, are less likely to stop without help, and often have a history of depression.[47]

What Causes Alcohol Dependence and Abuse

Although the exact cause of alcohol dependence and abuse is not known, certain factors—including biochemical imbalances in the brain, heredity, cultural acceptability, and stress—all seem to play a role. They include the following:

- *Genetics.* Scientists who are working toward mapping the genes responsible for addictive disorders have not yet been able to identify conclusively a specific gene that puts people at risk for alcoholism. However, epidemiological studies have shown evidence of heredity's role. An identical twin of an alcoholic is twice as likely as a fraternal twin to have an alcohol-related disorder. The incidence of alcoholism is four times higher among the sons of Caucasian alcoholic fathers, regardless of whether they grow up with their biological or adoptive parents. The sons of alcoholic fathers have characteristic changes in brain wave activity.

- *Stress and traumatic experiences.* Many people start drinking heavily as a way of coping with psychological problems. About half of all individuals who abuse or are dependent on alcohol also have another mental disorder. Alcohol often is linked with depressive and anxiety disorders. Men and women with these problems may start drinking in an attempt to alleviate their anxiety or depression.

- *Parental alcoholism.* According to researchers, alcoholism is four to five times more common among the children of alcoholics, who may be influenced by the behavior they see in their parents. The sons and daughters of alcoholics share certain characteristics, including early onset of problem drinking with severe social consequences, an unstable family, poor academic and social performance in school, and antisocial behavior.

- *Drug abuse.* Alcoholism is also associated with the abuse of other psychoactive drugs, including marijuana, cocaine, heroin, amphetamines, and various antianxiety medications. Adults under age 30 and adolescents are most likely to use alcohol plus several drugs of abuse, such as marijuana and cocaine. Middle-aged men and women are more likely to combine alcohol with benzodiazepines, such as antianxiety medications or sleeping pills, which may be prescribed for them by a physician. Whatever the reason they start, some people keep drinking out of habit. Once they develop physical tolerance and dependence—the two hallmarks of addiction—they may not be able to stop drinking on their own.

Types of Alcoholism

Mental health professionals have developed different theoretical models to explain alcoholism. Although these models are used mainly by researchers and clinicians, they offer individuals with drinking problems and those close to them some insight into various personality and drinking patterns.

According to one long-established model, there are two primary types of alcoholics. *Type I,* or milieu-limited, alcoholics generally start heavy drinking, often in response to setbacks, losses, or other external circumstances, after age 25. They can abstain for long periods of time and frequently feel loss of control, guilt, and fear about their alcoholism. They also have characteristic personality traits: they tend to be anxious, shy, pessimistic, sentimental, emotionally dependent, rigid, reflective, and slow to anger. Because alcohol reduces their anxiety level, it serves as a positive reinforcer for continued use and contributes to the development of alcohol dependence.

Type II alcoholics are close relatives of an alcoholic male and become heavy drinkers before age 25. They drink regardless of what is going on in their lives; have frequent fights and arrests; and do not usually experience guilt, fear, or loss of control over their drinking. Unlike Type I alcoholics, they are impulsive and aggressive risk-takers, curious, excitable, quick-tempered, optimistic, and independent. Alcohol reinforces their feelings of euphoria and pleasant excitement. Often they abuse drugs as well as alcohol.

Newer research on male and female alcoholics classifies alcoholics as *Type A* or *Type B.* Type A alcoholism is a milder form, characterized by onset later in life, fewer childhood risk factors, less severe dependence, fewer alcohol-related physical and social consequences, fewer symptoms of other mental disorders, and less interference with work and family. Type B alcoholism is linked with childhood and familial risk factors, begins at an earlier age, involves more severe dependence and abuse of other substances, leads to more serious consequences, and often occurs along with other mental disorders. Type B alcoholics are younger, more inclined to experiment with other drugs and are more anxious, and of lower occupational status than Type A alcoholics.

Medical Complications of Alcohol Abuse and Dependence

Excessive alcohol use adversely affects virtually every organ system in the body, including the brain, the digestive tract, the heart, muscles, blood, and hormones. In addition, because alcohol interacts with many drugs, it can increase the risk of potentially lethal overdoses and harmful interactions. Among the major risks and complications are:

- *Liver disease.* Because the liver is the organ that breaks down and metabolizes alcohol, it is especially vulnerable to its effects. Chronic heavy drinking can lead to alcoholic hepatitis (inflammation and destruction of liver cells) and, in the 15% of people who continue drinking beyond this stage, cirrhosis (irreversible scarring and destruction of liver cells). (See Figure 15-5.) The liver eventually may fail completely, resulting in coma and death.

- *Cardiovascular system.* Heavy drinking can weaken the heart muscle (causing cardiac myopathy), elevate blood pressure, and increase the risk of stroke. The combined use of alcohol and tobacco, or heavy drinking greatly increases the likelihood of damage to the heart.

- *Cancer.* Heavy alcohol use may contribute to cancer of the liver, stomach, and colon, as well as malignant melanoma, a deadly form of skin cancer. Alcohol, in combination with tobacco use, also increases the risk of cancer of the mouth, tongue, larynx, and esophagus. Several major studies have implicated alcohol as a possible risk factor in breast cancer, particularly in young women, although the degree of danger remains unclear.

- *Brain damage.* Chronic brain damage resulting from alcohol consumption is second only to Alzheimer's disease as a cause of cognitive deterioration in adults. Long-term heavy drinkers may suffer memory losses, be unable to think abstractly or recall names of common objects, and not be able to follow simple instructions. Further cognitive deterioration can be stopped if drinking stops.

- *Vitamin deficiencies.* Alcoholics often tend to have very poor nutrition. Alcoholism is associated with vitamin deficiencies, especially of thiamine (B_{12}), which may be responsible for certain diseases of the neurological, digestive, muscular, and cardiovascular systems. Lack of thiamine, caused by alcoholism, may result in Wernicke's syndrome, a serious disease characterized by a "clouding" of consciousness and paralysis of eye nerves. Korsakoff's syndrome, a rare form of amnesia caused by alcohol-associated thiamine deficiency, is characterized by disorientation, memory failure, confabulation, and hallucinations, and can be disabling enough to require lifelong custodial care.

- *Digestive problems.* Alcohol triggers the secretion of acids in the stomach, which irritate the mucous lining and cause gastritis. Chronic drinking may result in peptic ulcers (breaks in the stomach lining) and bleeding from the stomach lining.

- *Reproductive and sexual dysfunction.* Alcohol interferes with male sexual function and fertility through direct effects on testosterone and the testicles. In half of alcoholic men, increased levels of female hormones lead to breast enlargement and a feminine pubic hair pattern. Damage to the nerves in the penis by heavy drinking can lead to impotence.[48] In women who drink heavily, a drop in female hormone production may cause menstrual irregularity and infertility.

- *Fetal alcohol syndrome.* The risk of this condition, discussed earlier in the chapter, is greatest if a mother-to-be drinks 3 ounces or more of pure alcohol (the equivalent of six or seven cocktails) a day. Consumption of lower quantities of alcohol can lead to fetal alcohol effects, including low birth weight, irritability in a newborn, and permanent mental impairment. Because no one knows how much—if any—alcohol is safe during pregnancy, the National Institute of Alcohol Abuse and Alcoholism recommends that pregnant women not drink at all.[49]

- *Accidents and injuries.* Alcohol may contribute to almost half of the deaths caused by car accidents, burns, falls, and choking. Nearly half of those convicted and jailed for criminal acts committed these crimes while under the influence of alcohol.

- *Higher mortality.* The mortality rate for alcoholics is two to three times higher than that for nonalcoholics of the same age. The leading alcohol-related cause of death is injury, chiefly in auto accidents involving a drunk driver. The second leading cause of alcohol-related deaths is digestive disease, most notably cirrhosis of the liver. In addition, alcohol plays a role in about 30% of all suicides. Alcoholics who attempt suicide may have other risk factors, including major depression, poor social support, serious medical illness, and unemployment.

- *Withdrawal dangers.* Withdrawal can be life-threatening when accompanied by medical problems, such as grand mal seizures, pneumonia, liver failure, or gastrointestinal bleeding.

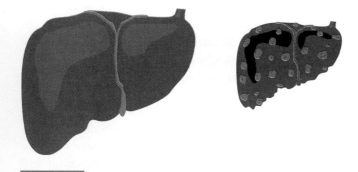

Figure 15-5

A normal liver (left) compared to one infected with cirrhosis of the liver.

Alcohol Treatments

Almost 600,000 Americans undergo treatment for alcohol-related problems every year. Until recent years, the only options for professional alcohol treatment were, as one expert puts it, "intensive, extensive and expensive," such as residential programs at hospitals or specialized treatment centers. Today individuals whose drinking could be hazardous to their health may choose from a variety of approaches. Treatment that works well for one person may not work for another. As research into the outcomes of alcohol treatments has grown, more attempts have been made to match individuals to approaches tailored to their needs and more likely to help them overcome their alcohol problems.[50]

Detoxification

The first phase of treatment for alcohol dependence focuses on **detoxification**, the gradual withdrawal of alcohol from the body. For 90 to 95% of alcoholics, withdrawal symptoms are mild to moderate. They include sweating; rapid pulse; elevated blood pressure; hand tremor; insomnia; nausea or vomiting; malaise or weakness; anxiety; depressed mood or irritability; headache; and temporary hallucinations or illusions.

Those who have drunk heavily for a prolonged period may develop more severe symptoms, including seizures or alcohol withdrawal delirium, commonly known as **delirium tremens**, or **DTs**, characterized by agitated behavior, delusions, rapid heart rate, sweating, vivid hallucinations, trembling hands, and fever. This problem is most likely to develop in chronic heavy drinkers who also suffer from a physical illness, fatigue, depression, or malnutrition. The symptoms usually appear over several days after heavy drinking stops. Individuals frequently report terrifying visual hallucinations, such as seeing insects all over their bodies. With treatment, most cases subside after several days, although delirium tremens has been known to last as long as four or five weeks. In some cases, complications such as infections or heart arrhythmias prove fatal.

Medications

Antianxiety and antidepressive drugs are sometimes used in early treatment for alcoholism, especially for those with underlying mental disorders. Several medications, including certain antidepressant drugs that increase the neurotransmitter serotonin, are being studied as medical interventions to reduce cravings or pre-vent relapses. Vitamin supplements, especially thiamine and folic acid, can help overcome some of the nutritional deficiencies linked with alcoholism.

The drug disulfiram (Antabuse), given to deter drinking, causes individuals to become nauseated and acutely ill when they consume alcohol. Antabuse interrupts the removal of acetaldehye by the liver, so this toxic substance accumulates and causes nausea or vomiting. If individuals taking Antabuse drink at all or consume foods with alcoholic content, they become extremely ill. They must avoid foods cooked or marinated in wine and cough syrup preparations containing alcohol. Some individuals have reactions to the alcohol in after-shave lotion. A large amount of alcohol can make them dangerously ill; fatalities have occurred. Side effects are usually mild and include drowsiness, bad breath, skin rash, and temporary impotence. Because Antabuse does not reduce cravings for alcohol, psychotherapy and support groups remain a necessary part of treatment.

Inpatient or Residential Treatment

In the past, 28-day treatment programs in a medical or psychiatric hospital or a residential facility were the cornerstone of early recovery treatment. According to outcome studies, inpatient treatment was effective, with as many as 70% of "graduates" remaining abstinent or stable, nonproblem drinkers for five years after. However, because of cost pressures from the insurance industry, the length of stay has been reduced, and there's been increasing emphasis on outpatient care.

Outpatient Treatment

Outpatient treatment may involve group therapy, individual supportive therapy, marital or family therapy, regular attendance at Alcoholics Anonymous (AA) or another support group, brief interventions, and relapse prevention. According to outcome studies, intensive outpatient treatment at a day hospital (with individuals returning home every evening) are as effective as inpatient care.[51] Outpatient therapy continues for at least a year, but many individuals continue to participate in outpatient programs for the rest of their lives.

Brief Interventions

These methods include individual counseling, group therapy and training in specific skills—such as assertiveness—all packed into a six- to eight-week period. Offered at a growing number of centers, brief interventions may be most helpful for problem drinkers who are not physically dependent on alcohol. The University of Michigan's DrinkWise program offers clients the options of one-on-one therapy, group sessions, or telephone counseling. In its first year of operation, DrinkWise reported a success rate of 90% in helping clients quit or control their drinking.

Moderation Training

Highly controversial, this approach uses cognitive-behavioral techniques, such as keeping a diary to chart drinking patterns and learning "consumption management" techniques, such as never having more than one drink an hour. "We tell our clients that there is no such thing as no-risk drinking," says Keith Bruhnsen, manager of DrinkWise, "What we offer are guidelines for low-risk drinking."[52] The upper limits are nine drinks a week for women, with no more than three drinks on any one day, and twelve drinks a week for men, with a one-day maximum of four drinks.

Treatment programs in other countries, such as Great Britain and Canada, have long offered moderation training for problem drinkers who consume too much alcohol. However, most experts agree that the best—and perhaps only—hope for recovery for chronic alcoholics who are physically dependent on alcohol is complete abstinence. Because support is critical for maintaining moderation as well as abstinence, those trying to cut back on alcohol can turn to a new support network called Moderation Management. Aimed at problem drinkers rather than alcoholics, it teaches members how to use alcohol responsibily. After a period of abstinence, members follow drinking guidelines that restrict the number of drinks they have per day and the number of days per week that they drink.[53]

Self-Help Programs

The best-known and most commonly used self-help program for alcohol problems is Alcoholics Anonymous (AA), which was founded more than 60 years ago and which has grown into an international organization that includes 2 million members and 185,000 groups worldwide. Acknowledging the power of alcohol, AA offers support from others struggling with the same illness, from a sponsor available at any time of the day or night, and from fellowship meetings that are held every day of the year. Because anonymity is a key part of AA, it has been difficult for researchers to study its success, but it is generally believed to be a highly effective means of overcoming alcoholism and maintaining abstinence. Its

12 steps, which emphasize honesty, sobriety, and acknowledgment of a "higher power," have become the model for self-help groups for other addictive behaviors, including drug abuse (discussed in Chapter 14) and compulsive eating.

The average age of entry into AA is 30; about 60% of the members are men. Members encompass a wide range of ages, occupations, nationalities, and socioeconomic classes. People generally attend 12-step meetings every day when they first begin recovery; most programs recommend 90 meetings in 90 days. Many people taper off to one or two meetings a week as their recovery progresses. No one knows exactly how 12-step programs help people break out of addictions. Some individuals stop their drinking, or other destructive behavior, simply on the basis of the information they get at meetings. Others bond to the group and use it as a social support and refuge while they explore and release their inner feelings—a process similar to what happens in psychotherapy.

Alternatives to AA

Secular Organizations for Sobriety (SOS) was founded in 1986 as an alternative for people who couldn't accept the spirituality of AA. Like AA, SOS holds confidential meetings, celebrates sobriety anniversaries, and views recovery as a one-day-at-a-time process.

Rational Recovery, which also emphasizes anonymity and total abstinence, focuses on the self rather than spirtuality. Members use reason instead of prayer and learn to control the impulse to drink by learning how to cotnrol the emotions that lead them to drink. Women for Sobriety (WFS), discussed earlier in the chapter, addresses the unique needs of women with drinking problems.

Recovery

Recovery from alcoholism is a lifelong process of personal growth and healing. The first two years are the most difficult, and relapses are extremely common. By some estimates, more than 90% of those recovering from substance use will use alcohol or drugs in any one 12-month period after treatment. However, approximately 70% of those who get formal treatment stop drinking for prolonged periods. Even without treatment, 30% of alcoholics are able to stop drinking for long periods. Those most likely to remain sober after treatment have the most to lose by continuing to drink: they tend to be employed, married, and upper-middle class.

Most recovering alcoholics experience urges to drink, especially during early recovery when they are likely to feel considerable stress. These urges are a natural consequence of years of drinking and diminish with time. Mood swings are common during recovery, and individuals typically describe themselves as alternately feeling relieved or elated and then discouraged or tearful. Such disconcerting ups and downs also decrease over time. Patience—learning to take "one day at a time"—is crucial.

Increasingly, treatment programs focus on **relapse prevention**, which includes the development of coping strategies and learning techniques that make it easier to live with alcohol cravings and rehearsal of various ways of saying "no" to offers of a drink. According to outcomes research, social skills training—a combination of stress management therapy, assertiveness and communication skills training, behavioral self-control training, and behavioral marital therapy—has proven effective in decreasing the duration and severity of relapses after one year in a group of alcoholics.

Strategies for Prevention

Preventing Relapses

✔ Exercise, which provides an outlet for aggression, enhances self-image, and reduces mild depression.

✔ Lifestyle changes, including developing a network of nondrinking friends; removing alcohol from the house; and avoiding high-risk situations, such as stopping at a bar.

✔ Refusal training; rehearsing various ways of saying "No."

✔ Stress reduction, to ease the desire to drink; learning to live with craving.

The Impact on Relationships

Alcoholism shatters families and creates unhealthy patterns of communicating and relating. Separation and divorce rates are high among alcoholics. Another common occurrence is **codependence**, a term used to described the behavior of close family members or friends who act in ways that enable their spouses, parents, or friends to continue their self-destructive behavior. (Codependence also is discussed in Chapter 12.)

Codependence and Enabling

Codependent spouses of alcoholics follow a predictable pattern of behavior: While trying to control the drinkers, they act in ways that enable the drinkers to keep drinking. If an alcoholic finds it hard to get up in the morning, his wife wakes him up, pulls him out of bed and into the shower, and drops him off at work. If he is late, she makes excuses to his boss. By helping him evade his responsibilities, his wife is helping him continue drinking. Indeed, he might not be able to keep up his habit without her cooperation.

Such behavior is harmful for individuals who are dependent on alcohol because it reinforces their denial. They do not feel out of control or powerless over alcohol because the person or persons closest to them are constantly protecting them from the consequences of their actions. Every crisis—a missed deadline, a forgotten appointment, a child's disappointment when a parent doesn't come to an important event—should be seen as a chance for the individual to recognize what alcohol is doing to the lives of all those close to him or her. If family members let their loved one experience the consequences of drinking, the person may be able to come to the moment of truth concerning alcohol.

Like alcoholics, codependents try to rationalize or deny their own behavior, often using excuses such as, "The reason I stayed home was to catch up on my reading, not to keep an eye on my partner." In time, the worlds of the alcoholic and the codependent become smaller and smaller, with the codependents losing sight of everything but their loved one. They feel that if they can only solve this person's problems, everything will be fine.

Codependents often need help in acknowledging their own feelings and needs. National self-help organizations, such as Al-Anon, help adult family members recognize dysfunctional behaviors in their relationships and start looking at their own problems. Similar self-help groups, such as Alateen, provide support for the teenaged children of alcoholics. These organizations also help family members cope with their loved one's alcoholism—whether or not codependence is a problem.

Strategies for Change

Recognizing Signs of Codependence

If you're involved with someone with an addictive behavior, read through the following list of characteristics of codependence. If you identify with some of the statements, you may wish to visit a self-help group in your area:

✔ "Covering" for another person's alcohol or drug use, eating disorders, gambling, sexual escapades, or general behavior.

✔ Spending a great deal of time talking about—and worrying about—other people's behavior/problems/future instead of living your own life.

✔ Marking or counting bottles, searching for a hidden "stash," or in other ways monitoring someone else's behavior.

✔ Taking on more responsibility at home or in a relationship—even when you resent it.

✔ Ignoring your own needs in favor of meeting someone else's.

✔ Worrying that if you leave a relationship, the other person will fall apart.

✔ Self-esteem that depends on what others say and think.

✔ Growing up in a family where there was little communication, where expressing feelings was not acceptable, and where there were either rigid rules or none at all.

Growing Up with an Alcoholic Parent

An estimated 7 million youngsters in the United States live with an alcoholic parent—an experience that often leads youngsters to play certain roles: The adjuster or "lost child" does whatever the parent says. The responsible child, or "family hero," typically takes over many household tasks and responsibilities. The acting-out child, or "scapegoat," shows his or her anger early in life by causing problems at home or in school and taking on the role of troublemaker. The "mascot" disrupts tense situations by focusing attention on himself or herself, often by clowning. Regardless of which roles they assume, the children of alcoholics are prone to learning disabilities, eating disorders, and addictive behavior.

Numerous studies have linked child abuse and neglect to parental drinking. Children of women who are problem drinkers have 2.1 times the risk of serious injury as children of mothers who don't drink. Children with two parents who are problem drinkers are at even higher risk. As teenagers, children of alcoholics are more likely to report early sexual intercourse and face a greater risk of adolescent pregnancy.[54]

Adult Children of Alcoholics

Growing up with an alcoholic parent can have a long-lasting effect. Adult children of alcoholics are at risk for many problems. Some try to fill the emptiness inside with alcohol, drugs, or addictive habits. Others find themselves caught up in destructive relationships that repeat the patterns of their childhood. They are likely to have difficulty solving problems, identifying and expressing their feelings, trusting others, and being intimate. In addition to their own increased risk of addictive behavior, they are likely to marry individuals with some form of addiction and keep on playing out the roles of their childhood. They may feel inadequate, not know how to set limits or recognize normal behavior, be perfectionistic, and want to control all aspects of their lives. However, not all adult children are alike or necessarily suffer from psychological problems or face an increased risk of substance abuse themselves.[55]

Because the impact of alcoholism can be so enduring, support groups—such as Adult Children of Alcoholics, Children of Alcoholics, and Adult Children of Dysfunctional Families—have spread throughout the country in the last decade. These organizations provide adult children of alcoholics a mutually supportive group setting to discuss their childhood experiences with alcoholic parents and the emotional consequences they carry into adult life. Through such groups or other forms of therapy, individuals may learn to move beyond anger and blame, see the part they themselves play in their current state of unhappiness, and create a future that is healthier and happier than their past.

Strategies for Change

If Someone Close to You Drinks Too Much

✔ Try to remain calm, unemotional, and factually honest in speaking about the drinker's behavior. Include the drinker in family life.

✔ Discuss the situation with someone you trust: a member of the clergy, social worker, friend, or someone who has experienced alcoholism directly.

✔ Be patient; live one day at a time.

✔ Never cover up or make excuses for the drinker, or shield him or her from the consequences of drinking. Assuming the drinker's responsibilities undermines his or her dignity and sense of importance.

✔ Refuse to ride with the drinker if he or she is driving while intoxicated.

✔ Encourage new interests and participate in leisure-time activities that the drinker enjoys.

✔ Try to accept setbacks and relapses calmly.

Making This Chapter Work for You
Responsible Drinking

■ When comparing amounts and types of alcohol, assume that one drink contains the equivalent of 1/2 ounce of 100% ethyl alcohol. The percentage of alcohol in a person's blood, or blood-alcohol concentration, is the measurement used by law enforcement officers to determine whether someone is legally drunk.

■ The rate of alcohol absorption depends on many factors: the strength of the drink; the drinker's size, sex, age, and race; family history of alcoholism; whether there's food in the drinker's stomach; and the drinker's expectations and tolerance for alcohol.

■ Moderate amounts of alcohol may have a positive effect on the cardiovascular system. In excess, however, alcohol can weaken the heart muscle, increase blood pressure, increase the risk of stroke, and inhibit the production of white and red blood cells.

■ Alcohol, a central nervous system depressant, also impairs thinking, vision, motor skills, hearing, smell and taste, pain perception, sense of time and space, speech, and sexual response and performance. When combined with other drugs, alcohol can have serious adverse effects.

■ About half (52%) of American adults drink, with little variation among the races with respect to quantity, frequency, and amount of alcohol consumed. Men generally drink more, in quantity and frequency, than women. Children are beginning to experiment with alcohol at a younger age than in the past.

■ Patterns of drinking vary greatly, from complete abstinence to infrequent drinking to moderate drinking. None of these patterns poses a current or future threat to a drinker's well-being. Problem drinking refers to any kind of drinking that interferes with a major aspect of life, such as sleep, energy, family relationships, health, or safety. A drinking binge consists of having five or more drinks at a single sitting for a man and four drinks at a single sitting for women.

■ Alcohol is the substance most commonly used by college students. Drinking by college women and binge drinking have increased on campuses. Alcohol abuse by students has led to violence, sexual assaults, and other dangers, which have triggered a backlash among students who drink little or no alcohol.

■ Women drink for different reasons and in different ways than men. Because of their smaller bodies and lack of a stomach enzyme that neutralizes alcohol, they feel its impact much more quickly and severely than men do. Breast cancer, infertility, and osteoporosis are among the possible special health risks that women face. Many respond best to treatments tailored to the unique needs of women, such as Women for Sobriety, a national network of self-help groups.

■ Although there has been a successful campaign against drunk driving, this dangerous crime continues to kill thousands of Americans. Families of the victims of drunk drivers continue to work to change the way America treats its drunk drivers and to keep drunk drivers off the road.

■ There is a spectrum of alcohol problems that range from problem drinking to alcohol dependence or abuse. The difference is one of degree and of loss of control over one's craving for alcohol.

■ Alcohol abuse, as defined by the American Psychiatric Association's *Diagnostic and Statistical Manual of Mental Disorders*, 4th edition *(DSM-IV)*, involves continued use of alcohol despite awareness of social, occupational, psychological, or physical problems related to drinking, or to drinking in dangerous ways or situations (before driving, for instance).

■ Alcohol dependence is a separate disorder in which individuals develop a strong craving for alcohol because it produces pleasurable feelings or relieves stress or anxiety. Over time they experience physiological changes that lead to tolerance ; if they abruptly stop drinking, they suffer withdrawal, a state of acute physical and psychological discomfort.

■ Although the exact cause of alcohol dependence or abuse isn't known, certain factors—including a biochemical imbalance in the brain, heredity, cultural acceptability, and stress—may play a role in the development of this disease.

Health Online

Drinking: A Student's Guide http://www.glness.com/ndhs

This Web site is exclusively oriented to the questions and concerns students have about drinking. Their online quiz can help you determine if you might be at risk for developing an alcohol problem. In addition there are sections on alcohol facts, binge drinking, drinking and health, drinking and women, and drinking and drugs.

Think about it ...

- According to this quiz, are you at risk for developing an alcohol problem? If so, does this concern you?

- What do you think are the special risks college students face regarding alcohol use that set them apart from other young adults?

- Do you know someone who you think may have an alcohol problem based on these criteria? How has alcohol use affected that person's life?

■ In the past, alcoholics were categorized as Type 1, who generally start heavy drinking, reinforced by external circumstances, after age 25; and Type 2, who typically become heavy drinkers before age 25 and drink regardless of external circumstances.

■ Newer research classifies alcoholics as Type A or Type B. Type A alcoholism develops later in life and involves less severe dependence, fewer alcohol-related problems, and less distress in the areas of work and family. Type B alcoholism, linked with childhood and familial risk factors, starts earlier and involves greater dependence and more serious complications.

■ Chronic heavy drinking can cause severe liver damage, hepatitis, or cirrhosis. Vitamin deficiencies, which commonly occur with alcoholism, can result in severe neurological, muscular, digestive, and cardiovascular diseases. Excessive alcohol consumption can damage the brain, causing mental deterioration, and is also associated with heart damage and several types of cancer.

■ Treatments for alcohol problems include detoxification, medications, inpatient care, outpatient treatment, and brief interventions. Problem drinkers who have not become dependent on alcohol may be able to learn to control their alcohol intake through moderation training.

■ Self-help groups, including AA, Rational Recovery,

Secular Organizations for Sobriety, and Women for Sobriety, can offer ongoing support to individuals recovering from alcohol problems as they build a new alcohol-free life.

■ Individuals with addictive behaviors or dependence on drugs or alcohol, and the children or partners of such people, are especially likely to find themselves in dysfunctional relationships that do not promote healthy communication, honesty, and intimacy.

■ Children of an alcoholic parent are vulnerable to learning disabilities, eating disorders, and addictive behavior. Adult children of parents with addictive behaviors are more likely to have difficulty solving problems, identifying and expressing their feelings, trusting others, and being intimate. They may develop some form of addiction themselves or marry someone with addictive behavior patterns.

■ Support groups, such as Al-Anon, Codependents Anonymous, and Adult Children of Dysfunctional Families, can help family members and adults who grew up in unhealthy homes come to terms with their past and prepare for a happier future.

■ For people with alcohol dependence and abuse, recovery is a lifelong process of change rather than a one-time treatment. Through therapy, education, and a reevaluation of what's meaningful in life, they can find hope for a better way of living. Relapses are so common that therapists believe they may be part of the process of recovery. Although painful, they may serve a purpose in developing the insight and motivation needed to break out of a self-destructive pattern once and for all.

Responsible drinking is a matter of you controlling your drinking, rather than the drinking controlling you. The Serenity Prayer, written by Protestant theologian Reinhold Niebuhr, summarizes the attitudes and values that can help people break free from their addictions and find purpose and meaning in life:

> *God grant me the Serenity*
> *to accept the things I cannot change;*
> *Courage to change the things I can; and*
> *Wisdom to know the difference.*

Key Terms

The terms listed here are used within the chapter. Page numbers are included for each term. A definition of each term is given in the green Glossary pages at the end of this book.

absorption *479*

alcohol abuse *495*

alcohol dependence *495*

alcoholism *496*

blood-alcohol concentration (BAC) *478*

codependence *501*

delirium tremens (DTs) *499*

detoxification *499*

ethyl alcohol *478*

fetal alcohol effects (FAE) *493*

fetal alcohol syndrome (FAS) *493*

intoxication *483*

proof *478*

relapse prevention *501*

Review Questions

1. How does alcohol affect the body's various systems?

2. What is alcoholism? How can you tell if someone is an alcoholic?

3. What are the negative consequences of being an alcoholic? How does alcoholism affect our society?

4. Can alcoholism be prevented? What are some common treatments? Which are the most effective?

5. What are some possible adverse effects of drinking during pregnancy? Describe a child born to a mother who has continued to drink throughout her pregnancy.

6. How is BAC relevant to the drunk-driving laws in your state? At what BAC level are you considered to be legally drunk?

7. What cultural views or customs might influence an individual's alcohol consumption? What physiological differences might increase or decrease alcohol's effect on these individuals?

Personal Health
15.2
INTERACTIVE

Critical Thinking Questions

1. Driving home from his high school graduation party, 18-year-old Rick has had too much to drink. As he crosses the dividing line on the two-lane road, the driver of an oncoming car—a young mother with two young children in the backseat—swerves to avoid an accident. She hits a concrete wall and dies instantly; but her children survive. Rick has no record of drunk driving. Should he go to prison? Is he guilty of manslaughter? How would you feel if you were the victim's husband? if you were Rick's friend?

2. Some groups concerned about alcohol abuse advocate greater restrictions on availability, such as prohibiting the sale of alcoholic beverages in supermarkets, convenience stores, and gas stations. They would like to see a ban on advertisements, especially those aimed at young people. Opponents argue that laws have never been effective in controlling alcohol abuse. Do you think our society is too permissive in the way we allow alcohol to be promoted or sold? Would you support anti-alcohol laws? Why or why not?

3. What effects has alcohol use had in your life? Try making a list of the positive and negative effects your own alcohol use has had. Be specific. If you continue to drink at your current rate, what positive and negative effects do you think it will have on your future? What effects has other people's drinking had on your life? List family members and friends who drink regularly, and how their drinking has affected you.

 ## Connections to Personal Health Interactive

To enhance your understanding of the material covered in this chapter, check out the following study aids on the **Personal Health Interactive CD-ROM**. *Each numbered icon within the chapter corresponds to an appropriate activity listed here.*

15.1 Personal Insights: How Do You Feel About Alcohol?

15.2 Chapter 15 Review

References

1. Winerip, Michael. "Binge Nights: The Emergency on Campus." *New York Times Education Life*, January 4, 1998.
2. Archer, Loran, et al. "What If Americans Drank Less? The Potential Effect on the Prevalence of Alcohol Abuse and Dependence." *American Journal of Public Health*, Vol. 85, No. 1, January 1995.
3. Whitcomb, David, and Geoffrey Block. "Association of Acetaminophen Hepatotoxicity with Fasting and Ethanol Use." *Journal of the American Medical Association,* Vol. 272, No. 23, December 21, 1994. Sherlock, Sheila. "Alcoholic Liver Disease." *Lancet*, Vol. 345, No. 8944, Jan 28, 1995.
4. Johnson, Patrick. "Alcohol Expectancies and Reaction Expectancies: Their Impact on Student Drinking." *Journal of Alcohol & Drug Education*, Vol. 40, No. 1, Fall 1994. de Boer, Mieke, et al. "The Effects of Alcohol, Expectancy, and Alcohol Beliefs on Anxiety and Self-Disclosure in Women: Do Beliefs Moderate Alcohol Effects?" *Addictive Behaviors*, Vol. 19, No. 5, September–October 1994.
5. Thun, Michael, et al. "Alcohol Consumption and Mortality Among Middle-aged and Elderly U.S. Adults." *New England Journal of Medicine*, Vol. 337, No. 24, December 11, 1997.
6. American Psychiatric Association. *Diagnostic and Statistical Manual of Mental Disorders*, 4th edition *(DSM-IV)*. Washington, D.C.: American Psychiatric Press, 1994.
7. Urbano-Marquez, Alvaro, et al. "The Greater Risk of Alcoholic Cardiomyopathy and Myopathy in Women Compared with Men." *Journal of the American Medical Association,* Vol. 274, No. 2, July 12, 1995.
8. Tracy, Joseph, and Marsha Bates. "Models of Functional Organization as a Method for Detecting Cognitive Deficits: Data from a Sample of Social Drinkers." *Journal of Studies on Alcohol*, Vol. 55, No. 6, November 1994.
9. Skelly, Flora Johnson. "The Drinking Diagnosis." *American Medical News*, May 11, 1992.
10. "Bibulous America: Over Half of All Adults Are Drinkers." *Dialogue*, Vol. 5, No. 1, February 1995.
11. Centers for Disease Control and Prevention. "Frequent Alcohol Consumption Among Women of Childbearing Age." *Journal of the American Medical Association*, Vol. 271, No. 23, June 15, 1994.
12. "Bibulous America."
13. Urberg, Kathryn, et al. "Close Friend and Group Influence on Adolescent Cigarette Smoking and Alcohol Use." *Developmental Psychology*, Vol. 130, No. 5, September 1997.
14. Connolly, Gary, et al. "Alcohol in the Mass Media and Drinking by Adolescents: A Longitudinal Study." *Addiction*, Vol. 89, No. 10, October 1994.
15. Sanchez-Craig, Martha, et al. "Empirically Based Guidelines for Moderate Drinking: One-Year Results from Three Studies with Problem Drinkers." *American Journal of Public Health*, Vol. 85, No. 6, June 1995.
16. Moore, Laurence, et al. "Binge Drinking: Prevalence, Patterns, and Policy." *Health Education Research*, Vol. 9, No. 4.
17. Cohen, Adam. "Battle of the Binge." *Time*, September 8, 1997.
18. Douglas, Kathy, et al. "Results from the 1995 National College Health Risk Behavior Survey." *Journal of American College Health*, Vol. 46, September 1997.
19. Kassel, Jon. Presentation, Association for the Advancement of Behavior Therapy, November 1997.
20. Arenson, Karen. "Fraternity Leaders Display Least Restraint in Drinking." *New York Times*, December 15, 1997.
21. Gleason, Nancy. "College Women and Alcohol: A Relational Perspective." *Journal of American College Health*, Vol. 42, No. 6, May 1994.
22. Svenson, Lawrence, et al. "Gender and Age Differences in the Drinking Behaviors of University Students." *Psychological Reports*, Vol. 75, No. 1, August 1994.
23. Wright, Deborah, and Paul Heppner. "Examining the Wellbeing of Nonclinical College Students: Is Knowledge of the Presence of Parental Alcoholism Useful?" *Journal of Counseling Psychology*, Vol. 40, No. 3, July 1993.
24. Winerip, Michael. "Binge Nights: The Emergency on

Campus." *New York Times Education Life,* January 4, 1998.

25. *Time,* December 19, 1994.

26. Rivinus, Timothy, and Mary Larimer. "Violence, Alcohol, Other Drugs, and the College Student." *Journal of College Student Psychotherapy,* Vol. 8, No. 1–2, 1993.

27. Nathan, Peter. "Unanswered Questions About Distressed Faculty, Staff and Students: Why Won't They Let Us Help Them?" In *Alcohol Use and Misuse by Young Adults,* Notre Dame, IN: University of Notre Dame Press, 1994. Kinney, Jean. "A Model Comprehensive Alcohol Program for Universities." In *Alcohol Use and Misuse by Young Adults.* Notre Dame, IN: University of Notre Dame Press, 1994.

28. Ross, Helen, and Gordon Tisdall. "Identification of Alcohol Disorders at a University Mental Health Center Using the CAGE." *Journal of Alcohol & Drug Education,* Vol. 39, No. 3, Spring 1994. Presley, Cheryl, et al. "Development of the Core Alcohol and Drug Survey: Initial Findings and Future Directions." *Journal of American College Health,* Vol. 42, No. 6, May 1994.

29. Gose, Ben. "Colleges Try to Curb Excessive Drinking by Saying Moderation Is Okay." *Chronicle of Higher Education,* Vol. 44, No. 9, October 24, 1997. Piombo, Maria, and Melinda Piles. "The Relationship Between College Females' Drinking and Their Sexual Behavior." *Women's Health Issues,* Vol. 6, No. 4, July–August 1996. Wilsnack, Sharon, et al. "Childhood Sexual Abuse and Women's Substance Abuse." *Journal of Studies on Alcohol,* Vol. 58, No. 5, May 1997.

30. Centers for Disease Control and Prevention. "Frequent Alcohol Consumption Among Women of Childbearing Age." *Journal of the American Medical Association,* Vol. 271, No. 23, June 15, 1994.

31. Svikis, Dace, et al. "Genetic Aspects of Alcohol Use and Alcoholism in Women." *Alcohol Health & Research World,* Vol. 18, No. 3, Summer 1994. Kendler, Kenneth, et al. "A Population-Based Twin Study of Alcoholism in Women." *Journal of the American Medical Association,* October 14, 1992.

32. Wilsnack, Sharon. Personal interview. Wilsnack, Sharon, et al. "How Women Drink: Epidemiology of Women's Drinking and Problem Drinking." *Alcohol Health & Research World,* Vol. 18, No. 3, Summer 1994.

33. Thorp, John, and Susanne Hiller-Sturumhofel. "The Obstetrician/Gynecologist." *Alcohol Health & Research World,* Vol. 18, No. 2, 1994.

34. Grodstein, Francine, et al. "Infertility in Women and Moderate Alcohol Use." *American Journal of Public Health,* Vol. 84, No. 9, September 1994.

35. Stewart, Donna, and David Streiner. "Alcohol Drinking in Pregnancy." *General Hospital Psychiatry,* Vol. 16, No. 6, November 1994. Eliason, Michele, and Anne Skinstad. "Drug/Alcohol Addictions and Mothering." *Alcoholism Treatment Quarterly,* Vol. 12, No. 1, 1995. Drug and alcohol abuse also can affect a woman's mothering. See Eliason, Michele, and Anne Skinstad. "Drug/Alcohol Addictions and Mothering." *Alcoholism Treatment Quarterly,* Vol. 12, No. 1, 1995.

36. Urbano-Marquez, Alvaro, et al. "The Greater Risk of Alcoholic Cardiomyopathy and Myopathy in Women Compared with Men." *Journal of the American Medical Association,* Vol. 274, No. 2, July 12, 1995.

37. McDonough, Russell, and Lori Russell. "Alcoholism in Women: A Holistic, Comprehensive Care Model." *Journal of Mental Health Counseling,* Vol. 16, No. 4, October 1994. Elsie Shore. "Outcomes of a Primary Prevention Project for Business and Professional Women." *Journal of Studies on Alcohol,* Vol. 55, No. 6, November 1994.

38. Kirkpatrick, Jean. Personal interview.

39. National Highway Safety Administration.

40. Castaneda, Carol, and Paul Hoversten. "War of Attrition on Drunken Driving." *USA Today,* May 23, 1997.

41. Hoversten, Paul. "Most Repeat Offenders Are Beer-Drinking Men." *USA Today,* May 23, 1997.

42. Bruhnsen, Keith. Personal interview.

43. Lester, David. "The Effect of Alcohol Consumption on Marriage and Divorce at the National Level." *Journal of Divorce and Remarriage,* Vol. 27, Nos. 3–4, November–December 1997.

44. American Psychiatric Association.

45. Ibid.

46. "Bibulous America."

47. Ibid.

48. Schiavi, Raul, et al. "Chronic Alcoholism and Male Sexual Function." *The American Journal of Psychiatry,* Vol. 152, No. 7, July 1995.

49. Hankin, Janet. "FAS Prevention Strategies: Passive and Active Measures." *Alcohol Health & Research World,* Vol. 18, No. 1, 1994.

50. McCaul, Mary, and Janice Furst. "Alcoholism Treatment in the United States." *Alcohol Health & Research World,* Vol. 18, No. 4, 1994.

51. Ibid.

52. Bruhnsen, Keith. Personal interview.

53. Kishline, Audrey. *Moderate Drinking: The Moderation Management Guide for People Who Want to Reduce their Drinking.* New York: Crown Publishers, 1995.

54. Chandy, Joseph, et al. "Female Adolescents of Alcohol Misusers: Sexual Behaviors." *Journal of Youth & Adolescence,* Vol. 23, No. 6, December 1994.

55. Mintz, Laurie, et al. "Relations Among Parental Alcoholism, Eating Disorders, and Substance Abuse in Non Clinical College Women: Additional Evidence Against the Uniformity Myth." *Journal of Counseling Psychology,* Vol. 42, No. 1, January 1995.

CHAPTER 16

TOBACCO USE, MISUSE, AND ABUSE

After studying the material in this chapter, you should be able to:

Describe today's typical tobacco smoker and the common reasons why he or she smokes.

List the health effects of smoking tobacco or using smokeless tobacco.

List the health problems that can be prevented by quitting smoking.

List the health effects of passive, or secondhand, tobacco smoke.

Discuss several recommended ways to quit smoking.

Plan a strategy for keeping your personal environment smoke-free.

Imagine living in a smoke-free society. No one would light up at the table next to yours at a restaurant. There wouldn't be clouds of smoke in bus and train terminals, airports, conference rooms, or theater lobbies. Parks and beaches wouldn't be littered with cigarette butts. Billboards and magazine ads wouldn't portray a deadly habit as glamorous and enticing.

A generation ago the very idea would have seemed like a fantasy. Now in many places around the country, such scenes are a reality. Nationwide, nonsmokers now outnumber smokers by a ratio of two to one. Half the men and nearly half the women who ever smoked in this country have quit—90% of them on their own, usually after several failed attempts to break the habit. The Food and Drug Administration (FDA), American Medical Association (AMA), and other health groups have targeted nicotine as a dangerous addictive drug and have called for an all-out campaign against this devastating killer.[1]

At the same time, some groups—particularly white teenage girls—are lighting up at earlier ages than in the past. An estimated 4.5 million children and adolescents smoke, and the average age of a child who tried cigarettes is 11.6 years.[2] If young smokers continue to smoke throughout their lives, half will die as a result of smoking-related diseases, losing an average of 22 years of life expectancy.[3] (See Figure 16-1, "How Smokers Will Die.")

Tobacco use is the single leading preventable cause of death in the United States. It kills more than 400,000 Americans every year—more people than AIDS, car accidents, alcohol, murders, illegal drugs, suicides, and fires, combined.[4] Even people who don't use tobacco face danger from others' smoke, and the enormous costs of tobacco's ill effects are something we all share. If current trends continue, smoking's annual death toll worldwide will rise to 10 million people.[5] (By contrast, the bubonic plague of the fourteenth century killed 20 million people over four years.)

This chapter discusses the effects of tobacco on the body, smoking patterns, tobacco dependence, quitting smoking, and passive smoking. The information it provides may help you to breathe easier today—and may help ensure cleaner air for others to breathe tomorrow.

HOW SMOKERS WILL DIE

For every 1000 20-year-olds who smoke, here's a look ahead at how they will die:

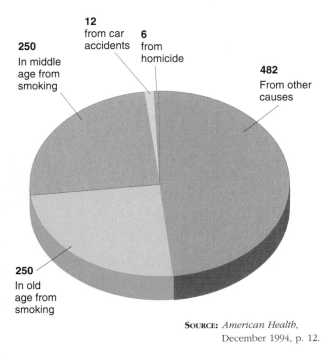

250
In middle age from smoking

12
from car accidents

6
from homicide

482
From other causes

250
In old age from smoking

Source: *American Health*, December 1994, p. 12.

Figure 16-1

Tobacco and Its Effects

Tobacco was introduced to Western civilization more than 300 years ago. Until the twentieth century, there was no medical objection to its use, although fundamentalist religious groups crusaded against it. Over time, tobacco smoking gained snob appeal among educated and cultured Europeans and Americans, who then were imitated by the so-called common man and, later, woman. Only in recent decades has society begun to frown—or cough—in the presence of smokers.

Tobacco, an herb that can be smoked or chewed, directly affects the brain. While its primary active ingredient is nicotine, there are almost 400 other compounds and chemicals in tobacco smoke, including gases, liquids, particles, tar, carbon monoxide, cadmium, pyridine, nitrogen dioxide, ammonia, benzene, phenol, acrolein, hydrogen cyanide, formaldehyde, and hydrogen sulfide. See Figure 16-2 for a summary of their physiological effects.

Nicotine

A colorless, oily compound, **nicotine** is poisonous in concentrated amounts. If you inhale while smoking, 90% of the nicotine in the smoke is absorbed into your body. Even if you draw smoke only into your mouth and not into your lungs, you still absorb 25% to 30% of the nicotine. The FDA has concluded that nicotine is a dangerous, addictive drug that should be regulated.

Nicotine stimulates the cerebral cortex, the outer layer of the brain that controls complex behavior and mental activity and enhances mood and alertness. Nicotine also acts as a sedative. How often you smoke and how you smoke determine nicotine's effect on you. If you're a regular smoker, nicotine will generally stimulate you at first, then tranquilize you. Shallow puffs tend to increase alertness, because low doses of nicotine facilitate the release of the neurotransmitter *acetylcholine,* which makes one feel alert. Deep drags, on the other hand, relax the smoker, because high doses of nicotine block the flow of acetylcholine.

Nicotine stimulates the adrenal glands to produce adrenaline, a hormone that increases blood pressure, speeds up the heart rate by 15 to 20 beats a minute, and constricts blood vessels (especially in the skin). Nicotine also inhibits the formation of urine, dampens hunger, irritates the membranes in the mouth and throat, and dulls the taste buds, so foods don't taste as good as they would otherwise. Nicotine is a major contributor to heart and respiratory diseases.

Tar

As it burns, tobacco produces **tar**, a thick, sticky dark fluid made up of several hundred different chemicals—many of them poisonous, some of them *carcinogenic* (enhancing the growth of cancerous cells). As you inhale tobacco smoke, tar and other particles settle in the forks of the branchlike bronchial tubes in your lungs, where precancerous changes are apt to occur. In addition, tar and smoke damage the mucus and the cilia in the bronchial tubes, which normally remove irritating foreign materials from your lungs.

Carbon Monoxide

Smoke from cigarettes, cigars, and pipes also contains **carbon monoxide**, the deadly gas that comes

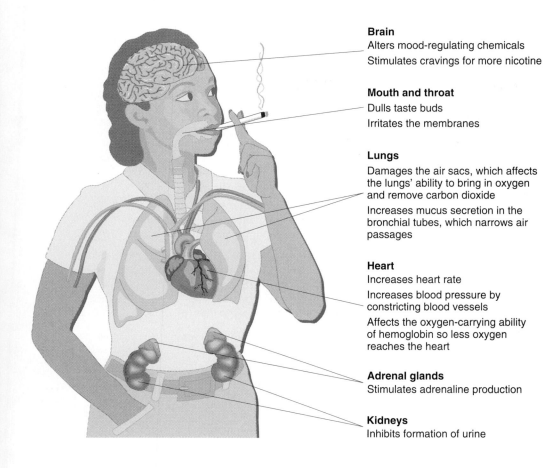

Brain
Alters mood-regulating chemicals
Stimulates cravings for more nicotine

Mouth and throat
Dulls taste buds
Irritates the membranes

Lungs
Damages the air sacs, which affects
the lungs' ability to bring in oxygen
and remove carbon dioxide
Increases mucus secretion in the
bronchial tubes, which narrows air
passages

Heart
Increases heart rate
Increases blood pressure by
constricting blood vessels
Affects the oxygen-carrying ability
of hemoglobin so less oxygen
reaches the heart

Adrenal glands
Stimulates adrenaline production

Kidneys
Inhibits formation of urine

Figure 16-2
Some effects of smoking
on the body.

out of the exhaust pipes of cars, in levels 400 times those considered safe in industry. Carbon monoxide interferes with the ability of the hemoglobin in the blood to carry oxygen, impairs normal functioning of the nervous system, and is at least partly responsible for the increased risk of heart attack and strokes in smokers.

The Impact of Tobacco

Smoking tobacco is the largest and most preventable cause of mortality in the United States, causing more than 430,000 deaths among smokers and another 50,000 deaths among nonsmokers exposed to environmental tobacco smoke.[6] Americans who die of smoking-related causes before age 65 lose a total of 949,924 years of potential life. Moreover, smoking-related diseases account for $22 billion in health-care costs and $43 billion in lost productivity each year.[7]

Health Effects of Cigarette Smoking

Tobacco is the ultimate underlying cause of nearly one of every five deaths in the United States every year.[8] If you're a smoker who inhales deeply and started smoking before the age of 15, you're trading a minute of future life for every minute you now spend smoking. Smoking not only eventually kills, it also ages you: Smokers get more wrinkles than nonsmokers. But the effects of smoking are far more than skin-deep. A cigarette smoker is 10 times more likely to develop lung cancer than a nonsmoker and 20 times more likely to have a heart attack. Those who smoke two or more packs a day are 15 to 25 times more likely to die of lung cancer than are nonsmokers. Moreover, the danger of lung cancer skyrockets when smokers are also exposed to other carcinogens, such as asbestos. This double threat increases the risk of lung cancer to as much as 92 times that for nonsmokers not exposed to asbestos.

Self-Survey

Are You Addicted to Nicotine?

Answer the following questions as honestly as you can by placing a check mark in the appropriate column:

	Yes	No
1. Do you smoke every day?	____	____
2. Do you smoke because of shyness and to build up self-confidence?	____	____
3. Do you smoke to escape from boredom and worries or while under pressure?	____	____
4. Have you ever burned a hole in your clothes, carpet, furniture, or car with a cigarette?	____	____
5. Have you ever had to go to the store late at night or at another inconvenient time because you were out of cigarettes?	____	____
6. Do you feel defensive or angry when people tell you that your smoke is bothering them?	____	____
7. Has a doctor or dentist ever suggested that you stop smoking?	____	____
8. Have you ever promised someone that you would stop smoking, then broken your promise?	____	____
9. Have you ever felt physical or emotional discomfort when trying to quit?	____	____
10. Have you ever successfully stopped smoking for a period of time, only to start again?	____	____
11. Do you buy extra supplies of tobacco to make sure you won't run out?	____	____
12. Do you find it difficult to imagine life without smoking?	____	____
13. Do you choose only those activities and entertainments during which you can smoke?	____	____
14. Do you prefer, seek out, or feel more comfortable in the company of smokers?	____	____
15. Do you inwardly despise or feel ashamed of yourself because of your smoking?	____	____
16. Do you ever find yourself lighting up without having consciously decided to?	____	____
17. Has your smoking ever caused trouble at home or in a relationship?	____	____
18. Do you ever tell yourself that you can stop smoking whenever you want to?	____	____

	Yes	No
19. Have you ever felt that your life would be better if you didn't smoke?	____	____
20. Do you continue to smoke even though you are aware of the health hazards posed by smoking?	____	____

If you answered Yes to one or two of these questions, there's a chance that you are addicted or are becoming addicted to nicotine. If you answered Yes to three or more of these questions, you are probably already addicted to nicotine.

Source: Nicotine Anonymous World Services, San Francisco.

Making Changes ....

Breaking the Habit

Here's a six-point program to help you or someone you love quit smoking. (*Caution*: Don't undertake the quit-smoking program until you have a two- to four-week period of relatively unstressful work and study schedules or social commitments.)

1. *Identify your smoking habits.* Keep a daily diary (a piece of paper wrapped around your cigarette pack with a rubber band will do) and record the time you smoke, the activity associated with smoking (after breakfast, in the car), and your urge for a cigarette (desperate, pleasant, or automatic). For the first week ot two, don't bother trying to cut down; just use the diary to learn the conditions under which you smoke

2. *Get support.* It can be tough to go it alone. Phone your local chapter of the American Cancer Society, or otherwise get the names of some ex-smokers who can give you support.

3. *Begin by tapering off.* For a period of one to four weeks, aim at cutting down to, say, 12 or 15 cigarettes a day; or change to a lower-nicotine brand, and concentrate on not increasing the number of cigarettes you smoke. As indicated by your diary, begin by cutting out those cigarettes you smoke automatically. In addition, restrict the times you allow yourself to smoke. Throughout this period, stay in touch, once a day or every few days, with your ex-smoker friend(s) to discuss your problems.

4. *Set a quit date.* At some point during the tapering-off period, announce to everyone—friends, family, and ex-smokers—when you're going to quit. Do it with flair. Announce it to coincide with a significant date, such as your birthday or anniversary.

5. *Stop.* A week before Q-day, smoke only five cigarettes a day. Begin late in the day, say after 4:00 P.M. Smoke the first two cigarettes in close succession. Then, in the evening, smoke the last three, also in close succession, about 15 minutes apart. Focus on the negative aspects of cigarettes, such as the rawness in your throat and lungs. After seven days, quit and give yourself a big reward on that day, such as a movie or a fantastic meal or new clothes.

6. *Follow up.* Stay in touch with your ex-smoker friend(s) during the following two weeks, particularly if anything stressful or tense occurs that might trigger a return to smoking. Think of the person you're becoming—the very person cigarette ads would have you believe smoking makes you. Now that you're quitting smoking, you're becoming healthier, sexier, more sophisticated, more mature, and better looking—and you've earned it!

SOURCES: American Cancer Society; National Cancer Institute.

Heart Disease and Stroke

Although a great deal of publicity has been given to the link between cigarettes and lung cancer, heart attack is actually the leading cause of deaths for smokers. Smoking doubles the risk of heart disease, and smokers who suffer heart attacks have only a 50% chance of recovering. Smokers have a 70% higher death rate from heart disease than do nonsmokers, and those who smoke heavily have a 200% higher death rate. Even aerobic exercise, which generally protects the heart's health, cannot overcome the negative effects of smoking, especially on cholesterol levels.[9]

The federal Office of the Surgeon General blames cigarettes for one out of every ten deaths attributable to heart disease. Smoking is more dangerous than are the two most notorious risk factors for heart disease: high blood pressure and high cholesterol. If smoking is combined with one of these, the chances of heart attack are four times greater. Women who smoke and use oral contraceptives have a ten times higher risk of suffering heart attacks than women who do neither.

Smoking also causes a condition called *cardiomyopathy,* which weakens the heart's ability to pump blood and results in the death of about 10,000 people a year. Although researchers don't know precisely how smoking poisons the heart muscle, they speculate that either nicotine or carbon monoxide has a direct toxic effect. Other coronary diseases may be associated with smoking. *Aortic aneurysm* is a bulge in the aorta (the large artery attached to the heart) caused by a weakening of its walls. *Pulmonary heart disease* is a heart disorder caused by changes in blood vessels in the lungs. (See Chapter 12 for further discussion of heart disease.)

Even people who have smoked for decades can reduce their risk of heart attack if they quit smoking. However, recent studies indicate some irreversible damage to blood vessels. Progression of atherosclerosis—hardening of the arteries—among past smokers contin-ues at a faster pace than among those who never smoked.[10]

In addition to contributing to heart attacks, cigarette smoking increases the risk of stroke two to three times in men and women, even after other risk factors are taken into account. According to one study of middle-aged men, giving up smoking leads to a considerable decrease in the risk of stroke within five years of quitting, particularly in smokers of less than 20 cigarettes a day. Those with hypertension show the greatest benefit. The risk for heavy smokers declines but never reverts back to that of men who never smoked.[11]

Cancer

The American Cancer Society estimates that tobacco smoking is the cause of 28% of all deaths from cancer and the cause of more than 85% to 90% of all cases of lung cancer. The more people smoke, the longer they smoke, and the earlier they start smoking, the more likely they are to develop lung cancer.

Smokers of two or more packs a day have lung cancer mortality rates 15 to 25 times greater than nonsmokers. If smokers stop smoking before cancer has started, their lung tissue tends to repair itself, even if there were already precancerous changes. Former smokers who haven't smoked for 15 or more years have lung cancer mortality rates only somewhat above those for nonsmokers.

Chemicals in cigarette smoke and other environmental pollutants switch on a particular gene in the lung cells of some individuals. This gene produces an enzyme that helps manufacture powerful carcinogens, which set the stage for cancer. The gene seems more likely to be activated in some people than others, and people with this gene are at much higher risk of developing lung cancer. However, smokers without the gene still remain at risk, because other chemicals and genes also may be involved in the development of lung cancer.

Smokers who are depressed are more likely to get cancer than nondepressed smokers. Although researchers don't know exactly how smoking and depression may work together to increase the risk of cancer, one possibility is that stress and depression cause biological changes that lower immunity.

Despite some advances in treating lung cancer, the prognosis for sufferers is not good. Even with vigorous therapy, fewer than 10% survive for five years after diagnosis. This is one of the lowest survival rates of any type of cancer. And if the cancer has spread from the lungs to other parts of the body, only 1% survive for five years after diagnosis. (See Chapter 13 for further discussion of cancer.)

Respiratory Diseases

Smoking quickly impairs the respiratory system. Even some teenaged smokers show signs of respiratory difficulty—breathlessness, chronic cough, excess phlegm production—when compared with nonsmokers of the same age. Cigarette smokers are up to 18 times more likely than are nonsmokers to die of noncancerous diseases of the lungs.

Cigarette smoking is the major cause of chronic obstructive lung disease (COLD), which includes emphysema and chronic bronchitis, in men and women. COLD is characterized by progressive limitation of the flow of air into and out of the lungs. In emphysema, the limitation of airflow is the result of disease changes in the lung tissue, affecting the bronchioles (the smallest air passages) and the walls of the alveoli (the tiny air sacs of the lung) (see Figure 16-3). Eventually, many of the air sacs are destroyed, and the lungs become much less able to bring in oxygen and remove carbon dioxide. As a result, the heart has to work harder to deliver oxygen to all organs of the body.

In chronic bronchitis, the bronchial tubes in the lungs become inflamed, thickening the walls of the bronchi, and the production of mucus increases. The result is a narrowing of the air passages. Smoking is more dangerous than any form of air pollution, at least for most Americans, but exposure to both air pollution and cigarettes is particularly harmful. Although each may cause bronchitis, together they have a synergistic effect—that is, their combined impact exceeds the sum of their separate effects.

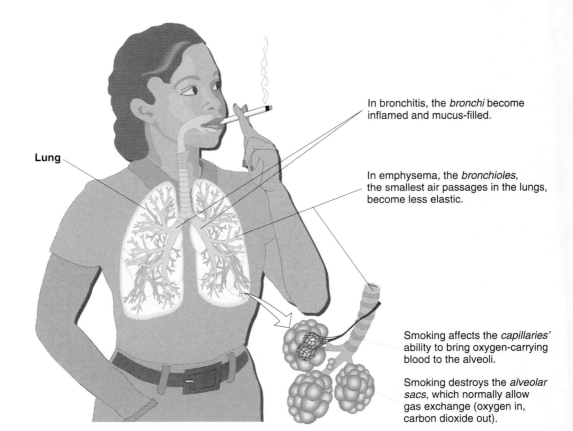

Figure 16-3

How smoking affects the lungs.

Lung

In bronchitis, the *bronchi* become inflamed and mucus-filled.

In emphysema, the *bronchioles*, the smallest air passages in the lungs, become less elastic.

Smoking affects the *capillaries'* ability to bring oxygen-carrying blood to the alveoli.

Smoking destroys the *alveolar sacs*, which normally allow gas exchange (oxygen in, carbon dioxide out).

Other Smoking-Related Problems

Smokers are more likely than nonsmokers to develop gum disease, and they lose significantly more teeth. Even those who quit have worse gum problems than people who never smoked at all. Smoking may also contribute to the loss of teeth and teeth supporting bone, even in individuals with good oral hygiene. (See Chapter 20 for more on oral health.)

Cigarette smoking is associated with stomach and duodenal ulcers; mouth, throat, and other types of cancer; and cirrhosis of the liver. Smoking may worsen the symptoms or complications of allergies, diabetes, hypertension, peptic ulcers, and disorders of the lungs or blood vessels. Some men who smoke ten cigarettes or more a day may experience sexual impotence. Cigarette smokers also tend to miss work one-third more often than do nonsmokers, primarily because of respiratory illnesses. In addition, each year cigarette-ignited fires claim thousands of lives.

Smoking and Medication

Smokers use more medications—aspirin, painkillers, sleeping pills, tranquilizers, antihistamines, cough medicines, stomach medicines, laxatives, diuretics, and antibiotics—than nonsmokers do. According to the American Pharmaceutical Association, nicotine and other tobacco ingredients speed up the process by which the body uses and eliminates drugs, so they may not be able to do what they're intended to do. As a result, smokers may have to take a medication more frequently than do nonsmokers. If you smoke, let your physician know so that he or she can adjust any prescriptions, if necessary.

Among the drugs affected by smoking are antianxiety drugs (including Valium), painkillers (including Darvon), tricyclic antidepressants (including Elavil), anti-blood-clotting medications (such as heparin), antiasthmatic drugs (including theophylline), and the cardiovascular drugs known as beta blockers (such as propranolol).

The Financial Cost of Smoking

The total costs of cigarette smoking to American society include greater work absenteeism, higher insurance premiums, disability payments, and training costs to replace employees who die prematurely from smoking. In the course of a lifetime, the average smoker can expect to spend $10,000 to $20,000 on cigarettes—but that's only the beginning. The potential costs for medical services for a man between the ages of 35 and 39 who smokes heavily may be as high as $60,000. But the greatest toll—the pain and suffering of cancer victims and their loved ones—obviously cannot be measured in dollars and cents.

Strategies for Prevention

Why Not to Light Up

Before you start smoking—before you ever face the challenge of quitting—think of what you have to gain by *not* smoking:

✔ A significantly reduced risk of cancer of the larynx, mouth, esophagus, pancreas, and bladder.

✔ Half the risk of heart disease that smokers face.

✔ A lower risk of stroke, chronic obstructive lung disease (COLD), influenza, ulcers, and pneumonia.

✔ A lower risk of having a low-birth-weight baby.

✔ A longer life span.

✔ Potential savings of tens of thousands of dollars that you would otherwise spend on tobacco products and medical care.

Smoking in America

Tobacco use remains the most serious and widespread addictive behavior in the world and the major cause of preventable deaths in our society. Although smoking by adults has declined, many young teenagers—particularly white girls—are smoking as much or more than they were ten years ago.

Who Smokes?

About 46 million Americans smoke, and another 44 million are ex-smokers. According to the American Academy of Pediatrics, one in ten eighth-graders and nearly one in five of our high school seniors smoke daily.[12] This early age is an ominous sign, since most

CAMPUS FOCUS: COLLEGE STUDENTS & SMOKING

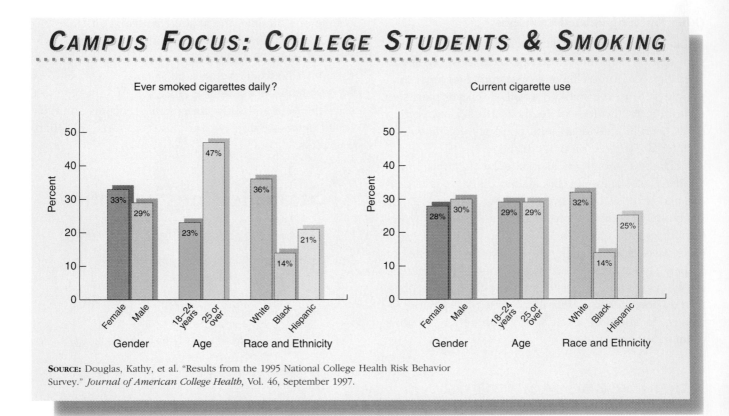

Source: Douglas, Kathy, et al. "Results from the 1995 National College Health Risk Behavior Survey." *Journal of American College Health*, Vol. 46, September 1997.

adults who currently smoke began to do so before the age of 19, at an average age of 12.5 years, and most were regular smokers by the age of 14. Among high school smokers who thought they wouldn't be smoking in five years, 73% still are.[13]

It is no coincidence that so many people start to smoke early in life. According to investigations reported in 1998, the tobacco industry deliberately targeted young teenagers by many means, including advertising in magazines with large youth readerships.[14] Researchers estimate that the tobacco industry's promotional activities in the late 1990s will influence 17% of those who turn 17 years old each year to experiment with cigarettes.[15]

There are dramatic racial differences in teen smoking patterns. African-American and Latino adolescents smoke much less than white teens, with fewer than 5% of African-American teenagers describing themselves as regular smokers—compared with 22.9% of whites.[16] As Campus Focus: "College Students and Smoking" shows, 28% of college women and 30% of college men currently use cigarettes. In the national survey of college students' health habits and risk behavior, 17.7% of the women and 14.9% of the men describe themselves as frequent smokers.[17]

Why People Start Smoking

The two main factors linked with the onset of a smoking habit are age and education. The vast majority of white men (93%) with less than a high school education are current or former daily cigarette smokers. White women with similar educational backgrounds are also very likely to smoke or to have smoked every day. Latino men and women without a high school education are less likely to be or become daily smokers.[18]

Most Americans are aware that there is a health risk associated with smoking, but many don't know exactly what that risk is or how it might affect them. Other factors associated with starting smoking are discussed in the following sections.

Heredity

Researchers speculate that genes may account for about 50% of smoking behavior, with environment playing an equally important role. Studies have shown that identical twins, who have the same genes, are more likely to have matching smoking profiles than fraternal twins. If one identical twin is a heavy smoker, the other is also likely to be; if one smokes only occasionally, so does the other.[19]

Parental Role Models

Children who start smoking are 50% more likely than youngsters who don't smoke to have at least one smoker in their families. A mother who smokes seems a particularly strong influence on making smoking seem acceptable. The majority of youngsters who smoke say that their parents also smoke and are aware of their own tobacco use.

Adolescent Experimentation and Rebellion

Young people who are trying out various behaviors may take up smoking because they're curious or because they want to defy adults. Others simply want to appear grownup or cool. In a 1998 poll by University of Michigan researchers, about 30% of 2000 high school seniors reported that they had their first cigarettes in or before the sixth grade. The majority of teens surveyed—88%—said they have at least a few friends who smoke; only 59% felt that they would definitely not smoke themselves. At least from the teens' perspective, little is done to discourage smoking by young people. Fewer than half reported that teachers and administrators attempted to prevent smoking, while more than half said they believed there are no health consequences or only mild health consequences from smoking.[20] Whatever the reason for starting may be, teens often misjudge the addictive power of cigarettes. Many, sure that they'll be able to quit any time they want, figure that smoking for a year or two won't hurt them. But when they try to quit, they can't.[21] Like older smokers, most young people who smoke have tried to quit at least once. The American Cancer Society has found that young smokers tend to become heavy smokers and that the longer anyone is exposed to smoke, the greater the health dangers.

Limited Education

People who have graduated from college are much less likely to smoke than are high school graduates; those with fewer than 12 years of education are most likely to smoke. An individual with 8 years or less of education is 11 times more likely to smoke than someone with postgraduate training.

Weight Control

Smokers burn up an extra 100 calories a day compared with nonsmokers—the equivalent of walking a mile—probably because nicotine increases metabolic rate. Once they start smoking, many individuals say they can-not quit because they fear they'll gain weight. The CDC estimates that women who stop smoking gain an average of eight pounds, while men put on an average of six pounds. One in eight women and one in ten men who stop smoking put on 29 pounds or more. The reasons for this weight gain include nicotine's effects on metabolism as well as emotional and behavioral factors, such as the habit of frequently putting something into one's mouth. Yet as a health risk, smoking a pack and a half to two packs a day is a greater danger than carrying 60 pounds in extra weight.

Weight gain for smokers who quit is not inevitable, however. Aerobic exercise helps increase metabolic rate; and limiting alcohol and foods high in sugar and fat can help smokers control their weight as they give up cigarettes.[22]

Aggressive Marketing

Cigarette companies spend billions each year on advertisements and promotional campaigns, with manufacturers targeting ads especially at women, teens, minorities, and the poor. Most controversial are cigarette advertisements in magazines and media aimed at teenagers and even younger children. As part of a nationwide antismoking campaign, health and government officials have called for restrictions on cigarette ads, and manufacturers have agreed not to aim their sales efforts at children and teens.

Stress

In studies that have analyzed the impact of life stressors, depression, emotional support, marital status, and income, researchers have concluded that an individual with a high stress level is approximately 15 times as likely to be a smoker than a person with low stress. About half of smokers identify workplace stress as a key factor in their smoking behavior.[23]

Why People Keep Smoking

Whatever the reasons for lighting up that first cigarette, very different factors keep cigarettes burning pack after pack, year after year. In national polls, four out of five smokers say that they want to quit but can't. The reason isn't a lack of willpower. Medical scientists have recognized tobacco dependence as an addictive disorder that may be more powerful than heroin dependence and that may affect more than 90% of all smokers.

Pleasure

According to the American Cancer Society, 87.5% of regular smokers find smoking pleasurable. Nicotine—the addictive ingredient in tobacco—is the reason. Researchers have shown that nicotine reinforces and strengthens the desire to smoke by acting on brain chemicals that influence feelings of well-being. This drug also can improve memory, help in performing certain tasks, reduce anxiety, dampen hunger, and increase pain tolerance.

Relief of Depression

Some people with depression use the mood-altering properties of nicotine to relieve depressive symptoms. According to new research, depressed and nondepressed people who smoke to improve their mood may do so because of their genetic makeup.[24] Previous studies have shown that people with a history of depression are significantly more likely to be smokers and to be diagnosed as nicotine-dependent. Smokers are more likely than nonsmokers to report depressive symptoms—and these symptoms may interfere with quitting.

According to researchers, the likelihood of quitting smoking is about 40% lower among depressed than nondepressed smokers.

Dependence

Nicotine has a much more powerful hold on smokers than alcohol does on drinkers. Whereas about 10% of alcohol users lose control of their intake of alcohol and become alcoholics, as many as 80% of all heavy smokers have tried to cut down on or quit smoking but cannot overcome their dependence.

Nicotine causes dependence by at least three means:

- It provides a strong sensation of pleasure.
- It leads to fairly severe discomfort during withdrawal.
- It stimulates cravings long after obvious withdrawal symptoms have passed (see Figure 16-4).

Few drugs act as quickly on the brain as nicotine does. It travels through the bloodstream to the brain in seven seconds—half the time it takes for heroin injected into a blood vessel to reach the brain. And a pack-a-day smoker gets 200 hits of nicotine a day—73,000 a year.

Figure 16-4

The effects of nicotine, a fast-acting and potent drug, on the body.

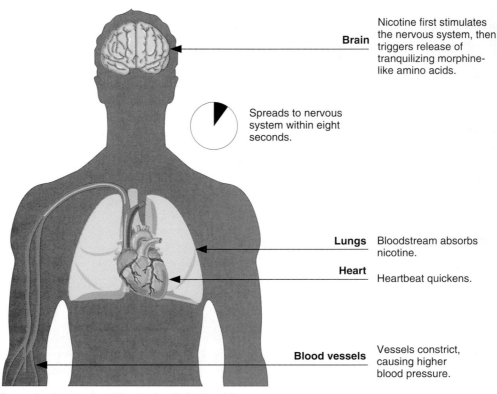

Brain — Nicotine first stimulates the nervous system, then triggers release of tranquilizing morphine-like amino acids.

Spreads to nervous system within eight seconds.

Lungs — Bloodstream absorbs nicotine.

Heart — Heartbeat quickens.

Blood vessels — Vessels constrict, causing higher blood pressure.

Sources: American Lung Association, American Medical Association

After a few years of smoking, the most powerful incentive for continuing to smoke is to avoid the discomfort of withdrawal. Generally, ten cigarettes a day will prevent withdrawal effects. For many who smoke heavily, signs of withdrawal, including changes in mood and performance, occur within two hours after smoking their last cigarette. (See the Self-Survey: "Are You Addicted to Nicotine?") Smokeless tobacco users also get constant doses of nicotine. However, absorption of nicotine by the lungs is more likely to lead to dependence than absorption through the linings of the nose and mouth. As with other drugs of abuse, continued nicotine intake results in tolerance (the need for more of a drug to maintain the same effect), which is why only 2% of all smokers smoke just a few cigarettes a day, or smoke only occasionally.

Use of Other Substances

Many smokers also drink or use drugs. According to the Addiction Research Foundation in Canada, tobacco smokers say cigarettes are harder to abandon than other drugs, even when they find them less pleasurable than their preferred drug of abuse. Individuals who drink excessively also find their cigarette habit a hard one to break. In a study of 3977 men and women, those who drank heavily or in binges were more likely to smoke more—and to find it harder to quit.[25]

Women and Smoking: Special Risks

The World Health Organization (WHO) reports that 20% to 30% of women in wealthy nations smoke, compared with 2% to 10% of women in the developing nations. In the United States, 26% of women smoke, and more young women than men are starting the habit. This is a troubling trend because, once women start, they often find it difficult to quit, in part because they fear gaining weight.[26]

Lung cancer now claims more women's lives than breast cancer. The risk of heart attack in women who smoke 25 or more cigarettes a day is more than 500% greater than the risk in women who don't smoke. Even smoking just one to four cigarettes a day doubles the risk. Women who smoke low nicotine cigarettes are four times more likely to have a first heart attack than women who don't smoke—the same risk as for those who smoke high-nicotine cigarettes.

Smoking directly affects women's reproductive organs and processes. Women who smoke are less fertile and experience menopause one or two years earlier than women who don't smoke. Smoking also boosts a woman's likelihood of developing cervical cancer and greatly increases the possible risks associated with taking oral contraceptives. Older women who smoke are weaker, have poorer balance, and are at greater risk of physical disability than nonsmokers.[27]

Women who smoke also are more likely to develop osteoporosis (discussed in Chapter 18). They tend to be thin, which is a risk factor for osteoporosis, and they enter menopause earlier, thus extending the period of jeopardy from estrogen loss.

An estimated 19 to 27% of women smoke during pregnancy, thereby increasing their risk of miscarriage and pregnancy complications, including bleeding, premature delivery, and birth defects such as cleft lip or palate.[28] Women who smoke are twice as likely to have an ectopic pregnancy (in which a fertilized egg develops in the fallopian tube rather than in the uterus) and to have babies of low birth weight as those who have never smoked. However, women who stop smoking before pregnancy reduce their risk of having a low-birth-weight baby to that of women who don't smoke. Even those who quit three or four months into the pregnancy have babies with higher birth weights than those who continue smoking throughout pregnancy. (See Chapter 10 for more information on the health risks associated with smoking during pregnancy.)

Other Forms of Tobacco

Other ways of ingesting tobacco may be less deadly than smoking cigarettes, but all are dangerous. Smoking clove cigarettes, cigars, and pipes, and chewing or sucking on smokeless tobacco all put the user at risk of cancer of the lip, tongue, mouth, and throat—as well as other diseases and ailments.

Clove Cigarettes

Sweeteners have long been mixed into tobacco, and clove, a spice, is the latest ingredient to be added to the recipe for cigarettes. Clove cigarettes typically contain two-thirds tobacco and one-third cloves. Consumers of these cigarettes are primarily teenagers and young adults.

Many users believe that clove cigarettes are safer than regular ones because they contain less tobacco, but this isn't necessarily the case. The CDC reports that people who smoke clove-containing cigarettes may be at risk of serious lung injury. Smoking clove cigarettes during a mild upper respiratory tract illness can lead to severe breathing difficulty. And clove cigarette smokers, like other cigarette smokers, can become addicted to the tobacco.

Clove cigarettes may actually be more harmful than conventional cigarettes. Puff for puff, they deliver twice as much nicotine, tar, and carbon monoxide as moderate-tar American brands. Moreover, eugenol, the active ingredient in cloves (which dentists have used as an anesthetic for years), deadens sensation in the throat, allowing smokers to inhale more deeply and hold smoke in their lungs for a longer time. Close chemical relatives of eugenol can produce the kind of damage to cells that may eventually lead to cancer.

Cigars

Cigar-smoking has become a widespread fad, particularly among men. Total cigar consumption in the United States totals approximately 4.5 billion cigars, and consumption of larger cigars increased by 44.5% from 1993 to 1996. Although this trend may have started among adult men, it has spread to adolescents. In various state surveys, approximately 27 to 28% of high school students reported having smoked at least one cigar in the previous 30 days.[29] A national survey of high schoolers found that approximately 6 million students had smoked a cigar in the previous year.[30] Although federal and state laws prohibit sale of cigars and other tobacco products to minors, many young people, including ninth graders, reported no difficulty in making such purchases.

Many cigar smokers of all ages assume that because they do not inhale the smoke, they are not at risk for heart disease or lung cancer. This has not been proven. And it has been shown that cigars, like cigarettes, greatly increase the risk of cancer of the mouth, larynx, throat, and esophagus.[31]

Pipes

Many cigarette smokers switch to pipes to reduce their risk of health problems. But former cigarette smokers may continue to inhale, even though pipe smoke is more irritating to the respiratory system than cigarette smoke. People who have only smoked pipes and who do not inhale are much less likely to develop lung and heart disease than are cigarette smokers. However, they are as likely as cigarette smokers to develop—and die of—cancer of the mouth, larynx, throat, and esophagus.

Smokeless Tobacco

Other tobacco products may be taking the place of cigarettes in the mouths of Americans. The sale and consumption of smokeless tobacco products are rising, particularly among young males. These substances include snuff, finely ground tobacco that can be sniffed or placed inside the cheek and sucked, and chewing tobacco, which consists of tobacco leaves mixed with flavoring agents such as molasses. With both, nicotine is absorbed through the mucous membranes of the nose or mouth.

Although not as deadly as cigarette smoking, the use of smokeless tobacco is dangerous. It can cause cancer and noncancerous oral conditions and lead to nicotine addiction and dependence. Smokeless tobacco users are more likely than nonusers to become cigarette smokers.[32] Powerful carcinogens in smokeless tobacco include nitrosamines, polycyclic aromatic hydrocarbons, and radiation-emitting polonium. Its use can lead to the development of white patches on the mucous membranes of the mouth, particularly on the site where the tobacco is placed (see Figure 16-5); these can develop into cancer. Cancers of the lip, pharynx, larynx, and esophagus have all been linked to smokeless tobacco.

An estimated 7 to 22 million people, many of them young, use snuff and chewing tobacco. In a national survey of 5894 men and women from 72 colleges and universities, 22% of college men and 2% of college women used smokeless tobacco. The lowest percentage was in the Northeast, the highest, in the Southcentral region. In different regions, 8 to 36% of male high school students are regular users.[33] Many are emulating professional baseball players who keep wads of tobacco jammed in their cheeks. Even when they spot lesions in their mouths, most do not seek medical help but continue to use smokeless tobacco.[34]

In recent years, there has been a decline in chewing tobacco, but an increase in the use of moist snuff, a product that is higher in nicotine and potential cancer-causing chemicals.[35] The use of snuff increases the like-

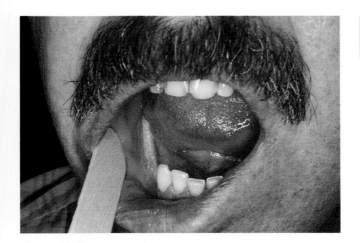

Figure 16-5

Chewing smokeless tobacco can damage the tissues of the mouth. In addition to causing oral cancer, the use of smokeless tobacco can lead to cancer of the larynx, esophagus, kidney, pancreas, and bladder.

lihood of oral cancer by more than four times. Other effects include bad breath, discolored or missing teeth, cavities, gum disease, and nicotine addiction.

Strategies for Change

How to Stop Using Smokeless Tobacco

✔ Keep a record of when, where, and why you're most likely to use smokeless tobacco. Identify high-risk situations, such as while playing softball with your friends.

✔ Gradually reduce the amount of time you keep a wad of chewing tobacco or snuff in your cheek. As soon as you remove it, rinse your mouth with mouthwash or, if possible, brush your teeth. Use breath mints if you can't rinse or brush.

✔ Substitute sugarless chewing gum for chewing tobacco or snuff.

✔ If you're a young man (as most users of smokeless tobacco are), ask some of the women you know what they think of guys who chew tobacco or suck on snuff.

✔ When you're ready to quit, have your teeth cleaned. Talk to your dentist about staining, gum disease, and other hazards of smokeless tobacco.

✔ Drink a lot of fluids and exercise regularly to cleanse your system of nicotine.

Environmental Tobacco Smoke

Maybe you don't smoke—never have, never will. That doesn't mean you don't have to worry about the dangers of smoking, especially if you live or work with people who smoke. **Environmental tobacco smoke**, or secondhand cigarette smoke, the most hazardous form of indoor air pollution, ranks behind cigarette smoking and alcohol as the third-leading preventable cause of death. Its annual toll in lives lost: 53,000.[36]

Mainstream and Sidestream Smoke

On the average, a smoker inhales what is known as **mainstream smoke** eight or nine times with each cigarette, for a total of about 24 seconds. However, the cigarette burns for about 12 minutes, and everyone in the room (including the smoker) breathes in what is known as **sidestream smoke**.

According to the American Lung Association, incomplete combustion from the lower temperatures of a smoldering cigarette makes sidestream smoke dirtier and chemically different from mainstream smoke. It has twice as much tar and nicotine, five times as much carbon monoxide, and 50 times as much ammonia. And because the particles in sidestream smoke are small, this mixture of irritating gases and carcinogenic tar reaches deeper into the lungs. If you're a nonsmoker sitting next to someone smoking seven cigarettes an hour, even in a ventilated room, you'll take in almost twice the maximum amount of carbon monoxide set for air pollution in industry—and it will take hours for the carbon monoxide to leave your body.

New research indicates that environmental tobacco smoke is even more dangerous than previously thought. According to the Centers for Disease Control and Prevention (CDC), every year environmental tobacco smoke causes 3000 deaths from lung cancer.[37] In a Harvard University study that tracked 10,000 healthy women who never smoked over ten years, regular exposure to other people's smoke at home or work almost doubled the risk of heart disease. On the basis of their findings, the researchers estimated that up to 50,000 Americans may die of heart attacks from environmental tobacco smoke every year, while 3000 to 4000 die of other forms of heart disease.[38] As a cancer-

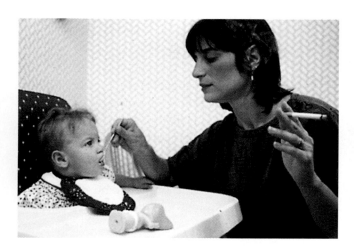

Innocent victims. Children whose parents or caregivers smoke are exposed to passive (or secondhand) smoke, the most hazardous form of indoor air pollution.

causing agent, secondhand smoke may be twice as dangerous as radon gas and more than a hundred times more hazardous than outdoor pollutants regulated by federal law.

Families of Smokers: Living Dangerously

The most vulnerable nonsmokers are the spouses and children of smokers. Numerous epidemiological and autopsy studies have linked environmental tobacco smoke with lung cancer and other disorders. The nonsmoking spouses of smokers, for instance, are 30% more likely to die of heart disease than other nonsmokers.[39]

Environmental tobacco smoke also poses great danger to young children. According to a 1997 study of more than 7000 youngsters, those who breathe environmental tobacco smoke suffer from more asthma, wheezing, and bronchitis than children in smoke-free homes. Children regularly exposed to tobacco smoke also face increased risk of lung cancer, heart disease, and stroke.

Infants of parents who smoke are hospitalized for bronchitis and pneumonia more often than are youngsters in nonsmoking households. In addition, environmental tobacco smoke may increase the risk of sudden infant death syndrome (SIDS). Infants who died of SIDS were more likely to have been exposed to environmental tobacco smoke from their mothers, fathers, or careproviders. Infants of mothers who smoked during pregnancy also were more likely to die of SIDS.[40]

Among children of parents who smoke, 74% worry that their parents' smoking is harming others in the family, including themselves; 48% worry about a possible fire caused by smoking; and 48% object to the odor of cigarette smoke in the house and on their clothes and hair.[41]

The Politics of Tobacco

More than three decades after government health authorities began to warn of the dangers of cigarette smoking, tobacco remains a politically hot topic. In 1997 the tobacco industry and attorneys general from nearly 40 states reached an historic settlement. Major tobacco countries agreed to pay $368.5 billion to settle smoking-related lawsuits filed by states, to finance antismoking campaigns, to restrict marketing, to permit federal regulation of tobacco, and to pay fines if tobacco use by minors does not decline. In return, the industry would be protected against most tobacco-related lawsuits and the awarding of punitive damages. The Food and Drug Administration (FDA) would have regulatory control over the way cigarettes are manufactured and packaged (see Figure 16-6).

In the course of congressional hearings on this settlement, investigators discovered documents indicating that tobacco manufactures had been aware of nicotine's addictive potential and had deliberately directed advertising campaigns at adolescents and at African Americans. One marketing objective revealed in a memo was "to ensure increased and long-term growth penetration among the 14–24 age group...which represents tomorrow's cigarette business."[42] Other documents showed that cigarette makers deliberately targeted blacks, particularly in inner cities, by means of advertising in magazines, on billboards, and on buses and through special promotions.[43] As this textbook goes to press, the "historic settlement" between government and tobacco companies had collapsed.

Other groups are fighting smoking on different fronts. The federal government has launched a seven-year grass-roots antismoking coalition called Americans Stop Smoking Intervention Study (ASSIST) to combat cigarette smoking. Community leaders in some neighborhoods have whitewashed billboard ads for cigarettes. Some civic and consumer associations have proposed boycotting athletic events sponsored by tobacco companies. In some states, tough antismoking campaigns, financed by taxes on cigarettes, have led to impressive declines in cigarette sales.

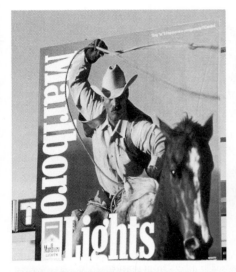

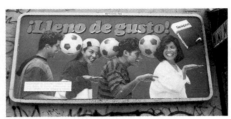

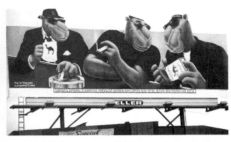

Figure 16-6
The tobacco settlement put strong limits on advertising aimed at children.

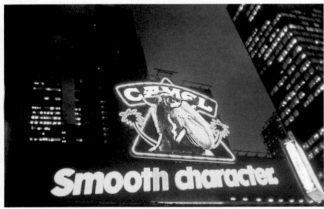

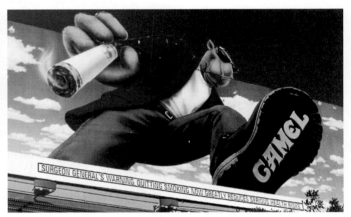

The Fight for Clean Air

Nonsmokers, realizing that their health is being jeopardized by environmental tobacco smoke, have increasingly turned to legislative and administrative measures to clear the air and protect their rights. (See Figure 16-7.) More than 1000 cities, towns, and counties now restrict smoking in public places or regulate the sale of tobacco to minors.[44] Nationally, the airlines have banned smoking on domestic flights. Minnesota prohibits smoking indoors virtually everywhere except in bars, private homes, and one-person offices. In San Francisco, city employers must resolve conflicts in favor of nonsmokers, even if only one nonsmoking employee complains. Many institutions, including medical centers and some universities, no longer allow smoking on their premises.

Supporters of smoking restrictions argue that no one should be subjected involuntarily to the dangers of environmental tobacco smoke. They point out that other people's smoke can cause headaches or hoarseness, and

may pose more serious health hazards. In addition, smokers jeopardize nonsmokers by increasing the danger of fire.

Opponents of smoking restrictions contend that banning smoking on the job might impair rather than enhance productivity, because employees would take more frequent breaks to go to lounges where smoking is permitted—or else would suffer the negative effects of nicotine withdrawal. Others argue that restaurants and bars would lose business if they had to clamp down on smoking.

Strategies for Change
....
How Nonsmokers Can Clear the Air

✔ Let people know your feelings in advance by putting up "No Smoking" signs in your office, home, or car. If you're in a car and someone pulls out a cigarette, ask

Figure 16-7

Nonsmoker's bill of rights.

Nonsmoker's Bill of Rights

Nonsmokers Help Protect the Health, Comfort, and Safety
of Everyone by Insisting on the Following Rights:

The Right to Breathe Clean Air

*Nonsmokers have the right to breathe clean air, free from harmful and irritating
tobacco smoke. This right supersedes the right to smoke when the two conflict.*

The Right to Speak Out

*Nonsmokers have the right to express — firmly but politely — their discomfort
and adverse reactions to tobacco smoke. They have the right to voice their objections
when smokers light up without asking permission.*

The Right to Act

*Nonsmokers have the right to take action through legislative means — as
individuals or in groups — to prevent or discourage smokers from polluting the
atmosphere and to seek the restriction of smoking in public places.*

politely if the smoker can hold off until you reach your destination or stop for a break.

✔ When giving a party, designate a smoking room. Suggest that friends do the same for parties at their houses.

✔ If you're about to participate in a long meeting or class, suggest regular smoking breaks to avoid a smoke-filled room.

✔ At restaurants, always ask for a table in the nonsmoking section or, if there is none, one in a well-ventilated part of the restaurant.

✔ If someone's smoke is bothering you, speak up. Be polite, not pushy. Say something like, "Excuse me, but smoke bothers me."

Quitting

Tobacco dependence may be the toughest addiction to overcome. One-third of smokers try to quit annually, but fewer than 10% succeed. Most people who eventually quit on their own have already tried other methods.

According to therapists, quitting usually isn't a one-time event but a "dynamic process" that may take several years and four to ten attempts. The good news is that half of all living Americans who ever smoked have managed to quit. And thanks to new products and programs, it may be easier now than ever before to become an ex-smoker.

Quitting on Your Own

More than 90% of former smokers quit on their own—by throwing away all their cigarettes, by gradually cutting down, or by first switching to a less potent brand. One characteristic of successful quitters is that they see themselves as active participants in health maintenance and take personal responsibility for their own health.[45] Often they experiment with a variety of strategies, such as learning relaxation techniques. In women, exercise has proven especially effective for quitting and avoiding weight gain.[46] (See Pulsepoints: "Ten Ways to Kick the Habit" for tips on how to smoke less—and less dangerously.)

Stop-Smoking Groups

Joining a support group doubles your chances of quitting for good. The American Cancer Society's FreshStart

Pulsepoints

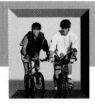

Ten Ways to Kick the Habit

1. Use delaying tactics. Have your first cigarette of the day 15 minutes later than usual, then 15 minutes later than that the next day, and so on.

2. Distract yourself. When you feel a craving for a cigarette, talk to someone, drink a glass of water, or get up and move around.

3. Establish nonsmoking hours. Instead of lighting up at the end of a meal, for instance, get up immediately, brush your teeth, wash your hands, or take a walk.

4. Never smoke two packs of the same brand in a row. Buy cigarettes only by the pack, not by the carton.

5. Make it harder to get to your cigarettes. Lock them in a drawer, wrap them in paper, or leave them in your coat or car.

6. Change the way you smoke. Smoke with the hand you don't usually use. Smoke only half of each cigarette.

7. Keep daily records. Chart your daily cigarette tally to see what progress you're making.

8. Stop completely for just one day at a time. Promise yourself 24 hours of freedom from cigarettes; when the day's over, make the same commitment for one more day. At the end of any 24

hour period, you can go back to smoking and not feel guilty.

9. Spend more time in places where you can't smoke. Take up bike-riding or swimming. Shower often. Go to movies or other places where smoking isn't allowed.

10. Go cold turkey. If you're a heavily addicted smoker, try a decisive and complete break. Smokers who quit completely are less likely to light up again than those who gradually decrease their daily cigarette consumption, switch to low-tar and low-nicotine brands, or use special filters and holders.

Program runs about 1500 stop-smoking clinics, each with about eight to eighteen members meeting for eight 2-hour sessions over four weeks. Instructors explain the risks of smoking, encourage individuals to think about why they smoke, and suggest ways of unlearning their smoking habit. A quitting day is set for the third or fourth session.

The American Lung Association's Freedom from Smoking Program consists of eight 1- to 2-hour sessions over seven weeks. The approach is similar to the American Cancer Society's, but smokers keep diaries and team up with buddies. Ex-smokers serve as advisers on quitting day. Both groups estimate that 27% or 28% of their participants successfully stop smoking.

Stop-smoking classes are also available through health-science departments and student-heath services on many college campuses, as well as through community public health departments. The Seventh-Day Adventists sponsor a four-week Breathe Free Plan, in which smokers commit themselves to clean living (no smoking, alcohol, tea, or coffee, along with a balanced diet and regular exercise). Many businesses sponsor smoking-cessation programs for employees, which generally follow the approaches of professional groups. Motivation may be even higher in these programs than

in programs outside the workplace, however, because some companies offer attractive incentives to participants, such as lower rates on their health insurance.

Some smoking-cessation programs rely primarily on **aversion therapy**, which provides a negative experience every time a smoker has a cigarette. This may involve taking drugs that make tobacco smoke taste unpleasant, undergoing electric shocks, having smoke blown at you, or rapid smoking (the inhaling of smoke every six seconds until you're dizzy or nauseated).

Nicotine Replacement Therapy

This approach uses a variety of products that supply low doses of nicotine in a way that allows smokers to taper off gradually over a period of months. They include nicotine gum (available in two doses) and slow-release skin patches. Although still experimental, a nasal spray also has shown promise.[47]

In research studies, nicotine replacement is the only treatment for nicotine addiction that has proven clearly beneficial. When measured against a look-alike placebo treatment, nicotine gum and patches have doubled the initial quitting rate and the numbers of smokers who remain abstinent six months to one year later. However, even with these approaches, only about one smoker in four quits completely; about half of these remain abstinent over the long term. Sales of nicotine patches, which rose rapidly after its introduction in 1992 to $600 million, have declined to $200 million annually.[48]

Nicotine Gum

Nicotine gum, sold as Nicorette, contains a nicotine resin that's gradually released as the gum is chewed. Absorbed through the mucous membrane of the mouth, the nicotine doesn't produce the same rush as a deeply inhaled drag on a cigarette. However, the gum maintains enough nicotine in the blood to diminish withdrawal symptoms. A month's supply of Nicorette costs roughly $45. (See Figure 16-8.)

Although this gum is lightly spiced to mask nicotine's bitterness, many users say that it takes several days to become accustomed to its unusual taste. Its side effects include mild indigestion, sore jaws, nausea, heartburn, and stomachache. Also, because Nicorette is heavier than regular chewing gum, it may loosen fillings or cause problems with dentures. Drinking coffee or other beverages may block absorption of the nicotine in the gum; individuals trying to quit smoking shouldn't ingest any substance immediately before or while chewing nicotine gum.

Nicotine in any form is harmful, and nicotine gum should not be used during pregnancy or by people with heart disease. Most people use nicotine gum as a temporary crutch and gradually taper off it until they can stop chewing it relatively painlessly. However, 5% to 10% of users transfer their dependence from cigarettes to the gum. When they stop using Nicorette, they experience withdrawal symptoms, although the symptoms tend to be milder than those prompted by quitting cigarettes. Intensive counseling to teach smokers coping methods can greatly increase the success rates.

Nicotine Patches

Nicotine transdermal delivery system products, or patches, provide nicotine, their only active ingredient, via a patch attached to the skin by an adhesive. Like nicotine gum, the nicotine patch minimizes withdrawal symptoms, such as intense craving for cigarettes. Some insurance programs pay for patch therapy. (See Figure 16-9.) Nicotine patches, which cost between $3.25 and $4 each, are replaced daily during therapy programs that run between 6 and 16 weeks. However, there is no evidence that continuing their use for more than eight weeks provides added benefit.[49]

Some patches deliver nicotine around the clock and others for just 16 hours (during waking hours). Those most likely to benefit from nicotine patch therapy are people who smoke more than a pack a day, are highly motivated to quit, and participate in counseling programs. However, the nicotine patch is not a cure for a smoking habit. While using the patch, 37% to 77% of people are able to abstain from smoking. But the patch doesn't affect the psychological dependence that makes quitting smoking so hard. That's why the key to long-term success in quitting smoking is getting support. When combined with counseling, the patch can be about twice as effective as a placebo, enabling 26% of smokers to abstain for six months.[50]

Because nicotine is a powerful, addictive substance, the use of nicotine patches for a prolonged period is not advised. Pregnant women and individuals with heart disease shouldn't use them. Patch wearers who smoke or use more than one patch at a time can experience a nicotine overdose; some users have even suffered heart attacks. Occasional side effects include redness, itching, or swelling at the site of the patch application; insomnia; dry mouth; and nervousness.

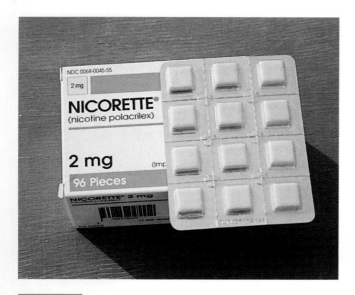

Figure 16-8

Nicorette gum, when chewed, gradually releases a nicotine resin and helps some smokers break their habit. Nicorette is now available without a prescription.

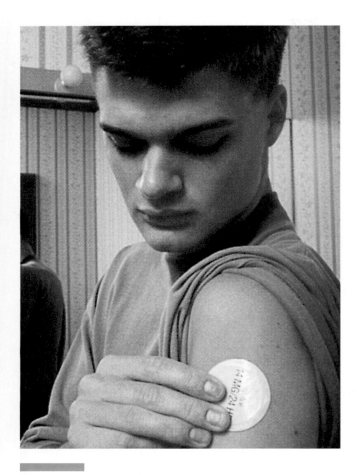

Figure 16-9

A nicotine patch releases nicotine transdermally (through the skin) in measured amounts, which are gradually decreased over time.

Smoke-Free Days

Since 1976, a November day has been set aside in the United States for the annual Great American Smoke-Out, an idea promoted by the American Cancer Society to encourage smokers to give up cigarettes for 24 hours. As many as 36% of American smokers have given up cigarettes on Smoke-Out Day; about 5 to 6% have quit permanently; 15% reduced smoking for extended periods.[51] In addition, the World Health Organization has established World No-Tobacco Days in May to call on nations to urge tobacco users to abstain for at least one day and perhaps quit for good.

Other Ways to Quit

Hypnosis may help some people quit smoking. Hypnotherapists use their techniques to create an

atmosphere of strict attention and give smokers in a mild trance positive suggestions for breaking their cigarette habit.

Acupuncture, in which a circular needle or staple is inserted in the flap in front of the opening to the ear, has also had some success. When smokers feel withdrawal symptoms, they gently move the needle or staple, which may increase the production of calming chemicals in the brain.

Making This Chapter Work for You
Clearing the Air

■ Many people have stopped smoking because of the health risks associated with tobacco use and because, as a social behavior, smoking has become unpopular. However, smoking is increasing among young white teens.

■ Smokers may continue to smoke because they find smoking pleasurable or because the nicotine in cigarettes relieves feelings of depression. Most become dependent on nicotine, which is powerfully addictive. If they don't receive regular daily doses, smokers suffer withdrawal symptoms, such as irritability, anxiety, headache, and changes in performance.

■ Nicotine affects mood, hunger, blood pressure, heart rate, and the performance of certain mental tasks. It also contributes to heart and respiratory diseases. The tar in cigarettes is carcinogenic and can damage the respiratory system.

■ The incidence of heart attack and cardiomyopathy is high among smokers, possibly because of the effects of nicotine, which increases blood pressure and constricts blood vessels, and carbon monoxide, which diminishes oxygen received by the heart. In the United States, more people die of lung cancer, usually caused by smoking, than of any other type of cancer. Smoking also contributes to the development of other cancers, including cancer of the mouth and larynx, esophagus, bladder and kidney, and pancreas.

■ Besides causing lung cancer, smoking can cause two types of chronic obstructive lung disease—emphysema and chronic bronchitis. Cigarette smoking is also

Health Online

The Quitnet   http://www.quitnet.org

This site is dedicated to helping smokers kick the habit. It contains many interactive exercises, including quizzes to determine why you smoke and where you are in the quitting process. There are also features to help you set a quit date and make a behavior change plan, and an online support forum to allow you to chat with others who are trying to stop smoking. If you want further references on tobacco use, turn to the library, links, or news features.

Think about it ...

- If you are currently a smoker, would this Web site make it easier for you to quit? What features would be most helpful to you?

- Do you have any friends or family members who are smokers? How do you feel about their smoking? Do you know if they have ever tried to quit?

- What strategies does this site offer that might apply to other behaviors you would like to change in your life?

associated with ulcers, liver disease, and gum disease and dental problems.

- Women who smoke face the additional risk of developing reproductive disorders such as cervical cancer. A pregnant woman who smokes has a high risk of miscarriage, ectopic pregnancy, or losing her baby shortly before, during, or after birth. Her baby may be born prematurely or underweight; with poor respiration, heart rate, muscle tone, or color; or with respiratory or heart disease.

- Clove cigarettes may be more dangerous than conventional cigarettes because they contain more nicotine, tar, and carbon monoxide. People who chew tobacco or use snuff are at risk of nicotine addiction, teeth and gum conditions, and cancer of the mouth and throat.

- Environmental, or secondhand, smoke is a dangerous carcinogen. Nonsmokers constantly exposed to cigarette smoke are at risk of many illnesses, including lung cancer and heart disease. The spouses and children of smokers are at greatest risk of developing lung cancer, heart disease, and other ailments.

- Quitting cigarettes often requires four to ten attempts, but 90% of those who quit eventually succeed on their own. The health benefits of quitting smoking include longer life span and greatly reduced risk of heart disease, cancer, and other diseases. One approach to quitting smoking is gradually reducing the number of cigarettes smoked per day. Another is stopping all at once. People who need help to stop smoking can try stop-smoking groups or programs, aversion therapy, nicotine replacement (with gum or patches), hypnosis, and acupuncture.

Learning to live without tobacco requires great commitment. If you smoke and want to stop, don't think of quitting as giving up something pleasant, but rather as beginning something even more pleasant. With every healthy breath you take, you're renewing yourself, becoming better—making a new you.

Key Terms

The terms listed here are used within the chapter. Page numbers are included for each term.
A definition of each term is given in the green Glossary pages at the end of this book.

aversion therapy *525*   **nicotine** *510*   **sidestream smoke** *521*

carbon monoxide *510*   **mainstream smoke** *521*   **tar** *510*

**environmental tobacco
   smoke** *521*

Review Questions

1. Who is likely to be today's tobacco smoker? Why do young people start to smoke?

2. How does smoking tobacco affect a person's health? What are the health effects of using smokeless tobacco?

3. What health problems can be prevented by quitting smoking?

4. Describe some methods smokers use to quit smoking. Which are the most effective?

5. What is sidestream, or secondhand, smoke? How does it affect the health of nonsmokers?

6. What are some ways you can keep your personal environment smoke-free? What are the advantages of doing so?

Critical Thinking Questions

1. Has smoking become unpopular among your friends or family? What social activities continue to be associated with smoking? Can you think of any situations in which smoking might be frowned upon?

2. How would you motivate someone you care about to stop smoking? What reasons would you give for them to stop? Describe your strategy.

3. According to the chapter, environmental tobacco smoke is even more dangerous than mainstream smoke. If you're a nonsmoker, how would you react to someone who's smoking in the same room as you? Define the rights of smokers and nonsmokers.

Connections to Personal Health Interactive

To enhance your understanding of the material covered in this chapter, check out the following study aids on the **Personal Health Interactive CD-ROM**. *Each numbered icon within the chapter corresponds to an appropriate activity listed here.*

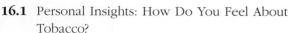

16.1 Personal Insights: How Do You Feel About Tobacco?

16.2 Chapter 16 Review

References

1. Hilts, Philip. "Tobacco Held to Be Drug That Must Be Regulated." *New York Times*, July 13, 1995.

2. "Things You Should Know About Children and Tobacco Use." *American Academy of Pediatrics Fact Sheet*, 1997.

3. Voelker, Rebecca. "Young People May Face Huge Tobacco Toll." *Journal of the American Medical Association*, Vol. 274, No. 3, July 19, 1995.

4. "Things You Should Know About Children and Tobacco Use."

5. "The Plague Years." *American Health*, December 1994.

6. "New APA Position Statement Urges Action to Reduce High Rates of Nicotine Dependence." *Psychiatric Services*, Vol. 46, No. 2, February 1995.

7. American Cancer Society.

8. Koop, C. Everett, et al. "Reinventing American Tobacco Policy." *Journal of the American Medical Association*, Vol. 279, No. 7, February 18, 1998.

9. "Smoking Found to Snuff Out the Benefits of Exercise." *American Medical News*, April 6, 1992.

10. Howard, George, et al. "Cigarette Smoking and Progression of Atherosclerosis." *Journal of the American Medical Association*, Vol. 279, No. 2, January 14, 1998.

11. Wannamethee, S. Goya, et al. "Smoking Cessation and the Risk of Stroke in Middle-Aged Men." *Journal of the American Medical Association*, Vol. 274, No. 2, July 12, 1995.

12. Cunningham, Health "Daily Tobacco Use Among Young People at Epidemic Level." *American Academy of Pediatrics News*, October 10, 1997.

13. "Youth and Tobacco Addiction." CDC's Tobacco Information & Prevention Sourcepage, www.cdc.gov., 1998.

14. King, Charles, et al. "Adolescent Exposure to Cigarette Advertising in Magazines." *Journal of the American Medical Association*, Vol. 279, No. 7, February 18, 1998.

15. Pierce, John, et al. "Tobacco Industry Promotion of Cigarettes and Adolescent Smoking." *Journal of the American Medical Association*, Vol. 279, No. 7, February 18, 1998.

16. Hilts, Philip, "Black Teen Agers Are Turning Away from Smoking, But Whites Puff On." *New York Times*, April 19, 1995.

17. Douglas, Kathy, et al. "Results from the 1995 National College Health Risk Behavior Survey." *Journal of American College Health*, Vol. 46, September 1997.

18. Centers for Disease Control and Prevention. Kemper, Vicki. "Where the Action Is." *Common Cause Magazine*, Vol. 21, No. 1, Spring 1995. Spector, Rosanne. "White Men with Limited Education Almost Certain to Smoke; Hispanics Less Likely." Stanford University Medical Center, August 8, 1995.

19. Benowitz, Neal. "The Genetics of Drug Dependence: Tobacco Addiction." *New England Journal of Medicine*, September 17, 1992.

20. Hales, Dianne. "Smoking Earlier." *Parade*, March 1, 1998.

21. Centers for Disease Control and Prevention. "Reasons for Tobacco Use and Symptoms of Nicotine Withdrawal Among Adolescent and Young Adult Tobacco Users." *Journal of the American Medical Association*, Vol. 272, No. 21, December 7, 1994. Gibbons, Frederick, et al. "Prevalence Estimates and Adolescent Risk

Behavior: Cross-Cultural Differences in Social Influence." *Journal of Applied Psychology*, Vol. 80, No. 1, February 1995.

22. Talcott, Gerald, et al. "Is Weight Gain After Smoking Cessation Inevitable?" *Journal of Consulting & Clinical Psychology*, Vol. 63, No. 2, April 1995.

23. Sheahan, Sharon, and Melissa Latimer. "Correlates of Smoking, Stress, and Depression Among Women." *Health Values*, Vol. 19, No. 1, January–February 1995.

24. Lerman, Caryl, et al. "Depression and Self-Medication with Nicotine: The Modifying Influence of the Dopamine D4 Receptor Gene." *Health Psychology*, Vol. 17, No. 1, January 1998.

25. Murray, Robert, et al. "Level of Involvement with Alcohol and Success at Smoking Cessation in the Lung Health Study." *Journal of Studies on Alcohol*, Vol. 56, No. 1, January 1995.

26. "Nicotine Addiction in Female Smokers." *American Family Physician*, Vol. 51, No. 7, May 15, 1994.

27. Helson, Heidi, et al. "Smoking, Alcohol and Neuromuscular and Physical Function of Older Women." *Journal of the American Medical Association*, Vol. 272, No. 23, December 21, 1994.

28. Morbidity and Mortality Weekly Report (MMWR). "Medical Care Expenditures Attributable to Cigarette Smoking During Pregnancy." *Journal of the American Medical Association*, Vol. 278, No. 23, December 17, 1997.

29. Morbidity and Mortality Weekly Report (MMWR). "Cigar Smoking Among Teenagers." *Journal of the American Medical Association*, Vol. 278, No. 1, July 2, 1997.

30. Morbidity and Mortality Weekly Report (MMWR). "Cigar Smoking Among Teenagers—United States, Massachusetts and New York." Vol. 46, No. 20, May 23, 1997.

31. Cowley, Geoffrey. "Are Stogies Safer Than Cigarettes?" *Newsweek*, July 21, 1997.

32. Federal Trade Commission. *Smokeless Tobacco Report 1997*.

33. Darmody, Donna, and Beverly Ehrich. "Snuffing It Out: A Smokeless Tobacco Intervention with Athletes at a Small Private College." *Journal of American College Health*, Vol. 43, July 1994.

34. Daughety, Virginia, et al. "Surveying Smokeless Tobacco Use, Oral Lesions and Cessation Among High School Boys." *Journal of the American Dental Association*, Vol. 125, No. 2, February 1994.

35. "Dipping into Nicotine Content in Snuff." *Science News*, Vol. 147, No. 19, May 13, 1995. Tilashalski, Ken, et al. "Assessing the Nicotine Content of Smokeless Tobacco Product." *Journal of the American Dental Association*, Vol. 125, No. 5, May 1994.

36. Glantz, Stanton, and William Parmley. "Passive Smoking and Heart Disease." *Journal of the American Medical Association*, Vol. 273, No. 13, April 5, 1995.

37. Centers for Disease Control and Prevention (CDC). "State-specific Prevalence of Cigarette Smoking Among Adults, and Children's and Adolescents Exposure to Environmental Tobacco Smoke." *Journal of the American Medical Association*, Vol. 278, No. 23, December 17, 1997.

38. Grady, Denise. "Study Finds Second-hand Smoke Doubles Heart Disease." *New York Times*, May 2, 1997.

39. Steenland, Kyle. "Passive Smoking and the Risk of Heart Disease." *Journal of the American Medical Association*, January 1, 1992.

40. "Klonoff-Cohen, Hillary, et al. "The Effect of Passive Smoking and Tobacco Exposure Through Breast Milk on Sudden Infant Death Syndrome." *Journal of the American Medical Association*, Vol. 273, No. 10, March 8, 1995.

41. Gergen, Peter, et al. "Environmental Tobacco Smoke: A Hazard to Children." *Pediatrics*, February 1997.

42. Stapleton, Stephanie. "Papers Deal Another Blow to Tobacco." *American Medical News*, Vol. 41, No. 5, February 2, 1998.

43. Meier, Barry. "Data on Tobacco Show a Strategy Aimed at Blacks." *New York Times*, February 6, 1998.

44. Siegel, Michael, et al. "Preemption in Tobacco Control." *Journal of the American Medical Association*, Vol. 278, No. 10, September 10, 1997.

45. Cooper, Thomas. *New Hope for Heavy Smokers*. Lexington, KY: SBC, 1992.

46. Marcus, Bess, et al. "Exercise Enhances the Maintenance of Smoking Cessation in Women." *Addictive Behaviors*, Vol. 20, No. 1, January–February 1995.

47. Apgar, Barbara, et al. "Effect of Nicotine Nasal Spray on Smoking Cessation." *Archives of Internal Medicine*, November 28, 1994.

48. Thorndike, Anne, et al. "National Patterns in the Treatment of Smokers by Physicians." *Journal of the American Medical Association*, Vol. 279, No. 8, February 25, 1998.

49. Franklin, John. "Addiction Medicine." *Journal of the American Medical Association*, Vol. 273, No. 21, June 7, 1995.

50. Buttaro, Marissa. "Staying on Top of Transdermal Drug Patches." *Nursing*, Vol. 24, No. 11, November 1994.

51. Morbidity and Mortality Weekly Report. "Impact of Promotion of the Great American Smokeout and Availability of Over-the-Counter Nicotine Medications." *Journal of the American Medical Association*, Vol. 278, No. 23, December 17, 1997.

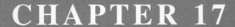

CHAPTER 17

PROTECTING YOURSELF

After studying the material in this chapter, you should be able to:

List and **explain** factors that increase the likelihood of an accident or injury.

Describe safety procedures for road, residential, worksite, and outdoor safety.

Define sexual victimization, sexual harassment, and sexual coercion, and **explain** how each can develop.

List the different types of rape, and **describe** recommended actions for preventing rape.

Explain the consequences of sexual violence, and **describe** how they can be treated.

Describe the abuse pattern, and **explain** how it relates to child abuse and partner abuse.

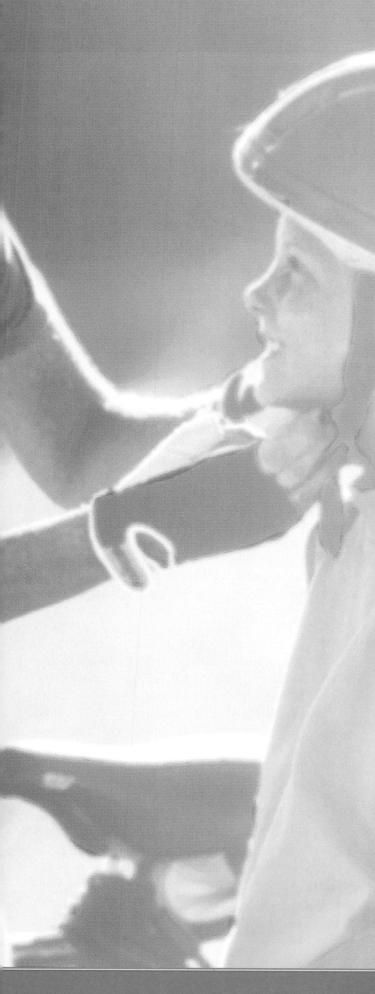

The major threats to the well-being of most college students aren't illnesses but injuries. Accidents, especially motor-vehicle crashes, kill more college-age men and women than all other causes combined; the greatest number of lives lost to accidents is among those 21 years of age.[1] In recent years, another threat has claimed the lives of tens of thousands of Americans of all ages: violence. Each year 40,000 men, women, and children die and 100,000 are injured by firearms.[2] Violent crime—murders, rapes, robberies, aggravated assaults—victimize some 4.4 million Americans a year.[3]

Recognizing the threat of intentional and unintentional injury is the first step to ensuring your personal safety. You may think that the risk of something bad happening is simply a matter of chance, of being in the wrong place at the wrong time. That's not the case. Certain behaviors, such as alcohol and drug use (which are involved in many fatal car accidents and violent crimes), greatly increase risk and threaten safety. Ultimately, you have more control over such risks than anyone or anything else in your life.

This chapter is a primer in self-protection that could help safeguard—perhaps even save—your life. Included are recommendations for common sense safety on the road, at home, outdoors, and on the job. This chapter also explores other serious threats to personal safety in our society—violence, both public and domestic, and sexual victimization.

Unintentional Injury: Why Accidents Happen

You may assume that most accidents happen without any warning. Yet often an accident is the unfortunate result of a series or combination of events. The more you know about the factors that increase the likelihood of an accident or injury, the more you can do to prevent it. (See Self-Survey: "Are You Doing Enough to Prevent Accidents?")

Unsafe Attitudes

Where do you feel safest? Chances are you'll answer by naming the places that are most familiar to you: your room, your home, your car. Yet that's where you're most likely to have an accident—often because you let your guard down. While listening to the morning news, you may forget to shut off a burner on the stove. Since there usually isn't much traffic on your street, you may back out of your driveway without looking both ways. Most of the time you, or someone with you, is able to correct such dangerous situations before a fire or collision occurs. But you can't count on always being so lucky.

Keep in mind that *feeling* safe is not the same as *being* safe. Away from home, unsafe attitudes can set the stage for unsafe behaviors. If you're overly confident in your driving skills, you may speed on a winding or wet road. If you're daydreaming, you may trip and fall as you hike. Keeping your wits about you is essential to keeping yourself safe.

Individual Risk Factors

Many factors influence an individual's risk of accident or injury, including those discussed in the following sections.

Age and Gender

The very young and the very old are the most susceptible to serious injury. Children may not recognize the danger of running into the street or jumping into a pool. In older people, a combination of factors—poor health, vision and hearing impairments, a faltering sense of balance, decreased agility, slower reflexes, and reduced resilience—make accidents a greater threat. Most victims of fatal accidents victims are males, often in their teens and twenties. Feeling full of life and energy, they may take dangerous risks because they think they're invulnerable.

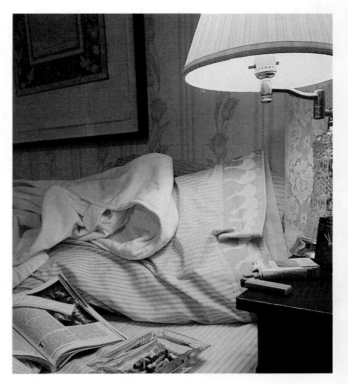

Home is a dangerous place. Many accidents happen at home—perhaps because we let down our guard there.

Alcohol and Drugs

An estimated 40% of Americans are involved in an alcohol-related accident sometime during their lives. In nearly half of motor-vehicle deaths, either the driver or a pedestrian was intoxicated at the time of the crash.[4] Other drugs also affect driving ability by impairing judgment and perceptions. (See Chapters 14 and 15.)

Stress

In times of tension and anxiety, we all pay less attention to what we're doing. We rush about; we don't take time to relax or rest. One common result is an increase in accidents during busy or stressful periods. If you find yourself having a series of small mishaps or "near-misses," it's important to do something to lower your stress level, rather than wait for something more harmful to happen. (See Chapter 2 on stress.)

Situational Factors

Some situations—such as driving on a curvy, wet road in a car with worn tires—are so inherently dangerous that they greatly increase the odds of an accident. But even when there's greater risk, you can lower the danger—for instance, you can't make the road dry, but you can make sure your tires and brakes are in good condition.

Self-Survey

Are You Doing Enough to Prevent Accidents?

Accidents frequently result in serious injury, and a large number of deaths.

The following questions are designed to test how well you protect yourself and your family from accidental injury. The first group of questions concentrates on guarding against possible hazards in and around your house or apartment. The second group deals with safety measures that should be taken against accidents that might happen to you or your family on the road, whether in a vehicle or as pedestrians. The third group is concerned mainly with safety on vacations, when unfamiliar surroundings and activities present special hazards.

Group 1: Safety at Home
Answer Yes or No to the following questions:

1. Do you make it a point never to smoke in bed?
2. If you have fireplaces, do you keep screens around them?
3. When cooking, do you guard against accidental hot spills by positioning pan handles so that they don't extend outward?
4. Do you keep electrical cords out of the reach of children and avoid overloading electrical outlets?
5. Are you careful never to leave small children unsupervised in the kitchen or bathroom?
6. Are nightclothes and soft toys labeled to show that they're made of nonflammable materials?
7. Are medicines in your house kept in a secure place, out of children's reach and away from beds?
8. Are you careful never to store drugs or dangerous chemicals (bleach, paint-stripper, and so on) within children's reach or in incorrectly labeled containers?
9. If you own a gun, do you keep it unloaded, separate from the ammunition, and locked away?
10. Do you make a point of preventing your children from playing with objects small enough to be swallowed or inhaled?
11. Do you keep plastic bags away from your children?
12. When working around the house, do you wear safety glasses, earplugs, and protective clothing such as sturdy shoes?
13. Are your carpets firmly fixed, with no ragged spots or edges, and are loose rugs placed to minimize the risk of sliding or tripping?
14. Are your stairs, halls, and other passages lit brightly enough to read a newspaper?
15. Is it a rule in your house that nothing gets left on the stairs?
16. If you spill or drop something on the floor that might be slippery, do you always clean it up right away?
17. Do you keep nonslip mats both in and alongside the bath or shower?

Group 2: Safety on the Road
Answer Yes or No to the following questions:

18. Have you taught your children exactly how, when, and where to cross streets safely?
19. Have your children been taught the basic rules of the road to use when bicycling?
20. When walking in streets or open roads at twilight or in the dark, do all members of your family carry a flashlight, or wear a markedly visible outer garment, such as a white or luminous jacket?
21. Do you always drive within the speed limit and defensively?
22. Are you always careful not to drink if you're going to drive a car soon afterward?
23. Do you avoid driving when you feel unusually tired or ill, or if you're taking drugs (such as antihistamines) known to impair alertness?
24. Do you have your car fully serviced, including checking the lights, tires, windshield washer and wipers, brakes, and steering, either every 6000 miles (10,000 km) or at least every six months?
25. Do you check at least once a week to make sure that your car windows, lights, mirrors, and reflectors are clean?
26. When driving, do you always try to keep a gap between your car and the one in front of you of at least a yard (or meter) for each mile-per-hour you're traveling?
27. Do you always make sure that you and all passengers in your car use available seatbelts?
28. Are any infants or toddlers riding in your car securely strapped into infant car seats?

Group 3: Safety on Vacations
Answer Yes or No to the following questions:

29. Are all members of your family able to swim or in the process of learning how to swim?
30. Do you test the depth of the water and go in feet first?
31. In a boat, does everyone always wear a life jacket?
32. If you do any skiing, hiking, or climbing, do you always go properly prepared with the right clothing and equipment?
33. When going on an excursion for a day or longer, do you tell someone what your route is and when you expect to return?
34. Do you and your family take full safety precautions and have the proper equipment when you engage in contact and other possibly dangerous sports?

35. Before taking up a new and potentially dangerous activity, such as hang gliding, do you make sure you get proper instruction?

36. During a vacation, do you make sure you get adequate rest and relaxation?

Evaluation

A No answer to any of the above questions indicates that you're not doing all you can to minimize your risk of accidents. You can and should take all the protective steps suggested by the questions.

Making Changes ······························
Staying Safe

Staying safe is a matter of attitude, awareness of potential danger, and attention to what's happening around you. Here are some suggestions to keep you on the safe side:

- Look for accidents waiting to happen, such as newspapers and cans piled on the stairs, or an empty coffee pot or electric hair curler left on. Try to develop the habit of looking around your room or home regularly to check for potential dangers.

- Don't be so sure that an accident could never happen to you. If you think that accidents only affect other people, you may take risks that jeopardize your well-

being, such as diving head-first into unfamiliar waters. Everyone needs to be aware of potential risks.

- During busy or stressful periods, think of minor injuries, such as a finger cut in the kitchen or a fender-bender in a parking lot, as warning signs of stress overload. Try to keep certain aspects of your life—morning rituals, a relaxing dinnertime, daily exercise—unchanged. Also, incorporate some of the stress-management strategies discussed in Chapter 2 into your daily schedule.

- In dangerous situations, such as driving on a snowy road on a foggy night, do whatever you can to lower the risks. For instance, put chains on your tires and drive much more slowly than usual. The best way to protect yourself from external dangers is to identify potential threats and take protective action before an accident occurs.

- Don't abuse alcohol or drugs. Substance abuse plays a major role in all types of accidents. Alcohol is involved in nearly half of all motor-vehicle fatalities; other drugs, including cocaine, also affect driving ability by impairing judgment and perceptions. Drug abuse also increases the danger of work-related injuries.

SOURCE: Kunz, Jeffrey, and Asher Finkel, eds. *The AMA Family Medical Guide.* New York: Random House, 1987.

Thrill-Seeking

Some people crave the sensation of danger. To them, activities that others might find terrifying—such as skydiving or parachute-jumping—are stimulating. The reason may be that they have lower than normal levels of the brain chemicals that regulate excitement. Because the stress of potentially hazardous sports may increase the levels of these chemicals, they feel pleasantly aroused rather than scared. However, their desire for this sensation could lead them to ignore safety precautions and jeopardize their safety.[5]

Left-Handedness

America's 33 million left-handed individuals, or "lefties," have nearly two accidents for every one suffered by right-handers. While left-handers are at greater risk in various situations and activities, driving seems especially dangerous for them. Left-handers are 85% more likely to have an accident-related injury when driving than are right-handers; the risk is greatest for left-handed men. According to Stanley Coren, author of *The Left-Hander Syndrome,* left-handers face more dangers because "the world was primarily designed by right-handers for the comfort and convenience of right-handers."[6]

Strategies for Prevention
·····················
Coping with Emergencies

Life-threatening situations rarely happen more than once or twice in any person's life. When they do, you must think and act quickly to prevent disastrous consequences.

✔ *Don't panic.* Your immediate response to an emergency may be overwhelming fear and anxiety. Take several deep breaths. Start by assessing the circumstances. Shout for help if you're in a public place. Look for any possible dangers to you or the victim, such as a live electrical wire or a fire. Seek medical assistance as quickly as possible. Don't attempt rescue techniques, such as cardiopulmonary resuscitation (CPR), unless you're trained. (For advice on what to do in case of a heart attack, see Chapter 12 and the "Emergency!" section at the back of this book.)

✔ *Don't wait for symptoms to go away or get worse.* If you suspect that someone is having a heart attack or stroke, or has ingested something poisonous, *phone for help immediately.* A delay could jeopardize the person's life. Stay on the line long enough to give your name, address, and a brief description of the emergency.

✔ *Don't move a victim.* The person may have a broken neck or back, and attempting to move him or her could cause extensive damage or even death.

✔ *Don't drive.* Even if the hospital is just ten minutes away, you're better off waiting for a well-equipped ambulance with trained paramedics who can deliver emergency care on the spot. People rushing to emergency rooms are more likely to get into accidents themselves.

✔ *At home, keep a supply of basic first-aid items in a convenient place.* Make sure that emergency telephone numbers (ambulance service, police and fire departments, poison control center, your doctor and neighbors) are handy. If you can't find a number quickly, call the operator.

✔ *Don't do too much.* Often well-intentioned Good Samaritans make injuries worse by trying to tie tourniquets, wash cuts, or splint broken limbs. Also, don't give an injured person anything to eat or drink. (See "Emergency!" in the Hales Health Almanac at the back of this book for more on first-aid and emergency care.)

Safety on the Road

Although the number of deaths and injuries from car crashes has declined in recent years, motor-vehicle accidents remain the leading cause of death among Americans aged 1 to 34, and the third most significant cause of lost years of potential life (after heart disease and can-

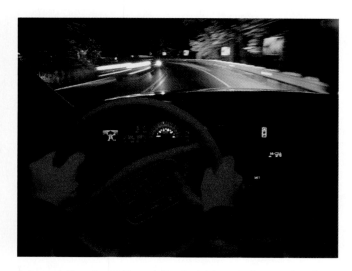

Asleep at the wheel? Especially at night, and when you're alone, falling asleep while driving can be particularly dangerous. Sleep-related vehicle accidents are second only to alcohol-related accidents.

cer). As shown in Campus Focus: "College Students and Road Safety," many college students also take risks on the road: 12.3% of men and 6.6% of women rarely or never buckle up; 33.2% of men and 22.8% of women have driven after drinking; among those who rode motorcycles in the previous year, 31.1% of men and 37% of the women rarely or never wore helmets.[7]

Defensive Driving

Basic precautions can greatly increase your odds of reaching a destination alive. Number one is not driving after drinking. In recent years, there has been a decline in the number of fatalities caused by drunk driving, particularly among young people. The National Highway Traffic Safety Administration attributes this decline to increases in the drinking age from 18 to 21 in all 50 states and the District of Columbia, to educational programs aimed at reducing and driving by teens, to the formation of Students Against Driving Drunk (SADD) and similar groups, and to changes in state laws that penalize drivers younger than age 21 for driving with even lower blood-alcohol concentration levels than were previously acceptable (from 0.01% to 0.05%). (See Chapter 15 for more information on blood-alcohol concentrations and drunk driving.)

Falling asleep at the wheel is second only to alcohol as a cause of serious motor-vehicle accidents. According to the National Commission on Sleep Disorders Research, each year 200,000 sleep-related motor-vehicle accidents claim more than 5000 lives, cause hundreds of thousands of injuries, and lead to billions of dollars in indirect costs.

The best lifesavers for drivers and passengers are seatbelts, which are now required for children and adults in many states. Because of changes in federal law, beginning with 1998 models, all new cars will be equipped with air bags. Safety officials recommend that people shopping for a new car invest in vehicles with dual air bags in front and lap-shoulder belts for the rear as well as the front seats.

Although air bags can save adults' lives, they may be hazardous to infants and young children. In 1998, the national Highway Traffic Safety Administration gave automobile owners permission to deactivate air bags. However, the American Academy of Pediatrics, which has argued that deactivation may pose an even greater risk by jeopardizing the safety of older children, teenagers, and adult passengers, has recommended that children be placed in the backseat, whether or not the car is equipped with an air bag.[8]

CAMPUS FOCUS:
COLLEGE STUDENTS AND ROAD SAFETY

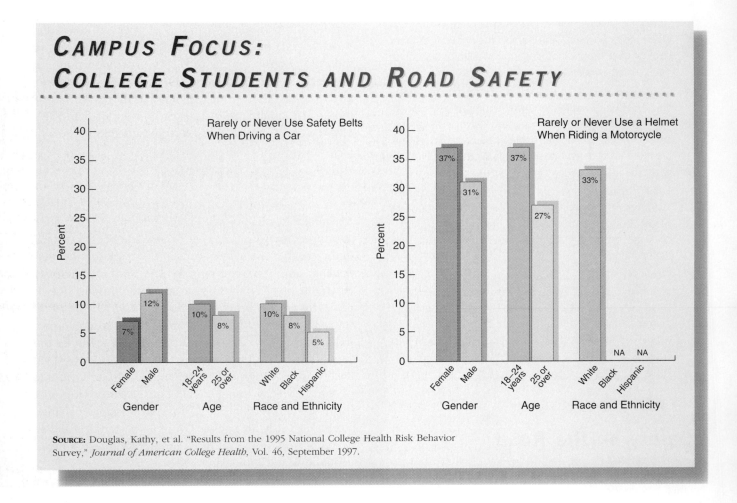

SOURCE: Douglas, Kathy, et al. "Results from the 1995 National College Health Risk Behavior Survey," *Journal of American College Health*, Vol. 46, September 1997.

Road Rage

According to a recent study by the AAA Foundation for Traffic Safety, "violent aggressive driving"—a deliberate attempt to harm another driver after a traffic dispute—is rising by 7% per year. "The violent incidents that make the papers are still relatively rare," says Phil Berardelli, author of *The Driving Challenge*. "But what's equally horrible is the everyday climate of driving, the basic level of aggression that almost everyone participates in. The majority of drivers, women and men, drive more discourteously than they should."[9]

This habitual hostility can and often does erupt into the emotional outbursts known as road rage—a factor, says the National Highway Traffic Safety Administration, in as many as two-thirds of all fatal car crashes and one-third of nonfatal accidents.[10] Psychologist Arnold Nerenberg of Whittier, California, a specialist in motorway mayhem, estimates that there may be 1.78 billion episodes of road rage a year, resulting in more than 28,000 deaths and 1 million injuries.[11]

What transforms perfectly polite, well-mannered Joe and Jane Jekylls into hell-bent Mr. and Mrs. Hydes behind the wheel? Terror, says Stephanie Faulk of the AAA Foundation for Traffic Safety. "If someone darts in front of you, for a second you think you are going to die, and the fight or flight impulse kicks in. People are more likely to fight in a car because they're encased in a steel shell and they feel safe. And the other driver is anonymous. You can't see his face or hear his voice so you don't have any social cues to guide you. You think, 'I'll show him,' because the consequences seem remote." This isn't necessarily so. Road rage has led to deadly races, confrontations, and shootings.[12] Some strategies for reducing road rage include the following:

- *Lower the stress in your life.* Take a few moments to breathe deeply and relax your shoulders before putting the key in the ignition.

- *Consciously decide not to let other drivers get to you.* Decide that whatever happens, it's not going to make your blood pressure go up.

- *Slow down.* If you're going five or ten miles over the speed limit, you won't have the time you need to react to anything that happens.

- *Modify bad driving habits one at a time.* If you tend to tailgate slow drivers, spend a week driving at twice your usual following distance. If you're a habitual horn honker, silence yourself.

- *Be courteous—even if other drivers aren't.* Don't dawdle in the passing lane. Never tailgate or switch lanes without signaling. Don't use your horn or high beams unless absolute necessary.

- *Never retaliate.* Whatever another driver does, keep your cool. Count to ten. Take a deep breath. If you yell or gesture at someone who's upset with you, the conflict may well escalate.

- *If you do something stupid, show that you're sorry.* On its web site, the AAA Foundation for Traffic Safety solicited suggestions for automotive apologies. The most popular: slapping yourself on your forehead or the top of your head to indicate that you know you goofed. Such gestures can soothe a miffed motorist—and make the roads a slightly safer place for all of us to be.

Strategies for Prevention

How to Drive Safely

Don't drive while under the influence of alcohol or other drugs, including medications that may impair your reflexes, cause drowsiness, or affect your judgment. Never get into a car if you suspect the driver may be intoxicated or affected by a drug.

✔ Remain calm when dealing with drivers who are reckless or rude. Be alert and anticipate possible hazards. Don't let yourself be distracted by conversations, children's questions, arguments, food or drink, or scenic views. If you become exhausted, pull over and rest.

✔ Don't get too comfortable. Alertness matters. Use the rearview mirror often. Don't let passengers or packages obstruct your view. Use the turn signals when changing lanes or making a turn. If someone cuts you off, back off to a safe distance. When you can, drive so that you have enough space around you.

✔ Make sure small children are in safety seats. Unless pets are trained to ride quietly in a car, keep them in carrying cases.

✔ Drive more slowly if weather conditions are bad. Avoid driving at all during heavy rain, snow, or other conditions that affect visibility and road conditions. If you must drive in hazardous conditions, make sure that your car has the proper equipment, such as chains or snow tires, and that you know how to respond in case of a skid.

✔ Maintain your car properly, replacing windshield wipers, tires, and brakes when necessary. Keep flares and a fire extinguisher in your car for use in emergencies.

✔ To avoid a head-on collision, generally veer to the right—onto a shoulder, lawn, or open space. Steer your way to safety; avoid hitting the brakes hard once you leave the pavement. If you have to hit something stationary, look for a "soft" target—bushes, parked cars, woodframe buildings—as opposed to "hard" boulders, brick walls, trees, concrete abutments, and so on.

Safe Cycling

Mile for mile, motorcycling is far more risky than automobile driving. The most common motorcycle injury is head trauma, which can lead to physical disability, including paralysis and general weakness, as well as problems reading and thinking. It can also cause personality changes and psychiatric problems, such as depression, anxiety, and uncontrollable mood swings and anger. Some improvement may occur naturally as swelling diminishes and the brain heals. However, complete recovery from head trauma can take four to six years, and the costs can be staggering. Head injury can also result in permanent disability, coma, and death. To

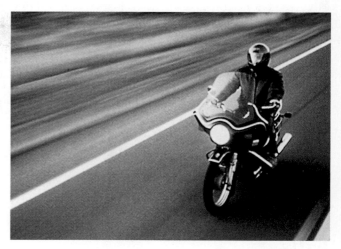

Use your head. Head trauma is the most common motorcycle injury—and one of the most preventable.

prevent head trauma, motorcycle helmets are required in most states. Federal law dictates that a certain percentage of highway construction funds be reallocated for safety programs in states that don't require motorcycle helmets.

Bicycling injuries cause almost 200,000 head injuries each year; they account for 70% to 80% of all bicycle fatalities. According to CDC estimates, safety helmets—now required by law in some states—reduce the risk of head injury by 85% and could prevent one death every day and one head injury every four minutes.[13]

In the past, many cyclists resisted wearing helmets because of their appearance or bulk. However, new designs are both attractive and lightweight. Today's average helmet weighs a pound or less; new ultralight models weigh as little as 8.5 ounces. Made of very dense foam with no outer shell, they're cool and comfortable but may not be as durable as conventional helmets. Helmets should meet the standards set by the American National Standards Institute (ANSI) or the Snell Memorial Foundation, and should be replaced every five years because the materials deteriorate under the stress of regular wear and exposure to heat.

In addition to wearing helmets, cyclists should know and follow traffic rules: yield right-of-way appropriately, signal turns properly, obey stop signs, and so on. They should use bike lanes if they're available, and avoid weaving in and out of traffic or riding in the center of the street or against the flow of traffic. Bikes should have reflectors on the front, back, and both wheels, as well as taillights and headlights for night use.

TABLE 17-1 CAUSES OF FATAL ACCIDENTS

Age	Cause	Deaths per 100,000
Overall	Motor-vehicle accidents	18.8
	Falls	5
	Poison[a]	2
Under 1 year	Suffocation	6.1
	Motor-vehicle accidents	4.9
	Choking on food or an object	4.2
1–4	Motor-vehicle accidents	6.3
	Drowning	3.8
	Fires and/or burns	3.7
5–14	Motor-vehicle accidents	5.9
	Drowning	1.4
	Fires and/or burns	0.9
15–24	Motor-vehicle accidents	34.1
	Drowning	2.5
	Firearm injuries	1.4
25–44	Motor-vehicle accidents	20.5
	Poison	4
	Drowning	1.8
45–64	Motor-vehicle accidents	18.6
	Falls	3.2
	Poison	1.7
65–74	Motor-vehicle accidents	18.6
	Falls	9
	Medical complications	3.5
75+	Falls	59
	Motor-vehicle accidents	30
	Choking on food or an object	12.5

[a] Solid or liquid, including drug overdoses.
SOURCE: *American Health*, June 1994, p. 54.

Safety at Home

Every year home accidents claim more than 24,000 lives and cause nearly 25 million injuries. Common dangers are poisoning, falls, and burns. Half a million children swallow poisonous materials each year; 90% are under age 5. Adults may also be poisoned by mistakenly taking someone else's prescription drugs or taking medicines in the dark and swallowing the wrong one (see Table 17-1). In most cities, you can call a poison control center for advice. (See "Emergency!" in the Hales Health Almanac for first-aid advice for poisoning.)

Falls

Falls are the leading cause of fatal accidents at home. High heels or worn footgear, poor lighting, slippery or uneven walkways, broken stairs and handrails, loose or worn rugs, or objects left where people walk all increase the likelihood of a slip. Falls are an especially serious health risk for the elderly. Each year about one-third of all people 65 years of age or older who live at home fall; 6% to 10% of these falls result in injury, including fractures, muscle injuries, sprains, lacerations, and dislocations. Fearing another fall, older people may limit their activity, becoming less independent and fit.

Strategies for Prevention

Staying Safe at Home

 Wear gloves when using household cleaning products. Read labels carefully, and use the products only in well-

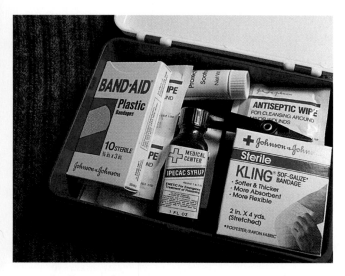

Your home first-aid kit should include (at minimum) bandages, sterile gauze pads, adhesive tape, scissors, cotton, antibiotic ointment, a needle, safety pins, calamine lotion, syrup of ipecac to induce vomiting, and a thermometer.

ventilated rooms. Never combine cleaning products; doing so could produce a dangerous chemical reaction.

✔ Maintain oil- and natural-gas-fired furnaces in good working order to avoid emission of carbon monoxide and fire hazards. Use kerosene heaters only if people are at home and awake. If such heaters malfunction, they can suffocate sleepers.

✔ Post the number of the local emergency service and poison control center near each phone in the house.

✔ Light stairways well. Remove clutter, cords, wires, and furniture from walking paths in living areas. Make sure carpets are attached firmly and area rugs are secure. Install nonskid mats in bathtubs and showers.

✔ Carry only loads you can see over. Clean up spills immediately, or mark the spill with a paper towel or wastebasket until you get a chance to clean it up. If you must walk over wet or slippery surfaces, take short steps to keep your center of balance beneath you. Slow down.

✔ To avoid shocks, be careful about anything involving electricity and water. Avoid using power tools in the rain; be careful with electrical heaters and other appliances, such as radios and hair dryers, in the bathroom; and use tools with nonconducting handles.

✔ Keep a first-aid kit at home.

Microwave Ovens

Microwave ovens have made cooking faster and easier than ever, but they've also created some new safety haz-

ards, including burns, fire and shock. Improper or careless use of microwaves is the primary cause of injuries.

To avoid problems, be sure your oven is properly installed and grounded. Be careful of heating food on paper or plastic plates, which can ignite when overheated. Glass containers not specifically designed for microwave use can explode. If you cover a dish with plastic wrap to help hold in moisture, steam can build up during the heating process. Be extremely careful removing the covering, because a gush of steam can cause a painful burn; use a long-handled wooden spoon rather than your hand to lift lids or coverings. When taking containers out of microwave ovens, use a pot holder. Be careful when taking the first few bites of any food you've just heated up. Since the plate may not be very hot, you may underestimate the temperature of the food and burn yourself.

Fires

You can prevent fires from occurring by making sure that the three ingredients of fire—fuel, a heat source, and oxygen—don't get a chance to mix. Almost anything can act as fuel for fire, including paper, wood, and, of course, flammable liquids such as oils, gasoline, and some paints. A heat source can be a spark from a lighted match, pilot light, or an electrical wire. Oxygen is necessary for the chemical reaction between the fuel and heat source that causes combustion.

If a fire starts and it's small, you may be able to put it out with a portable fire extinguisher before it spreads. However, if the fire does get out of control, you might have only two to five minutes to get out of the house or building alive. A fire-escape plan can save time and lives. Sketch a plan of your house, apartment building, dormitory, or fraternity or sorority house. Identify two ways out of each room or apartment. Make sure everyone is familiar with these escape routes. Designate an area outside where all family members or dorm residents should meet after escaping from a fire.

If a fire breaks out in your dorm room, get out as quickly as possible, but don't run. Before opening a room door, place your hand on it. If it's hot, don't open it. If the door feels cool, open it slightly to check for smoke. If there's none, leave by your planned escape route. If you're on an upper floor and your escape routes are blocked, open a window (top and bottom, if possible) and wait or signal from the window for help. Never try to use an elevator in a fire.

If you can't leave your room safely during a fire, call for help and turn off the air-conditioning or heating systems. To block smoke, press sheets and towels (wet, if possible) around and under the door. Keep as close to the floor as possible (where there's likely to be more oxygen), and place a wet washcloth over your face to filter out smoke particles.

Strategies for Prevention

Staying Safe from Fires

✔ Keep gasoline, paint, oily rags, newspapers, plastics, glues, and lightweight materials away from pilot lights, heaters, and other sources of heat. Store flammables in metal cans. Clean up grease on stoves.

✔ Don't overload electrical circuits, use worn wiring, or use portable heaters that have no cutoff feature if they tip over.

✔ Keep matches and cigarette lighters out of children's reach. Don't smoke in bed.

✔ Check to see that at least one smoke detector has been installed on each floor of your dorm or home. Make sure that you have a multipurpose fire extinguisher available to put out small fires.

✔ Close bedroom doors when you sleep. Closed doors slow the spread of fire. Keep a flashlight by each bedside to light the way out at night.[14]

On-the-Job Safety

The workplace is second only to the home as the most frequent site of accidents. The industries with the highest fatality rates are mining; transportation, communication, and public utilities; construction; and agriculture, forestry, and fishing. Whatever your job, find out about potential hazards and learn the proper safety regulations. (Chapter 12 discusses some potential environmental hazards at work, including noise, toxic substances, and video display terminals.)

Working with Computers

A new concern among many workers is **repetitive motion injury (RMI)**, which has surpassed back and neck injuries as the number one claim for workers compensation injuries. Repeated motions—such as the hand and arm movements made while using a computer key-

board—all day, every day, can result in muscle and tendon strain and inflammation. Symptoms include pain, swelling, and numbness and weakness in the hands or the arms. If these problems are identified early, permanent damage can generally be avoided by altering the work environment and allowing for more breaks during the day. If you work at a computer, good posture and correct positioning of the computer screen and keyboard can help prevent repetitive motion injuries, eyestrain, and back strain (see Figure 17-1). Here are some additional tips:

• Place the keyboard so that your elbows are bent at a 90° angle and you don't have to bend your wrists to type.

• Use a chair that provides ample back support. Keep your thighs parallel to the floor and your feet on the floor. If your feet don't reach the floor, use a footrest.

• If you experience neck strain, place a document holder next to your screen so that you can view the materials you are typing more easily.

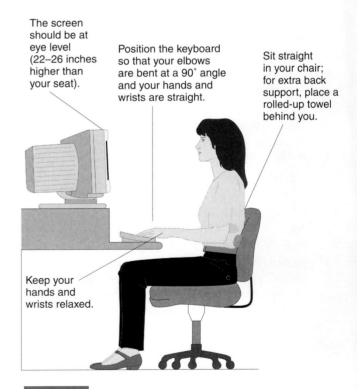

The screen should be at eye level (22–26 inches higher than your seat).

Position the keyboard so that your elbows are bent at a 90° angle and your hands and wrists are straight.

Sit straight in your chair; for extra back support, place a rolled-up towel behind you.

Keep your hands and wrists relaxed.

Figure 17-1

Safe computing. By paying attention to your posture and your computer's position, you can help protect yourself from repetitive motion injury, back strain, and eyestrain.

- Every 15 minutes take a 30-second break, stretch your arms, and walk around the office. Take a 15-minute break at least once every two hours.

Working with Chemicals

Many different types of workers, from laboratory technicians to professional artists, must use dangerous chemicals to perform their jobs. Employers and manufacturers of these chemicals are required by federal law to inform workers about any potential hazards, as well as first-aid measures in case they're accidentally exposed.

Here are some safety guidelines to follow if you work with dangerous substances:

- Make sure your work space is adequately ventilated. This doesn't mean a fan, which just blows dust and fumes around, but the equivalent of a filtered vacuum cleaner at the source of the toxic material.

- Be careful with the storage and handling of flammable solvents. Label all toxic materials clearly and carefully. Store them in nonbreakable containers. Discard them according to the manufacturer's instructions.

- Wash yourself thoroughly with soap and water before taking a break. Don't sweep up: vacuum or wet mop.

- Do not eat or smoke when using toxic materials. Wear appropriate protective gear: air respirators, goggles, gloves, earplugs, and so on.

- If you're pregnant or planning to conceive, check with your doctor about any potential risks to an unborn child.

Recreational Safety

When you want to take a break, exercise, or simply enjoy yourself, you probably go outside. But if you aren't careful, even a simple stroll or swim can turn into a hazardous event. According to a study by the Johns Hopkins School of Public Health, every year 750,000 Americans are injured during recreational activities such as horseback riding, skiing, sledding, snowboarding, skating, and playground activities; 82,000 suffer head injuries requiring emergency room or hospital treatment. Two dangers on the increase are in-line skating (rollerblading) and skateboarding. Public health experts urge helmet use for sports such as rollerblading and skateboarding because such activities combine high speeds with exposure to traffic.[15]

Handling Heat

Each year as many as 1000 Americans die from heat-caused illnesses that are almost always preventable. Two common heat-related maladies are **heat cramps** and **heat stress**. Heat cramps are caused by hard work and heavy sweating in the heat. Heat stress may occur simultaneously or afterward, as the blood vessels try to keep body temperature down. **Heat exhaustion**, a third such malady, is the result of prolonged sweating with inadequate fluid replacement. (See Table 17-2.)

The first step in treating the above conditions is to stop exercising, move to a cool place, and drink plenty of water. Don't resume work or activity until all the symptoms have disappeared; see a doctor if you're suffering from heat exhaustion. **Heat stroke** is a life-threatening medical emergency caused by the breakdown of the body's mechanism for cooling itself. The treatment is to cool the body down: Move to a cooler environment; sponge down with cool water, and apply ice to the back

TABLE 17-2   HEAT DANGERS

Illness	Symptoms	Treatment
Heat cramps	Muscle twitching or cramping; muscle spasms in arms, legs, and abdomen.	Stop exercising; cool off; drink water.
Heat stress	Fatigue, pale skin, blurred vision, dizziness, low blood pressure.	Stop exercising; cool off; drink water.
Heat exhaustion	Excessive thirst, fatigue, lack of coordination, increased sweating, elevated body temperature.	See a doctor.
Heat stroke	Lack of perspiration, high body temperature (over 105°F), dry skin, rapid breathing, coma, seizures, high pulse.	Cool the body; sponge; get medical help.

of the neck, armpits, and groin. Immersion in cold water could cause shock. Get medical help immediately.

Coping with Cold

The tips of the toes, fingers, ears, nose, chin, and cheeks are most vulnerable to exposure to high wind speeds and low temperatures, which can result in **frostnip**. Because frostnip is painless, you may not even be aware of it occurring. Watch for a sudden blanching or lightening of your skin. The best early treatment is warming the area by firm, steady pressure with a warm hand; blowing on it with hot breath; holding it against your body; or immersing it in warm (not hot) water. As the skin thaws, it becomes red and starts to tingle. Be careful to protect it from further damage. Don't rub the skin vigorously or with snow, as you could damage the tissue.

More severe is **frostbite**. There are two types of frostbite, *superficial* and *deep*. Superficial frostbite, the freezing of the skin and tissues just below the skin, is characterized by a waxy look and firmness of the skin, although the tissue below is soft. Initial treatment should be to slowly rewarm the area. As the area thaws, it will be numb and bluish or purple, and blisters may form. Cover the area with a dry, sterile dressing, and protect the skin from further exposure to cold. See a doctor for further treatment. Deep frostbite, the freezing of skin, muscle, and even bone, requires medical treatment. It usually involves the tissues of the hands and feet, which appear pale and feel frozen. Keep the victim dry and as warm as possible on the way to a medical facility. Cover the frostbitten area with a dry, sterile dressing.

The gradual cooling of the center of the body may occur at temperatures above, as well as below, freezing—usually in wet, windy weather. When body temperature falls below 95°F, the body is incapable of rewarming itself because of the breakdown of the internal system that regulates its temperature. This state is known as **hypothermia**. The first sign of hypothermia is severe shivering. Then the victim becomes uncoordinated, drowsy, listless, confused, and is unable to speak properly. Symptoms become more severe as body temperature continues to drop, and coma or death can result.

Hypothermia requires emergency medical treatment. Try to prevent any further heat loss: Move the victim to a warm place, cover him or her with blankets, remove wet clothing, and replace it with dry garments. If the victim is conscious, administer warm liquids, not alcohol.

Strategies for Prevention

Protecting Yourself from the Cold

✔ Dress appropriately. Choose several layers of loose clothing made of wool, cotton, down, or synthetic down. Make sure your head, feet, and hands are well protected. A pair of cotton socks inside a pair of wool socks will keep your feet warm.

✔ Don't go out in the cold after drinking. Alcohol can make you more susceptible to cold (see Chapter 15) and can impair your judgment and sense of time.

✔ When snowshoeing or cross-country skiing, always let a responsible person know where you're heading and when you expect to be back. Stick to marked trails.

✔ Carry a small emergency kit that includes waterproof matches, a compass, a map, high-energy food, and water.

✔ Don't eat snow; it could lower your body temperature.

Drowning

Drowning claims more than 6000 lives a year, according to the National Safety Council. Toddlers under age 4 and teenage boys between 15 and 19 are at greatest risk. Among young children, 90% of drownings occur in residential swimming pools.[16]

The causes of drowning, in order of frequency, are becoming exhausted, being swept into deep water, losing support, becoming trapped or entangled, having a cramp or other attack, and striking an underwater

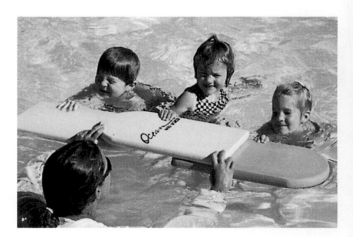

Water safety training can begin in early childhood. Swimming, treading water, and engaging in safe water practices are all important to preventing drownings.

object. Many drowning victims were strong swimmers. Most drownings occur at unorganized facilities, such as ponds or pools with no lifeguard present. Health officials believe that pool fencing alone, along with adequate gates and latches, could prevent as many as half of all drownings or near-drownings of children.

Alcohol also increases the dangers of swimming and boating accidents. Among the college students who reported swimming or boating in the previous year, 30.5% had used alcohol before going into or on the water. More than a third of the men—35.2%—said they had drunk alcohol when boating or swimming.[17]

Strategies for Prevention

How to Enjoy the Water Safely

✔ Learn "drownproofing," or ways of treading water or moving with minimal output of energy. Know your limits as a swimmer, and don't try to swim beyond your depth or capability.

✔ Don't swim after drinking.

✔ Don't swim in the dark, especially in the ocean. Find out about currents, undertows, or sharp underwater rocks before swimming in a strange place. Never dive before knowing the depth of the water below you.

✔ Always use a buddy system, even when swimming with a group. Even a strong swimmer can suffer a cramp or another problem that can jeopardize his or her ability to stay afloat.

✔ Don't swim in boating or fishing areas. If thrown from a boat or canoe, stay with the craft and use it for support. Wear a personal flotation device whenever you're boating, rafting, or canoeing.

✔ Be careful when diving into waves, and pay attention to the undertow, which could pull you out to sea.

▌Intentional Injury: ▌Violence in America

Crime in the United States has declined throughout the 1990s. Experts cite many reasons: an improved economy, an older population, more police, longer prison sentences, a decline in the use of crack cocaine and other drugs.[18] But crime still touches many people's lives. For every 1000 persons age 12 or older, the public experiences two rapes or attempted rapes, two assaults with serious injury, and five robberies. According to the Bureau of Justice Statistics, U.S. residents age 12 or older experience approximately 39.6 million crimes a year. About 29 million are property crimes, 9.9 million are crimes of violence, and 396,000 are personal thefts. In the mid-1990s, the violent crime rate declined about 10% a year, and property crimes continued a 16-year decline.[19]

The best approach to criminal violence, as to other public health problems, is prevention. As an initial step, the Centers for Disease Control and Prevention (CDC) have called upon parents to prevent unsupervised access to guns by their children and have developed pilot community programs for youngsters in high-crime areas. The American Medical Association has proposed greater restrictions on gun ownership, including strict registration and licensing. The Public Health Service is advocating a reduction in weapon-carrying by adolescents and in weapons-related injuries and deaths. The American Psychological and American Psychiatric Associations have called for decreased violence in the media.

All of these steps could make a difference. In the view of psychologists and sociologists, violence far from being "random, uncontrollable, or inevitable," can be prevented. Early intervention is critical, because aggression in childhood typically escalates into violence and other harmful behaviors. Ideally, programs should teach young children skills for managing anger, solving problems, thinking of alternative solutions, and seeing another person's perspective. Equally important are programs that enhance positive interactions between children and adults. Such relationships may act as protective factors that can lower the risk of aggressive and violent behavior.[20]

The Roots of Aggression and Violence

While anger is considered a normal, sometimes inevitable emotion, aggression—behavior with the intent to control or dominate—is a threat to individuals and to society. Angry people may want to push or punch someone; aggressive people carry through on such impulses and become violent. Why? The reasons, discussed in the following sections, are complex.

Biological Causes

Traumatic brain injury, which can lead to violent outbursts of explosive anger, is one of many medical factors associated with violence (Table 17-3). As many as 70% of those who suffer head injuries report some degree of irritability or explosive rage. The use of alcohol or drugs before or after a head injury may increase the likelihood of such problems. Illnesses that affect the brain—stroke and neurologic diseases, brain tumors, infectious illnesses, epilepsy, metabolic disorders (such as hyperthyroidism or hypothyroidism), multiple sclerosis, and systemic lupus erythematosus—can also lead to aggressive behavior.[21]

Certain medications—painkillers, antianxiety agents, steroids, antidepressants, and over-the-counter sedatives (which may produce delirium)—can trigger aggression. Alcohol abuse, which lowers inhibitions against violent behavior and interferes with judgment, and many street drugs, including amphetamines, cocaine, and hallucinogens, are also associated with violence.

In searching for other biological abnormalities that may be linked with violence, neuroscientists have noted low levels of the neurotransmitter serotonin in men convicted of homicide. Serotonin is involved in the control

TABLE 17-3 BIOLOGICAL CAUSES OF AGGRESSIVE BEHAVIOR

Illnesses

- Alzheimer's disease
- Brain injury
- Brain tumors
- Delirium
- Hormonal disorders (such as hyperthyroidism or hypothyroidism)
- Infectious illnesses
- Multiple sclerosis
- Parkinson's, Huntington's or Wilson's disease
- Seizure disorders
- Stroke and other neurologic disease
- Systemic lupus erythematosus
- Vitamin deficiencies

Substances

- Alcohol
- Antianxiety agents (barbiturates, benzodiazepines)
- Antidepressants
- Over-the-counter sedatives (which may produce delirium)
- Painkillers (opiates and other narcotics)
- Steroids

of impulses, particularly toward violent or self-destructive acts. Other neurotransmitters also may play important roles in aggression, and the relations among these chemicals ultimately may prove more critical than the levels of any single one of them.

Sex chromosome abnormalities have been investigated but do not seem to lead to a greater tendency toward violence in, for example, men with an extra Y chromosome. The role of the male sex hormone testosterone also has been investigated. The highly competitive men most likely to dominate a situation or group—whether it's a seminar or a street gang—tend to have higher testosterone levels than other men. But testosterone in itself does not make men aggressive. Rather, scientists explain, it is only one of many contributing factors.

According to recent research, individuals with serious mental disorders may be somewhat more violent than the general population. Individuals with a serious mental illness (such as schizophrenia) report having been violent much more often than those with no mental disorder. However, alcohol and drug users are, as a group, more violent than individuals with serious mental illnesses.[22]

Developmental Factors

Many developmental factors—childrearing practices, parental discipline, relations to peers, sex-role socialization, economic inequality, lack of opportunity, and media influences—contribute to violence. Parents who reject their youngsters, who are physically abusive, or who have a criminal history are most likely to have children with early signs of aggressive behavior. As discussed later in this chapter, violence in the home, especially when it is experienced at a young age, breeds more violence. Brutalized children learn to be brutal themselves. The reason for this may be that such children haven't learned effective ways to relate to others, or they may suffer from emotional and cognitive disorders.

Exposure to community violence also may have an effect. In a study of nearly 150 grade schoolers, NIMH researchers found that 14% of first and second-graders had seen someone shot, stabbed, or raped; 30% had seen a mugging or someone being chased by a gang. Among these young witnesses to crime, about 30% developed behavior problems or signs of depression and fear. In other cases, for a variety of reasons, children never seem to learn effective ways of handling frustration. Instead, they lash out violently, which can lead to punishment by adults and rejection by peers. Doing poorly at school or feeling ostracized as "dumb" increases the likelihood of aggression.[23]

Violence in the Media

The media's portrayal of aggressive acts can stimulate violence. A riot, cross-burning, or grisly television murder sometimes triggers similar forms of violence. The average American youth is exposed to 40,000 deaths and hundreds of thousands of incidents of other mayhem while growing up. Researchers estimate that, if television had never been invented, there would be 10,000 fewer murders, 70,000 fewer rapes, and 700,000 fewer assaults each year in the United States. Studies in the United States, Australia, Finland, Israel, and Poland have found that more aggressive children watch more television, prefer violent programs, identify with violent TV characters, and perceive violence as more real than less aggressive youngsters. They also grow up to be more aggressive adults, with a higher likelihood of being convicted for serious crimes and for aggressive behavior in public and in their own homes. [24]

Guns

Almost half of all homes in the United States contain at least one firearm, which may be kept for self-defense, hunting, target shooting, or collecting. An estimated 3 to 4 million handguns are circulating in the United States; an estimated 100,000 students carry a gun to school.[25] In eight states, firearms kill more people than motor-vehicle accidents. Across the country, they are quickly becoming the leading cause of traumatic brain injury and traumatic death.[26] For each fatal shooting, there are an estimated 2.6 injuries. The price tag for treating firearms-related injuries has been estimated at $20 billion a year.[27]

Young men in their teens and early twenties, especially those who are African American, are most likely to suffer both fatal and nonfatal gunshot wounds.[28] In the inner cities, gunshot wounds are the leading cause of death in teenage boys. Gang membership multiplies the danger, and gang members are three times more likely to commit aggravated assault or murder than those who are not in gangs. However, arguments lead to many more acts of violence.

Ease of access to a gun has consistently been found to increase homicide rates since, with a gun at hand, an assault, rape, robbery, or fight may well result in murder. It also increases the risk of suicide and accidental shootings by adults and children. Several states have passed Child Accident Prevention laws that make it a crime to leave a loaded firearm within easy reach of a child.[29]

Social Factors

Extreme poverty, deprivation, unemployment, prejudice, discrimination, involvement with gangs, and repeated exposure to actual violence all contribute to aggressive and violent behavior. The risk of violence increases for those who can find few, if any, economic and social opportunities in mainstream society. Violence is most common among the poor, regardless of race. Most people of color, including those who grow up with poverty, discrimination, and family disruptions, do not engage in violence and are more likely to be victims of violent crime than white Americans.

Strategies for Prevention
Ways to Stop Violence

✔ Object to jokes about racism, women, rape, minorities, or nationalities.

✔ Watch your own anger—talk it out, write it out, sing it out—but don't act on it.

✔ Refuse to hate.

✔ Don't retaliate.

✔ Volunteer at a shelter for battered women or runaway youths.

✔ Write a letter protesting a violent movie or television program.

✔ Support a tax on guns and ammunition that would help pay for health care.

✔ Avoid a conflict. It's usually not worth it to argue.

✔ Be charitable toward rude people—they don't know better.

✔ Don't get discouraged. Hope grows the way a path does in the country. As more people walk it, it turns into a road.

Crime on Campus

Once considered havens from the meanness of America's streets, colleges and universities have seen a dramatic rise in crime in recent years. In a survey of more than 2400 schools, there were 30 murders, almost 1000 rapes and more than 1800 robberies, along with 32,127 burglaries and 8981 car thefts.[30] Under the Federal Student Right to Know and Campus Security Act, all colleges and universities receiving federal funds must publish and make readily available the number of campus killings, assaults, sexual assaults, robberies, burglaries and other crimes, and their security policies.[31] (See discussions of sexual harassment and assault later in this chapter.)

As the national College Health Risk Behavior Survey found, the majority of college students are not violent. (See Campus Focus: "College Students and Violence.") Yet a not-significant minority—14.2% of the men—reported being involved in at least one physical fight during the previous year, and 13.8% of the men said they had carried a weapon (gun, knife, or club) at least once during the preceding 30 days.[32]

Because of concerns about safety on campus, more schools are taking tougher stands on student behavior. Many have established codes of conduct barring the use of alcohol and drugs, fighting, and sexual harassment. Many also have instituted policies requiring suspension or expulsion for students who violate this code.[33]

Many campuses have set up public safety programs, which include late-night shuttle buses and escorts, student bicycle patrols, outdoor emergency phones, and increased numbers of police and security guards. Sexual-assaults services provide counseling, crisis intervention, and educational programs. Students are urged to walk in groups, lock doors and windows, and limit alcohol consumption. Freshman orientation often includes mandatory sessions on campus safety and sexual assault.[34]

Domestic Violence

Violence doesn't stop at the front doors of America's homes. According to the Federal Bureau of Investigation, the most common and least-reported violent crimes are attacks in which the victim and the perpetrator knew each other at the time of or before the incident. One-third of all murders occur within families. Physical violence may occur in 20% to 30% of all American households.[35]

Partner Abuse

Every nine seconds a woman is battered by her partner. During their lifetime, at least one of every five women will be assaulted by a partner or ex-partner. Domestic violence is the single most common cause of injury to women—more common than car accidents, muggings, and rapes combined—and accounts for 42% of female murders.[36]

Battered women (who outnumber battered men ten to one) are victims of severe, deliberate, and repeated physical assaults, often accompanied by psychological abuse and threats on their lives. A significant proportion of women who visit emergency departments seek help for symptoms related to ongoing abuse, yet only 5% are identified as victims of domestic violence by the physicians who treat them. In one study, when women seeking emergency services for any reason were specifically asked about abuse, 54.2% said they had been assaulted, threatened, or made to feel afraid by partners at some point in their lives.[37]

The primary factors contributing to physical abuse are the degree of frustration and stress a man is under, his use of alcohol (involved in up to 60% of battering cases), and whether he was raised in an abusive home. Only one in twenty men who beat their partners are violent outside the home; nine in ten refuse to admit that they have a problem. In homes where a wife is beaten, children also may be abused. The primary risk factors for domestic murder are poverty and household crowding; the lower a family's socioeconomic status—regardless of its racial or ethnic background—the greater the risk of deadly violence.[38]

Abused wives and children are often trapped in terror. Wives may stay with abusive husbands because of love, financial dependence, shame, guilt, fear of being pursued, harmed, or killed if they leave, or a sense of responsibility to their children. The incidence of alcoholism, substance abuse, depression, and suicide attempts is higher in battered women than others. (See Personal Voices: "Why Does She Stay?")

Child Abuse

Severe child abuse occurs an estimated 1.7 million times each year and claims the lives of as many as 5000 children a year. Parents in every economic, social, educational, religious, and racial group abuse children, but poverty is a significant factor in abuse. Mistreatment is seven times more likely in families with incomes under $15,000.

Abuse can take many forms: physical, psychological, or sexual. Physical abuse often leaves visible marks. However, emotional abuse—rejection, verbal cruelty such as constant berating and belittling, serious threats of harm, frequent tension in the home, and violent arguments among parents—can be just as devastating to a child.

Sexual abuse of children involves *any* sexual contact, whether it is sexually suggestive conversation, prolonged kissing, petting, oral sex, or intercourse, between an adult and child. Because children are not intellectually or emotionally mature enough to consent to sexual involvement, any such action is illegal and a violation of a child's rights.

Pedophilia, or child molestation, refers to abuse by individuals—teachers, babysitters, neighbors, and so

Personal Voices   Why Does She Stay?

I could be your sister, your daughter, your mother. I could be you. I am a victim of domestic violence.

Battered women are the product of the crime of domestic violence—not the cause. Until the only man I ever loved enough to marry beat me, I was a person, a woman. As a result of his crimes against me, I am now a battered woman. My behavior is simply reacting to what he did to me. My being a battered woman is about him, not me.

I fell in love with a man who charmed and impressed and romanced me. I loved him more than any man I had ever dated, and I married him. However, I did not know who he was. Batterers know that if they present their true selves no one would ever talk to them, so they don't. They act, they con, they deceive—we fall in love. Then, when we start seeing who they really are, we can't believe it. We want to believe anything but the truth. And the truth is that these men trick and woo us and then commit crimes of violence upon us.

We are confused and shocked by what we have seen and experienced. They tell us that they don't know what happened, they lost control, they were drunk, we made them do it. We want to believe anything other than that they meant to do this terrible thing to us. it is not in our capacity to understand that their acts of violence are deliberate, but they are. As long as we believe that we have the power to get the man with whom we fell in love back, as long as we believe that this is caused by something we can fix, as long as we believe anything but the truth, we will stay.

We know he does not have to be this way; he acted entirely different when we met and fell in love. We know we can get him back. I remember pleading with my new husband: "You are not the man I married; you are his evil twin. What have you done with him?" And later in anger: "How dare you show me how wonderful you can be and then not be that way."

When we start to give up hope, the man we feel in love with comes back. We are constantly off balance because he keeps changing from the man we fell in love with to monster boy. When do we leave? When things are wonderful and the man we fell in love with is loving us? No, life is too wonderful, and everything is fixed and right with the world. When we are battered? No, we don't have the strength or desire to live, much less fight. So we give up. We give in. we disappear. Our only existence is keeping him happy so he won't hurt us. He begs us to cheer up, he makes promises, he woos us back.

Eventually, many of us reach a point where we no longer have hope for the relationship or our fear of being injured or killed becomes too great, or we see our children being damaged, or in some cases our children, sometimes very small children, save our lives by calling 911…whatever it is that happens, something in us changes. We decide we can't or won't take the abuse, and we decide to leave. It can take seconds, or it can take years. And the most dangerous time for a battered woman is while she is leaving or after she has left, according to countless studies. This is when most of us are killed.

He begs us to stay; when it doesn't work, he threatens to kill us and our children. My batterer threatened to kill my parents in front me, then torture me until I prayed for death. He told me he could have someone else kill me and he could be 100 miles away having dinner with witnesses who would back him up. We are hostages; still, we are safer on the streets than in our own homes.

The first time that I called a crisis hotline, I found out that domestic violence happens to millions of women every year in this country. This means that millions of husbands and boyfriends beat up their wives and girlfriends every year. There isn't an entity called domestic violence that is doing the battering. It is men. Men who say that they love us and can't live without us. I learned that four to six women a day are killed in this country by their husbands and boyfriends. I learned that we have thousands of shelters for women and children to hide from their husbands, boyfriends and fathers. I was outraged. Not in this country, not in America.

I was married for nine months. I knew my ex-husband for nine months before that. He was convicted of eight felonies, two with great bodily injury enhancements. Two of these felonies are for threatening to kill me and worse if I ever told or if he ever spent a day in jail. He was sentenced to 12 years in prison. He will serve six years and eight months. He gets out in six months. I am terrified and have spent the past six years preparing for this.

Why does she stay? Because if she leaves, the chances increase that he may kill her. And if she wins in court, all she does is buy some time. I left. I won. Do you envy me?

Butler, Pam. "Why Does She Stay?"
San Francisco Chronicle, Sept. 26, 1997.

---

on—who are not related to the child. **Incest** is sexual contact between two people who are closely related, including siblings as well as children and parents, grandparents, uncles, and aunts. Abuse—emotional, physical, or sexual—can affect every aspect of a child's life. Youngsters may develop physical symptoms, such as headaches, stomachaches, and sleep problems, and run into academic and social difficulties in school. Since children often blame themselves for whatever happened and assume they are responsible, they may develop a sense of hopelessness, shame, and pessimism. Some become clinically depressed or develop other mental or emotional problems that may continue into adolescence and adulthood, including more reports of headaches, depression, insomnia, obesity, and fatigue.

Abusing parents are not necessarily sick. Only 10% have mental disorders. Many other factors play a role: ignorance about childrearing, absence of role models,

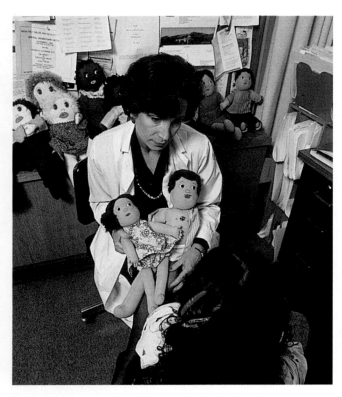

Child sexual abuse. Specialists in the field of child sexual abuse may use anatomically correct dolls to educate children about "okay" touches. These dolls may also be used in discussions with very young victims to clarify the nature of the abuse that has occurred.

teenage parenthood, lack of a partner or supportive family network, and the stress of poverty. However, most abusive parents share a similar psychological history. As youngsters, they felt misunderstood, unrewarded, criticized, and denied the right to behave like children. Sometimes they were abused themselves, physically or psychologically, so they grew up feeling so worthless and unlovable that as adults they continue to search for mothering and love. Often such an individual will marry a person with problems similar to his or her own. When the new relationship cannot meet their psychological needs, they feel rejected. Their children may seem the last resort in obtaining the love they crave, and children who do not—cannot—live up to these unrealistic expectations in turn become the victims of abuse. In other cases, parents who cannot cope with daily stress may feel pushed beyond their ability to cope and end up abusing their children.

Many abusive families can be helped with appropriate treatment. Usually, this involves counseling for the entire family. Within the family structure, the abusive par-

ent must learn to trust, to establish healthy intimate relationships, and to ask for help when it's needed. Parents must learn to view their children realistically; their children must realize that it's permissible to act like children.

The effects of any form of child abuse can be life-long. Sexual abuse survivors suffer deep psychological wounds, including a profound sense of betrayal and loss. As adults, many find it hard to form intimate adult relationships and experience sexual difficulties. Other common problems include depression, feelings of guilt or shame, inability to trust, drug and alcohol abuse, and a vulnerability to other forms of victimization.[39]

Helping the Victims of Violence

As their numbers have grown and their anguish has been recognized, the victims of violence have received greater attention. In the last decade, hundreds of shelters for battered wives and their children have been set up across the country. They offer physical and psychological treatment, and a haven where women can begin to rebuild their shattered self-esteem, as well as their daily lives. Rape counseling and crisis centers on college campuses and in the community provide various forms of assistance to victims of rape. In many cities, the telephone directory lists hot lines and resources. More than 400 victims' advocacy groups have been set up across the country to advise those hurt by crime. Support organizations help many survivors deal with the emotional aftermath of their experiences. (See the "Yellow Pages" at the back of this book for listings.)

Strategies for Change

··
How to Help Victims of Violence

Sometimes well-intentioned friends and relatives add to the stress felt by the victims of violence. Here's how to offer comfort without implying criticism:

✔ Don't blame the victim. Even when no one doubts that the victim is completely innocent, individuals may be plagued by regrets and self-accusation: Why didn't I lock the windows? Why did I park on that dark street? Any second-guessing or implied criticism adds to this burden of blame and shame.

✔ Don't try to deny that it happened. Although it may be hard to talk about—or even listen to—what happened, the reality of the event must not be ignored. Denial makes victims doubt their own experience and question themselves at a time when they crave reassurance.

✔ Don't pressure the victim to talk—or not to talk. Some individuals need to go over every detail of what happened, again and again, until they work out their feelings of outrage and become ready to get on with their lives. Others find going into details too humiliating. Let the victim set the tone and limits for disclosure. Don't pry or prod.

✔ Don't try to rush the victim to leave the past behind and get on with his or her life. Recovery from any traumatic event takes time, and only the victim knows the appropriate pace. If, however, months pass without any lessening of symptoms or improvement in day-to-day functioning, family members and friends shouldn't hesitate to recommend that their loved one see a mental health professional.

Sexual Victimization and Violence

Sexual victimization refers to any situation in which a person is deprived of free choice and forced to comply with sexual acts. It is not only a woman's issue; in fact, men are also victimized. In recent years, researchers have come to view acts of sexual victimization along a continuum, ranging from behaviors such as street hassling, grabbing, and obscene telephone calls to rape, battering, and incest (see Table 17-4).

What Causes Sexual Victimization and Violence?

While obscene comments or calls may seem minor annoyances compared with acts of sexual violence, all

TABLE 17-4 CONTINUUM OF VIOLENCE AGAINST WOMEN (IN INCREASING ORDER OF SEVERITY)

Action	Description	Action	Description
Street hassling	Comments, whistles, stares, or catcalls, generally of a sexual nature, that make a woman feel embarrassed, coerced, and fearful.		explicit photographs/films. Again, the women may appear to be free agents but are frequently subjected to behind-the-scenes violence and control.
Grabbing	Unwanted physical contact, usually from a stranger and in public, designed to touch a woman's body without her consent.	Sexual harrassment	Actions, often committed in a campus harassment or work setting, that subject a woman to sexual coercion, comments, and advances from individuals in positions of power.
Obscene telephone calls	Calls, usually aggressive and/or sexual and made at night, that provoke feelings of fear and powerlessness.	Abuse by professionals	Acts committed in the context of a professional relationship in which a male professional uses his position of trust to coerce sexual favors from a client, patient, student, or parishioner.
Voyeurism	"Peeping Toms" or hidden males violating a woman's privacy by attempting to view her undressing, nude, or in intimate situations.		
Indecent exposure	An unwanted display of a man's sexual organs.	Rape	Sexual activity forced upon a woman against her will by a stranger or acquaintance through threats or assault.
Lesbian baiting	Verbal and physical acts designed to hurt or offend women because of their sexual orientation.	Battering	Physical and psychological abuse (often brutal) of a wife, girlfriend, or cohabiting woman by a husband, boyfriend, or cohabiting man that is designed to intimidate, control, or coerce.
Prostitution	Women, usually under the control of a male pimp, offering sexual acts to men for money. Although the illusion is that the women are under their own control, they are often victimized by pimps, customers, and police.	Incest	Coercive sexual acts instigated by a trusted older family member (usually male) and forced upon a financially, physically, and emotionally dependent child (usually female).
Pornography	Women paid to participate in sexually		

SOURCE: Leidig, Marjorie Whittaker. "The Continuum of Violence Against Women: Psychological and Physical Consequences," *Journal of American College Health*, January 1992.

forms of sexual victimization attack a person's integrity. The roots of this problem extend beyond individuals to our society and the beliefs and assumptions—many of them false—that it engenders:

- *Acceptance of myths about sexual conduct.* Our culture, consciously and unconsciously, teaches women not to make sexual advances and to limit sexual intimacy to love relationships. At the same time, men are encouraged to pursue sexual encounters with numerous partners and to view sex as an achievement. Men who accept these gender roles—particularly those who admit to using force or deception to obtain sex—may believe that women who say no really mean yes, and that women like to lead men on. They may also feel that coercion is legitimate in certain situations—for example, if a woman asks a man out or comes to his apartment or home.[40]

- *Acceptance of male aggression.* Boys in our culture learn at early ages that "real men" are aggressive and powerful and are expected to make sexual conquests. Researchers have found that men who are predisposed to sexual violence typically want to avoid acting in any way that might be seen as feminine or sissy; strive for power, status, and control; act tough and unemotional; and tend to be aggressive and take risks. These collective attitudes, sometimes dubbed the "masculine mystique," are used to justify aggressive behavior by reducing women to sex objects.[41]

- *The uncontrollable male sex drive.* Both men and women often believe—erroneously—that young men, once stimulated, cannot control their sexual appetites. Yet, as educators have pointed out, any college-age man would be able to stop immediately if his partner's parents walked into the room. A related myth is that stopping sexual activity is in some way harmful to a male; it isn't.

- *Blaming the victim.* Although victims of thefts, carjackings, and other crimes aren't blamed for what happened to them, women are often held responsible for "provoking" sexual attacks by wearing tight clothing, flirting, or going to a bar alone.

- *Trivializing.* Many acts of sexual victimization, such as the use of verbal slurs when talking about women's bodies, are treated as jokes or pranks rather than serious offenses. This makes such behaviors seem acceptable and denies the very real distress they cause.

- *Exposure to sexually violent material.* Repeated exposure to magazines, books, movies, and videos that link sex and violence may desensitize men to violence toward women so that they come to think of it as normal and acceptable. As they become more callous in their attitudes toward women, men are less inclined to view forced sexual activity, including rape, as wrong and are more likely to admit that they would commit rape if they could get away with it.

Increasingly, researchers have come to view rape, an extreme and violent form of sexual victimization, more as the result of socialization within our "normal" culture than as a sign of an individual's psychopathology. Anthropologists have noted that rape-prone societies, such as ours, encourage boys and men to be aggressive and tolerate—even glorify—male violence. Men in such societies tend to have more economic and political power than women, and often demean woman's judgments and domestic responsibilities. By comparison, in rape-free societies, men and women share power and authority and contribute equally to the community.

Sexual Harassment

All forms of sexual harassment or unwanted sexual attention—from the display of pornographic photos to the use of sexual obscenities to a demand for sex by anyone in a position of power or authority—are illegal. (See Pulsepoints: "Ten Ways to Prevent Sexual Victimization.")

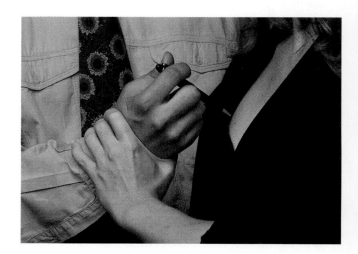

Sexual harassment on the job can take many forms, from remarks, unwelcome attention, and violations of personal space to the extreme of sexual assault.

Pulsepoints 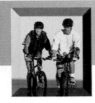 Ten Ways to Prevent Sexual Victimization

1. Challenge gender stereotypes. Just because you're male doesn't mean you have to act in a macho, sexually aggressive way. Just because you're female doesn't mean you have to be passive and accepting of male behavior.

2. Don't tolerate inappropriate language or behavior. If you find someone's sexually crude language offensive, say so. If you don't like to be touched by casual acquaintances, back away, and keep your distance.

3. Be careful of your sexual signals. Men often assume that women who smile, make conversation, and flirt are signaling sexual availability. Women typically think they're just being friendly. Make sure you know the message you want to send—and don't assume you can tell what someone else is trying to signal.

4. Choose safe settings. If you're going out with someone you don't know well or have reservations about being alone with, suggest meeting in a public place or participating in a group activity.

5. Think about your sexual expectations for a relationship. What are you willing to do? How much sexual activity is enough? Where do you want to draw the line? Remember, your partner will be making decisions about the same things.

6. Talk about sex. Using the communication guidelines in Chapters 8 and 9, bring up the topic of sexual involvement. Let your date know from the beginning how you feel about sexual activity on first, second, third, or twentieth dates.

7. Think ahead. Rather than letting yourself get carried away by passion, anticipate what could happen if, for instance, you agree to go to your date's apartment for a drink or park in an isolated spot. State your feelings clearly.

8. Say "no" clearly when you mean it, and accept "no" when you hear it. If you're the one saying no, use a firm, even loud voice, and back up what you say with body language. If you're on the receiving end of a no, pay attention. A "no"—even if said quietly and shyly—still means no.

9. Keep your wits about you. Alcohol and other drugs can affect your judgment and inhibitions. You may become more sexually aggressive under their influence, or you may greatly increase your risk of being victimized.

10. Call it like it is. If you're the target of sexual taunts or unwanted propositions on campus or at work, say, "What you're doing is sexual harassment, and I'm going to report it." If a date or acquaintance won't respect your limits, one of the most effective defensive tactics is saying, "This is rape, and I'm calling the cops."

Sexual Harassment on the Job

The issue of sexual misconduct on the job exploded into the national consciousness at the confirmation hearings for Supreme Court Justice Clarence Thomas in 1991. "Anita Hill's testimony [in which she described comments about pornographic movies and pubic hair on Coke bottles] sensitized women to things they didn't think about as sexual harassment before," says Barbara Gutek, Ph.D., author of *Sex and the Workplace* and a professor of psychology and business at the University of Arizona.[42] Various surveys have found rates of sexual harassment ranging from 42% to 66%. Overall, only 5% of sexual harassment victims are men—and their harassers are more likely to be other men than women. The incidence is not limited to low-paying jobs or any particular segment of the workforce. Several recent studies have revealed high rates of harassment in medical settings. In one survey of 133 physicians, 73% of the women and 22% of the men reported experiencing sexual harassment during their residency training.[43]

As defined by the Equal Employment Opportunity Commission, sexual harassment takes two basic forms: in **quid pro quo** harassment, a person in power or authority makes unwanted sexual advances as a condition for receiving a job, a promotion, or another type of favor; in harassment by means of a **hostile or offensive environment**, supervisors or coworkers engage in persistent inappropriate behaviors that make the workplace hostile, abusive, or otherwise unbearable.

"There's a spectrum of verbal, nonverbal and physical acts, ranging from making off-color remarks to grabbing someone's breast or buttocks," says consultant Susan L. Webb of Seattle, author of *Step Forward: Sexual Harassment in the Workplace.* "But sexual harassment always involves behavior that is related to or based on sex, that is deliberate or repeated, and that is not welcome, not asked for, and not returned."[44] Sexual comments, propositions, dirty jokes, suggestive looks or remarks, displays of pinups or pornography, "accidental" touches, pats, squeezes, pinches, fondling and ogling are all potentially offensive.[45]

"There isn't always a clear line," says Webb. "Each sexual harassment case has to be considered in its own context." The standard the courts use is whether a reasonable person would consider the behavior or environment abusive or hostile. Since most targets of sexual harassment are women, that usually translates into what a reasonable *woman* would think—which may be quite different from a man's view. Psychologist Gutek once asked 1200 men and women how they would view a sexual proposition in the workplace. About 67% of the men said they would find it flattering, while 63 percent of the women said they would be insulted.[46]

Sexual harassment can affect employees in many ways—financially, psychologically, even physically. If they are fired because they refuse to endure sexual harassment, they may jeopardize their own and their family's economic security. Common psychological effects include crying spells, loss of self-esteem, anger, humiliation, shame, alienation, helplessness, and degradation. Many victims also suffer physical symptoms that stem directly from pressures associated with sexual harassment, including headache, stomach ailments, decreased appetite, weight loss, back and neck pain decreased sleep, and other stress-related problems.[47]

Workers who feel victimized by sexual harassment should document their complaints by writing down specific incidents (including dates, times, places, and what happened). It sometimes helps initially to confront the harasser, either in person or by writing a note, and state that you're not interested in his or her attention. Many companies have established grievance procedures for handling sexual harassment complaints. The courts have awarded substantial payments of both punitive and compensatory damage to victims of physical and verbal harassment and have held companies liable for failing to halt offensive actions.

Strategies for Change

· ·

Gender Etiquette on the Job

✔ Be polite and respectful. Whenever possible, rely on courtesy rather than contact. Offer a handshake instead of a hug; an encouraging word, not a pat on the back.

✔ Use the same-sex standard. If you're not sure whether a comment is appropriate, think of what you would do with a colleague of the same sex.

✔ Give compliments based on merit, not appearance. "Men will compliment a woman on what she's wearing, rather than the report she wrote," says Webb. "This

puts her gender and looks above her status as a coworker."

✔ Think of how a loved one would react. If you're a man, before making a comment or telling a joke, imagine how your mother, sister, or daughter would respond. If you're a woman, think of the impact your words might have on a father, brother, or son.

✔ Speak up. If you don't like your boss to rub your neck or you don't appreciate tasteless jokes on your e-mail, say, "I find your behavior offensive, and I'd appreciate your stopping it." Focus on the behavior, not the person, to take the emotion out of the interaction.

Sexual Harassment on Campus

Sexual harassment starts early. In a survey conducted by the American Association of University Women, 81% of students in grades 9 through 11 said they had been harassed at least once. Of these, 76% of girls and 56% of boys reported that on at least one occasion they had been targets of sexual comments, jokes, or gestures; 65% of the girls and 42% of the boys said they had been touched, grabbed, or pinched in a sexual way.[48]

As many as a third to a half of female undergraduates and 20% of males have experienced some form of sexual harassment. Professors or supervisors may pressure students into sexual involvement for the sake of a grade, recommendation, or special opportunity. If a student tries to end a sexual relationship, they may threaten reprisals. Most harassment comes from male faculty members, but both men and women report having been harassed by either male or female faculty. (See Figure 17-2.) Overall, 94% of female students reportedly had been harassed by men; 15% by women; 79% of male students reportedly had been harassed by women and 55% by men.

Sexual harassment can undermine students' well-being and academic performance. Its effects include diminished ambition and self-confidence, reduced ability to concentrate, sleeplessness, depression, physical aches, and ailments. Some students avoid classes or work with certain faculty members because of the risk of sexual advances. However, few file official grievances.

Because college administrations can be held legally responsible for allowing a hostile or offensive sexual environment, many schools have set up committees to handle such student reports and to take action against faculty members. Universities also are discouraging and, in some cases, restricting consensual relationships between teachers and students, especially any dating of

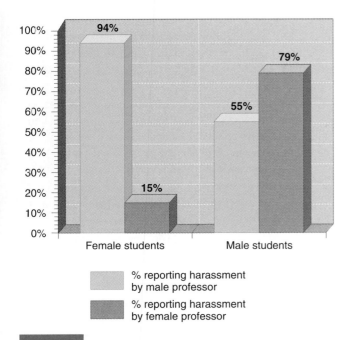

Figure 17-2

Sexual harassment does happen on campus, to both women and men. Such harassment can affect self-esteem and academic performance.

students by their academic professors or advisers. Although such relationships may seem consensual, in reality they may not be because of the power faculty members have to determine students' grades and futures. In some cases, students have sued their universities for failing to protect them from professors who pressured them into sexual liaisons.

If you encounter sexual harassment as a student, report it to the department chair or dean. If you don't feel that you're getting an adequate response to your complaint, talk with the campus representatives who handle matters involving affirmative action or civil rights. Federal guidelines prevent any discrimination against you in terms of grades or the loss of a job or scholarship if you report harassment. Schools that do not take measures to remedy harassment could lose federal funds.[49]

Sexual Coercion and Rape

At a bar on a weekend night, a group of intoxicated young men grab a woman and squeeze her breasts as she struggles to get free. At a party, a man offers his date drugs and alcohol in the hope of lowering her resistance to sex. Although some people don't realize it, such

actions are forms of sexual coercion (forced sexual activity), which is very common, on and off college campuses. In fact, 20.4% of college women report being forced to have sexual intercourse.

Sexual coercion can take many forms, including exerting peer pressure, taking advantage of one's desire for popularity, threatening an end to a relationship, getting someone intoxicated, stimulating a partner against his or her wishes, or insinuating an obligation based on the time or money one has expended. Men may feel that they need to live up to the sexual stereotype of taking advantage of every opportunity for sex. Women are far more likely than men to encounter physical force.

Rape refers to sexual intercourse with an unconsenting partner under actual or threatened force. Sexual intercourse between a male over the age of 16 and a female under the "age of consent" (which ranges from 12 to 21 in different states) is called *statutory* rape. In *acquaintance* rape, or *date* rape, discussed in depth later in this chapter, the victim knows the rapist; in stranger rape, the rapist is an unknown assailant. Both stranger and acquaintance rapes are serious crimes that can have a devastating impact on their victims.

The motives of rapists vary. Those who attack strangers often have problems establishing intimate relationships, have poor self-esteem, feel inadequate, and may have been sexually abused as children. Some rapists report a long history of fantasizing about rape and violence, generally while masturbating. Others commit rape out of anger that they can't express toward a wife or girlfriend. The more sexually aggressive men have been, the more likely they are to see such aggression and violence as normal and to believe rape myths, such as that it's impossible to rape a woman who doesn't really want sex. Sexually violent and degrading photographs, films, books, magazines, and videos may contribute to some rapists' assaultive behaviors.[50] Hardcore pornography depicting violent rape has been strongly associated, not only with judging oneself capable of sexual coercion and aggression, but also with engaging in such acts.[51]

Alcohol and drugs also play a major role. About 25% of both men and women report unwanted sexual experiences as a result of alcohol use. Many rapists drink prior to an assault, and alcohol may interfere with a victim's ability to avoid danger or resist attack.

For many years, the victims of rape were blamed for doing something to bring on the attack. Researchers have since shown that women are raped because they encounter sexually aggressive men, not because they look or act a certain way. However, while no woman is immune to attack, women who were sexually abused as children are at greater risk than others. Scientists are exploring the reasons for this greater vulnerability.

Women who successfully escape rape attempts do so by resisting verbally and physically, usually by yelling and fleeing. In a study of 150 rapes or attempted rapes, women who used forceful verbal or physical resistance (screaming, hitting, kicking, biting, running, etc.) were more likely to avoid rape than women who tried pleading, crying, or offering no resistance.[52]

Strategies for Prevention

Reducing the Risk of Stranger Rape

Rape prevention consists primarily of making it as difficult as possible for a rapist to make you his victim:

✔ Don't advertise that you're a woman living alone. Use initials on your mailbox and in the phone book; even add a fictitious name.

✔ Install and use secure locks on doors and windows, changing door locks after losing keys or moving into a new residence. A peephole in your front door can be particularly helpful.

✔ Don't open your door to strangers. If a repairman or public official is at your door, ask him to identify himself and call his office to verify that he is a reputable person on legitimate business.

✔ In public, demonstrate self-confidence through your body language and speech to communicate that you won't be intimidated. Rapists often select as victims women who exhibit passivity and submissiveness.

✔ Lock your car when it's parked, and drive with locked car doors. Should your car break down, attach a white

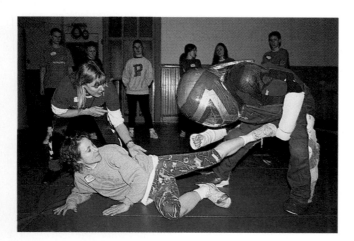

Model mugging courses train women to actively resist assault and rape.

cloth to the antenna and lock yourself in. If someone other than a uniformed officer stops to offer help, ask this person to call the police or a garage but do not open your locked car door.

✔ Avoid dark and deserted areas, and be aware of the surroundings where you're walking. This may help if you need an opportunity to escape. Should a driver ask for directions when you're a pedestrian, avoid approaching his car. Instead, call out your reply from a safe distance.

✔ Have house or car keys in hand before coming to the door, and check the back seat before getting into your car.

✔ Wherever you go, it can be very helpful to carry a device for making a loud noise, like a whistle or, even better, a small pint-sized compressed air horn available in many sporting goods and boat supply stores. Sound the noise alarm at the first sign of danger.

✔ Take a self-defense class to learn techniques of physical resistance that can injure the attacker or distract him long enough for you to escape.

Types of Rape

Although rape has long been viewed as an act of violence and domination, recent studies indicate that not all rapes fit into a single pattern. Within the broad category of rape are specific, but not mutually exclusive, subcategories of the crime, including anger rape, power rape, sadistic rape, gang rape, and sexual gratification rape.[53]

Anger rape, is an unplanned, violent physical attack, usually on a total stranger, motivated by hatred and a desire for revenge for the rejection the rapist feels he's suffered from women. Anger rapists often harbor long-standing hostility toward women, use far more physical violence than is needed for submission, and usually don't find the rape sexually gratifying.

Power rape is a generally premeditated attack motivated by a desire to dominate and control another person. Power rapists, unable to deal with stress and their sense of failure, may rape to regain a sense of power. They use only as much force as needed to make their victims submit and may find the rape sexually gratifying, even though that's not their primary motive.

Sadistic rape is a premeditated assault that often involves bondage, torture, or sexual abuse. Sadistic rapists find power and anger sexually arousing, and may subject victims to rituals of humiliation or torture. They're often preoccupied with violent pornography; their motives are more complex and difficult to understand than those of other types of rapists.

Gang rape involves three or more rapists. Men in

close groups that drink and party together—such as fraternities or athletic teams— are more likely to participate in such assaults. The reasons may go beyond aggression and sexual gratification to the excitement and camaraderie the men feel while sharing the experience.

Sexual gratification rape is a usually impulsive attack by someone willing to use physical coercion for the sake of sex. These rapists generally use no more force than needed to get a partner to submit and may stop the attack if it becomes clear they'll have to use extreme violence to overcome resistance. Many acquaintance rapes fit into this category.

Acquaintance or Date Rape

Most rapes are committed by someone who is known to the victim. Both women and men report having been forced into sexual activity by someone they know. Many college students are in the age group most likely to face this threat: women aged 16 to 25 and men under 25. Women are most vulnerable and men are most likely to commit assaults during their senior year of high school and their first year of college. In several surveys of college students, 79.7% to 97.5% of the women and 62.1% to 93.5% of the men reported that they had been coerced into some unwanted sexual behavior.[54]

Often women who describe incidents of sexual coercion that meet the legal definition of rape don't label it as such. Often they have a preconceived notion that true "rape" consists of a blitzlike attack by a stranger.[55] Or they may blame themselves for getting into a situation in which they couldn't escape, or they may feel some genuine concern for others who would be devastated if they knew the truth (for example, if the rapist were the brother of a good friend or the son of a neighbor).

Men who admit to being sexually aggressive don't see themselves as would-be rapists. The reasons stem from our society's ambivalence about sexual violence and standards for "normal" interactions between potential sexual partners. According to various studies, 25% to 60% of college men have engaged in some form of sexual coercion. Most often these men simply ignored a woman when she said no or protested. In addition, many college men report engaging in sexual activity against their own wishes, most often because of male peer pressure or a desire to be popular.

The same factors that lead to other forms of sexual victimization can set the stage for date rape. Socialization into an aggressive role, acceptance of rape myths, and a view that force is justified in certain situations increase the likelihood of a man's committing date rape. Other factors can also play a role, including the following:

- *Personality and early sexual experiences.* Psychological studies haven't found that date rapists are more disturbed than other men. However, certain factors may predispose individuals to sexual aggression, including first sexual experience at a very young age, earlier and more frequent than usual childhood sexual experiences (both forced and voluntary), hostility toward women, irresponsibility, lack of social consciousness, and a need for dominance over sexual partners.

- *Situational variables (what happens during the date).* Men who initiate a date, pay all expenses, and provide transportation are more likely to be sexually aggressive, perhaps because they feel that they can call all the shots. For instance, a man may drive to an isolated area and park his car, setting the stage for a sexual assault.

- *Acceptance of sexual coercion.* Some social groups, such as fraternities or athletic teams, may encourage the use of alcohol; reinforce stereotypes about masculinity; and emphasize violence, force, and competition. The group's shared values, including an acceptance of sexual coercion, may keep individuals from questioning their behavior. In studies comparing self-admitted date rapists with college men who had not sexually victimized women, the rapists were more likely to have taken advantage of women—for example, by saying that they loved them—for the sake of sex. They also were much more likely to have friends who viewed rough sex and rape as justified—or even as something that would enhance their reputation among their peers.

- *Drinking.* Alcohol use is one of the strongest predictors of acquaintance rape. Men who've been drinking may not react to subtle signals, may misinterpret a woman's behavior as come-ons, and may feel more sexually aroused. At the same time, drinking may impair a woman's ability to communicate her wishes effectively and to cope with a man's aggressiveness. Alcohol also affects the way rape is perceived: Assailants suffer less blame when drunk than when sober, while victims may be considered more responsible for the rape if they were drunk.

- *Date Rape Drugs.* As discussed in Chapter 14, at least two drugs—Rohypnol (roofie, La Rocha, rope, Mexican Valium, Rib Roche, R-2), a tranquilizer used overseas, and gammahydroxybutrate of GHB (Liquid X), a depressant with potential benefits for people with narcolepsy—have been implicated in cases of

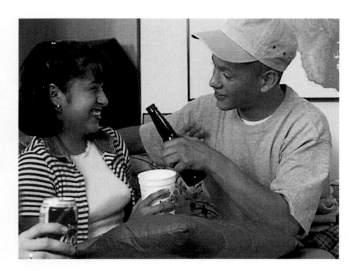

Acquaintance rape and alcohol use are very closely linked.   Both men and women may find their judgment impaired or their communications unclear as a result of drinking.

acquaintance or date rape. Since both are odorless and tasteless, a woman has no way of knowing whether her drink has been tampered with. The subsequent loss of memory leaves her with no explanation for where she's been or what's happened in the hours before she regains consciousness. Women have reported waking up naked in college fraternity houses or in the apartments of dates or casual acquaintances with no recall of what happened.[56]

Rohypnol can cause impaired motor skills and judgment, lack of inhibitions, dizziness, confusion, lethargy, very low blood pressure, coma, and death.[57] Its use has been outlawed in this country; rapists found guilty of giving this drug to one of their victims can get an additional 20 years tacked on to their prison sentences. Deaths also have been attributed to GHB overdoses.

• *Gender differences in interpreting sexual cues.* In research comparing college men and women, the men typically overestimated the woman's sexual availability and interest, seeing friendliness, revealing clothing, and attractiveness as deliberately seductive. In one study of date rapes, the men reported feeling "led on," in part because their female partners seemed to be dressed more suggestively than usual. They didn't define their behavior as rape, placed equal responsibility on their partners for what happened, and said that they'd behave similarly again. They also disagreed with their victims about the amount of force used and viewed the women's protests as token resistance.[58]

Strategies for Prevention

Preventing Date Rape

For men:

✔ Remember that it's okay not to "score" on a date.

✔ Be aware of your partner's actions. If she pulls away or tries to get up, understand that she's sending you a message—one you should acknowledge and respect.

✔ Don't assume that a sexy dress or casual flirting is an invitation to sex.

✔ Be aware of drinking, drug use, or other behaviors (such as hanging out with a group known to be sexually aggressive in certain situations) that could affect your judgment and ability to act responsibly.

✔ Think of the way you'd want your sister or a close woman friend to be treated by her date. Behave in the same manner.

For women:

✔ Be wary if the man calls all the shots (ordering for you at restaurants, planning what to do on your date); he may do the same when it comes to sex. If he pays for all expenses, he may think he's justified in using force to get "what he paid for." If you cover some of the costs, he may be less aggressive.

✔ Back away from a man who pressures you into other activities you don't want to engage in on a date, such as chugging beer or drag racing with his friends.

✔ Avoid misleading messages and avoid behavior that may be interpreted as sexual teasing. Don't tell him to stop touching you, talk for a few minutes, and then resume petting. If you know or feel at the onset of a relationship that you don't want to have sex with this person, say so.

✔ If, despite direct communication about your intentions, your date behaves in a sexually coercive manner, use a strategy of escalating forcefulness—direct refusal, vehement verbal refusal, and, if necessary, physical force.

✔ Avoid using alcohol or other drugs when you definitely do not wish to be sexually intimate with your date.

Male Rape

No one knows how common male rape is because men are less likely to report such assaults than women. However, in recent years, there have been more frequent reports of male rape by both other men and by women. Researchers estimate that the victims in about 10% of acquaintance rape cases are men. These "hidden victims" often keep silent because of embarrassment, shame, or humiliation and their own feelings and fears about homosexuality and conforming to conventional sex roles.

Although many people think that men who rape other men are always homosexuals, most male rapists consider themselves to be heterosexual. Young boys aren't the only victims. The average age of male rape victims is 24. Rape is a serious problem in prison, where men may experience brutal assaults by men who usually resume sexual relations with women once they're released.

There have been reports of men forced by women to participate in sexual intercourse. Typically, these men feel very upset afterward because they functioned sexually in circumstances that they thought should have made it impossible to obtain an erection. They suffer a post-assault syndrome comparable to the rape trauma syndrome women experience, including psychological and sexual difficulties. Men raped by other men also suffer extreme emotional distress after an attack.

The Impact of Rape

Only a small percentage of college women who are raped report their assaults to the police; many don't even tell a close friend or relative about the assault. However, women who survive a rape can benefit from the support of others. If you are raped, call a friend or rape crisis center. Before you take a bath or shower, go to a doctor; you may later decide to report the rape. If you must go to a hospital, remember that you don't necessarily have to talk to the police. Talk to a counselor or health-care workers at the hospital about testing and antibiotics for sexually transmitted diseases and post-intercourse contraception (discussed in Chapter 10).

Sexual violence has both a physical and a psychological impact. Rape-related injuries include unexplained vaginal discharge, bleeding, infections, multiple bruises, and fractured ribs. Victims of sexual violence often develop chronic symptoms, such as headaches, backaches, high blood pressure, sleep disorders, pelvic pain, and sexual fertility problems.

The psychological scars of a sexual assault take a long time to heal. Therapists have linked sexual victimization with hopelessness, low self-esteem, high levels of self-criticism, and self-defeating relationships. Some have described a "rape trauma syndrome," similar to posttraumatic stress disorder, in which women suffer both acute symptoms, such as crying, shortly after the rape and long-term symptoms, which can persist for years and often include deeply disturbing flashbacks in which they "relive" the rape.

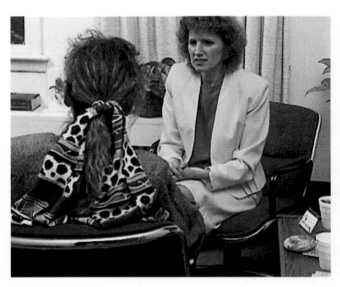

Counseling from a trained professional can help ease the trauma suffered by a rape victim.

Acquaintance rape may cause fewer physical injuries but greater psychological torment. The victims of date rape are less likely to notify the police, in part because they fear that no one will believe their stories. Often too ashamed to tell anyone what happened, they may suffer alone, without skilled therapists or sympathetic friends to reassure them. Women raped by acquaintances blame themselves more, see themselves less positively, question their judgment, have greater difficulty trusting others, and have higher levels of psychological distress. Nightmares, anxiety, and flashbacks are common. The women may avoid others, become less capable of protecting themselves, and come to accept victimization as part of being a woman.

According to some researchers, victims of acquaintance rape rate themselves as less recovered than women raped by strangers for up to three years after the assault. Years after a rape, victims of date rape may still be struggling with rage against men and having problems establishing trusting relationships. Women who remain haunted by the sexual violence should seek professional help. A therapist can help them begin the slow process of healing.[59]

What to Do in Case of Rape

If a woman has been raped, she will have to decide whether to report the attack to the police. Even an unsuccessful rape attempt should be reported because the information a woman may provide about the attack—the assaulter's physical characteristics, voice, clothes, car, even an unusual smell—may prevent another woman from being raped. A woman shouldn't bathe or change her clothes before calling the police. Semen, hair, and material under her fingernails or on her apparel all may be useful in identifying the man who raped her. Many rape victims find it very helpful to contact a rape crisis center, where qualified staff members assist in dealing with the trauma. Many colleges, universities, and large urban communities in the United States have such programs. Friends and family members should remember that many women will mistakenly blame themselves for the rape. However, the victim hasn't committed a crime—the man who raped her has.

Strategies for Prevention

What to Do in Threatening Situations Involving Strangers

When a woman is approached by a man or men who may intend to rape her, she will have to decide what to do. Each situation, assailant, and woman is unique. There are no absolute rules, but the following can serve as guides:

✔ Run away if you can.

✔ Resist if you can't run. Make it difficult for the rapist. Many men, upon locating a potential victim, test her to see if she's easily intimidated. Shout; kick; cause a scene; run away; fight back.

✔ Ordinary rules of behavior do not apply. Vomiting, screaming, or acting crazy—whatever you're willing to try—can be appropriate responses to an attempted rape.

✔ Stall to give yourself a chance to devise an escape plan or another strategy. Get the attacker to start talking ("What has happened to make you so angry?") or to negotiate ("Let's take time to talk about this").

✔ Remain alert for an opportunity to escape—for example, if a passerby approaches.

Sexual Abuse of Children

Pedophilia, or child molestation, refers to abuse by individuals—teachers, babysitters, neighbors, and the like—who aren't related to the child. (Sexual abuse by family members is discussed earlier in this chapter.) Researchers find it difficult to make accurate estimates about the prevalence of child molestation. Many victims of childhood sexual abuse are under age 7 and may not realize that an adult's behavior is improper, or may not

know how to distinguish between affection and inappropriate sexual contact. Older children may feel ashamed and not confide in their parents for fear of being punished. Even when they do inform them, the parents may not believe them, may be unable to handle the emotional trauma of finding out that some adult they love would "do that," or may not want to subject the child to the stress of a criminal investigation. Counseling can help the entire family.

Parents should explain to children at an early age the differences between okay touches, such as snuggles and hugs, and touches that are not okay (touches under clothes, touches to areas of the body that would be covered by a bathing suit, or any other touches that make a child feel uncomfortable or confused), and the differences between okay kisses and not-okay kisses (prolonged, tongue in mouth). Children also need to understand that they have rights, including the right to control their bodies and say no to being touched in a way that makes them uncomfortable. They should have a talk about strategies adults may use to get children to go along with their wishes, such as saying they're "teaching" them something that will make them feel good. Parents also should let children know that it's okay to scream, yell, run away, or get assistance from a trusted adult if they're in a situation that makes them feel uncomfortable. Youngsters should be encouraged to tell someone right away if an adult has touched them or done anything to make them feel uncomfortable. Stress that you will not be angry with them and that they will not get into trouble. Instruct them to tell anyone who tries to touch them that they will tell a responsible adult.

Halting Sexual Violence: Prevention Efforts

Sexual violence has its roots in social attitudes and beliefs that demean women and condone aggression. As colleges and universities have become more aware of the different forms of sexual danger, many have taken the lead in setting up primary prevention programs (including newspaper articles; seminars in dormitories, fraternities, and sororities; and lectures) to help students examine their attitudes and values, understand cultural influences, and develop skills for avoiding or escaping from dangerous situations. All men and women should understand the impact of socialization on their willingness to tolerate or participate in sexual victimization, recognize misleading rape myths, and develop effective

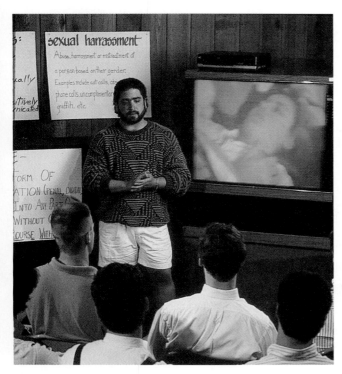

All-male workshops can generate discussion about gender roles, violence, and other societal ideas. These discussions may also provide positive pressure against rape and other forms of aggression against women.

ways of communicating to avoid misinterpretation of sexual cues. Students should also know where they can turn to learn more about and seek help for sexual victimization: counselors, campus police, deans of student affairs, fraternity or sorority representatives, campus ministers, and so on.

Discussion groups led by campus leaders and facilitated by students are very effective in producing positive peer pressure against rape and modeling alternatives to sexist male behaviors. Some campuses have found that all-male workshops are best at creating a safe environment in which men can talk with other men about gender-role expectations, expressing anger without violence, communication skills, and power and control issues.

In addition, practical institutional steps—such as providing adequate lighting, escort services, and clear policies against both violence and drug and alcohol abuse—can help. Some campuses offer self-defense classes, which teach women how to avoid becoming victims either by escaping or protecting themselves. Individuals who advocate such training believe that it can strengthen women's physical capacities and encourage them to be less passive in encounters with potential victimizers. Others, however, view self-defense behav-

iors as violent actions in themselves, and are concerned that they may lead to an increased risk of injury or death. Followup studies of college women have found that self-defense training increased their feelings of self-improvement, a sense of control over their life, confidence, security, independence, and physical prowess.[60]

Campuses are also providing "secondary prevention" by getting help to victims of sexual violence as soon as possible through rape crisis teams and emergency mental-health services; and "tertiary prevention" by working with victims to ameliorate the long-term effects of their experience through psychotherapy, educational services, and medical care.

Making This Chapter Work for You
Staying Alive and Healthy

- The major threats to the well-being of most college students are unintentional and intentional injuries. Accidents, especially motor-vehicle crashes, kill more college-age men and women than all other causes combined. Young people also are at risk of becoming victims of physical and sexual violence.

- The risk factors that increase the likelihood of accidents include unsafe attitudes and behaviors, alcohol and drug use, stress, age and gender, environmental conditions, and thrill-seeking.

- The most common causes of fatal accidents for Americans are motor-vehicle injuries. Using seat belts, practicing defensive driving, and being extra cautious and wearing a helmet when on a motorcycle or bicycle can increase your odds of staying safe on the road.

- The risk of accidents is greatest in the home. Falls are a common cause of injury, particularly for the elderly. Fires, another serious threat, can often be prevented by eliminating hazards, using caution with flammable materials, and knowing the proper way to use and maintain electrical appliances, including microwave ovens.

- Work-related risks range from obvious hazards, such as toxic chemicals, to more subtle dangers, such as trauma from repetitive motions like typing.

- Recreational safety demands common sense and proper planning. Anyone who exercises or spends a great deal of time outdoors should be aware of the early warning signs of problems related to temperature—whether they're caused by excess heat or

Health Online

Rate Your Risk   http://www.Nashville.Net/~police/risk/

This site, courtesy of the Nashville Police Department, will allow you to rate your chances of becoming a crime victim. There are detailed questionnaires that measure your risk of being raped, assaulted, murdered, or burglarized, including feedback on what your risk factors are and how you might change them.

Think about it ...

- According to these quizzes, are you at high risk for becoming a victim of a crime? If so, what steps could you rake to lower your risk?

- Can you list five risk factors for violence that a person could change (i.e., varying their daily routine) and five that couldn't be easily changed (i.e., living in an urban area)?

- What special risks might college students face for becoming victims of crime?

extreme cold. Even strong swimmers are at risk of drowning, especially if they drink before diving into the water or ignore safety precautions.

- Health officials have declared violence a national emergency that threatens the well-being of all Americans. Homicide has become the tenth leading killer in the nation; among African-American youth, homicide is the most common cause of death. The costs to the economy total in the billions of dollars each year.

- Many factors contribute to aggression and violence: biological causes, such as traumatic brain injury, certain medications, and the abuse of drugs or alcohol; developmental factors, such as harsh parental discipline, relations to peers, sex-role socialization, economic inequality, and lack of opportunity; exposure to violence in the media; the widespread availability of guns; and social factors, such as extreme poverty, deprivation, unemployment, prejudice, discrimination, involvement with gangs, and repeated exposure to actual violence.

- There has been a dramatic increase in crime on college and university campuses. Federal law requires disclosure of school crime statistics and security policies. Many campuses have set up safety programs, which include late-night shuttle buses and escorts, patrols, outdoor emergency phones, and increased numbers of guards.

- Physical violence may occur in 20% to 30% of all American households. Domestic violence is the single most common cause of injury to women—more common than car accidents, muggings, and rapes combined. Severe child abuse occurs an estimated 1.7 million times each year and claims the lives of as many as 5000 children. Abusive partners or parents may have been abused themselves, and have low self-esteem and little sense of empathy. Abuse occurs within families of every racial, social, and economic group and takes many forms, including physical, sexual, and psychological abuse. All can cause long-term emotional distress.

- Sexual victimization refers to any situation in which a person is deprived of free choice and is forced to comply with sexual acts. At its root are false beliefs and callous attitudes that stem from myths about sexual conduct, acceptance of male aggression, trivialization of the impact of sexual misconduct, blame of the victim, and exposure to sexually violent material.

- Any unwanted sexual attention by a teacher, counselor, boss, coworker, or other authority figure constitutes sexual harassment and is illegal. The two basic forms are "quid pro quo" harassment, in which a person in power or authority makes unwanted sexual advances as a condition for receiving a job, a promotion, or another type of favor, and creation or tolerance of a "hostile or offensive environment," in which supervisors or coworkers engage in persistent inappropriate behaviors that make the workplace hostile, abusive, or otherwise unbearable.

■ Sexual coercion (forced sexual activity) is common on college campuses. Both men and women report that they have performed sexual acts because of peer pressure, a desire for popularity, a threatened end to a relationship, intoxication, obligation, or unwanted physical stimulation.

■ Rape refers to sexual intercourse with an unconsenting partner, who may be a stranger or an acquaintance, under actual or threatened force. The different types of rape include anger rape, an unplanned violent physical attack, usually on a total stranger; power rape, a generally premeditated attack motivated by a desire to dominate and control; sadistic rape, which often involves bondage, torture, and sexual abuse; gang rape, involving three or more rapists; and sexual gratification rape, usually an impulsive attack by someone willing to use force to obtain sex.

■ Date or acquaintance rape, usually committed for the sake of sexual gratification, stems from the same factors that lead to other forms of sexual victimization, including male socialization into an aggressive role, widespread acceptance of rape myths, early sexual experiences (both forced and voluntary), the acceptance of sexual coercion, drinking, and gender differences in interpreting verbal and nonverbal sexual cues.

■ Sexual violence has both a physical and a psychological impact and can lead to chronic symptoms, such as pain in the head, stomach, back, or chest, as well as depression, low self-esteem, and self-defeating relationships. Victims of date rape, who may feel too ashamed to tell anyone what happened, may blame themselves more than those raped by strangers, see themselves less positively, question their judgment, have greater difficulty trusting others, and experience higher levels of psychological distress. Male rape victims, whether they're forced into sexual activity by a woman or another man, also suffer emotionally after an attack.

Because so many dangers exist in our society, you may feel that there's little you can do to ensure your safety. That's not true. Most accidents, injuries, and acts of violence don't happen randomly. The more aware you are of the risks surrounding you, the more you can do to reduce or eliminate them. If you proceed with caution on the road, watch out for potential hazards at home, follow safety guidelines outdoors and at work, and recognize and avoid potential dangers, you can learn to live on the safe side—always the healthiest place to be.

▶ Key Terms

The terms listed here are used within the chapter. Page numbers are included for each term. A definition of each term is given in the green Glossary pages at the end of this book.

Review Questions

1. What factors increase the likelihood of accident or injury?

2. What can you do to increase safety on the road, at home, outdoors, and at work?

3. What is sexual victimization? Why does it occur? What are the consequences?

4. What is sexual harassment? How can it be prevented or discouraged?

5. Describe the typical pattern of abuse. How does it apply to partners and to children?

6. List the different types of rape. What are the characteristics of date rape? What should a person do if she or he is raped? Where can someone who has been raped seek help?

Critical Thinking Questions

1. Can you name two risk factors in your daily life that might increase the likelihood of accidental injury? What actions have you taken to keep yourself safe? Are there any additional risk factors you haven't taken action to minimize or eliminate? What might you do about them?

2. A friend of yours, Eric, frequently makes crude or derogatory comments about women. When you finally call him on it, his response is, "I didn't say anything wrong. I like women." What might you say to him?

3. At one college, women raped by acquaintances or dates scrawled the names of their assailants on the walls of women's rest rooms on campus. Several young men whose names appeared on the list objected, protesting that they were innocent and were being unfairly accused. How do you feel about this method of fighting back against date rape? Do you think it violates the rights of men? How do you feel about naming women who've been raped in news reports? Are there circumstances in which a woman's identity should be revealed? Would fewer women report a rape if not assured of privacy?

Connections to Personal Health Interactive

To enhance your understanding of the material covered in this chapter, check out the following study aids on the **Personal Health Interactive CD-ROM**. *Each numbered icon within the chapter corresponds to an appropriate activity listed here.*

17.1 Personal Insights: How Well Are You Protected?
17.2 Chapter 17 Review

References

1. Sarvela, Paul, Derek Holcomb, and Justin Odulana. "Designing a Safety Program for a College Health Service." *Journal of American College Health*, March 1992.

2. "America the Violent." *American Medical News*, July 17, 1995.

3. "Handgun Use Rose in 1993, Report Shows." *New York Times*, July 10, 1995.

4. Randall, Teri. "Driving While Under Influence of Alcohol Remains Major Cause of Traffic Violence." *Journal of the American Medical Association*, July 15, 1992.

5. Roberts, Paul. "Risk!" *Psychology Today*, Vol. 27, No. 6, November–December 1994.

6. Coren, Stanley. *The Left-Hander Syndrome.* New York: Free Press, 1992.

7. Douglas, Kathy, et al. "Results from the 1995 National College Health Risk Behavior Survey." *Journal of American College Health*, Vol. 46, September 1997.

8. National Highway Traffic Safety Administration, American Academy of Pediatrics.

9. Berardelli, Phil. *The Driving Challenge.* McLean, VA: EPM Publishers, 1998.

10. AAA Foundation for Traffic Safety.

11. Nerenberg, Arnold. Personal interview.

12. Faulk, Stephanie. Personal interview.

13. "Bicycle Helmets Policy." *Pediatrics*, April 1995.

14. National Safety Council.

15. National Safe Kids Campaign. "Skate Smart and Safeboard Safe." May, 1995. "Skateboard Injuries." *Pediatrics*, April 1995.

16. National Safety Council.

17. Douglas, et al., "Results from the 1995 National College Health Risk Behavior Survey."

18. Butterfield, Fox. "Drop in Homicide Rate Linked to Crack's Decline." *New York Times*, October 27, 1997.

19. Bureau of Justice Statistics.

20. Reiss, Albert, and Jeffrey Roth (eds). *Understanding and Preventing Violence.* Washington, D.C.: National Academy Press, 1993.

21. Yudofsky, Stuart, and Robert Hales. *Textbook of Neuropsychiatry.* (2nd ed.). Washington, D.C.: American Psychiatric Press, 1994.

22. Hales, Dianne, and Robert Hales. *Caring for the Mind.* New York: Bantam Books, 1995.

23. Reiss, Albert, and Jeffrey Roth. Anderson, Elijah. "The Code of the Streets" *The Atlantic*, May 1994.

24. "America the Violent."

25. Kellerman, Arthur, et al. "Weapon Involvement in Home Invasion Crimes." *Journal of the American Medical Association*, Vol. 273, No. 22, June 14, 1995.

26. Marwick, Charles. "A Public Health Approach to Making Guns Safer." *Journal of the American Medical Association*, Vol. 273, No. 22, June 14, 1995. Sosin, Daniel, et al. "Trends in Death Associated with Traumatic Brain Injury, 1979 Through 1992." *Journal of the American Medical Association*, Vol. 273, No. 22, June 14, 1995.

27. Annest, Joseph, et al. "National Estimates of Nonfatal Firearm-Related Injuries." *Journal of the American Medical Association*, Vol. 273, No. 22, June 14, 1995.

28. Kizer, Kenneth. "Hospitalization Charges, Costs, and Income for Firearm Related Injuries at a University Trauma Center." *Journal of the American Medical Association*, Vol. 273, No. 22, June 14, 1995.

29. Saunders, Carol. "Safe at Home?" *American Health*, November 1994.

30. McLarin, Kimberly. "Fear Prompts Self-Defense as Crime Comes to College." *New York Times*, September 7, 1994.

31. Kirtley, Jane. "Shedding Light on Campus Crime," American Journalism Review, Vol. 19, No. 6, July–August 1997.

32. Douglas, et al., "Results from the 1995 National College Health Risk Behavior Survey."

33. Lewin, Tamar. "Schools Are Moving to Police Students' Off-Campus Lives." *New York Times*, February 6, 1998.

34. Whitaker, Leighton, and Jeffrey Pollard. "Campus Violence: Kinds, Causes and Cures." *Journal of American College Health*, Vol. 43, No. 2, September 1994.

35. Hyman, Ariela, et al. "Laws Mandating Reporting of Domestic Violence." McAfee, Robert. "Physicians and Domestic Violence." *Journal of the American Medical Association*, Vol. 273, No. 22, June 14, 1995.

36. Correia, Felicia Collins. "Domestic Violence Can Be Cured." *USA Today* (Magazine), Vol. 126, No. 2630, November 1997.

37. Abbott, Jean, et al. "Domestic Violence Against Women." *Journal of the American Medical Association*, Vol. 273, No. 22, June 14, 1995.

38. Centerwall, Brandon. "Race, Socioeconomic Status, and Domestic Homicide." *Journal of the American Medical Association*, Vol. 273, No. 22, June 14, 1995.

39. Leidig, Marjorie Whittaker. "The Continuum of Violence Against Women: Psychological and Physical Consequences." *Journal of American College Health*, January 1992.

40. Berkowitz, Alan. "College Men as Perpetrators of Acquaintance Rape and Sexual Assault: A Review of Recent Research." *Journal of American College Health*, January 1992.

41. Benson, Dennis, Catherine Charlton, and Fem Goodhart. "Acquaintance Rape on Campus: A Literature Review." *Journal of American College Health*, January 1992.

42. Gutek, Barbara. Personal interview.

43. Langelan, Martha. *Back Off! How to Confront and Stop Sexual Harassment and Harassers.* New York: Fireside, 1993.

44. Fisher, Anne. "After All This Time, Why Don't People Know What Sexual Harassment Means?" *Fortune*, Vol. 137, No. 1, January 12, 1998.

45. Susan Webb. Personal interview.

46. Gutek, Barbara.

47. Charney, D. and Russell, R. "An Overview of Sexual Harassment." *American Journal of Psychiatry*, Vol. 151, 1994.

48. Cleary, Jane, et al. "Sexual Harassment of College Students: Implications for College Health Promotion" *Journal of College Health*, Vol. 43, July 1994.

49. Crooks, Robert, and Karla Baur. *Our Sexuality*, 7th ed. Pacific Grove, CA: Brooks/Cole, 1999.

50. Crooks and Baur, 1999.

51. Boeringer, Scot. "Pornography and Sexual Aggression." *Deviant Behavior*, Vol. 15, 1994.

52. Zoucha-Jensen, J., and Coyne, A. "The Effects of Resistant Strategies on Rape." *American Journal of Public Health*, Vol. 83, 1993.

53. Crooks and Baur, 1999.

54. Ibid.

55. Ibid.

56. Crooks and Baur, 1999.

57. Horowitz, Josh. "Date-Rape Drug Scare." *New York Times Education Life*, January 4, 1998.

58. Berkowitz, Alan. "College Men as Perpetrators of Acquaintance Rape."

59. Santello, Mark and Harold Leitenberg. "Sexual Aggression by an Acquaintance: Methods of Coping and Later Psychological Adjustments. " *Violence & Victims*, Vol. 8, No. 2, Summer 1993.

60. Cummings, Nina. "Self-Defense Training for College Women." *Journal of American College Health*, January 1992.

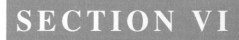

THE CIRCLE OF LIFE

To a great extent, we all live for today. Inevitably, though, tomorrow catches up with us—a fact many of us don't realize when we're young and healthy. However, sooner or later we come to understand that we're not alone, that we are part of all who came before us and all who will come after us. This section examines the state and fate of the planet on which we live, the changes that come with time, and the prospect of dying and death.

CHAPTER 18

LIVING LONGER AND BETTER

After studying the material in this chapter, you should be able to:

Explain the impact of aging on major body systems and on mental health.

Discuss the influence of social and cultural factors on aging.

List factors that increase life expectancy.

List and **explain** major health and health-related problems faced by older people in our society.

Identify some strategies for preventing osteoporosis.

America is turning gray. By the year 2010, one in four Americans—some 74.1 million people—will be over age 55; one in seven will be 69 or older. The most rapidly growing group of elders are those over age 100. In 1950, there were 4475 Americans 100 years or older. Today there are more than 54,000 centenarians, and their numbers are growing.[1] By the midpoint of the 21st century, 80 million Americans—one in five—will be seniors (65 or older).[2] (See Figure 18-1.)

People are not only surviving longer, but from a physiological standpoint, they're staying younger longer too. Couples are having babies in their forties. Men and women are hiking, biking, heading back to school, or launching new careers in their fifties, sixties, and beyond. Eighty- and ninety-year-olds are climbing mountains and competing in marathons.

Aging—the characteristic pattern of normal life changes that occurs as humans, plants, and animals grow older—clearly isn't what it used to be. Although the process of aging remains inevitable, you can do a great deal to influence the impact that the passage of time has on you. At any age, at any stage of life, at any level of physical fitness, you can get better instead of merely getting older. As a result of the preventive steps you take now, you can expand your "health span"—your years of health and vitality—as well as possibly extend your lifespan. This chapter gives you a preview of the future of the changes age brings, of the steps you can take to age healthfully, and of ways to make the most of all the years of your life.

Living in a Graying Society

In the last 100 years, the United States and other developed nations have experienced a greater increase in life expectancy than in all of recorded history prior to 1900. Today the elderly account for 13% of the American population.[3] The ranks of the elderly will grow even more in the next few decades, as the 75 million "baby boomers" conceived from 1946 to 1964 pass their 65th birthdays.

Regardless of your age, you will be affected by this "graying" of the American population. This is one reason why it's important to bridge the gap in understanding and information between younger and older Americans. A survey of 1200 men and women by the American Association of Retired Persons (AARP) revealed many misconceptions: 46% of respondents said that most older people could not adapt to change; 65% felt that most older people are lonely; 71% thought that one of every ten elderly Americans lives in an institution (the actual percentage, according to the AARP, is 1 in 20).[4] Such negative assumptions may reflect **ageism**, a form of discrimination based on myths about aging and the elderly. As with other forms of discrimination, the best way to confront ageism is to seek accurate information, challenge stereotypes, and get involved in overcoming barriers to understanding.

Throughout your life, you will confront a variety of issues related not just to your age, but also to that of the aging American population. These include:

- *Retirement costs.* Unless the retirement age is raised or other changes are made to decrease the demand on the Social Security system, Social Security taxes on workers may have to be increased.

- *Health costs.* Some experts argue that health costs will soar because people over age 65 use more health services and require more medical care than younger ones. However, others contend that nations with a large elderly population do not necessarily spend more of their national wealth on health care.

- *The daughter track.* American women will spend an average of 17 years raising children and 18 years helping aged parents, according to a U.S. House of Representatives study. Many may have to switch from full-time to part-time jobs to provide the care their parents need; some have to give up work entirely. Because they postponed childbearing, many couples will find themselves sandwiched between caring for children and caring for aging parents.

- *Gray-power politics.* Senior citizens go to the polls in larger numbers than younger voters. With such voting power, programs for the elderly may make up a larger share of future federal budgets.

- *Antiaging gimmicks.* As the population ages, health hucksters push an ever-growing number of unproven antiaging treatments, such as melatonin or the hormone DHEA. Because some preparations have the potential to harm, as a consumer, you should be wary of all claims to turn back or slow down the biological clock. (Chapter 20 offers advice on avoiding health quackery.)

Figure 18-1

Tracking the baby-boom generation in the United States.

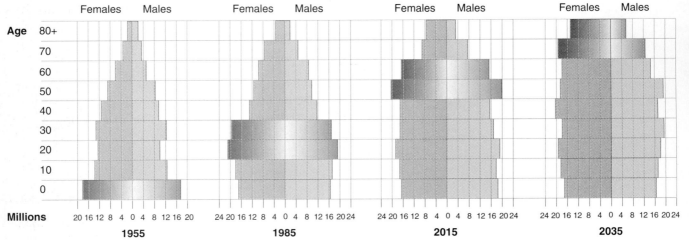

Sources: Population Reference Bureau and U.S. Census Bureau

How Long Can You Live?

According to the National Center for Health Statistics, life expectancy in the United States now averages about 75 years. Many researchers expect to see discoveries in our lifetimes that will slow aging and stretch life to its outer limits.[5] (See Spotlight on Diversity: "The Crossover Effect.")

Antioxidants Versus Aging

Some researchers believe aging is the result of cellular damage caused by harmful free radicals, proteins that oxidize and slowly damage body tissue, particularly cell membranes, sabotaging the body's immune and repair systems. Antioxidants—substances including vitamins A, C, and E and the mineral selenium—combine with free radicals to neutralize their effects. Increasing the body's supply of antioxidants, in theory, would slow age-related changes and damage, but there's no proof that this, in fact, happens. (See Chapter 6 for further discussion of antioxidants.)

Eat Less, Live Longer?

An alternative route to longer life and better health stems from the principle that less is more. In this case, less food may mean longer life—in theory, at least. Numerous studies with rats, mice, and simpler animals have found that a significant reduction in food intake can lengthen life, prevent disease, and slow down the aging process. Although most laboratory mice live about 36 months, for example, those on a restricted diet have lived up to 55 months. Studies are under way to determine what effect calorie restriction might have on humans. Some researchers believe that weight loss is the best method for reducing the risk of heart disease in overweight middle-aged and older individuals.[6]

Replacing Hormones

Aging brings changes in the delicate balance of **hormones**, chemical messengers produced by our bodies and brains that influence the way we think, look, feel, and act. Levels of a naturally occurring substance called *human growth hormone (HGH)* decline over time. About 30% of those over age 60 produce little or no HGH. Some of the changes attributed to normal aging,

such as loss of muscle mass and strength and of bone mineral density, may be a consequence of diminished HGH. Preliminary studies suggest that replacing HGH can change body composition, increase muscle mass, and lower weight. However, scientists don't yet know how much promise—or how many perils—growth hormone therapy for adults might hold. Potential side effects include an increased risk of heart disease, muscle disorders, and certain cancers.[7] Despite these risks, a black market has sprung up for HGH, which athletes and bodybuilders view as an alternative to steroids.

Wearing Out or Rusting Out?

The finite length of the human life maybe built into our cells. According to one scientific theory, the number of cell doublings needed to replace dead cells may be finite in the average lifespan of each species. Human cells were long thought to double about 50 times; after that, new cells fail to grow, even though nutrients and other conditions remain the same.

When a cell divides, its DNA splits down the middle. With each division, a small bit at the end of one strand, called the telomere, gets progressively shorter. Eventually, the telomere shrinks so much that the cell can no longer divide.[8] Time on the biological clock runs out; the cell "ages," stops dividing, and eventually dies. But this may not be inevitable.

In 1998, scientists discovered that the enzyme telomerase—which some scientists have called a "cellular fountain of youth"—causes human cells grown in the laboratory to continue to divide long past the time when they normally would stop. In effect, they have figured out how to overcome the mechanisms that control cellular aging and extend the lifespan of human cells.[9] However, it will take a great deal of time and research to apply this new understanding. While scientists are enthusiastic about extending cellular lifespans, they note that one danger may be the sort of uncontrolled proliferation that occurs in a disease like cancer.

Strategies for Prevention

How to Live to Be 100 Years Old

The Committee for an Extended Lifespan, in San Marcos, California, collected information on 100 men and women who lived 100 years or more. Here's what they can teach us about how to survive for a century:

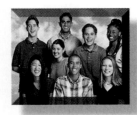

Spotlight on Diversity
The Crossover Effect

Until about age 75, African Americans and Native Americans are at greater risk of dying than Caucasians. However, those who live for three-quarters of a century have superior health and longevity. African Americans now make up a sizable percentage of the fastest-growing portion of the very old: While they account for only about 12% of the entire population, they constitute as much as 21% of those age 100 and over. Researchers refer to this phenomenon as "the crossover effect."

Some researchers believe that these statistics are deceptive, possibly the result of exaggerations about actual age. Yet Census Bureau experts who've analyzed millions of records of Medicare recipients believe that the crossover effect is too common and consistent to be a fluke.

How might race affect long-term longevity? Some scientists suggest that older African Americans and Native Americans are hardier than those who die at earlier ages—and hardier than elderly whites. According to this survival-of-the-fittest theory, overcoming the hardships of the early and middle ages of their lives might somehow equip individuals to live longer. Yet there is little evidence to back this theory up.

One physiological racial difference that may make a difference in longevity is cardiovascular disease. African Americans and Native Americans are more susceptible to high blood pressure, which can lead to death at an earlier age. Whites, on the other hand, are more prone to atherosclerosis, the buildup of plaque in the coronary arteries that is most likely to prove deadly later in life. African Americans who keep their blood pressure under control (see Chapter 12) may remain heart-healthy for a longer time than those with hypertension—and than whites.

Another, possibly key, racial difference is social. In their youth, African Americans—especially African-American males—face a greater threat from violence than do their white counterparts. But when they're old and ill, African Americans may receive more social support. For instance, they are more likely to live with their families, whereas whites are more likely to be in nursing homes. The love and care of family may help elderly African Americans survive longer than other senior citizens.

SOURCES: Park, Alice. "How to Live to Be 120." *Time*, March 6, 1995. Wray, Linda. "Health Policy and Ethnic Diversity in Older Americans." *Western Journal of Medicine*, September 1992. *Minority Elders: Longevity, Economics and Health*. Washington, DC: Gerontological Society of America. 1992.

✔ *Do nothing in excess.* The centenarians who drink do so in moderation. Few are fat. They aren't given to binges of any kind.

✔ *Get up early.* The centenarians are early risers. Usually, this means they go to bed early, too.

✔ *Have faith in some higher power.* A high proportion have led what they consider a spiritual life.

✔ *Keep busy.* Few are dreamers or loungers. The majority attribute their long survival to hard work.

✔ *Take care of yourself.* Centenarians are as self-sufficient as possible.

As Time Goes By

For years, **gerontologists**—specialists in the interdisciplinary field that studies aging—viewed the process of getting older only in terms of deterioration, frailty, the grinding away of time. Today, instead of focusing on the minority of the elderly who go into a steady decline, they are studying the majority of men and women who remain vital and resilient in their later years. The term *optimal aging* refers to the new focus on ways to enhance the well-being and preserve the abilities of older people. Its goal is to enable people to live through old age with the best possible quality of life and the least possible premature disability.

The Impact of Age

From a purely physiological standpoint, the body's finest years come in youth, when lung capacity is greatest, grip is firmest, motor responses are quickest, and physical endurance is longest. After age 30, the body's powers gradually decline. Between the ages of 20 and 80, the percentage of body fat typically increases from 15% to 35% or 40% in men and from 20% to 40% in women.

Many of the changes time brings, however have more to do with how you look than how you feel. At age 30, you'll have a few lines on your forehead. At age 40, you'll find "crow's feet" (from squinting) at the corners of your eyes and arcs (from smiling) linking your nostrils to the sides of your mouth. At age 50, these lines will look more pronounced, and the skin at your cheeks may sag; and at age 60, excess skin and fat deposits may form bags under your eyes. At age 70, your skin will be rougher, your face wrinkled, and your earlobes will droop about a quarter-inch lower than they did at age 20. (See Figure 18-2.)

After age 30, the heart's ability to pump blood decreases about 1% each year. At age 30, your heart pumps 3.6 quarts of blood per minute, but at age 70, only 2.6 quarts per minute. Blood pressure rises; circulation slows. These changes simply mean that the average 70-year-old can't compete with a 30-year-old in wrestling or running, but has sufficient energy and stamina for day-to-day functioning. (See Figure 18-3.)

Aerobic capacity—the amount of oxygen the body can use and the best measure of ability to do work—declines with age. By age 75, a man's aerobic capacity is less than half what it was at age 17; a woman's is about one-third what it was in her twenties.

Strength also diminishes slowly. Between the ages of 30 and 70, muscle strength declines about 12% to 15%, and the speed of muscle contraction and coordination drops 25%. Each decade after age 25, men and women lose 3% to 5% of their muscle mass, which often is replaced by fatty tissue.

As you get older, bones lose minerals and become softer and shorter. Your muscles weaken and your back slumps. The disks between the bones of the spine also deteriorate, moving those bones closer together. As a result, after 30, both men and women shrink by as much as half an inch in total height with each decade. Basal metabolism—the fundamental chemical process of living—slows down because the aging body requires less upkeep. The rate at which the body turns food into energy declines about 3% every ten years.[10]

As we age, the brain becomes smaller, but mental abilities do not diminish. Aging nerve cells, however, result in slower reaction times and slower movement, and we process information more slowly. A grandfather playing a video game with his 14-year-old grandson will lose every time. However, on tests that involve real-life experience and acquired knowledge, he has the edge. (See Self-Survey: "What Is Your Aging IQ?")

How Men and Women Age

People of both genders go through numerous physiological changes at midlife. Men experience a decrease in the level of the male sex hormone testosterone, leading to a slowing of the sexual response. Changes in the prostate gland also cause increased urinary urgency, particularly at night (the condition may be alleviated with foods rich in zinc, such as whole grains and milk); the risk of developing prostate cancer grows. (For more information on prostate problems and male midlife changes, see Chapter 9.)

For women, the changes at midlife, especially physical ones, can be even more profound. The period from the mid-forties through the mid-sixties is called the *climacteric;* its most obvious change is the onset of *menopause,* the end of ovulation and menstruation. (See Chapter 9.)

An estimated 10 to 15% of women sail through menopause without any significant complaints. At the other end of the spectrum, a similar percentage develop symptoms that make it difficult, if not impossible, for them to function as usual. The majority of women—70 to 80%—are somewhere in between. Most can take advantage of new insight into the processes involved

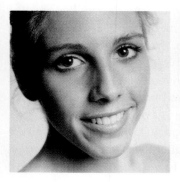
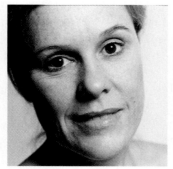
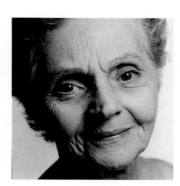

Figure 18-2

The appearance of age. The stages of life are reflected in our faces.

Figure 18-3

The effects of aging on the body.

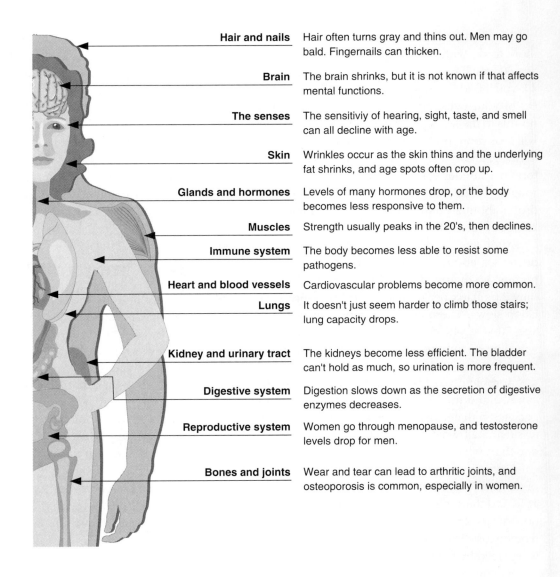

Hair and nails   Hair often turns gray and thins out. Men may go bald. Fingernails can thicken.

Brain   The brain shrinks, but it is not known if that affects mental functions.

The senses   The sensitiviy of hearing, sight, taste, and smell can all decline with age.

Skin   Wrinkles occur as the skin thins and the underlying fat shrinks, and age spots often crop up.

Glands and hormones   Levels of many hormones drop, or the body becomes less responsive to them.

Muscles   Strength usually peaks in the 20's, then declines.

Immune system   The body becomes less able to resist some pathogens.

Heart and blood vessels   Cardiovascular problems become more common.

Lungs   It doesn't just seem harder to climb those stairs; lung capacity drops.

Kidney and urinary tract   The kidneys become less efficient. The bladder can't hold as much, so urination is more frequent.

Digestive system   Digestion slows down as the secretion of digestive enzymes decreases.

Reproductive system   Women go through menopause, and testosterone levels drop for men.

Bones and joints   Wear and tear can lead to arthritic joints, and osteoporosis is common, especially in women.

in menopause and new approaches to relieving its symptoms.

"Thirty years ago menopause research involved about a half dozen experts around the world," says gynecologist Wulf Utian, M.D., founder of the North American Menopause Society (NAMS). "I would go to meetings, and no one was talking about it. I felt I was a lone voice in the wilderness."[11] Now annual NAMS meetings draw thousands of attendees from around the world for a newsmaking array of renowned speakers, heated debates, and hot research findings. New information has fostered new understanding—and new attitudes. In a recent NAMS poll, more than half of women between 45 and 60 viewed menopause as a positive phase in their lives. Of those who'd completed menopause, eight in ten expressed relief to be done with menstruation; six in ten did not associate

menopause with a lessened willingness to try new things or with becoming less attractive.

The most serious health hazard associated with menopause is an increased risk of heart disease (see Chapter 12). Throughout a woman's reproductive years, estrogen keeps her arteries supple, prevents blood clots, boosts levels of beneficial high density lipoproteins (HDL), and decreases harmful low density lipoproteins (LDL). As estrogen falls at menopause, a woman's heart becomes as vulnerable as a man's. Her HDL slumps; her LDL increases; her risk of blood clots grows; atherosclerotic plaque builds up in her arteries. After age 45, one in nine women has a least one symptom of heart disease. By 65, this figure rises to one in three.

Also at risk are a woman's bones. Although the process of bone loss begins in a woman's thirties, it speeds up to as much at 2 to 5% annually in the first five

Self-Survey

What Is Your Aging IQ?

Mark each of the following statements True or False.

	True	False
1. Everyone becomes senile sooner or later, if he or she lives long enough.	___	___
2. American families have by and large abandoned their older members.	___	___
3. Depression is a serious problem for older people.	___	___
4. The numbers of older people are growing.	___	___
5. The vast majority of older people are self-sufficient.	___	___
6. Mental confusion is an inevitable, incurable consequence of old age.	___	___
7. Intelligence declines with age.	___	___
8. "Sex" urges and activity normally cease between ages 55 and 60.	___	___
9. If a person has been smoking for thirty or forty years, it does no good to quit.	___	___
10. Older people should stop exercising and should rest.	___	___
11. As you grow older, you need more vitamins and minerals to stay healthy.	___	___
12. Only children need to be concerned about calcium for strong bones and teeth.	___	___
13. Extremes of heat and cold can be particularly dangerous to older people.	___	___
14. Many older people are hurt in accidents that could have been prevented.	___	___
15. More men than women survive to old age.	___	___
16. Deaths from stroke and heart disease are declining.	___	___
17. Older people on the average take more medications than younger people.	___	___
18. Snake-oil salesmen are as common today as they were on the frontier.	___	___
19. Personality changes with age, as do hair color and skin texture.	___	___
20. Sight declines with age.	___	___

Answers

1. False. Even among those who live to be 80 years of age or older, the majority do not develop Alzheimer's disease or forms of brain disease. Senility is a medically meaningless term.

2. False. The American family is still the number-one caretaker of older Americans. Most older people live close to their children and see them often; many live with their spouses. Eight out of ten men and six out of ten women live in family settings.

3. True. Depression, loss of self-esteem, loneliness, and anxiety can become more common as older people face retirement, the deaths of relatives and friends, and other such crises—often at the same time. Fortunately, depression is treatable.

4. True. By the year 2030, one out of every five people will be over 65 years of age.

5. True. Only 5% of the older population live in nursing homes; the rest are basically healthy and self-sufficient.

6. False. Mental confusion and serious forgetfulness in old age can be caused by Alzheimer's disease or other conditions that cause incurable damage to the brain, but a hundred other problems can cause the same symptoms. A minor head injury, a high fever, poor nutrition, adverse drug reactions, and depression can all be treated, and the confusion will go away.

7. False. Intelligence per se doesn't decline without reason. Most people maintain or improve their intellect as they grow older.

8. False. Most older people can lead an active, satisfying sex life.

9. False. Stopping smoking at any age reduces the risk of cancer and heart disease, and leads to healthier lungs.

10. False. Many older people enjoy, and benefit from, exercises such as walking, swimming, and bicycle riding. Exercise at any age can help strengthen the heart and lungs, and lower blood pressure.

11. False. Although certain requirements, such as that for "sunshine" vitamin D, may increase slightly with age, older people need the same amounts of most vitamins and minerals as do younger people. Older people, in particular, should eat nutritious foods and cut down on sweets, salty snack foods, high-calorie drinks, and alcohol.

12. False. Older people require fewer calories, but adequate intake of calcium for strong bones can become more important as you grow older. This is particularly

true for women, whose risk of osteoporosis increases after menopause. Milk and cheese are rich in calcium, as are cooked dried beans, collards, and broccoli. Some people need calcium supplements as well.

13. True. The body's thermostat tends to function less efficiently with age, and the older person's body may be less able to adapt to heat or cold.

14. True. Falls are the most common cause of injuries among the elderly. Good safety practices, including proper lighting and nonskid carpets, can help prevent serious accidents.

15. False. Women tend to outlive men by an average of eight years. There are 150 women for every 100 men over age 65, and nearly 250 women for every 100 men over age 85.

16. True. Fewer men and women are dying of stroke or heart disease. This has been a major factor in the increase in life expectancy.

17. True. The elderly consume 25% of all medications and, as a result, have many more problems with adverse drug reactions.

18. True. Medical quackery is a $10 billion business in the United, States. People of all ages are commonly duped into quick cures for aging, arthritis, and cancer.

19. False. Personality doesn't change with age. Therefore, all old people can't be described as rigid and cantankerous. You are what you are for as long as you live. But you can change what you do to help yourself enjoy good health.

20. False. Although changes in vision become more common with age, any dramatic change in vision, regardless of age, may be related to a specific disease.

Making Changes ....
Staying Younger Longer

As the above answers indicate, many common beliefs about aging simply aren't true. In fact, you have a great deal of control over how you age; and by changing your health habits, you may be able to buy yourself extra years of life and health. Here are some guidelines that can extend both your "health span"—your active, healthy years —and your lifespan:

- Don't smoke. If you smoke two or more packs of cigarettes a day, you are essentially trading a minute of life for a minute of smoking. You can expect to lose 8.3 years of life you might have lived as a nonsmoker.

- If you drink, don't overdo it. Drinking excessive amounts of alcohol can lead to cirrhosis of the liver, car accidents, pneumonia, high blood pressure, diabetes, and many other life-threatening conditions.

- Eat a lowfat, balanced diet. Some believe a bad diet can decrease the average lifespan six to ten years. Certainly, diet may have a lot to do with your risk of heart disease, colon or breast cancer, and other disorders.

- Watch your weight. Whether or not you're overweight can make a difference in your predisposition to heart attacks, strokes, kidney disease, diabetes, and other disorders.

- Exercise regularly. Exercise may add six to nine years to your life. The fitter you are, the longer you can expect to live.

- Learn to manage stress effectively. Establish a good balance of work and play in your life. Try to keep stress within reasonable limits. Excessive stress can make intense demands on the body and may make some people prone to heart attacks. Learning to manage and control stress effectively can lessen the toll it takes on well-being.

SOURCE: U.S. Department of Health and Human Services. Bethesda, MD: Government Printing Office, 1986.

years after menopause. Women with small bones, smokers, and those with a family history of bone problems are at increased risk of fractures and the bone-thinning disease known as osteoporosis, which strikes more than a third of older women (discussed later in this chapter).

"One in five women continues to make enough estrogen that she doesn't need replacement estrogen," says Marianne Legato, M.D., the director of the Partnership for Women's Health at Columbia University.[12] The other four have to weigh the potential benefits with the possible risks.[13]

Hormone replacement therapy (HRT) is synthetic estrogen, often combined with progesterone, and given in the form of a pill or a patch to postmenopausal women. It often relieves symptoms of menopause and provides health benefits. The most compelling reason to take replacement hormones is to protect the heart. "Regardless of when a postmenopausal woman starts HRT or for how long she takes it, there is an association with lower incidence of coronary artery disease," says Dr. Legato. "If a woman has coronary artery disease, HRT may extend her lifespan by two-and-a-half years. If she doesn't have heart disease, estrogen won't prolong her life, but it will lower her risk of developing cardiovascular problems."

HRT also protects a woman's bones. However, the benefits last only as long as the woman takes estrogen, and doctors are still debating whether it's best to start HRT immediately after menopause of later in life. Women who start HRT within five years of menopause decreased their risk of hip, wrist, and nonspinal fractures when compared with women who have never used estrogen. Yet once they stop HRT, bone loss proceeds at the same rate as in early menopause. Some argue that older women in the sixties and seventies, whose low bone density puts them at greater immediate risk of fractures, might benefit most from HRT.[14] But hormone replacement is no longer a woman's only option for strengthening bones. New treatments, such as the drugs known as biphophonates, may prove to be good alternatives.[15]

In addition to these long-term benefits, replacement estrogen relieves hot flashes, improves sleep, alleviates sexual symptoms, makes intercourse more comfortable, and lessens urinary tract problems. Women on HRT report that they think better, remember more, and feel more energetic. They're less prone to many age-related problems, such as tooth loss and driving accidents (possibly a consequence of improved concentration). They also live longer. Compared with women who never used replacement hormones, women who take HRT are less likely to die of what researchers call "all-cause mortality" (that is, for any and every reason). In one analysis of 40,000 postmenopausal women followed for 16 years, the risk of death in those taking estrogen was 37% lower than those who had never taken HRT. The risk of fatal heart disease was 53% lower.[16]

Hormone replacement also entails side effects and risks: Some women who try HRT gain weight, become depressed (particularly if they had a similar reaction to birth control pills), develop gall stones, and experience a worsening of migraines, fibroids, or endometriosis. These problems may explain why, at least in the past, as many as half of women who began HRT stopped within two years. Many women find that the progestin component of combination hormone treatment is most problematic; switching to a natural progesterone or a different dosing schedule sometimes helps.

However, the number-one reason why women are wary of HRT is the risk of breast cancer. According to one survey, 25% of women who refuse hormones and 20% of women who stop their use do so because of concern about breast cancer. Is this fear justified? The answer isn't clear.

Although there have been contradictory findings, breast cancer rates do generally increase among women who take replacement hormones for prolonged periods. (In various studies, these have extended for five, seven, or ten or more years.)[17] Based on this evidence, physicians may advise against HRT for women who've had breast cancer or who are at high risk for this disease. But for other women, the potential benefits of HRT may outweigh the dangers. Even among those at high risk of breast cancer, the presence of even one risk factor for heart disease tips the balance in favor of HRT.[18] "Women are ten times more likely to die of heart disease than breast cancer," notes Legato. "For many, the risks of not taking HRT are far greater than its use."

In the future, women's choice may be easier, thanks to the development of selective estrogen receptor modulators (SERMS), like raloxifene, that are tailor-made to act only on certain targets, such as the heart and bones, rather than the breast or uterine lining.[19] However, it is not yet known if these agents will relieve hot flashes and lower the risk of Alzheimer's. And it will be years, perhaps decades, before we have data on their long-term safety and efficacy.[20]

There are other drugs as well as lifestyle alternatives for women who cannot or do not want to rely on HRT. Clonidine, a drug that reduces blood pressure and heart rate, may relieve hot flashes; testosterone creams, used in the vagina, can help with dryness and irritation. Some women report relief from hot flashes, fatigue, depression, and other menopausal symptoms with vitamin E or B-6 or ginseng (which has some estrogen in it), although there are no scientific studies supporting this effect. Moreover, many postmenopausal women relieve their symptoms and lower their risk of future health problems by making lifestyle changes. Exercise can lower the risk of heart disease and strengthen bones; calcium-rich foods and supplements can also help keep bones strong.

Making the Most of Middle Age

People used to think of middle age as the beginning of the end, but these days it's merely the end of the beginning. Men and women of age 40 or 50 certainly aren't the boys and girls they used to be, but they've often not yet become the individuals they might be. Millions of

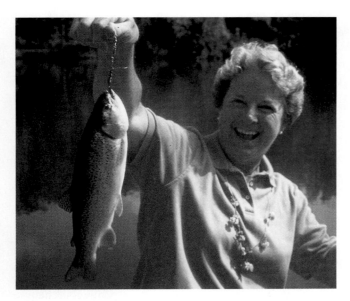

We can view midlife as "the end of the beginning," when we've mastered the major tasks of life. The way is clear to realize the potential of adulthood.

men and women consistently say, "Older is better." As writer Gail Sheehy, author of the best-seller *New Passages*, contends, middle age is beginning later and serving as a transition into a "second adulthood" for more and more Americans.[21]

Midlife can be the most fruitful time of life, if marriage and career bring fulfillment, and health and vigor remain strong. The reordering of priorities that most people do in their forties and fifties often paves the way to richer, more satisfying relationships, a deeper emotional life, and greater compassion, concern for others, and altruism.

By middle age, most men and women have learned a great deal about what they can and cannot do. According to many reports, women's happiness rises dramatically through middle age, reaching a preliminary peak at around age 57, when it then soars still higher. Men, too, discover greater life satisfactions as they age. New potentials and special strengths frequently emerge between ages 45 and 60, including the following:

- A relaxation of gender roles; greater assertiveness in women and greater expressiveness in men.
- The freedom to pick up and go, again.
- More time and money for yourself.
- Greater opportunities for companionship with your mate.
- Opportunities to meet your children again as friends.
- Opportunities to contribute to your community, history, and culture.

Strategies for Change

Starting in the Middle

If you're a nontraditional student who's returned to school in your thirties or later, or if you're interested in looking ahead to future decisions, consider the following suggestions for midlife corrections of your life course:

✔ *Take time to sort out what you want.* Society tends to make us shuffle along in lockstep, and many people never get breathing space to figure out who they are. Your life will be richer if you search out your identity before moving on to your own second act.

✔ *Pursue the interests that give you pleasure.* Freed from the pressure to prove themselves, at midlife many people return to skills and hobbies they thought they had no time for in their twenties and thirties.

✔ *Reach out to others.* Again and again, people find new meaning in life by focusing not on their own needs but on those of others with greater problems. Get involved with political and social causes, as well as with conventional charitable work.

✔ *Follow your instincts.* Many people use their heads to plot out "Act I" of their lives, carefully charting their way up the ladder of success. However, if they're knocked off the ladder or if they don't like what they find at the top, their hearts often lead them to better choices.

✔ *Focus on the future.* Life inevitably brings setbacks, losses, and disappointments. Try to realize that the loss of the familiar always opens up possibilities for something new and maybe even more rewarding.

Good News About Getting Older

The key to staying vital and healthy in old age is maintaining healthful behaviors throughout life. As many as half of the losses linked to age may be the result not of time's passage but of disuse. "If you don't use it, you lose it," says Dr. James Fries, a Stanford University professor who's done extensive research on aging.

Heredity's Role

Genes aren't destiny, but they have a continuing impact throughout the lifespan. Yet even individuals with genes that contribute to fast aging can modify their impact.

Pulsepoints

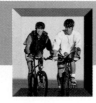

Ten Ways to Live Longer

1. Exercise regularly. By improving blood flow, staving off depression, warding off heart disease, and enhancing well-being, regular workouts help keep mind and body in top form.

2. Don't smoke. Every cigarette you puff can snuff out seven minutes of your life, according to the Centers for Disease Control and Prevention.

3. Watch your weight and blood pressure. Increases in these vital statistics can increase your risk of hypertension, cardiovascular disease, and other health problems.

4. Eat more fruits and vegetables. These foods, rich in vitamins and protective antioxidants, can reduce your risk of cancer and damage from destructive free radicals. (See Chapter 6.)

5. Cut down on fat. Fatty foods can clog the arteries (Chapter 12) and contribute to various cancers. (See Chapter 13.)

6. Limit drinking. Alcohol can undermine physical health and sabotage mental acuity. (See Chapter 15.)

7. Cultivate stimulating interests. Elderly individuals with complex and interesting lifestyles are most likely to retain sharp minds and memories beyond age 70.

8. Don't worry; be happy. At any age, emotional turmoil can undermine well-being. Relaxation techniques, such as meditation, help by reducing stress.

9. Reach out. Try to keep in contact with other people of all ages and experiences. Make the effort to invite them to your home or go out with them. On a regular basis, do something to help another person.

10. Make the most of your time. Greet each day with a specific goal—to take a walk, write letters, visit a friend.

What you do to stop the genes that speed up aging is less important than what you do to cooperate with the genes that slow it down. (See Pulsepoints: "Ten Ways to Live Longer.")

Exercise: An Antiaging Pill

Staying in bed for three weeks has the same effect on fitness as aging 30 years. At any age, the unexercised body—though free of the symptoms of illness—will rust out long before it could ever wear out. Inactivity can make anyone old before his or her time. Just as inactivity accelerates aging, activity slows it down. The effects of ongoing activity are so profound that gerontologists sometimes refer to exercise as "the closest thing to an antiaging pill." Exercise can reverse many of the changes that occur with age, including increases in body fat and decreases in muscle strength. The bottom line: What you *don't* do may matter more than what you do do.

Exercise—resistance, balance, and so on—also reduces the number of falls in the elderly. Each year about 30% of men and women over age 65 sustain a fall; about half have multiple falls. About 10% to 15% of falls result in serious injuries, ranging from hip fractures to other fractures to soft-tissue injuries. Unintentional injury is the sixth leading cause of death in persons over 65; most such injury involves falls.[22]

The Aging Brain

Ten years ago, scientists thought that the aging brain, once worn out, could never be fixed. They've since learned that the brain can and does repair itself. When **neurons** (brain cells) die, the surrounding cells develop "fingers" to fill the gaps and establish new connections, or synapses, between surviving neurons. Although self-repair occurs more quickly in young brains, the process continues in older brains. Even victims of Alzheimer's disease, the most devastating form of senility, have enough healthy cells in the diseased brain to regrow synapses. Scientists hope to develop drugs that someday may help the brain repair itself. (See the section on Alzheimer's disease later in this chapter.)

Mental ability does not decline along with physical vigor. Researchers have been able to reverse the supposedly normal intellectual declines of 60- to 80-year-olds by tutoring them in problem solving. Reaction time, intellectual speed and efficiency, nonverbal intelligence, and maximum work rate for short periods may diminish

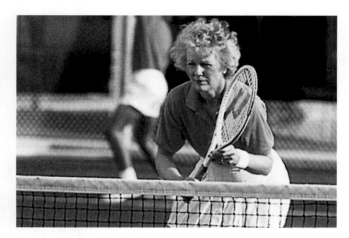

Older athletes know that the passage of time doesn't necessarily mean a loss of abilities and skills.

by age 75. However, understanding, vocabulary, ability to remember key information, and verbal intelligence remain about the same.

There are gender differences in the aging of the brain. From ages 18 to 45, neurons in a male brain die three times faster than in the female. By middle age, a man's frontal lobes and hippocampus shrink so much that they reach approximately the same size as a woman's. "If you look at men from young adulthood to middle age, you see a steady decline in abilities, particularly attention," says neuropsychologist Ruben Gur, Ph.D., of the University of Pennsylvania. "You don't even see a trend in women the same age toward any deterioration of abilities or brain volume." The consequences of this shrinkage include poorer verbal memory, diminished ability to pay attention, and increased irritability.[23]

Why do men's brain age so rapidly? The reason may have to do with fuel efficiency. The female brain is able to reduce its metabolic rate—its utilization of brain glucose—as it loses tissue with aging, whereas the brains of older men continue to metabolize glucose at the same rate as when they were younger. Women, in other words, gear down to a more fuel-efficient cruising speed, while male brains keep revving the engine—possibly because of testosterone's influence. Brain regions with abundant androgen receptors during fetal development seem especially susceptible to the effects of aging later in life.

"Women seem to be able to reduce the rate of neuronal activity in proportion to the tissue that they lose, whereas men continue to overdrive their neurons," says Gur. "Even though women too lose tissue as they age,

they seem to be riding hard on what's left." This difference, he speculates, may be part of the reason that females generally outlive males—in our species as well as many others.

Estrogen, the hormone that protects a woman's heart and bones, also seems to strengthen her mind and memory by building and maintaining the densest possible network of the microscopic dendrites connecting nerve cells to one another. But with estrogen's decline at menopause, a woman's brain becomes increasingly vulnerable to aging's toll. As some neuroscientists describe it, the female brain, like an overzealous gardener, may thin out synaptic interconnections, perhaps leaving cells more vulnerable to deterioration and death.

The decline of estrogen may also reduce production of acetylcholine, which allows messages to leap from one neuron to the next. These changes may explain why women's brains, though more durable in midlife, eventually become three times more prone to Alzheimer's disease. Despite the recognition of estrogen's potential benefits, experts believe that the research studies that have been done are too small and methodologically flawed to serve as a basis for estrogen replacement's use to prevent or treat mental deterioration in women.[24]

Memory

Although some memory skills, particularly the ability to retrieve names and process information quickly, inevitably diminish over time, there are highly effective ways of compensating for such age-related losses. "The aging brain is like the aging body: It's not the same as it used to be," says psychologist Denise Park, Ph.D., of the University of Georgia in Augusta. "Your muscle mass and cardiovascular stamina decline with age, but if you stay fit, you can function at a very high level. The same is true for memory. With a little effort, you can remember what you want and need to know."[25]

What normal changes should you expect? Here is a preview:

- *Recalling information takes longer.* As individuals reach their mid- to late sixties, the brain slows down. "This may just be a matter of milliseconds, but when you're processing thousands of bits of information— as you must when driving on a busy, unfamiliar freeway and trying to remember the turn-off—it can add up to a significant delay," says Park. "Whenever you put young and old individuals in equally novel environments, the younger ones will adapt faster." But as long as they're not rushed, older adults eventually adapt and perform just as well.

- *Distractions become more disruptive.* Teenagers can study and listen to the stereo at the same time. Thirty-something moms can soothe the baby, field her baby's big brother's questions on homework, and put together a dinner all at once. But as individuals pass age 50, they find it much more difficult to divide their attention or to remember details of a story after having switched their attention to something else. "Concentration becomes crucial," says social worker Lynn Stern, who advises turning off the TV and giving 100 percent of your attention to whatever you want to recall.[26]

- *"Accessing" names gets harder.* "The ability to remember names—especially those that you don't use frequently—diminishes by as much as 50% between ages 25 and 65," says psychologist Thomas Crook, Ph.D., who advises preventive strategies, such as repeating a person's name when introduced, writing down the name as soon as possible and making obvious associations (the Golden Gate for a man named Bridges).[27]

- *Learning new information is harder.* "It's not the quality of memory that changes, just the speed at which we receive, absorb and react to information," says Crook. That's why strategies like taking notes or outlining material—techniques you may never have needed before—become critical for older "students," especially when learning brand-new skills. However, adding to existing knowledge remains as easy as ever.

- *Wisdom matters.* In any memory test involving knowledge of the world, vocabulary or judgment, older people outperform younger ones.

While such changes are common, some minds hold up better than others. In longitudinal studies that have followed thousands of men and women in Baltimore and Seattle from middle age into their nineties, more than a quarter retained strong minds and memories past age 70. The factors that researchers have linked with long-lasting memory and mental ability include: above-average level of education, stimulating interests, and marriage to a smart spouse.[28]

At any age, occasional forgetfulness, memory lapses, and misplacing everyday objects are common. What's *not* normal are any of the following:

- Frequent difficulty completing a sentence because of forgetting what you want to say or the words with which to say it.

- Misplacing important items, such as money or bank records.

- Frequent confusion.

- Forgetting how to use common items or perform simple tasks.

- Getting lost or disoriented in familiar places, especially at home.

- Difficulty identifying the month or season.

- Dizzy spells or severe headaches accompanying memory loss.

A number of illnesses, including depression, kidney disease, alcoholism, and Alzheimer's disease, can cause these symptoms. Only thorough medical and neurological examinations can pinpoint the specific problem.

Strategies for Prevention

How to Stay Sharp

✔ *Watch your blood pressure.* Over time hypertension can take a significant toll on recall. In studies that followed elderly men and women for 15 years, psychololgists at the University of Maine found that the longer individuals lived with elevated blood pressure, the more their memory suffered. The reason, they theorize, may be that high blood pressure interferes with the brain's oxygen supply or blood flow.[29]

✔ *Be flexible.* Men and women who settle into wellworn ruts in middle age, researchers have found, are more likely to end up with less supple minds and memories.

✔ *Organize.* Try to set up simple routines, such as always putting certain things in certain places, so you can spare yourself the effort of tracking them down.

✔ *Write it down.* In a survey of memory experts, their top technique for not forgetting was the simplest: making notes. Especially when you're trying to take in complex information—directions to an unfamiliar address, for instance—writing forces you to focus attention and provides a backup in case your memory fails.

Mental Health

Optimal aging demands a redefinition of who a person is and what makes his or her life worthwhile. Some sources of satisfaction, such as physical challenges or professional achievements, diminish later in life. Yet older people in general feel psychologically better than young people, with fewer worries about themselves and how they look to other people, higher self-esteem, and less loneliness.[30]

The secret of emotional well-being in old age does-n't seem to be professional success or a happy marriage but the ability to cope with life's setbacks without blame or bitterness. In general, psychiatric disorders do not occur more frequently in the elderly. Even depression—which is not uncommon among the elderly—strikes less often in old age than at earlier stages of the life cycle. Those most likely to become depressed often have lost a spouse and have few social supports. The social ties of the elderly are most likely to fray as they retire, move, or lose spouses and close friends.[31]

Intimacy and Sexual Activity

Sexual activity typically decreases in the elderly, but it doesn't end. According to a 1995 national survey by Mark Clements Research, Inc., about 55% of those between ages 65 and 69 remain sexually active. This percentage declines with age—to 48% of those between 70 and 74, 28% of those 75 to 79, 21% of those 80 to 84, and 13% of those over age 85.[32]

Aging does cause some changes in sexual response: Women produce less vaginal lubrication, and it takes longer for an older man to achieve an erection or orgasm and longer to attain another erection after ejacu-lating. Both men and women experience fewer contrac-tions during orgasm. However, none of these changes reduces sexual pleasure or desire.

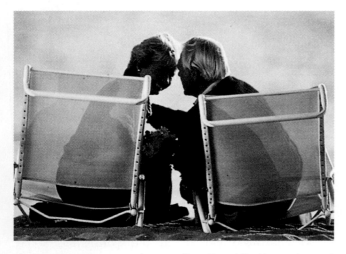

Many senior citizens remain sexually active. Affection and sexual intimacy may increase as the pressures of child-raising and careers ease.

Problems of the Elderly

Sadly, life's final decades aren't always golden. Senior citizens may face physical, economic, social, and psychological challenges during what one therapist describes as "the season of loss." They may have to give up many things: gratifying work, cherished friendships, financial and physical independence. Millions are economically vulnerable: A serious illness, the loss of their home in a fire or flood, or other unexpected catastrophes could easily plunge them into poverty. A lack of money limits the options of the elderly and can impair their health. They may not be able to afford nutritious food, regular health checkups, new eyeglasses or hearing aids, or the small pleasures that make life enjoyable. The cumulative impact of such challenges, one often following the other before individuals have a chance to adjust or cope, can take a toll on physical and emotional well-being.

Health Problems

With the passage of time, many people develop serious diseases such as arthritis, atherosclerosis, and cancer. In the past, elderly men and women often were not treated as aggressively for some conditions, such as cancer, as younger patients. But research has shown that older patients can respond well to aggressive therapeutic approaches and benefit just as much as younger individuals.[33]

Nutritional Needs

Among the elderly, nutritional deficiencies are a serious problem; being underweight can be as great a health risk as being overweight. About 16% of Americans over age 65 consume fewer than 1000 calories a day—too little to provide an adequate supply of vitamins and minerals. Common causes of malnutrition in old age include medications, emotional depression, loss of teeth, swallowing and absorption disorders, lack of money, and difficulties shopping and preparing food. Many nutritionists recommend multivitamin and mineral supplements for the elderly, although they caution against overdosing or taking any single vitamin or mineral without medical supervision.

Osteoporosis

One common problem, especially among elderly women, is **osteoporosis**, a condition in which losses in bone density become so severe that a bone will break after even slight trauma or injury (see Figure 18-4). Among those who live to age 90, 32% of women and 19% of men will suffer a hip fracture as a result of osteoporosis.[34] Women, who have smaller skeletons, are more vulnerable than men; in extreme cases, their spines may become so fragile that just bending causes severe pain. "Osteoporosis is a terrible crippler and killer," says endocrinologist Joseph Goldzieher, M.D., professor emeritus at Baylor College of Medicine. "The life expectancy for a woman over 70 who breaks her hip is only six months."[35]

Osteoporosis doesn't begin in old age. In fact, the best time for preventive action is early in life. Increased calcium intake, particularly during childhood and the growth spurt of adolescence, can produce a heavier, denser skeleton and reduce the risk of the complications of bone loss later in life. College-age women also can strengthen their bones and reduce their risk of osteoporosis by increasing their calcium intake and physical activity. Adequate dietary calcium in adulthood can help maintain bone density for years.

Various factors can increase a woman's risk of developing osteoporosis, including family history (a mother, grandmother, or sister with osteoporosis, fractures, height loss, or humped shoulders); petite body structure; white or Asian background; menopause before age 40; smoking; heavy alcohol consumption; loss of ovarian function through chemotherapy, radiation, or hysterectomy; low calcium intake; and a sedentary lifestyle.

Among the tests that can detect low bone density are:

- DXA (or DEXA) Dual Energy X-ray Absorptiometry, the most accurate and advanced technique now available. DXA uses a double beam from an X-ray source, and spine, hip, and total body examinations take less than 20 minutes to perform. Peripheral DXA (PDXA) assesses hand or heel bones.

- DPA Dual Photon Absorptiometry, an older test now in limited use, employs a double beam from a radioactive energy source. Spine, hip, and total body examinations take approximately 40 minutes.

- SXA Single Energy X-ray Absorptiometry relies on a very low dose X-ray source to measure the bones of the wrist or heel. SPA Single Photon Absorptiometry is an earlier generation of SXA utilizing a single beam from an energy source that passes through water. The process takes less than 15 minutes.

- QCT Quantitative Computed Tomography uses a conventional CT (computed tomography) software. Effective in measurement of the spine, this method emits a comparatively higher dose of radiation than DXA and is usually more costly than other methods.

- RA Radiographic Absorptiometry, also called photodensitometry, relies on X-rays of the hand and small metal wedge to calculate bone density.[36]

As an alternative to HRT, new treatments, such as the medication alendronate, have proven effective in increasing bone mass and reducing fractures, deformities, and height loss in postmenopausal women with osteoporosis.[37, 38]

Personal Health
18.3
INTERACTIVE

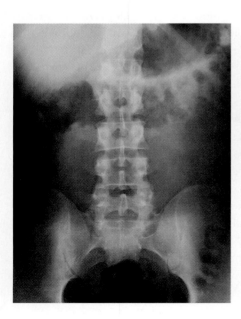 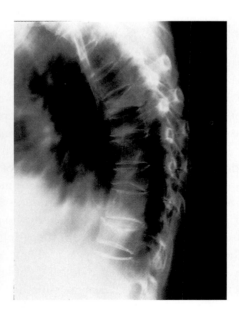

Figure 18-4

Comparison of a normal backbone (left) to one with osteoporosis (right).

Strategies for Prevention

Lowering Your Risk of Osteoporosis

Regardless of your age and gender, you can prevent future bone problems by taking some protective steps now. The most important guidelines are as follows:

✔ Make sure you get adequate calcium. Most researchers recommend 500–800 mg a day. Two excellent sources of calcium are nonfat milk (275 mg in an 8-ounce glass) and sardines (370 mg in 3 ounces with bones). (See Chapter 5 for further discussion of calcium.)

✔ Exercise regularly. Both aerobic exercise and weight training can help preserve bone density.[39]

✔ Watch your caffeine intake, and put some nonfat milk in your coffee. Extra caffeine increases the amount of calcium lost in urine by 65%; milk helps compensate for the loss.

✔ Drink alcohol only moderately. More than two or three alcoholic beverages a day impairs intestinal calcium absorption.

✔ Don't smoke. Smokers tend to be thin (a risk factor for osteoporosis) and enter menopause earlier, thus extending the period of jeopardy from estrogen loss.

✔ Let the sunshine in (but don't forget your sunscreen). Vitamin D, a vitamin produced in the skin in reaction with sunlight, boosts calcium absorption.

Substance Misuse and Abuse

Misuse and abuse of prescription and over-the-counter medications occur frequently among the elderly. In part this is because people over age 65 consume one-quarter of all drugs prescribed in the United States. Moreover, many older people have multiple health problems, requiring several medications at the same time. The drugs may interact and cause a confusing array of symptoms and reactions.

The most commonly misused drugs are sleeping pills, tranquilizers, pain medications, and laxatives. Sometimes a person innocently uses more than the prescribed dose or takes several prescriptions simultaneously. Other older people are aware of their overreliance on drugs, but don't like how they feel when they don't take the pills.

Problems remembering, concentrating, and thinking are the most common psychiatric side effects of drugs in the elderly. As people age, their bodies take longer to metabolize drugs, so medications like sleeping pills build up in the body. Almost any amount of alcohol can make mental confusion and memory problems worse. Whenever older people become confused, forgetful, or paranoid, family members should find out which medications they've been taking.

Alcohol abuse can be particularly harmful for older men and women because it increases the likelihood of malnutrition, liver disease, heart damage, digestive problems, cognitive impairment, and dementia. Depending on the severity of the problem, older individuals may require close supervision in a hospital during withdrawal.

Psychological Problems

As men and women end their careers, and as friends and loved ones become ill or die, loneliness can become a chronic problem. Women, who generally outlive their husbands, are most likely to find themselves living alone. Whereas seven out of ten men age 75 or older are still married and living with their spouses, seven out of ten women in that age group are widowed. "We have our children and grandchildren and friends," says one woman in her eighties who lives in an apartment complex for elderly widows. "But we do miss our men."

Depression

According to a report by the National Institutes of Health Consensus Development Panel on Depression in Later Life, about 15% of men and women over 65 living in the community experience depression. In nursing homes, the rate is higher: 15% to 25%. Moreover, recurrences are common, with 40% of older persons suffering repeat bouts with depression.[40]

Late-life depression can be particularly hard to spot because older men and women often do not display the typical symptoms, or their symptoms are mistaken for normal signs of aging.[41] Elderly people with physical problems are most prone to depression. Some classic signs of depression—appetite changes, a gain or loss of 5% of body weight in a month, insomnia or excessive sleep, fidgeting or extremely slow movements or speech, fatigue, or loss of energy—may be attributed to medical problems, medications, or old age itself. Depression that develops following an illness or injury, if not identified and treated, can hinder recovery.

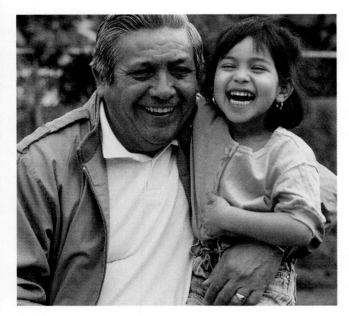

Family ties are extremely important to young and old alike.

The consequences of not recognizing and treating depression late in life can be tragic. Older Americans have the highest suicide rates in our society, with some 8500 elderly persons killing themselves every year. The suicide rate is five times higher for those aged 65 than for younger individuals. And depressed older men and women are also more likely to die of other causes. However, late-life depression can be overcome. With treatment, more than 70% of the depressed elderly improve dramatically. Since loneliness and loss are often important contributing factors, psychiatrists often combine counseling, such as brief psychotherapy, with medication. Because of various physiological differences in the elderly, they usually respond more slowly to antidepressants than younger persons, and the benefits thus may not be apparent for 6 to 12 weeks.[42]

Mental Deterioration

About 15% of older Americans lose previous mental capabilities, a brain disorder called **dementia**. Sixty percent of these—a total of 4 million men and women over age 65—suffer from the type of dementia called **Alzheimer's disease**, a progressive deterioration of brain cells and mental capacity.

Women are more likely to develop Alzheimer's than men. By age 85, as many as 28 to 30% of women suffer from Alzheimer's, and women with this form of dementia perform significantly worse than men in various

visual, spatial, and memory tests. Estrogen replacement—despite the risks and concerns discussed earlier—may help keep women's brains healthy as they age, particularly for those at high genetic risk for Alzheimer's. In various studies of postmenopausal women, those taking replacement hormones were up to 40% less likely to develop Alzheimer's. And women who do develop Alzheimer's show less mental deterioration if they are taking estrogen.[43]

Major advances have been made in unraveling the keys to Alzheimer's, a disease that can rob individuals of their memories, their intellects, their personalities, and eventually their lives. Scientists have traced this dementia to particular genetic defects, and these breakthroughs may help in identifying individuals at risk and pointing the way to new, more effective treatments.[44]

Often the illness progresses slowly, stealing bits of a person's mind and memory a little at a time. Its victims may withdraw into a world of their own, become quarrelsome or irritable, and say or do inappropriate things. The personalities of individuals with Alzheimer's often change. Some become more stubborn or impulsive; others may become increasingly apathetic, withdrawn, irritable, or suspicious, accusing others of thefts, betrayal, or plotting against them. As cognitive impairment worsens, inhibitions often loosen; they may masturbate or take off their clothes in public. Some become aggressive or violent. Eventually, individuals may forget the names of their close relatives, their own occupations, occasionally even their own names.[45]

The early signs of dementia—insomnia, irritability, increased sensitivity to alcohol and other drugs, and decreased energy and tolerance of frustration—are usually subtle and insidious. Diagnosis requires a comprehensive assessment of an individual's medical history, physical health, and mental status, often involving brain scans and a variety of other tests.[46] In 1997 the American Association for Geriatric Psychiatry, the Alzheimer's Association, and the American Geriatrics Society developed guidelines for the diagnosis and treatment of Alzheimer's.[47]

Even though no one can restore a brain that is in the process of being destroyed by an organic brain disease like Alzheimer's, medications can control difficult behavioral symptoms and enhance or partially restore cognitive ability. Often physicians find other medical or psychiatric problems, such as depression, in these patients; recognizing and treating these conditions can have a dramatic impact. Most people with Alzheimer's do best in consistent, familiar surroundings, with daily routines, prominently displayed clocks and calendars, nightlights, checklists, and diaries.

Many hospitals provide outpatient day therapy that seems to help Alzheimer's patients orient themselves. Staff members use large clocks and calendars to remind the patients of the time and day, provide photographs of themselves and the group to help the patients recall faces, label cupboards so items can more easily be found, and so on. Alzheimer's can take an enormous toll on the relatives of victims of the disease. Often they must watch helplessly as a loved one slowly becomes a stranger to them. Many hospitals and community mental health centers provide counseling and support groups for spouses and children of Alzheimer's patients.

Nursing Homes

Many older people need help from another person in performing some daily living activity, such as dressing, walking, bathing, or shopping. In the past, aging parents tended to live with their children's families. That's changed dramatically—not only because children live farther away, or may be separated or divorced, but also because the older parents seem to prefer their independence. Problems can develop, however, when declining health or increasing disability makes it more difficult for the elderly to manage on their own. Home-care services, day care, and foster homes help growing numbers of the elderly by filling the gap between living at home and entering a nursing home.

More than 1.5 million elderly Americans currently live in nursing homes, and their numbers are certain to grow in the coming decades. But such care is expensive and can be substandard, if not abusive. Families of elderly patients mistreated in nursing homes have successfully sued the homes, not for acts that led to death or disability, but for neglect, such as leaving residents in a smelly room or not bathing them, or verbal abuse.[48]

Making This Chapter Work for You
Getting Older and Better

■ Lifespans and life expectancy for Americans are growing. Although the process of aging—the characteristic pattern of normal life changes that occurs as humans, plants, and animals grow older—is

inevitable, individuals can do a great deal to influence the impact of the passage of time.

■ By the year 2020, one of five Americans will be older than age 65—a fact that will affect everyone in the country in many ways, including dealing with issues such as retirement benefits, health costs, and caring for aging parents.

■ Breakthroughs in longevity research have sparked hope that the human lifespan can be expanded, perhaps by means of antioxidants, replacement hormone therapy, and dietary restriction. However, scientists still disagree as to the limits of human life, and no single substance or program has been conclusively proven effective in stopping or turning back the clock.

■ Gerontologists do know that, whether or not we can add years to our lives, we can add life to our years. The key to optimal aging—living through old age with the best possible quality of life and the least possible premature disability—is having good health habits throughout life.

■ Many of the physical changes that accompany aging—such as the decline in heart and lung functioning, slowing of circulation and metabolism, loss of muscular strength, and slowing of reaction time—can be delayed by regular exercise and a nutritious diet.

■ Most intellectual abilities don't diminish with age, although some, such as the ability to remember names and newly learned information, do decline. Sexual interest need not fade with age, although sexual activity may decrease because of physical illness or a lack of partners.

■ The elderly face physical and psychological challenges, including a greater likelihood of illness and disability. Osteoporosis, a major health problem for elderly people, can be prevented by exercise and increased calcium intake. Depression, which is not uncommon in the elderly, responds well to treatment with drugs and psychotherapy.

■ One of the greatest fears about aging is that we will lose our memories and our minds. Diminished mental capacity can be the result of a brain tumor, abnormal thyroid activity, drug side effects, depression, or Alzheimer's disease, a progressive condition in which the mind slowly deteriorates. Although there are no

Health Online

Family Caregiver Alliance   http://www.caregiver.org/

This site provides information and support to those who care for older family members of friends. It includes information on finding in-home help, selecting an assisted living or residential care facility, respite resources, balancing work, family, and caregiving, medical information, online support, and much more.

Think about it ...

- Have you or your parents ever been called on to help care for an older person? What kinds of decisions were involved? What was the impact of caregiving on your family?

- What kinds of decisions could you or your parents make now that will make growing older easier on your family.

- If you are called on to help care for an older relative, what resources do you have to help you? Consider friends and family, and community, government, financial, and technological resources. What personal qualities do you have that you could bring to the situation?

cures for this form of dementia, treatments can sometimes relieve symptoms and enhance mental abilities.

■ Many older Americans lack the financial resources for basic necessities such as regular health care and a nutritious diet. Because of illness or disability, many older adults need assistance in performing the activities of daily living. The number of elderly men and women requiring long-term care is certain to increase dramatically in the coming decades.

Right now aging may seem like something that happens to your grandparents, parents, teachers, bosses, or neighbors. But stop and ask yourself: How are you changing with the years? What do you think you will be like in 20, 30, or 40 years? What can you do to ensure that you'll remain healthy and active as long as you possibly can? Just as you were a different person ten years ago, you will undoubtedly be a different person decades from now. And, to a remarkable degree, you can shape who that person will be.

 ## Key Terms

The terms listed here are used within the chapter. Page numbers are included for each term.
A definition of each term is given in the green Glossary pages at the end of this book.

ageism   *570*

aging   *569*

Alzheimer's disease   *585*

dementia   *585*

gerontologist   *572*

hormone   *571*

hormone replacement therapy
  (HRT)   *576*

neuron   *579*

osteoporosis   *582*

Review Questions

1. What kinds of physiological changes take place as you age?

2. What does it mean to be middle-aged? What are some of the physical changes and psychological issues associated with middle age?

3. How does exercise affect the aging process?

4. What are some of the health problems faced by the elderly? How can these problems be alleviated or prevented?

5. What percentage of the population over age 65 develops symptoms of mental deterioration? What is Alzheimer's disease? Why is this disease so devastating?

6. What is the best age at which to prevent osteoporosis? What are some things you can do now to help prevent osteoporosis?

Critical Thinking Questions

1. If you had to choose between an extremely long life and an extremely satisfying or happy one, which would you choose? What can you do now to ensure that you will live as long and as well as you'd like?

2. For years your parents fed, sheltered, clothed, and nurtured you. Someday they may need this care from you as much as you once needed it from them. Think ahead to the time when your parents will be 75, 85, or even older. What if they need constant care? What would be your responsibility? What options will you have? Can you do anything now to prepare for your parents' later years?

3. What are three fears you have about aging? What are three reasons for positive anticipation of aging?

Connections to Personal Health Interactive

To enhance your understanding of the material covered in this chapter, check out the following study aids on the **Personal Health Interactive CD-ROM**. *Each numbered icon within the chapter corresponds to an appropriate activity listed here.*

18.1 U.S. Population Patterns

18.2 Personal Insights: How Long Do You Think You Are Going to Live?

18.3 Parkinson's Disease

18.4 Chapter 18 Review

References

1. Marwick, Charles. "Longevity Requires Policy Revolution." *Journal of the American Medical Association,* Vol. 273, No. 17, May 3, 1995.

2. U.S. Bureau of the Census. *How We're Changing.* Washington, DC: U.S. Bureau of the Census, 1995. "New Census Report Details Graying of U.S." *HealthSpan,* Vol. 6, No.1, Summer 1995.

3. Steel, Knight. "Research on Aging: An Agenda for All Nations Individually and Collectively." *Journal of the American Medical Association,* Vol. 278, No. 16, October 22/29, 1997.

4. Stock, Robert. "Senior Class." *New York Times,* June 1, 1995.

5. Katzel, Leslie, et al. "Effects of Weight Loss vs. Aerobic Exercise Training on Risk Factors for Coronary Disease in Healthy Obese, Middle-Aged and Older Men." *Journal of the American Medical Association,* Vol. 274, No. 24, December 27, 1995. "Gerontology Researchers Sharpen Focus But Face More Complex Challenges as 21st Century Looms." *Journal of the American Medical Association,* Vol. 273, No.17, May 3, 1995.

6. "Can You Live Longer?" *Consumer Reports,* January 1992. Masoro, E. J., et al. "Retardation of the Aging Processes in Rats by Food Restriction." *Annals of the New York Academy of Sciences,* Vol. 621, 1992.

7. Brody, Jane. "Restoring Ebbing Hormones May Slow Aging." *New York Times,* July 18, 1995. Kaiser, Fran. "Aging and Malnutrition: Growth Hormone Therapy Shows Promise." *Geriatrics,* March 1992.

8 de lange, Titia. "Telomeres and Senescence: Ending the Debate." *Science,* Vol. 279, No. 5349, January 16, 1998.

9. Bodnar, Andrea, et all. "Extension of Life-span by Intro-

duction of Telomerase into Normal Human Cells." *Science*, Vol. 279, No. 5349, January 16, 1998.

10. "Can You Live Longer?" *American Health,* August 1994.

11. Utian, Wulf. Personal interview.

12. Legato, Marianne. Personal interview.

13. Nemecek, Sasha. "Hold the Hormones?" *Scientific American*, Vol. 277, No. 3, September, 1997.

14. "Who Benefits Most from HRT?" *Harvard Heart Letter*, Vol. 8, No. 3, November, 1997.

15. Delmas, Pierre, et al. "Effects of Raloxifene on Bone Mineral Density, Serum Cholesterol Concentrations, and uterine Endometrium in Postmenopausal Women." *New England Journal of Medicine*, Vol. 337, No. 23, December 4, 1997.

16. Stewart, Donna, and Gail Robinson. *A Clinician's Guide to Menopause*. Washington, DC: Health Press, 1997.

17. "Breast Cancer and Hormone Replacement Therapy: Collaborative Reanalysis of Data from 51 Epidemiological Studies of 52, 705 Women with Breast Cancer and 108,411 Women Without Breast Cancer." *Lancet*, Vol. 350, No. 9084, October 11, 1997.

18. LaCroix, Andrea, and Wylie Burke. "Breast Cancer and Hormone Replacement Therapy." *Lancet*, Vol. 350, No. 9084, October 11, 1997.

19. Hdajj, Fuleihan, and Ghada El. "Tissue-specific Estrogens—the Promise for the Future." *New England Journal of Medicine*, Vol. 337, No. 23, December 4, 1997. Rubin, Rita. "Fight Osteoporosis; Cut Side Effects—Can a New Drug Also Prevent Heart Disease?" *U.S. News & World Report*, Vol. 124, No. 6, February 16, 1998.

20. Mestel, Rosie. "A Safer Estrogen: Would You Take It?" *Health*, Vol. 11, No. 8. November–December 1997.

21. Sheehy, Gail. *New Passages*: New York: Random House, 1995.

22. Province, Michael, et al. "The Effects of Exercise on Falls in Elderly Patients." *Journal of the American Medical Association,* Vol. 273, No. 17, May 3, 1995. Hadley, Evan. "The Science of the Art of Geriatric Medicine." *Journal of the American Medical Association,* Vol. 273, No. 17, May 3, 1995.

23. Gur, Reubenl. Personal interview.

24. Yaffe, Kristine, et al. "Estrogen Therapy in Post-menopausal Women." *Journal of the American Medical Association*, Vol. 279, No. 9, March 4, 1998.

25. Park, Denise. Personal interview. Park, Denise. "Aging, Cognition, and Work." *Human Performance*, Vol. 7, No. 3, 1994.

26. Stern, Lynn. Personal interview.

27. Crook, Thomas. Personal interview. Larrabee, Glenn, and Thomas Crook. "Estimated Prevalence of Age-Associated Memory Impairment Derived from Standardized Tests of Memory Function." *International Psychogeriatrics*, Vol. 6, No. 1, Spring 1994.

28. Neimark, Jill. "It's Magical. It's Malleable. It's Memory." *Psychology Today*, January–February 1995.

29. Robbins, Michael, et al. "Unmedicated Blood Pressure Levels and Quality of Life in Elderly Hypertensive Women." *Psychosomatic Medicine*, Vol. 56, No. 3, May–June 1994.

30. Sheehy, *New Passages*.

31. Hales, Dianne, and Robert Hales. *Caring for the Mind*. New York: Bantam Books, 1995.

32. Mark Clements Research, Inc. "Sex over 65 Survey." August 1995.

33. American Cancer Society. Doll, R., et al. (eds.). *Trends in Cancer Incidence and Mortality*. Plainview, NY: Cold Spring Harbor Laboratory Press, 1994. Skolnick, Andrew. "Leader in War on Cancer Looks Ahead: Talking with Vincent T. DeVita, Jr., M.D." *Journal of the American Medical Association*, Vol. 273, No.7, February 15, 1995.

34. Krall, Elizabeth, et al. "Bone Mineral Density and Biochemical Markers of Bone Turnover in Healthy Elderly Men and Women." *Journal of Gerontology*, Vol. 52, No. 2, March 1997.

35. Goldzieher, Joseph. Personal interview.

36. Rizzoli, Rene, and Jean-Phillippe Bonjour. "Hormones and Bones." *Lancet*, Vol. 349, No. 9052, March 1, 1997.

37. Walling, Anne. "Effect of Alendronate in Postmenopausal Fractures." *American Family Physician*, Vol. 55, No. 4, March 1997.

38. Kessenich, Cathy. "Preventing and Managing Osteoporosis." *American Journal of Nursing*, Vol. 97, No. 1, January 1997.

39. Chrebet, Jennifer. "More Ways to Keep Bones Strong." *American Health*, June 1995.

40. Blazer, Dan. "Depression in Late Life." *Health in Mind & Body*, Vol. 2, No., 1, January 1998.

41. Valan, N. M., and Dm Hilty. "Depression in the Elderly Not Always What It May Seem" *Health in Mind & Body*, Vol. 2, No. 1, January 1998.

42. Hales and Hales, *Caring for the Mind*.

43. Gilman, Sid. "Alzheimer's Disease" *Perspectives in Biology and Medicine*, Vol. 40, No. 2, Winter 1997.

44. Gatz, Margaret, et al. "Heritability for Alzheimer's Disease: The Study of Dementia in Swedish Twins." *Journal of Gerontology*, Vol. 52, No. 2, March 1997.

45. Lawlor, Brian. *Behavioral Complications in Alzheimer's Disease*. Washington, DC: American Psychiatric Press, 1995.

46. Rebok, George, and Marshal Folstein. "Challenges in Diagnosing and Treating Alzheimer's Disease." *Psychiatric Times*, February 1994.

47. Small, Gary, et al. "Diagnosis and Treatment of Alzheimer Disease and Related Disorders." *Journal of the American Medical Association*, Vol. 278, No. 16, October 22/29, 1997.

48. "New Census Report Details Graying of U.S." *HealthSpan*, Vol. 6, No.1, Summer 1995. Kane, Robert. "Improving the Quality of Long-Term Care." *Journal of the American Medical Association*, Vol. 273, No. 17, May 3, 1995.

CHAPTER 19

WHEN LIFE ENDS

After studying the material in this chapter, you should be able to:

Define death and **explain** the stages of emotional reaction experienced in facing death.

Explain the controversy surrounding the right to die, including the influence of culture on life-and-death decisions.

Describe the impact of death on the grieving survivors.

List and **explain** factors affecting the length and intensity of grief.

Explain the purposes of a living will and a holographic will.

No one gets out of this life alive. Death is the natural completion of things, as much a part of the real world as life itself. If you're in your teens or twenties, death may seem remote, even unimaginable. That's normal: At all ages, we struggle to deny the reality of death. Yet we never escape it. We lose grandparents, aunts and uncles, parents, friends, coworkers, teachers, and neighbors. With every loss, part of us dies; yet each loss also reaffirms how precious life is.

The death that most fascinates and frightens us is our own. We hope that it won't come for a long, long time. We also hope that when it does come, we'll be able to face it with dignity and courage, and we wonder what, if anything, waits beyond death. This chapter explores the meaning of death, describes the process of dying, provides practical information on medical and legal arrangements, and offers advice on comforting the dying and helping their survivors.

Understanding the Meaning of Death

In our society, death isn't a part of everyday life, as it once was. Because machines can now keep alive people who, in the past, would have died, the definition of death has become more complex. Death has been broken down into the following categories:

- *Functional death.* The end of all vital functions, such as heartbeat and respiration.
- *Cellular death.* The gradual death of body cells after the heart stops beating. If placed in a tissue culture or, as is the case with various organs, transplanted to another body, some cells can remain alive indefinitely.
- *Cardiac death.* The moment when the heart stops beating.
- *Brain death.* The end of all brain activity, indicated by an absence of electrical activity (confirmed by an *electroencephalogram, or EEG*) and a lack of reflexes. The notion of brain death is bound up with what we consider to be the actual person, or self. The destruction of a person's brain means that his or her personality no longer exists; the lower brain centers controlling respiration and circulation no longer function.
- *Spiritual death.* The moment when the soul, as defined by many religions, leaves the body.

When does a person actually die? The traditional legal definition of death is failure of the lungs or heart to function. However, because modern medicine is often able to maintain respiration and circulation by artificial means, most states have declared that an individual is considered dead only when the brain, including the brain stem, completely stops functioning. Brain-death laws prohibit a medical staff from "pulling the plug" if there is any hope of sustaining life.[1]

Denial and Death

Most of us don't quite believe that we're going to die. A reasonable amount of denial helps us focus on the day-to-day realities of living. However, excessive denial can be life-threatening. Many drivers, for instance, refuse to buckle their seat belts, because they refuse to acknowledge that a drunk driver might collide with them. Similarly, cigarette smokers deny that lung cancer will ever strike them, and people who eat high-fat meals deny that they'll ever suffer a heart attack.

One important factor in denial is the nature of the threat. It's easy to believe that death is at hand when someone's pointing a gun at you; it's much harder to think that cigarette smoking might cause your death 20 or 30 years down the road. (See the Self-Survey: "How Do You Feel About Death?") Yet as Elisabeth Kübler-Ross, a psychiatrist who has extensively studied the process of dying, writes in *Death: The Final Stage of Growth:*

> It is the denial of death that is partially responsible for people living empty, purposeless lives; for when you live as if you'll live forever, it becomes too easy to postpone the things you know that you must do. You live your life in preparation for tomorrow or in the remembrance of yesterday,—and meanwhile, each today is lost. In contrast, when you fully understand that each day you awaken could be the last you have, you take the time that day to grow, to become more of who you really are, to reach out to other human beings.[2]

Emotional Responses to Death

Kübler-Ross has identified five typical stages of reaction that a person goes through when facing death (see Figure 19-1).

1. *Denial ("No, not me").* At first knowledge that death is coming, a terminally ill patient rejects the news. The denial overcomes the initial shock, and allows the person to begin to gather together his or her resources. Denial, at this point, is a healthy defense mechanism. It can become distressful, however, if it's reinforced by the relatives and friends of the dying patient.

2. *Anger ("Why me?").* In the second stage, the dying person begins to feel resentment and rage regarding

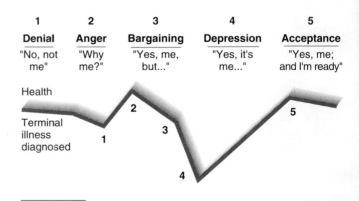

Figure 19-1

Kübler-Ross's five stages of adjustment to death.

Self-Survey

How Do You Feel About Death?

This questionnaire isn't designed to test your knowledge. Instead, it should encourage you to think about your present attitudes toward death and how these attitudes may have developed. Answer the questions, to the best of your knowledge, by circling the appropriate letter.

1. Who died, in your first personal involvement with death?
   a. Grandparent or great-grandparent
   b. Parent
   c. Brother or sister
   d. Friend or acquaintance
   e. Stranger
   f. Public figure
   g. Animal

2. To the best of your memory, at what age were you first aware of death?
   a. Under 3 years
   b. 3–5 years
   c. 5–10 years
   d. 10 years or older

3. When you were a child, how was death talked about in your family?
   a. Openly
   b. With some sense of discomfort
   c. Only when necessary, and then with an attempt to exclude children
   d. As though it were a taboo subject
   e. Don't recall any discussion

4. Which of the following best describes your childhood conceptions of death?
   a. Heaven-and-hell concept
   b. Afterlife
   c. Death as sleep
   d. Cessation of all physical and mental activity
   e. Mysterious and unknowable
   f. Something other than the above
   g. No conception
   h. Can't remember

5. To what extent do you believe in a life after death?
   a. Strongly believe in it
   b. Tend to believe in it
   c. Uncertain
   d. Tend to doubt it
   e. Convinced it doesn't exist

6. Regardless of your belief about life after death, what is your wish about it?
   a. I strongly wish that there were a life after death.
   b. I am indifferent about life after death.
   c. I definitely prefer that there not be a life after death.

7. Has there been a time in your life when you wanted to die?
   a. Yes, mainly because of great physical pain
   b. Yes, mainly because of great emotional upset
   c. Yes, mainly to escape an intolerable social or interpersonal situation
   d. Yes, mainly because of great embarrassment
   e. Yes, for a reason other than one above
   f. No

8. What does death mean to you?
   a. The end, the final process of life
   b. The beginning of a life after death, a transition, a new beginning
   c. A joining of the spirit with a universal cosmic consciousness
   d. A kind of endless sleep, rest, and peace
   e. An interim period before being born again
   f. Termination of this life but survival of the spirit
   g. Don't know
   h. Other (specify)

9. What aspect of your own death is the most distasteful to you?
   a. I could no longer have any experiences.
   b. I'm afraid of what might happen to my body after death.
   c. I'm uncertain about what might happen to me if there is a life after death.
   d. I could no longer provide for my dependents.
   e. It would cause grief to my relatives and friends.
   f. All my plans and projects would come to an end.
   g. The process of dying might be painful.
   h. Other (specify)

10. How do you rate your present physical health?
    a. Excellent
    b. Very good
    c. Moderately good
    d. Moderately poor
    e. Extremely poor

11. How do you rate your present mental health?
    a. Excellent
    b. Very good
    c. Moderately good
    d. Moderately poor
    e. Extremely poor

12. Based on your present feelings, what is the probability of your taking your own life in the near future?
    a. Extremely high (feel very much like killing myself)
    b. Moderately high
    c. Between high and low
    d. Moderately low
    e. Extremely low (very improbable that I would kill myself)

13. In your opinion, at what age are people most afraid of death?
    a. Up to 12 years
    b. 13–19 years
    c. 20–29 years
    d. 30–39 years
    e. 40–49 years
    f. 50–59 years
    g. 60–69 years
    h. 70 years and over

14. When you think of your own death (or when circumstances make you realize your own mortality), how do you feel?
    a. Fearful
    b. Discouraged
    c. Depressed
    d. Purposeless
    e. Resolved, in relation to life
    f. Pleasure, in being alive
    g. Other (specify)

15. What is your present orientation to your own death?
    a. Death-seeker
    b. Death-hastener
    c. Death-accepter
    d. Death-welcomer
    e. Death-postponer
    f. Death-fearer

16. If you were told that you had a terminal disease and a limited time to live, how would you want to spend your time until you died?
    a. I would make a marked change in my lifestyle to satisfy hedonistic needs (travel, sex, drugs, or other experiences).
    b. I would become more withdrawn—reading, contemplating, or praying.
    c. I would shift from my own needs to a concern for others (family and friends).
    d. I would attempt to complete projects, to tie up loose ends.
    e. I would make little or no change in my lifestyle.
    f. I would try to do one very important thing.
    g. I might consider committing suicide.
    h. I would do none of the above.

17. How do you feel about having an autopsy done on your body?
    a. Approve
    b. Don't care one way or the other
    c. Disapprove
    d. Strongly disapprove

Making Changes
Facing the Reality of Death

Examine your attitudes toward death and discuss your feelings with classmates, friends, and family. Although we read about death in the newspapers every day, we rarely come in close contact with it. Our society tends to reinforce the denial of death. By completing this questionnaire, you're taking an important step toward facing the reality of death.

SOURCE: Shneidman, Edwin. "You and Death Questionnaire." *Psychology Today*, August 1970.

imminent death. The anger may be directed at God or at the patient's family and caregivers, who can do little but try to endure any expressions of anger, provide comfort, and help the patient on to the next stage.

3. *Bargaining ("Yes, me, but...").* In this stage, a patient may try to bargain, usually with God, for a way to reverse, or at least postpone, dying. The patient may promise, in exchange for recovery, to do good works or to see family members more often. Alternatively, the patient may say, "Let me live long enough to see my grandchild born" or "to see the spring again."

4. *Depression ("Yes, it's me").* In the fourth stage, the patient gradually realizes the full consequences of his or her condition. This may begin as grieving for health that has been lost, and then become anticipatory grieving for the loss that is to come of friends, loved ones, and life itself. This is perhaps the most difficult time: the dying person should not be left alone during this period. Neither should one try to cheer the patient, however, who must be allowed to grieve.

5. *Acceptance ("Yes, me; and I'm ready").* In this last stage, the person has accepted the reality of death: The moment looms as neither frightening nor painful, neither sad nor happy—only inevitable. The person who waits for the end of life may ask to see fewer visitors, to separate from other people, or perhaps to turn to just one person for support.

Several stages may occur at the same time and some may happen out of sequence. Each stage may take days or only hours or minutes. Throughout, denial may come

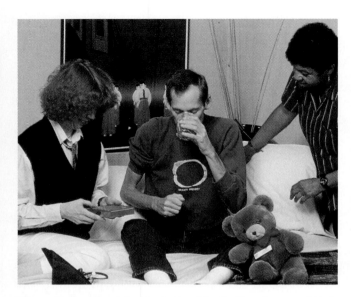

Humanitarian caregiving for both critically ill patients and their loved ones can help to take some of the fear out of death.

back to assert itself unexpectedly—and hope for a medical breakthrough or a miraculous recovery is forever present.

Some experts dispute Kübler-Ross's basic five-stage theory as too simplistic, and argue that not all people go through such well-defined stages in the dying process. The way a person faces death is often a mirror of the way he or she has faced other major stresses in life: Those who have had the most trouble adjusting to other crises will have the most trouble adjusting to the news of their impending death.

An individual's will to live can postpone death for a while. In a study of elderly Chinese women, researchers found that their death rate decreased before and during a holiday during which the senior women in a household play a central role; it increased after the celebration. A similar temporary drop occurs among Jews at the time of Passover. However, different events may have different effects. In a study of 2,745,149 deaths, researchers at the University of California, San Diego, found that the prospect of an upcoming birthday postpones death in women but hastens it in men. The women were more likely to die in the week following their birthdays than in any other week during the year—and less likely in the week before. Among the men, however, mortality peaked shortly before their birthdays. The reason for this gender difference, the researchers speculated, may be that many people use birthdays to take stock of their ambitions versus their accomplishments. Men, who in our society often base

their self-esteem on professional achievement, may be more likely to evaluate themselves in negative terms.[3]

The family of a dying person experiences a spectrum of often wrenching emotions. Family members, too, may deny the verdict of death, rage at the doctors and nurses who can't do more to save their loved one, bargain with God to give up their own health if necessary, sink into helplessness and depression, and finally accept the reality of their anticipated loss.

One way of reducing the mystery and fear of death is to learn more about it. **Thanatology**, a term derived from the Greek god of death, Thanatos, refers to "the discipline of humanitarian caregiving for critically ill patients and their grieving family members and friends." Such care, which may be provided by physicians, nurses, social workers, psychologists, and others, helps ensure that terminally ill patients receive the compassionate, respectful care they deserve. The more we all learn about the process of dying and about what can be done to help more people die more peacefully, the better we can understand, and offer support to, the terminally ill.

Personal Health
19.1
INTERACTIVE

Ethical Dilemmas

Modern medicine can do more to delay or defeat death than was once thought possible. However, the ability to sustain life in patients with no hope of recovery has created wrenching medical and moral dilemmas. Increasingly, lawyers, ethicists, and consumer advocates are arguing that health-care providers must recognize a fundamental right of patients: the right to die.

Health economists, noting that more than half of U.S. health-care dollars are spent in the last year of life, have questioned "heroic" measures to prolong the life of chronically ill elderly patients or those with fatal diseases. Policies on such aggressive measures vary from hospital to hospital and state to state. Some health-care facilities require that staff members try to resuscitate any patient whose heart stops unless a do-not-resuscitate (DNR) order has been written, usually with the family's permission. (DNR documents are discussed later in this chapter.) In other cases, physicians may decide against resuscitation despite the family's wishes if they think that treatment would be futile and that the family's objections are not based on the patient's values or best interests. However, the wishes of dying patients often go unheeded. Even when patients have specified that they do not want high-tech treatments or life support, physicians may continue to order such care.[4]

Another major ethical concern is the fate of an estimated 5,000 to 10,000 unconscious Americans who are being kept alive by artificial means. Some are in a **coma**, a state of total unconsciousness. They may have no sense of where they are, no memory, and no experience of pain. Others are in a **persistent vegetative state**, in which they're awake and yet unaware. They open their eyes; their brain waves show the characteristic patterns of waking and sleep. They can usually breathe on their own after a few weeks on artificial respiration; they can cough; the pupils of their eyes respond to light; but they do not respond to pain.

The questions about the rights of individuals in comas or persistent vegetative states are complex. Two decades ago, the removal of a respirator, water, or food from a patient who was not brain-dead was not accepted medical practice. In 1976 the courts allowed the removal of the ventilator thought to be keeping Karen Ann Quinlan, who had lived in a coma for seven years, alive. In the 1980s court cases allowed the withdrawal of water and nourishment from chronically unconscious patients who were not terminally ill. In the 1990s there have been "wrongful life" suits by those resuscitated or kept alive against their wishes.

In one landmark case, the parents of Nancy Cruzan went all the way to the Supreme Court for permission to stop artificial feeding of their daughter, so that she could die after existing for eight years in a vegetative state. The Court denied the family's plea, saying that the state had the right to require more evidence of a patient's wishes. The family went back to a lower court with new evidence, including testimony from friends, that their daughter would not want to be kept alive. The court ultimately gave permission for her artificial feeding to stop. However, the questions of when to use and when to discontinue artificial means of life support remain among the most challenging ethical dilemmas facing health-care workers and the families of critically ill patients. (See Spotlight on Diversity: "Deciding on Life or Death.")

Preparing for Death

Throughout this book we have stressed the ways in which you can determine how well and how long you live. You can also make decisions about the end of your life, particularly its impact on other people. In order to clarify your thinking on this difficult subject, ask yourself the following questions:

- Would I prefer to receive or not to receive any specific treatments if I were unconscious or incapable of voicing my opinion?

- Would I like my bodily systems to be kept functioning by extraordinary life-sustaining measures, even though my natural systems had failed? If I could not survive without mechanical assistance, would I want to be kept alive or resuscitated if my heart were to stop?

- Would I like the state to decide how to distribute my property or provide for my children (if any), or my family to decide how to handle my funeral arrangements?

- Would I care to give someone else, by donating my organs, the same possibilities for life that I have had?

You can assure that your wishes are heeded by several means, including advance directives, such as health-care proxies and living wills; a holographic will; and an organ donation card.

Advance Directives

Every state and the District of Columbia have laws authorizing the use of **advance directives** to specify the kind of medical treatment individuals want in case of a medical crisis. However, very few Americans, including only 4 to 24% of men and women have any type of advance directive. These documents are important because, without clear indications of a person's preferences, hospitals and other institutions often make decisions on an individual's behalf, particularly if family members are not available or disagree.[5]

According to the Patient Self-Determination Act, which went into effect in 1991, health-care facilities that receive Medicare or Medicaid reimbursements (see Chapter 2 for an explanation of these programs) must advise patients of their rights to sign advance directives for health-care decisions, such as whether they want to be kept alive by artificial means. These statements allow medical professionals to know and follow an individual's wishes, or the wishes of a person to whom the patient has given authority to make decisions on his or her behalf. However, as mentioned earlier, they often are ignored by physicians and other hospital workers committed to sustaining life at all costs.[6]

A *health-care proxy* is an advance directive that gives someone else the power to make decisions on your behalf. (See Figure 19-2.) People typically name a relative or close friend as their agent. Let family and

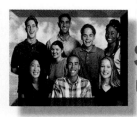

Spotlight on Diversity
Deciding on Life or Death

Nothing more can be done. A family member, critically ill or injured, will almost certainly die if artificial means of sustaining life were disconnected. How does a family make the wrenching decision of whether to pull the plug?

Many factors—religious values, political beliefs, past experiences—influence relatives as they struggle with the difficult decision of what to do for a parent, partner, sibling, or child. One of the major, yet often unrecognized, influences on life-and-death decisions is cultural background. Only recently have researchers begun to explore the ways in which culture shapes decisions about dying. A 1995 study found ethnic differences in what patients want to know about terminal illness. In the study, black and white respondents were much more likely than Korean Americans or Mexican Americans to feel that seriously ill patients should be told about the severity of illness and the possibility of dying and given the right to decide about the use of artificial means of sustaining life. Here are some insights into the decision-making dynamics of different ethnic and racial groups.

• **African Americans**   In general, African Americans want life-support measures to be continued for their loved ones. This attitude stems in part from the fact that African Americans as a group are more religious and more devout than various other groups. Because of their religious convictions, many believe it would be wrong to discontinue life-support measures, and would feel tremendous guilt about doing so. In addition, African Americans place a high value on their elders, a long life (even if an individual is suffering), and a person's will to survive. Concerns stemming from racial discrimination also play a role: Since African Americans often have less access to health services and receive less intense care, they may be distrustful of the medical establishment and fear that physicians may act prematurely in discontinuing life support.

• **Chinese Americans**   Many religious traditions—Confucianism, Taoism, Buddhism—as well as Marxism, have influenced the Chinese, who value not just life, but living in an ideal way. Many Chinese-American patients and their families believe that nature should be allowed to take its course, especially when a person is suffering. Chinese philosophy includes the right to choose death, and most Chinese approve of dyathanasia, or passive euthanasia. In addition, many Chinese Americans wouldn't want their care to be a

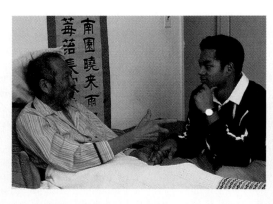

Cultural attitudes and beliefs can greatly influence life-and-death decisions.

financial burden for their families, and know that others would hold them in high esteem for deciding to forego life support so that their family will not suffer.

• **Iranian Americans**   Whether they're Muslims or Christians, Iranian patients usually oppose stopping life support in any situation. The predominant code of Iran is based on Islamic tradition, which views life and death as controlled by God. Because God alone can decide when someone dies, life support is viewed as an obligation, not an option. Instituting therapy is viewed as an appropriate use of the gift of medical technology. Removing supportive measures is viewed negatively as "playing God."

• **Korean Americans**   Most Korean Americans are religious, with Buddhism and Protestantism the dominant influences. Many Korean Americans see stopping life support as interfering with God's will, although starting such measures is not. Also important is the concept of loyalty to one's parents, especially by the oldest son, who is obliged to preserve his father's and mother's lives at all cost. Agreeing to stop life support, even if a parent wishes it, may dishonor the family member in the eyes of the community or other relatives.

• **Mexican Americans**   The Mexican culture includes customs and beliefs based on native traditions as well as the influence of Spain and the neighboring United States. Mexican-American families tend to be strong and close. When faced with a decision on life support, religious values are critical. More than 85% of Mexican Americans are Roman Catholics and oppose any means of hastening death. In addition, Mexican Americans often view health as a gift from God and illness or injury as a punishment or as part of God's plan for an individual—one that shouldn't be interfered with. For them, enduring physical suffering is a sign of strength that inspires respect. Others may see illness as being caused by evil spirits or the devil and believe that a native healer (*curandero*) will be able to help when traditional medicine cannot.

SOURCE: Koenig, Barbara, and Jan Gates-Williams. "Understanding Cultural Differences in Caring for Dying Patients." *The Western Journal of Medicine*, Vol. 163, No. 3, September 1995. Mydans, Seth. "Should Dying Patients Be Told? Ethnic Pitfall Is Found." *New York Times*, September 13, 1995. Klessig, Jill. "The Effects of Values and Culture on Life-Support Decisions." *Western Journal of Medicine*, September 1992.

Except in California, where they must be renewed every five years, living wills are effective until they're revoked. Still, it's considered a good idea to initial and date your living will every few years to show that it still expresses your wishes.

"Imminent" is used on many living wills to express the inevitability and timing of death, but it's open to varying interpretations. A recent Virgina court decision found that it doesn't necessarily mean "immediately, at once, within a few days," and that a comatose person who's within a few months of death falls within the definition.

Except in California, Idaho, and Oregon, living wills have a space to specify treatment you do or don't want. Ask your physician what to include here. You can:

• Ask for or prohibit use of artificial feeding tubes, cardiopulmonary resuscitation, antibiotics, dialysis, and respirators.

• Ask for pain medication to keep you comfortable.

• State whether you would prefer to die in the hospital or at home.

• Designate a proxy—someone to make decisions about your treatment when you're unable.

• Donate organs or other body parts.

If your directions are contrary to state law, they'll be ignored, but the rest of the document will stand.

DIRECTIVE TO PHYSICIANS

Directive made this _____day of_____ (month, year). I, _____being of sound mind, willfully and voluntarily make known my desire that my life shall not be artificially prolonged under the circumstances set forth below, and do hereby declare:

If at any time I should have an incurable condition caused by injury, disease, or illness certified to be a terminal condition by two physicians, and where the application of life-sustaining procedures would serve only to artificially prolong the moment of death and where my attending physician determines that my death is imminent whether or not life-sustaining procedures are utilized, I direct that such procedures be withheld or withdrawn, and that I be permitted to die naturally.

In the absence of my ability to give directions regarding the use of such life-sustaining procedures, it is my intention that this directive shall be honored by my family and physicians as the final expression of my legal right to refuse medical or surgical treatment and accept the consequences from such refusal.

If I have been diagnosed as pregnant and that diagnosis is known to my physician, this directive shall have no force or effect during the course of my pregnancy.

Other directions:
This directive shall be in effect until it is revoked. I understand the full import of this directive, and I am emotionally and mentally competent to make this directive. I understand that I may revoke this directive at any time.

Signed _____

City, County, and State of Residence _____

The declarant has been personally known to me and I believe him/her to be of sound mind. I am not related to the declarant by blood or marriage, nor would I be entitled to any portion of the declarant's estate on his/her decease, nor am I the attending physician of the declarant or an employee of the attending physician or a health facility in which the declarant is a patient, or a patient in the health care facility in which the declarant is a patient, or any person who has a claim against any portion of the estate of the declarant upon his/her decease.

Witness _____ Witness _____

SOURCE: Adapted from "Guide to the Living Will." *Hippocrates*, May–June 1988.

"Life-sustaining procedures" are those that only prolong the process of dying. Most states include feeding and hydration tubes in this definition.

In some states a physician who will not carry out a patient's wishes must make a "good faith effort" to locate a doctor who will; other states require the physician to actually find someone and specify penalties—in some cases, jail terms—for failure to do so.

In some states the living will is valid for pregnant women. Others exclude women during all or part of their pregnancy, although that has been challenged on the grounds that a woman's right to privacy doesn't end when she becomes pregnant.

You can revoke or amend your living will at any time simply by making a statement to a physician, nurse, or other health-care worker.

Several states provide for the appointment of a proxy. In others decisions may be delegated through a document called a Durable Power of Attorney.

In some states, your signature must be notarized. Elsewhere, the signature of the witnesses is adequate although if you're in a hospital or nursing home in some states you may need as an additional witness the chief of staff or medical director.

Figure 19-2
Preparing a living will, or physician's directive.

friends know your thoughts about treatments and life-support. You also should let your primary physician know about the type of care you would or wouldn't want to receive in various circumstances, such as an accident that results in an irreversible coma, but you should not designate your doctor as your agent. Many states prohibit this. Even when allowed, it is not a good idea because your doctor's primary responsibility is to administer care.

It also is possible to sign an advance directive specifying that you do not want to be resuscitated in case your heart stops beating or that you want to be allowed to die naturally.[7] **Do-not-resuscitate (DNR)** orders apply mainly to hospitalized, terminally ill patients. However, in some states, it is possible to complete a "nonhospital DNR" form that specifies an individual's wish not to be resuscitated at home. Patients in the final stages of advanced cancer or AIDS may choose to use such forms to protect their rights in case paramedics are called to their home.[8]

Whereas a health-care proxy allows you to name someone to make health-care decisions for you, a power of attorney designates someone to make financial decisions on your behalf. An aging parent might give a son or daughter the power to file tax returns, pay bills, or handle other financial matters. One partner might give similar authorization to another. Power-of-attorney forms are sold at many large stationery or office supply stores. Some experts advise consulting with an attorney to make sure your power of attorney is "durable"— meaning that it remains in effect even if you should become mentally incapacitated.

The Living Will

Living wills aren't just for people who don't want to be kept alive by artificial means. Individuals can also use these advance directives to indicate that they want all possible medical treatments and technology used to prolong their lives. Most states recognize living wills as legally binding, and a growing number of health-care professionals and facilities are offering patients help in drafting living wills. You can obtain state-specific forms for living wills and health-care proxies free from an organization called Choice in Dying (1-800-989-WILL). Computer software for preparing such documents also is available. (See Figure 19-3.)

Once the forms are completed, make copies of your living will and other advance directives and give them to anyone who might have input in decisions on your behalf. Also give copies to your physician or health-care organization, and ask that they be made part of your medical record.

The Holographic Will

Perhaps you think that only wealthy or older people need to write wills. However, if you're married, have children, or own property, you should either hire a lawyer to draw up a will, or write a **holographic will** yourself, specifying who you wish to raise your children or who should have your property. If you die *intestate* (without a will), the state will make these decisions for you. Even a modest estate can be tied up in court for a long period of time, depriving family members of money when they need it most.

Many states will recognize a handwritten (not typed) statement by you, through which you can accomplish the following:

- Name a family member or friend as the executor, the person who sees that your wishes are carried out.

- List the things you own and to whom you want them to go; include addresses and telephone numbers, if possible.

- Select a guardian for your children (if any), presumably someone whose ideas about raising children are similar to your own. Be sure that they are willing and able to accept this responsibility before writing them into your will.

- Specify any funeral arrangements.

- Be sure to keep the will in a safe place, where your executor, family members, or closest beneficiary can get to it quickly and easily; tell them where it is.

The Gift of Life

If you're at least 18 years old, you can fill out a donor card (see Figure 19-4), agreeing to designate, in the event of your death, any organs or tissues needed for transplantation. Corneas may help a blind person see, for example. Kidneys, or even a heart, may be transplanted. The donation takes effect upon your death and is a generous way of giving others the possibilities for life that you have had yourself. The card should be filled out and signed; some must be signed in the presence of two witnesses. Attach the donor card to the back of your driver's license or I.D. card. (Whole-body donations may require other arrangements.)

A LIVING WILL

To My Family, Doctors, and All Those Concerned with My Care:

I, _____, being of sound mind, make this statement as a directive to be followed if I become unable to participate in decisions regarding my medical care.

If I should have an incurable or irreversible mental or physical condition with no reasonable expectation of recovery. I direct my attending physician to withhold or withdraw treatment that merely prolongs my dying. I further direct that treatment be limited to measures to keep me comfortable and to relieve pain.

This declaration sets forth your directions regarding medical treatment.

These directions express my legal right to refuse treatment. Therefore, I expect my family, doctors, and everyone concerned with my care to regard themselves as legally and morally bound to act in accord with my wishes, and in so doing to be free of any legal liability for having followed my directions.

You have the right to refuse treatment you do not want, and you may request the care you do want.

I especially do not want _____
_____
_____
_____
_____
_____
_____

You may list specific treatment you do not want (for example, cardiac resuscitation, mechanical respiration, artificial feeding/fluids by tube); otherwise, your general statement, top left, will stand for your wishes.

Other instructions/comments: _____
_____
_____
_____

You may want to add instructions or care you do want—for example, pain medication, or that you prefer to die at home if possible.

Proxy Designation Clause: Should I become unable to communicate my instructions as stated above, I designate the following person to act on my behalf:

Name _____

Address _____

If the person I have named above is unable to act on my behalf, I authorize the following person to do so:

Name_____

Address_____

This living will declaration expresses my personal treatment preferences. The fact that I may have also executed a document in the form recommended by state law should not be construed to limit or contradict this living will declaration, which is an expression of my common-law and constitutional rights.

If you want, you can name someone to see that your wishes are carried out, but you do not have to do this.

Signed: _____ Date: _____

Witness:_____ Witness:_____

Address:_____ Address:_____

Keep the assigned original with your personal papers at home. Give signed copies to doctors, family, and proxy. Review your declaration from time to time: initial and date it to show it still expresses your intent.

Sign and date here in the presence of two adult witnesses, who should also sign.

Fig 19-3
A sample form for a living will.

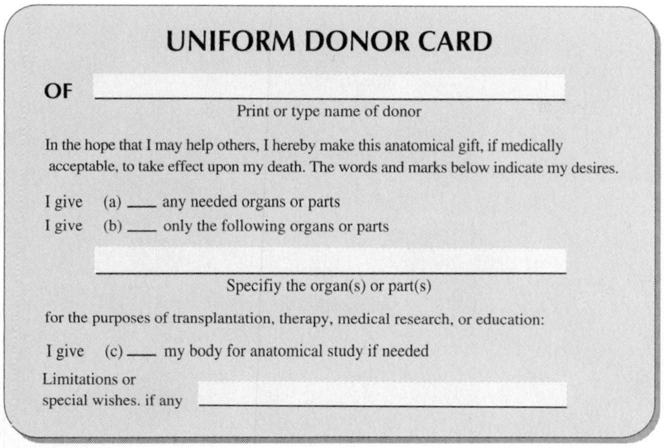

UNIFORM DONOR CARD

OF _____
Print or type name of donor

In the hope that I may help others, I hereby make this anatomical gift, if medically acceptable, to take effect upon my death. The words and marks below indicate my desires.

I give   (a) ____ any needed organs or parts
I give   (b) ____ only the following organs or parts

_____
Specifiy the organ(s) or part(s)

for the purposes of transplantation, therapy, medical research, or education:

I give   (c) ____ my body for anatomical study if needed

Limitations or
special wishes. if any _____

Figure 19-4

Example of a uniform donor card.

The Process of Dying

Most people who have a fatal or **terminal illness** prefer to know the truth about their health and chances for recovery. (See Table 19-1) Even when they're not officially informed by a doctor or relative, most fatally ill people know or strongly suspect that they're dying. Dying people usually make it clear whether they want to talk about death and to what extent. The most frequent concern is how much time is left. Usually physicians can give only a rough estimate, such as "several weeks or months."[9]

Because of the emphasis on high-tech treatments in modern training, physicians often are uncomfortable talking about death with their patients. "We have lost the ability to talk openly about what death is, what our needs are, and the best way to provide what we have euphemistically come to call the 'good' death," says Sherwin Nuland, M.D., author of *How We Die*, who asserts that dying patients have three common needs: to know that they will not die alone, that no extraordinary means will be used to artificially prolong life, when "nature of the disease has decreed that there is no possibility of doing this without a great deal of suffering," and to be reassured that they will be remembered and will live on through those they leave behind. The people who are close to dying patients need to let them know what their lives have meant to them, Nuland contends. It is the final gift loved ones can offer.[10]

Life Before Death

Most older Americans do not die isolated, alone, and in great pain. They spend their last days at home and die peacefully. According to a study of nearly 4000 individuals over age 65 who died, more than half were in good to excellent health a year before death. About a fourth were still in good health a month before they died. Eighty percent were mentally alert; 60% were mobile. More than half died in their sleep.

Older people frequently have several serious health problems, rather than any single condition that leads to

---

TABLE 19-1   ATTITUDES TOWARD THE DYING

Percent of ethnic group who believe:	Korean Americans	Mexican Americans	African Americans	European Americans
A patient should be told diagnosis of metastatic cancer.	47%	65%	89%	87%
A patient should be told of terminal prognosis.	35	48	63	69
A patient should decide about the use of life support.	28	41	60	65

SOURCE: *The University of Southern California*

their demise. In one 1998 report, 20 variables—including age, sex, income, cardiovascular abnormalities, smoking, lack of exercise, and impaired cognitive function—contributed to mortality.[11] But, as medical experts emphasize, what is less important than the predictors of death is the quality of life before death.[12]

Strategies for Change
....
How to Help a Dying Person

✔ Don't worry about what to say. Your words matter less than your presence. Just being there, holding hands, is a comfort.

✔ Listen. Dying people often need someone to listen as they talk through their feelings. Such discussions don't make them more upset but help them come to terms with what's happening.

✔ Be genuine. Don't try to look or act cheerful. Your loved one will see through you and feel more isolated than before. It's better to let your sadness and concern show.

✔ Don't try to explain or rationalize what has happened. Offer consolation and reassurance.

Pain Relief

In the past, medical professionals often gave drugs to a terminal patient on an as-needed basis—that is, when the pain got so bad that the person asked for relief. However, because this approach can result in the person's last hours being a cycle of anxiety, anger, and pain, drugs are now often given on a regular, timed basis, beginning with a small dose and gradually increasing until the patient is pain-free, with each subsequent dose given before the previous one has worn off. In addition to standard pain medication, researchers have also experimented with such restricted drugs as marijuana (for the relief of nausea in cancer patients undergoing chemotherapy) and heroin (as a painkiller for people who don't respond well to other narcotics).

Hospice: Caring When Curing Isn't Possible

A **hospice** is a homelike health-care facility or program that helps dying men and women who can afford such care to live their final days to the fullest, as free as possible from disabling pain and mental anguish. Hospice

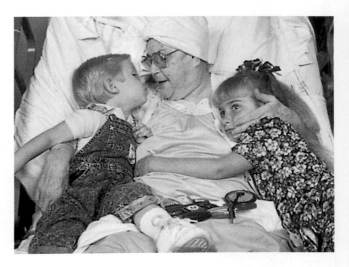

A hospice provides care and support and helps people die with comfort and dignity.

workers generally work in teams, usually consisting of a nurse, physician, social worker, chaplain, and trained volunteers. Other professionals, such as a physical therapist, may join the team when needed. These workers provide the comfort, support, and care dying patients need until they do die.

Hospice programs offer a combination of medical and emotional care that involves not only the patient but also the family members or others concerned with caring for the patient. Most hospice patients have life expectancies of six months or less, and are no longer receiving treatments aimed at curing their diseases. When someone is available to provide care, patients remain in their own homes. Hospice nurses regularly visit all home patients and are available around the clock.

For patients requiring care that the family cannot provide, round-the-clock care is available at the hospice facility. Unlike a traditional hospital, where the focus is on diagnosis, cure, and treatment, a hospice works to make what is left of life pain-free and comfortable. Visiting hours for relatives and friends are flexible, with no restrictions on visits by children and grandchildren. Hospice services are covered, in full or in part, by most major insurance companies.[13]

Near-Death Experiences

In recent years, the number of reports of **near-death experiences** has grown, thanks largely to advances in emergency medical care. Most such experiences are remarkably similar, whether they occur in children or adults, whether they're the result of accidents or illnesses, even whether the individuals actually are near death or only think they are. Some individuals who have survived a close brush with death report **autoscopy** (watching, from several feet in the air, resuscitation attempts on their own bodies) or **transcendence** (the sense of passing into a foreign region or dimension). Some see light, often at the end of a tunnel. Their vision seems clearer; their hearing, sharper. Some recall scenes from their lives or feel the presence of loved ones who have died. Many report profound feelings of joy, calm, and peace. Fewer than 1% of those who've reported near-death experiences described them as frightening or distressing, although a larger number recall transitory feelings of fear or confusion.[14]

Are near-death encounters truly a glimpse of life beyond? Are they the result of physiological changes caused by drugs or the process of dying? Or are they psychological reactions to the prospect of death? Numerous studies of individuals who've reported near-death experiences have found these persons to be, as one researcher put it, "psychologically unremarkable." The individuals' own religious beliefs and their awareness (or ignorance) of reports of similar encounters had no demonstrable effect on their experiences. Cross-cultural studies have documented a consistent pattern in reports about almost dying, regardless of the individuals' belief systems or life experiences.

Many near-death experiences occur in individuals who've been sedated or given other medications; however, many others do not. Several studies have shown that individuals who received medication or anesthesia were actually less likely to remember near-death experiences than those who hadn't had any drugs.[15] Some scientists have speculated that lack of oxygen, changes in blood gases, altered brain functioning, or the release of neurotransmitters (messenger chemicals in the brain) may play a role in near-death experiences. However, there's little solid evidence that physiological events are responsible. There's also no proof that wishful thinking, cultural conditioning, post-traumatic stress, or other psychological mechanisms may be at work. For now, the most that scientists can say for sure about this medical mystery is that it needs further study.

Suicide

Suicide is among the ten leading causes of death in the United States; each year 25,000 to 55,000 people kill themselves. And for every completed suicide, there are 10 to 40 unsuccessful attempts. (Chapter 5 presents a detailed discussion of the risk factors and warning signs of suicide.)

One of the main factors leading to suicide is illness, especially terminal illness. Approximately three-fourths of those who commit suicide consult a physician, most with medical complaints, within the six-month period prior to their deaths. Disease, medication, and the fear of pain or of being a burden to one's family can breed depression, a primary factor among those who attempt suicide.[16] Fatally ill individuals who talk about suicide should be taken seriously; family physicians can arrange for them to talk with psychotherapists. (Physician-assisted suicide is discussed below.)

"Rational" Suicide

An elderly widow suffering from advanced cancer takes a lethal overdose of sleeping pills. A young man with several AIDS-related illnesses shoots himself. A woman in her fifties, diagnosed as having Alzheimer's disease, asks a doctor to help her end her life. Are these suicides "rational" because these individuals used logical reasoning in deciding to end their lives?

The question is intensely controversial. Advocates of the right to "self-deliverance" argue that individuals in great pain or faced with the prospect of a debilitating, hopeless battle against an incurable disease can and should be able to decide to end their lives. As legislatures and the legal system tackle the thorny questions of an individual's right to die, mental health professionals worry that, even in those with fatal diseases, suicidal wishes often stem from undiagnosed depression.

In one classic study of 44 terminally ill individuals, 34 had never been suicidal or wished for death. The remaining ten (seven who did desire early death and three who specifically considered suicide) all had severe depression. Their despair and preoccupation with dying may well have contributed to their willingness to consider suicide. Numerous studies have indicated that most patients with painful, progressive or terminal illnesses do not want to kill themselves. The percentage of those who report thinking about suicide ranges from 5% to 20%; most of these have major depressions. Many mental health professionals argue that what makes patients with severe illnesses suicidal is depression, not their physical condition.[17]

Because depression may indeed warp the ability to make a rational decision about suicide, mental health professionals urge physicians and family members to make sure individuals with chronic or fatal illnesses are evaluated for depression and given medication, psychotherapy, or both. It is also important for everyone to allow enough time—an average of three to eight weeks—to see if treatment for depression will make a difference in their desire to keep living.

Physician-Assisted Suicide

If patients have a right to die, should doctors help them end their lives? Physicians have been willing to stop any extraordinary efforts to sustain life (for example, by withholding oxygen or ending intravenous feedings); such actions are referred to as passive **euthanasia**, or **dyathanasia**. Euthanasia, the active form of so-called mercy killing, has generally been viewed as illegal and unethical. Euthanasia has been tolerated for years in the Netherlands, but it is not technically legal there.

In 1994, Oregon passed the "Death with Dignity" act and became the first state to legalize physician-assisted suicide for terminally ill patients. However, federal courts have ruled the act unconstitutional because it unfairly discriminates against the terminally ill by excluding them from safeguards that apply to others.[18] The issue of whether physicians should aid in patients' suicide remains highly controversial.[19]

Jack Kevorkian, M.D., a Michigan pathologist, has stirred public debate by using a "suicide machine" to help end the life (at their request) of dozens of people suffering from chronic, but not necessarily fatal, illnesses. He was accused of murder, but a judge dismissed the charges. The Michigan Supreme Court has since ruled physician-assisted suicide a "common law felony." Some medical groups, such as the American Medical Association, oppose as unethical any physician's involvement in euthanasia. Others argue that individuals have the right to end their own lives and that physicians who provide prescriptions for lethal doses of certain drugs are acting out of compassion.[20]

The Practicalities of Death

At a time of great emotional pain, grieving family members must cope with medical, legal, and practical concerns, including obtaining a medical certificate of the cause of death, registering the death, and making funeral arrangements. They may also want to arrange for organ donations and, in some circumstances, an autopsy.

Funeral Arrangements

Memorial societies are voluntary groups that help people plan in advance for death. They obtain services at moderate cost, keep the arrangements simple and dignified, and—most importantly, perhaps—ease the emotional and financial burden on the rest of the family when death finally does come.

A body can be either buried or cremated. Burial requires the purchase of a cemetery plot, which many families do decades before death. If the body is to be cremated, you must comply with some additional formalities, with which the funeral director can help you. After a cremation (incineration of the remains), you can either collect the ashes to keep, bury, or scatter yourself, or ask the crematorium to dispose of them.

The tradition of a funeral may help survivors come to terms with the death, enabling them both to mourn their loss and to celebrate the dead person's life. Alternatively, the body may be disposed of immediately, through burial, cremation, or bequeathal to a medical school, and a memorial service held later.

Funerals are usually held two to four days after the death. Many have two parts: a religious ceremony at a church or funeral home, and a burial ceremony at the grave site. In a memorial service, the body is not present, which may change the focus of the service from the person's death to his or her life.

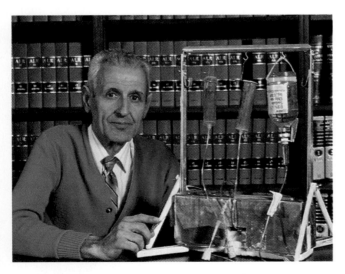

Dr. Jack Kevorkian designed this suicide machine to enable patients with fatal or incurable diseases to take their own lives.

Personal Voices One Man's Grief

*I*n the following essay, a college student describes what it's like to lose a close friend:

On a December night, Gary was shot and killed on the street. It happened during our junior year of college. For nearly sixteen years, we had been companions and confidantes, passing through childhood, adolescence, and early adulthood together. Each of us had always provided the other a word of encouragement, an available ear, a shoulder to lean on. In school, sports, and play, we competed as equals; and as our lives unfolded, our friendship developed with the same equality.

Staring at his body in the funeral home left me bewildered: Where had Gary gone? This had happened just as he and I thought we had begun to untangle some of life's intricacies. I was 20 years old, and the confrontation with mortality left me breathless, robbed of my desire to fight.

I went through the motions of being back in school. Each day I attended classes and meals, but every morning I faced the same sadness and anger: Why had I awakened? Couldn't I just die in my sleep? One night I had a dream in which Gary was comforting me. His words were assuaging the pain: "Death is friendly. It doesn't hurt. I promise you, I never felt the bullets. I'll see you again someday." I wrapped that dream around my shivering soul.

Then one morning in April, I awoke to the sun pouring into my room and the sound of birds singing outside. Something about awakening that morning was different. A realization drifted up slowly from within: I was glad to be alive.

That was the most painful, wonderful discovery. I knew it meant that I would go on with my life, that I was ready and wanted to continue living; but it also confirmed the knowledge that Gary was dead. I finally understood the contradiction: Gary would always be with me; yet I would have to go on living without him.

SOURCE: "One Man's Grief," *Journal of the American Medical Association*, March 23–30, 1984.

Autopsies

An autopsy is a detailed examination of a body after death, also called a postmortem exam. There are two types:

1. *Medicolegal.* This is an autopsy performed to establish the cause of death and to gather information about the death for use as evidence in any legal proceedings. It is done to detect any crimes and to help identify the proper person for prosecution, to investigate possible industrial hazards or contagious diseases that may endanger the public health, or to establish the cause of death for insurance purposes.

2. *Medical/educational.* This is an autopsy performed, usually in the hospital where the person died, to increase medical knowledge and to determine a more exact cause of death. It may be requested by the attending physician or the family, but it cannot be performed without the family's permission.

Autopsies can be extremely valuable in establishing an accurate cause of death, revealing a different diagnosis that might have led to a change in therapy and prolonged survival in about 10% of cases. Thirty years ago about 50% of patients who died in hospitals were autopsied. However, the autopsy rate in the United States has been steadily declining, and today about 10 to 20% of deaths in teaching hospitals are autopsied. Physicians are arguing for an increase in autopsies as the best method for establishing the cause of death, helping to spot infectious diseases, aiding medical education, and helping assure the high quality of medical practice.[21]

Grief

An estimated 8 million Americans lose a member of their immediate families each year. The death of a loved one may be the single most upsetting and feared event in a person's life.

The death of a family member produces a wide range of reactions, including anxiety, guilt, anger, and financial concern. Many see the death of an old person as less tragic (usually) than the death of a child or young person. A sudden death is more of a shock than one following a long illness (see Personal Voices: "One Man's Grief"). A suicide can be particularly devastating, because family members may wonder whether they could have done anything to prevent it. The cause of death can also affect the reactions of friends and acquaintances. Some people express less sympathy and support when individuals are murdered or take their own lives.

Encountering death can make us feel alone and vulnerable. The most common and one of the most painful experiences is the death of a parent. When both parents die, individuals may feel like orphaned children. They

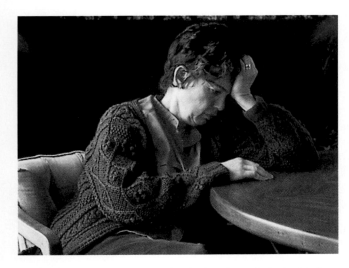

Grief can take an enormous physical and psychological toll on family members and loved ones.

mourn, not just for the father and mother who are gone, but for their lost role of being someone's child.

The death of a child can be even more devastating. Grieving may continue for many years. Eventually parents may be able to resolve their grief and accept the death as "God's will" or as "something that happens." Time erases their pain, and they feel a desire to get on with their lives, consciously putting the loss behind them. Others deal with their grief by keeping busy, or by substituting other problems or situations to take their minds off their loss. Yet many parents who lose a child continue to grieve for many years. Although the pain of their loss diminishes with time, they view it as part of themselves and describe an emptiness inside—even though most have rich, meaningful, and happy daily lives.

The loss of a mate can also have a profound impact, although men's and women's responses to the death— and their subsequent health risks—may depend on how their spouses died. Men whose wives die suddenly face a much greater risk of dying themselves than those whose wives die after a long illness. On the other hand, women whose husbands die after a long illness face greater risk than other widows. The reason may be that men whose wives were chronically ill learned how to cope with the loss of their nurturers, while women who spend a long time caring for an ill husband may be at greater risk because of the combined burdens of caregiving and loss of financial support.

All grieving people continue to need support for many months. The anniversary of a death or the first several holidays spent alone can be particularly difficult.

(See Pulsepoints: "Ten Ways to Cope with Grief".) For individuals who remain intensely distressed, or whose grief does not ease over time, therapy and medication may be enormously helpful—and potentially life-saving. Grieving parents, partners, or adult children are at increased risk of serious physical and mental illness, suicide, and premature death. The family members of a suicide victim are especially likely to need, and benefit from, professional help in sorting out their feelings of failure, anger, and sorrow.

The Effects of Grief

Men and women who lose partners, parents, or children endure so much stress that they're at increased risk of serious physical and mental illness, and even of premature death. Studies of the health effects of grief have found the following:

- Grief produces changes in the respiratory, hormonal, and central nervous systems, and may affect functions of the heart, blood, and immune systems.
- Grieving adults may experience mood swings between sadness and anger, guilt and anxiety. They may feel physically sick, lose their appetites, sleep poorly, or fear that they're going crazy because they "see" the deceased person in different places.
- Friends and remarriage offer the greatest protection against health problems.
- Some widows may have increased rates of depression, suicide, and death from cirrhosis of the liver. The greatest risk factors are poor previous mental and physical health, and a lack of social support.[22]

Methods of Mourning

Grief is a psychological necessity, not self-indulgence. Psychotherapists refer to grief as work, and it is—slow, tedious, and painful. Yet only by working through grief, by dealing with feelings of anger and despair, and adjusting emotionally and intellectually to the loss, can bereaved individuals make their way back to the living world of hope and love.[23]

Some widows and widowers move through the grieving process without experiencing extreme distress. Others stop somewhere in the midst of normal grieving and become clinging and overreliant, continue to pine for the deceased, or show signs of denial, avoidance, or anxiety. Individuals who lose children or spouses in car accidents are particularly likely to remain depressed and anxious years later. One of the most devastating losses is the death of a child killed by a drunk driver. Many years

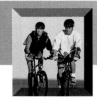

Pulsepoints   Ten Ways to Cope with Grief

1. Accept your feelings—sorrow, fear, emptiness, whatever—as normal.

2. Don't try to deny emotions such as anger, guilt, despair, or relief.

3. Let others help you—by bringing you food, by taking care of daily necessities, by providing companionship and comfort. (It will make them feel better, too.)

4. Express your feelings—through tears, recollections, and talking with others—so that you can accept the loss.

5. Don't feel that you must be strong and brave and silent, though you have every right to keep your grief private.

6. Face each day as it comes. Let yourself live in the here-and-now until you're ready to face the future.

7. Give yourself time—perhaps more than you ever imagined—for the pain to ebb, the scars to heal, and your life to move on.

8. Commemorate. A funeral or memorial service can help you come to terms with a loved one's death and provides an opportunity to celebrate the dead person's life.

9. Don't think there's a right or wrong way to grieve. Mourning takes many forms, and there's no set timetable for working through the various stages of grief.

10. Seek professional counseling if you remain intensely distressed for more than six months or your grief does not ease over time. Therapy can be enormously helpful—and can help prevent potentially serious physical and psychological problems.

---

afterward parents often cannot find any "meaning" in what happened.[24]

Childhood Losses

The poet Edna St. Vincent Millay once described childhood as "the kingdom where nobody dies." Until about age 3, children have no concept of death. By age 9, most understand that death is the end of life and is inevitable.

When death does invade the magical world of childhood, its effects can be so traumatic that they last a lifetime. Because they may not be able to verbalize their grief, young children often "act out" their feelings. Parents and teachers should watch for danger signs, such as repeated aggressive or hostile behavior toward others, a prolonged drop in school performance, or regressive or insecure behaviors (bed-wetting, thumb-sucking, or clinging to a blanket or toy). These behaviors may continue for some time after the actual loss.

Strategies for Change

Helping a Child Cope with Death

✔ Don't hide your own sadness, because a child can often sense unexpressed feelings and will feel excluded. However, you should try not to convey a sense of anxiety about the future.

✔ Communicate with the child at his or her level. Offer clear, simple information.

✔ Give the child every opportunity to ask questions about the death. Some children may feel that they did something wrong or were responsible for the death. They need frequent reassurance to the contrary.

✔ To establish feelings of stability and security, try to avoid other major changes in the child's life for about six months.

Helping Survivors

Although we grieve for the dead, the living are the ones who need our help. Bereavement is such an intense state that survivors may be too numb or too stunned to ask for help. Family and friends must take the initiative and spend time with them, even if that means sitting together silently. Offer empathy and support, and let the grieving person know with verbal and nonverbal expressions that you care and wish to help. Simply being there is enough to let your friend know you care.

You may also wish to write a simple note expressing your sympathy. A phrase, such as "I want to let you know I'm thinking of you and praying for you," can mean a great deal. A small gift, such as a book or plant, is also thoughtful. Or you can invite your friend to do

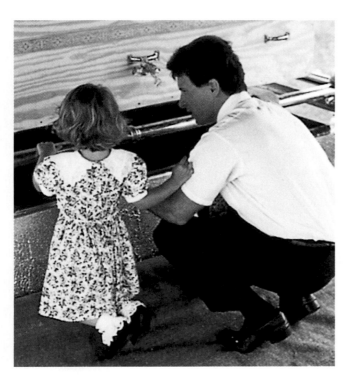

Openness, honest communication, and concern for the child's feelings and needs are all important in helping a child deal with death.

something with you. Choose something you know your friend might enjoy—a walk in the country or a concert. And don't just give your help over the first few days or weeks and then withdraw. Grieving people continue to need support for many months. The first anniversary of a death or the first holiday spent alone can be particularly difficult.

Most bereaved people don't need professional psychological counseling. In most instances, sharing their feelings with friends is all that's needed. However, you should urge a friend or relative to seek help if he or she shows no sign of grieving, or exhibits as much distress a year after the loss as during the first months. The family members of a suicide victim are those most likely to need, and benefit from, professional help in sorting out their feelings of failure, anger, and sorrow.

Making This Chapter Work for You
Understanding the Meaning of Death

■ Many states define death as the end of all functioning of the brain, including those parts of the brain that control breathing and circulation. But while death itself is an end, dying can be a long, complex process.

■ Individuals with fatal illnesses may go through various emotional stages: denial, anger, bargaining, depression, and acceptance.

■ The ability to sustain life by artificial means has created agonizing dilemmas for health-care professionals and the families of individuals in vegetative states. The courts have upheld an individual's right to refuse treatment and have allowed patients with no hope of recovery to be removed from ventilators and feeding tubes.

■ You can assure that your wishes concerning heroic treatments are heeded by several means, including "advance directives," such as health-care proxies and living wills. They allow individuals to state their wishes for treatment options and to designate a friend or relative to make decisions for them.

■ In many states, a handwritten holographic will is considered a legal document.

■ People over 18 years of age can designate that in the event of their death, their organs are to be donated to others.

■ Dying patients often share common physical and mental symptoms, whether they die in a hospital or at home.

■ Hospice care provides comfort, support, and needed treatment for the terminally ill in a home or home-like setting.

■ Many individuals with deadly or severe illnesses may consider suicide. Often they are suffering from untreated depression.

■ Euthanasia involves active participation in ending a dying person's life. Dyathanasia refers to passive willingness to withhold or stop any extraordinary measures to sustain life.

■ Some lawmakers and patient advocates no longer believe that it's unethical for doctors to aid in the suicide of a rational patient, but physician-assisted suicide has raised many thorny legal and ethical issues.

■ When a loved one dies, individuals must deal with many practical matters, including funeral and burial arrangements. They may be asked their approval for an autopsy to determine the cause of death or to advance medical knowledge or training.

■ Grief encompasses many feelings, including sadness, anger, guilt, despair, confusion, relief, and fear, and has profound effects on the body. Various individuals mourn in different ways, depending on the cause of

Health Online

Crisis, Grief, and Healing   http://www.webhealing.com/

This site is a resource for anyone suffering from grief. Perhaps the most remarkable section of this page is A Place to Honor Grief, in which you can remember a person in your life who has died by writing about him or her, and read about others who have experienced similar losses. There is also an online discussion forum and links to information on death and bereavement.

Think about it...

- Have you ever experienced the death of a loved one? If so, do you think writing about the experience would help you heal from the loss?

- Read some of the entries on this site by people who have lost friends and family members. What do their stories have in common? What are some of the different reactions you find?

- What would you do if you found out you had a short time left to live? What does your answer say about your feelings toward life and death?

the death, the age and health of the person who died, and the survivor's age and life circumstances.

Thinking about death can be difficult. It can also be peaceful, depending on how we envision what is beyond. Realizing that life won't go on forever can be a frightening thought. However, the realization that our lives have limits is what makes every day, every minute, of living so very precious.

Key Terms

The terms listed here are used within the chapter. Page numbers are included for each term. A definition of each term is given in the green Glossary pages at the end of this book.

advance directives *596*
autoscopy *603*
coma *596*
do-not-resuscitate (DNR) *599*
dyathanasia *604*

euthanasia *604*
holographic will *599*
hospice *602*
living wills *599*
near-death experiences *602*

persistent vegetative state *596*
terminal illness *601*
thanatology *595*
transcendence *603*

Review Questions

1. How is death defined?

2. What are the five stages of a person's emotional reaction to a terminal illness, as described by Elisabeth Kübler-Ross?

3. What is euthanasia?

4. How does death affect the survivor? What are some of the physiological responses associated with grief?

5. What determines the length and intensity of grief? Can you name some strategies for dealing with grief?

6. What is the difference between a living will and a holographic will? What might a living will contain?

Critical Thinking Questions

1. Do you think that coming to terms with mortality allows an individual to live each day to its fullest, rather than putting off what he or she would like to do until tomorrow? How does this concept affect your own life? Explain. Do you believe in a next life or a greater reality? If so, how does this affect your view of life and death?

2. In 20 cases over the last 50 years, family members accused of mercy killings of fatally ill relatives have gone to trial. One was a father who held off hospital workers with a pistol while he unplugged his baby's respirator. Another was a man who suffocated his wife, who had Alzheimer's disease, with a pillow. Only three of the defendants were sentenced to jail. Do you think these individuals should have been put on trial? Should all have been punished? Are there circumstances that would make mercy killing a crime in some cases but not in others?

3. As many as 10,000 people in this country are chronically unconscious, kept alive by artificial respirators and feeding tubes. What if you were in an accident that left you in a vegetative state? Would you want doctors to do everything possible to fight for your life? Would you want to spend months or even years totally unaware of your surroundings? Should healthcare professionals have the right to declare that anyone is too old, too ill, or too frail to try to save? Should they have the right to insist that someone live on even if that person isn't experiencing much of a "life"?

Connections to Personal Health Interactive

To enhance your understanding of the material covered in this chapter, check out the following study aids on the **Personal Health Interactive CD-ROM** *. Each numbered icon within the chapter corresponds to an appropriate activity listed here.*

19.1 Personal Insights: How Do You Feel About Death?

19.2 Chapter 19 Review

References

1. Dyer, Kristi. "Reshaping Our Views of Death and Dying." *Journal of the American Medical Association*, March 4, 1992.

2. Kübler-Ross, Elisabeth. *Death: The Final Stage of Growth.* Englewood Cliffs, NJ: Prentice-Hall, 1975.

3. Phillips, David, et al. "The Birthday: Lifeline or Deathline?" *Psychosomatic Medicine*, September–October 1992.

4. Lo, Bernard. "Improving Care near the End of Life: Why Is It So Hard?" *Journal of the American Medical Association*, Vol. 274, No. 20, November 22–29, 1995. SUPPORT Principal Investigators "A Controlled Trial to Improve Care for Seriously Ill Hospitalized Patients" *Journal of the American Medical Association*, Vol. 274, No. 20, November 22–29, 1995.

5. Carney, Maria, and Sean R. Morrison. "Advance Directives: When, Why, and How to Start Talking." *Geriatrics*, Vol. 52, No. 4, April 1997.

6. Parkman, Cynthia, and Barbara Calfee. "Advance Directives: Honoring Your Patient's End-of-Life Wishes." *Nursing*, Vol. 27, No. 4, April 1997.

7. Thomas, William, et al. "Advance Directives in the Perioperative Setting." *AORN Journal*, Vol. 66, No. 4, October 1997.

8. Hill, T. Patrick. "Last Rights." *American Health*, November 1993.

9. McCue, Jack. "The Naturalness of Dying." *Journal of the American Medical Association*, Vol. 273, No. 13, April 5, 1995. McCormick, Thomas, and Becky Conley. "Patients' Perspectives on Dying and the Care of Dying Patients." *The Western Journal of Medicine*, Vol. 163, No. 3, September 1995.

10. Mitchell, Deborah. "The 'Good' Death." *Geriatrics*, Vol. 52, No. 8, August 1997.

11. Fried, Linda, et al. "Risk Factors for 5-year Mortality in Older Adults." *Journal of the American Medical Association*, Vol. 279, No. 8, February 26, 1998.

12. Barrett-Connor, Elizabeth, and Cynthia Stuenkel. "Questions of Life and Death in Old Age." *Journal of the American Medical Association*, Vol. 279, No. 8, February 26, 1998.

13. McNeilly, Dennis, and Kristine Hillary. "The Hospice Decision: Psychosocial Facilitators and Barriers." *Omega—The Journal of Death and Dying*, Vol. 35, No. 2, September 1997.

14. Wrenn, Robert. "The Near Death Experience," *Omega—The Journal of Death and Dying*, Vol. 35, No. 4, December 1997.

15. Greyson, B., and N. E. Bush. "Distressing Near-Death Experiences." *Psychiatry*, February 1992. Morse, Melvin, and Paul Perry. *Transformed by the Light*. New York: Tillard, 1992.

16. Hendin, Herbert. *Suicide in America*, New and revised edition. New York: W. W. Norton, 1995.

17. Hales, Dianne, and Robert Hales. *Caring for the Mind*. New York: Bantam Books, 1995.

18. Kaveny, M. Cathleen. *Assisted Suicide, the Supreme Court, and the Constitutive Function of the Law*. Hastings Center Report, September–October 1997.

19. Roberts, Patricia. "Doctor-Assisted Suicide Stirs Physicians' Fears." *Christianity Today*, Vol. 41, No. 14, December 8, 1997.

20. Mariner, Wendy. "Physician Assisted Suicide and the Supreme Court: Putting the Constitutional Claim to Rest." *American Journal of Public Health*, Vol. 87, No. 12, December 1997.

21. "Pathologists Request Autopsy Revival." *Journal of the American Medical Association*, Vol. 273, No. 24, June 28, 1995.

22. Prigerson, Holly et al. "Complicated Grief and Bereavement-Related Depression as Distinct Disorders." *American Journal of Psychiatry*, Vol. 152, No. 1, January 1995.

23. Smith-Stoner, Marilyn, and Amy Lynn Frost. "Coping with Grief and Loss: Bringing Your Shadow Self into the Light." *Nursing*, Vol. 28, No. 2, February 1998.

24. Viederman, Milton. "Grief: Normal and Pathological Variants." *American Journal of Psychiatry*, Vol. 152, No. 1, January 1995.

CHAPTER 20

TAKING CHARGE OF YOUR HEALTH

After studying the material in this chapter, you should be able to:

Define *self-care,* and **describe** appropriate self-care actions.

Describe different types of health-care professionals, and explain what to consider in selecting a health-care professional.

Describe the different types of health-care facilities.

Explain how medical treatments are evaluated.

Discuss the issues facing the U.S. health-care system today.

List and **explain** the most common methods of paying for medical care.

*H*ealth care in the United States is among the best in the world. Our physicians are well trained; our hospitals are modern; our technology is state-of-the-art. Americans use more health services, see more physicians, undergo more surgery, take more prescription drugs, and spend more time in hospitals than the citizens of any other nation. We also spend more on health-care services. Medical costs are higher in the United States than in any other country: almost $1 trillion a year.[1]

Despite such enormous expense, not every American receives good, or even adequate, medical care. Consumers have long complained about insensitive treatment, lack of comprehensive care, and far too little emphasis on the prevention of disease. Because of recent efforts to curb spending, health-care providers may now seem to pay greater attention to cost than caring. And because of a lack of insurance, millions of people have limited, if any, access to needed health services.

Because of the dramatic changes in the American health-care system described in this chapter, now more than ever you have to be a savvy, informed, and involved health-care consumer. The reason for learning how to take charge of your health care is simple: No one cares more about your health than you do, and no one will fight harder on your behalf.

Personal Health Care

Knowing how to spot health problems, what to expect from health-care professionals, and where to turn for appropriate treatment can help you keep your own costs down while ensuring the best possible care.

Self-Care

Most people do treat themselves. You probably prescribe aspirin for a headache, chicken soup or orange juice for a cold, or a weekend trip to unwind from stress. At the very least, you should know what your **vital signs** are and how they compare against normal readings (see Figure 20-1).

Some simple tests, such as examinations of the skin, breasts, and testicles for changes that might be an early indication of cancer, require no special equipment and should be part of your normal health routine (see Chapter 18). Other tests require diagnostic equipment, such as digital blood pressure cuffs that inflate automatically and print out the reading, date, and time; ovulation pre-

dictors; and home pregnancy tests. Home testing can be useful, but it is not a substitute for medical evaluation. An essential part of taking good care of yourself is knowing when to seek professional care.

Self-care also can mean getting involved in the self-help movement, which has grown into a major national trend involving an estimated 25 million Americans. Initially criticized for implicitly blaming victims rather than changing society, many self-help groups have become more politicized and are working not just to address specific needs of individuals, but to transform social structures.

The internet has had a tremendous impact. According to some experts, it "may represent the most powerful new element in self-help's future," primarily by providing person-to-person communication and support.[2] For example, an estimated 40,000 people with diabetes share information and experience via chat rooms and other web sites. The American Self-Help Clearinghouse has an information hotline and a directory of more than 700 self-help groups; the Clearinghouse and many of the groups are (listed in the Yellow Pages at the back of this book).

Figure 20-1

What's normal? How to check your vital signs.

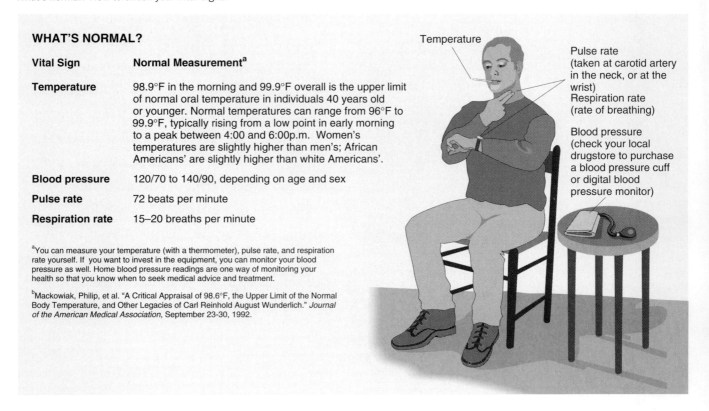

WHAT'S NORMAL?

Vital Sign	Normal Measurement[a]
Temperature	98.9°F in the morning and 99.9°F overall is the upper limit of normal oral temperature in individuals 40 years old or younger. Normal temperatures can range from 96°F to 99.9°F, typically rising from a low point in early morning to a peak between 4:00 and 6:00p.m. Women's temperatures are slightly higher than men's; African Americans' are slightly higher than white Americans'.
Blood pressure	120/70 to 140/90, depending on age and sex
Pulse rate	72 beats per minute
Respiration rate	15–20 breaths per minute

[a]You can measure your temperature (with a thermometer), pulse rate, and respiration rate yourself. If you want to invest in the equipment, you can monitor your blood pressure as well. Home blood pressure readings are one way of monitoring your health so that you know when to seek medical advice and treatment.

[b]Mackowiak, Philip, et al. "A Critical Appraisal of 98.6°F, the Upper Limit of the Normal Body Temperature, and Other Legacies of Carl Reinhold August Wunderlich." *Journal of the American Medical Association*, September 23-30, 1992.

Temperature

Pulse rate (taken at carotid artery in the neck, or at the wrist)
Respiration rate (rate of breathing)

Blood pressure (check your local drugstore to purchase a blood pressure cuff or digital blood pressure monitor)

Dental Care

The good news is that, thanks to fluoridated water and toothpaste, and improved dental care, Americans' teeth are healthier than in the past. Today's children have far less tooth decay than their parents had, and adults are keeping their teeth longer. Thirty years ago, 64% of adults between ages 36 and 64 were toothless, compared with 26% today—thanks primarily to advances in the prevention and treatment of oral disease.[3] The bad news is that, without good self-care, you can—and probably will—lose some teeth to decay and gum disease. The best way to prevent such problems is through proper and regular brushing and flossing.

Gum, or periodontal, **disease**, is an inflammation that attacks the gum and bone that hold your teeth in place. The culprit is **plaque**, the sticky film of bacteria that forms on teeth. More than 300 species of bacteria live under the gum-line, and about half a dozen have been linked to serious gum problems. The early stage of gum disease is called **gingivitis**. If untreated, it develops into a more serious form known as **periodontitis**, in which plaque moves down the tooth to the roots, which then become infected. In advanced periodontitis, the infection destroys the bone and fibers that hold teeth in place.

Symptoms of gum disease include bleeding during brushing or flossing, redness and puffiness of gums, tenderness or pain, persistent bad breath or a bad taste in the mouth, receding gums, shifted or loosened teeth, and changes in the way your teeth fit together when you bite. Treatments include scraping plaque and tartar off the crown and root of the tooth, followed by scaling or smoothing the surfaces of the root, or **flap surgery**, in which the gum is lifted and diseased tissue and bone removed.

Strategies for Prevention
······································
Taking Care of Your Mouth

✔ Brush your teeth every morning and every night. Oral bacteria reach their highest count during sleep because fluids in the mouth accumulate. Nighttime cleaning reduces the bacterial population; morning cleaning lets you reduce the buildup.

✔ Use a toothpaste that has the American Dental Association (ADA) seal of acceptance and a toothbrush with soft, rounded bristles. Replace your toothbrush every three months.

✔ Hold the brush at a 45-degree angle from your gums.

Pay particular attention to the space between your teeth and gums, especially on the inside, toward your tongue. Brush for two to five minutes. Don't brush too vigorously. If you scrub as hard as you can, you may cause damage to teeth and gums. Abrasion—a problem for more than half of American adults—erodes tooth surfaces, weakens teeth, and increases sensitivity to hot and cold foods.

✔ Because brushing can't reach plaque and food trapped between teeth, daily flossing is essential. Using waxed or unwaxed floss, start behind the upper and lower molars at one side of your mouth and work toward the other side. (See Figure 20-2.)

✔ See your dentist twice a year for routine cleaning and examination. To find a dentist, call a local dental school, which may have a public clinic, or check with your county dental society. Ask for information regarding fees, hours, and after-hour emergency service. Your dentist should take a complete **medical history** from you and update it every six months, examine your mouth for signs of cancer, and thoroughly outline all treatment options.

✔ Make sure that everyone who works on the inside of your mouth wears a mask and rubber gloves to reduce the risk of disease transmission (i.e., bacterial and viral infections, such as hepatitis, herpes, and HIV).

✔ Check out your family's dental insurance coverage. About 40% of employed Americans have dental plans, which generally cover all costs for regular six-month checkups and cleanings and a percentage of the costs for fillings, gum treatment, root canals, and so on.[4]

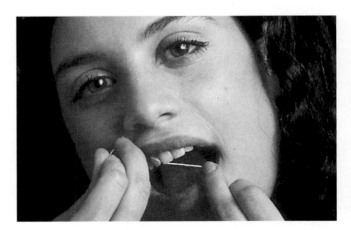

Figure 20-2

Flossing every day helps prevent gum disease. Although brushing keeps your teeth clean, it can't reach the plaque or food trapped between them. Using a gentle sawing motion, work the floss down to your gum-line. Move the floss up and down to scrape the sides of each tooth. In this way, clean between all your teeth, using a fresh section of floss for each tooth.

Self-Survey

Do You Know Your Medical Rights?

You or someone you love is sick. You're anxious and apprehensive, and you want your doctors and nurses to provide the best possible care. The last thing you may be thinking about is the fact that you have rights—as a patient, parent, spouse, or relative. These include legal rights, which would definitely or probably be backed by law if a case went to court, and human rights, which are recognized as critical to human dignity even without formal legal recognition. The first step to making sure your medical rights are protected and respected is knowing what they are. The following quiz is a good way to start. To complete it, simply answer Yes or No to the following questions:

1. Your 8-year-old son is injured in a ball game and rushed to the hospital. At the emergency room, staff members ask you to step outside while they examine the frightened, sobbing boy. Do you have to leave? ____

2. You're going to the hospital for an operation, and you want your partner to be with you through all tests and consultations and to be able to visit you at any time of the day or night. Can the hospital refuse? ____

3. You're moving to another city, and you ask your physician for copies of your medical records. He refuses, but agrees to send them to your new doctor. Do you have the right to see them yourself? ____

4. Upon entering a hospital, you're asked to sign a blanket consent form, allowing physicians to administer whatever treatments they deem necessary and relieving the hospital and your doctor of all liability for your care. Do you have to sign it? ____

5. While on a weekend trip out of your home state, you're seriously injured in a car accident. At the nearest emergency room, you're asked for proof of insurance coverage; you have none. Can the hospital refuse to treat you? ____

6. You have a complex medical problem, and your doctor recommends that you enter a large teaching hospital that provides training for doctors, nurses, and other health professionals. You're afraid that you won't have any privacy. Can you refuse to be interviewed or examined by anyone but your own physician? ____

7. You're hesitant about a treatment your physician strongly recommends. You'd like to seek a second opinion and spend more time discussing your options, but you're afraid that your doctor might drop you as a patient if you consulted another doctor or demanded more attention. Can a physician drop a patient for challenging him or her? ____

8. Hospital staff members routinely call you by your first name or a nickname, such as "Sweetie" or "Sonny," which makes you feel childlike and powerless. Can you insist on more respectful treatment? ____

9. As you prepare to leave the hospital, you're informed that you won't be released until you pay all charges not covered by your insurance policy. Can the hospital keep you until you ante up? ____

10. You agreed to participate in a research test of an experimental drug, mainly because you didn't want to say no to your doctor. However, the side effects are much worse than you anticipated. Can you drop the study? ____

11. When you get a bill from your doctor or hospital, you're stunned by the total amount and can't make sense of the specific items. Can you refuse to pay it? ____

12. You've had a biopsy, and you think your overly protective family doesn't want your doctor to tell you if you have cancer. You'd rather know the facts, however upsetting they might be. Do you have a right to insist that your doctor tell you the whole truth? ____

Answers

Compare your answers with those below. A high total of correct replies (ten or more) indicates that you're well prepared to deal with the health-care system. The lower your score, the more you may need to learn about protecting your medical rights.

1. *No.* Parents have a right to stay with a child 24 hours a day, in either a hospital or a doctor's office. Health professionals can't stop you from remaining with your child during all tests and treatments, or from being in the recovery room when your child regains consciousness after surgery. You can be forced to leave your child alone with health-care providers under only two circumstances: if they suspect child abuse by a parent or guardian or if you're interfering with medical treatment (for example, getting in the way during a diagnostic test).

2. *No.* Adult patients have the right to request that a spouse, grown child, relative, or friend stay with them during an exam, diagnostic test, or treatment. As long as your partner doesn't get in the way, he or she can remain with you and act as your advocate, asking for information and making sure you understand what's happening.

3. *That depends on your state's law.* In most states patients are entitled by law to copies of their medical records. All they have to do is sign a release form and pay a copying fee. Other states guarantee patients access to their records only under certain conditions, such as if

they show good cause for wanting to see them, or exclude lab reports, X rays, prescriptions, and technical information. Some states require patients to obtain access through an attorney or physician.

4. *No.* Legally, you have the right not to sign. However, unless you require emergency care, a hospital can refuse to admit you unless you provide some sort of authorization. Remember that the actual content of hospital forms is not set by law, but by the hospital, and you can challenge or change it. Some consumer advocates suggest signing the blanket form to give consent for routine hospital procedures, such as taking blood pressure, and asking for a separate consent form for each invasive procedure, such as certain diagnostic tests or surgery.

5. *No.* A hospital with emergency facilities cannot turn away anyone requiring immediate treatment, regardless of ability to pay. It doesn't matter whether you actually have insurance but no proof or have no insurance at all. You still have a legal right to prompt attention in a medical emergency (any situation that is likely to cause death, disability, or serious illness if not attended to immediately).

6. *Yes.* Patients always have the right to refuse to be examined by anyone not involved directly in their care. However, in a teaching hospital, you will have more people treating you than in a smaller community hospital. Your own doctor (your "attending" physician) will be in charge, but recent medical school graduates (interns and residents) will provide most of your day-to-day care. In addition, as part of their training, medical students also regularly examine patients. By law, they must identify themselves as students.

7. *No.* Doctors can't drop patients because they sought another opinion or didn't follow their advice. According to the American Medical Association's Principles of Medical Ethics, doctors must comply with a patient's request for a second opinion or a referral to a specialist. Many insurance carriers now require a second opinion for hospitalization or surgery, and most physicians consider them routine.

8. *Yes.* The Joint Commission for the Accreditation of Hospitals (JCAH), which licenses the nation's hospitals, recognized a patient's "right to considerate, respectful care at all times and under all circumstances, with recognition of his personal dignity." Rude, patronizing, or indifferent treatment is not only disrespectful but demeaning and demoralizing.

9. *No.* Anyone can leave the hospital at any time—even against medical advice or without paying the bill. Trying to keep patients against their will for any reason represents false imprisonment.

10. *Yes.* You always have the right to say no or stop any treatment, whether or not it is experimental. You don't have to provide any justification. By law, a physician or hospital can never administer a treatment against your will.

11. *Yes.* Regardless of who is paying for their care, patients have the right to receive and examine an itemized, detailed bill for all services rendered in a doctor's office or hospital. If the charges seem exorbitant, it's recommended that you write a letter to the doctor, clinic, or hospital stating that you are withholding payment (which is your right) until you get an explanation of the charges. If the explanation is unsatisfactory, document the reasons why you believe the charges to be exorbitant. For instance, compile a list of comparable charges for the same services from other health-care providers.

12. *Yes.* By law, physicians must tell patients what their diagnosis and prognosis are—and in language they can understand. The only exceptions are when the patients specifically say that they don't want to know and when the doctor has good reason to believe that the patient could be harmed by the information (for instance, if a patient is extremely depressed and might consider suicide after learning of a fatal disease).

Making Changes
Protecting Your Rights

- Request records from doctors, hospitals, and laboratories to check for any errors regularly. If you've been hospitalized or have had surgery, don't put off checking your records too long. They tend to get lost as time passes.

- Keep your own set of family medical records. Include notes on every doctor's visit, test, procedures, prescriptions, recommended treatments, and so on. Maintaining your own records can help you understand more about your condition and treatment and can also safeguard your legal rights.

- Be very wary of any forms allowing release of your records for insurance reimbursement or for a preemployment physical. Specify exactly which items of information in your record can be released.

- If asked to participate in a research study, find out exactly what the scientists are studying and their motive, why they think you might be a good candidate for the study, how you might benefit, what risks you face, and what are the advantages and disadvantages of not participating.

- Select someone (a "proxy") to make decisions on your behalf in case you can't speak for yourself, and name an alternate in case that person can't be reached. You can simply draw up a document stating that you give so-and-so the power to make medical decisions on your behalf, and have it witnessed by two people.

- Draw up a living will, a document that spells out your wishes on artificial life support. In 39 states, living wills are legally binding. (See Chapter 19 for an in-depth discussion of living wills.)

SOURCE: *American Health,* December 1994.

Health-Care Practitioners

Fewer than 10% of health-care practitioners are physicians; other types of health professionals are assuming more important roles in delivering primary, or basic, health services. As a consumer, you should be aware of the range and special skills of the most common types of health-care providers.

Physicians

A medical doctor (M.D.) trained in American medical schools usually takes at least three years of premedical college courses (with an emphasis on biology, chemistry, and physics) and then completes four (but sometimes three or five) years of medical school. The first two years of medical school are devoted to the study of human anatomy, embryology, pharmacology, and similar basic subjects. During the last two years, students work directly with physicians in hospitals. Medical students who pass a series of national board examinations then enter a one-year internship in a hospital, followed by another two to five years of residency (depending on their specialty), which leads to certification in a particular field, or specialty.

About 500,000 of the nation's 700,000 physicians are specialists or subspecialists, who focus on a specific part of the body, organ system, type of disease, or type of treatment. (For a listing of medical specialties and subspecialties, see Table 20-1.) Traditionally, they have had greater status and earned much larger incomes than primary care physicians—family practitioners, pediatricians, and internists—who provide preventive care, regular checkups, and routine treatments of uncomplicated medical conditions. However, in recent years, changes in health policy (such as increases in Medicare payments to primary care physicians) and in the delivery of services have given a more prominent role to primary care physicians. They now often function as "gatekeepers" who decide whether a patient needs to see a medical specialist (Figure 20-3). In 1995, for the first time in many years, more than half of U.S. medical school seniors said they planned to enter primary care rather than a medical specialty.[5]

Nurses

A registered nurse (R.N.) graduates from a school of nursing approved by a state board and passes a state board examination. R.N.s may have a bachelor's or an associate degree and may specialize in certain areas, such as intensive care or nurse-midwifery. Nurse practitioners, R.N.s with advanced training and experience, may run community clinics or provide screening and preventive care at group medical practices. Some have independent practices.

Licensed practical nurses (L.P.N.s), also called licensed vocational nurses, are licensed by the state. After graduating from state-approved schools of practical nursing, they must take a board exam. They work under the supervision of R.N.s or physicians. Nursing aides and orderlies assist registered and practical nurses in providing services directly related to the comfort and well-being of hospitalized patients.

Specialized and Allied-Health Practitioners

More than 60 different types of health practitioners work with physicians and nurses in providing medical services. Some, such as *occupational therapists,* have at least a bachelor's degree. Allied-health professionals may specialize in a variety of fields. *Clinical psychologists,* for example, have graduate degrees and provide a wide range of mental health services but don't prescribe medications—as do *psychiatrists. Optometrists,* trained in special schools of optometry, diagnose visual abnormalities and prescribe lenses or visual aids; however, they don't prescribe drugs, diagnose or treat eye diseases, or perform surgery—functions performed by *ophthalmologists. Podiatrists* are specially trained, licensed health-care professionals who specialize in problems of the feet. (For a partial listing of allied-health professionals, see Table 20-2.)

Dentists

Most dental students earn a bachelor's degree and then complete two more years of training in the basic sciences and two years of clinical work before graduating with a degree of D.D.S. or D.M.D. (Doctor of Dental Surgery or Doctor of Medical Dentistry). To qualify for a license, graduates must pass both a written and a clinical examination. Dentists may work in general practice or choose a specialty, such as *orthodontics* (straightening teeth).

Chiropractors

Chiropractors hold the degree of Doctor of Chiropractic (D.C.), which signifies that they have had two years of college-level training, plus four years in a health-care school specializing in **chiropractic**, a method of treatment based on the theory that most human diseases are caused by misalignment of the bones *(subluxation).* In particular, chiropractic theory holds that the misalign-

TABLE 20-1 MEDICAL SPECIALTIES

Specialties

Allergy/Immunology	Nuclear Medicine	Plastic Surgery
Anesthesiology	Obstetrics-Gynecology	Preventive Surgery
Colon/Rectal Surgery	Ophthalmology	Psychiatry and Neurology
Dermatology	Orthopedic Surgery	Radiology
Emergency Medicine	Otolaryngology	Surgery
Family Practice	Pathology	Thoracic Surgery
Internal Medicine	Pediatrics	Urology
Neurological Surgery	Physical Medicine and Rehabilitation	

Subspecialties

Blood Banking	Gynecologic Oncology	Nuclear Medicine
Cardiovascular Disease	Hand Surgery	Pediatric Cardiology
Child and Adolescent Psychiatry	Hematology	Pediatric Endocrinology
Critical Care Medicine	Immunology	Pediatric Hematology-Oncology
Diagnostic Laboratory	Infectious Disease	Pediatric Surgery
Endocrinology and Metabolism	Maternal and Fetal Medicine	Pulmonary Disease
Forensic Pathology	Medical Microbiology	Reproductive Endocrinology
Gastroenterology	Medical Oncology	Rheumatology
General Vascular Surgery	Neonatal-Perinatal Medicine	Surgical Critical Care
Geriatric Medicine	Nephrology	

ment of individual vertebrae in the backbone leads to pressure on nerve tissue, which in turn affects other parts of the body. Chiropractors emphasize wellness and healing without drugs or surgery. Although chiroprac-tors may use X rays in making diagnoses, chiropractic treatment consists solely of the manipulation of bones. Spinal manipulation has proven effective in relieving certain types of lower-back pain.

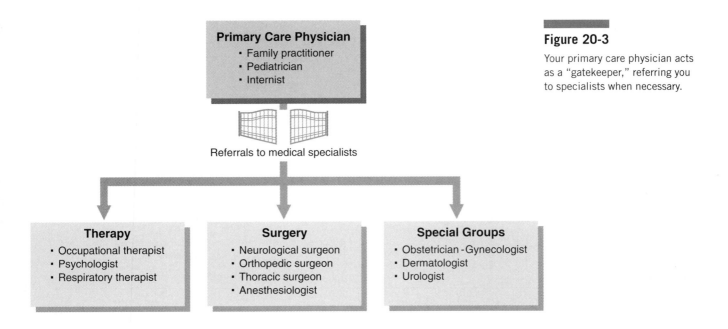

Figure 20-3

Your primary care physician acts as a "gatekeeper," referring you to specialists when necessary.

Table 20-2 Partial Listing of Allied-Health Professionals

Health Workers	Description
Dental hygienists	Provide services for the maintenance of oral health, including cleaning and scaling teeth.
Emergency medical technicians (E.M.T.s)	Licensed to provide immediate care in emergency situations.
Home health aides	Provide personal-care services and some nursing to homebound sick and disabled. Homemakers provide household services under similar circumstances.
Licensed vocational nurses (L.V.N.s)	Trained and licensed to provide hands-on nursing care under the supervision of registered nurses or doctors.
Medical records personnel	Responsible for keeping patients' records complete, accurate, up-to-date, and confidential.
Medical technologists	Perform laboratory tests to help in the diagnosis of disease and to determine its extent and possible causes.
Nurses' aides, orderlies, and attendants	Assist nurses in hospitals, nursing homes, and other settings.
Occupational therapists	Work with disabled patients to help them adapt to their disabilities. This may involve relearning skills needed for daily activities and modifying the physical environment.
Opticians	Fit corrective glasses and manufacture lenses.
Optometrists	Measure vision for corrective lenses and prescribe glasses.
Orthodontists and prosthetists	Prepare and fit braces and artificial limbs.
Paramedics	Provide care in emergency situations; more highly trained than E.M.T.s.
Pharmacists	Trained and licensed to dispense medications in accordance with a doctor's prescription.
Physical therapists	Provide services designed to prevent loss of function and to restore function in the disabled. Exercise, heat, cold, and water are among the agents they use.
Physician's assistants (P.A.s)	Perform physical examinations, provide counseling, and prescribe certain medications under a doctor's supervision.
Podiatrists	Prevent, diagnose, and treat diseases, injuries, and abnormalities of the feet. The only health-care practitioners other than physicians and dentists who may use drugs and surgery to treat illness.
Psychologists	Trained in the study of human behavior; provide counseling and testing in areas related to mental health; also provide individual and group therapy.
Radiologic technicians	Prepare patients for X rays and take and develop X-ray photographs.
Recreational therapists	Provide services to improve patients' well-being through music, dance, and other artistic activities.
Registered dietitians (R.D.s)	Licensed to apply dietary principles to the maintenance of health and the treatment of disease.
Respiratory therapists	Treat breathing disorders, according to a doctor's directions; assist in postoperative rehabilitation.
Social workers	Help patients with finances, insurance, discharge plans, placement, housing, and other social and family programs arising out of illness or disability; also do individual and group counseling and therapy.
Speech pathologists and audiologists	Measure hearing ability and treat disorders of verbal communications.

Source: Columbia University College of Physicians and Surgeons. *Complete Home Medical Guide,* Rev. Ed. New York: Crown, 1989.

The nation's 45,000 chiropractors are licensed by the state. Many insurance programs, including Medicaid, cover chiropractic care. After a long struggle for recognition and respect, chiropractic now ranks as the third largest primary health-care profession in the United States (after medicine and dentistry). An estimated one in twenty Americans visits a chiropractor every year; in all, Americans spend $2.4 billion a year on chiropractic care.

Health-Care Facilities

As a prospective patient, you can choose from various options: a physician's office, a clinic, an emergency room, or a hospital. Most **primary care**—also referred to as ambulatory or outpatient care—is provided by a physician in an office, emergency room, or clinic. *Secondary care* usually is provided by specialists or subspecialists in either an outpatient or inpatient (hospital) setting. *Tertiary care*, available at university-affiliated hospitals and regional referral centers, includes special procedures such as kidney dialysis, open-heart surgery, and organ transplants.

College Health Centers

The American College Health Association estimates that about 1500 institutions of higher learning provide direct health services. Student health centers range in size from small dispensaries staffed by nurses to large-scale, multispecialty clinics that provide both inpatient and outpatient care and are fully accredited by the Joint Commission on Accreditation of Healthcare Organizations. Some serve only students; others provide services for faculty, staff, and family members.

On some campuses, health educators work with the student health centers to provide counseling on such topics as nutrition; tobacco, drug, and alcohol abuse; exercise and fitness; sexuality; and contraception. Some college health centers provide psychological counseling, as well as dental, pharmacy, and optometric services. Some campuses also provide sports-medicine services for student athletes. Services are paid for by various combinations of prepaid health fees, general university funds, fee-for-service charges, and health-insurance reimbursements.

Outpatient Treatment Centers

Increasingly, procedures that once required hospitalization, such as simple surgery, are being performed at outpatient centers, which may be freestanding or affiliated with a medical center. Patients have any necessary tests performed beforehand, undergo surgery or receive treatment, and return home after a few hours to recuperate. Outpatient centers can handle many common surgical procedures, including cataract removal, tonsillectomy, breast biopsy, dilation and curettage (D and C), vasectomy, and face-lifts.

Without the high overhead costs of a hospital, outpatient surgery costs run only about 30% to 50% of standard hospital fees. Today, 70% of hospitals do outpatient, or "in-and-out," surgery. To cut health-care costs, insurance companies are encouraging, or in some cases requiring, their policyholders to choose outpatient surgery. However, operations requiring prolonged general anesthesia (such as abdominal surgery) or extensive postoperative care (such as heart surgery) must still be performed on an inpatient basis.

Freestanding emergency centers (those not part of a hospital) claim that they deliver high-quality medical treatment with maximum convenience in minimal time. Critics dismiss them as impersonal and mechanized, and refer to them as "Big Mac" medicine. Nevertheless, many customers seem pleased. Rather than going to crowded hospital emergency rooms when they slice a finger in the kitchen, they can go to a freestanding emergency center and receive prompt attention.

Hospitals and Medical Centers

Different types of hospitals offer different types of care. The most common type of hospital is the *private*, or community, *hospital*, which may be run on a profit or a nonprofit basis, generally contains 50 to 400 beds, and provides more personalized care than public hospitals do. The quality of care individual patients receive depends mostly on the physicians themselves. *Public hospitals* include city, county, public health service, military, and Veterans Administration hospitals. The quality of patient care depends on the overall quality of the institution.

Of the more than 6500 hospitals nationwide, about 300 are major *academic medical centers* or teaching hospitals. Affiliated with medical schools, they generally provide the most up-to-date and experienced care, because staff physicians must stay current in order to teach their students. These centers, with the best equipment, researchers, and resources, have been described as representing "the high-technology care that many U.S. citizens associate with worldwide leadership in the quality of their medical care."[6]

Such care comes at a price, however: the cost of treatment at all teaching hospitals averages approximately 20% higher than at nonteaching hospitals. At major teaching hospitals with large graduate training programs for physicians and other health providers, the costs are as much as 45% higher than those at non-teaching hospitals. Faced with declining revenues as a result of the advent of managed care (discussed later in this chapter), teaching hospitals have been forced to make major cutbacks in personnel and patient services. Many are forming networks with other hospitals and developing less costly methods (such as home health services) to deliver health care.[7]

In January 1998 a panel, appointed by the U.S. Department of Health and Human Services to examine the state of federally subsidized university medical centers, recommended that the centers, comprised of medical schools and their affiliated teaching hospitals, collaborate more fully with government, the public, and the insurance industry to set goals that promote public health and provide quality medical care within their home regions. The panel also identified potential threats to the centers, including the growth of managed care plans and shrinking federal funding.[8]

The Joint Commission on the Accreditation of Healthcare Organizations (JCAH) reviews all hospitals every three years. Eighty percent of hospitals qualify for JCAH accreditation. If you have to enter a hospital and your health insurance or plan allows a choice, try to find out as much as you can about the alternatives available to you:

• Talk to your physician about a hospital and why he or she recommends it.

• As a cost-cutting strategy, many hospitals have cut back on the use of registered nurses. Check with the local nursing association about the ratio of patients to nurses, and the ratio of R.N.s to licensed practical, or vocational, nurses.

• Find out room rates and charges for ancillary services, including tests, lab work, X rays, and medications. Check with your health plan to see whether you need preapproval for any of these costs and ask what you will be expected to pay.

• Ask how many times in the past year the hospital has performed the procedure recommended for you, and what the success and complication rates have been. Ask about the hospital's nosocomial (hospital-caused) infection rate and accident rate. You also have the right to information on the number and types of malpractice claims filed against a hospital.

• If possible, go on a tour of the hospital. Does the setting seem comfortable? Is the staff courteous? Does the hospital seem clean and efficiently run?

Emergency Services Hospital emergency rooms should be used only in a true emergency. Most are overwhelmed, understaffed, and underfinanced—particularly in big cities. Patients usually see a different physician each time; he or she deals with their main complaints but doesn't have time for a full examination. Extensive tests and procedures are difficult to arrange in an emergency room, and patients who don't have truly urgent problems may have to wait for a long time. Emergency-room fees are higher than those for standard office visits and are not always covered by medical insurance.

Inpatient Care Inpatient hospital care remains the most expensive form of health care. Health-insurance companies and health-care plans (described below) often demand a second opinion or make their own evaluation before approving coverage of an elective, or non-emergency, hospital admission. As another means of controlling costs, health insurers (including Medicare) may limit hospital stays or pay for hospital care on the basis of **diagnostic-related groups**, or **DRGs**. Under this system, hospitals are paid according to a patient's diagnosis—for example, a set number of dollars for every appendectomy. If the hospital can treat and discharge patients more quickly than the national average for that DRG, it makes money. On the other hand, if a patient develops unexpected complications or is slow to recover, the hospital loses money.

Because hospital stays are shorter than in the past, patients often leave "quicker and sicker"—after a shorter stay and not as far along in their recovery. Nevertheless, the benefits of shorter hospital stays, including reduced complications and more rapid resumption of normal life activities, may outweigh the slightly increased risks associated with early discharge.

The Risks of a Hospital Stay

Hospitals are places where lives are both saved and lost, and the quality of care varies greatly. A report on 14,000 patients in five states found that large hospitals in big cities provide better care and have lower death rates than small, rural hospitals with fewer than 100 beds.[9] Overall, medical therapy in a hospital results in injuries to an estimated 1.3 million people every year, two-thirds of which could be avoided.[10]

The risks associated with hospitalization include what health workers call the "terrible I's": infection; inac-

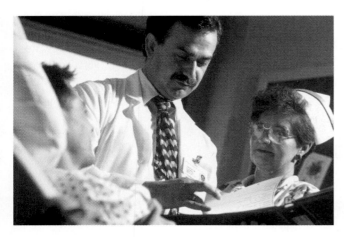

A healthy hospital stay. Read consent forms carefully and ask for more information if you don't understand. Talk to the staff and pay attention to your care routine.

tivity; incorrect actions; and the inherent risks of drugs, X rays, and false lab tests. The simplest method for preventing hospital-acquired infection—handwashing—is often ignored by health-care providers, according to a 1995 American Medical Association report. Only 14 to 59% of physicians wash their hands regularly, as do 25 to 45% of nurses and 23 to 73% of other health-care workers.[11]

Surgical and medication mistakes are another hazard. In highly publicized cases, hospital physicians have amputated a patient's healthy leg, operated on the wrong side of a woman's brain, and administered deadly doses of cancer drugs. As hospitals cut back on staff and services in order to control costs, the likelihood of such errors may increase.

Strategies for Prevention

How to Survive a Hospital Stay

✔ Make sure the name on your wristband is spelled correctly and clearly. Talk to everyone who brings you a pill or performs a test or procedure. Patient charts can get mixed up, and you don't want to undergo a treatment intended for someone else.

✔ Know which medicines you're supposed to get and what they look like. If you're uncertain that a medication is the right one for you, ask someone to double-check.

✔ Make sure the people caring for you wash their hands. A polite reminder won't offend good professionals—and could prevent infection.

✔ Be sure to bring along any recent test results or X rays

that your physician feels may be helpful. You may be able to avoid some repeat testing.

✔ If you're asked to sign a consent form, read it carefully. If you want more information, ask before signing. Don't feel pressured to sign if you want to discuss something with your physician first.

Home Health Care

With hospitals discharging patients sooner, **home health care**—the provision of equipment and services to patients in the home to restore or maintain comfort, function, and health—has become a major industry. Advances in technology have made it possible for treatments once administered only in hospitals—such as kidney dialysis, chemotherapy, and traction—to be performed at home at 10% to 40% of the cost. The physician's house call, once considered an anachronism, has also come back in fashion. According to various surveys, the majority of primary care physicians see patients in their homes.

Hospital discharge planners usually arrange home health care for patients who've been hospitalized. Families can also contact health aides, nurses, and other needed professionals on their own. According to the Health Insurance Association of America, most private insurance policies offer some coverage for these home health care costs.

The Doctor-Patient Relationship

Once the family doctor was indeed part of the family. The family doctor brought babies into the world, shepherded them through childhood, comforted and counseled them, stood by their bedside in their darkest hours. Patients entrusted the doctor with their cares, their confidences, their very lives. In the twentieth century, with dramatic breakthroughs in diagnosing and treating illness, the focus in medicine shifted from the family physician to the specialist, from basic caring to high-tech medical care. Patients today are more likely to be cured of a vast array of illnesses than those of a century ago. However, they often complain of insensitive, uncaring physicians who focus on their diseases rather than on them as individuals.[12]

As more physicians have joined managed-care organizations (discussed later in this chapter), which emphasize efficiency, they sometimes feel pressure to

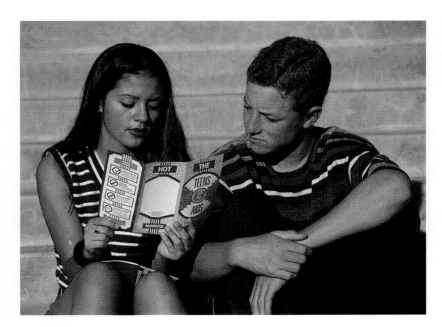

You can improve your health education. Today's physicians are pressured to spend less time with each patient. You can make better use of your physician visits by actively educating yourself about health and health care.

see more patients a day, to spend less time with each, and to discourage expensive tests and treatments. Because physicians have less time and less autonomy, patients today must do more. Your first step should be learning more about your body, any medical conditions or problems you develop, and your options for treatment. You can find a great deal of information available via computer on-line services (which often have discussion groups or "chat rooms" dedicated to a particular medical topic), patient advocacy and support organizations (see the Health Directory at the end of this book for listings), and libraries.

This information can help you know what questions to ask and how to evaluate what your doctor says. But you have to be willing to speak up. "Too many patients are so respectful of—and intimidated by—doctors that they don't realize that they have a right and an obligation to be assertive about their health situation," say Richard Podell, M.D., and William Proctor, authors of *When Your Doctor Doesn't Know Best.* Their advice: Be courageous.

"To be effective as a patient in the current health-care environment, you must have the guts to stand up to your doctor and ask pointed questions. The alert—and safe—patient is the one who can be assertive, even aggressive, with physicians. The goal isn't to pick a fight but to work instead toward an active collaboration. Done smartly and effectively, being an alert patient should improve, not harm, your relationship with your doctor."[13] (See Pulsepoints: "Ten Ways to Get Good Health Care".)

Your "Primary" Physician

The primary care physicians who are playing increasingly important roles in American health care include family practitioners, general internists, and pediatricians. Obstetrician-gynecologists serve as the primary providers of health care for more than half of all women.[14] If you're a woman and your gynecologist is the only physician you see, make sure that he or she performs other tests, such as measuring your blood pressure, in addition to a pelvic and breast exam. If you develop other symptoms or health concerns, ask for an appropriate referral.

At college health centers, clinics, and some health-care organizations, consumers may be assigned to a primary physician or restricted to certain doctors. Even if your choices are limited, don't suspend your critical judgment. If you feel that your assigned physician does not listen to your concerns or is not providing adequate care, you can—and should—request another physician. Your rapport with your primary physician and the feelings of mutual trust and respect that develop between you can have as much of an impact on your well-being as your doctor's technical expertise.

When consumers can freely choose their physicians, they often do so, not just on the basis of qualifications, but also because of the physician's gender, race, or ethnic background. Frustrated by what they see as insensitive treatment by male physicians, many women are turning to female physicians—especially for gynecologic care. For other health services, women say that what

Pulsepoints   Ten Ways to Get Good Health Care

1. Trust your instincts. You know your body better than anyone else. If something is bothering you, it deserves medical attention. Don't let your health-care provider—or your health plan administrator—dismiss it without a thorough evaluation.

2. Inform yourself. Go to the library or an on-line information service and find articles that describe what you're experiencing. The more you know about possible causes of your symptoms, the more likely you are to be taken seriously.

3. Find a good primary care physician who listens carefully and responds to your concerns. Look for a family doctor or general internist who takes a careful history, performs a thorough exam, and listens and responds to your concerns.

4. See your doctor regularly. If you're in your twenties or thirties, you may not need an annual exam, but it's important to get checkups at least every two or three years, not so much for the sake of finding hidden disease, but so you and your doctor can get to know each other and develop a trusting, mutually respectful relationship.

5. Get a second opinion. If you are uncertain of whether to undergo treatment or which therapy is best, see another physician and listen carefully for any doubts or hesitation about what you're considering.

6. Challenge medical judgments based on personal circumstances. Insist that your doctor base any diagnosis on a thorough medical evaluation, not on a value judgment about you or your lifestyle.

7. Seek support. Patient support and advocacy groups can offer emotional support, information on many common problems, and referral to knowledgeable physicians. (See the Hales Health Directory at the back of the book for numbers and addresses.)

8. If your doctor cannot or will not respond to your concerns, get another one. Regardless of your health coverage, you have the right to replace a physician who is not meeting your health-care needs.

9. Speak up. If you don't understand, ask. If you feel that you're not being taken seriously or being treated with respect, say so. Sometimes the only difference between being a patient or becoming a victim is making sure your needs and rights are not forgotten or overlooked.

10. Bring your own advocate. If you become intimidated or anxious talking to physicians, ask a friend to accompany you, to ask questions on your behalf, and to take notes.

---

matters most is having a caring physician who makes them feel comfortable and secure and invites them to participate in treatment decisions.[15]

As the number of minority physicians has increased (up 124 percent for African-American physicians and 335 percent for Asian-American physicians from 1970 to 1980), more racial and ethnic minority group members are seeking out physicians with similar backgrounds. Often they see them as role models for their children. They may also feel that these professionals will have a natural empathy for their needs and concerns. According to a 1995 report in the *Journal of the American Medical Association,* nonwhite physicians provide more care to racial and ethnic minority patients as well as to poorer and sicker patients.[16] Language also affects patient choices. Some individuals, such as Mexican-American and Puerto Rican patients, find it easier to communicate with Spanish-speaking physicians.[17]

One key to making the health-care system work for you lies in choosing a good physician. After seeing your primary care physician, ask yourself the following questions to evaluate the quality of care you are getting.

- Did your physician take a comprehensive history? Was the physical examination thorough?

- Did your physician explain what he or she was doing during the exam?

- Did he or she spend enough time with you?

- Did you feel free to ask questions? Did your physician give you straight answers? Did he or she reassure you when you were worried?

- Does your physician seem willing to admit that he or she doesn't know the answers to some questions?

- Does your physician hesitate to refer you to a specialist even when you have a complex problem that warrants such care?

Look back at your answers. If they make you feel uneasy, have a talk with your physician. Or, find a physician or a health plan that provides better service.

What to Expect in a Medical Exam

Most physicians believe that you don't need annual checkups if you're young and feel well. However, certain types of screening tests should be performed periodically, particularly if you're 45 or older, or if you are at a higher-than-average risk of developing a particular disease, such as high blood pressure (discussed in Chapter 12) or colon cancer (discussed in Chapter 13).

Your physician will want a past medical history, including major illnesses, surgery, and treatments. Report any allergies you have, particularly to drugs, and the medications you take, including aspirin, antacids, sleeping pills, oral contraceptives, and recreational drugs, even if illegal. Your physician may also want to know about topics you consider private, such as sexually transmitted diseases. Remember that he or she is attempting to gather all the information needed to provide you with comprehensive treatment. Note, too, that a physician must report certain information—for example, certain sexually transmitted diseases—to health authorities.

After the physician has asked you questions about your complaints, medical history, and lifestyle, he or she will probably perform the standard tests described below. During the examination, point out any pains, lumps, or skin growths you've noticed. If you feel pain when the physician palpates (feels) any part of your body, say so.

- *Head.* Using a flashlightlike instrument called an *ophthalmoscope,* the physician will look at the lens, retina, and blood vessels of your eyes. For patients over 40, he or she may test for a treatable eye disease called *glaucoma* (a disorder characterized by increased pressure within the eye), which can cause blindness if not detected early. The physician simply presses against the surface of each eye a soft instrument that measures the pressure within the eye and checks to see if the reading is normal. He or she will also examine your ears, mouth, tongue, teeth, and gums.

- *Neck.* Feeling around your neck, the physician will check for enlarged lymph glands (a sign of infection), for lumps in the thyroid gland, and for warning signs of stroke in the neck arteries.

- *Chest.* With a *stethoscope,* the physician will listen to the sounds made by your heart, to detect heart murmurs and irregular contractions, and by your lungs, to detect asthma or emphysema. By tapping on your chest and back with his or her fingers, the physician can tell the size and shape of your heart, which may reveal some forms of heart disease, and whether any fluid has collected in your lungs. The physician will also check for abnormal lumps in a woman's breasts.

- *Abdomen.* Here the physician uses his or her fingers to probe for tender spots and malformations of the liver and other organs, that may reveal signs of alcoholism, hepatitis, or hernias.

- *Rectum and genitals.* With a gloved hand, the physician can feel in the rectum for growths and hemorrhoids. A rectal examination can also reveal enlargement of the male's prostate gland. The physician will check male testicles and spermatic cords for abnormalities.

- *Pelvic examination.* During a pelvic examination, a woman lies on her back, with her heels in stirrups at the end of the examining table and her legs spread out to the sides. The physician inspects the labia, clitoris, and vaginal opening. Using two gloved, lubricated fingers, the physician will check for abnormalities in the vagina, uterus, fallopian tubes, and ovaries. Many physicians will also perform a rectal or rectovaginal (one finger in the rectum and one in the vagina) examination. A nurse or other health-care worker should be present throughout the exam.

The *speculum* is a medical instrument that's used to spread the walls of the vagina so that the inside may be seen. The physician will gently scrape cells from the cervix for a **Pap smear**, a procedure that identifies abnormal cells, that may indicate an infection or, more seriously, cervical cancer, a slow-growing cancer that's usually curable if detected early (see Chapter 13). All women should start having regular Pap smears once they begin having intercourse, or at age 18. While there has been debate about how often women should have Pap smears, many health-care providers recommend Pap smears every year for women who are sexually active or have other risk factors, such as infection with the human papilloma virus (see Chapter 11).

- *Extremities.* The physician may check your knees and other joints for reflexes, which may indicate nerve disorders, and look for tremors in outstretched hands or in the face. The color, elasticity, and wetness or dryness of your skin may alert him or her to nutritional problems, or may indicate diabetes, skin cancer, and the like. Hair and nails may give indications of internal health, such as blood disorders.

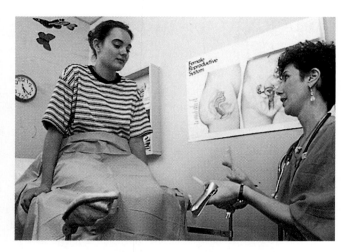

Many women choose female health-care practitioners to provide gynecologic services.

Swelling of the ankles can be an indication of heart, kidney, or liver disease.

- *Pulse and blood pressure.* Your physician may check your pulse in various places, looking for signs of poor circulation. The rhythm and speed of the heart may also signal diseases of the heart or thyroid gland. High blood pressure can be an early warning sign of possible heart attack, stroke, or kidney damage.

Medical Tests

Besides all the diagnostic tests listed above, the physician may order some laboratory and other tests, including the following: (See also the Hales Health Almanac at the back of this book for a comprehensive guide to medical tests.)

- *Chest X ray.* A chest X ray can reveal abnormalities of the heart and lungs; if you're a smoker, the physician may insist on one.

- *Electrocardiogram.* The *electrocardiogram* is a test performed while you're at rest that records the electrical activity of your heart. It can show irregularities in heart rhythm or muscle damage, as well as hardening of the arteries.

- *Urinalysis.* Your urine may be analyzed by a medical laboratory. If sugar (glucose) is found in your urine, your physician may order a separate blood test to check for diabetes. The presence of blood cells may indicate infection of the bladder or kidneys. Abnormal amounts of albumin (protein) in the urine may also suggest kidney disease.

- *Blood tests.* The physician or laboratory technician may draw blood to do a blood cell count. An excess of white blood cells may be an indication of infection or, occasionally, leukemia. A deficiency of red blood cells may indicate anemia. A sample of your blood may also be analyzed to measure the levels of its various components. High levels of glucose may indicate diabetes, and high levels of uric acid may mean gout or kidney stones. A high cholesterol level may indicate cardiac risk (see Chapter 12).

Strategies for Prevention
································
The Whats, Whys, and Hows of Testing

✔ Before undergoing any test, find out why you need it. Get a specific answer, not a "just in case" or "for your peace of mind." If you've had the test before, could the earlier results be used? Would a followup exam be just as helpful?

✔ Get some practical information as well: Are there specific things you should do before the test (such as not eat for a specified period)? How long will the test take? What will the test feel like? Will you need help getting home afterward?

✔ Check out the risks. Any invasive test—one that penetrates the body with a needle, tube, or viewing instrument—involves some risk of infection, bleeding, or tissue damage. Tests involving radiation also present risks. In addition, some people develop allergic reactions to the materials used in testing.

✔ Get information on the laboratory that will be evaluating the test. Ask how often **false positives** or **false negatives** occur. (False positives are abnormal results indicating that you have a particular condition when you really don't; false negatives indicate that you don't have a particular condition when you really do.) Find out about civil or criminal **negligence** suits filed against the laboratory on charges such as failing to diagnose cervical cancer because of incorrect reading of Pap smears.

✔ You'll also want to know what happens when the test indicates a problem: Will the test be repeated? Will a different test be performed? Will treatment begin immediately? Could any medications you're taking (including nonprescription drugs, like aspirin) affect the testing procedures or results?

Developing a Treatment Plan

After your exam, the physician will report his or her findings about your health and complaints, and advise you as to treatment. Depending on your problem, your physician may recommend an **over-the-counter (OTC)** drug, such as aspirin or an antihistamine; prescribe a medication; or recommend more invasive treatment, such as surgery.

Once a treatment recommendation has been made, you face a decision: Do you follow the advice? Be sure you understand fully the consequences of what you do—or don't do. You may be risking harm if, for instance, you don't take the antibiotics prescribed for your strep throat, or if you stop taking them in midtreatment (strep throat can lead to heart damage). For major nonemergency procedures, get more than one physician's opinion. Eight out of ten operations are elective, meaning that they don't have to be performed to save the patient's life.

Your Medical Rights

As a consumer, you have basic rights that help ensure that you know about any potential dangers, receive competent diagnosis and treatment, and retain control and dignity in your interactions with health-care professionals. Many hospitals publish a patient's bill of rights, including your rights to know whether a procedure is experimental; to refuse to undergo a specific treatment; to designate someone else to make decisions about your care if and when you cannot; and to leave the hospital, even against your physician's advice. (See the Self-Survey:, "Do You Know Your Medical Rights?")

You have the right to be treated with respect and dignity, including being called "Mr." or "Ms." or whatever you wish, rather than by your first name. Make clear your preferences. If you feel that health-care professionals are being condescending or inconsiderate in any way, say so—in the same tone and manner that you would like others to use with you. If you're hospitalized, find out if there's a patient advocate or representative at your hospital. These individuals can help you communicate with physicians, make any special arrangements, and get answers to questions or complaints.

You have the right to give consent to donate an organ while alive, or have your organs removed in the event of an accident, injury, or illness that leaves you brain-dead. (See Chapter 19 for definitions of death.) However, you cannot agree to donate a body part for money or other compensation. Congress has prohibited the marketing of organs; any attempt to do so is a felony punishable by up to five years in jail and a $50,000 fine.

Your Right to Information

By law, a patient must give consent for hospitalization, surgery, and other major treatments. **Informed consent** is a right, not a privilege. Use this right to its fullest. Ask questions. Seek other opinions. Make sure that your expectations are realistic and that you understand the potential risks, as well as the possible benefits, of a prospective treatment. Informed consent is required for research studies, but patients often don't realize that they have the right not to participate and to get complete information on the purpose and nature of the study.

Your Medical Records

You have a right to know what is in your medical records. Some states have laws assuring patient access to records. Consumer advocates advise that you routinely request records from physicians, hospitals, and laboratories—first verbally, then in writing. Privacy has become an increasing concern as patients' records have been computerized in large databases. The Medical Information Bureau (MIB) (see the Health Directory for its address and number) obtains information on individuals' medical claims and conditions from about 750 life insurance companies and combines it into the equivalent of a credit report. Anytime you fill out an application for insurance or file a claim for disability or reimbursement, your insurance company or health-care plan can contact MIB to review every medical claim you've made in the previous seven years.[18]

To protect your privacy, don't routinely fill out medical questionnaires or histories. Always ask the purpose and find out who will have access to it. Specifically ask if your history may be entered into a computer database.[19] Tell your physician or health-care group that you do not want your records to leave their offices without your approval. Put it in writing. When you do have to authorize the release of your records, limit the information to a specific condition, physician, and hospital rather than authorizing release of all your records. Contact the MIB to find out if there is a file on you and ask to review it. Be sure to correct any inaccuracies.[20]

Your Right to Good, Safe Care

Concern about **malpractice** suits provides an incentive for physicians to provide high-quality care. The essence of a malpractice suit is the claim that the physician failed to meet the standard of care required of a reasonably skilled and careful medical doctor. Although physicians don't have to guarantee good results to their patients and aren't held liable for unavoidable errors, they are required to use the same care and judgment in treatment that other physicians in the same specialty would use under similar circumstances. To protect themselves financially, physicians, particularly those in surgical specialties who are most likely to be sued, pay tens of thousands of dollars a year in malpractice-insurance premiums. Some of this cost is passed on to patients.

Most lawsuits are based on negligence and assert that a physician failed to render diagnosis and treatment with appropriate professional knowledge and skill. Other cases are brought for failure to provide information, obtain consent, or respect a patient's confidentiality. However, analysis of malpractice cases has shown that, in 70% to 80%, a doctor's attitude and inability to communicate effectively—by devaluing patients' views, delivering information poorly, failing to understand patients' perspectives, or displaying an air of superiority—also played a role.[21]

The Public Citizen Health Research Group has compiled a national directory of "questionable physicians," which lists physicians disciplined by state medical boards or the federal government for offenses ranging from overprescribing drugs to sexual misconduct to negligent or substandard care. Some of these physicians committed minor misdeeds, such as failing to complete continuing medical education requirements. Consumer advocates urge patients to find out why a particular name appears on the list by calling the state licensing board. At the federal level, the agencies most involved in ensuring quality health care are the Food and Drug Administration (FDA), which approves the production and labeling of drugs; and the Federal Trade Commission (FTC), which oversees advertising and prohibits deceptive or false claims.

The American Health-Care System: A Revolution in Progress

In the past, getting health care was fairly simple. When people were sick, they went to their family physician and paid in cash. If they didn't have enough money, the physician would still provide care. Health insurance did not become common as a standard benefit until World War II, when the government imposed wage controls and businesses offered free health-insurance policies to lure prospective employees. For the next 50 years, patients went to the physicians of their choice, with insurance companies usually paying part or all of their fees.

As technological breakthroughs, such as magnetic resonance imaging (MRI) and bone-marrow transplants, transformed modern medicine, subspecialists multiplied, and medical costs spiraled upward. Finally, in the 1990s, health policymakers and the employers that had footed the bills agreed that health costs, which had grown to almost 14% of the gross domestic product, had to be controlled.[22]

The first Clinton administration's plan to reform health-care failed to meet with congressional approval in 1994. However, other attempts to reduce health-care costs have continued, including the movement toward **managed care**, a new way of delivering and paying for health-care services. Managed care organizations provide health- care of health-care insurance at lower costs to employers. The tradeoff for such savings is that a third party makes the final decision on when or if a medical visit or treatment is necessary.[23] This differs from traditional *fee-for-service* medicine, in which patients decide when to seek care and choose which physician to see. (See Figure 20-4.)

Both fee-for-service and managed-care systems have drawbacks. Fee-for-service medicine errs on the side of doing too much and providing unneeded tests and therapies. Managed-care organizations are more likely to do too little so they can keep costs low. "The more care you're given by a private physician, the more money he or she can make," note Richard Podell, M.D., and William Proctor, authors of *When Your Doctor Doesn't Know Best*. In some managed-care plans, by comparison, your primary care doctor "may have funds deducted from his or her income each time you're referred to a specialist."[24]

Traditional Health Insurance

In the past, most working Americans relied on conventional **indemnity** insurance policies to pay major medical expenses. Policyholders paid a percentage (generally 20%) of hospitalization costs and a deductible (a minimum paid out each year before the insurance company pays anything). While indemnity insurance gave patients freedom to choose physicians and hospitals, it often failed to cover routine physical exams and screening tests. Individuals with "preexisting" conditions often

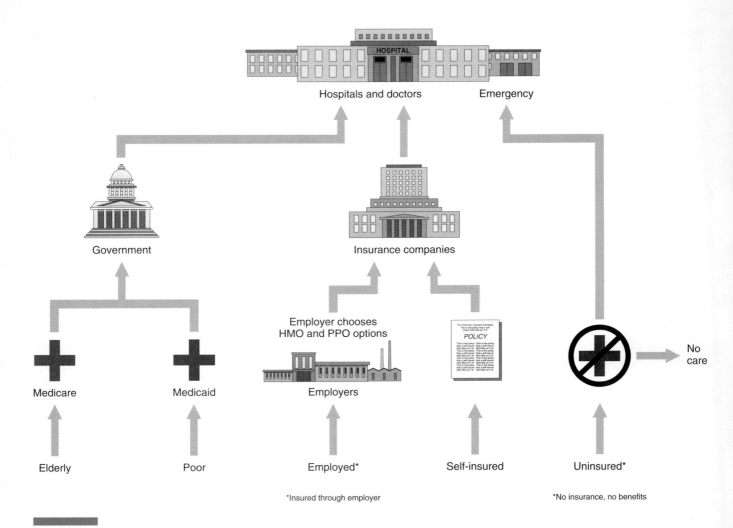

Figure 20-4

Medical coverage in the United States is complex; you and your doctor are connected through a bureaucracy of policies and agencies.

could not qualify for coverage or were not reimbursed for treatments related to these conditions. In the last decade, as health-care costs skyrocketed, insurers increasingly refused to pay claims, canceled groups with high medical bills, or denied coverage to people in high-risk occupations.

Managed Care

There has been a dramatic shift away from indemnity insurance to managed-care plans, which cost less but also offer less freedom and flexibility. (See Table 20-3.) Managed-care organizations, which take various forms, deliver care through a network of physicians, hospitals, and other health-care professionals who agree to provide their services at fixed or discounted rates.

Consumers in a managed-care group must follow certain procedures in advance of seeking care (for example, getting prior approval for a test or treatment) and must abide by a limit on reimbursement for certain services. Some procedures may be deemed unnecessary and not be covered at all. Patients who choose to see a physician who is not a participating member of the medical-insurance coverage group may have to pay the entire fee themselves.[25]

Managed-care plans have been criticized for pressuring providers to "undertreat" patients—for example, sending them home from the hospital too soon or denying them costly tests or treatments. Some members complain of long waits, the need to switch primary physicians if their doctor leaves the plan, difficulty getting approval for needed services, and a sense that

TABLE 20-3 THE GROWTH OF MANAGED CARE

Year	Managed Care	Fee-for-Service
1988	29%	71%
1992	55%	45%
1996	74%	26%

SOURCE: KPMG Peat Marwick LLP Survey of Employer Sponsored Health Benefits, 1996; 1995; 1994; 1993; 1992.

providers pay more attention to the bottom line than to their health needs. There have been increasing demands for government regulation of managed-care plans.[26]

Health Maintenance Organizations (HMOs)

Health maintenance organizations, or **HMOs**, are managed-care plans that emphasize routine care and prevention by providing complete medical services in exchange for a predetermined monthly payment. HMOs deliver health care to more than 25% of the population.[27]

In a *group-model* HMO, physicians provide care in offices at a clinic run by the HMO. In an *individual practice association (IPA)*, or network HMO, independent physicians provide services in their own offices.

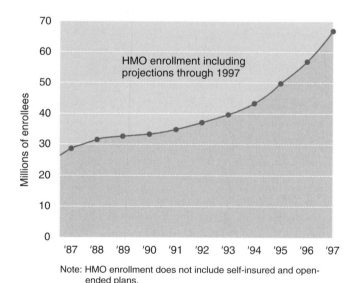

Figure 20-5

HMOs are becoming a primary source of medical care, with membership doubling from 1987 to 1997.

IPAs comprise 65% of all HMOs and serve almost half of HMO patients.[28] HMOs generally pay a fixed amount per patient to a physician or hospital, regardless of the type and number of services actually provided. This is called *capitation.*

Members of HMOs pay a regular, preset fee that usually includes diagnostic tests, routine physical exams, and vaccinations as well as treatment of illnesses. HMOs usually do not require a deductible, and copayments for medications or services are small. The primary drawback of standard HMOs is that the consumer is limited to a particular health-care facility and staff. *Open-ended* or *point-of-service* HMOs charge more but let members seek treatment elsewhere if they prefer. These "hybrid" plans have proven the most popular, with total enrollment reaching 10 million members in 1995. However, members must pay a deductible and a 20% to 30% copayment for hospitalization outside the system, and dissatisfaction rates for both enrollees and employers have been higher than for other HMOs or conventional insurance.[29]

Preferred Provider Organizations (PPOs)

In a **preferred provider organization (PPO)**, a third party—a union, an insurance company, or a self-insured business—contracts with a group of physicians and hospitals to treat members at a discount. PPO members may choose any physician within the network, and usually pay a 10% copayment for care within the system and a higher percentage (20%–30%) for care elsewhere. PPOs generally require prior approval for expensive tests or major procedures.

A *point-of-service (POS)* plan is a PPO that permits patients to use physicians outside the network. Consumers pay the difference between the preferred provider's discounted fee and the outside physician's fee. A *gatekeeper* plan requires members to choose a primary physician, as in an HMO, who must approve all referrals to specialists.

Government-Financed Insurance Plans

The government provides two major forms of health financing: Medicare and Medicaid. Under Medicare, the federal government pays 80% of most medical bills, after a deductible fee, for people over age 65. Medicare doesn't cover drugs, eyeglasses, or dental work.

Medicaid, a federal and state insurance plan that protects people with very low or no incomes, is the chief source of coverage for the unemployed. However, many unemployed Americans don't qualify because their family incomes are above the poverty line. Publicly insured patients are more likely than those with private insurance to receive inadequate care and to experience adverse health outcomes.

The public sector also is switching to managed care. The number of Medicaid managed-care plans more than tripled between 1983 and 1994, and Medicaid enrollments in HMOs are expected to grow throughout the nineties. There has been concern that quality of care for the poor could be jeopardized if uniform standards are not assured in managed-care plans.[30]

The Uninsured

As many as 42 million Americans lack health insurance; many others are underinsured, meaning that they don't have adequate coverage.[31] (See Table 20-4.) Uninsured patients have shorter hospital stays, cannot undergo costly therapies, and have a greater risk of dying in the hospital than insured patients. About 85% of uninsured Americans are from families in which the head of the family works but can't get insurance through his or her employer. Some of these people work part-time and do

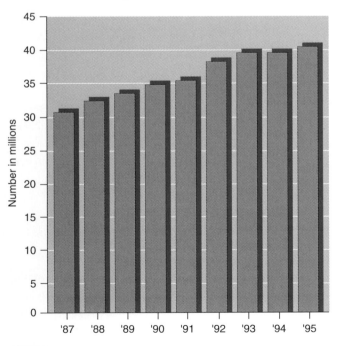

The Growing Number of Uninsured in the U.S.

Table 20-4

not qualify for insurance. Others work for businesses too small to qualify for group insurance. The availability of insurance affects both access to care and the way care is delivered.

Evaluating Health Care

How do you know you're getting quality health care? Answering this question can be tricky. Some patients criticize a physician who won't give them penicillin for their colds, even though it is sound practice not to overuse antibiotics. Others may feel relieved if a physician doesn't perform an awkward procedure, such as a rectal examination. However, by avoiding a moment's awkwardness, the physician could be missing an early sign of malignancy.

Medical research is the only way that anyone, physician or consumer, can assess the quality of diagnostic methods, medications, or surgical treatments. The principal rule of science is that nothing works until it's been proven.

Making Sense of Medical Research

Researchers rely on a variety of studies to determine whether a new approach to prevention, diagnosis, or treatment works. These include:

- *Epidemiological studies*, in which scientists assess the health status of a large, defined group of people, such as the population of a country or region. They may look at various health habits, such as alcohol consumption, to determine whether those who practice these habits have a higher likelihood of developing certain diseases.

- *Animal studies*, or *preclinical trials*, in which scientists administer a drug or try a procedure on various laboratory animals to assess its safety and determine its effects.

- *Clinical trials*, in which volunteers agree to act as test subjects—"human guinea pigs," as it were. Patients must give written permission in order to participate. Clinical trials generate data for the purpose of evaluating one or more diagnostic or therapeutic approaches in a population. Well-designed clinical trials, which must have strict eligibility criteria, a standardized intervention, followup, and measures of outcome, set the "gold standard" for new diagnostic tests or medical or surgical treatments.

In *controlled studies,* the group receiving an experimental drug or treatment is compared with a group receiving no treatment or standard therapy. In *single-blind studies,* the subjects don't know whether they're receiving the experimental drug or treatment, or an inactive substance. In *double-blind studies,* neither the subjects nor the researchers have this information. In *prospective studies,* patients are selected, assessed, participate in the trial, and are then followed for a preset period. In *retrospective studies,* investigators look back at their past experiences with a certain group of patients.

The results of even the most careful studies aren't considered conclusive in and of themselves. The FDA reviews every new drug, as well as the research methods used to test it, before it's allowed on the market. And a new therapy is widely accepted (or rejected) only after publication of study results in a *peer-reviewed* journal (one in which scientists in the same field critique the research methods before accepting the paper) and *replication* (the repetition of the same investigation by other researchers with similar results). In recent years, a technique called **meta-analysis**, which summarizes and reviews research in a particular area, has been used to evaluate the results of several large trials in a uniform manner.

One reason why study results must be confirmed is that, no matter what treatment patients receive, one-third to one-half of all patients improve temporarily. This well-documented but little-understood phenomenon is called the *placebo effect.* Scientific trials of a new treatment must show that the patients receiving the experimental medication or therapy improve *more* than those receiving a sugar pill or mock procedure (the placebo).

Strategies for Change

Before You Participate in a Clinical Trial

These are the questions patients should ask in considering whether to participate in a trial of a new diagnostic or therapeutic method:

✔ What is the purpose of the study?

✔ What does the study involve? What kinds of tests and treatments will I undergo?

✔ What is likely to happen in my case with or without this new treatment?

✔ What are my other alternatives and their advantages and disadvantages?

✔ How could the study affect my daily life?

✔ What side effects might I expect?

✔ How long will the study last?

✔ Will treatment be free? Will I have any costs?

✔ If I am harmed in any way, what treatment would I be entitled to?

✔ What type of long-term followup care is part of this study?[32]

Outcomes Research

As part of the nationwide effort to cut costs while maintaining quality care, more research has focused on **outcomes**—the ultimate impact of treatment. The questions that outcomes research is designed to answer include: Is treatment better or worse than no treatment? Is one treatment better than another? If a treatment is effective, is a little just as good as a lot? Does quality of life change because of treatment? Are the benefits of treatment worth the cost or the risks to the patient?

Studies of outcomes look at how patients fared with or without a specific treatment, the costs involved, and the impact of undergoing or not undergoing treatment on the patients' quality of life. Outcomes research can help determine which of several therapies or approaches provides the best results at the most reasonable costs. In the future, health-care purchasers, such as employers and insurance companies, hope to use studies of outcomes to hold health plans accountable for providing appropriate, cost-effective care.[33]

Clinical Practice Guidelines

In an effort to provide consistent quality of care, federal agencies and professional medical groups have developed **clinical practice guidelines** for problems ranging from depression to cataracts to congestive heart failure. These treatment recommendations help physicians choose the most appropriate therapies—and help patients determine whether they are getting state-of-the-art, scientifically proven care. (Free practice guidelines and patient guides can be ordered from the Agency for Health Care Policy and Research at 800-358-9295.)[34]

Evaluating Health News and Online Medical Advice

Cure! Breakthrough! Medical miracle! These are the words headlines are made of. But remember that although medical breakthroughs and cures do occur, most scientific progress is made one small step at a time. And even though medicine is considered a science, some experts estimate that no more than 15% of medical interventions can be supported by reliable scientific evidence.[35]

Medical opinions invariably change over time, sometimes going from one extreme to another. For instance, several decades ago the treatment of choice for breast cancer was radical mastectomy—removal of the woman's breast, lymph nodes, and chest wall. Since then much less extensive surgery (lumpectomy), coupled with chemotherapy or radiation, or both, has proven equally effective. Once individuals who'd suffered heart attacks were advised to limit all physical activity. Today a progressive exercise program is a standard component of rehabilitation.

Health researchers are struggling to find better ways of assessing what they know and need to know in order to offer more complete and balanced information to consumers. However, sometimes the only certainty is uncertainty. Rather than putting your faith in the most recent report or the hottest trend, try to gather as much background information and as many opinions as you can. Weigh them carefully—ideally with a trusted physician—and make the decision that seems best for you.

In recent years the Internet has become a major source of health information—and misinformation. More than 10,000 health-related web sites offer ways for patients to educate themselves about medical problems and options for treatment and share experiences with other people with similar conditions. The Internet also permits ease of access to cutting-edge medical knowledge and bridges the communication gap created by high-tech medicine.

However, there also are serious drawbacks. Because information on web sites is unregulated, there is no regulation of accuracy or reliability. Many sites are used to promote products or people. Some chat rooms can lead to encounters with unpleasant people. Even when information is technically precise, laypeople may not know how to interpret it properly.[36]

Whenever using the Internet for medical guidance, always check the sponsor of a site. Is it a hospital, a research institute, a drug manufacturer, or a distributor for an herbal remedy? Look for references to peer-reviewed medical journals. Beware of endorsements of miracle products that claim to cure various diseases and flashy sites that may have little substance behind them. Always verify any information before you act on it with organizations such as the American Medical Association or the National Institutes of Health.

Strategies for Change

How to Evaluate Health News

When reading a newspaper or magazine story or listening to a radio or television report about a medical advance, look for answers to the following questions:

✔ Who are the scientists involved? Are they recognized, legitimate health professionals? What are their credentials? Are they affiliated with respected medical or scientific institutions? Be wary of individuals whose degrees or affiliations are from institutions you've never heard of, and be sure that the person's educational background is in a discipline related to the area of research reported.

✔ Where did the scientists report their findings? The best research is published in peer-reviewed professional journals, such as the *New England Journal of Medicine*. Research developments also may be reported at meetings of professional societies.

✔ Is the information based on personal observations? Does the report include testimonials from cured patients or satisfied customers? If the answer to either question is yes, be wary.

✔ Does the article, report, or advertisement include words like *amazing*, *secret*, or *quick*? Does it claim to be something the public has never seen or been offered before? Such sensationalized language is often a tip-off to a dubious treatment.

✔ Is someone trying to sell you something? Manufacturers who cite studies to sell a product have been known to embellish the truth.

✔ Does the information defy all common sense? Be skeptical. If something sounds too good to be true, it probably is.

Alternative Forms of Therapy

Modern medicine, with its emphasis on technology and highly specialized treatments, is most successful in fighting disease rather than preventing illness or dealing with lifestyle problems such as stress, addiction, and obesity. As a consequence, as many as 50% of Americans have turned to alternative or nontraditional health-care approaches.[37]

Alternative therapies appeal to people for many reasons. They often cost less. They cause fewer side effects. Practitioners spend more time with and listen more attentively to patients. In addition, they often emphasize the connection between mind and body, and the body's own healing powers, thereby giving individuals a greater sense of control over their health. One danger, say their critics, is that people who turn to alternative therapies may ignore or refuse conventional medicines that could improve their health or even save their lives.

At present, alternative medicine is exactly that: an option to be considered as carefully as any more widely known and accepted medical therapy. If you're considering a nontraditional treatment, first compare what traditional medical science has to offer and what the alternatives claim. Avoid practitioners who insist that their brand of healing is the only effective approach. Check practitioners' credentials as carefully as possible. Some "doctors" in white coats have questionable degrees, often in fields that are not at all related to health. Remember that you are ultimately responsible for your well-being: Don't entrust it to anyone who doesn't deserve your trust.

The National Institutes of Health, (NIH), noting that "treatments considered unconventional today may become conventional in the future," has begun investigating such practices, including those discussed in the following sections.[38] Although there has been some controversy in traditional scientific and medical circles about the NIH's move, there is increasing recognition of the need for such research.[39]

Acupuncture

An ancient Chinese form of medicine, **acupuncture** is based on the philosophy that a cycle of energy circulating through the body controls health. Pain and disease are the result of a disturbance in the energy flow, which can be corrected by inserting long, thin needles at specific points along longitudinal lines, or *meridians,* throughout the body. Each point controls a different corresponding part of the body. Once inserted, the needles are rotated gently back and forth or charged with a small electric current for a short time. Western scientists aren't sure exactly how acupuncture works, but some believe that the needles alter the functioning of the nervous system.

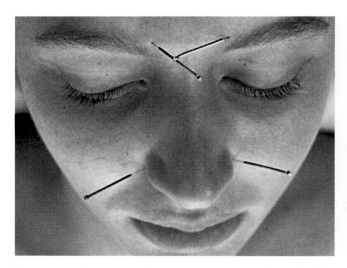

The ancient Chinese practice of acupuncture produces healing through the insertion and manipulation of needles at specific points throughout the body. The procedures are not painful.

In *acupressure,* the therapist uses his or her finger and thumb to stimulate certain points, relieve pain, and relax muscles. *Reflexology* is based on the theory that massaging certain points on the foot or hand relieves stress or pain in corresponding parts of the body. These methods seem most effective in easing chronic pain, arthritis, and withdrawal from nicotine, alcohol, or drugs.

An NIH consensus development panel that evaluated current research into acupuncture concluded that there is "clear evidence" that acupuncture can control nausea and vomiting in patients after surgery or while undergoing chemotherapy and relieve postoperative dental pain. The panel said that acupuncture is "probably" also effective in the control of nausea in early pregnancy and that there were "reasonable" studies showing that the use of acupuncture, by itself or as an adjunct to other therapies, resulted in satisfactory treatment of a number of other conditions, even though there was not "firm evidence of efficacy at this time." These conditions include addiction to illicit drugs and alcohol (but not to tobacco), stroke rehabilitation, headache, menstrual cramps, tennis elbow, general muscle pain, low back pain, carpal tunnel syndrome, and asthma.[40]

Ayurveda

Considered alternative here, **ayurveda** is a traditional form of medical treatment in India, where it has evolved over thousands of years. Its basic premise is that illness stems from incorrect mental attitudes, diet, and posture.

Practitioners use a discipline of exercise, meditation, herbal medication, and proper nutrition to cope with such stress-induced conditions as hypertension, the desire to smoke, and obesity. The best known advocate of ayurvedic medicine in the United States is Deepak Chopra, M.D., an endocrinologist (specialist in hormone-related disorders) who has written several books on ayurveda and the intimate relationship between consciousness and health.

Biofeedback

A marriage of technology and mysticism, biofeedback uses machines that measure temperature or skin responses and relays (or feeds back) this information to the subject. In this way, people can learn to control usually involuntary functions, such as circulation to the hands and feet, tension in the jaws, and heartbeat rates. Biofeedback has been used to treat dozens of ailments, including asthma, epilepsy, pain, and *Reynaud's disease* (a condition in which the fingers become painful and white when exposed to cold). Many health insurers now cover biofeedback treatments.

Bodywork

Numerous techniques focus on manipulation of the body. The *Alexander technique,* popular among actors and dancers, coaches people to improve their posture to relieve tension and pain. *Hellerwork* uses deep massage to eliminate pain and tension. Practitioners of *therapeutic touch* move their hands above the body; as they do, they sense blockages in a person's "life energy" and redirect energy to promote healing.

Herbal Medicine

Herbal medicine, or **herbology**, an ancient form of treatment, uses substances derived from trees, flowers, ferns, seaweeds, or lichens to treat disease. Many manufactured drugs are made from plants, or are synthetic recreations or modifications of naturally occurring substances. However, advocates of herbal medicine feel that herbs work differently on the body than purified drugs, with fewer side effects and faster healing.[41]

Herbal treatments have been developed for practically all known diseases from corns and callouses to anemia and hypertension. While plant extracts can be beneficial, many producers don't monitor the purity or potency of herbal products, which may contain insect parts, pollen, molds, and toxins such as lead and arsenic

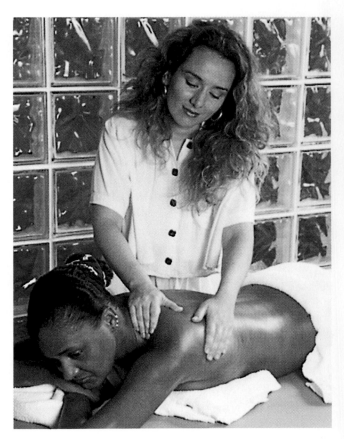

Bodywork practitioners use touch and massage to relieve tension and improve energy flow, thereby enhancing the body's own healing power.

acquired from the soil. Never use more than the recommended amounts, and don't continue to take an herbal remedy for prolonged periods of time or if you're pregnant or using a prescription drug. Watch out for allergic reactions to herbs, including herbal teas. And always seek medical care if symptoms persist or worsen over time.

Homeopathy

Homeopathy is based on three fundamental principles: Like cures like; treatment must always be individualized; and less is more—increasing dilution (lowering the dosage) can increase efficacy. By administering doses of animal, vegetable, or mineral substances to a large number of healthy people to see if they all develop the same symptoms, homeopaths determine which substances may be given, in small quantities, to alleviate the symptoms. Some of these substances are the same as those used in conventional medicine: nitroglycerin for certain heart conditions, for example, although the dose is minuscule.

The FDA hasn't demanded proof of efficacy for homeopathic remedies because they aren't considered harmful. However, some consumer groups are petitioning the FDA to require that homeopathic products be proven safe and effective before they're marketed. These products amount to about $250 million in annual sales; most popular are products for insomnia, coughs, and colds.[42]

Naturopathy

Naturopathic physicians (who are not M.D.s) emphasize natural remedies, such as sun, water, heat, and air, as the best treatments for disease. Therapies might include dietary changes (such as more vegetables and no salt or stimulants), steam baths, and exercise. Some work closely with medical doctors in helping patients.

Visualization

Carl Simonton, M.D., a cancer specialist, developed the technique of creative **visualization**, or imaging, to help heal cancer patients, including some diagnosed as terminally ill. On the premise that positive and negative beliefs and attitudes have a great deal to do with whether people get well or die of disease, patients imagine themselves getting well—they "see," for instance, their immune-system cells marching to conquer the cancer cells. Others use visualization in different ways—for example, to create a clear idea of what they want to achieve, whether the goal is weight loss or relaxation.

Quackery

Every year millions of Americans go searching for medical miracles that never happen. In all, they spend more than $10 billion on medical **quackery**, unproven health products and services. Those who lose only money are the lucky ones. Many also waste precious time, during which their conditions worsen. Some suffer needless pain, along with crushed expectations. Far too many risk their lives on a false hope—and lose.

The peddlers of such false hopes are quacks, who, by definition, promote for profit worthless or unproven treatments. A quack's greatest skill is telling people what they want to hear. Quackery's most recent disguise has been in the form of untested treatments for cancer, HIV infection and AIDS, and other life-threatening conditions. Many men and women who aren't ill or in pain take various powders and extracts to enhance their health or delay aging. Some see lifestyle or self-care

approaches, such as taking megadoses of vitamins or eating special foods, as a means of staying in control of their bodies and preventing disease or deterioration.

Sometimes individuals with certain diseases, such as arthritis or multiple sclerosis, who try unproven remedies do indeed improve. "If someone with arthritis starts feeling better the day after getting a copper bracelet, the bracelet will get the credit," says one physician. "Yet it's just coincidence." This is one reason scientists put little stock in enthusiastic testimonials from people who genuinely believe they have been helped by a new drug or treatment. Their heartfelt stories can be persuasive but are scientifically meaningless. The satisfied patient may not actually have had the disease in the first place, may have gotten other treatments too, or may be responding to a remedy that masks the symptoms without treating the disease.

Strategies for Prevention

Protecting Yourself Against Quackery

✔ Arm yourself with up-to-date information about your condition or disease from appropriate organizations, such as the American Cancer Society or the Arthritis Foundation, which keep track of unproven and ineffective methods of treatment.

✔ Ask for a written explanation of what a treatment does and why it works, evidence supporting all claims (not just testimonials), and published reports of the studies that have been done, including specifics on numbers treated, doses, and side effects. Be skeptical of self-styled "holistic practitioners," treatments supported by crusading groups, and endorsements from so-called authorities.

✔ Don't part with your money quickly. You need to be especially careful because insurance companies won't reimburse for unproven therapies.

✔ Don't discontinue your current treatment without your physician's approval. Many physicians encourage supportive therapies—such as relaxation exercises, meditation, or visualization—as a supplement to standard treatments.

Making This Chapter Work for You
Smart Health-Care Decisions

■ The American health-care system, though considered among the best in the world, is complex and

Health Online

A Guide to Health Care Reform for Young Americans
http://www.iuma.com/rtv/

The current health care crisis is likely to affect your generation the most. This site, designed especially for younger Americans, outlines the issues that our health care system faces and what you can do about it. There are stories about young people entangled with the system and how their plight illustrate larger social issues. In the Resources section, there are ideas for how you can write to your political representatives to urge them to make changes to the system.

Think about it ...

- Have you or a friend or family member ever faced a medical crisis without health insurance? Why wasn't this person insured?

- Do the stories told on this Web site make health care issues seem more personal and urgent to you? What special health care issues do young people face?

- If you were in charge of overhauling the American health care system, what changes would you make?

changing, and people must become savvy consumers in order to ensure that they get the best possible care.

- Self-care is an important aspect of maintaining good health and preventing disease. Home tests and equipment can identify any suspicious signs that require professional care.

- Proper dental care includes regular brushing and flossing, which can reduce the risk of cavities and of gum or periodontal disease.

- As a consumer, you may turn to physicians, nurses, and any number of specialists and allied-health professionals.

- Health-care facilities include student health centers, clinics, hospitals, outpatient surgery centers, and freestanding emergency centers.

- Most primary care is provided by a physician in an office, emergency room, or clinic. Secondary care usually is provided by specialists or subspecialists in either an outpatient or inpatient, or hospital, setting. Tertiary care, available at university-affiliated hospitals and regional referral centers, includes special procedures such as kidney dialysis, open-heart surgery, and organ transplants.

- Increasingly, primary care physicians are playing an

important role in providing basic care and serving as "gatekeepers" who determine if a patient should see a specialist.

- A thorough medical evaluation includes a medical history and a physical examination that evaluates all systems of the body and includes appropriate screening and medical tests.

- As a consumer, you have the right of information about possible treatments, access to your records, respectful treatment, and safe, quality care. A health professional also can be sued for malpractice if a patient believes that the care received was substandard or that the health-care provider was negligent.

- The effort to control health-care costs has led to dramatic changes in how we pay for health care. Fewer Americans now have conventional indemnity health insurance policies, which pay physicians and hospitals for the services they perform.

- Managed-care plans, which now dominate the health-care system, offer lower costs by providing services through an organized network of providers, who receive a fixed or discounted rate for their services.

- Health maintenance organizations, or HMOs, are managed care groups that emphasize preventive health care. Preferred provider organizations, or

PPOs, allow consumers to choose from a preselected list of physicians and facilities.

■ The government helps defray medical expenses through two programs: Medicare, for people over age 65, and Medicaid, for people unable themselves to pay for health care.

■ Evaluating health care is a complex process. The best information comes from scientific research, which may involve laboratory tests, animal experiments, and clinical trials. To provide consistent quality care, government agencies and medical specialty groups are developing clinical practice guidelines for specific conditions and studying the outcomes of different treatments.

■ Millions of Americans, often disillusioned by conventional therapists and therapies, have tried alternative forms of healing, which are undergoing assessment by the National Institutes of Health. Alternative therapies include acupuncture, biofeedback, homeopathy, naturopathy, visualization, and other approaches that stress the mind-body connection.

■ Quackery is worthless, fraudulent, or unproven treatment for incurable diseases, longer life, better health, or delayed aging.

The more you know about your body and your health, the better decisions you can make about health care. Here are a few simple steps you can take to form a partnership with the health-care professionals you see:

■ Realize that what you have to say is worth the health expert's time. Think of each professional as a highly paid consultant who's there to perform a service for you. Don't be intimidated if a health-care worker seems busy or restless. If you don't understand his or her explanations, say something like, "Please tell me about the procedure again. I'm not sure I understood everything you said."

■ Be as specific as possible in describing symptoms. Ask questions whenever you're doubtful. Try not to be rude or disagreeable. Physicians, nurses, dentists, and other health-care workers are human beings. Just like the rest of us, they pull away from confrontations with unpleasant people.

■ Inform your primary care physician about what everyone else is doing as part of your treatment. Don't assume specialists, hospital nurses, physical therapists, and others are all in contact.

■ Never leave a physician's office uncertain about the diagnosis or recommended treatment. Ask about anything that's unclear, and repeat the answers in your own words. If your physician is unwilling to talk with you or is incapable of communicating clearly, find another.

■ Your health is your most important asset. Consider the time and effort you spend learning about your body and caring for your health an investment in your future.

▶ Key Terms

The terms listed here are used within the chapter. Page numbers are included for each term. A definition of each term is given in the green Glossary pages at the end of this book.

acupuncture *635*
ayurveda *635*
chiropractic *618*
clinical practice guidelines *633*
diagnostic-related group (DRG) *622*
false negative *627*
false positive *627*
flap surgery *615*
gingivitis *615*
gum disease *615*
health maintenance organization (HMO) *631*

herbal medicine *636*
herbology *636*
home health care *623*
homeopathy *636*
indemnity *629*
informed consent *628*
malpractice *628*
managed care *629*
medical history *615*
meta-analysis *633*
negligence *627*
outcomes *633*
over-the-counter (OTC) *628*

Pap smear *626*
periodontitis *615*
plaque *615*
preferred provider organization (PPO) *631*
primary care *621*
quackery *637*
visualization *637*
vital signs *614*

Review Questions

1. What does self-care mean? What actions are involved in practicing self-care?

2. Name some different types of health-care professionals and their responsibilities. What criteria should you use in selecting a health-care professional?

3. List and describe the different types of health-care facilities and the services they provide.

4. Do medical patients have rights? If so, what are they?

5. How are new treatments evaluated before they are available to the public?

6. What are the most common methods of payment for medical care?

Critical Thinking Questions

1. Think about an experience you've had with a medical practitioner. How did you feel during the physical examination? Did you trust the practitioner? Were you comfortable with the level of communication? Evaluate your experience and give your opinion of the value of the checkup.

2. What nontraditional or alternative approaches to health care are you aware of? How do you feel about alternative care? Do you feel confident in knowing the difference between alternative care and quackery?

3. If you're young and healthy, you'll have little problem getting health insurance. However, if you develop a chronic illness, sustain serious injuries in an accident, or simply get older, you may find insurance harder to get and more expensive to keep. What is your insurance coverage? Do you believe insurance companies have the right to turn down applicants with preexisting conditions, such as high blood pressure? Do they have the right to require screening for potentially serious health problems, such as HIV infection, or to cancel the policies of individuals who have run up high medical bills in the past?

4. What do you see as the solution to America's health-care crisis? What role should the government play? What should be done so that all Americans have access to necessary health services?

Connections to Personal Health Interactive

To enhance your understanding of the material covered in this chapter, check out the following study aids on the **Personal Health Interactive CD-ROM**. *Each numbered icon within the chapter corresponds to an appropriate activity listed here.*

20.1 Personal Insights: Are You in Control of Your Health?

20.2 Chapter 20 Review

References

1. Lundberg, George. "The Failure of Organized Health System Reform—Now What?" *Journal of the American Medical Association*, Vol. 273, No. 19, May 17, 1995.
2. "The Future of Self-Help." Social Policy, Vol. 27, No. 3, Spring 1997.
3. Little, Wayne. "Research Centers Established to Improve Minority Oral Health." *NIH News & Features*, Spring 1995.
4. Sharp, David. "Watch Your Mouth." *Health*, December/January 1992.
5. Weiss, Barbara. "Managed Care: There's No Stopping It Now." *Medical Economics*, April 1995.
6. Epstein, Arnold. "U.S. Teaching Hospitals in the Evolving Health Care System." *Journal of the American Medical Association*, Vol. 273, No. 15, April 19, 1995.
7. Marwick, Charles. "Federal Report on Academic Research Funding." *Journal of the American Medical Association*, Vol. 278, No. 11, September 17, 1997.
8. Campbell, Paulette Walker. "Study Urges New Philosophy

on Federal Support for Academic Health Centers." *Chronicle of Higher Education*, Vol. 44, No. 21, January 30, 1998.

9. Keeler, E. B., et al. "Hospital Characteristics and Quality of Care." *Journal of the American Medical Association*, October 7, 1992.

10. Leape, Lucian, et al. "Systems Analysis of Adverse Drug Events." *Journal of the American Medical Association,* Vol. 274, No. 1, July 5, 1995.

11. Shelton, Deborah. "Doctors Get a Reminder: Wash Your Hands." *American Medical News*, July 17, 1995.

12. Hathaway, Stacey. "the Intelligent Patient's Guide to the Doctor-Patient Relationship: Learning How to Talk So Your Doctor Will Listen." *Library Journal*, Vol. 122, No. 16, October 1, 1997.

13. Podell, Richard and William Proctor. *When Your Doctor Doesn't Know Best.* New York: Simon & Schuster, 1995.

14. Hale, Ralph. "The Obstetrician and Gynecologist: Primary Care Physician or Specialist." *American Journal of Obstetrics and Gynecology*, Vol 171, No. 4, April 1995. Gerbie, Albert. "The Obstetrician-Gynecologist: Specialist and Primary Care Physician."*American Journal of Obstetrics and Gynecology*, Vol. 171, No. 4, April 1995.

15. "It's My Body and I'll Care If I Want to." *Psychology Today*, January–February 1995.

16. Moy, Ernest, and Barbara Bartman. "Physician Race and Care of Minority and Medically Indigent Patients." *Journal of the American Medical Association*, Vol. 273, No. 19, May 17, 1995.

17. Garb, Maggie. "Like Doctor, Like Patient." *American Medical News*, September 14, 1992.

18. Gellman, Robert. "Fair Health Information Practices." *Behavioral Healthcare Tomorrow*, January–February 1995. Anthony, Joseph. "Who's Reading Your Medical Records?" *American Health*, July–August 1993.

19. Turkington, Richard. "Medical Record Confidentiality Law, Scientific Research, and Data Collection in the Information Age." *Journal of Law, Medicine & Ethics*, Vol. 25, No. 2-3, Summer–Fall 1997.

20. Woodward, Beverly. "Medical Record Confidentiality and Data Collection: Current Dilemmas." *Journal of Law, Medicine & Ethics*, Vol. 25, No. 2–3, Summer-Fall 1997.

21. McCormick, Brian. "Seeking a Way Out." *American Medical News*, January 9, 1995. Levinson, Wendy. "Physician-Patient Communication: A Key to Malpractice Prevention." *Journal of the American Medical Association*, Vol. 272, No. 20, November 23/30, 1994. Hickson, Gerald, et al. "Obstetricians' Prior Malpractice Experience and Patients' Satisfaction with Care." *Journal of the American Medical Association*, Vol. 272, No. 20, November 23/30, 1994.

22. Lundberg, George. "The Failure of Organized Health System Reform—Now What?" *Journal of the American Medical Association*, Vol. 273, No. 19, May 17, 1995.

23. Barron, Bruce. "The Price of Managed Care." *Commentary*, Vol. 103, No. 5, May 1997.

24. Podell, Richard, and William Proctor. "Watching Out for Yourself." *Remedy*, March–April 1995. Vladeck, Bruce. "Managed Care and Quality." *Journal of the American Medical Association*, Vol. 273, No. 19, May 17, 1995. McCann, Karen. *Take Charge of Your Hospital Stay: A "Start Smart" Guide for Patients and Care Partners.* New York: Insight Books, Plenum Press, 1994.

25. Barron, "The Price of Managed Care."

26. Carey, Mary Agnes. "Managed Care Faces Showdown over Federal Regulation. *Congressional Quarterly Weekly Report*, Vol. 55, No. 46, November 22, 1997.

27. Evans, M. Stanton. "If You're in an HMO, Here's Why." *Consumer Research Magazine*, Vol. 80, No. 12, December 1997.

28. "The Changing HMO Scene." *Medical Economics*, April 1995.

29. Freudenheim, Milt. "The New Breed of Insurance." *New York Times*, July 28, 1995.

30. Voelker, Rebecca. "Quality Care for the Poor." *Journal of the American Medical Association*, Vol. 273, No. 20, May 24–31, 1995.

31. "Health Care Services." *Forbes*, Vol. 161, No. 1, January 12, 1998.

32. Trimble, Edward, and Robert Park. "What You Should Know about Clinical Trials." *Contemporary Ob/Gyn*, May 1995.

33. Voelker, Rebecca. "Creating a Basis for Good Outcomes." *Journal of the American Medical Association*, Vol. 273, No. 18, May 10, 1995. Headrick, Linda, et al. "Quality Health Care." *Journal of the American Medical Association*, Vol. 273, No. 21, June 7, 1995.

34. Zinman, David. "Keeping Score." *American Health*, April 1993.

35. Nuland, Sherwin. "Medical Fads: Bran, Midwives and Leeches." *New York Times*, June 25, 1995. Richardson, W. Scott, et al. "Users' Guides to the Medical Literature." *Journal of the American Medical Association*, Vol. 273, No. 20, May 24–31, 1995.

36. Parrish, Michael. "On-Line Medical Advice." *American Health*, October 1996.

37. Elder, Nancy. "Use of Alternative Health Care by Family Practice Patients." *Journal of the American Medical Association*, Vol. 278, No. 1, July 2, 1997.

38. Wadman, Meredith. "Row over Alternative Medicine's Status at NIH." *Nature*, Vol. 389, No. 6652, October 16, 1997.

39. Micozzi, Marc. "The Need for Research on 'Complementary' Medicine." *Chronicle of Higher Education*, Vol. 44, No. 14, November 28, 1997.

40. Marwick, Charles. "Acceptance of Some Acupuncture Applications." *Journal of the American Medical Association*, Vol. 278, No. 231, December 3, 1997.

41. Tyler, Varro. "The Herbal Remedies Market." *Chemtech*, May 1997.

42. Katzenstein, Larry. "Protesting Homeopathic Products." *American Health*, May 1995.

CHAPTER 21

WORKING TOWARD A HEALTHY ENVIRONMENT

After studying the material in this chapter, you should be able to:

List and **explain** the major hazards to the survival of our planet.

List and **explain** the major types of indoor pollution.

Explain the hazardous impact of chemicals on air, land, and water.

Describe ways to protect your ears from noise-induced hearing loss.

Define *electromagnetic fields,* and **describe** the recommended procedures to protect yourself from their dangers.

Explain the risks of radiation.

*I*n some ways, this is both the best and the worst of times for the planet we call home. Never before has global attention focused so sharply on the fate of the world. Never before have scientists known so much about the complexities of life on earth. Yet, at the same time, the threats to our planet have never seemed so great nor the quest for solutions so challenging.

The World Health Organization (WHO) has stated that "a healthy environment is not only a need, it is also a right," a right that everyone—governments, businesses, research institutions, communities, and individuals—is responsible for upholding.[1] If you, as a citizen of the world, don't become part of the solution, you end up as part of the problem. And, the fact is, you *can* help find solutions. The first step is realizing that you have a personal responsibility for safeguarding the health of your environment and, thereby, your own well-being.

This chapter explores the complex interrelationships between your world and your well-being. It discusses the major threats to the environment—including overpopulation; atmospheric changes; depletion of resources; air, water, and noise pollution; chemical risks; and radiation—and provides specific guidance on what you can do about them.

The State of the Environment

The planet earth—once taken for granted as a ball of rock and water that existed for our use for all time—now is seen as a single, fragile **ecosystem** (a community of organisms that share a physical and chemical environment). Our environment is a closed ecosystem, powered by the sun. The materials needed for the survival of this planet must be recycled over and over again. Increasingly, we're realizing just how important the health of this ecosystem is to our own well-being and survival.

Centuries ago the English poet John Donne observed that no man is an island. Today, on an increasingly crowded and troubled planet, these words seem truer than ever. Directly or indirectly, the problems of the environment (including such threats as overpopulation, atmospheric changes, and the depletion of resources) affect the well-being of all who inhabit the earth—now and in the future.

The Fight to Save the Planet

Concern over the future of our environment has brought the nations of the world together in a search for solutions. One problem is the great chasm between rich countries, concentrated in the northern hemisphere, and poor nations, mainly in the south. Affluent nations have more cars, more heavy industry, and higher energy consumption. For instance, the United States, with only 5% of the world's population, uses a much greater percentage of the earth's resources than any other region of the world. Poor countries tend to blame the industrialized nations for environmental problems, whereas the rich nations fear that the high birth rates and rapid industrialization of developing nations may jeopardize the progress that has been made in limiting pollution and protecting the environment.

Increasingly, all nations are recognizing the need to abandon destructive practices in favor of "sustainable" development—that is, economic growth that doesn't cause irreparable damage to the environment. Ever since the United Nations Conference on Environment and Development, also called the Earth Summit, in 1992 the International Conference on Population and Development in Cairo in 1994, and the Kyoto Conference on Global Warming in 1997, some 150 countries have been working toward both economic and political solutions

to environmental woes. For instance, they've agreed that polluters ought to bear the cost of the damage they cause to the environment, that family planning should be promoted, that special priority should be given to the needs of developing countries, and that emissions of certain dangerous gases should be cut back to 1990 levels by the end of the decade.[2]

The United States has taken steps to clean up the environment by enacting tougher environmental legislation and working with business and industry leaders to develop innovative ways of protecting the environment. Scientists and engineers are coming up with new approaches to recycling, waste management, and alternative energy sources. Various organizations and agencies are working to protect and help environmental quality. Some, citing the undeniable progress that has been made, have become increasingly optimistic about the future of the earth. Others fear that Americans are becoming too complacent or cost-conscious to follow through on their commitment to environmental initiatives.[3]

Formed in 1970 and often under fire for being too lax or too tough, the Environmental Protection Agency (EPA) has helped enforce laws to ensure clean air and water; manage solid waste; and control toxic substances, pesticides, radiation, and other potential dangers. In addition, many private groups, such as Friends of the Earth and the Audubon Society, have been working to preserve and restore natural resources. Although no one denies that the environment is in peril, there is also great promise in working together at community, corporate, national, and international levels to overcome the threats to the planet.

Overpopulation

In the year 1800, about 1 billion people lived on earth. The world's population grew to 2 billion in the next 130 years (1930); to 3 billion in 30 years (1960); to 4 billion in 15 years (1975); to 5 billion in 12 years (1987); to 6 billion in just 10 years (1997). The world population is now growing more slowly, and experts now believe that the population could stabilize at 8 billion by the year 2025 (the point at which the number of births equals the numbers of deaths is called **zero population growth**). However, in 1997, the Population Institute warned that the population crisis is far from over. In that year, more than 30% of all births took place in one country: India. Although India's fertility rate fell sharply from 1986 to

Self-Survey

Are You Doing Your Part for the Planet?

You may think that there is little you can do, as an individual, to save the earth. But everyday acts can add up and make a difference in helping or harming the planet on which we live.

	Almost Never	Sometimes	Always
1. Do you walk, cycle, car pool, or use public transportation as much as possible to get around?	_____	_____	_____
2. Do you recycle?	_____	_____	_____
3. Do you reuse plastic and paper bags?	_____	_____	_____
4. Do you try to conserve water by not running the tap as you shampoo or brush your teeth?	_____	_____	_____
5. Do you use products made of recycled materials?	_____	_____	_____
6. Do you drive a car that gets good fuel mileage and has up-to-date emission control equipment?	_____	_____	_____
7. Do you turn off lights, televisions, and appliances when you're not using them?	_____	_____	_____
8. Do you avoid buying products that are elaborately packaged?	_____	_____	_____
9. Do you use glass jars and waxed paper rather than plastic wrap for storing food?	_____	_____	_____
10. Do you take brief showers rather than baths?	_____	_____	_____
11. Do you use cloth towels and napkins rather than paper products?	_____	_____	_____
12. When listening to music, do you keep the volume low?	_____	_____	_____
13. Do you try to avoid any potential carcinogens, such as asbestos, mercury, or benzene?	_____	_____	_____
14. Are you careful to dispose of hazardous materials (such as automobile oil or antifreeze) at appropriate sites?	_____	_____	_____
15. Do you follow environmental issues in your community and write you state or federal representative support "green" legislation?	_____	_____	_____

Making Changes ....

Count the number of items you've checked in each column. If you've circled 10 or more in the "always" column, you're definitely helping to make a difference. If you've circled 10 or more in the "never" column, read this chapter carefully, particularly the "Strategies for Change" to find out how and why you should make some changes. If you've mainly circled "sometimes," you're moving in the right direction, but you need to be more consistent and more conscientious.

1997, it is still expected to overtake China as the world's most populous country by the middle of the 21st century. At least 74 countries—including Ethiopia, El Salvador, Nigeria, Iran, Iraq, and Syria—are expected to double their populations in the next 30 years.[4]

Birth control has become a critical public health issue, as well as a personal concern, around the world. Yet according to the Alan Guttmacher Institute, a nonprofit research and public education agency, approximately one in six women of reproductive age—nearly 230 million in all—do not have access to effective, reversible contraception and voluntary sterilization. More than one in four of the 190 million pregnancies to women worldwide every year end in abortion; many women say their last birth was unwanted or mistimed. In most countries, there is a gap between the number of children women want and the number they have. Around the world, women spend half to three quarters of their childbearing years trying to avoid pregnancy. No matter where she lives in the world, a woman must use some form of effective contraception for at least 20 years of her life if she wants to limit her family size to two children.[5]

Strategies for Change

How to Slow Population Growth

Policymakers suggest that the following social and political changes are critical in preventing global overpopulation:

■ Improve the quality of reproductive services and family planning services around the globe.[6]

■ Meet current needs for contraception. This alone could cut the population projections for the year 2100 by nearly 2 billion.[7]

■ Increase access to education for girls and opportunities for women. Educated women with recognized status—whether because of paid jobs or positions of respect within the community—have fewer and healthier children.[8]

■ Involve men. Men who share equally in childrearing in the family take more responsibility for family planning.

Pollution

You may not think of **pollution** or global warming as health issues, but they are. The term *environment* refers to the conditions under which a person lives—the air you breathe, the water you drink, the sounds you hear—all of which have an enormous impact on your health. In turn, your decisions and actions—the method of transportation you choose, the products you use, the waste you create—have an impact on the environment. Health depends on our ability to understand and manage the interaction between human activities and our physical and biological environment. As Table 21-1 shows, pollution can have an enormous impact on health, killing at least 2.7 million people around the world every year.

Any change in the air, water, or soil that could reduce its ability to support life is a form of pollution. Natural events, such as smoke from fires triggered by lightning, can cause pollution.

However, most pollution is a byproduct of human activities. In 1997 the combination of fires deliberately set to clear lands in Indonesia and Malaysia, severe urban pollution from cars and factories, and a persistent drought led to fires so widespread that much of Southeast Asia was blanketed in toxic smoke. Schools were closed, and residents were warned to stay indoors, drink plenty of fluids, and take special precautions for the very young and the very old.[9] The effects of pollution depend on the concentration (amount per unit of air, water, or soil) of the **pollutant**, how long it remains in the environment, and its chemical nature. An *acute effect* is a severe immediate reaction, usually after a single, large exposure. For example, pesticide poisoning can cause nausea and dizziness, even death. A *chronic effect* may take years to develop or may be a recurrent or continuous reaction, usually after repeated exposures. The development of cancer after repeated exposure to a pollutant such as asbestos is an example of a chronic effect.

Environmental agents that trigger changes, or **mutations**, in the genetic material, the DNA, of living cells are called **mutagens**. The changes that result can lead to the development of cancer. As previously discussed, a substance or agent that causes cancer is a *carcinogen:* all carcinogens are mutagens; most mutagens are carcinogens (see Chapter 13). Furthermore, when a mutagen affects an egg or a sperm cell, its effects can be passed on to future generations. Agents that can cross the placenta of a pregnant woman and cause a spontaneous abortion or birth defects in the fetus are called **teratogens**.

Toxic substances can enter the human body in three ways: (1) through the skin, (2) through the digestive system, and (3) through the lungs. The combined interaction of two or more hazards can produce an effect greater than that of either one alone. Pollutants can affect an organ or organ system directly or indirectly.

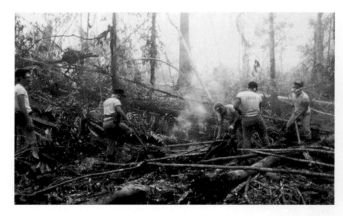

Forest fires in Southeast Asia in 1997 created pervasive clouds of smoke that threatened the health of tens of millions of people.

TABLE 21-1   AIR POLLUTION TAKES ITS TOLL

According to the World Health Organization, at least 2.7 million people die each year from illnesses caused by air pollution.		**Indoor Pollution** Caused primarily by smoke from cooking and heating fires.		**Outdoor Pollution** Largely attributed to industrial and automobile emissions.	
Region	**Deaths:**	**Rural**	**Urban**	**Urban**	**Total Deaths**
India		496,000	93,000	84,000	673,000
Sub-Saharan Africa		490,000	32,000	*	522,000
China		320,000	53,000	70,000	443,000
Other Asian and Pacific countries		363,000	40,000	40,000	443,000
Latin America and Caribbean		180,000	113,000	113,000	406,000
Former socialist economies of Europe		*	*	100,000	100,000
Established market economies		0	32,000	47,000	79,000
Middle East		*	*	57,000	57,000
Total Deaths		1,849,000	363,000	511,000	2,723,000

*Not Available.

SOURCE: *New York Times*, November 29, 1997.

Among the health problems that have been linked with pollution are the following:

- Headaches and dizziness.

- Eye irritation and impaired vision.

- Nasal discharge.

- Cough, shortness of breath, and sore throat.

- Constricted airways.

- Chest pains and aggravation of the symptoms of colds, pneumonia, bronchial asthma, emphysema, chronic bronchitis, lung cancer, and other respiratory problems.

- Birth defects and reproductive problems.

- Nausea, vomiting, and stomach cancer.[10]

Changes in the Atmosphere and Climate

According to one still-controversial theory, the use of carbon (fossil) **fuels** such as oil and gas, the burning of tropical forests, and methane emissions (produced mainly by cattle and the cultivation of rice) have led to a buildup of the so-called *greenhouse gases* (principally, carbon dioxide, methane, and nitrous dioxide). The **greenhouse effect**—an environmental phenomenon in which the buildup of greenhouse gases leads to warming of the planet—has already led to record warmth.[11] In the future it may increase global temperatures by 1°C within 30 years and by 3°C within 100 years. (See Figure 21-1.) No one can predict exactly what effects a continuing temperature rise may have, but some experts have predicted severe drought and a rise in ocean levels of 2 to 20 feet—conditions that will affect everyone on earth. Ways to prevent these consequences include increasing the globe's tree cover (which accelerates carbon dioxide removal) and reducing fossil fuel combustion.

The **ozone layer** is a region of the upper atmosphere where ozone, created by the energy of sunlight acting on ordinary oxygen, repels the most dangerous ultraviolet radiation from the sun. *Chlorofluorocarbons (CFCs)*, which are gases used in fire extinguishers,

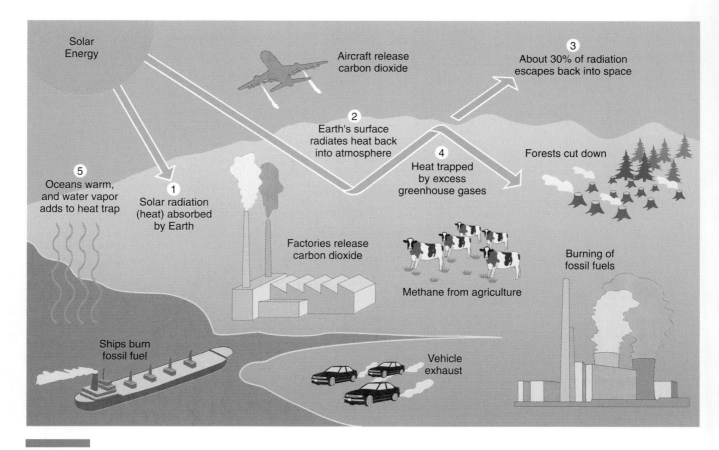

Figure 21-1

The buildup of carbon dioxide and other greenhouse gases in the atmosphere could result in the greatest climatic change in human history. A combination of factors, including the burning of fossil fuels and deforestation, is causing the atmosphere to retain heat. Scientists estimate that the world will be as much as 3°C warmer within a hundred years—the hottest it's been in two million years.

refrigerators, air-conditioning units, and styrofoam, rise into the atmosphere and damage this protective layer. In the past, products in aerosol cans contained high levels of CFCs, but all aerosols now sold in the United States must not exceed legal limits for CFC levels. However, because these products can still contribute to the destruction of the ozone layer, consumers are advised to switch to nonaerosol sprays.

One result of the shrinking of the ozone cover has been a dramatic increase in skin cancer, particularly its deadliest form: malignant melanoma (see also Chapter 13). In 1930 the average person's risk of melanoma was one in 1500. By the year 2000, it will be one in 75.[12] Most of the world's industrialized nations have agreed to cut their production and use of ozone-destroying chemicals and to provide funds to help developing countries obtain alternatives to these substances. In the future, developing countries will be crucial to planetary well-being. Although Asia now produces only 17% of green-

house gases, its carbon dioxide emissions are rising at four times the world average.[13]

Depletion of the Earth's Resources

A major concern is the loss of tropical rainforests, which play a vital role in regulating climate. As tropical rainforests shrink, their capacity to absorb carbon dioxide declines, hastening the onset and increasing the extent of global warming. Each year 40 to 50 million acres of trees worldwide—an area the size of the state of Washington—are cut up for timber or to clear land for agriculture and other development.

The decrease in rainforests has led to the extinction of many species of plants and wildlife. But the loss of life forms isn't confined to rainforests. As development continues in the next half-century, about 25% of the estimated 250,000 known plant species may become extinct. Three-fourths of the world's bird species are declining or facing extinction, as are a third of North America's freshwater fish and two-thirds of the world's 150 primate species.

The world's oceans are also threatened. Many U.S. coastal fishing grounds are contaminated with *polychlorinated biphenyls (PCBs)* from insulation and electronics manufacturing. These chemicals can cause cancer in fish, and the birds who eat them may be unable to reproduce or may produce damaged eggshells. (See the further discussion of PCBs later in this chapter.)

The Haves and Have-Nots

As the planet has become more crowded, the divisions between economic groups have widened. With only 22% of the world's population, the developed nations use two-thirds of all resources consumed and generate 75% of all pollutants and wastes. Without a reduction in population growth and changes in consumption of resources, there may be, according to a 1995 statement from the U.S. National Academy of Sciences and the Royal Society of London put it, "either irreversible degradation of the environment or continued poverty for much of the world."[14]

Overall, hunger has declined in the last 20 years, largely because of improvements in Asia. However, hunger has worsened in Latin America, Africa, and the Near East. More than 700 million people—one in eight—do not have enough to eat. Even though world grain production has risen dramatically and food prices have declined steadily, most of the world's hungry have no money to pay for food. It is not clear whether food production will be able to keep pace with population growth in the coming decades.[15]

The Homeless

They appear on streets in cities and towns across the country. By some estimates, more than a million Americans don't have a place to call home. Families with children—more than a third of the homeless—end up on the street or in shelters for many reasons: separation or divorce, firing or layoffs, illness, economic misfortunes or miscalculations, floods, fires, or other acts of God. For the urban poor, the roots of homelessness include a lack of affordable housing because developers have razed low-rent neighborhoods. For military veterans, who make up nearly a third of the homeless population, the causes of homelessness include unemployment; loss of social, medical, and economic support; and drug abuse. The homeless are more vulnerable to substance abuse, addiction, and serious infectious illnesses. Many have criminal records, but few are hard-core criminals; about 25% suffer from severe mental illness.

Public support for the homeless has been strong. More than half of Americans have said they would be willing to pay more taxes to help the homeless. Most favor increased job training and building more low-cost housing rather than increasing welfare spending. However, in some cities, citizens seem to be losing sympathy, and police have cracked down on homeless "street people," forcing them out of public areas.

What You Can Do to Protect the Planet

By the choices you make and the actions you take, you can improve the state of the world. No one expects you to sacrifice every comfort or spend great amounts of money. However, for almost everyone, there's plenty of room for improvement. If enough people make small individual changes, they can have an enormous impact. (See the Self-Survey: "Are You Doing Your Part for the Planet?")

Going "Green"

As a consumer, you have a great deal of influence on manufacturers and distributors. When making purchases, consider their environmental impact. A simple switch—from plastic wrap to wax paper, for example—can make a difference. However, it can be difficult to know which choice is best for the environment. For years, for example, environmental and consumer groups have differed about disposable versus cloth diapers. Disposable diapers, though convenient, don't break down; cloth diapers can be reused, but laundering them requires energy and produces wastewater and air pollution. One compromise that suits some parents is using cloth diapers at home and disposable diapers when out. (See Pulsepoints "Ten Ways to Protect the Planet" for other practical suggestions for protecting the planet.)

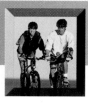

Pulsepoints

Ten Ways to Protect the Planet

1. Plant a tree. Even a single tree helps absorb carbon dioxide and produces cooling that can reduce the need for air-conditioning.

2. Look for simply packaged items. Whenever possible, choose items packed in recycled materials or something recyclable.

3. Bring your own bag. Whenever possible, avoid using plastic or paper bags for items you could carry in a cloth or string carry all.

4. Hit the switch. Turn off all electrical appliances (TVs, CD players, radios, lights) when you're not in the room or paying attention to them.

5. Avoid disposables. Use a mug instead of a paper or Styrofoam cup, a sponge instead of a paper towel, a cloth napkin instead of a paper one.

6. Be water wise. Turn off the tap while you shave or brush your teeth. Install water-efficient faucets and shower heads. Wash clothes in cold water.

7. Cancel junk mail. It consumes 100 million trees a year. To get off mailing lists, write: Mail Preference Service, Direct Marketing Association, 11 East 42nd St., PO. Box 3861, New York, NY 10163-3861.

8. Spare the seas. If you live near the coast or are picnicking or hiking near the ocean, don't use plastic bags (which are often blown into the water) or plastic six-pack holders (which can get caught around the necks of sea birds).

9. Don't buy products made of endangered substances. Examples include coral, ivory, tortoise shell, or wood from endangered forests (teak, mahogany, ebony, rosewood).

10. Speak out. Write to your senators and congressional representatives, who vote on pollution controls, budgets for the enforcement of safety regulations, and the preservation of forests and wildlife. Identify the particular bill or issue you're addressing. Be as specific, brief, and to the point as possible, and make sure you have the correct addresses:

Hon. [Your District's Congressperson]
House Office Building
Washington, DC 20515
or
Senator [Your State's Senator]
Senate Office Building
Washington, DC 20510

You can even have an impact on problems that seem remote, such as the devastation of the rainforests: Look for products whose manufacturers provide support for the rainforests. Some companies use nuts or plants from the rainforests in an ecological way, or give a percentage of their profits to environmental groups working to save the rainforests. For a minimum donation of $10, the Natural Resources Defense Council will plant a tree in a Hawaiian rainforest. For $25, you can become a Guardian of the Amazon through the World Wildlife Fund, which uses the money to set aside land, hire local people to fence it, and help tribes protect their land from deforestation. (For the addresses of both groups, see "Your Health Directory" at the back of this book.)

Precycling and Recycling

One basic principle of buying green is **precycling**: buying products packaged in recycled materials. According to Earthworks, a consumer group, packaging makes up a third of what Americans throw away. When you precycle, you consider how you're going to dispose of a product and the packaging materials before purchasing it. For example, you might choose eggs in recyclable cardboard packages rather than plastic ones and look for refillable bottles.

Recycling—collecting, reprocessing, marketing, and using materials once considered trash—has become a necessity for several reasons. We've run out of space for all the garbage we produce, waste sites are often health and safety hazards, recycling is cheaper than landfill storage or incineration (which is a major source of air pollution), and recycling helps save energy and natural resources. Different communities take different approaches to recycling. Many provide regular curbside pickup of recyclables, which is so convenient that a majority of those eligible for such services participate. Most programs pick up bottles, cans, and newspapers—either separated or mixed together. Other communities have drop-off centers where consumers can leave recyclables. Conveniently located and sponsored by community organizations (such as charities or schools), these centers accept beverage containers, newspapers, cardboard, metals, and other items.

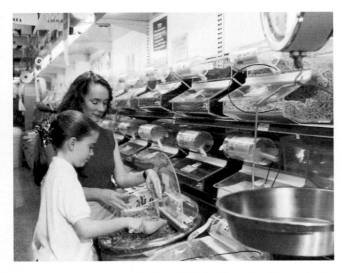

Reduce; reuse; recycle. Buying bulk foods, using fewer plastic bags, and taking canvas carryalls for your groceries all help reduce the amount of paper and plastic that must be recycled.

Buy-back centers, usually run by private companies, pay for recyclables. Many centers specialize in aluminum cans, which offer the most profit. Some operate in supermarket parking lots; other centers have regular hours and staff members who carefully weigh and evaluate recyclables. In some places, "reverse vending machines" accept returned beverage containers and provide deposit refunds, in the form of either cash or vouchers. Enthusiasm and support for recycling has grown, and, thanks to these efforts along with new manufacturing techniques and other technological advances, Americans are consuming some natural materials, such as aluminum and steel, at lower rates.[16]

With composting—which some people describe as nature's way of recycling—the benefits can be seen as close as your backyard. Organic products, such as leftover food and vegetable peels, are mixed with straw or other dry material and kept damp. Bacteria eat the organic material and turn it into a rich soil. Some people keep a compost pile (which should be stirred every few days) in their backyards; others take their organic garbage (including mowed grass and dead leaves) to community gardens or municipal composting sites.

Strategies for Change
....
Becoming Environmentally Responsible

✔ Wear sweaters, socks, or other warm clothes in cooler temperatures rather than turning up the heat.

✔ Use glass or reusable plastic containers rather than plastic wrap or aluminum foil. In supermarkets try leaving vegetables and fruit loose, or bundling items such as carrots or asparagus with rubber bands.

✔ Use compact fluorescent bulbs, which require 75% less energy than incandescent light bulbs. Use lamps rather than overhead lights for reading.

✔ Use cold water for laundry and rinsing dishes—or anything that doesn't require hot water. Use rechargeable batteries rather than disposable ones.

✔ Don't buy items designed to be thrown away after a few uses, such as disposable razors or one-serving drink containers.

✔ Buy unbleached or oxygen-bleached paper towels, toilet paper, and other paper products. The chlorine used to make products bright white has been linked to dioxin (a toxin discussed later in this chapter).

Clearing the Air

The good news is that, in most places in the United States, you can breathe easier today than you might have a quarter-century ago. Smog has declined by about a third, although there are now 85% more vehicles being driven 105% more miles a year. In Los Angeles, smog has decreased by almost 50%, even though the city's vehicle population has risen 65%. Several urban areas, such as Detroit and Kansas City, have been removed from the federal smog watch list, and none has been added. Current model automobiles emit an average of 80% less pollution per mile than was emitted by new cars in 1970, and the fuel efficiency of new cars has reduced the typical car's average annual gasoline consumption by around 300 gallons—more than enough fuel to take the average driver across the United States and back again.[17]

The bad news is that air quality still is far from optimal in many places (see Figure 21-2). According to the Harvard School of Public Health, living in a city with even moderately sooty air may shorten your life span by about a year.[18] In fact, air pollution can be as harmful to breathing capacity as smoking. Residents of polluted cities are exposed to some of the same toxic gases, such as nitrogen oxide and carbon monoxide, found in cigarettes.[19] In countries where heavy industries operated without controls for decades, such as the former Soviet Union, pollution has caused serious

HOW SAFE IS YOUR AIR?

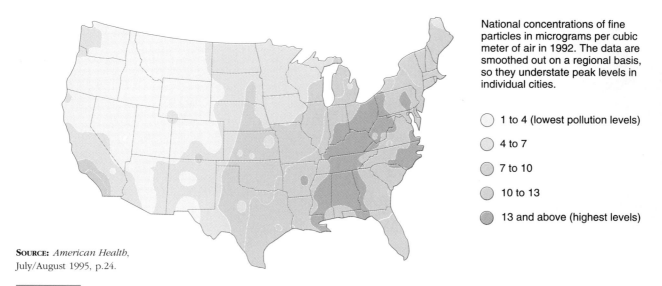

National concentrations of fine particles in micrograms per cubic meter of air in 1992. The data are smoothed out on a regional basis, so they understate peak levels in individual cities.

- 1 to 4 (lowest pollution levels)
- 4 to 7
- 7 to 10
- 10 to 13
- 13 and above (highest levels)

SOURCE: *American Health*, July/August 1995, p.24.

Figure 21-2

health problems and shortened life expectancies in addition to destroying forests and water supplies.[20]

Air pollution of any sort can cause numerous ill effects. As pollutants destroy the hairlike cilia that remove irritants from the lungs, individuals may suffer chronic bronchitis, characterized by excessive mucus flow and continuous coughing. Emphysema may develop or worsen, as pollutants constrict the bronchial tubes and destroy the air sacs in the lungs, making breathing more difficult. In addition to respiratory diseases, air pollution also contributes to heart disease, cancer, and weakened immunity. For the elderly and people with asthma or heart disease, polluted air can be life-threatening. Even healthy individuals can be affected, particularly if they exercise outdoors during high-pollution periods.

Strategies for Change

Doing Your Part for Cleaner Air

✔ Drive a car that gets high gas mileage and produces low emissions. Keep your speed at or below the speed limit.

✔ Keep your tires inflated and your engine tuned. Recycle old batteries and tires. (Most stores that sell new ones will take back old ones.)

✔ Turn off your engine if you're going to be stopped for more than a minute.

✔ Collect all fluids that you drain from your car (motor oil, antifreeze) and recycle or dispose of them properly.

✔ Car-pool, bicycle, or take public transportation whenever you can.

Smog

A combination of smoke or gases and fog, **smog** is made up of chemical vapors from auto exhaust and industrial and commercial pollutants that react with sunlight, including volatile organic compounds, carbon monoxide, nitrogen oxides, sulfur oxides, particulate, and ozone. The most obvious sources of these pollutants are motor vehicles, industrial factories, electric utilities plants, and wood-burning stoves.

Gray-air, or *sulfur-dioxide*, smog, often seen in Europe and much of the eastern United States, is produced by burning oil of high sulfur content. Among the cities that must deal with gray-air smog are Chicago, Baltimore, Detroit, and Philadelphia. Like cigarette smoke, gray-air smog affects the cilia in the respiratory passages; the lungs are unable to expel particulate, such as soot, ash, and dust, which remain and irritate the tissues. This condition is hazardous to people with the chronic respiratory problems described in Chapter 18.

Brown-air, or *photochemical*, smog is found in large

traffic centers such as Los Angeles, Salt Lake City, Denver, Mexico City, and Tokyo. This type of smog results principally from nitric oxide in car exhaust reacting with oxygen in the air, forming nitrogen dioxide, which produces a brownish haze and, when exposed to sunlight, other pollutants. One of these, *ozone*, the most widespread pollutant, can impair the body's immune system and cause long-term lung damage. (Ozone in the upper atmosphere protects us by repelling harmful ultraviolet radiation from the sun; but ozone in the lower atmosphere is itself a harmful component of air pollution.) Automobiles also produce carbon monoxide, a colorless and odorless gas that diminishes the ability of red blood cells to carry oxygen. The resulting oxygen deficiency can affect breathing, hearing, and vision.

Acid Rain

The burning of fossil fuels, such as oil and gas, and the smelting of certain ores, such as copper and nickel, can produce **acid rain**—rain, sleet, snow, mist, fog, and clouds containing sulfuric acid, and nitric acid. These pollutants are carried through the atmosphere long distances from their sources and fan to earth when it rains. Acid rain, which is believed to be declining in some regions, has damaged buildings, monuments, and other structures.

Indoor Pollutants

Because people in industrialized nations spend more than 90% of their time in buildings, the quality of the air they breathe inside can have an even greater impact on

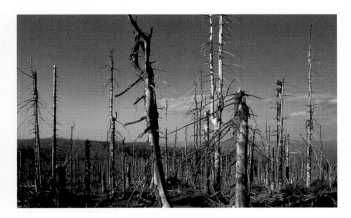

The effects of acid rain on a forest.

their well-being than outdoor pollution.[21] The most hazardous form of indoor air pollution is cigarette smoke. Passive smoking—inhaling others' cigarette smoke—may rank behind active smoking and alcohol use as the third-leading preventable cause of death. Each year secondhand cigarette smoke kills 53,000 nonsmokers. (See Chapter 16 for a complete discussion of smoke's harmful effects.)[22]

Formaldehyde

Unlike outdoor contaminants from exhaust pipes or smokestacks, indoor pollutants come from the very materials the buildings are made of and from the appliances inside them.[23] For instance, formaldehyde, commonly used in building materials, carpet backing, furniture, foam insulation, plywood, and particle board, can cause nausea, dizziness, headaches, heart palpitations, stinging eyes, and burning lungs. Formaldehyde has been shown to cause cancer in animals. Most manufacturers have voluntarily quit using it, but many homes already contain materials made with urea-formaldehyde, which can seep into the air. To avoid formaldehyde exposure, buy solid wood or nonwood products whenever possible; and ask about the formaldehyde content of building products, cabinets, and furniture before purchasing them.

Asbestos

Asbestos, a mineral widely used for building insulation, has been linked to lung and gastrointestinal cancer among asbestos workers and their families, although it may take 20 to 30 years for such cancer to develop. If fibers from asbestos home insulation or fireproofing become airborne, they can cause progressive and deadly lung diseases, including cancer. By the year 2000, an estimated 300,000 American workers will have died from asbestos-linked diseases, including lung cancer. The danger may be greatest for those who smoke and are also exposed to asbestos.[24]

If you're concerned about asbestos in your home, don't waste money searching for asbestos in the air. The results of such tests are meaningless. To check a building material for asbestos, put three small pieces in a film canister and send it to an EPA-approved laboratory. The cost for testing is usually $25 to $75 per sample. If you find asbestos in your house, sealing it may be safer than removing it. Contact your state or city health department for advice. If asbestos must be removed, have it done by professionals.

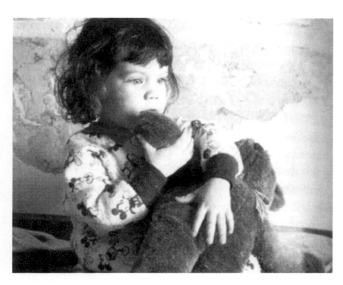

Lead-based paint poses a hazard, especially to young children, who can be poisoned from ingesting even small amounts of paint chips.

Lead

A danger both inside and outside our homes is lead, which lurks in some 57 million American homes, most built before 1960, with walls, windows, doors, and banisters coated with more than 3 million metric tons of lead paint.[25] One out of every six youngsters—as many as 4 million American boys and girls—may have toxic levels of lead in their bodies; millions more are at risk of poisoning from lead in the air they breathe or the water they drink. (See Personal Voices: "An Invisible Threat.") "In terms of the number of children affected, the number at risk and the dire effects of exposure, lead is the number-one environmental threat to our youngsters," says pediatrician John Rosen, M.D., chairman of the advisory committee on childhood lead poisoning for the CDC.[26]

Fetuses and children under age 7 are particularly vulnerable to lead because their nervous systems are still developing and because their body mass is so small that they ingest and absorb more lead per pound than adults. Even 10 micrograms (millionths of a gram) of lead per deciliter of blood—the CDC standard for lead poisoning—can kill a child's brain cells and cause poor concentration, reduced short-term memory, slower reaction times, and learning disabilities. Workers exposed to lead may become sterile or suffer irreversible kidney disease, anemia, damage to their central nervous system, stillbirths, or miscarriages.

The CDC and the American Academy of Pediatrics recommend annual testing of blood levels of lead in all children from age 9 months to 6 years, regardless of where they live. High-risk youngsters—those who live or play in older housing (especially if a building is in poor condition or undergoing renovation); those who live with someone who uses lead for a job or hobby; and those who live near a lead smelter, a processing plant, or a heavily traveled road or highway—should be screened every two or three months until age 3 and every six months until age 6.

Mercury

While free of lead, some popular, easy-to-use latex paints may contain potentially hazardous mercury, which manufacturers routinely added until a 1990 ban to prevent the growth of mold and mildew. The threat of mercury poisoning is greatest during painting and immediately after. Symptoms of mercury poisoning include a racing heartbeat, sweating, aching limbs, kidney problems, hand tremors, peeling skin, and emotional problems.

Carbon Monoxide and Nitrogen Dioxide

Carbon monoxide (CO) gas, which is tasteless, odorless, colorless, and nonirritating, can be deadly. Produced by the incomplete combustion of fuel in space heaters, furnaces, water heaters, and engines, it reduces the delivery of oxygen in the blood. Every year an estimated 10,000 Americans seek treatment for CO inhalation; at least 250 die because of this silent killer. Those most at risk are the chronically ill, the elderly, pregnant women, and infants. Typical symptoms of CO poisoning are headache, nausea, vomiting, fatigue, and dizziness. A blood test can measure CO levels; inhaling pure oxygen speeds removal of the gas from the body. Most people who don't lose consciousness as a result of CO poisoning recover completely.[27]

Another dangerous gas, nitrogen dioxide, can reach very high levels if you use a natural gas or propane stove in a poorly ventilated kitchen. This gas may lead to respiratory illnesses. Pilot lights are a steady source of nitrogen dioxide; to reduce exposure, switch to spark ignition.

Radon

Radioactive radon—which diffuses from rock, brick, and concrete building materials and natural soil deposits under some homes—produces charged decay products that cling to dust particles, which often lodge in the lungs. Once trapped inside, radon can reach levels that may increase the risk of lung cancer. EPA estimates that the inhalation of indoor radon is responsible for approx-

Personal Voices An Invisible Threat

ickie will never forget the phone call that, as she puts it, "shattered everything in our lives." In stunned silence, she listened as her pediatrician reported that her nine-month-old daughter Cassandra had a dangerously high level of lead in her blood. Like 17% of American youngsters, little Cassie had been poisoned by an ubiquitous substance that can stunt growth, lower IQ, damage major organs, and permanently sabotage a child's potential.

"How could this have happened?" asked Nickie, a medical assistant, and her physician husband Charles. From the day they'd brought their newborn daughter home to their "nice flat in a nice two-family house in a nice neighborhood" in a small town outside Boston, they'd done everything they could to ensure her safety. They never realized that every time they mixed a bottle of powdered formula with tap water—either warm or boiled—they were poisoning Cassie with lead. If they didn't live in Massachusetts, the only state that requires lead screening for all children, they might never have discovered the problem—at least not until it

was too late to do anything about it.

Cassie, whose initial blood lead level was 43 micrograms per deciliter—more than four times the amount considered safe—underwent nine hours of chelation, in which a drug that leaches lead molecules from the body was injected into her tiny veins. It didn't work. For a year, she took tablets of penicillamine, a medicine that, as her doctor puts it, "is wonderful because it's highly effective but terrible because it smells bad, tastes bad and causes side-effects." Cassie hated it. "The only way we could get her to take it was by giving it to her in the middle of the night," Nickie recalls, "She had to have blood drawn every two to four weeks, which was painful. It's terrible to watch a child go through this ordeal. I worry all the time about what the long-term effects may be. And every day I face the guilt of wondering, 'Is this my fault?'"

As millions of Americans have sadly discovered, no family—regardless of race, education or income—is immune to lead damage. One of every six youngsters—as many as 4 million American boys and girls—may have toxic levels of lead in their bodies; millions more are at

risk of poisoning from lead in the air they breathe or the water they drink.

In terms of the number of children affected, the number at risk and the dire effects of exposure, lead is the number-one environmental threat to our youngsters. Invisible and insidious, it invades a child's brain and body bit by bit, drop by drop, breath by breath. In amounts as small as 10 micrograms (or millionths of a gram) per deciliter of blood—the new CDC standard for lead poisoning—lead can kill brain cells. The greatest danger lurks in some 57 million American homes, most built before 1960, with walls, windows, doors and banisters coated with more than 3 million metric tons of lead paint.

"Parents and pediatricians have taken an ostrich attitude," says Michael Shannon, M.D., a specialist in lead and toxicology at Boston's Children's Hospital. "Because they haven't looked for lead in their own homes, they don't realize that it's there. They think that lead is only a threat in inner cities and that kids can only be poisoned by eating paint chips. That's not the case."

imately 14,000 lung cancer deaths per year.[28] Radon levels tend to be highest in areas with granite and black shale topped with porous soil. If you live in a high-radon area, don't panic. Your hypothetical risk of dying from radon-caused lung cancer is about equal to the known risk of dying in a home fire or fall. Check with the geology department at the nearest university or with your state health department to find out if they've performed radon tests in your area. If there may be danger, you can buy a radon detector. In most homes, the readings turn out to be low. If not, your state health department can provide guidelines for bringing them down.[29]

Strategies for Prevention
....

Protecting Yourself from Indoor Air Pollution

✔ If you live in a formaldehyde-insulated home, keep heat and humidity down, because formaldehyde vapors increase in hot, humid weather. Air conditioning and dehumidifiers reduce such emissions. An air-to-air heat exchanger can increase the circulation of outside air

without sharply increasing heating costs. Treatment with specially formulated sealants can cut formaldehyde emissions from wood products to 1% of their original level.

✔ Before renovating your home, inspect pipe and furnace coverings and insulation in attics and crawlspaces for signs of cracking, flaking, or loose asbestos.

✔ To minimize lead exposure, watch out for peeling or chipping lead paint, particularly from window sills and frames, which can release dust contaminated with lead. Watch out when scraping or sanding lead-based paint. Water flowing through lead pipes, brass faucets, or pipes connected with lead solder can contain lead. Imported products sold in cans may contain lead that leaches in from the solder. (Most domestic cans do not use lead solder.) Lead in the glaze used for ceramic dishes or cookware can leach into food.

✔ To prevent carbon monoxide poisoning, provide adequate ventilation when using wood stoves, space heaters, and fireplaces. Make sure that your furnace has adequate air intake. Don't use ovens or gas ranges to heat your home, or operate gasoline-powered engines in confined spaces. Never burn charcoal inside a home, recreational vehicle, or tent. The Consumer Product Safety Commission recommends installing at least one CO detector, which sounds an alarm before the gas reaches hazardous levels, in all homes.[30]

✔ Limit your use of cleaners and aerosols that fill the air with chemicals, and ventilate your house immediately after their use. Air your house daily or as often as possible—particularly in the winter, when pollutants build up inside.

Protecting Your Hearing

Noise is the most pervasive pollutant on the planet. Wherever you go, whatever you do, you may not be able to escape the roar of traffic, the blast of boom boxes, the screech of airplanes, the babble of voices. Of course, sound can be a soothing source of beauty and pleasure. But once the volume reaches the discomfort zone, sound turns into noise. Any noise loud enough to damage the sensitive structures of the inner ear can produce irreversible hearing loss.

More than 20 million Americans are exposed to hazardous levels of noise at home, on the job, and during recreation. About 10 million have already suffered hearing loss at least in part because of exposure to loud sounds. Noise-induced hearing loss can occur at any age, including early infancy, and can range from mild to profound. Increasingly, people are showing signs of damaged hearing as early as in their teens and twenties.

Sensitivity to noise varies greatly from person to person. Beginning in their teens, men, who tend to have greater exposure to loud noise, have poorer hearing than women. Damage to the ear is cumulative and so gets worse over time. By age 65, one in three Americans suffers hearing loss serious enough to interfere with communication. However, aging isn't the culprit. In quieter societies, many elderly people have little impairment in hearing.

How Loud Is Too Loud?

Loudness, or the intensity of a sound, is measured in **decibels (dB)**. A whisper is 20 decibels; a conversation in a living room is about 50 decibels. On this scale, 50 isn't two and a half times louder than 20, but 1000 times

louder: Each 10-dB rise in the scale represents a tenfold increase in the intensity of the sound.

Sounds under 75 dBs don't seem harmful. However, prolonged exposure to any sound over 85 dBs (the equivalent of a power mower or food blender) or brief exposure to louder sounds can harm hearing. The noise level at rock concerts can reach 110–140 dBs—about as loud as an air raid siren. Personal sound systems (boom boxes) can blast sounds of up to 115 dBs. Cars with extremely loud music systems, known as boom cars, can produce an earsplitting 145 dBs—louder than a jet engine or thunderclap.

Most hearing loss occurs on the job. The people at highest risk are firefighters, police, military personnel, construction and factory workers, musicians, farmers, and truck drivers. Other sources of danger include live or recorded high-volume music, recreational vehicles, airplanes, lawn-care equipment, woodworking tools, some appliances, and chain saws (see Figure 21-3).

The Effects of Noise

The healthy human ear can hear sounds within a wide range of frequencies (measured in **hertz**), from the low-frequency rumble of thunder at 50 hertz to the high-frequency overtones of a piccolo at nearly 20,000 hertz. High-frequency noise damages the delicate hair cells that serve as sound receptors in the inner ear. Damage first begins as a diminished sensitivity to frequencies around 4000 hertz—the highest notes of a piano. Early symptoms of hearing loss include difficulty understanding speech and tinnitus (ringing in the ears). Brief, very loud sounds, such as an explosion or gunfire, can produce immediate, severe, and permanent hearing loss. Longer exposure to less intense but still hazardous sounds, such as those common at work or in public places, can impair hearing gradually, often without the individual's awareness.

Conductive hearing loss, often caused by ear infections, cuts down on perception of low-pitched sounds. Sensorineural loss involves damage or destruction of the sensory cells in the inner ear that convert sound waves to nerve signals.

Noise can harm more than our ears: High-volume sound has been linked to high blood pressure and other stress-related problems that can lead to heart disease, insomnia, anxiety, headaches, colitis, and ulcers. Noise frays the nerves; people tend to be more anxious, irritable, and angry when their ears are constantly barraged with sound. Even unborn babies respond to sounds; some researchers speculate that noise, particularly if it stresses the mother, may be hazardous to the fetus.

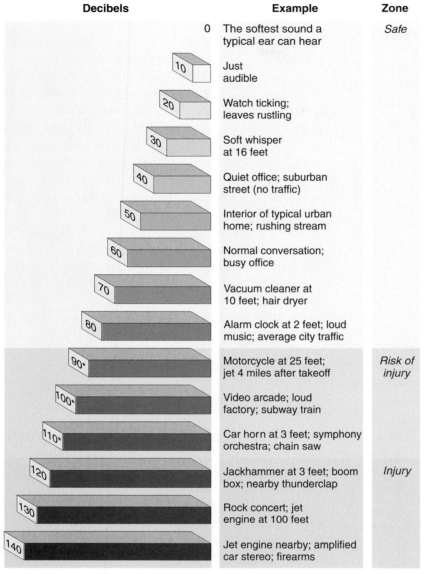

Decibels	Example	Zone
0	The softest sound a typical ear can hear	Safe
10	Just audible	
20	Watch ticking; leaves rustling	
30	Soft whisper at 16 feet	
40	Quiet office; suburban street (no traffic)	
50	Interior of typical urban home; rushing stream	
60	Normal conversation; busy office	
70	Vacuum cleaner at 10 feet; hair dryer	
80	Alarm clock at 2 feet; loud music; average city traffic	
90*	Motorcycle at 25 feet; jet 4 miles after takeoff	Risk of injury
100*	Video arcade; loud factory; subway train	
110*	Car horn at 3 feet; symphony orchestra; chain saw	
120	Jackhammer at 3 feet; boom box; nearby thunderclap	Injury
130	Rock concert; jet engine at 100 feet	
140	Jet engine nearby; amplified car stereo; firearms	

Figure 21-3

Loud and louder. The human ear perceives a 10-decibel increase as a doubling of loudness. Thus, the 100 decibels of a subway train sounds much more than twice as loud as the 50 decibels of a rushing stream.

*Note: The maximum exposure allowed on the job by federal law, in hours per day, is as follows: 90 decibels–8 hours; 100 decibels–2 hours; 110 decibels–1/2 hour.

Strategies for Prevention

Sound Safety

✔ If you must live or work in a noisy area, wear hearing protectors to prevent exposure to blasts of very loud noise. Don't think cotton or facial tissue stuck in your ears can protect you; foam or soft plastic earplugs are more effective. Wear them when operating lawn mowers, weed trimmers, or power tools.

✔ Soundproof your home by using draperies, carpets, and bulky furniture. Put rubber mats under washing machines, blenders, and other noisy appliances. Seal cracks around windows and doors.

✔ When you hear a sudden loud noise, press your fingers against your ears. Limit your exposure to loud noise. Several brief periods of noise seem less damaging than one long exposure.

✔ Be careful if you wear Walkman-type stereos. The volume is too high if you can feel the vibrations.

✔ Beware of large doses of aspirin. Researchers have found that eight aspirins a day can aggravate the damage caused by loud noise; twelve aspirins daily can cause ringing in the ears (tinnitus).

✔ Don't drink in noisy environments. Alcohol intensifies the impact of noise and increases the risk of lifelong hearing damage.

Is Your Water Safe to Drink?

According to various EPA reports, as many as 37% of public water-supply systems contains measurable and possibly dangerous quantities of man-made chemicals. Some make water look or taste funny. Others have lethal effects at very high concentrations. Some contaminants enter the water as a result of natural processes, such as the decay of vegetation. Others are the result of urban development, industrial activity, and agricultural runoff. In 1995, the drinking water supply of some 21 million Americans violated one or more public health standards.[31]

Many toxic chemicals and heavy metals—including lead, mercury, cadmium, and chromium that can cause kidney and nervous system damage and birth defects—accumulate in fish and shellfish, which can pass them on to humans. Several states have had to ban fishing in specific areas because the contamination level posed a significant risk of cancer or other health effects.

Each year the CDC reports an average of 7400 cases of illness related to the water people drink. (See Chapter 11 on infectious diseases.) The most common culprits include parasites, bacteria, viruses, chemicals, and lead. Health officials suggest having your water tested if you live near a hazardous waste dump or industrial park, if the pipes in your house are made of lead or joined together with lead solder, if your water comes from a well, or if you purchase it from a private company. Check to see if your state health department or local water supplier will provide free testing. If not, use a state-certified laboratory that tests water in accordance with EPA standards.

Is bottled water better? That's what consumers have often assumed. Yet in the past, the Food and Drug Administration (FDA) simply defined bottled water as "sealed in bottles or other containers and intended for human consumption." Bottled water wasn't required to be "pure" or even to be tested for toxic chemicals. However, the FDA has called for federal monitoring of the purity of bottled water. Some states, including California and New York, have their own bottled-water safety standards to ensure that bottled water is at least as safe as drinking water. In cases where public drinking water has been contaminated (for instance, by a toxic spill) and health authorities advise using bottled waters, check the label to make sure that the brand you purchase has been tested or undergone purification treatment.

Fluoride

About half (53%) of Americans drink water containing fluoride, an additive to water and toothpaste that helps teeth resist decay. According to the American Dental Association (ADA), tooth decay is 50% to 70% lower in areas with fluoridated water. However, laboratory rats given fluoridated water have shown a high rate of bone cancer. The more fluoride they drank in their water, the more likely they were to develop this cancer. But this type of cancer is extremely rare in humans, and the estimated lifetime risk to any individual from drinking fluoridated water is less than one in 5000.

Federal health officials have found no evidence that fluoride causes cancer in humans and have concluded that its benefits far outweigh any risks. However, excessive fluoride can increase bone loss and fractures in pre- and postmenopausal women. Health professionals advise consumers to use only small amounts of fluoridated toothpastes, rinse thoroughly after brushing, and use fluoride supplements only when the home water supply is known to be deficient.[32]

Chlorine

Three-quarters of the American population drinks water treated with chlorine to kill disease-causing bacteria. The Council on Environmental Quality has warned that people drinking chlorinated water have a 53% greater risk of getting colon and bladder cancer and a 13%–93% greater risk of getting rectal cancer than those not drinking chlorinated water. There may even be a link between soft water and a higher rate of cardiovascular disease, perhaps because soft water in some areas tends to have more sodium in it.

Lead

Long recognized as a hazard in paint and dust, lead can also leach from pipes into the drinking supply. According to a 1992 EPA report, lead in drinking water exceeds permissible levels in nearly 20% of the nation's largest cities. The highest risk exists in cities with older housing and lead pipes or water lines.

Strategies for Prevention

Water Safety

 Carefully examine a glass of water from your faucet: Does it have a red or orange hue? Does it smell funny?

Unusual colors or smells may indicate contamination. If you have any reason to be suspicious of your tap water, switch to bottled water until you can have it checked.

✔ Whenever the faucet hasn't been used for several hours, let water run for three to five minutes before drinking or cooking with it. This lowers lead content.

✔ Don't use hot tap water for drinking, cooking, or mixing baby formulas. Hot water dissolves lead more quickly than does cold water and is likely to have a higher lead concentration.

✔ Never pour toxic materials down the kitchen drain. Store them until you can take them to a hazardous waste collection center.

Chemical Risks

Each year, a thousand new chemicals join the 50,000–75,000 already in common use. In most cases, little is known about their potential ill effects. However, scientists have identified the types that may pose the greatest risk. An estimated 50,000–70,000 U.S. workers die each year of chronic diseases related to past exposure to toxic substances, including lung cancer, bladder cancer, leukemia, lymphoma, chronic bronchitis, and disorders of the nervous system.

Pesticides

The chemical agents used to destroy unwanted insects, plants, and fungi save billions of dollars of valuable crops from pests; at the same time, they may endanger human health and life. **Chlorinated hydrocarbons** include several high-risk substances—such as DDT, kepone, and chlordane—that have been restricted or banned because they may cause cancer, birth defects, neurological disorders, and damage to wildlife and the environment. They are extremely resistant to breakdown.

Organic phosphates, including chemicals such as malathion, break down more rapidly than do the chlorinated hydrocarbons. Most chlorinated hydrocarbons are highly toxic, causing cramps, confusion, diarrhea, vomiting, headaches, and breathing difficulties. Higher levels in the blood can lead to convulsions, paralysis, coma, and death. Farm workers and those in the surrounding communities are at greatest risk for pesticide exposure.

Strategies for Prevention
Using Pesticides Safely

✔ If you must use a pesticide or household chemical rather than a safer alternative, read the label carefully. Make sure you understand the directions for use, precautions, and first-aid instructions.

✔ Store these products in a locked place, out of the reach of children and pets.

✔ Don't measure chemicals with food-preparation utensils. Don't mix different chemicals unless their labels tell you to do so. Wear rubber gloves when using chemicals, and store them only in their manufacturer's container.

✔ If you have your house commercially fumigated for termites, hire licensed exterminators. Make sure that they don't use chlordane or spray into heating or cooling vents. Find out which chemicals they use. To check these out, call the EPA hotline. Keep everyone out of the house while the exterminators are working. If possible, sleep elsewhere for a few days after a full-scale fumigation.

Toxic Chemicals, Metals, and Wastes

The family of 75 chemicals called **dioxins** can linger in the body for years. In sunlight, dioxins break down

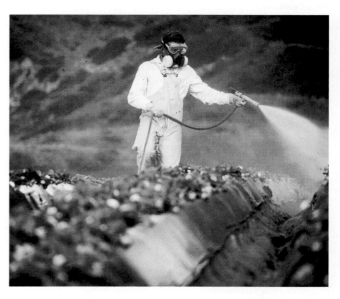

Pesticides protect crops from harmful insects, plants, and fungi but may endanger human health.

fairly quickly into less toxic compounds. However, when they get into the upper layers of the soil, they retain their original structure. Long-term exposure to dioxin—a chemical linked to birth defects, tumors, and skin problems—may damage the body's immune system and may increase the risk of infections or possibly cancer.

Agent Orange, a herbicide containing dioxin, was used to clear vegetation during the Vietnam War in the 1960s and early 1970s. Although some studies found no birth defects in children whose fathers served in Vietnam, others found a higher incidence of stillbirths and birth defects in children whose fathers might have been exposed to Agent Orange.

Polychlorinated biphenyls (PCBs) belong to a family of 209 chemical compounds that are widely used as coolants and lubricants in electrical equipment; in insulating fluids; and in the manufacture of common products such as plastics, adhesives, paints, and varnishes. PCBs made their way into the environment when industries discharged PCB-laden wastes into rivers and streams, or disposed of them in open landfills. A possible human carcinogen, PCB is no longer commercially produced in the United States, but high levels of PCB remain in certain parts of the country, and in eggs, poultry, and fish.

In the United States, exposure to the heavy metal cadmium results mainly from inhaling cigarette smoke or city air. Cadmium may be linked to high blood pressure and heart disease. The use of beryllium, a metal with many industrial uses (fluorescent bulb manufacture, for example), has increased 500% over the past 25 years. According to the EPA, beryllium can cause severe respiratory problems, including bronchitis and lung cancer.

Before the environmental laws of the last two decades, industry dumped most of its waste into open pits, abandoned mines, or nearby rivers. The EPA has identified thousands of potentially dangerous dumps, pits, ponds, and landfills across the nation (Figure 21-4). Many of these are designated industrial-waste sites, but even the local landfill can be a danger.

The burning of garbage and industrial waste in the country's toxic-waste incinerators has created a new problem: emissions containing dangerous pollutants, such as lead, which can damage children's central nervous systems, and cancer-causing dioxins.[33] Toxic waste dumps often end up near low-income areas, placing those populations at greatest risk. Other sources of pollution are the 2 million or more storage tanks containing gasoline, petroleum, and other chemicals, which are buried underground at gas stations, factories, and other sites around the country. The EPA estimates that 10% to 30% of these may be leaking their contents into the water supply. New laws are requiring the replacement of some tanks.

Figure 21-4

Hazardous waste dumps. Each dot represents a hazardous waste dump that poses a serious threat to life. These are sites on the EPA's priority list for cleanup, but there are many other dangerous waste dumps in the United States.

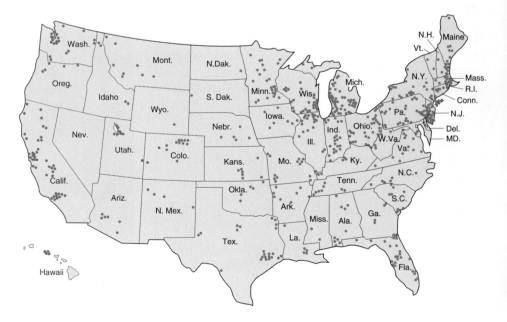

Invisible Dangers

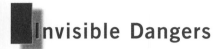

Among the unseen threats to health are various forms of radiation.

Electromagnetic Fields

Any electrically charged conductor generates two kinds of invisible fields: electric and magnetic. Together they're called **electromagnetic fields (EMFs)**. For years, these fields, produced by household appliances, home wiring, lighting fixtures, electric blankets, and overhead power lines, were considered harmless. Although epidemiological studies have shown a link between exposure to high-voltage lines and cancer (especially leukemia, a blood cancer) in electrical workers and children, this association remains controversial.

Laboratory studies on animals have shown that alternating current, which changes strength and direction 60 times a second (and electrifies most of North America), emits fields that may interfere with the normal functioning of human cell membranes, which have their own electromagnetic fields. The result may be mood disorders, changes in circadian rhythms (our inner sense of time), miscarriage, developmental problems, or cancer. Researchers have documented an increase in breast cancer deaths in women who worked as electrical engineers, electricians, or in other high-exposure jobs and a link between EMF exposure and an increased risk of leukemia and possibly brain cancer.[34]

Many scientists disagree about the threat posed by EMFs. Almost 20 years of research into the effects of electromagnetic fields have revealed no strong link between these fields and cancer. In a 1997 study of more than 1000 children, researchers actually measured electromagnetic levels in the children's homes, rather than estimating the exposure on the proximity to power lines, and found no adverse effects.[35] However, there is continued debate about the effects of relatively low exposure levels, with a focus on cellphones and TV transmitters.[36]

Appliances that are used only briefly, such as hair dryers, are probably less dangerous than electric blankets, which people sleep under for an entire night. Expectant mothers who often use electric blankets or heated water beds during winter have a higher miscarriage rate than nonusers; babies conceived in the winter by electric blanket-users grow more slowly in the womb and tend to have a lower birth weight than others. Federal officials urge "prudent avoidance" of electric blankets for women who are pregnant or hoping to conceive.

Strategies for Prevention

Protecting Yourself from Electromagnetic Fields

✔ Sit at least 3 feet from a 19-inch television screen, and even farther from a larger screen. Sit at least 13 inches from the computer screen. Install a special screen on your computer that can block out some of the radiation.

✔ If you use a plug-in electric alarm clock, which produces strong magnetic fields, keep it at least 3 feet away from your head at night. Some experts suggest switching to a battery-powered or wind-up clock.

✔ Use electric blankets only to warm the bed. Unplug the blanket or remove it before climbing under the covers. Children and pregnant women should avoid using them entirely.

Video Display Terminals (VDTs)

Chances are there's a **video display terminal (VDT)** in your life—at the school library, at the office where you work, or maybe in your home. Is it a health hazard? The answer is a definite maybe. Although VDTs have been blamed for increases in reproductive problems, miscarriages, low infant birthweights, and cataracts, repeated measurements of radiation from VDTs have shown that leakage is well below present standards for safe occupational exposure. However, VDTs emit electromagnetic fields from all sides, not just the screen, and the strongest emissions are from the sides, backs, and tops of monitors. At least in theory, working next to someone using a computer may be more hazardous than using one yourself. Scientists are continuing to investigate possible links between VDT use and health hazards.

Microwaves

Microwaves (extremely high frequency electromagnetic waves) increase the rate at which molecules vibrate; this vibration generates heat. There's no evidence that existing levels of microwave radiation encountered in the environment pose a health risk to people, and all home microwave ovens must meet safety standards for leakage.

Another concern about the safety of microwave ovens stems from the chemicals in plastic wrapping and containers used for them, which may leak into food. Some, such as DEHA, a chemical that makes plastic more pliable, can cause cancer in mice in high concentrations. Consumers should be cautious about using clingy plastic wrap when reheating leftovers, and plastic-encased metal "heat susceptors" included in convenience foods such as popcorn and pizza. Although these materials seem safe when tested in conventional ovens at temperatures of 300°F–350°F, microwave ovens can boost temperatures to 500°F.

Ionizing Radiation

Radiation that possesses enough energy to separate electrons from their atoms, leaving charged ions, is called **ionizing radiation**. Its effects on health depend on many factors, including the amount, length of exposure, type, part of the body exposed, and the health and age of the individual.

We're surrounded by low-level ionizing radiation every day (see Table 21-2). Most comes from cosmic rays and radioactive minerals, which vary according to geography. (Denver has more than Atlanta, for instance, because of its altitude.) Man-made sources, including medical and dental X rays, account for approximately 18% of the average person's lifetime exposure.

TABLE 21-2   RADIATION EXPOSURE AND RISKS

Sources of Radiation	Exposure and Percentage of Total Annual Dose
Natural	
Radon	200 millirems (55%)
Internal exposure	40 millirems (11%)
Rocks and soil	28 millirems (8%)
Cosmic	27 millirems (8%)
Man-made	
Medical X rays	39 millirems (11%)
Nuclear medicine	14 millirems (4%)
Consumer products	10 millirems (3%)
Others	Less than 1%

Toxic levels	Effects
50 rads	A few people develop radiation sickness, which is characterized by nausea and vomiting, diarrhea, hair loss, hemorrhaging, and bone-marrow damage; some develop leukemia later in life.
150 rads	About half of those exposed become ill; some die.
300 rads	Half of those exposed die within thirty days.
650 rads	All of those exposed die within thirty days.

SOURCE: National Council on Radiation Protection and Measurement.

Radiation exposure in humans is measured in units called rads and rems. A *rad (radiation absorbed dose)* is a measure of the energy deposited by ionizing radiation when it's absorbed by an object. A *rem (roentgen equivalent man)* is a measure of the biological effect of ionizing radiation. Different types of radiation cause different amounts of damage. The rem measurement takes this into account. For X rays, rads and rems are equivalent. A quantity of 1 rad or 1 rem is a substantial dose of radiation. Smaller doses are measured in *millirads (thousandths of a rad)* or *millirems (thousandths of a rem)*. The average annual radiation exposure for a person in the United States is about one-tenth of a rem.

Although high levels of radiation are most dangerous, even low-level radiation can be harmful to health. According to the National Research Council, the risk of getting cancer from small amounts of radiation is four times more than had been previously estimated, and there's much greater danger of mental retardation among babies exposed to radiation in the womb from eight to fifteen weeks after conception.

Diagnostic X Rays

The EPA estimates that 30% to 50% of the 700 million X rays taken every year in the United States are unnecessary. However, doctors sometimes prescribe X rays or newer imaging techniques involving radiation, such as CT scans, to protect themselves from malpractice suits, and hospitals benefit financially from the heavy use of X-ray equipment.

Dental X rays involve little radiation, but many people receive so many so often that they're second only to chest examinations in frequency. Dentists typically obtain radiographs of all the teeth at the beginning of a patient's care, and again every three to five years. However, you can cut down on total X rays by bringing previous films with you or having your dentist forward copies when you switch dentists.

Always ask why an X ray is being ordered. Don't give your consent unless there's a clear need. Keep a record of the date and location of every X ray exam. Some of these X rays may someday provide information that would make more X rays unnecessary. Ask the radiologist to explain specifically how much radiation you'll be exposed to, and be sure to wear a protective leaded apron. There's no sense in refusing a needed medical X ray just because you're afraid of the radiation exposure. Under certain circumstances, the benefits far outweigh the risks.

Frequent Flying

The Department of Transportation has identified a new radiation risk: air travel. While the occasional traveler faces slight danger, the radiation that penetrates the thin metal "skins" of airplanes can increase the risk of cancer in airline crews and very frequent fliers. Those flying at higher altitudes and over the earth's North or South Pole are at greater risk. Among 100,000 crew members who spend 20 years aloft on the high-risk routes, radiation could cause 1000 "premature cancer deaths." Pregnant women crew members may face a slightly increased risk of birth defects, especially from the eighth to fifteenth week after conception.

Radioactivity

The emission of nuclear radiation by radioactive materials is called radioactivity. The degree of damage it causes depends on the particular type of radioactivity, as well as the dosage. The following are the three major kinds of radioactivity:

1. *Alpha particles.* The slowest and least penetrating; cannot pass through the skin and are not a health hazard unless the emitting material is ingested or inhaled.
2. *Beta particles.* Can penetrate slightly into the body; if the emitting material is ingested, can affect the bones and thyroid.
3. *Gamma rays.* Similar to X rays and the most hazardous; can pass right through the human body.

Irradiated Foods

The use of radiation on food, from either radioactive substances or devices that produce X rays, is known as **irradiation**. It doesn't make the food radioactive; its primary benefit is to prolong the food's useful life. Like the heat in canning, irradiation can kill all the microorganisms that might grow in a food; the sterilized food can then be stored for years in sealed containers at room temperature without spoiling. In addition, low-dose irradiation can inhibit the sprouting of vegetables such as potatoes and onions, and delay the ripening of some fruits, such as bananas, mangoes, tomatoes, pears, and avocados—cost-saving benefits of great appeal to the food industry.

Irradiated foods are believed to be safe to eat, and the federal government has approved their distribution. Most research has focused on low-dose irradiation to

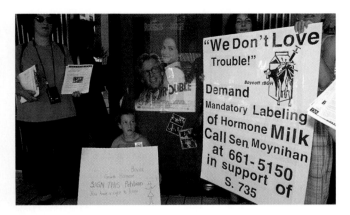

Irradiated foods are believed to be safe and to retain nutritional value. Nevertheless, irradiation of food is controversial, and many consumers have lobbied for labeling of irradiated products.

delay ripening and destroy insects. Nutritional studies have shown no significant decreases in the quality of the foods, but high-dose treatments may cause vitamin losses similar to those that occur during canning. It's also possible that the ionizing effect of radiation creates new compounds in foods that may be mutagenic/carcinogenic.[37]

Nuclear Reactors and Radioactive Wastes

In the United States, nuclear power hasn't become a major energy source. One reason is the fear of a possibly catastrophic accident, such as those that occurred at Three Mile Island in Pennsylvania in 1979 and at Chernobyl in the former Soviet Union in 1986. At Three Mile Island, as a result of operator mistakes, design flaws, and mechanical failures (a stuck valve), the nuclear reactor destroyed itself by overheating to 2500°F. At Chernobyl, while the operators of the nuclear plant were testing the plant's turbines to examine how they might be used in an emergency, they deactivated several safety systems. During the test, the reactor's temperature soared to 5000°F, and an enormous steam explosion blew the roof off the building. The radioactive uranium core melted, giving off many radioactive isotopes that eventually circled the globe. Even if no accidents occur, a nuclear plant is expected to be safe for only about 30 years. After that, parts of the reactor mechanism are so weakened by radioactivity that they must be removed and the plant shut down.

More than 23,000 tons of highly radioactive waste materials—sometimes called *radwaste*—have accumulated around the 111 operating nuclear power plants in the United States. Each year the world produces about 1 million cubic feet of intermediate and high-level waste—that's equal to a cube about 100 feet on each side. Researchers have documented higher than normal rates of cancer among those who live near nuclear facilities.

Most nuclear wastes haven't found a permanent home. Military radwaste—some 380,000 cubic meters' worth, equivalent to a giant cube 240 feet wide—is scattered across the nation, in liquid vats or underwater barrels. The U.S. Congress has allocated $3 billion to the cleanup of hazardous wastes surrounding weapons stores, plants, and bases. Some radioactive byproducts must be stored for periods of 10 to 20 times their half-lives (the time it takes the radioactivity to reduce to one-half its original amount). This means that it will be tens of thousands of years before the radioactivity of these byproducts reaches safe levels.

Making This Chapter Work for You
Creating a Healthier World

- The term *environment* refers to the conditions under which you live—including the air you breathe, the water you drink, the sounds you hear. Decisions you make everyday—about what you buy, use, and throw away—have an impact on the environment. Your health depends on the interaction between the environment's impact on your well-being and your impact on your environment.

- The earth is a closed ecosystem or community of organisms sharing a physical and chemical environment that depends on materials that must be recycled over and over again.

- Threats to the environment include overpopulation, atmospheric changes, and the depletion of resources. In recent decades, both the United States and other nations have joined together to take steps to protect planetary well-being.

- As the world's population continues to soar, family planning has become a global public health issue. The critical steps to slowing population growth include improving the quality of reproductive and family planning services, meeting current needs for contraception, increasing access to education for girls, and involving men in family planning.[38]

Health Online

The Sierra Club   http://www.sierraclub.org/

Are you concerned about our environment? Do you want to get involved? The Sierra Club's Web site offers information on how to help influence environmental policy. It contains guidelines on how to write an effective letter to the editor, how to write or e-mail your congressional representative, and how to track down the voting record of your representative on environmental issues.

Think about it...

• Many people are concerned about environmental issues but never take the time to write to an elected official. Why do you think this is? What might help people to get involved?

• How do your local congressional representatives stand on environmental issues? Do you agree or disagree with their stands? Pick one who you disagree with and write a letter outlining your concerns.

• What environmental issues are most important to your community? Are there groups at your school that are working on these issues?

■ Pollution—any change in the air, water, or soil that could reduce its ability to support life—can have acute, or immediate, effects as well as chronic, or long-term, ones. Pollutants that trigger changes, or mutations, in the genetic material, the DNA, of living cells are called mutagens.

■ Atmospheric changes, such as the warming of the planet because of a buildup of gases and the depletion of the protective ozone layer, can have an impact on the well-being of everyone on earth. Most of the world's industrialized nations have agreed to take steps to stop or limit environmentally destructive practices.

■ Other environmental concerns include the widening gap between rich and poor in and among nations, poverty, homelessness, and hunger.

■ Individuals can make environmentally responsible decisions by precycling, recycling, and choosing products that do not harm the environment.

■ In most places in the United States, air quality has improved in the last 25 years. However, it remains less than optimal in many places, and living in a city with even moderately sooty air may shorten your life span by about a year.

■ Indoor air pollutants include environmental tobacco smoke, formaldehyde, asbestos, lead, carbon monoxide gas, nitrogen dioxide, and radioactive radon.

■ The most widespread form of environmental pollution is invisible: noise. Sounds above 85 decibels can damage sound receptors in the inner ear, resulting in hearing problems. Rock concerts and powerful stereos can produce sounds as loud as—and sometimes louder than—jackhammers and jet planes.

■ Air pollution may be caused by natural events, such as dust storms or forest fires; or it may be man made, as is smog, which may cause or worsen emphysema, chronic bronchitis, lung and stomach cancer, and heart disease.

■ The water that we drink may also be dangerous because of additives such as fluoride and chlorine, and contamination by toxic chemicals.

■ Chemical threats to health include industrial wastes, pesticides, lead, dioxin, PCBs, and heavy metals, such as cadmium and beryllium.

■ Electromagnetic fields produced by appliances, electrical wires, televisions, and VDTs may cause biological changes in body tissues in humans and animals.

■ Sources of potentially harmful ionizing radiation include X rays, food irradiation, radioactive wastes, and nuclear power plants. Even low levels of radiation can damage the genetic material in the body's cells and result in cancer and birth defects.

Environmental problems can seem so complex that you may think there's little you can do about them. That's not the case. This world can be made better instead of worse. The job isn't easy, and all of us have to do our part. Just as many diseases of the previous century have been eradicated, so, in time, we may be able to remove or reduce many environmental threats. Your future—and our planet's future—may depend on it.

Key Terms

The terms listed here are used within the chapter. Page numbers are included for each term. A definition of each term is given in the green Glossary pages at the end of this book.

acid rain *653*
chlorinated hydrocarbons *659*
decibel (dB) *656*
dioxins *659*
ecosystem *644*
electromagnetic fields
 (EMFs) *661*
fuels *647*
greenhouse effect *647*
hertz *656*
ionizing radiation *662*

irradiation *663*
microwaves *662*
mutagen *646*
mutation *646*
organic phosphates *659*
ozone layer *646*
pollutant *646*
pollution *646*
polychlorinated biphenyls
 (PCBs) *660*

precycling *650*
recycling *650*
smog *652*
teratogen *646*
video display terminal
 (VDT) *661*
zero population growth
 (ZPG) *644*

Review Questions

1. What is an ecosystem?

2. What are some major hazards to the survival of our planet? Why are they considered hazards? What are their potential effects?

3. What is indoor pollution? How is it created, and what forms does it take?

4. Describe how chemicals can affect the air, water, and land around us. How can chemicals cause pollution?

5. How does one develop a noise-induced hearing loss? What steps can a person take to protect against such loss?

6. What risks are associated with exposure to electromagnetic fields? What procedures should be followed to minimize the risk of exposure?

Critical Thinking Questions

1. How do you personally contribute to environmental pollution? How might you change your practices to protect the environment instead?

2. In the past few years, we've witnessed the end of the Cold War era in which nuclear war was often considered the ultimate health threat. Do you feel that nuclear war is still the number-one threat to health, or have other issues replaced it? What, in your opinion, is the number-one health threat?

3. In one Harris poll, 84% of Americans said that, given

a choice between a high standard of living (but with hazardous air and water pollution and the depletion of natural resources) and a lower standard of living (but with clean air and drinking water), they would prefer clean air and drinking water and a lower standard of living. What about you? What exactly would

you be willing to give up: air conditioning, convenience packaging and products, driving in your own car rather than using public transportation? Do you think that most people are willing to change their lifestyles to preserve the environment?

 ## Connections to Personal Health Interactive

To enhance your understanding of the material covered in this chapter, check out the following study aids on the **Personal Health Interactive CD-ROM**. *Each numbered icon within the chapter corresponds to an appropriate activity listed here.*

21.1 Personal Insights: How Healthy Is Your Environment?

21.2 Chapter 21 Review

 ## References

1. Population Reference Bureau, World Population Data Sheet, 1995.
2. Stevens, William. "In Kyoto, the Subject Is Climate; The Forecast Is for Storms." *New York Times*, December 1, 1997.
3. Dowie, Mark. *Losing Ground: American Environmentalism at the Close of the Twentieth Century*. Cambridge, MA: MIT Press, 1995.
4. Holmes, Steven. "Global Crisis in Population Still Serious, Group Warns." *New York Times*, December 31, 1997. "Poverty Kills—in More Ways Than You Think." *Facts of Life: An Issue Briefing for Health Reporters*, Vol. 3, No. 1, January–February 1998.
5. Alan Guttmacher Institute. *Hopes and Realities: Closing the Gap Between Women's Aspirations and Their Reproduction Experiences*. New York: Alan Guttmacher Institute, 1995.
6. Andruh, Jain, and Judith Bruce. "Quality: The Key to Success." In *Beyond the Numbers: A Reader on Population, Consumption and the Environment*. Washington, DC: Island Press, 1994.
7. Bongaarts, John. "Population Policy Options in the Developing World." *Science*, Vol. 263, February 11, 1994.
8. Bruce, Judith. "Population Policy Must Encompass More Than Family Planning Services." In *Beyond the Numbers: A Reader on Population, Consumption and the Environment*. Washington, DC: Island Press, 1994.
9. Mydans, Seth. "Southeast Asia Chokes as Indonesian Forests Burn." *New York Times*, September 25, 1997.
10. Committee on Curriculum Development in Environmental Medicine. Landrigan, Philip. "Commentary: Environmental Disease—A Preventable Epidemic." *American Journal of Public Health*, July 1992. Heam, Wayne. "Fighting a

Growing Menace." *American Medical News*, October 26, 1992.
11. Stevens, William. "Ever-so-slight Rise in Temperatures Led to a Record High in 1997." *New York Times*, January 9, 1998.
12. Whited, Johen, and Grichnik, James. "Does This Patient Have a Mole or Melanoma?" *Journal of the American Medical Association*, Vol. 279, No. 9, March 4, 1998.
13. Kristof, Nicholas. "Asian Pollution Is Widening Its Deadly Reach." *New York Times*, November 29, 1997.
14. Worldwatch Institute. *Vital Signs 1995: The Trends That Are Shaping Our Future*. New York: W. W. Norton, 1995.
15. Bongaarts, John. "Can the Growing Human Population Feed Itself?" *Scientific American*, March 1994.
16. DeLeon, Iser G., and R. W. Fuqua. "The Effects of Public Commitment and Group Feedback on Curbside Recycling." *Environment & Behavior*, Vol. 27, No. 2, March 1995.
17. Easterbrook, Gregg. "Here Comes the Sun." *The New Yorker*, April 10, 1995.
18. "When Fresh Air Kills." *American Health*, July–August 1995.
19. Witherell, Mary. "Lung Damage: Pollution May Rival Smoking." *American Health*, October 1994.
20. Specter, Michael. "Plunging Life Expectancy Puzzles Russia." *New York Times*, August 2, 1995.
21. American Lung Association et al. *Indoor Air Pollution: An Introduction for Health Professionals*. Washington, DC: Environmental Protection Agency, 1995.
22. Glantz, Stanton, and William Parmley. "Passive Smoking and Heart Disease." *Journal of the American Medical Association*, Vol. 273, No. 13, April 5, 1995.
23. Robinson, John, and Tibbett Speer. "The Air We

Breathe." *American Demographics*, Vol. 17, No. 6, June 1995.

24. Ileman, James, and Brooke Mossman. "Asbestos Revisited." *Scientific American*, Vol. 277, No. 1, July 1997.

25. Morrison, Dorothy. "Lead-based Paint Hazards: Funding Opportunities Provide Control." *Public Management*, Vol. 80, No. 1, January 1998.

26. Rosen, John. Personal interview.

27. Witherell, Mary. "Danger: Indoor Air." *American Health*, December 1994.

28. Greenwald, Judith. "A Multimedia Approach to Radon." *Environment*, Vol. 39, No. 5, June 1997.

29. Committee on Residential Radon. "ACOEM Position Statement on Residential Radon Exposure." *Journal of Medicine*, October 1992.

30. Margolis, Dawn. "Carbon Monoxide: Invisible Killer." *American Health*, January–February 1994.

31. Luong, Christine. "Can You Drink the Water?" *NEA Today*, Vol. 15, No. 9, May 1997.

32. "Uses of Dietary Reference Intakes." *Nutrition Reviews*, Vol. 55, No. 9, September 1997.

33. Pearch, Fred. "Errors of Emission." *New Scientist*, Vol. 155, No. 2102, October 4, 1997.

34. Wartik, Nancy. "Killing Fields?" *American Health*, December 1994.

35. Linet, Martha et al. "Residential Exposure to Magnetic Fields and Acute Lymphoblastic Leukemia in Children." *New England Journal of Medicine*, Vol. 337, No. 1, July 3, 1997.

36. Beale, Ivan. "The Effects of Electromagnetic Fields on Mental and Physical Health." *Journal of Child and Family Studies*, Vol. 6, No. 3, September 1997.

37. Hileman, Bette. "New Rules, Devices Advance Food Irradiation." *Chemical & Engineering News*, Vol. 75, No. 48, December 1, 1997.

38. "Progress Review: Environmental Health." Department of Health & Human Services, Public Health Service, March 12, 1997.

HALES HEALTH

ALMANAC

- ▷ HEALTH INFORMATION ON THE INTERNET
- ▶ EMERGENCY!
- ▶ A CONSUMER'S GUIDE TO MEDICAL TESTS
- ▶ COUNTING YOUR CALORIES AND FAT
- ▶ YOUR HEALTH DIRECTORY

HEALTH INFORMATION ON THE INTERNET

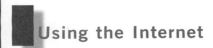

Using the Internet

The Internet: A Gateway to Health Information

What are the very latest statistics on the incidence of AIDS? Are any new drugs in the works for the treatment of diabetes? How can I get in touch with others who suffer from asthma? Is it possible to make a low-fat chocolate cake? These are the kinds of questions you can answer from your home or computer lab, with the help of the Internet. The Internet is a gold mine of information for the student of health. It can help you with research for your schoolwork, and also with personal questions and concerns about your own health. But the Internet is not comprehensively catalogued, and finding the information you need can be daunting. This guide will introduce you to health resources on the Internet and how to find them.

When you first start to explore the world of the Internet, it can seem overwhelming. What are the practical uses of the Internet for the student of health and the health care consumer?

- *Educational resources.* Most colleges and universities now have Internet hosts and World Wide Web sites. Faculty often post course information and syllabi on line, and some courses are even offered entirely on line. Some instructors require students to do tutorials or other projects on the Internet, or to do research using the Internet. In addition, you may be able to get general information about your school, its policies, programs, graduation requirements, and faculty on the Net.

- *Research.* The Internet is a repository for many health journals, government statistics, archives, and other sources of scholarly information. In addition, subscribing to a mailing list or posting to a newsgroup in an area of interest can yield new sources of information that would be hard to get elsewhere.

- *Graduate school and career information.* The Internet is a great resource for those interested in a career in a health-related field. Most graduate schools have Web sites that list their programs, entrance requirements, faculty profiles, and other information of interest to prospective students. And once you get that degree you can consult on line listings of jobs available in many areas of health care.

- *Self-help and support.* The Internet is a good way of providing information and support to people who might not otherwise have access to it. There are dozens of newsgroups and mailing lists that offer support and advice for people dealing with all kinds of health-related issues, from Alzheimer's caregivers to people with eating disorders to athletes comparing training programs.

- *Goods and services.* As many people have discovered, the Web can serve as an electronic shopping mall. For people with concerns about health it can be a place to order books, software, or journals of interest, sign up for classes or conferences, or even get online professional consultations (though we're not recommending that).

The World Wide Web

The World Wide Web is an information retrieval system designed to offer a user-friendly graphical interface with the Internet. You can surf the Web using any one of a number of different programs called browsers, such as Netscape or Microsoft Explorer. Many Web sites now offer exciting capabilities, such as audio, video, animation clips, and interactivity. Each Web site has its own unique address, or URL. URLs often begin with the characters http://. To go to a Web site, you can either type its URL into the box at the top of your browser, or click on a hyperlink from another page that will take you to the new site. Hyperlinks often appear as color or underlined text, and offer links to other Web sites that may be of interest.

There are thousands of sites related to health and wellness on the World Wide Web. As a starting point, you can try using any of the sources listed in the Resources section of this appendix. Or you can try to look for specific information by doing a Web search.

Bookmarks

When you find a website you will want to return to again in the future, you can "bookmark" it. To bookmark a site, go to that site and choose "bookmark" from your menu bar. Your browser will record the address of that site in your bookmark folder. Anytime you want to return to that site, you simply open the bookmark folder and click on the title of that website.

Tips for Using the World Wide Web

- *Be patient.* Accessing a website can take time depending on how elaborate the site is, how fast your modem can download the information, and what time of day you are surfing. You can speed things up a bit by turning off the "auto load image" option in your browser.

- *Keep in mind that glitches can occur in the transfer process.* Sometimes the server of the website you are trying to reach may be down, there may be a lot of activity on that site, or there may be line noise. Just try again to load the website, or try again later.

- *Because the Web is so dynamic, sites and links change every day.* You might find some links on webpages that go nowhere, if the link has moved their pages to a new server or address.

- *Remember that while the Web is a great source of information, not everything on it is true.* It is up to you to evaluate the information you get from the Web; see the section on Thinking Critically about Health Information on the Internet.

Searching the Web

How do you go about finding Web sites that might interest you? One way is to use one of the popular directories on the Web called search engines. A search engine allows you to type in keywords on the topic that you are interested in, and it will retrieve sites that contain those words. Some of the larger and more popular search engines are:

- **Yahoo!**
  http://www.yahoo.com

- **Alta Vista**
  http://altavista.digital.com

- **Excite**
  http://www.excite.com

- **Hot Bot**
  http://www.hotbot.com

- **Lycos**
  http://www.lycos.com

- **Infoseek**
  http://www.infoseek.com

- **WebCrawler**
  http://webcrawler.com

To use a search engine, type in one of the URLs listed above. When the home page for the site comes up you will notice a "search" box in which you can type one or more key words or phrases. The engine will then search all the sites in its index and return a list to you, with hyperlinks and sometimes short descriptions, of those that contain your keywords.

There is no single search engine that contains all the contents of the Internet. After connecting to a search engine for the first time, it is a good idea to read the tool's description, search options, and rules and restrictions. Each engine offers a different "view" of the Web and you'll want to tailor your query to make the best use of that system. Some search engines contain indexes to huge amounts of online information, so it pays to make precise queries so you don't get thousands of sites returned to you. It is also possible to make queries that are too precise and retrieve no results.

The key to an effective search is picking the right keywords. Commonly used words make poor search keywords; try to find distinctive words or combinations of words. If you use several keywords, separate them with one of these three operators: AND, OR, and NOT. Using the word AND actually narrows the results you obtain in a search. For example, if you search for "pregnancy AND teen," you will get back only sites that contain both these keywords. The word "OR" broadens the search results. You may try searching "pregnancy AND teen OR adolescent," to find sites that refer to teen or adolescent pregnancy. To limit your results, you can use the word NOT. Searching for "pregnancy AND teen NOT United States" might help you find sites that deal with teen pregnancy in other countries.

Now that you have done your search, you may end up with hundreds or even thousands of results—or only a few. If you have more results than you can handle, try making the keywords in your search more precise. See if you can think of words that uniquely identify what you are looking for, and use several relevant keywords. If you have too few results, try another search engine, using synonyms or variations on your keywords, or be less specific in your query.

Newsgroups

Newsgroups are a way of discussing topics over the Internet with other people who share the same interests or concerns. They are a popular way to establish an online community, share information, and give and receive support. For example, a person suffering from a relatively rare disorder may not know anyone else with the same problems and concerns on campus or in town, but he or she can frequent a newsgroup specifically for people with that disorder to learn about other peoples' experiences, the latest treatments, and just to commiserate. Or a person who is trying to quit smoking can participate in a newsgroup to share frustrations, tips, and successes. But, as always, be aware that not everything posted to a newsgroup is necessarily true; you must be a critical thinker.

Many commercial online services offer members-only newsgroups to their subscribers, but there are many other newsgroups available to anyone. To find a newsgroup on a topic of interest to you, try looking on the Deja News Web page, http://www.dejanews.com, which lists hundreds of newsgroups. Some health-related newsgroups are listed in the Resources section of this appendix.

Newsgroup addresses are grouped into several broad categories called hierarchies. Listed below are some of the standard hierarchies that relate to health.

- **alt**
  groups generally alternative in nature (i.e., alt.sex)

- **bionet**
  groups discussing biology and biological sciences (i.e., bionet.immunology)

- **misc**
  groups that don't fit into other categories (i.e., misc.fitness)

- **rec**
  groups discussing hobbies, sports, music, and art (i.e., rec.food)

- **sci**
  groups discussing subjects related to science and scientific research (i.e., sci.epidemiology)

- **soc**
  groups discussing social issues including politics, social programs, etc. (i.e., soc.college)

- **talk**
  public debating forums on controversial issues (i.e., talk.abortion)

Before you make a posting to a newsgroup, you may want to "lurk" for awhile, that is, read the discussion without contributing your own posting. Lurking will give you a sense of the kinds of postings that are appropriate for that newsgroup and what the newsgroup culture is like. It is also a good idea to read the newsgroup's "FAQ," or list of answers to frequently asked questions.

Postings to many newsgroups are

updated frequently, so if an item is of interest to you, you should print it or save it to your computer since it may be gone the next day. After lurking for awhile, you can join in the discussion by posting a message to the newsgroup. You may also want to reply only to the originator of a certain message. You may want to join in on the discussion of an already-existing topic, or start your own "thread."

Mailing Lists

Mailing lists (or listservs) are groups of people who "get together" via e-mail to discuss a specific topic. Mailing lists offer a way to participate in lively discussions, stay up on current research, or find out answers to burning questions. There are mailing lists on nearly every topic imaginable. Mailing lists are similar to newsgroups in that they are forums for discussion, but the messages are delivered to your e-mail account instead of to a public bulletin board. Here's how it works:

- First, find a mailing list dealing with a subject you are interested in discussing with others (i.e., attention deficit disorder). A good list of health-related mailing lists can be found on the Good Health Web site, http://www.social.com/health/mlists.html.

- In order to get involved in a discussion group, you have to subscribe to it. To subscribe, send an e-mail to that mailing list's "subscribe" address with the word "subscribe" in the subject line and in the main body of the text. Also include your e-mail address.

- Usually, the listserv will then subscribe you to the list and send you instructions on how to "post" to the group. "Posting" means that you send out a comment to the entire mailing list that you have subscribed to.

- Every time any member posts to the listserv, all the subscribers get that posting as an e-mail message in their mailbox.

- Once you have subscribed you will begin to receive e-mail messages from the mailing list. Be careful though: some discussion groups have a large

following and you may find your mailbox filling up faster than you can read the messages.

- Again, evaluate carefully any information you get from a mailing list to make sure it is accurate.

Thinking Critically About Health Information on the Internet

Unlike information in most books and journals, anyone can post information or advice on the Internet. Some of this information can be misleading or downright harmful, so it is important to use your best critical thinking skills to evaluate health information you find on the Internet. When evaluating information on the Net, ask yourself the following questions.

- *Who is the author or sponsor of the information?* The author of the site is usually listed at the top or bottom of a site's home page. Be very wary of any anonymous site. Sites that are maintained by established schools or universities, government agencies, professional organizations, or other established organizations like the American Cancer Society are probably trustworthy. Sites created by individuals or other groups may or may not contain valid information; see if you can verify their information in other places. And keep in mind that many sites contain links to other pages which may be maintained by other less (or more) reliable sources.

- *Is it current?* Many sites post the date of their most recent modification. Look for sites where you can determine when the information was created or modified; many of the best sites are updated weekly or even daily.

- *What is the purpose of the site?* The hidden purpose of some health Web sites is to sell products or act as a vehicle for advertisements. Be wary of any site that tries to sell you things or get your money. Also beware of sites that seem to be trying to persuade you of things, promote "miracle cures" or anything that seems too good to be true. There are also people who use newsgroups and other chat forums to

sell or persuade. Be skeptical and use your common sense.

- *Who is the intended audience?* Some Internet information is intended for doctors and other health care professionals; although the information may be accurate, it may be too difficult for a layperson to interpret on their own. Other Web sites or Internet forums are targeted toward people with specific problems or disorders, students, or the general public.

- *Is the information verifiable?* To get a better perspective on information from the Internet, see if you can verify it with other sources. Before you follow any health advice you get from the Net, check it out with your physician.

Health Resources on the Internet

General Health Resources

Centers for Disease Control and Prevention
http://www.cdc.gov

National Health Information Center (NHIC)
http://www.nhic-nt.health.org/

Yahoo Health Directory
http://www.yahoo.com/health

Achoo Health Directory
http://www.achoo.com/health

American Medical Association
http://ama-assn.org

Go Ask Alice
http://www.columbia.edu/cu/health-wise/all.html

Healthfinder
http://www.healthfinder.gov/

Health A to Z
http://www.HealthAtoZ.com

Duke University Diet and Fitness Center Home Page
http://dmi-www.duke.edu/dfc/home.html

Healthy People 2000
http://odphp.osophs.dhhs.gov/pubs/hp2000/

Mental, Emotional, and Spiritual Health

National Institute of Mental Health (NIMH)
http://www.nimh.hih.gov/home.htm

Psych Central: Dr. John Grohol's Mental Health Page
http://www.coil.com/~grohol/

Internet Mental Health
http://www.mentalhealth.com/

American Psychological Association
http://www.apa.org

National Depressive/Manic-Depressive Association
http://www.ndmda.org/

Stress Management
http://www.ivf.com/stress.html

Stress Busters
http://stressrelease.com/strssbus.html

Stress, Depression, Anxiety, Sleep Problems, and Drug Use
http://www.teachhealth.com/

Trauma Info Pages
http://gladstone.uoregon.edu/~dvb/trauma.htm

The International Society for Traumatic Stress Studies
http://istss.com

Newsgroups
- alt.support.anxiety-panic
- alt.support.depression
- alt.support.loneliness
- alt.support.sleep-disorders
- soc.support.depression.crisis
- soc.support.dpression.family
- soc.support.depression.manic
- soc.support.depression.misc
- soc.support.depression.seasonal
- soc.support.depression.treatment
- alt.support.ocd
- alt.support.schizophrenia
- alt.support.shyness

Fitness

The Fitness Partner Connection Jumpsite
http://www.primusweb.com/fitnesspartner/

The Internet's Fitness Resource
http://rampages.onramp.net/~chaz/

President's Council on Physical Fitness and Sports
http://www.hoptechno.com/book11.htm

Worldguide Online
http://www.worldguide.com/Fitness/

Stretching Information
http://www.cs.huji.ac.il/papers/rma/stretching_1.html

American College of Sports Medicine (ACSM)
http://www.a1.com/sportsmed/

Newsgroups
- misc.fitness
- misc.fitness.aerobic
- rec.fitness

Nutrition and Eating Issues

FDA Center for Food Safety and Applied Nutrition
http://vm.cfsan.fda.gov/list.html

USDA Food and Nutrition Information Center
http://www.nalusda.gov/fnic/

Diet Analysis Web Page
http://dawp.futuresouth.com/

Fast Food Finder
http://www.olen.com/food/

Virtual Vegetarian
http://www.vegetariantimes.com/

Ask the Dietitian
http://www.hoptechno.com/rdindex.htm

Center for Science in the Public Interest
http://www.cspinet.org/

Meals Online
http://www/meals.com

The Overeaters Recovery Group
http://www..hiwaay.net/recovery/

Overeaters Anonymous
http://www.overeatersanonymous.org/

Cyberdiet
http://www.cyberdiet.com/

Light Cooking
http://www.lightcooking.com/

Eating Disorders
http://www.something-fishy.com/ed.htm

Ask the Dietitian/Overweight
http://www.hoptechno.com/overweig.htm

Newsgroups
- sci.med.nutrition
- alt.support.diet
- alt.support.obesity
- alt.support.big-folks
- alt.support.eating-diord

Sexuality

Planned Parenthood
http://www.ppfa.org/ppfa/

Ultimate Birth Control Links Page
http://gnspages.com/ultimate/

Association of Voluntary and Safe Contraception International
http://www.avsc.org/avsc/

National Abortion Federation
http://www.prochoice.org/naf/

National Abortion and Reproductive Rights League
http://www.naral.org/

National Right to Life Committee
http://www.nrlc.org/

Labor and Birth Resources
http://www.childbirth.org/articles/labor.html

International Council on Infertility Information Dissemination
http://www.mnsinc.com/inciid.html

National Coalition for Birthing Alternatives
http://www.ptw.com/~troytash/

Pregnancy, Reproduction, and Health Education
http://www.childbirth.org/

It's Just Another Baby
http://www.westnet.com/~crywalt/pregnancy/

The Kinsey Institute for Research in Sex, Gender, and Reproduction
http://www.indiana.edu/~kinsey/

The Institute for Advanced Study of Human Sexuality
http://www.netaccess.on.ca/~sexorg/

Sexology Netline
http://www.netaccess.on.ca/~sexorg/

Sexuality Information and Education Council of the United States (SIECUS)
http://www.siecus.org/

The Johns Hopkins University STD Page
http://www.med.jhu.edu/jhustd/

American Foundation for the Prevention of Venereal Disease
http://www.iacnet.com/health/09112524.htm

The Safer Sex Page
http://www.safersex.org/

American Social Health Association
http://sunsite.unc.edu/ASHA

Newsgroups
- sci.med.midwifery
- sci.med.obgyn
- alt.infertility.primary
- alt.infertility.secondary
- misc.health.infertility
- soc.support.pregnancy.loss
- alt.support.breastfeeding
- alt.support.childfree

- talk.abortion
- alt.support.abortion
- alt.support.herpes
- alt.sex.safe

Diseases and Disorders

CDC National AIDS Clearinghouse
http://www.cdcnac.org/

The CDC HIV/AIDS Page
http://www.cdc.gov/diseases/hivqa.html

Harvard AIDS Institute
http://www.hsph.harvard.edu/Organizations/hai/home_pg.html

HIV InSite
http://www.hivinsite.ucsf.edu/

HIV Infoweb
http://carebase2.jri.org/infoweb/

Newsgroups
- sci.med.aids
- misc.health.aids
- clari.tw.health.aids
- alt.sex.safe

American Cancer Society
http://www.cancer.org

National Cancer Institute
http:www.nci.nih.gov/

Cancer-related links
http://users.aol.com/ronmairrag/rcancer.html

Med Help International/Cancer Library
http://medhlp.netusa.net/general/cancer2/cancerpt.htm

OncoLink/The University of Pennsylvania Cancer Center Resource
http://cancer.med.upenn.edu/

Newsgroups
- sci.med.diseases.cancer
- alt.support.cancer
- alt.support.cancer.prostate
- alt.support.cancer.testicular

American Heart Association
http://www.amhrt.org

Heart and Stroke Foundation of Canada
http://www.hsf.ca/

Determining Your Risk of Heart Disease
http://207.69.209.38/detrskm.htm

The Heart: An Online Exploration
http://www.fi.edu/biosci/heart.html

Cardiovascular Disease in Minority Populations
http://www.uvm.edu/~vdouglas/project.htm

Cut to the Heart
http://www.pbs.org/wgbh/pages/nova/heart/

Newsgroups
- sci.med.cardiology
- alt.support.heart

Drug Use, Misuse, and Abuse

Alcoholics Anonymous
http://www.alcoholics-anonymous.org

National Institute on Alcohol Abuse and Alcoholism
http://www.niaaa.nih.gov/

National Association for Children of Alcoholics
http://www.health.org/nacoa/

Web of Addictions
http://www.well.com/user/woa

Al-Anon/Alateen
http://solar.rtd..utk.edu/~al-anon/

Habitsmart
http://www.cts.com/~habtsmrt//

Newsgroups
- alt.recovery
- clari.news.alcohol

National Institute on Drug Abuse
http://www.nida.hih.gov

Higher Education Center for Alcohol and Other Drug Prevention
http://www.edc.org/hec/

Cocaine Anonymous World Services
http://www.ca.org/

Narcotics Anonymous
http://users.aol.com/na4napa/na1.html

National Organization for the Reform of Marijuana Laws
http://www.natlnorml.org/

CDC's Tobacco Information and Prevention Sourcepage
http://www/cdc.gov/tobacco/

Prevention Online
http://www.health.org/

NicNet: Nicotine and Tobacco Network
http://www.acsc.arizona.edu/nicnet/

Tobacco Control Resource Center
http://www.tobacco.neu.edu/

The Quitnet
http://www.quitnet.org/

Smokescreen Tobacco Central Network
http://www.Smokescreen.org

Medicine OnLine/environmental tobacco smoke
http://www.com/mol/env_smk.html

Newsgroups
- alt.support.stop-smoking

- alt.support.non-smokers
- alt.support.non-smokers.moderated
- clari.news.smoking
- sci.med.cannabis
- alt.support.recovery.na
- alt.drugs
- clari.news.drugs
- talk.politics.drugs

Planning for Tomorrow

American Environmental Health Foundation
http://www.aehf.com/

The Envirolink
http://envirolink.org/start_web.html

Directory of Sites in Occupational and Environmental Health
http://www.ed.ac.uk/hew/links/

Environmental Protection Agency
http://www.epa.gov/

Community Environmental Action Web
http://www.commpages.com/globe/

MedAccess
http://www.medaccess.com

MedScape
http://www.medscape.com/

Idea Central Health Policy Page
http://epn.org/idea/health.html

The Alternative Medicine Homepage
http://www.pitt.edu/~cbw/altm.html

Caregiver Survival Resources
http://www.caregiver911.com/

Administration on Aging
http://www.aoa.dhhs.gov/

The Alzheimer's Page
http://

The National Council on the Aging
http://www.ncoa.org/

University of Texas Medical Branch Center on Aging
http://www.utmb.edu/aging/

Choice in Dying
http://www.choices.org/

The Compassionate Friends
http://www.jjt.com/~tcf_national/

Hospice Hands
http://gator.net/~jnash/hospice.html

Newsgroups
- clari.news.aging
- alt.support.alzheimers
- bionet.neuroscience.amyloid
- alt.support.grief
- soc.support.pregnancy.loss

EMERGENCY!

By definition, an emergency is a situation in which you have to think and act fast. Start by assessing the circumstances. Shout for help if you're in a public place. Look for any possible dangers to you or the victim, such as a live electrical wire or a fire. Seek medical assistance as quickly as possible. Dial 911, the operator, or a local emergency phone number, and keep it near every phone in your house. Don't attempt rescue techniques, such as cardiopulmonary resuscitation (CPR), unless you are trained. If you have a car, be sure you know the shortest route from your home to the nearest 24-hour hospital emergency department.

Supplies

Every home should have a kit of basic first aid supplies kept in a convenient location out of the reach of children. Stock it with the following:

- Bandages
- Sterile gauze pads and bandages
- Adhesive tape
- Scissors
- Cotton balls or absorbent cotton
- Cotton swabs
- Thermometer
- Syrup of ipecac to induce vomiting
- Antibiotic ointments
- Sharp needle
- Safety pins
- Calamine lotion

Keep a similar kit in your car or boat. You might want to add some extra items from your home, such as a flashlight, soap, blanket, paper cups, and any special equipment that a family member with a chronic illness may need.

Bleeding

Blood loss is frightening and dangerous. Direct pressure stops external bleeding. Since internal bleeding can also be life-threatening, you must be aware of the warning signs.

For an Open Wound

1. Apply direct pressure over the site of the wound. Cover the entire wound.

2. Use sterile gauze, a sanitary napkin, a clean towel, sheet, or handkerchief or, if necessary, your washed bare hand. Ice or cold water in a pad will help stop bleeding and decrease swelling.

3. Apply firm, steady pressure for five to fifteen minutes. Most wounds stop bleeding within a few minutes.

4. If the wound is on a foot, hand, leg, or arm, use gravity to help slow the flow of blood. Elevate the limb so that it is higher than the victim's heart.

5. If the bleeding doesn't stop, press harder.

6. Seek medical attention if the bleeding was caused by a serious injury, if stitches will be needed to keep the wound closed, or if the victim has not had a tetanus booster within the last ten years.

For Internal Bleeding

1. Suspect internal bleeding if a person coughs up blood, vomits red or brown material that looks like coffee grounds, passes blood in urine or stool, or has black, tarlike bowel movements.

2. Do not let the victim take any medication or fluids by mouth until seen by a doctor, because surgery may be necessary.

3. Have the victim lie flat. Cover him or her lightly.

4. Seek immediate medical attention.

For a Bloody Nose

1. Have the victim sit down, leaning slightly forward so the blood does not run down his or her throat. The person should spit out any blood in his or her mouth.

2. Use the thumb and forefingers to pinch the nose. If the victim can do the pinching, apply a cold compress to the nose and surrounding area.

3. Apply pressure for ten minutes without interruption.

4. If pinching does not work, gently pack the nostril with gauze or a clean strip of cloth. Do not use absorbent cotton, which will stick. Let the ends hang out so you can remove the packing easily later. Pinch the nose, with the packing in place, for five minutes.

5. If a foreign object is in the nose, do not attempt to remove it. Ask the person to blow gently. If that does not work, seek medical attention.

6. The nose should not be blown or irritated for several hours after a nosebleed stops.

Breathing Problems

If a person appears to be unconscious, approach carefully. The victim may be in contact with electrical current. If so, make sure the electricity is shut off before touching the victim. The first function you should check is respiration. Tap or shake the victim's shoulder gently, shouting, "Are you all right?" Look for any signs of breathing: Can you hear breath sounds? Can you feel breath on your cheek? If the person is breathing, do not perform mouth-to-mouth resuscitation.

If you aren't certain if the victim is breathing, or if there are no signs of breath, follow these steps:

1. Lay the person on his or her back on the floor or ground. Roll the victim over if necessary, being careful to turn the head with the remainder of the body as a unit to avoid possible neck injury. Loosen any tight clothing around the neck or chest.

2. Check for any foreign material in the mouth or throat and remove it quickly.

3. Open the airway by tilting the head back and lifting the chin up.

4. Pinch the nostrils shut with your thumb and index finger.

5. Take a deep breath, open your mouth wide and place it securely over the victim's, and give two slow breaths, each lasting 1 to 10 seconds. Remove your mouth, turn your head, and check to see if the victim's chest rises and falls. If you hear air escaping from the victim's mouth and see

the chest fall, you know that you are getting air into the lungs.

6. Repeat once every five seconds (twelve breaths per minute) until professional help takes over, or the victim begins breathing on his or her own. It may take several hours to revive someone. If you stop, the victim may not be able to breathe on his or her own. Once the person does begin to breathe independently, always get professional help.

7. If air doesn't seem to be entering the chest, or the chest doesn't fall between breaths, tilt the head further back. If that doesn't work, follow the directions for choking emergencies later in this section.

8. If the victim is a child, do not pinch the nose shut. Cover both the mouth and nose with your mouth, and place your free hand very lightly on the child's chest. Use small puffs of air rather than big breaths. Feel the chest inflate as you blow, and listen for exhaled air. Repeat once every three seconds (twenty breaths per minute).

Broken Bones

If you suspect that a person has broken a leg, do not move him or her unless there is immediate danger.

1. Check for signs of breathing. If there is none or breathing is very weak, administer mouth-to-mouth resuscitation.

2. If the person is bleeding, apply direct pressure on the site of the wound.

3. Try to keep the victim warm and calm.

4. Do not try to push a broken bone back into place if it is sticking out of the skin. You can apply a moist dressing to prevent it from drying out.

5. Do not try to straighten out a fracture.

6. Do not allow the victim to walk.

7. Splint unstable fractures to prevent painful motion.

Burns

1. If fire caused the burn, cool the affected area with water to stop the burning process.

2. Remove the victim's garments and jewelry and cover him or her with clean sheets or towels.

3. Call for help immediately.

4. If chemicals caused the burn, wash the affected area with cool water for at least twenty minutes. Chemical burns of the eye require immediate medical attention after flushing with water for twenty minutes.

Choking

A person with anything stuck in the throat and blocking the airway can stop breathing, lose consciousness, and die within four to six minutes. A universal signal of distress because of choking is clasping the throat with one or both hands. Other signs are an inability to talk and noisy, difficult breathing. You need to take immediate action, but *NEVER* slap the victim's back. This could make the obstruction worse.

If the victim can speak, cough, or breathe, do not interfere. Coughing alone may dislodge the foreign object. if the choking continues without lessening, call for medical help.

If the victim cannot speak, cough, or breathe but is conscious, use the Heimlich maneuver, as follows

1. Stand behind the victim (who may be seated or standing) and wrap your arms around his or her waist.

2. Make a fist with one hand and place the thumb side of your fist against the victim's abdomen, just above the navel. Grasp your fist with your other hand and press into his or her abdomen with a quick, upward thrust. Do not exert any pressure against the rib cage with your forearms.

3. Repeat this procedure until the victim is no longer choking or loses consciousness.

4. If the person is lying facedown, roll the victim over. Facing the person, kneel with your legs astride his or her hips. Put the heel of one hand below the rib cage and place your other hand on top. Press into the abdomen with a quick, upward thrust. Repeat thrusts as needed.

5. If you start choking when you're by yourself, place your fist below your rib cage and above your navel. Grasp this fist with your other hand and press into your abdomen with a quick, upward thrust. You also can lean over a fixed, horizontal object, such as a table edge or chair back, and press your upper abdomen against it with a quick, upward thrust. Repeat as needed until you dislodge the object.

If the Victim Is Unconscious

1. Place him or her on the ground and give mouth-to-mouth resuscitation as described earlier.

2. If the victim does not start breathing and air does not seem to be going into his or her lungs, roll the victim onto his or her back and give one or more manual thrusts: Place one of your hands on top of the other with the heel of the bottom hand in the middle of the abdomen, slightly above the navel and below the rib cage. Press into the abdomen with a quick, upward thrust. Do not push to either side. Repeat 6 to 10 times as needed.

3. Clear the airway. Hold the victim's mouth open with one hand and use your thumb to depress the tongue. Make a hook with the index finger of your other hand and, using a gentle, sweeping motion, reach into the victim's throat and feel for a swallowed foreign object in the airway.

4. Repeat the following steps in this sequence:

   –00 Six to ten abdominal thrusts
   • Probe in mouth
   • Try to inflate lungs
   • Repeat

5. If the victim suddenly seems okay, but no foreign material has been removed, take him or her directly to the hospital. A foreign object, such as a fish or chicken bone or other jagged object, could do internal damage as it passes through the victim's system.

If the Victim Is a Child

1. If the child is coughing, do nothing. The coughing alone may dislodge the object.

2. If the airway is blocked and the child is panicky and fighting for breath, do *NOT* probe the airway with your fingers to clear an unseen foreign object. You might push the material back into the airway, worsening the obstruction.

3. For an infant younger than a year, hang the child over your arm so that the head is lower than the trunk. Using the heel of your hand, administer four firm blows high on the back between the shoulder blades. For a bigger child, follow the same procedure, but invert the child over your knee rather than your arm.

4. After four back blows, perform four chest thrusts (the Heimlich maneuver as described above).

Drowning

A person can die of drowning four to six minutes after breathing stops. Although prevention is the wisest course, follow these steps in case of a drowning emergency:

1. Get the victim out of the water fast. Be extremely cautious, because a drowning person may panic and grasp at a rescuer, endangering that individual as well. If possible, push a branch or pole within the victim's reach.

2. If the victim is unconscious, use a flotation device if at all possible. Carefully place the person on the device. Once out of the water, place the victim on his or her back.

3. If the victim is not breathing, start mouth-to-mouth resuscitation Continue until the person can breathe unassisted or help arrives. (Note that it may take an hour or two for a drowning victim to resume independent breathing.) Do not leave the victim alone for any reason.

4. Once the person is breathing without assistance, even if he or she is still coughing, you need only stay nearby until professional help arrives.

Electrical Shock

1. If you suspect that an electrical shock has knocked a person unconscious,

approach very carefully. Do not touch the victim unless the electricity has been turned off.

2. Shut off the power at the plug, circuit breaker, or fuse box. Simply shutting off an appliance does not remove the shock hazard. Use a dry stick to move a wire or downed power line from the victim. Keep in mind that you also are in danger until the power is off.

3. If the person's breathing is weak or has stopped, follow the steps for mouth-to-mouth resuscitation.

4. Even if the victim returns to consciousness, call for medical help. While waiting, cover the victim with a blanket or coat to keep him or her warm. Place a blanket underneath the body if the surface is cold. Be sure the person lies flat if conscious, with legs raised. If the victim is unconscious, place him or her on one side, with a pillow supporting the head. Do not give the victim anything to eat or drink.

5. Electrical burns can extend deep into the tissue, even when they appear minor. Do not put butter, household remedies, or sprays on burns without a doctor's instruction. Do not use ice or cold water on an electrical burn that is more than two inches across.

Heart Attack

Chest pain can be caused by indigestion, strained muscles, or lung infections. The warning signs of a heart attack are:

- Intense pain that lasts for more than two minutes, produces a tight or crushing feeling, is centered in the chest, or spreads to the neck, jaw, shoulder, or arm
- Shortness of breath that is worse when the person lies flat and improves when the person sits
- Heavy sweating
- Nausea or vomiting
- Irregular pulse
- Pale or bluish skin or lips
- Weakness
- Severe anxiety, feeling of doom

If an individual develops these symptoms:

1. Call for emergency medical help immediately.

2. Have the person sit up or lie in a semi-reclining position. Loosen tight clothing. Keep him or her comfortably warm.

3. If the person loses consciousness, turn on his or her back and check for breathing and pulse. If vomiting occurs, turn the victim's head to one side and clean the mouth.

4. If the person has medicine for angina pectoris (chest pain) and is conscious, help him or her take it.

5. If the person is unconscious, and you are trained to perform cardiopulmonary resuscitation (CPR), check for a pulse at the wrist or neck. If there is none, begin CPR in conjunction with mouth-to-mouth resuscitation. Do not attempt CPR unless you are trained. It is not a technique you can learn from a book.

Poisoning

Many common household substances, including glue, aspirin, bleaches, and paint, can be poisonous. Make sure you know the emergency numbers for the Poison Control Center and Fire Department Rescue Squad. Keep them near your telephone. Be prepared to provide the following information:

- The kind of substance swallowed and how much was swallowed
- If a child or adult swallowed the substance
- Symptoms
- Whether or not vomiting has occurred
- Whether you gave the person anything to drink
- How much time it will take to get to an emergency room

The Poison Control Center or rescue team will tell you whether or not to induce vomiting or neutralize a swallowed poison. Here are some additional guidelines:

1. Always assume the worst if a small child has swallowed or might have swallowed something poisonous. Call the local Poison Control Center or emergency number (911 in many

areas). Keep the suspected item or container with you to answer questions.

2. Do not give any medications unless a physician or the Poison Control Center instructs you to do so.

3. Do not follow the directions for neutralizing poisons on the container unless a doctor or the Poison Control Center confirms that they are appropriate measures to take.

4. If the child is conscious, give moderate doses of water to dilute the poison.

5. If a poisoning victim is unconscious, make sure he or she is breathing. If not, give mouth-to-mouth resuscitation. Do not give anything by mouth or attempt to stimulate the person. Call for emergency help immediately.

6. If the person is vomiting, make sure he or she is in a position in which he or she cannot choke on what is brought up.

7. While vomiting is the fastest way to expel swallowed poisons from the body, never try to induce vomiting if the person has swallowed any acid or alkaline substance, which can cause burns of the face, mouth, and throat (examples include ammonia, bleach, dishwasher detergent, drain and toilet cleaners, lye, oven cleaners, or rust removers), or petroleum-like products, which produce dangerous fumes that can be inhaled during vomiting (examples include floor polish, furniture wax, gasoline, kerosene, lighter fluid, turpentine, and paint thinner).

A CONSUMER'S GUIDE TO MEDICAL TESTS

✔ **What They Tell the Doctor**

✔ **How Often You Need Them**

✔ **What to Do About Abnormal Results**

Do you wonder what the doctor sees when he looks into your eyes with that little light, or what it means when your blood or urine test is normal? In this section we cover some of the most common tests your doctor does, what they tell, and how often they should be done.

General Information

- Always ask your doctor what tests are being done, why they are being ordered, what they involve, and what the results mean.
- No test is foolproof. If a result is unexpected, whether normal or abnormal, your doctor should repeat the test before making any decisions.
- Modern X-ray machines expose you to a minuscule amount of radiation. Nevertheless, be sure to tell the physician or X-ray technician if there is even a chance you may be pregnant.
- Often a doctor orders a test because that is the only way to prove you do *not* have a disease.

Allergy Skin Testing

- Skin testing is still the most reliable method.

- The physician either pricks your skin twenty to forty or more times to introduce a tiny bit of potentially allergic material or injects a small amount.
- Children who are frightened by multiple needle sticks and are unlikely to sit still for as long as necessary may have blood (RAST) tests instead.

What results mean

If you develop redness or a hivelike bump around an area, you are probably allergic to the injected substance. Sometimes you can avoid the offending material, but things like pollen and dust are everywhere. Your allergist may recommend desensitizing shots to reduce your reaction. Note that the results of skin tests won't be reliable if you take antihistamines within 48 hours of the test.

How often to be tested

Skin tests are necessary only if you cannot get allergy relief from other measures such as over-the-counter medications, reducing mold and dust in the house, and staying away from animals.

Blood-Pressure Reading

- High blood pressure, a major cause of stroke and heart attacks, usually causes no symptoms.
- The upper number in a reading—the systolic—refers to peak amount of pressure generated when your heart pumps blood, the lower number—the diastolic—measures the least amount of pressure.

What results mean

Most doctors today think the lower the pressure the better, which means a reading of 120/80 or less. Because the mere anxiety of having your blood pressure taken can cause a mild elevation, your doctor will want to repeat an abnormal test, ideally on a different day, before diagnosing high blood pressure.

How often to be tested

Everyone—no matter how healthy—should have a blood-pressure reading taken at least once a year, more often if you have high blood pressure

Blood Tests

- Blood may be taken from either a finger prick or, more commonly, a vein in your arm.
- See below for information on cholesterol testing, which is also done from a blood sample.

Complete Blood Count (CBC)

This is the most commonly performed of all blood tests.

What results mean

A *low red-cell count,* called anemia, can be caused by something as simple as too little iron in your diet, as complex as an abnormality in your digestion, or as serious as a bone marrow problem or silent bleeding. Iron deficiency is the most frequent cause, with women who menstruate and limit their intake of red meat at the greatest risk. If your doctor diagnoses this problem, ask about making dietary changes as well as taking iron supplements.

A high white-cell count, a measure of the body's defenses against infection, usually indicates some kind of infection. Depending on the type of cell that predominates, your doctor may be able to identify whether you have a bacterial or viral infection.

Platelets, the first participants in blood clotting, may be decreased because of a viral infection, abnormal bleeding, or for no identifiable reason.

Chemistry Panels (Chem 12 or 18, SMA 12 or 24)

Kidney, bone, liver, pancreas, prostate, and some glandular functions are screened by these tests.

What results mean

An abnormality may signal a problem that needs treatment. Because accuracy decreases when many tests are run together, any specific abnormal test should be repeated, especially if unexpected.

CAT (Computerized Axial Tomography) Scan

- A CAT scan is 100 times more sensitive than an X-ray.

- You lie as motionless as possible in a large tube while an X ray beam travels 360 degrees around you. The test takes about an hour.

What results mean

The test can help diagnose such conditions as tumors, blood clots, cysts, and bleeding in the brain as well as in various other organs.

Cholesterol Test

- Anyone can have a high cholesterol level, but you are more apt to be at risk if there is a family history of early heart attacks, strokes, or high cholesterol tests.

- Your doctor will look at not only total cholesterol but also the levels of high-density lipoprotein (HUL), the "good" cholesterol that prevents cholesterol from sticking to your blood vessels, and low-density lipoprotein (LDL), the "bad" cholesterol that does the reverse.

What results mean

Experts today think optimum cholesterol levels are below 200 mg/ml of blood. The following chart shows the risk by age of various cholesterol levels.

Cholesterol Risk Chart

Age	Moderate Risk	High Risk
20–29	200–220 mg/ml	Over 220
30–39	220–240	Over 240
Over 40	240–260	Over 260

Persistently high cholesterol values will prompt your doctor to advise dietary and lifestyle changes—less fat intake, more exercise—and perhaps medication. This will particularly be the case if LDL levels also are high (less than 130 mg/ml is considered desirable, 130–159 is borderline risk, and over 160 is high risk).

How often to be tested

If your cholesterol level is under 200 and your LDL level is under 130, repeat the test every five years. if your test is borderline, repeat it annually. (Note that the test should be taken when you have not eaten for at least twelve hours.)

If you have a family history of cholesterol problems, have your children tested annually from age 2; if you don't, have them tested around age 10 and every few years thereafter. Children under 2 should not be given a low-cholesterol diet; they need extra fat to make brain tissue and hormones for growth.

Fundoscopy

- The doctor looks into your eye with a little light.

What results mean

The beginnings of cataracts may be visible, as well as irregularities in the blood vessels that indicate damage from high cholesterol (fatty deposits in the blood vessels), high blood pressure (narrowing and notching), diabetes, or other diseases. If the optic nerve is swollen, there may be excess pressure inside your skull.

What your doctor *cannot* see are the early signs of glaucoma, which can lead to blindness if not treated. Over age 20, have a pressure check for glaucoma from an opthalmologist or optometrist every three years—or every year if you have a family history of glaucoma.

Heart Tests

- The tollowing tests are listed from the simplest through the most complicated.

- Also see listings for blood pressure read!ings, cholesterol tests, and pulse.

Electrocardiogram (EKG, ECG)

- A machine amplifies the electrical signals from your heart and records them on paper.

What results mean

An EKG can detect such things as an enlarged heart, abnormal levels of potassium or calcium, disease of the small vessels of the heart, and where an abnormal heart rhythm originates. It is a nonspecific test, however, and more advanced studies should be done if serious disease is suspected.

Echocardiogram

This is a painless test in which sound waves are used to produce a picture of the heart in action on a TV-type screen.

What results mean

The test investigates the size of the heart chambers, the thickness of the walls, how the four heart valves are working, and the condition of the membrane surrounding the heart. Mitral valve prolapse, a common minor abnormality, often shows up on this test, as well as more serious problems.

Stress Test

Your heart rate, blood pressure, and EKG are constantly monitored as you exercise on a treadmill that goes faster and faster with a steeper and steeper incline. This test—also called an exercise tolerance test or treadmill test—should be performed in the presence of a cardiologist and in or near a hospital in case the strain causes heart problems that need emergency treatment. The test should be stopped immediately if you experience any lightheadedness, chest pain, nausea, or palpitations.

What results mean

The changes that an increasing strain on the heart causes can tell your doctor if you are at risk of a heart attack. This is because a blockage in the coronary arteries—the blood vessels that feed your heart muscle—may show up only during exercise.

Angiography

A dye is injected into various arteries, and X rays are taken.

What results mean

The doctor can detect blockages in the blood vessels that can lead to heart attack or stroke, as well as aneurysms (weakened spots in the blood-vessel walls). The test carries some risk of causing stroke.

Kidney Tests

- The tests noted here involve taking X rays. In addition, ultrasound (similar to an echocardiogram) can be used to outline the kidneys.

Intravenous Pyelogram (IVP)

After an iodine-containing substance is injected into a vein, X rays are taken at five-minute intervals to show the outlines of the kidney, ureter, and bladder.

What results mean

Tumors, kidney stones, and swelling of the kidney tissue can be seen, as well as blockage to urine flow or a mass that may be pressing on the kidney. A kidney that is not functioning will not appear on the X ray, and one in an abnormal position can be found.

Voiding Cystourethrogram (VCUG)

A technician will fill your bladder with a dye injected through a catheter and take X rays while you urinate.

What results mean

If you have recurrent urinary-tract infections, the test will show if there is a significant backup of urine from the bladder into the ureter, in which case daily antibiotics may be needed to prevent infection. Investigating recurrent urinary tract infections is particularly important for children.

Magnetic Resonance Imaging (MRI)

- MRI uses no radiation but produces pictures of the brain that are much more detailed than those of a CAT scan.

What results mean

In addition to locating bleeding or tumors, as a CAT scan does, the test picks up subtle signs such as those of Parkinson's disease and multiple sclero-

sis in the brain or a herniated disc in the spinal column.

Mammography

- Only a small amount of radiation is used to take the mammogram. You usually stand up and put your breast on a photographic plate where it is compressed with a plastic shield or balloonlike device. It shouldn't hurt. If your breasts are tender at certain times in your menstrual cycle, schedule your mammogram when they are least sensitive.
- Mammograms can detect breast abnormalities at easily treated stages before you can feel them, but they are not foolproof. Examine your breasts monthly.

What results mean

Mammograms can detect cysts, abscesses, and tumors. Whether a mass is benign or malignant is hard to tell in the early stages, so abnormalities usually need to be biopsied or removed totally to determine treatment.

How often to be tested

Although there is controversy over the benefits of mammography for women under 50, many experts still recommend having a first mammogram between ages 35 and 40, followed by one every two years between 40 and 50, and yearly thereafter. If your mother or sister has had breast cancer, consult your doctor for an appropriate schedule. And if you have a lump, pain, or nipple discharge, have a mammogram right away, no matter what your age.

You also should have a breast examination by a doctor at least every three years between ages 20 and 40, and every year after 40.

Pap Smear

- A routine part of every gynecological examination.
- Your doctor takes a painless swab from the cervix and vaginal walls and sends it to a lab for analysis.

What results mean

Pap smears can detect not only cervical cancer but also inflammation and many infections, minor and more serious; they

also provide important information about the state of your female hormones. A normal test is termed class 1, and abnormal results are graded by degree into four classifications, with only the most severe—a class V test—signifying outright cancer. Treatment depends on the diagnosis and may range from doing nothing for a minor inflammation to, in rare cases, a hysterectomy for cancer. Because the error rate of Pap smears is high, the doctor should always repeat an abnormal test.

How often to be tested

Women who are on birth control pills and are sexually active should have a Pap smear every six months; other women should be checked every year,

Physical Examination

- The routine physical exam generally includes a pulse and blood-pressure reading, measure of height and weight, blood tests (including a cholesterol test), fundoscopy, and sometimes other tests as well, such as a stool test for blood.

What results mean

A physical exam serves as a general measure of health and sometimes picks up early signs of disease.

How often to have a physical exam

Most doctors no longer recommend yearly physicals for everybody. A good schedule to follow instead is to have a complete checkup every four or five years under age 40, every three years between 40 and 50, every two years between 50 and 60, and every year after that. At any age, you should have more frequent examinations if you have chronic medical problems such as diabetes or high blood pressure, are obese, or smoke cigarettes.

Pulse

- To take your own pulse, press two fingertips over the artery in your wrist, just below the base of the thumb. Count the beats in 20 seconds, then multiply by 3.

What results mean

The normal pulse rate—the speed at

which your heart pumps blood—is 60–80 beats a minute; it should be regular, without skipped or extra beats. Abnormal rates can be due to thyroid problems (too high causes a fast rate, too low a slow one), heart problems, anxiety (even the stress of a physical exam), or weakness from an illness such as the flu or other problems.

The character of your pulse is also important. A discrepancy between the strength of the pulse on one side of the neck and the other may mean you are in danger of a stroke. A pulse that is abnormally strong and bounding can signal a problem with a heart valve. if the pulse is weak, you may have blockages in your blood vessels from diabetes, atherosclerosis (hardening of the arteries), or a variety of other disorders.

Stomach and Intestinal Tests

- Though most of these tests are uncomfortable, they generally are not painful.

Barium Enema

Barium, a radioactive material, is instilled in your large intestine through a tube inserted into your anus. Because barium is constipating, drink fluids afterward. Don't be alarmed if you have white stools for a day or two.

What results mean

The doctor will be able to see tumors or polyps, any obstructions, and other abnormalities.

Gastroscopy and Proctoscopy

In gastroscopy, for which you will be sedated, the doctor looks into the stomach with a flexible tube that goes through your mouth. The procedure is essentially the same for protoscopy, except that the doctor looks into your large intestine through a tube inserted into your anus.

What results mean

Your doctor can see where bleeding comes from, remove a polyp, or biopsy a mass.

Upper GI Series

You will be asked to down a drink of barium so that X rays can be taken of the esophagus, stomach, duodenum, and sometimes the small intestine.

What results mean

Your doctor can diagnose swallowing disorders, hiatus hernias, ulcers, tumors, and some inflammations of the stomach and small bowel.

Stool Test for Occult Blood

A small sample of stool that remains on the doctor's glove after a rectal exam or that is collected by you at home is tested for blood that is invisible to the eye.

What results mean

This test is done routinely as part of a regular checkup to detect the earliest sign of cancer of the colon. it is also part of an investigation of anemia or abdominal pain. If your test is positive, tell your doctor if you recently ate radishes, turnips, or red meat, took large doses of vitamin C or iron pills, or had a nosebleed. All of these things can produce misleading results.

Urinalysis

- Urine can tell about the health not only of the kidneys but also of other organ systems.

What results mean

Specific gravity is the degree to which your urine is concentrated or diluted. If it is persistently too dilute, your doctor may ask for a first morning sample to see how well your kidneys concentrate your urine overnight. Urine that is too concentrated may indicate poor fluid intake, decreased kidney function, or dehydration from vomiting and diarrhea.

pH or acidity or alkalinity is useful information when there is a history or possibility of kidney stones, urinary-tract infection, or kidney disease.

Glucose or sugar in the urine may mean you have diabetes. You will need a blood test to confirm the diagnosis, as some families filter sugar easily through their kidneys but do not have any disease. Inflammation of the pancreas and

thyroid problems also may cause sugar in the urine.

Blood in the urine may mean infection, a stone, or an inflammation of the kidney. Excessive exertion such as running sometimes causes some blood to leak into the urine; this usually disappears after resting.

Protein molecules are large and under normal conditions should not filter into the urine. However, they may appear in small amounts in the urine after strenuous exercise or an illness, especially one with a fever. In large amounts, protein in the urine warrants a search for an underlying kidney problem.

Nitrites, substances produced when bacteria multiply, may be the earliest or only sign of an infection.

White blood cells may be present because of a urinary-tract or vaginal infection.

X Ray

- The simple X ray is a nonspecific test that is being replaced more and more by CAT scans, magnetic resonance imaging, and other tests.

What results mean

An X ray can detect such things as an enlarged heart, a broken bone, a sinus infection, or pneumonia.

COUNTING YOUR CALORIES AND FAT

*T*otal calorie values for each item in this table were rounded to the nearest 5 calories (calories from fat and fat grams were not). The portion sizes are given in common household units and in grams. The portion size shown may not be the amount that you eat. If you choose larger or smaller portions than listed, increase or decrease the calorie and fat counts accordingly. Check nutrition labels on foods for additional information, including saturated fat, cholesterol, and sodium content.

Breads, Cereals, and Other Grain Products

BREADS	CALORIES	FAT GRAMS	CALORIES FROM FAT
Bagel			
plain, 1, 3-1/2 inch diameter	195	1	10
oat bran, 1, 3-1/2 inch	180	1	8
poppy seed, 1, Sara Lee	190	1	9
Cracked-wheat bread, 1, 25g slice	65	1	9
French bread, 1, 25g slice	70	1	7
Pita bread			
white, 1, 6-1/2 inch diameter	165		6
whole wheat, 1, 6-1/2 inch diameter	170		15
Pumpernickel, 1, 32g slice	80	1	9
Raisin, 1, 26g slice	70	1	10
Rye, 1, 32g slice	85	1	10
White			
regular, 1, 25g slice	65	1	8
Wonder bread light, 2 slices, 45g	80	1	9
Whole wheat			
regular, 1, 25g slice	70	1	11
Wonder bread, 2 slices, 45g	80	<1	14
ROLLS			
Croissant, prepared w/butter, 1, 57g	230	12	108
Dinner, 1, 28g	85	2	19
Frankfurter or hamburger, 1, 43g	125	2	20
French, 1, 38g	105	2	15
Hard, 1 3-1/2 inch, 57g	165	2	22
QUICK BREADS, BISCUITS, MUFFINS, BREAKFAST PASTRIES			
Biscuit			
plain, 2-1/2 in diameter, 60g	210	10	88
from dry mix, 3 inch diameter, 57g	190	7	62
from refrig. dough, 2-1/2 diam., 27g	95	4	36
Banana bread, 1 slice, 60g	195	57	
Coffee cake			
cinnamon w/crumb topping, 63g	265	15	132
butter streusel, Sara Lee, 41g	160	7	63
Danish			
cheese, Sara Lee, individual, 36g	130	8	72
cheese-filled, Entenmann's, fat-free 54g	130	0	0
Doughnuts			
plain cake, 1, 47g	200	11	97
glazed, 1, 45g	190	10	93
English muffin, plain, 1, 57g	135	1	9
Muffin			
blueberry, 2-1/2 inch, 1, 57g	160	4	33
bran w/raisins, Dunkin' Donuts 1, 104g	310	9	81

	CALORIES	FAT GRAMS	CALORIES FROM FAT
Pancake			
plain, from dry mix, 1, 56g	200	1	9
plain, frozen Aunt Jemima, 3, 114g	185	2	22
Waffle			
plain, 7 inch diameter, 75g	220	11	95
blueberry, frozen, Eggo, 2, 78g	220	8	72
BREAKFAST CEREAL			
All-Bran, 1/2 cup, 30g	80	1	9
Bran flakes, 3/4 cup, 28g	100	1	9
Cheerios, 1-1/4 cup, 28g	110	2	18
Corn flakes, 1 cup, 30g	110	0	0
Cream of Wheat			
regular or instant, cooked, 2/3 cup, 168g	100	0	0
instant, cooked, 2/3 cup, 161g	100	<1	0
mix'n eat, 1 pkg., 28g	100	0	0
Frosted Flakes, 3/4 cup, 30g	120	0	0
Frosted Mini-Wheats, 1 cup, 55g	190	1	9
Grape-Nut Flakes, 1 cup, 28g	100	1	9
Granola, date nut, Erewhon, 1/4 cup, 28g	130	6	50
Oatmeal			
reg., quick, or instant, cooked, 1 cup, 234g	145	2	21
cinnamon & spice, Instant , 1 pkg., 46g	170	2	18
Raisin bran, 1 cup, 55g	170	1	9
Rice Chex, 1 cup, 31g	120	0	0
Rice Krispies, 1-1/4 cup, 30g	110	0	0
Shredded wheat, Quaker	220	2	14
Special K, 1 cup, 30g	110	0	0
Total, 1 cup, 28g	100	1	9
Wheaties, 1 cup, 28g	100	1	9
PASTA AND RICE			
Macaroni			
cooked, plain, 1/2 cup, 65g	95	<1	3
spinach, cooked, Ronzoni, 1/2 cup, 67g	105	<1	4
Pasta,			
fresh, cooked, plain, 1 cup, 170g	225	2	16
homemade w/egg, cooked, 1 cup, 170g	220	3	27
Ravioli, cheese, cooked, Contadina,			
1/3 container, 190g	270	11	99
Rice, cooked, 1/2 cup			
Brown, medium grain, 98g	110	1	7
White, glutinous, 120g	115	<1	2
White, long grain instant, 82g	80	<1	1
White, medium grain, 93g	120	<1	2
Wild rice, 82g	85	<1	3
Spaghetti, cooked, plain, 1 cup, 140g	155	<1	4
CRACKERS			
Cheez-it, Sunshine, 24 crackers, 32g	140	8	72
Finn-Crisp dark, 3 crackers, 15g	60	0	0
Matzo, plain, 1 (28g)	110	<1	4
Ritz, Nabisco, 4 crackers, 14g	70	4	36
Saltine, 10 crackers, 28g	120	4	36
Soup or oyster, 4 crackers, 14g	70	4	36
Triscuit, Nabisco, 6 crackers, 28g	120	4	36

Fruits

FRUITS	CALORIES	FAT GRAMS	CALORIES FROM FAT
(calories in cooked and canned fruit include both fruit and liquid)			
Apple, raw, sliced, 1/2 cup, 55g	30	<1	2

C O U N T I N G   Y O U R   C A L O R I E S   A N D   F A T

	CALORIES	FAT GRAMS	CALORIES FROM FAT
Applesauce, 1/2 cup			
sweetened, 128g	95	<1	2
unsweetened, 122g	50	<1	1
Apricots			
canned, heavy syrup, 3 halves, 85g	70	<1	1
canned, light syrup pack, 3 halves, 85g	55	<1	0
dried, cooked without sugar, 1/2 cup, 125g	105	<1	2
raw, 4 halves, 78g	35	<1	3
Avocados			
California, 3 inch, 1/2, 86g	155	15	135
Florida, 3-5/8 inch, 1/2, 152g	170	13	121
Banana, medium, 114g	105	1	5
Blueberries, 1/2 cup			
frozen, unsweetened, 78g	40	<1	4
frozen, sweetened, 115g	95	1	5
raw, 72g	40	<1	3
Cherries, 1/2 cup			
raw, sweet, 72g	50	1	6
sweet, frozen, sweetened, 130g	115	<1	2
sour red, frozen, unsweetened, 78g	35	<1	3
Cranberry sauce, sweetened, 1/4 cup, 70g	110	0	0
Dates, dried, 10, 83g	230	<1	3
Fruit cocktail, canned, 1/2 cup			
juice pack, 124g	55	<1	0
heavy syrup, 128g	95	<1	1
Grapefruit, raw, 3-3/4 inch, 1/2, 118g	40	<1	1
Melon, honeydew, cubed, 1/2 cup, 85g	30	<1	1
Oranges, 1/2 cup			
Mandarin, canned, light syrup, 122g	80	0	0
raw, sections, 90g	40	<1	1
Peaches			
Canned, in juice, 1/2 cup, 77g	55	0	0
canned, in light syrup, 1/2 cup, 77g	70	<1	1
Pears			
Canned, in light syrup, 1 half, 77g	35	<1	1
Dried, without added sugar, 1/2 cup, 128g	165	<1	4
Pineapple			
Canned. juice pack, 1/2 cup, 125g	75	<1	1
Raw, diced, 1/2 cup, 78g	40	<1	3
Plums			
canned, juice pack, 3, 95g	55	<1	0
raw, 2-1/8 inch diameter, 66g	35	<1	4
Prunes			
dried, cooked, without sugar, 1/2 cup, 106g	115	<1	2
dried, uncooked, 10, 84g	200	<1	4
Raisins, seedless, 1/4 cup, 41g	125	<1	2
Raspberries, 1/2 cup			
frozen, unsweetened, 125g	61	1	6
raw, 62g	30	<1	3
Rhubarb, cooked, sweetened, 1/2 cup, 120g	140	<1	1
Tangerines, sections, 1/2 cup, 98g	45	<1	2
Watermelon, 10 inches x 1 inch, 480g	155	2	19
JUICES			
Apple juice or cider, 1 cup, 249g	120	0	0
Apricot nectar, canned, 3/4 cup, 188g	105	<1	2
Cranberry juice cocktail, 3/4 cup, 190g	110	<1	2
Grape juice			
bottled, 3/4 cup, 188g	110	0	0
from frozen concentrate, 3/4 cup, 188g	96	<1	2
Grapefruit			
Lemonade, 3/4 cup			
homemade, prepared w/sugar, 186g	90	0	0
from frozen concentrate, 186g	75	<1	0

	CALORIES	FAT GRAMS	CALORIES FROM FAT
Orange juice, 3/4 cup			
fresh, 186g	85	<1	3
from frozen concentrate, 187g	85	<1	1
Pineapple juice, canned, 3/4 cup, 188g	105	<1	1
Prune juice, canned, 3/4 cup, 192g	135	<1	1
Snapple, 1 bottle			
Dixie peach, 295g	140	0	0
Lemonade, 240g	110	0	0
Passion supreme, 309g	160	0	0
Pink grapefruit cocktail, 249g	120	0	0
V-8 juice, canned, 3/4 cup, 182g	35	0	0
VEGETABLE			
Alfalfa sprouts, raw, 1 cup, 33g	10	<1	2
Artichoke, cooked, medium, 120g	60	<1	2
Asparagus, 1/2 cup			
canned, drained, 120g	25	1	7
cooked, drained, 90g	20	<1	3
Bean sprouts, Mung, raw, 1/2 cup, 52g	15	<1	1
Beet greens, cooked, drained, 1/2 cup, 72g	20	<1	1
Beets, 1/2 cup			
canned, sliced, drained, 85g	25	<1	1
cooked, sliced, drained, 85g	35	<1	1
Broccoli, 1/2 cup			
frozen florets, cooked, 71g	20	0	0
raw, chopped, 44g	10	<1	1
Brussels sprouts, cooked, drained, 1/2 cup, 78g	30	<1	4
Cabbage, 1/2 cup			
Chinese bok-choy, shredded, raw, 35g	5	<1	1
shredded, raw, 35g	10	<1	1
shredded, cooked, drained, 75g	15	<1	3
Carrots			
frozen, sliced, cooked, drained, 1/2 cup, 73g	25	<1	1
raw, 7-1/1 inches x 1-1/8 inch, 72g	30	<1	1
Cauliflower, 1/2 cup			
frozen, cooked, drained, 90g	15	<1	2
raw, 1 inch pieces, 50g	10	<1	1
Celery, raw			
cooked, drained, 1/2 cup, 75g	15	<1	1
raw, 7-1/2 in x 1-1/4 inch, 40g	5	<1	1
Corn, cooked			
canned, yellow, cream style, 1/2 cup, 128g	90	1	5
canned, solids & liquid, 1/2 cup, 128g	80	1	5
frozen, white, cooked, drained, 1/2 cup, 82g	65	<1	1
on the cob, drained, 1 ear, 140g	85	1	9
Cucumber, raw, sliced, 1/2 cup, 52g	10	<1	1
Eggplant			
cooked, drained, 1 inch pieces, 1/2 cup, 48g	15	<1	1
in tomato sauce, 1 cup, 231g	75	<1	3
Green beans, 1/2 cup			
canned, drained, 68g	25	0	0
cooked, drained, 62g	20	<1	2
frozen, French style 85g	25	0	0
raw, snap, 55g	15	<1	1
Kale, cooked, drained, 1/2 cup, 65g	20	<1	1
Lettuce			
Iceberg, 1/4 of a 6-inch head, 135g	20	<1	2
looseleaf, shredded, 1/2 cup, 28g	5	<1	1
Romaine, shredded, 1/2 cup, 28g	5	<1	4
Lima beans, cooked, drained, 1/2 cup, 85g	105	<1	2
Mushrooms			
canned, pieces, drained, 1/2 cup, 78g	20	<1	2
raw, whole, 1, 18g	5	<1	1
Shiitake, cooked, 1/2 cup, 73g	40	<1	1
Onions			
canned, solids & liquid, 1 inch, 63g	10	<1	1
raw, chopped, 1/2 cup, 80g	30	<1	1
Peas, green, 1/2 cup			

	CALORIES	FAT GRAMS	CALORIES FROM FAT
frozen, cooked, drained, 80g	60	<1	2
raw, 72g	50	<1	3
Peppers, sweet, red or green, 1/2 cup			
cooked, drained, 68g	20	<1	1
raw, 50g	15	<1	1
Potatoes			
baked, w/skin, 4-3/4 inch x 2-1/3 inch, 156g	220	<1	2
boiled, no skin, 2-1/2 inch diameter, 135g	115	<1	1
hash browns, Ore-Ida frozen, 1 patty, 85g	70	<1	0
mashed, w/whole milk, 1/2 cup, 105g	80	1	6
scalloped, frozen, Stouffer's, 1/2 pkg., 165g	135	6	52
Tater Tots, frozen, Ore-Ida, 1-1/4 cup, 85g	160	7	63
Spinach, 1/2 cup			
frozen, cooked, drained, 95g	25	<1	2
raw, chopped, 28g	5	<1	1
Squash, 1/2 cup			
Summer, cooked, drained, 90g	20	<1	3
Winter, baked cubes, 102g	40	1	6
Sweet potatoes			
baked in skin, 5 inches x 2 inches, 114g	115	<1	1
canned, mashed, 128g	130	<1	2
Tomato sauce, canned, 1/2 cup, 122g	35	<1	2
Tomatoes, 1/2 cup			
canned, stewed, 103	35	0	0
raw, chopped, 90g	20	<1	3
Turnip greens, cooked, drained, 1/2 cup, 72g	15	<1	2
Turnips, cooked, mashed, 1/2 cup, 115g	20	<1	1

Meat, Poultry, Fish, and Alternates

(Serving sizes are cooked, edible parts.)

BEEF

	CALORIES	FAT GRAMS	CALORIES FROM FAT
Beef liver, 3 oz, 85g			
braised	135	4	37
pan-fried	185	7	61
Corned beef, canned, 1 oz, 28g	70	4	38
Ground beef, broiled, medium, 3 oz, 85g			
extra lean	220	14	125
ground chuck	230	16	141
regular	245	18	158
Roast beef, 3 oz, 85g			
bottom round, lean & fat	160	6	56
eye of round, lean & fat	195	11	98
pot roast, lean & fat	280	20	182
rib, lean & fat	300	24	216
tip round, lean & fat	160	7	60
Sirloin, broiled, lean & fat, 30 oz, 85g	165	6	55
Veal, loin, lean only, roasted, 30z, 85g	150	6	53

LAMB

	CALORIES	FAT GRAMS	CALORIES FROM FAT
Ground lamb, broiled, 3 oz, 85g	240	17	150
Leg of lamb, lean & fat, roasted, 3 oz, 85g	250	18	158
Shoulder chop, lean & fat, braised, 3 oz, 85g	295	20	185

PORK

	CALORIES	FAT GRAMS	CALORIES FROM FAT
Bacon, thick, broiled, 1 slice, 10g	55	4	40
Bacon, Canadian, grilled, 1 slice, 23g	45	2	18
Ham			
center slice, 3 oz, 85g	170	11	99
canned, lean, 3 oz, 85g	100	4	35
canned, regular, 30 oz, 85g	190	13	116
Pork chop, loin, broiled, 3 oz, 85g	205	11	100
Pork loin ribs, braised, 3 oz, 85g	250	18	165
Pork roast, center loin, 3 oz, 85g	200	11	103
Pork roast, sirloin, 3 oz, 85g	175	8	72

	CALORIES	FAT GRAMS	CALORIES FROM FAT
Pork shoulder, roasted, 3 oz, 85	245	20	180

SAUSAGE AND LUNCHEON MEATS

	CALORIES	FAT GRAMS	CALORIES FROM FAT
Bologna, 1 slice, 28g			
beef & pork	90	8	72
turkey	55	4	40
Braunschweiger, 1 slice, 18g	65	6	52
Chicken breast			
Oscar Mayer, roasted, 1 slice, 28g	25	<1	3
Healthy Choice, roasted, 3 slices, 28g	30	<1	4
Ham, boiled, 1 slice, 21g	20	1	9
Salami			
beef, 1 slice, 23g	60	5	43
turkey, 10% fat, 1 oz, 28g	45	3	24
Sausage, summer, beef, 1 slice, 23g	70	6	54
Turkey			
Oscar Mayer, roasted, 1 slice, 28g	25	1	7
Oscar Mayer, fat free, smoked, 4 slices, 52g	40	<1	3

POULTRY

	CALORIES	FAT GRAMS	CALORIES FROM FAT
Chicken breast, 1/2 breast			
boneless, w/out skin, roasted, 86g	140	3	28
boneless, w/skin, flour fried, 98g	220	9	78
Chicken drumstick, 1			
w/out skin, roasted, 72g	75	2	22
w/skin, roasted, 81g	110	6	52
Chicken liver, simmered, 1/2 cup, 70g	110	4	34
Chicken, thigh, 1			
w/out skin, roasted, 71g	110	6	51
w/skin, roasted, 81g	155	10	86
Turkey, ground, cooked, 1 patty, 82g	195	11	97
Turkey, roasted			
dark meat w/out skin, diced, 1/2 cup, 64g	120	5	42
dark meat w/skin, 3 oz, 85g	190	10	88
light meat w/out skin diced, 1/2 cup, 64g	100	2	19
light meat w/skin, 3 oz, 85g	170	7	64
Turkey liver, simmered, 1/2 cup, 70g	120	4	38

FISH AND SHELLFISH

	CALORIES	FAT GRAMS	CALORIES FROM FAT
Anchovies, canned in oil, drained, 5, 20g	45	2	17
Clams, canned, drained, 1/2 cup, 80g	120	2	14
Fish fillets			
breaded, frozen, 2, 99g	280	19	171
breaded, Healthy Choice, 1, 99g	160	5	45
Flounder, cooked, dry heat, 3 oz, 85g	100	1	12
Halibut, cooked, dry heat, 3 0z, 85g	120	2	22
Salmon 3 oz, 85g			
Chinook, cooked, dry heat	195	11	102
Chum, cooked, dry heat	130	4	37
Coho, cooked, moist heat	155	6	57
Sardines, Atlantic, canned in oil, drained solids, 2, 24g	50	3	25
Sea Bass, cooked, dry heat, 3 oz, 85g	105	2	20
Shrimp, cooked			
breaded & fried, 4, 30g	75	4	33
moist heat, large, 4, 22g	20	<1	2
Tuna, light, canned in water, 1/2 cup, 74g	85	1	5

EGGS

	CALORIES	FAT GRAMS	CALORIES FROM FAT
Fried, whole, 1, 46g	90	7	62
Hard-cooked, whole, 1, 50g	80	5	48
Poached, whole, 1, 50g	75	5	45
Scrambled, w/marg. & whole milk, 1, 64g	105	8	7
Soft-boiled, whole, 1, 50g	80	6	50
Whites, raw, 1, 33g	15	0	0

BEANS AND PEAS

	CALORIES	FAT GRAMS	CALORIES FROM FAT
Baked beans, canned			
pork & beans, tomato sauce, 1/2 cup, 114g	100	1	13
w/pork, molasses & sugar, 1/2 cup, 126g	190	6	58

	Calories	Fat Grams	Calories from Fat
Black-eyed peas, 1/2 cup			
canned, solids & liquid, 120g	90	1	6
cooked, drained, 1/2 cup, 82g	80	<1	3
Chickpeas (garbanzos), canned, 1/2 cup, 120g	145	1	12
Black beans, cooked, 1/2 cup, 86g	115	<1	4
Kidney beans, cooked, 1/2 cup, 88g	110	<1	4
Lima beans, cooked, drained, 1/2 cup, 85g	105	<1	2
Navy beans, cooked, 1/2 cup, 91g	130	1	5
Refried beans, canned, 1/2 cup, 126g	135	1	12
NUTS AND SEEDS			
Almonds, unblanched			
dried, 3 Tbs., 28g	165	15	133
dry roasted, 3 Tbs., 26g	150	13	119
Cashews, dry roasted, 3 Tbs., 28g	165	13	118
Coconut, dried, sweetened, flaked, 2 Tbs., 9g	45	3	27
Peanut butter, 2 Tbs., 32g	190	14	126
Peanuts, roasted			
dry roasted, 3 Tbs., 28g	165	14	125
honey roasted, 3 Tbs., 28g	170	14	126
Pecans, dried, 1/2 cup, 28g	190	19	173
Pine nuts, dried, 1 Tbs., 10g	50	5	46
Pistachios, dry roasted, 3 Tbs., 28g	170	15	135
Sesame seeds			
Tahini, raw kernels, 1 Tbs., 15g	85	7	65
dried, kernels, 1 Tbs., 8g	45	4	39
Sunflower seeds, dry roasted, 3 Tbs., 28g	165	14	127
Walnuts, dried, 1/4 cup, 28g	180	18	158
MEAT SUBSTITUTES			
Burger, vegetarian			
Vege burger, Natural Touch, 1, 64g	140	6	54
Veggie Sizzler, nonfat, Soy Boy, 1, 85g	90	0	0
Hot dog, Not Dogs, 1, 43g	105	5	45
Tofu			
fried, 2-3/4 x 1 x 1/2 inch, 29g	80	6	53
regular, 1/2 cup, 124g	95	6	53

Dairy Products

CHEESE	Calories	Fat Grams	Calories from Fat
American, light, 1 slice, 28g	70	4	36
Blue, crumbled (not packed) 1/4 cup, 34g	120	10	87
Brie, 1 oz, 28g	95	8	70
Cheddar			
1-inch cube, 17g	70	6	51
light, 1 slice, 28g	70	4	36
Colby, 1oz, 28g	110	9	79
Cottage cheese, 1/2 cup			
creamed, large curd, 113g	115	5	46
dry curd, 73g	60	<1	3
lowfat, 1% fat, 113g	80	1	10
Cream cheese, 2 Tbs..			
light, Philadelphia brand, 28g	60	5	45
regular, 30g	105	10	94
whipped, Philadelphia brand, 28g	100	10	90
Feta, 1 oz, 28g	75	6	54
Mozzarella, 1 oz, 28g			
regular	80	6	54
part skim	70	4	40
Parmesan, grated, 1 Tbs.., 5g	25	2	14
Swiss			
1-inch cube, 15g	55	4	37

	Calories	Fat Grams	Calories from Fat
light, 1 slice, 28g	70	3	27
CREAM			
Half & half, 1 Tbs., 15g	20	2	16
Heavy, whipping, 1 Tbs., 15g	50	6	48
Sour cream			
cultured, 2 Tbs., 24g	50	5	45
light, 50% less fat, 2 Tbs., 30g	40	2	22
Whipped cream, pressurized, 1 Tbs., 3g	10	1	6
IMITATION CREAM PRODUCTS			
Coffee creamers			
non-dairy, liquid, Coffee Rich, 1 Tbs., 14g	25	1	13
non-dairy, liquid, Int'l Delight, 1 Tbs., 15g	45	2	14
Sour cream			
imitation, cultured, nondairy, 2 Tbs., 28g	60	5	49
imitation, non-butterfat, 2 Tbs., 24g	45	4	36
powdered, Coffee-Mate, 1 tsp., 2 g	10	1	6
Whipped topping			
non-dairy, pressurized, 2 Tbs., 9g	25	2	19
non-dairy, frozen, Cool Whip, 1 Tbs., 4g	10	1	7
MILK			
Buttermilk, 1% fat, 1 cup, 245g	100	2	19
Chocolate milk, 1 cup, 250g			
lowfat, 1% fat	160	2	22
whole	210	8	76
Condensed, sweetened, 2 Tbs., 38g	125	3	30
Evaporated, canned, 2 tbs., 32g			
lowfat	30	1	5
skim	25	<1	1
whole	40	2	21
Lowfat, 1% fat, 1 cup, 244g	100	3	23
Skim, 1 cup, 245g	85	<1	4
Whole, 3.3% fat, 1 cup, 244g	150	8	73
YOGURT			
Fruit flavors, custard, Yoplait, 1 cont., 170g	190	4	36
Fruit-on-the-bottom, lowfat, 1 cont., 226g	230	3	27
Plain, 1 cont., 226g			
lowfat	145	4	32
nonfat	125	<1	4

Soups

CANNED SOUPS	Calories	Fat Grams	Calories from Fat
(Canned, condensed soups are prepared with water, unless otherwise noted.)			
Bean & ham, Healthy Choice, 1/2 can, 228g	220	4	36
Beef broth, ready-to-serve, 1 cup, 240g	15	1	5
Black bean, Health Valley, 1 cup, 240g	110	0	0
Chicken broth, ready-to-serve, 1/2 can, 249g	30	3	27
Chicken noodle, Campbell's, 1 cup, 226g	60	2	18
Chicken rice, 1 cup, 241g	60	2	17
Clam chowder, New England			
frozen, Stouffer's, 1 cup, 227g	180	9	81
prepared w/skim milk, 1 cup, 233g	100	2	18
prepared w/water, Campbell's, 1 cup, 244g	80	2	20
Cream of Chicken, 1 cup, 244g	110	7	62
Cream of mushroom, 1 cup			
prepared w/water, 244g	130	9	81
prepared w/whole milk, 248g	205	14	122
Minestrone			
prepared w/water, 1 cup, 241g	80	3	23
ready-to-serve, Hain, 1/2 can, 270g	160	3	27
Tomato, 1 cup			
prepared w/water, 244g	85	2	17

A19

	CALORIES	FAT GRAMS	CALORIES FROM FAT
prepared w/whole milk, 248g	160	6	54
Vegetable			
prepared w/water, 1 cup, 241g	90	1	9
ready-to-serve, Pritikin, 1/2 can, 209g	70	0	0

DRIED OR DEHYDRATED SOUPS

	CALORIES	FAT GRAMS	CALORIES FROM FAT
Black bean, Nile Spice, 1 container, 309g	180	1	5
Chicken vegetable, 1 cup, 251g	50	1	7
Cream of chicken, 1 cup, 261g	105	5	48
Mushroom, 1 cup, 253g	95	1	44
Onion, 1 pkg., 7g	20	<1	4
Split pea, 1 cup, 271g	135	2	14
Tomato, 1 cup, 265g	105	2	22

Desserts, Snack Foods, and Candy

CAKES

	CALORIES	FAT GRAMS	CALORIES FROM FAT
Angel food, 1/12 of 10 inch tube, 50g	130	<1	1
Boston Cream Pie, 1/6 of 20 oz, 92g	230	8	70
Carrot cake, Sara Lee, snack size, 1, 52g	180	7	63
Cheesecake, plain, 1/6 of 17 oz, 80g	255	18	160
Cupcake, 1			
chocolate, Hostess, 46g	170	5	45
yellow, w/icing, 36g	130	4	34
Devil's food, w/icing, 1/6 of 9 inch, 69g	235	8	72
Fruitcake, 1 slice, 34g	140	4	35
Pound cake, Sara Lee, 1/10 of cake, 30g	130	7	63
Yellow cake, w/icing, 1/8 of 8 oz, 64g	240	9	84

COOKIES AND BARS

	CALORIES	FAT GRAMS	CALORIES FROM FAT
Brownies, chocolate			
frozen, Weight-Watchers, 1, 36g	100	3	27
from mix, 2 inch square, 33g	140	7	59
Chocolate chip			
Chips Ahoy!, 3, 32g	160	8	72
refrigerated, Pillsbury, 2, 31g	140	7	59
Creme sandwich, Nabisco, 2, 28g	140	6	54
Fig bar, 2, 31g	110	2	21
Gingersnaps, Sunshine, 6, 28g	120	4	36
Graham crackers, 4, 1-1/2 squares, 28g	120	2	18
Oatmeal raisin, Barbara's, 2, 38g	160	7	63
Oreo, Nabisco, 2, 28g	100	4	36
Shortbread, 1-5/8 inch square, 4, 32g	160	8	69
Vanilla wafers, Nabisco, 7, 28g	120	4	36

PIES

	CALORIES	FAT GRAMS	CALORIES FROM FAT
Apple, 1/8 of 9 inch pie, 155g	410	19	175
Blueberry, 1/8 of 9 inch, 147g	360	17	157
Cherry, 1/8 of 9 inch pie, 180g	485	22	198
Chocolate cream, 1/8 of 9 inch, 142g	400	23	206
Custard, 1/8 of 9 inch, 127g	260	11	102
Lemon meringue, 1/8 of 9 inch, 127g	360	16	147
Pumpkin, 1/8 of 9 inch, 155g	315	14	130

OTHER DESSERTS

	CALORIES	FAT GRAMS	CALORIES FROM FAT
Custard, baked, 1/2 cup, 141g	150	7	60
Frozen yogurt, vanilla, 1/2 cup			
Haagen-Dazs, 98g	160	2	22
Yoplait, soft, 72g	90	3	27
Gelatin, Jell-O, 1/2 cup, 140g	80	0	0
Ice cream, vanilla, 1/2 cup			
regular, 10% fat, 66g	135	7	65

	CALORIES	FAT GRAMS	CALORIES FROM FAT
Haagen-Dazs, 106g	260	17	153
Ice cream, chocolate, 1/2 cup			
regular, 10% fat, 66g	145	7	65
Haagen-Dazs, 106g	270	17	153
Ice milk sandwich, Weight Watchers, 78g	160	4	36
Juice bars			
Strawberry, Fruit'n Juice, Dole, 74g	70	0	0
Strawberry, Welch's, 85g	80	0	0
Puddings, from mix, prepared w/2% milk			
butterscotch, 1/2 cup, 148g	150	2	20
chocolate, 1/2 cup, 147g	150	2	20
tapioca, 1/2 cup, 141g	145	2	22
vanilla, 1/2 cup, 144g	140	2	20
Sherbet, 1/2 cup, 87g	135	2	17

SNACK FOODS

	CALORIES	FAT GRAMS	CALORIES FROM FAT
Corn chips, 3/4 cup, 28g	155	9	85
Crackers (see Crackers)			
Nuts (see Nuts and Seeds)			
Popcorn			
air-popped, 1 cup, 8g	30	<1	3
microwave, natural flavor, 1 cup, 8g	35	2	18
Potato chips, 1 cup, 28g	150	10	90
Pretzels			
Dutch, twisted, 2-3/4 inch, 2, 32g	120	1	10
Sticks, 2-1/2 x 1/8 inch, 60, 30g	115	1	9
Twists, thin, Rold Gold, 10, 28g	110	1	9

CANDY

	CALORIES	FAT GRAMS	CALORIES FROM FAT
Caramel, plain, 3/4 inch, 8g	30	1	6
Fudge, chocolate, 1 cu inch, 17g	65	1	13
Gum drops, 8, 28g	110	0	0
Hard candy, 5, 28g	105	0	0
Jellybeans, 10 large or 26 small, 28g	105	<1	1
Hershey's Kisses, 6, 28g	150	9	81
Lollipops, 1, 28g	110	0	0

Beverages

(Milk and juices are in Dairy Products and Fruits sections.)

CARBONATED SODAS

	CALORIES	FAT GRAMS	CALORIES FROM FAT
Cola, 1-1/2 cup, 370g	150	<1	0
Diet cola, w/aspartame, 1-1/2 cup, 355g	4	0	0
Gingerale, 1-12 cup, 366g	125	0	0
Grape soda, 1-12/ cup, 372g	160	0	0
Lemon-lime, 1-1/2 cup, 368g	145	0	0
Orange soda, 1-12/ cup, 372g	180	0	0
Root beer, 1-12/ cup, 370g	150	0	0

COFFEE AND TEA

	CALORIES	FAT GRAMS	CALORIES FROM FAT
Coffee			
brewed, 1 cup, 235g	5	<1	0
brewed, decaffeinated, 1 cup, 240g	3	0	0
instant, 1 cup, 240g	5	0	0
Tea, brewed, 1 cup 237g	2	<1	0
Tea, brewed herb, unflavored, 1 cup, 236g	2	<1	0
Tea, iced, instant, lemon flavored			
sweetened w/aspartame, 1 cup, 259g	2	0	0
sweetened w/sugar, made w/4 tsp., 23g	85	<1	0

ALCOHOLIC BEVERAGES

	CALORIES	FAT GRAMS	CALORIES FROM FAT
Beer, 1-1/2 cup, 355g			
light	100	0	0
regular	145	0	0
nonalcoholic	50	0	0

	CALORIES	FAT GRAMS	CALORIES FROM FAT
Gin, Rum, Whiskey, or Vodka, 80-proof, 1 jigger, 42g	95	0	0
Wine, 1 glass			
red, 147g	105	0	0
white, 147g	100	0	0
Wine cooler, 1 glass, 360g	175	<1	0
Wine, dessert, 1 glass			
dry, 59g	75	0	0
sweet, 59g	90	0	0

Fats, Oils, and Condiments

FATS AND OILS

	CALORIES	FAT GRAMS	CALORIES FROM FAT
Butter			
regular or unsalted, 1 tsp., 5g	35	4	37
whipped, 1 Tbs., 11g	80	9	80
Margarine			
spread, tub, 1 Tbs., 14g	75	9	75
stick, 1 Tbs., 14g	100	11	100
Oil			
corn, 1 Tbs., 14g	120	14	122
olive, 1 Tbs., 14g	120	14	122
vegetable spray, 1-1/4 seconds, 1g	5	1	5
Salad dressing			
blue cheese, 1 Tbs., 15g	75	8	72
French, 1 Tbs., 16g	65	6	57
French, low calorie, 1 Tbs., 16g	20	1	9
Italian, 1 Tbs., 15g	70	7	64
Italian, low calorie, 1 Tbs., 16g	15	1	12
mayonnaise-like, 1 Tbs., 15g	55	5	43
thousand island, 1 Tbs., 16g	60	6	50

CONDIMENTS

	CALORIES	FAT GRAMS	CALORIES FROM FAT
Barbecue sauce, 1 Tbs., 15g	15	<1	3
Catsup, 1 Tbs., 15g	15	<1	0
Gravy, canned			
au jus, 1/4 cup, 60g	10	<1	1
beef, 1/4 cup, 58g	30	1	12
chicken, 1/4 cup, 60g	45	3	30
turkey, 1/4 cup, 60g	30	1	11
Horseradish, prepared, 1 tsp., 5g	2	<1	0
Mustard, prepared, 1 tsp., 5g	4	<1	2
Olives			
black, canned, small, 3, 10g	10	1	9
green, medium, 4, 13g	15	2	14
green, stuffed, 10, 34g	35	4	34
Pickles			
dill, kosher spears, 1, 28g	5	0	0
sweet, gherkins, small, 2-1.2 inches, 2, 30g	40	<1	0
Relish, sweet pickle, 2 Tbs., 30g	40	<1	1
Soy sauce, tamari, 1 Tbs., 18g	10	<1	0
Tartar sauce, 1 Tbs., 14g	75	8	68

SUGAR, JAMS, AND JELLIES

	CALORIES	FAT GRAMS	CALORIES FROM FAT
Chocolate syrup			
fudge-type, 2 Tbs., 42g	145	6	51
thin-type, 2 Tbs., 38g	82	<1	3
Honey, 1 Tbs., 21g	65	0	0
Jams and preserves, 1 Tbs., 20g	50	<1	0
Jellies, 1 Tbs., 19g	50	<1	0
Maple syrup, 2 Tbs., 40g	105	<1	1
Sugar			
brown, unpacked, 1 cup, 145g	545	0	0
white, granulated, 1 tsp., 4g	15	0	0

Fast Foods

BURGERS AND SANDWICHES

	CALORIES	FAT GRAMS	CALORIES FROM FAT
Burger King			
Big Fish	700	41	370
Broiler Chicken	550	29	260
Double Cheeseburger with Bacon	640	39	350
Hamburger	330	15	140
Whopper	640	39	350
McDonald's			
Big Mac	530	28	250
Filet-O-Fish	360	16	150
Hamburger	270	10	90
MacLean Deluxe	350	12	110
McChicken	570	30	270
McGrilled Chicken	510	30	270
Wendy's			
Big Bacon Classic	610	33	290
Chicken Club	500	23	200
Grilled Chicken Sandwich	310	8	70
Hamburger, with everything	420	20	180

SALADS, FRIES, AND MISCELLANEOUS

(Salad values are given for salads without dressing.)

	CALORIES	FAT GRAMS	CALORIES FROM FAT
Burger King			
Broiled Chicken Salad	200	10	90
French fries, medium	370	20	180
Garden Salad	100	5	45
Salad dressing, 30g, thousand island	140	12	110
Salad dressing, 30g, ranch	180	19	170
Salad dressing, 30g, reduced calorie Italian	15	<1	5
McDonald's			
Chef Salad	210	11	100
Fajita Chicken Salad	160	6	60
French fries, large	450	22	200
French fries, small	210	10	90
Salad dressing, 1 pkg., blue cheese	190	17	150
Salad dressing, 1 pkg., lite vinaigrette	50	2	20
Salad dressing, 1 pkg., ranch	180	19	170
Pizza Hut			
Breadsticks, 5	770	25	223
Buffalo wings, 12	565	35	310
Cheese pizza, 1/8 of med., thin crust	205	8	75
Cheese pizza, 1/8 of med., pan pizza	260	11	98
Pepperoni pizza, 1/8 of med., thin crust	215	10	69
Veggie Lover's, 1/8 of med., thin crust	185	7	61
Wendy's			
Baked potato, plain	310	0	0
Baked potato w/chili and cheese	620	24	220
Baked potato w/sour cream and chives	380	6	60
Deluxe Garden Salad	110	6	50
Salad dressing, 2 Tbs., blue cheese	170	19	170
Salad dressing, 2 Tbs., fat-free French	30	0	0
Salad dressing, 2 Tbs., ranch	90	10	90

DESSERTS

	CALORIES	FAT GRAMS	CALORIES FROM FAT
Burger King			
Dutch apple pie	300	15	140
McDonald's			
Baked apple pie	260	13	120
Cookies	260	9	80
Pizza Hut			
Dessert pizza, 1/8 of med.	245	5	46
Wendy's			
Chocolate chip cookies, 1, 57g	270	11	100

YOUR HEALTH DIRECTORY

*I*n *An Invitation to Health*, I emphasize that you shoulder a great deal of responsibility for your health and the quality of your life. Given the complexity of our minds and bodies and the many social and environmental factors that affect us, this responsibility can be a very heavy burden. But your load can be made lighter if you know where to turn for health information, services, and support.

In this directory, you will find over 100 health-related topics and about 250 resources, including addresses, phone numbers, and websites for government agencies, community organizations, professional associations, recovery groups, and Internet sources. Many of these organizations and groups have toll-free 800 or 888 phone numbers, and an increasing number of them have websites (one caution: as you may have experienced, website addresses—like street addresses and phone numbers—do change on occasion). Much of the material available from these groups is free.

Also included in Your Health Directory are clearinghouses and information centers that are especially rich sources of health knowledge. Their main purpose is to collect, help manage, and disseminate information. Clearinghouses often perform other services as well, such as creating original publications and providing tailored responses to individual requests. These organizations also may provide referrals to other groups that can help you.

Many of the groups listed here have local offices or chapters. You can call, write, or visit the websites of these organizations to find out if there is a branch in your vicinity, or you can check your local telephone directory.

The purpose of this directory is to help you be in control of your health. If you know where to turn for answers to your questions and if you know what choices you have, you may find that you have more control over your life.

General Information Resources

Agency for Health Care Policy Research
2101 E. Jefferson Street, Suite 501
Rockville, MD 20852
(301) 594-1360

Go Ask Alice
http://www.columbia.edu/cu/health-wise/all.html

Internet Grateful Med
National Library of Medicine
(offers assisted searching in online databases of the NLM)
8600 Rockville Pike
Bethesda, MD 20894
(800) 638-8480
(301) 402-1076
http://igm.nlm.nih.gov

National Center for Health Statistics (NCHS)
(produces vital statistics and health statistics for the United States)
Data Dissemination Branch
6525 Belcrest Road, Room 1064
Hyattsville, MD 20782
(301) 436-8500
http://www.cdc.gov/nchswww/index.htm

ODPHP National Health Information Center
P.O. Box 1133
Washington, D.C. 20013-1133
(301) 565-4167
(800) 336-4797
http://odphp.oash.dhhs.gov

National Institutes of Health (NIH)
9000 Rockville Pike
Bethesda, MD 20892
(301) 496-4000
http://www.nih.gov

New York Online Access to Health
http://www.noah.cuny.edu

Tel-Med Health Information Service
(provides taped messages on health concerns) See white pages of telephone directory for listing

Yahoo Health Directory
http://www.yahoo.com/health

Resources By Topic

Abortion

National Abortion Federation
(provides information about abortion and referral for abortion services)
(202) 667-5881
(800) 772-9100
http://www.prochoice.org

Accident Prevention

Centers for Disease Control and Prevention
1600 Clifton Road N.E.
Atlanta, GA 30333
(404) 639-3311
http://www.cdc.gov

National Safety Council
1121 Spring Lake Drive
Itasca, IL 60143-3201
(630) 775-2056
(800) 621-7619
http://www.nsc.org

Adoption

Adoptees' Liberty Movement Association (ALMA) Society
(provides assistance for adopted children to locate natural parents and for natural parents to locate relinquished children)
P.O. Box 727
Radio City Station
New York, NY 10101-0727
(212) 581-1568
http://www.almanet.com

AASK (Adopt a Special Kid)
(provides assistance to families who adopt older and handicapped children)
1025 N. Reynolds Road
Toledo, OH 43615
(419) 534-3350
http://www.aask.org

Aging

American Association of Retired Persons
601 E Street N.W.
Washington, D.C. 20049
(800) 424-3410
(202) 434-2277
http://www.aarp.org

Gray Panthers
2025 Pennsylvania Avenue, N.W.
Suite 821
Washington, D.C. 20006
(800) 280-5362
(202) 466-3132

AIDS (Acquired Immunodeficiency Syndrome)

Gay Men's Health Crisis
119 West 24th Street
New York, NY 10011
(212) 807-6664
http://www.gmhc.org

National AIDS Hotline
(800) 342-2437

San Francisco AIDS Foundation
P.O. Box 426182
San Francisco, CA 94162-6182
(415) 487-3000
http://www.sfaf.org

Alcohol Abuse and Alcoholism

Al-Anon and Alateen
(support groups for friends and relatives of alcoholics)
1600 Corporate Landing Parkway
Virginia Beach, VA 23454
(757) 563-1600
http://www.al-anon-alateen.org
See white pages of telephone directory for listing of local chapter

Alcohol Hotline
(800) ALCOHOL

Alcoholics Anonymous
P.O. Box 459
Grand Central Station
New York, NY 10163
(212) 870-3400
http://www.alcoholics-anonymous.org
See white pages of telephone directory for listing of local chapter

National Association of Children of Alcoholics
11426 Rockville Pike
Suite 100
Rockville, MD 20852
(888) 55-4COAS
(301) 468-0985
http://www.health.org/nacoa

National Clearinghouse for Alcohol and Drug Information
P.O. Box 2345
Rockville, MD 20847-2345
(800) 729-6686
(301) 468-2600
http://www.health.org/index.htm

National Institute on Alcohol Abuse and Alcoholism
6000 Executive Boulevard
Willco Building
Bethesda, MD 20892-7003
(301) 443-3860
http://www.niaaa.nih.gov

Women for Sobriety, Inc.
(support groups for women with drinking problems)
P.O. Box 618
Quakertown, PA 18951-0618
(800) 333-1606
(215) 536-8026
http://www.mediapulse.com/wfs/

Alzheimer's Disease

Alzheimer's Association
919 N. Michigan Avenue
Suite 1000
Chicago, IL 60611
(800) 272-3900
(312) 335-8700

Arthritis

Arthritis Foundation
1330 West Peachtree Street
Atlanta, GA 30309
(800) 283-7800
(404) 872-7100
http://www.arthritis.org

Asthma

Asthma and Allergy Foundation of America
1125 15th Street N.W.
Suite 502
Washington, D.C. 20005
(800) 7-ASTHMA
(202) 466-7643
http://www.aafa.org/home.html

Lung Line
National Jewish Center for Immunology and Respiratory Medicine
(information and referral service)
1400 Jackson Street
Denver, CO 80206
(800) 222-5864
(303) 388-4461
http://www.njc.org/Markethtml/Lungline.html

Attention Deficit Disorder

National Attention Deficit Disorder Association (National ADDA)
P.O. Box 972
Mentor, OH 44061-0972
(800) 487-2282
http://www.add.org

Children and Adults with Attention Deficit Disorder (CHADD)
499 N.W. 70th Avenue
Suite 101
Plantation, FL 33317
(305) 587-3700

Learning Disabilities Association (LDA)
4156 Library Road
Pittsburgh, PA 15234
(412) 341-1515
http://www.ldanatl.org

Automobile Safety

American Automobile Association (AAA)
1000 AAA Drive
Heathrow, FL 37246
(407) 444-7000
http://www.aaa.com

See also white or yellow pages of telephone directory for listing of local chapter

Insurance Institute for Highway Safety
1005 North Glebe Road
Suite 800
Arlington, VA 22201
(703) 247-1500

National Highway Traffic Safety Association
Office of Publications
400 7th Street S.W.
Room 6123
Washington, D.C. 20590
(202) 366-2587
http://www.nhtsa.dot.gov

Auto Safety Hotline
(for consumer complaints about auto safety and child safety seats, and requests for information on recalls)
(800) 424-9393

Birth Control and Family Planning

Advocates for Youth
(offers programs aimed at reducing teenage pregnancy)

1025 Vermont Avenue N.W.
Suite 200
Washington, D.C. 20005
(202) 347-5700
http://www.advocatesforyouth.org

American College of Obstetricians and Gynecologists
(provides literature and contraceptive information)
409 12th Street S.W.
Washington, D.C. 20024
(202) 638-5577
http://www.acog.com

Association for Voluntary Surgical Contraception (AVSC)
(provides information and referrals to individuals concerning tubal ligation or vasectomy)
79 Madison Avenue
7th Floor
New York, NY 10016-7802
(212) 561-8000

Planned Parenthood Federation of America (PPFA)
810 Seventh Avenue
New York, NY 10019
(212) 541-7800
http://www.plannedparenthood.org

See also white or yellow pages of telephone directory for listing of local chapter

Birth Defects

Cystic Fibrosis Foundation (CFF)
6931 Arlington Road
Bethesda, MD 20814
(800) FIGHT-CF
(301) 951-4422
http://www.cff.org

March of Dimes Birth Defects Foundation
1275 Mamaroneck Avenue
White Plains, NY 10605
(888) 663-4637
(914) 428-7100
http://www.modimes.org

Blindness

American Foundation for the Blind
1 Penn Plaza
Suite 300
New York, NY 10001
(800) AFB-LINE
(212) 502-7600
http://www.afb.org

National Federation for the Blind
1800 Johnson Street
Baltimore, MD 21230
(800) 638-7518
(410) 659-9314
http://www.nfb.org

National Library Service for the Blind and Physically Handicapped
Library of Congress
1291 Taylor Street, N.W.
Washington, D.C. 20542
(800) 424-8567
(202) 707-5100
http://www.loc.gov/nls

Blood Banks

American Red Cross
431 18th Street N.W.
Washington, D.C. 20006
(202) 737-8300
http://www.redcross.org

See also white or yellow pages of telephone directory for listing of local chapter

Brain

Brain Research Foundation
208 S. LaSalle Street
Suite 1426
Chicago, IL 60604
(312) 782-4311

Breast Cancer

Reach to Recovery
(support program for women who have undergone mastectomies as a result of breast cancer)
American Cancer Society
1599 Clifton Road N.E.
Atlanta, GA 30329-4251
(800) ACS-2345
(404) 320-3333

Burn Injuries

National Burn Victim Foundation
246-A Madisonville Road
P.O. Box 409
Basking Ridge, NJ 07920
(201) 676-7700
http://www.nbvf.org

Phoenix Society for Burn Victims
(self-help organization for burn victims and their families)

11 Rust Hill Road
Levittown, PA 19056
(800) 888-BURN
(215) 946-BURN
http://www.firealert.com/phoenix.htm

Cancer

American Cancer Society
1599 Clifton Road N.E.
Atlanta, GA 30329
(800) 227-2345
(404) 320-3333
http://www.cancer.org

Cancer Information Service
National Cancer Institute
9000 Rockville Pike
Building 31, Room 10A16
Bethesda, MD 20892-0001
(800) 4-CANCER
(301) 496-4000
http://www.nci.nih.gov/hpage/cis.htm

Leukemia Society of America, Inc.
600 Third Avenue
New York, NY 10011
(800) 955-4LSA
(212) 573-8484
http://www.leukemia.org

National Coalition for Cancer Survivorship
1010 Wayne Avenue
Suite 505
Silver Spring, MD 20910
(301) 650-8868
http://www.cansearch.org

National Council on Independent Living
2111 Wilson Boulevard, Suite 405
Arlington, VA 22201
(703) 525-3406

R. A. Bloch Cancer Foundation (Cancer Connection)
(support group that matches cancer patients with volunteers who are cured, in remission, or being treated for the same type of cancer)
4435 Main Street
Suite 500
Kansas City, MO 64111
(800) 433-0464
(816) 932-8453
http://www.blochcancer.org

Child Abuse

National Center for Assault Prevention
(provides services to children, ado-lescents, mentally retarded adults, and elderly)
606 Delsea Drive
Sewell, NJ 08080
(800) 258-3189
(609) 582-7000
http://www.ncap.org

National Child Abuse Hotline
(800) 422-4453

National Committee for the Prevention of Child Abuse
(provides literature on child abuse prevention programs)
200 S. Michigan Avenue
17th Floor
Chicago, IL 60604
(312) 663-3520
http://childabuse.org

Parents Anonymous
(self-help group for abusive parents)
675 W. Foothill Blvd., Suite 220
Claremont, CA 91711-3475
(909) 621-6184
http://www.parentsanonymous-natl.org

Childbirth

American College of Nurse-Midwives
(RNs who provide services through the maternity cycle)
818 Connecticut Avenue N.W.
Suite 900
Washington, D.C. 20006
(202) 728-9860

American College of Obstetricians and Gynecologists
409 12th Street S.W.
P.O. Box 96920
Washington, D.C. 20090
(202) 638-5577
http://www.acog.com

Lamaze International
1200 19th Street N.W.
Suite 300
Washington, D.C. 20036-2422
(800) 368-4404
(202) 857-1128
http://www.lamaze-childbirth.com

International Childbirth Education Association
P.O. Box 20048
Minneapolis, MN 55420
(612) 854-8660
http://www.icea.org

National Association of Parents and Professionals for Safe Alternatives in Childbirth
(provides information and support for alternatives in birth experiences)
Route 1, Box 646
Marble Hill, MO 63764
(314) 238-2010

Parent Care
(resource for parents of premature and high-risk infants)
9041 Colgate Street
Indianapolis, IN 46268-1210
(317) 872-9913

Child Health and Development

National Center for Education in Maternal and Child Health
2000 15th Street, N.
Suite 701
Arlington, VA 22201
(703) 524-7802

National Institute of Child Health and Human Development
31 Center Drive, MSC-2425
Building 31/2A32
Bethesda, MD 20892-2425
(301) 496-5133
http://www.nih.gov/nichd

Chiropractic

American Chiropractic Association
1701 Clarendon Boulevard
Arlington, VA 22209
(800) 986-INFO
(703) 276-8800
http://www.amerchiro.org

Consumer Information

Consumer Information Catalog
(catalog of publications developed by federal agencies for consumers)
Department WWW
Pueblo, CO 81009
http://www.pueblo.gsa.gov

Consumer Information Center
(distributes publications developed by federal agencies for consumers)
18 F Street N.W.
Washington, D.C. 20405
(202) 501-1794

Consumer Product Safety Commission
Office of Information Services
(800) 638-2772
(301) 504-0000
http://www.cpsc.gov

Consumers Union of the United States
(tests quality and safety of consumer products; publishes *Consumer Reports* magazine)
101 Truman Avenue
Yonkers, NY 10703
(914) 378-2000
http://www.consumerreports.org

Council of Better Business Bureaus (CBBB)
4200 Wilson Boulevard
Suite 800
Arlington, VA 22203
(703) 276-0100
http://www.bbb.org

See also white or yellow pages of telephone directory for listing of local chapter

Food and Drug Administration (FDA)
Office of Consumer Affairs
Consumer Inquiries
5600 Fishers Lane (HFE-88)
Rockville, MD 20857
(301) 827-4420
http://www.fda.gov

Crime Victims

Crisis Prevention Institute, Inc.
(offers programs on non-violent physical crisis interventions)
3315-K N. 124th Street
Brookfield, WI 53005
(800) 558-8976
(414) 783-5787

National Association for Crime Victims Rights (NACVR)
P.O. Box 16161
Portland, OR 97216
(503) 252-9012

Death and Grieving

SHARE
(support group for parents who have suffered loss of newborn baby)
c/o St. John's Hospital
800 E. Carpenter Street
Springfield, IL 62729
(217) 544-6464

Dental Health

American Dental Association (ADA)
211 E. Chicago Avenue
Chicago, IL 60611
(312) 440-2500
http://www.ada.org

National Institute of Dental Research
Office of Communication
9000 Rockville Pike
Building 31, Room 2C35
Bethesda, MD 20892
(301) 496-4261
http://www.nidr.nih.gov

Depressive Disorders

Depressives Anonymous: Recovery from Depression (DARFD)
329 East 62nd Street
New York, NY 10021
(212) 689-2600

National Depressive and Manic Depressive Association (NDMDA)
730 N. Franklin
Suite 501
Chicago, IL 60610
(312) 642-0049
(800) 826-3632
http://www.ndmda.org

DES (Diethylstibestrol)

DES Action, USA
(support group for persons exposed to DES)
1615 Broadway, Suite 510
Oakland, CA 94612
(510) 465-4011
http://www.desaction.org

Diabetes

American Diabetes Association
National Center
1660 Duke Street
Alexandria, VA 22314
(800) ADA-DISC
(703) 549-1500
http://www.diabetes.org

Juvenile Diabetes Foundation International (JDFI)
120 Wall Street
New York, NY 10005-4001
(800) JDF-CURE
(212) 785-9500
http://www.jdfcure.org

National Diabetes Information Clearinghouse
1 Information Way
Bethesda, MD 20892-3560
(301) 654-3327
http://www.niddk.nih.gov

Digestive Diseases

National Digestive Diseases Information
Clearinghouse (NDDIC)
Box NDDIC
9000 Rockville Pike
Bethesda, MD 20892
(301) 654-3810

Domestic Violence

Batterers Anonymous
(self-help group designed to rehabilitate men who abuse women)
1850 N. Riverside Avenue, Suite 220
Rialto, CA 92376
(909) 355-1100

National Coalition Against Domestic Violence (NCADV)
P.O. Box 18749
Denver, CO 80218
(303) 839-1852

National Domestic Violence Hotline
(800) 799-SAFE

National Network to End Domestic Violence
701 Pennsylvania N.W.
Suite 900
Washington, D.C. 20004
(202) 347-9520

Down Syndrome

National Association for Down Syndrome (NADS)
P.O. Box 4542
Oak Brook, IL 60522-4542
(708) 325-9112
http://www.nads.org

National Down Syndrome Society (NDSS)
666 Broadway, 8th Floor
New York, NY 10012-2317
(800) 221-4602
(212) 460-9330
http://www.ndss.org

Drug Abuse

Cocaine Anonymous World Services
P.O. Box 2000
Los Angeles, CA 90049
(800) 347-8998
(310) 559-5833
http://www.ca.org

Narcotics Anonymous (NA)
(support group for recovering recent
narcotics addicts)
P.O. Box 999
Van Nuys, CA 91409
(818) 773-9999
http://www.wsoinc.com

See also white or yellow pages of tele-
phone directory for listing of local
chapter

National Cocaine Hotline
(800) COCAINE

**National Institute on Drug Abuse
Helpline**
(800) 662-4357
http://nida.nih.gov

**National Parents Resource Institute
for Drug Education (PRIDE)**
3610 Dekalb Technology Parkway
Atlanta, GA 30340
(770) 458-9900
http://www.prideusa.org

Substance Abuse Prevention
Alcohol, Drug Abuse, and Mental
 Health Administration
5600 Fishers Lane
Rockwall 11 Building
Rockville, MD 20852
(301) 443-0365

Drunk Driving Groups

Mothers Against Drunk Driving
511 E. John Carpenter Freeway
Suite 700
Irving, TX 75062
(800) GET-MADD
(214) 744-6233
http://www.madd.org

See also white pages of telephone
directory for listing of local chapter

Remove Intoxicated Drivers (RID)
P.O. Box 520
Schenectady, NY 12301
(518) 372-0034
(518) 393-HELP

**Students Against Drunk Driving
(SADD)**
200 Pleasant Street
Marlboro, MA 01752
(508) 481-3568

Eating Disorders

**American Anorexia/Bulimia
Association (AA/BA)**
(self-help group that provides information and referrals to physicians
and therapists)
165 West 46th Street, #1108
New York, NY 10036
(212) 575-6200
http://members.aol.com/amanbu/

**Anorexia Nervosa and Related
 Eating Disorders (ANRED)**
(provides information and referrals
for people with eating disorders)
P.O. Box 5102
Eugene, OR 97405
(541) 344-1144
http://www.anred.com

Environment

**Environmental Protection Agency
(EPA)**
Public Information Center
PM 211-B
401 M Street S.W.
Washington, D.C. 20460
(202) 260-2080
http://www.epa.gov

Greenpeace, USA
1436 U Street N.W.
Washington, D.C. 20009
(800) 326-0959
(202) 462-1177
http://www.greenpeaceusa.org

Natural Resources Defense Council
40 West 20th Street
New York, NY 10011
(212) 727-2700
http://www.nrdc.org

Sierra Club
85 2nd Street, 2nd Floor
San Francisco, CA 94105
(415) 977-5500
http://www.sierraclub.org

World Wildlife Fund
1250 24th Street N.W.
Washington, D.C. 20037
(202) 293-4800
http://www.wwfus.org

Epilepsy

Epilepsy Foundation of America
4351 Garden City Drive
Landover, MD 20785-2267
(800) EFA-1000
(301) 459-3700
http://www.efa.org

Gay and Lesbian
Organizations and Services

Human Rights Campaign
1101 14th Street N.W.
Washington, D.C. 20005
(202) 628-4160
http://www.hrc.org

**National Gay and Lesbian Task
Force (NGLTF)**
2320 17th Street N.W.
Washington, D.C. 20009
(202) 332-6483
http://www.ngltf.org

**Parents, Family, and Friends of
Lesbians and Gays (P-FLAG)**
1101 14th Street N.W.
Washington, D.C. 20005
(202) 638-4200
http://www.pflag.org

Handicapped and Disabled

**American Alliance for Health,
Physical Education, Recreation,
and Dance (AAHPERD)**
(provides information about recreation and fitness opportunities for
the handicapped)
1900 Association Drive
Reston, VA 20191
(703) 476-3400
http://www.aahperd.org

**National Council on Independent
Living**
2111 Wilson Boulevard, Suite 405
Arlington, VA 22201
(703) 525-3406

**National Library Service for the
Blind and Physically Handicapped**
Library of Congress
1291 Taylor Street, N.W.
Washington, D.C. 20542
(800) 424-8567
(202) 707-5100
http://www.loc.gov/nls

**Special Olympics International
(SOI)**
1325 G Street N.W.
Suite 500
Washington, D.C. 20005
(202) 628-3630
http://www.specialolympics.org

Hazardous Waste

**Environmental Protection Agency
(EPA)**
Public Information Center
PM 211-B
401 M Street S.W.
Washington, D.C. 20460
(202) 260-2080
http://www.epa.gov

**Hazardous Waste Hotline
Information**
(800) 424-9346

Health Care

**American Association for
Therapeutic Humor (AATH)**
(publishes a newsletter and sponsors
seminars for people in the helping
professions)
222 S. Merimac Street
Suite 303
St. Louis, MO 63105
(314) 863-6232
http://ideanurse.com/aath

American Medical Association
515 N. State Street
Chicago, IL 60610
(312) 464-5000
http://www.ama-assn.org

American Nurses Association
600 Maryland Avenue S.W.
Washington, D.C. 20024-2571
(800) 274-4ANA
(202) 651-7000
http://www.nursingworld.org

Medical Self-Care Magazine
P.O. Box 717
Inverness, CA 94937

Health Education

**Center for Health Promotion and
Education**
Centers for Disease Control and
Prevention
Mail Stop A34
1600 Clifton Road, N.E.
Atlanta, GA 30333
(404) 639-3534

Hearing Impairment

**American Society for
Deaf Children**
(resource group for parents of hard
of hearing and deaf children)
2848 Arden Way
Suite 210
Sacramento, CA 95825
(800) 942-ASDC
(916) 482-0120

Better Hearing Institute (BHI)
(provides educational and resource
materials on deafness)
Box 1840
Washington, D.C. 20013
(800) EAR-WELL
(703) 642-0580
http://www.betterhearing.org

Heart Disease

American Heart Association (AHA)
7272 Greenville Avenue
Dallas, TX 75231
(800) 242-8721
(214) 373-6300
http://www.amheart.org

**National Heart, Lung, and
Blood Institute**
(provides information on cardiovascular risk factors and disease)
4733 Bethesda Avenue, Suite 530
Bethesda, MD 20814
(301) 951-3260
http://www.nhlbi.nih.gov/nhlbi/nlhbi.
htm

Holistic Medicine

**American Holistic Medical
Association (NHMA)**
6728 Old McLean Village Drive
McLean, VA 22101
(703) 556-8729
http://www.ahmaholistic.com

Homeopathy

**National Center for Homeopathy
(NCH)**
801 N. Fairfax Street, Suite 306
Alexandria, VA 22314
(703) 548-7790
http://www.healthworld.com/nch

Hospice

National Hospice Organization
1901 N. Moore Street, Suite 901
Arlington, VA 22209
(703) 243-5900
http://nho.org

Immunization

**National Center for Prevention
Services**
Centers for Disease Control
1600 Clifton Road, N.E.
Atlanta, GA 30333
(404) 332-4559

Infant Care

American Red Cross
431 18th Street N.W.
Washington, D.C. 20006
(202) 737-8300
http://www.redcross.org

LaLeche League International
(provides information and support to
women interested in breast-feeding)
1400 N. Meacham Road
Schaumburg, IL 60173
(800) LA-LECHE
(847) 519-7730
http://www.lalecheleague.org

Infectious Diseases

**Centers for Disease Control and
Prevention**
1600 Clifton Road, N.E.
Atlanta, GA 30333
(404) 639-3534
http://www.cdc.gov

Infertility

Resolve, Inc.
(offers counseling, information, and
support to people with
problems of infertility)
1310 Broadway
Somerville, MA 02144-1779
(617) 623-0744
http://www.resolve.org

In-Vitro Fertilization
Eastern Virginia Medical School
Howard and Georgeanna Jones
Institute
for Reproductive Medicine
601 Colley Avenue
Norfolk, VA 23507
(804) 446-8948

Inherited Diseases

Alliance of Genetic Support Groups
(provides information about inherited diseases; publishes a directory of genetic counseling services)
35 Wisconsin Circle
Suite 440
Chevy Chase, MD 20815
(800) 336-GENE

Kidney Disease

American Kidney Fund (AKF)
(provides information on financial aid to patients, organ transplants, and kidney-related diseases)
6110 Executive Boulevard
Suite 1010
Rockville, MD 20852
(800) 638-8299
(301) 881-3052
http://www.akfinc.org

American Association of Kidney Patients (AAKP)
100 S. Ashley Dr.
Suite 280
Tampa, FL 33602-5346
(800) 749-2257
http://www.aakp.org/aakpteam.html

National Kidney Foundation (NKF)
30 East 33rd Street
Suite 1100
New York, NY 10016
(800) 622-9010
(212) 889-2210
http://www.kidney.org

Learning Disorders

Learning Disabilities Association of America (LDA)
4156 Library Road
Pittsburgh, PA 15234
(412) 341-1515

Liver Disease

American Liver Foundation (ALF)
1425 Pompton Avenue
Cedar Grove, NJ 07009
(800) 465-4837

Lung Disease

American Lung Association (ALA)
1740 Broadway
New York, NY 10019
(800) LUNG-USA
(212) 315-8700
http://www.lungusa.org

NHLBI Educational Program Information Center
(provides information on cardiovascular risk factors)
P.O. Box 30105
Bethesda, MD 20824
(301) 951-3260

National Jewish Center for Immunology and Respiratory Medicine
1400 Jackson Street
Denver, CO 80206
(303) 388-4461

Lupus Erythematosus

Lupus Foundation of America (LPA)
1300 Picard Drive
Suite 200
Rockville, MD 20850-4303
(301) 670-9292
(800) 558-0121
http://www.lupus.org/lupus/index.html

Marriage and Family

Women Work! The National Network for Women's Employment
(national advocacy group for women over 35 who have lost their primary means of support through death, divorce, or disabling of spouse)
1625 K Street N.W.
Suite 300
Washington, D.C. 20006
(202) 467-6346

Family Service of America
1701 K Street N.W.
Suite 200
Washington, D.C. 20006
(202) 223-3447
http://www.fsanet.org/main/

Stepfamily Association of America
(provides information and publishes quarterly newsletter)
650 J Street, Suite 205
Lincoln, NE 68508
(402) 477-7837
(800) 735-0329
http://www.stepfam.org

Medical Information

Medic Alert Foundation
(provides those with medical problems bracelets or neck chains with special emblems to alert medical or law enforcement personnel)
2323 Colorado Avenue
Turlock, CA 95382
(800) 825-3785

Medications (Prescriptions and Over-the-Counter)

Food and Drug Administration (FDA)
Office of Consumer Affairs Public Inquiries
5600 Fishers Lane (HFE-88)
Rockville, MD 20857
(301) 443-3170
http://www.fda.gov

Mental Health

American Psychiatric Association
1400 K Street N.W.
Washington, D.C. 20005
(202) 682-6000
http://www.psych.org

American Psychological Association
750 First Street N.E.
Washington, D.C. 20002
(202) 336-5500
http://www.apa.org

National Alliance for the Mentally Ill (NAMI)
(self-help advocacy organization for persons with schizophrenia and depressive disorders and their families)
200 N. Glebe Road
No. 1015
Arlington, VA 22201
(800) 950-NAMI
(703) 524-7600

National Institute of Mental Health
Information Resources and Inquiries Branch
5600 Fishers Lane
Room 15C05
Rockville, MD 20857
(301) 443-4515

National Mental Health Association (NMHA)
1021 Prince Street
Alexandria, VA 22314-2971
(800) 969-NMHA
(703) 684-7722
http://www.nmha.org

Recovery, Inc.
(self-help group for former mental patients)

Association of Nervous and Former
  Mental Patients
802 N. Dearborn Street
Chicago, IL 60610
(312) 337-5661

Mental Retardation

**Association for Retarded Citizens
(ARC)**
500 E. Border Street
Suite 300
Arlington, TX 76010
(817) 261-6003
http://www.thearc.org

Missing and Runaway Children

Child Find of America
(800) I-AM-LOST

**National Center for Missing and
Exploited Children (NCMEC)**
2101 Wilson Boulevard, Suite 550
Arlington, VA 22201
(703) 235-9000
(800) 843-5678
http://www.missingkids.org

Runaway Hotline
(800) 231-6946

Neurological Disorders

**National Institute of Neurological
and Communicative Disorders and
Stroke**
National Institutes of Health
9000 Rockville Pike
Bethesda, MD 20205
(301) 496-4000

Nutrition

American Dietetic Association
216 West Jackson Boulevard
Chicago, IL 60606-6995
(312) 899-0040
http://www.eatright.org

**American Institute of Nutrition
(AIN)**
9650 Rockville Pike
Bethesda, MD 20814-3990
(301) 530-7050

Food and Drug Administration (FDA)
Office of Consumer Affairs
Public Inquiries

5600 Fishers Lane (HFE-88)
Rockville, MD 20857
(301) 443-3170
http://www.fda.gov

Food and Nutrition Board
Institute of Medicine
2101 Constitution Avenue N.W.
Washington, D.C. 20418
(202) 334-1732

**Food and Nutrition Information
Center**
National Agricultural Library
Room 304
10301 Baltimore Avenue
Baltimore, MD 20705
(301) 504-5719
http://nalusda.gov/fnic/

Occupational Safety and Health

**Clearinghouse for Occupational
Safety and Health Centers for
Disease Control**
National Institute for Occupational
  Safety and Health
5600 Fishers Lane
Rockville, MD 20857
(202) 472-7134

Organ Donations

The Living Bank (TLB)
(provides information and acts as
registry and referral service for people wanting to donate organs for
research or transplantation)
P.O. Box 6725
Houston, TX 77265
(800) 528-2971
in Texas (713) 961-9431

Osteopathic Medicine

**American Osteopathic Association
(AOA)**
142 East Ontario Street
Chicago, IL 60611
(312) 280-5800
(800) 621-1773
http://www.am-osteo-assn.org

Parent Support Groups

**National Organization of Mothers
with Twin Clubs (NOMOTC)**
P.O. Box 23188
Albuquerque, NM 87192-1188
(505) 275-0955

Parents Anonymous
(self-help group for abusive parents)
675 W. Foothill Boulevard
Suite 220
Claremont, CA 91711-3416
(909) 621-6184

Parents Without Partners, Inc.
401 N. Michigan Avenue
Chicago, IL 60611
(312) 644-6610
http://www.parentswithoutpartners.org

Pesticides

**National Pesticides
Telecommunications Network**
Agricultural Chemistry Extension
Oregon State University
333 Weniger Hall
Corvallis, OR 97331
(800) 858-7378

Phobias

**Anxiety Disorders Association of
American (ADAA)**
(provides information about phobias
and referrals to therapists and support groups)
11900 Parklawn Drive
Suite 100
Rockville, MD 20852
(301) 231-9350
http://www.adaa.org

TERRAP Programs
(headquarters for national network of
treatment clinics for agoraphobia)
932 Evelyn Street
Menlo Park, CA 94025
(415) 327-1312
(800) 2-PHOBIA

Physical Fitness

*See local yellow and white pages of
telephone directory for listing of local
health clubs and YMCAs, YWCAs, and
Jewish Community Centers*

**Cooper Institute for Aerobics
Research**
12330 Preston Road
Dallas, TX 75230
(214) 701-8001

**President's Council on Physical
Fitness and Sports**
701 Pennsylvania Avenue N.W.
Suite 250
Washington, D.C. 20004
(202) 272-3430

Women's Sports Foundation
Eisenhower Park
East Meadow, NY 11554
(516) 542-4700
(800) 227-3988
http://www.lifetimetv.com/WoSport/

Poisoning

See emergency numbers listed in the front of your local phone directory

National Poison Hotline
(800) 962-1253

Pregnancy

National Center for Education in Maternal and Child Health
2000 15th Street N.
Suite 701
Arlington, VA 22201-2617
(703) 524-7802

Product Safety

Consumer Product Safety Commission
Washington, D.C. 20207
(800) 638-CPSC
http://www.cpsc.gov

Radiation Control and Safety

Center for Devices and Radiological Health
Office of Consumer Affairs
5600 Fishers Lane HFC-210
Rockville, MD 20857
(301) 443-4190
http://www.fda.gov/cdrh/index.html

National Institute of Environmental Health Sciences
P.O. Box 12233
Research Triangle Park, NC 27709
(919) 541-3345
http://www.niehs.nih.gov

Rape

See white pages of telephone directory for listing of local rape crisis and counseling centers

National Clearinghouse on Marital and Date Rape
(for-profit referral service)
2325 Oak Street
Berkeley, CA 94708
(510) 524-1582
http://members.aol.com/ncmdr/index.html

National Coalition Against Sexual Assault
912 N. 2nd Street
Harrisburg, PA 17102
(717) 232-6745
http://www.achiever.com/freehmpg.ncas/

Reye's Syndrome

National Reye's Syndrome Foundation
426 North Lewis
Bryan, OH 43506
(419) 636-2679
(800) 233-7393

Self-Care/Self-Help

National Self-Help Clearinghouse (NSHC)
(provides information about self-help groups)
25 West 43rd Street
Room 620
New York, NY 10036
(212) 354-8525

United Way of America
701 N. Fairfax Street
Alexandria, VA 22314
(703) 836-7100
http://www.unitedway.org

Sex Education

American Association of Sex Educators, Counselors, and Therapists (AASECT)
435 North Michigan Avenue
Suite 1717
Chicago, IL 60611
(312) 644-0828
http://www.aasect.org

Advocates for Youth
(develops programs and material to educate youth on sex and sexual responsibility)
1025 Vermont Avenue, N.W. Suite 200
Washington, D.C. 20005
(202) 347-5700

Planned Parenthood Federation of America (PPFA)
810 Seventh Avenue
New York, NY 10019
(212) 541-7800
http://www.plannedparenthood.org

Sex Information and Education Council of the U.S. (SIECUS)
(maintains an information clearinghouse on all aspects of human sexuality)
130 West 42nd Street
Suite 350
New York, NY 10036
(212) 819-9770
http://www.siecus.org

Sexual Abuse and Assault

National Center for Assault Prevention
(provides services to children, adolescents, mentally retarded adults, and elderly)
606 Delsea Drive
Sewell, NJ 08080
(609) 582-7000
(800) 258-3189

National Committee for Prevention of Child Abuse
332 S. Michigan Avenue
Suite 1600
Chicago, IL 60604
(312) 663-3520

Parents United International
(support group for individuals—and their families—who have experienced molestation as children)
615 15th Street
Modesto, CA 95354-2510
(408) 453-7616

Sexual Difficulties

Impotence Institute of America
(provides information on causes and treatment of impotence)
119 S. Ruth Street
Maryville, TN 37803
(423) 983-6092

Sexually Transmitted Diseases

Centers for Disease Control and Prevention
1600 Clifton Road, N.E.
Atlanta, GA 30333
(404) 639-3311
http://www.cdc.gov

Herpes Resource Center
American Social Health Association
P.O. Box 13827
Research Triangle Park, NC 27709
(919) 361-8488
http://www.ashastd.org/herpes/hrc.
html

National STD Hotline
(800) 227-8922

Sickle Cell Disease

Center for Sickle Cell Disease
Howard University
2121 Georgia Avenue N.W.
Washington, D.C. 20059
(202) 806-7930

Sickle Cell Disease Association of America
200 Corporate Pointe, Suite 495
Culver City, CA 90230
(310) 216-6363
(800) 421-8453

Skin Disease

National Psoriasis Foundation
6600 S.W. 92nd Avenue, Suite 300
Portland, OR 97223
(503) 244-7404
http://www.psoriasis.org

Sleep and Sleep Disorders

American Narcolepsy Association
1255 Post Street
Suite 404
San Francisco, CA 94109
(415) 788-4793

American Sleep Disorders Association
6301 Bandel Road
Suite 101
Rochester, MN 55901
(507) 287-6006
http://www.asda.org

Better Sleep Council
333 Commerce Street
Alexandria, VA 22314
(703) 683-8371

Smoking and Tobacco

Action on Smoking and Health (ASH)
(provides information on non-smokers' rights and related subjects)
2013 H Street N.W.
Washington, D.C. 20006
(202) 659-4310
http://ash.org

American Cancer Society
(provides information about quitting smoking and smoking cessation programs)
1599 Clifton Road, N.E.
Atlanta, GA 30329
(800) 227-2345
http://www.cancer.org

American Heart Association
(provides information about quitting smoking and smoking cessation programs)
7272 Greenville Avenue
Dallas, TX 75321
(800) 242-8721
(214) 373-6300
http://www.amhrt.org

American Lung Association
(provides information about quitting smoking and smoking cessation programs)
1740 Broadway
New York, NY 10019
(800) LUNG-USA
(212) 315-8700
http://www.lungusa.org

Americans for Nonsmokers' Rights
2530 San Pablo Avenue
Suite J
Berkeley, CA 94702
(510) 841-3032
http://www.no-smoke.org

Stress Reduction

Association for Applied Psychophysiology and Biofeedback (AABP)
10200 W. 44th Avenue
Suite 304
Wheat Ridge, CO 80033
(800) 477-8892
(303) 422-8436

Stroke

Council on Stroke
American Heart Association
7320 Greenville Avenue
Dallas, TX 75321
(214) 373-6300

National Institute of Neurological and Communicative Disorders and Stroke
National Institutes of Health
9000 Rockville Pike
Bethesda, MD 20892
(301) 496-4000

Stuttering

National Center for Stuttering
200 East 33rd Street
New York, NY 10016
(800) 221-2483
(212) 532-1460
http://www.stuttering.com

Sudden Infant Death Syndrome (SIDS)

SIDS Alliance
(provides information and referrals for families who have lost an infant because of SIDS)
1314 Bedford Avenue
Suite 210
Baltimore, MD 21208
(800) 221-7437
(410) 653-8226

Suicide Prevention

American Association of Suicidology (AAS)
4201 Connecticut Avenue N.W.
Suite 310
Washington, D.C. 20008
(202) 237-2280
http://www.cyberpsych.org/aas/index.
htm

National Runaway Switchboard
3080 N. Lincoln Avenue
Chicago, IL 60657
(800) 621-4000
(773) 880-9860
http://nrs.crisisline.org/about.htm

Suicide Prevention Hotline
(800) 827-7571

Surgery

National Second Surgical Opinion Program
(800) 638-6833
in Maryland (800) 492-6603

Terminal Illness

Choices in Dying—The National Council for the Right to Die (CID)
(promotes research on death and dying and works for the right of terminally ill persons to refuse extraordinary life-prolonging measures)
200 Varick Street, 10th Floor
New York, NY 10014-4810
(800) 989-1011
(212) 366-5540

Make-a-Wish Foundation of America (MAWFA)
(dedicated to granting the special wishes of terminally ill children)
100 W. Clarendon Avenue

Suite 2200
Phoenix, AZ 85013
(800) 722-9474
(602) 279-9474
http://www.wish.org

Make Today Count (MTC)
(self-help group for persons with terminal illness)
1235 E. Cherokee Street
Springfield, MO 65804
(800) 432-2273
(417) 885-3324

Weight Control

Overeaters Anonymous (OA)
6075 Zenith Court, N.E.
Rio Rancho, NM 87124-6424
(505) 891-2664

Take Off Pounds Sensibly (TOPS)
P.O. Box 07360
4575 S. Fifth Street
Milwaukee, WI 53207-0360
(800) 932-8677
(414) 482-4620

Weight Watchers International
175 Crossways Park West
Woodbury, NY 11797

(516) 949-0400
http://www.weight-watchers.com

Wellness

Wellness Associates
(publishes The Wellness Inventory)
121489 Orr Springs Road
Ukiah, CA 95482
(707) 937-2331

Women's Health

Boston Women's Health Book Collective
(authors of *The New Our Bodies, Ourselves*, a well-known book on women's health)
240A Elm Street
Somerville, MA 02144
(617) 625-0271

National Women's Health Network (NWHN)
514 10th Street N.W.
Suite 400
Washington, D.C. 20004
(202) 347-1140

TEXT AND PHOTOGRAPHY CREDITS

Program. For more information, call the National Heart, Lung, and Blood Institute at 1-800-575-WELL.

p. 126   Based on data from Douglas, Kathy et al, "Results from the 1995 National College Health Risk Behavior Study," Journal of American College Health, Vol. 46, September 1997.

p. 127   From American Health, November 1994. The quiz is adapted from The Lazy Person's Guide to Fitness. Reprinted by permission.

p. 152   Based on data from Douglas, Kathy et al., "Results from the 1995 National College Health Risk Behavior Study," Journal of American College Health, Vol. 46, September 1997.

p. 160   "Sources of Dietary Fiber" from The Wellness Encyclopedia. Copyright (c) 1991 by Health Letter Associates. Reprinted by permission of Houghton Mifflin Company. All rights reserved.

p. 178   From American Health, July/August 1995, p. 51, by Denise Webb. Reprinted by permission.

p. 186   From a quiz developed by Dr. Kelly Brownell, Director of the Yale University Center for Eating and Weight Disorders author of the Learn Program for Weight Control which appeared in American Health, November 1994. Reprinted by permission.

p. 193   Based on data from Douglas, Kathy et al., "Results from the 1995 National College Health Risk Behavior Study," Journal of American College Health, Vol. 46, September 1997.

p. 216   From Why Marriages Succeeed or Fail, by J. Gottman. Copyright (c) 1994 by Simon & Schuster, Inc.

p. 258   Based on data from Douglas, Kathy et al., "Results from the 1995 National College Health Risk Behavior Study," Journal of American College Health, Vol. 46, September 1997.

p. 259   From Sex In America: A Definitive Survey by Robert Michael et al. Boston: Little Brown, 1994.

p. 283   Based on data from Douglas, Kathy et al., "Results from the 1995 National College Health Risk Behavior Study," Journal of American College Health, Vol. 46, September 1997.

p. 287   Based on data from "Fertility, family planning, and Women's Health: New Data from the 1995 National Survey of Family Growth," by J.C. Abma, A. Chandra, W. D. Mosher, L. Peterson, and L. Piccinono. National Center for Health Statistics. Vital Health Stat 23(19). 1997.

p. 291   From "The Economic Value of Contraception," by James Trussell et al. American Journal of Public Health, Vol. 85, No. 4. April, 1995. Reprinted by permission.

p. 353   From "Development of a Three-Component STD Attitude Scale," by W.L. Yarber, M. R. Torabi, and C. H. Veenker, 1989, Journal of Sex Education and Therapy, 15, 36-39. Copyright (c) 1989 by . Reprinted by permission

p. 393   Reprinted by permission from American Health, © 1993 by Michele Turk.

p. 413   Reprinted by permission from American Health, © 1995 by Trina Chang.

p. 443   Reprinted from the Mayo Clinic Health Letter, April 1994 with permission of Mayo Foundation for Medical Education and Research, Rochester, Minnesota 55905. For subscription information call (800) 333-9038.

p. 453   Based on data from Douglas, Kathy et al., "Results from the 1995 National College Health Risk Behavior Study," Journal of American College Health, Vol. 46, September 1997.

p. 490   Based on data from Douglas, Kathy et al., "Results from the 1995 National College Health Risk Behavior Study," Journal of American College Health, Vol. 46, September 1997.

p. 516   Based on data from Douglas, Kathy et al., "Results from the 1995 National College Health Risk Behavior Study," Journal of American College Health, Vol. 46, September 1997.

p. 535   From The American Medical Association Family Medical Guide by American Medical Association. Copyright (c) 1982 by The American Medical Association. Reprinted by permission of Random House, Inc.

p. 538   Based on data from Douglas, Kathy et al., "Results from the 1995

National College Health Risk Behavior Study," Journal of American College Health, vol 46, September 1997.

p. 551   From "The Continuum of Violence Against Women: Psychological and Physical Consequences," by Marjorie Whittaker Leidig. Journal of American College Health, January 1992. Reprinted with permission of the Helen Dwight Reid Educational Foundation. Published by Heldref Publications. Copyright (c) 1982.

p. 574   From The New York Times, January 13, 1998. Reprinted by permission

p. 593   From Schneidman, Edwin, "You and Death" (questionnaire), Psychology Today, August 1970. Reprinted with permission from Psychology Today Magazine. Copyright (c) 1970 Sussex Publishers, Inc.

p. 598   Adapted from "Guide to the Living Will," Hippocrates, May/June 1988. Copyright (c) 1988 Hippocrates.

p. 605   "One Man's Grief," Journal of the American Medical Association, March 23-30, 1984, v. 251, p. 1551, (c) 1984 American Medical Association.

p. 614   From "A Critical Appraisal of 98.6 F, the Upper Limit of the Normal Body Temperature and Other Legacies of Carl Reinhold August Wunderlich," by Philip Mackowiak et al., Journal of the American Medical Association, Vol. 268, September 23-30, 1992, pp. 1578-80, (c) 1992 American Medical Association.

p. 620   From Complete Home Medical Guide, Revised Edition by Columbia University College of Physicians and Surgeons. Copyright (c) 1989 by the Trustees of Columbia University in the City of New York and the College of Physicians and Surgeons of Columbia University. Reprinted by permission of Crown Publishers, Inc.

abscess A localized accumulation of pus and disintegrating tissue.

absorption The passage of substances into or across membranes or tissues.

abstinence Voluntary refrainment from sexual intercourse.

acid rain Rain with a high concentration of acids produced by air pollutants emitted during the combustion of fossil fuels and the smelting of ores; damages plant and animal life and buildings.

acquired immunodeficiency syndrome (AIDS) The final stages of HIV infection, characterized by a variety of severe illnesses and decreased levels of certain immune cells.

acupuncture A Chinese medical practice of puncturing the body with needles inserted at specific points to relieve pain or cure disease.

acute injuries Physical injuries, such as sprains, bruises, and pulled muscles, which result from sudden traumas, such as falls or collisions.

adaptive response The body's attempt to reestablish homeostasis or stability.

addiction A behavioral pattern characterized by compulsion, loss of control, and continued repetition of a behavior or activity in spite of adverse consequences.

additive Characterized by a combined effect that is equal to the sum of the individual effects.

additives Substances added to foods to enhance certain qualities, such as appearance, taste, or freshness.

adjustment disorder An extraordinary response to a stressful event or situation.

adoption The legal process for becoming the parent to a child of other biological parents.

advance directives Documents that specify individual's preferences regarding treatment in a medical crisis.

aerobic circuit training Combining aerobic and strength exercises to build both cardiovascular fitness and muscular strength and endurance.

aerobic exercise Physical activity in which sufficient or excess oxygen is continually supplied to the body.

after-intercourse methods Treatments, such as large doses of oral contraceptives, menstrual extraction, or dilation and curettage, given after unprotected intercourse to prevent pregnancy.

ageism A form of discrimination based on myths about aging and the elderly.

aging The characteristic pattern of normal life changes that occur as an individual gets older.

alcohol abuse Continued use of alcohol despite awareness of social, occupational, psychological, or physical problems related to its use, or use of alcohol in dangerous ways or situations, such as before driving.

alcohol dependence Development of a strong craving for alcohol due to the pleasurable feelings or relief of stress or anxiety produced by drinking.

alcoholism A chronic, progressive, potentially fatal disease characterized by impaired control of drinking, a preoccupation with alcohol, continued use of alcohol despite adverse consequences, and distorted thinking, most notably denial.

allergy A hypersensitivity to a particular substance in one's environment or diet.

altruism Acts of helping or giving to others without thought of self-benefit.

Alzheimer's disease A progressive deterioration of intellectual powers due to physiological changes within the brain; symptoms include diminishing ability to concentrate and reason, disorientation, depression, apathy, and paranoia.

amenorrhea The absence or suppression of menstruation.

amino acids Organic compounds containing nitrogen, carbon, hydrogen, and oxygen; the essential building blocks of proteins.

amnion The innermost membrane of the sac enclosing the embryo or fetus.

amphetamine Any of a class of stimulants that trigger the release of epinephrine, which stimulates the central nervous system; users experience a state of hyper-alertness and energy, followed by a crash as the drug wears off.

anabolic steroids Drugs derived from testosterone and approved for medical use, but often used by athletes to increase their musculature and weight.

anaerobic exercise Physical activity in which the body develops an oxygen deficit.

androgynous Not tied to traditional gender roles, as in a marriage.

androgyny The expression of both masculine and feminine traits.

anemia A condition characterized by a marked reduction in the number of circulating red blood cells or in hemoglobin, the oxygen-carrying component of red blood cells.

angina pectoris A severe, suffocating chest pain caused by a brief lack of oxygen to the heart.

angioplasty Surgical repair of an obstructed artery by passing a balloon catheter through the blood vessel to the area of disease and then inflating the catheter to compress the plaque against the vessel wall.

anorexia nervosa A psychological disorder in which refusal to eat and/or an extreme loss of appetite leads to malnutrition, severe weight loss, and possibly death.

antagonistic Opposing or counteracting.

antibiotics Substances produced by microorganisms, or synthetic agents, that are toxic to other types of microorganisms; in dilute solutions, used to treat infectious diseases.

antidepressant A drug used primarily to treat symptoms of depression.

antioxidants Substances that prevent the damaging effects of oxidation in cells.

antiviral drug A substance that decreases the severity and duration of a viral infection if taken prior to or soon after onset of the infection.

anxiety A feeling of apprehension and dread, with or without a known cause; may range from mild to severe and may be accompanied by physical symptoms.

anxiety disorders A group of psychological disorders involving episodes of apprehension, tension, or uneasiness, stemming from the anticipation of danger and sometimes accompanied by physical symptoms, which cause significant distress and impairment to an individual.

aorta The main artery of the body, arising from the left ventricle of the heart.

appetite A desire for food, stimulated by anticipated hunger, physiological changes within the brain and body, the availability of food, and other environmental and psychological factors.

arrhythmia Any irregularity in the rhythm of the heartbeat.

arteriosclerosis Any of a number of chronic diseases characterized by degeneration of the arteries and hardening and thickening of arterial walls.

arthritis Inflammation of the joints.

artificial insemination The introduction of viable sperm into the vagina by artificial means for the purpose of inducing conception.

assertive Behaving in a confident manner to make your needs and desires clear to others in a nonhostile way.

asthma A disease or allergic response characterized by bronchial spasms and difficult breathing.

atherosclerosis A form of arteriosclerosis in which fatty substances (plaque) are deposited on the inner walls of arteries.

atrial fibrillation A condition characterized by an irregular, abnormally rapid heartbeat.

atrium (plural atria) Either of the two upper chambers of the heart, which receive blood from the veins.

attention deficit/hyperactivity disorder (ADHD) A spectrum of difficulties in controlling motion and sustaining attention, including hyperactivity, impulsivity, and distractibility.

autoimmune Resulting from the attack on body tissue by an immune system that fails to recognize the tissue as self.

autonomy The ability to draw on internal resources; independence from familial and societal influences.

autoscopy The sensation of ones self being outside its body, often experienced by individuals in near-death medical crises.

aversion therapy A treatment that attempts to help a person overcome a dependence or bad habit by making the person feel disgusted or repulsed by that habit.

axon The long fiber that conducts impulses from the neurons nucleus to its dendrites.

axon terminal The ending of an axon, from which impulses are transmitted to a dendrite of another neuron.

ayurveda A traditional Indian medical treatment involving meditation, exercise, herbal medications, and nutrition.

bacteria (singular, bacterium) One-celled microscopic organisms; the most plentiful pathogens.

bacterial vaginosis A vaginal infection caused by overgrowth and depletion of various microorganisms living in the vagina, resulting in a malodorous white or gray vaginal discharge.

barbiturates Antianxiety drugs that depress the central nervous system, reduce activity and induce relaxation, drowsiness, or sleep; often prescribed to relieve tension and treat epileptic seizures or as a general anesthetic.

barrier contraceptives Birth-control devices that block the meeting of egg and sperm, either by physical barriers, such as condoms, diaphragms, or cervical caps, or by chemical barriers, such as spermicide, or both.

basal body temperature The body temperature upon waking, before any activity.

basal metabolic rate (BMR) The number of calories required to sustain the body at rest.

behavior therapy Psychotherapy that emphasizes application of the principles of learning to substitute desirable responses and behavior patterns for undesirable ones.

benign hypertrophy Enlargement of the prostate gland, resulting in a pinching of the urethra.

benzodiazepines Antianxiety drugs that depress the central nervous system, reduce activity and induce relaxation, drowsiness, or sleep; often prescribed to relieve tension, muscular strain, sleep problems, anxiety, and panic attacks; also used as an anesthetic and in the treatment of alcohol withdrawal.

binge eating The rapid consumption of an abnormally large amount of food in a relatively short time.

biofeedback A technique of becoming aware, with the aid of external monitoring devices, of internal physiological activities in order to develop the capability of altering them.

bipolar disorder Severe depression alternating with periods of manic activity and elation.

bisexual Sexually oriented toward both sexes.

blended family A family formed when one or both of the partners bring children from a previous union to the new marriage.

blood-alcohol concentration (BAC) The amount of alcohol in the blood, expressed as a percentage.

body mass index (BMI) The percentage of fat in ones body.

bone-marrow transplantation A cancer treatment involving high doses of radiation or chemotherapy during which the marrow is destroyed and then replaced with healthy bone marrow.

botulism Possibly fatal food poisoning, caused by a type of bacterium, which grows and produces its toxin in the absence of air and is found in improperly canned food.

bradycardia An abnormally slow heart rate, under 60 beats per minute.

breech birth A birth in which the infant's buttocks or feet pass through the birth canal first.

bulimia nervosa Episodic binge eating, often followed by forced vomiting or laxative abuse, and accompanied by a persistent preoccupation with body shape and weight.

burnout A state of physical, emotional, and mental exhaustion resulting from constant or repeated emotional pressure.

caesarean delivery The surgical procedure in which an infant is delivered through an incision made in the abdominal wall and uterus.

calorie The amount of energy required to raise the temperature of 1 gram of water by 1 Celsius. In everyday usage related to the energy content of foods and the energy expended in activities, a calorie is actually the equivalent of a thousand such calories, or a Kilocalorie.

candidiasis An infection of the yeast Candida albicans, commonly occurring in the vagina, vulva, penis, and mouth and causing burning, itching, and a whitish discharge.

capillary A minute blood vessel that connects an artery to a vein.

carbohydrates Organic compounds, such as starches, sugars, and glycogen, that are composed of carbon, hydrogen, and oxygen, and are sources of bodily energy.

carbon monoxide A colorless, odorless gas produced by the burning of gasoline or tobacco; displaces oxygen in the hemoglobin molecules of red blood cells.

carcinogen A substance that produces cancerous cells or enhances their development and growth.

cardiopulmonary resuscitation (CPR) A method of artificial stimulation of the heart and lungs; a combination of mouth-to-mouth breathing and chest compression.

cardiovascular fitness The ability of the heart and blood vessels to circulate blood through the body efficiently.

celibacy Abstention from sexual activity; can be partial or complete, permanent or temporary.

cell-mediated The portion of the immune response that protects against parasites, fungi, cancer cells, and foreign tissue, primarily by means of T cells, or lymphocytes.

certified social worker A person who has completed a two-year graduate program in counseling people with mental problems.

cervical cap A thimble-sized rubber or plastic cap that is inserted into the vagina to fit over the cervix and prevent the passage of sperm into the uterus during sexual intercourse; used with a spermicidal foam or jelly, it serves as both a chemical and a physical barrier to sperm.

cervix The narrow, lower end of the uterus that opens into the vagina.

chanchroid A soft, painful sore or localized infection usually acquired through sexual contact.

chemoprevention The use of natural or synthetic substances to reduce the risk of developing cancer.

chiropractic A method of treating disease, primarily through manipulating the bones and joints to restore normal nerve function.

chlamydial infections A sexually transmitted disease caused by the bacterium *Chlamydia trachomatis*, often asymptomatic in women, but sometimes characterized by urinary pain; if undetected and untreated, may result in pelvic inflammatory disease (PID).

chlorinated hydrocarbons Highly toxic pesticides, such as DDT and chlordane, that are extremely resistant to breakdown; may cause cancer, birth defects, neurological disorders, and damage to wildlife and the environment.

cholesterol An organic substance found in animal fats; linked to cardiovascular disease, particularly atherosclerosis.

chronic fatigue syndrome (CFS) A cluster of symptoms whose cause is not yet known; a primary symptom is debilitating fatigue.

chronic obstructive lung disease (COLD) Any one of several lung diseases characterized by obstruction of breathing, including emphysema and chronic bronchitis.

circumcision The surgical removal of the foreskin of the penis.

cirrhosis A chronic disease, especially of the liver, characterized by a degeneration of cells and excessive scarring.

clinical practice guidelines Recommendations used by physicians to determine appropriate health care for specific conditions.

clitoris A small erectile structure on the female, corresponding to the penis on the male.

cocaine A white crystalline powder extracted from the leaves of the coca plant which stimulates the central nervous system and produces a brief period of euphoria followed by a depression.

codependence An emotional and psychological behavioral pattern in which the spouses, partners, parents, children, and friends of individuals with addictive behaviors allow or enable their loved ones to continue their self-destructive habits.

cognitive therapy A technique used to identify an individuals beliefs and attitudes, recognize negative thought patterns, and educate in alternative ways of thinking.

cohabitation Tow people living together as a couple, without official ties such as marriage.

coitus interruptus The removal of the penis from the vagina before ejaculation.

colpotomy Surgical sterilization by cutting or blocking the fallopian tubes through an incision made in the wall of the vagina.

coma A state of total unconsciousness.

companion-oriented marriage A marital relationship in which the partners share interests, activities, and domestic responsibilities.

complementary proteins Incomplete proteins that, when combined, provide all the amino acids essential for protein synthesis.

complete proteins Proteins that contain all the amino acids needed by the body for growth and maintenance.

complex carbohydrates Starches, including cereals, fruits, and vegetables.

conception The merging of a sperm and an ovum.

conditioning The gradual building up of the body to enhance one or more of the three main components of physical fitness: flexibility, cardiovascular or aerobic fitness, and muscular strength and endurance.

condom A latex sheath worn over the penis during sexual acts to prevent conception and/or the transmission of disease; some condoms contain a spermicidal lubricant.

congestive heart failure Inability of the heart to pump at normal capacity, resulting in decreased blood flow throughout the body, collection of blood fluids in the lungs, and pulmonary congestion.

constant-dose combination pill An oral contraceptive that releases synthetic estrogen and progestin at constant levels throughout the menstrual cycle.

contraception The prevention of conception; birth control.

coping mechanism Any of several conscious and unconscious mental processes that enable a person to cope with a difficult situation or problem; usually healthier, more mature, and more effective than a defense mechanism.

coronary angiography A diagnostic test in which a thin tube is threaded through the blood vessels of the heart, a dye is injected, and X rays are taken to detect blockage of the arteries.

coronary bypass Surgical correction of a blockage in a coronary artery by grafting an artery from the patients leg or chest wall onto the damaged artery to detour blood around the blockage.

corpus luteum A yellowish mass of tissue that is formed, immediately after ovulation, from the remaining cells of the follicle; it secretes estrogen and progesterone for the remainder of the menstrual cycle.

Cowpers glands Two small glands that discharge into the male urethra; also called bulbourethral glands.

crib death The unexplained death of an apparently healthy baby under one year of age during sleep; also called **sudden infant death syndrome** (SIDS).

cross-training Alternating two or more different types of fitness activities.

crucifers Plants, including broccoli, cabbage, and cauliflower, that contain large amounts of fiber, proteins, and indoles.

culture The set of shared attitudes, values, goals, and practices of a group that are internalized by an individual within the group.

cunnilingus Sexual stimulation of a womans genitals by means of oral manipulation.

cystitis Inflammation of the urinary bladder.

decibel (dB) A unit for measuring the intensity of sounds.

deleriants Chemicals, such as solvents, aerosols, glue, cleaning fluids, petroleum products, and some anesthetics, that produce vapors with psychoactive effects when inhaled.

delirium tremens (DTs) The delusions, hallucinations, and agitated behavior following withdrawal from long-term chronic alcohol abuse.

dementia Deterioration of mental capability.

dendrites Branching fibers of a neuron that receive impulses from axon terminals of other neurons and conduct these impulses toward the nucleus.

depression In general, feelings of unhappiness and despair; as a mental illness, also characterized by an inability to function normally

depressive disorders A group of psychological disorders involving pervasive and sustained depression.

dermatitis Any inflammation of the skin.

designer drugs Illegally manufactured psychoactive drugs that have dangerous physical and psychological effects.

detoxification The supervised removal of a poisonous or harmful substance (such as a drug) from the body; a therapy for alcoholics in which they are denied alcohol in a controlled environment.

diabetes mellitus A disease in which the inadequate production of insulin leads to failure of the body tissues to break down carbohydrates at a normal rate.

diagnostic-related group (DRG) A category of conditions requiring hospitalization for which the cost of care has been determined prior to a clients hospitalization.

diaphragm A bowl-like rubber cup with a flexible rim that is inserted into the vagina to cover the cervix and prevent the passage of sperm into the uterus during sexual intercourse; used with a spermicidal foam or jelly, it serves as both a chemical and a physical barrier to sperm.

diastole The period between contractions in the cardiac cycle, during which the heart relaxes and dilates as it fills with blood.

digestion The process of chemically and mechanically breaking down foods into compounds capable of being absorbed by body cells.

dilation and evacuation (D and E) A medical procedure in which the contents of the uterus are removed through the use of instruments.

dioxins A family of chemicals used in industry; some forms are believed to be extremely toxic.

distress A negative stress stage that may result in illness.

do-not-resuscitate (DNR) A directive expressing an individual's preference that resuscitation efforts not be made during a medical crisis.

drug Any substance, other than food, that when taken, affects bodily functions and structures.

drug abuse The excessive use of a drug in a manner inconsistent with accepted medical practice.

drug misuse The use of a drug for a purpose (or person) other than that for which it was medically intended.

dyathanasia The act of permitting death by the removal or ending of any extraordinary efforts to sustain life; passive euthanasia.

dysfunctional Characterized by negative and destructive patterns of behavior between partners or between parents and children.

dysmenorrhea Painful menstruation.

dyspareunia A sexual difficulty in which a woman experiences pain during sexual intercourse.

dysthymia Frequent, prolonged mild depression.

eating disorders Bizarre, often dangerous patterns of food consumption, including anorexia nervosa, bulimia nervosa, and bulimarexia.

e coli *Escherichia coli*, a bacteria often spread through undercooked or inadequately washed foods.

ecosystem A community of organisms sharing a physical and chemical environment and interacting with each other.

ectopic pregnancy A pregnancy in which the fertilized egg has implanted itself outside the uterine cavity, usually in the fallopian tube.

ejaculation The expulsion of semen from the penis.

ejaculatory duct The canal connecting the seminal vesicles and vas deferens.

electrocardiogram (ECG, EKG) A graphic record of the electric current associated with heartbeats.

electromagnetic fields (EMFs) The invisible electric and magnetic fields generated by an electrically charged conductor.

embryo An organism in its early stage of development; in humans, the embryonic period lasts from about the second to the eighth week of pregnancy.

emotional health The ability to express and acknowledge ones feelings and moods.

emotional intelligence A term used by some psychologists to evaluate the capacity of people to understand themselves and relate well with others.

endocrine system The group of ductless glands that produce hormones and secrete them directly into the blood for transport to target organs.

endometrium The mucous membrane lining the uterus.

endorphins Mood-elevating, pain-killing chemicals produced by the brain.

endurance The ability to withstand the stress of continued physical exertion.

enkephalins Naturally occurring opioids that the body uses to relieve pain and stress.

environmental tobacco smoke Secondhand cigarette smoke; the third leading preventable cause of death.

epididymis That portion of the male duct system in which sperm mature.

epidural block An injection of anesthesia into the membrane surrounding the spinal cord to numb the lower body during labor and childbirth.

epilepsy A variety of neurological disorders characterized by sudden attacks (seizures) of violent muscle contractions and unconsciousness.

erogenous Sexually sensitive.

estrogen The female sex hormone that stimulates female secondary sex characteristics.

ethyl alcohol The intoxicating agent in alcoholic beverages; also called ethanol.

eustress Positive stress, which stimulates a person to function properly.

euthanasia Any method of painlessly causing death for a terminally ill person.

failure rate The number of pregnancies that occur per year for every 100 women using a particular method of birth control.

fallopian tubes The pair of channels that transport ova from the ovaries to the uterus; the usual site of fertilization.

false negative A diagnostic test result that falsely indicates the absence of a particular condition.

false positive A diagnostic test result that falsely indicates the presence of a particular condition.

family A group of people united by marriage, blood, or adoption, residing in the same household, maintaining a common culture, and interacting with one another on the basis of their roles within the group.

fat-soluble vitamins Vitamins absorbed through the intestinal membranes, with the aid of fats in the diet or bile from the liver, and stored in the body.

fellatio Sexual stimulation of a mans genitals by means of oral manipulation.

fertilization The fusion of the sperm and egg nuclei.

fetal alcohol effects (FAE) Milder forms of FAS, including low birth weight, irritability as new-borns, and permanent mental impairment as a result of the mothers alcohol consumption during pregnancy.

fetal alcohol syndrome (FAS) A cluster of physical and mental defects in the newborn, including low birth weight, smaller-than-normal head circumference, intrauterine growth retardation, and permanent mental impairment-caused by the mothers alcohol consumption during pregnancy.

fetus The human organism developing in the uterus from the ninth week until birth.

fiber Indigestible materials in food that lower blood cholesterol or facilitate digestion and elimination.

flap surgery Surgical removal of diseased tissue and bone from under the gums of the teeth.

flexibility The range of motion allowed by ones joints; determined by the length of muscles, tendons, and ligaments attached to the joints.

food allergies Hypersensitivities to particular foods.

food toxicologists Specialists who detect toxins in food and treat the conditions toxins produce.

frostbite The freezing or partial freezing of skin and tissue just below the skin, or even muscle and bone; more severe than frostnip.

frostnip Sudden blanching or lightening of the skin on hands, feet, and face, resulting from exposure to high wind speeds and low temperatures.

fungi (singular, fungus) Organisms that reproduce by means of spores.

gallstones Clumps of solid material, usually cholesterol, that fom in bile stored in the gallbladder.

gamma globulin The antibody-containing portion of the blood fluid (plasma).

gender Maleness or femaleness, as determined by a combination of anatomical and physiological factors, psychological factors, and learned behaviors.

gene therapy A cancer treatment involving the insertion of genes into a patient.

general adaptation syndrome (GAS) The sequenced physiological response to a stressful situation; consists of three stagesalarm, resistance, and exhaustion.

generalized anxiety disorder (GAD) An anxiety disorder characterized as chronic distress.

generic Refers to products without trade names that are equivalent to other products protected by trademark registration.

gerontologist A specialist in the interdisciplinary field that studies aging.

gingivitis Inflammation of the gums.

glia Support cells for neurons in the brain and spinal cord that separate the brain from the bloodstream, assist in the growth of neurons, speed transmission of nerve impulses, and eliminate damaged neurons.

gonadotropins Gonad-stimulating hormones produced by the pituitary gland.

gonads The primary reproductive organs in a man (testes) or woman (ovaries).

gonorrhea A sexually transmitted disease caused by the bacterium *Neisseria gonorrhoeae*; symptoms include discharge from the penis; women are generally asymptomatic.

greenhouse effect An environmental phenomenon in which the buildup of carbon dioxide and other greenhouse gases leads to warming of the planet.

guided imagery An approach to stress control, self-healing, or motivating life changes by means of visualizing oneself in the state of calmness, wellness, or change.

gum disease Inflammation of the gum and bones that hold teeth in place.

hallucinogen A drug that causes hallucinations.

hashish A concentrated form of a drug, derived from the cannabis plant, containing the psychoactive ingredient TCH, which causes a sense of euphoria when inhaled or eaten.

health A state of complete well-being, including physical, psychological, spiritual, social, intellectual, and environmental components.

health maintenance organization (HMO) An organization that provides health services on a fixed-contract basis.

health promotion An educational and informational process in which people are helped to change attitudes and behaviors in an effort to improve their health.

heat cramps Painful muscle spasms caused by vigorous exercise accompanied by heavy sweating in the heat.

heat exhaustion Faintness, rapid heart beat, low blood pressure, an ashen appearance, cold and clammy skin, and nausea, resulting from prolonged sweating with inadequate fluid replacement.

heat stress Physical response to prolonged exposure to high temperature; occurs simultaneously with or after heat cramps.

heat stroke A medical emergency consisting of a fever of at least 105F, hot dry skin, rapid heartbeat, rapid and shallow breathing, and elevated or lowered blood pressure, caused by the breakdown of the bodys cooling mechanism.

helminth A parasitic roundworm or flatworm.

hemoglobin The oxygen-transporting component of red blood cells; composed of heme and globin.

hepatitis An inflammation and/or infection of the liver caused by a virus, often accompanied by jaundice.

herbal medicine An ancient form of medical treatment using substances derived from trees, flowers, ferns, seaweeds, and lichens to treat disease.

herbology The practice of herbal medicine.

hernia The abnormal protrusion of an organ or body part through the tissues of the walls containing it.

herpes simplex A condition caused by one of the herpes viruses and characterized by lesions of the skin or mucous membranes; herpes virus type 2 is sexually transmitted, and causes genital blisters or sores.

hertz A unit for measuring the frequency of sound waves.

heterosexual Primary sexual orientation toward members of the other sex.

holographic will A will wholly in the handwriting of its author.

home health care Provision of medical services and equipment to patients in the home to restore or maintain comfort, function, and health.

homeopathy A system of medical practice that treats a disease by administering dosages of substances that would in healthy persons produce symptoms similar to those of the disease.

homeostasis The bodys natural state of balance or stability.

homosexual Primary sexual orientation toward members of the same sex.

hormones Substances released in the blood that regulate specific bodily functions.

hormone replacement therapy (HRT) The use of supplemental hormones during and after menopause.

hospice A homelike health-care facility or program committed to supportive care for terminally ill people.

host A person or population that contracts one or more pathogenic agents in an environment.

hostile or offensive environment A workplace made hostile, abusive, or unbearable by persistent inappropriate behaviors of coworkers or supervisors.

human immunodeficiency virus (HIV) A type of virus that causes a spectrum of health problems, ranging from a symptomless infection to changes in the immune system, to the development of life-threatening diseases because of impaired immunity.

human papilloma virus (HPV) A pathogen that causes genital warts and increases the risk of cervical cancer.

humoral A portion of the immune response that provides lifelong protection against bacterial or viral infections, such as mumps, by means of antibodies whose production is triggered by the release of antigens upon first exposure to the infectious agent.

hunger The physiological drive to consume food.

hydrostatic weighing The weighing of a person in water to distinguish buoyant fat from denser muscle.

hypertension High blood pressure occurring when the blood exerts excessive pressure against the arterial walls.

hypothermia An abnormally low body temperature; if not treated appropriately, coma or death could result.

hysterectomy The surgical removal of the uterus.

hysterotomy A procedure in which the uterus is surgically opened and the fetus inside it removed.

immune deficiency Partial or complete inability of the immune system to respond to pathogens.

immunity Protection from infectious diseases.

implantation The embedding of the fertilized ovum in the uterine lining.

impotence A sexual difficulty in which a man is unable to achieve or maintain an erection.

incest Sexual relations between two individuals too closely related to contract a legal marriage.

incomplete proteins Proteins that lack one or more of the amino acids essential for protein synthesis.

incubation period The time between when a pathogen enters the body and the first symptom.

indemnity A form of insurance that pays a major portion of medical expenses after a deductible amount is paid by the insured person.

indoles Naturally occurring chemicals found in foods such winter squash, carrots, and crucifers; may help lower cancer risk.

induced abortion A procedure to remove the uterine contents after pregnancy has occurred.

infertility The inability to conceive a child.

infiltration A gradual penetration or invasion.

inflammation A localized response by the body to tissue injury, characterized by swelling and the dilation of the blood vessels.

inflammatory bowel disease (IBD) A digestive disease that causes frequent and intense diarrhea, abdominal pain, gas, fever, and rectal bleedingCrohns disease is an inflammation anywhere in the digestive tract, and ulcerative colitis causes severe ulcers in the inner lining of the colon and rectum.

informed consent Permission (to undergo or receive a medical procedure or treatment) given voluntarily, with full knowledge and understanding of the procedure or treatment and its consequences.

influenza Any number of a type of fairly common, highly contagious viral diseases.

inhalants Substances that produce vapors having psychoactive effects when sniffed.

intercourse Sexual stimulation by means of entry of the penis into the vagina; coitus.

interpersonal therapy (IPT) A technique used to develop communication skills and relationships.

intimacy A state of closeness between two people, characterized by the desire and ability to share ones innermost thoughts and feelings with each other either verbally or nonverbally.

intoxication Maladaptive behavioral, psychological, and physiologic changes that occur as a result of substance abuse.

intramuscular Into or within a muscle.

intrauterine device (IUD) A device inserted into the uterus through the cervix to prevent pregnancy by interfering with implantation.

intravenous Into a vein.

ionizing radiation A form of energy emitted from atoms as they undergo internal change.

irradiation Exposure to or treatment by some form of radiation.

irritable bowel syndrome A digestive disease caused by intestinal spasms, resulting in frequent need to defecate, nausea, cramping, pain, gas and a continual sensation of rectal fullness.

isokinetic Having the same force; exercise with specialized equipment that provides resistance equal to the force applied by the user throughout the entire range of motion.

isometric Of the same length; exercise in which muscles increase their tension without shortening in length, such as when pushing an immovable object.

isotonic Having the same tension or tone; exercise requiring the repetition of an action that creates tension, such as weight lifting or calisthenics.

kidney stones Formations of calcium salts or minerals that form in the kidneys; may be passed out of the body in urine, surgically removed, or decomposed by high-frequency sound waves.

labia majora The fleshy outer folds that border the female genital area.

labia minora The fleshy inner folds that border the female genital area.

labor The process leading up to birth: effacement and dilation of the cervix; the movement of the baby into and through the birth canal, accompanied by strong contractions; and contraction of the uterus and expulsion of the placenta after the birth.

lacto-vegetarians People who eat dairy products as well as fruits and vegetables (but not meat, poultry, or fish).

Lamaze method A method of childbirth preparation taught to expectant parents to help the woman cope with the discomfort of labor; combines breathing and psychological techniques.

laparoscopy A surgical sterilization procedure in which the fallopian tubes are observed with a laparoscope inserted through a small incision, and then cut or blocked.

laparotomy A surgical sterilization procedure in which the fallopian tubes are cut or blocked through an incision made in the abdomen.

licensed clinical social worker (LCSW). See certified social worker.

lifestyle An individuals way of life, as indicated and expressed by ones daily practices, interests, possessions, and so on.

lipoprotein A compound in blood that is made up of proteins and fat; a high-density lipoprotein (HDL) picks up excess cholesterol in the blood; a low-density lipoprotein (LDL) carries more cholesterol and deposits it on the walls of arteries.

living will A written statement providing instructions for the use of life-sustaining procedures in the event of terminal illness or injury.

lochia The vaginal discharge of blood, mucus, and uterine tissue that occurs after birth.

locus of control An individuals belief about the source of power and influence over ones life.

lumpectomy The surgical removal of a breast tumor and its surrounding tissue.

Lyme disease A disease caused by a bacterium carried by a tick; it may cause heart arrhythmias, neurological problems, and arthritis symptoms.

lymph nodes Small tissue masses in which some immune cells are stored.

mainstream smoke The smoke inhaled directly by smoking a cigarette.

mainstreaming The placement of disabled students into regular school classes with specialized attention given in the classroom or in separate sessions.

major depression Sadness that does not end.

male pattern baldness The loss of hair at the vertex, or top, of the head.

malpractice The failure of a doctor or other health-care professionals to provide appropriate and skillful medical or surgical treatment.

mammography X-ray examination of the breasts for early detection of cancer.

managed care Health-care services and reimbursement predetermined by third-party insurers.

marijuana The drug derived from the cannabis plant, containing the psychoactive ingredient THC, which causes a mild sense of euphoria when inhaled or eaten.

marriage and family therapist A psychiatrist, psychologist, or social worker who specializes in marriage and family counseling.

mastectomy The surgical removal of an entire breast.

masturbation Manual (or nonmanual) self-stimulation of the genitals, often resulting in orgasm.

medical history The health-related information collected during the interview of a client by a health-care professional.

meditation A group of approaches that use quiet sitting, breathing techniques, and/or chanting to relax, improve concentration, and become attuned to ones inner self.

menarche The onset of menstruation at puberty.

menopause The complete cessation of ovulation and menstruation for twelve consecutive months.

menstruation Discharge of blood from the vagina as a result of the shedding of the uterine lining at the end of the menstrual cycle.

mental disorder Behavioral or psychological syndrome associated with distress or disability or with a significantly increased risk of suffering death, pain, disability, or loss of freedom.

mental health The ability to perceive reality as it is, to respond to its challenges, and to develop rational strategies for living.

meta-analysis Summarization and review of research in a particular area to evaluate the results of several large clinical trials in a uniform manner.

metastasize To spread to other parts of the body via the bloodstream or lymphatic system.

microwaves Extremely high frequency electromagnetic waves that increase the rate at which molecules vibrate, thereby generating heat.

migraine headache Severe headache resulting from the constriction, then dilation of blood vessels within the brain; sometimes accompanied by vomiting and nausea.

mindfulness A method of stress reduction that involves experiencing the physical and mental sensations of the present moment.

minerals Naturally occurring inorganic substances, small amounts of some being essential in metabolism and nutrition.

minilaparotomy A surgical sterilization procedure in which the fallopian tubes are cut or sealed by electrical coagulation through a small incision just above the pubic hairline.

minipill An oral contraceptive containing a small amount of progestin and no estrogen, which prevents contraception by making the mucus in the cervix so thick that sperm cannot enter the uterus.

miscarriage A pregnancy that terminates before the twentieth week of gestation; also called spontaneous abortion.

mononucleosis An infectious viral disease characterized by an excess of white blood cells in the blood, fever, bodily discomfort, a sore throat, and kidney and liver complications.

mons pubis The rounded, fleshy area over the junction of the female pubic bones.

mood A sustained emotional state that colors ones view of the world for hours or days.

moral The internal standard of right and wrong by which one makes judgments and decisions.

multiphasic pill An oral contraceptive that releases different levels of estrogen and progestin to mimic the hormonal fluctuations of the natural menstrual cycle.

mutagen An agent that causes alterations in the genetic material of living cells.

mutation A change in the genetic material of a cell or cells that is brought about by radiation, chemicals, or natural causes.

myocardial infarction (MI) A condition characterized by the dying of tissue areas in the myocardium, caused by interruption of the blood supply to those areas; the medical name for a heart attack.

near-death experiences See autoscopy.

negligence The failure to act in a way that a reasonable person would act.

neoplasm Any tumor, whether benign or malignant.

nephrosis A cluster of symptoms indicating chronic damage to the kidneys.

neuron The basic working unit of the brain, which transmits information from the senses to the brain and from the brain to specific body parts; each nerve cell consists of an axon, an axon terminal, and dendrites.

neuropsychiatry The study of the brain and mind.

neurotransmitters Chemicals released by neurons that stimulate or inhibit the action of other neurons.

nicotine The addictive substance in tobacco; one of the most toxic of all poisons.

nocturnal emissions Ejaculations while dreaming; wet dreams.

noncompliance Failure to take a prescription drug according to the doctor's instructions.

nongonococcal urethritis (NGU) Inflammation of the urethra caused by organisms other than the gonococcus bacterium.

nonopioids Chemically synthesized drugs that have sleep-inducing and pain-relieving properties similar to those of opium and its derivatives.

norms The unwritten rules regarding behavior and conduct expected or accepted by a group.

nucleus The central part of a cell, contained in the cell body of a neuron.

nutrients Elements in food that the body cannot produce on its own, which are essential for growth, repair, and energy.

nutrition The science devoted to the study of dietary needs for food and the effects of food on organisms.

obesity The excessive accumulation of fat in the body; a condition of being 20% or more above the ideal weight for a person of that height and gender.

obsessive-compulsive disorder (OCD) An anxiety disorder characterized by obsessions and/or compulsions that impair ones ability to function and form relationships.

oncogene A gene that, when activated by radiation or a virus, may cause a normal cell to become cancerous.

opioids Drugs that have sleep-inducing and pain-relieving properties, including opium and its derivatives and nonopioid, synthetic drugs.

optimism The tendency to seek out, remember, and expect pleasurable experiences.

oral contraceptives Preparations of synthetic hormones that inhibit ovulation; also referred to as birth control pills or simply the pill.

organic phosphates Toxic pesticides that may cause cancer, birth defects, neurological disorders, and damage to wildlife and the environment.

organic Term designating food produced with, or production based on the use of, fertilizer originating from plants or animals, without the use of pesticides or chemically formulated fertilizers.

orgasm A series of contractions of the pelvic muscles occurring at the peak of sexual arousal.

osteoporosis A condition common in older people in which the bones become increasingly soft and porous, making them susceptible to injury.

outcomes The ultimate impacts of particular treatments or absence of treatment.

ovary The female sex organ that produces egg cells, estrogen, and progesterone.

over-the-counter (OTC) drugs Medications that can be obtained legally without a prescription from a medical professional.

overloading Method of physical training involving increasing the number of repetitions or the amount of resistance gradually to work the muscle to temporary fatigue.

overtrain Working muscles too intensely or too frequently, resulting in persistent muscle soreness, injuries, unintended weight loss, nervousness, and an inability to relax.

overuse injuries Physical injuries to joints or muscles, such as strains, fractures, and tendinitis, which result from overdoing a repetitive activity.

ovo-lacto-vegetarians People who eat eggs, dairy products, and fruits and vegetables (but not meat, poultry, or fish).

ovulation The release of a mature ovum from an ovary approximately 14 days prior to the onset of menstruation.

ovulation method A method of birth control based on the observation of changes in the consistency of the mucus in the vagina to predict ovulation.

ovum (plural, **ova**) The female gamete (egg cell).

ozone layer An upper layer of the earths atmosphere tha protects the earth from harmful ultraviolet radiation from the sun.

panic attack A short episode characterized by physical sensations of light-headedness, dizziness, hyperventilation, and numbness of extremities, accompanied by an inexplicable terror, usually of a physical disaster such as death.

panic disorder An anxiety disorder in which the apprehension or experience of recurring panic attacks is so intense that normal functioning is impaired.

Pap smear A test in which cells removed from the cervix are examined under a microscope for signs of cancer; also called a Pap test.

pathogen A microorganism that produces disease.

PCP (phencyclidine) A synthetic psychoactive substance that produces effects similar to other psychoactive drugs when swallowed, smoked, sniffed, or injected, but may also trigger unpredictable behavioral changes.

pedophilia Sexual contact between an adult and an unrelated child.

pelvic inflammatory disease (PID) An inflammation of the internal female genital tract, characterized by abdominal pain, fever, and tenderness of the cervix.

penis The male organ of sex and urination.

percutaneous transluminal coronary angioplasty (PTCA) A procedure for unclogging arteries; also called balloon angioplasty.

perimenopause The period from a womans first irregular cycles to her last menstruation.

perinatology The medical specialty concerned with the diagnosis and treatment of pregnant women with high-risk conditions and their fetuses.

perineum The area between the anus and vagina in the female and between the anus and scrotum in the male.

periodentitis Severe gum disease in which the tooth root becomes infected.

persistent vegetative state A state of being awake and capable of reacting to physical stimuli, such as light, while being unaware of pain or other environmental stimuli.

personality disorder An inflexible, maladaptive pattern of behavior that impairs an individuals ability to function.

phobia An anxiety disorder marked by an inordinate fear of an object, a class of objects, or a situation, resulting in extreme avoidance behaviors.

physical dependence The physiological attachment to, and need for, a drug.

physical fitness The ability to respond to routine physical demands, with enough reserve energy to cope with a sudden challenge.

phytochemicals Chemicals such as indoles, coumarins, and capsaicin, which exist naturally in plants and have disease-fighting properties.

placenta An organ that develops after implantation and to which the embryo attaches, via the umbilical cord, for nourishment and waste removal.

plaque The sludgelike substance that builds up on the inner walls of arteries.

pneumonia An inflammation of the lungs caused by infection or irritants.

pollutant A substance or agent in the environment, usually the by-product of human industry or activity, that is injurious to human, animal, or plant life.

pollution The presence of pollutants in the environment.

polyabuse The misuse or abuse of more than one drug.

polychlorinated biphenyls (PCBs) A family of chemical compounds, ranging from light, oily fluids to greasy or waxy substances, that have been widely used as industrial coolants and lubricants and in the manufacture of plastics, paints, and varnishes; a possible human carcinogen.

postpartum depression The emotional downswing that occurs after having a baby due to hormonal changes, physical exhaustion, and psychological pressures.

posttraumatic stress disorder (PTSD) The repeated reliving of a trauma through nightmares or recollection.

potentiating Making more effective or powerful.

preconception care Health care to prepare for pregnancy.

precycling The use of products that are packaged in recycled or recyclable material.

preferred provider organization (PPO) A group of physicians contracted to provide health care to members at a discounted price.

premature ejaculation A sexual difficulty in which a man ejaculates so rapidly that his partners satisfaction is impaired.

premature labor Labor that occurs after the twentieth week but before the thirty-seventh week of pregnancy.

premenstrual dysphoric disorder (PMDD) A disorder that causes symptoms of psychological depression during the last week of the menstrual cycle.

premenstrual syndrome (PMS) A disorder that causes physical discomfort and psychological distress prior to a womans menstrual period.

prevention Information and support offered to help healthy people identify their health risks, reduce stressors, prevent potential medical problems, and enhance their well-being.

primary care Ambulatory or outpatient care provided by a physician in an office, emergency room, or clinic.

progesterone The female sex hormone that stimulates the uterus, preparing it for the arrival of a fertilized egg.

progestin-only pill See minipill.

progressive relaxation A method of reducing muscle tension by contracting, then relaxing certain areas of the body.

promotion The process of enabling people to improve and increase control over their health in order to achieve a state of optimal health.

proof The alcoholic strength of a distilled spirit, expressed as twice the percentage of alcohol present.

prostate gland A structure surrounding the male urethra that produces a secretion that helps liquefy the semen from the testes.

prostatitis Inflammation of the prostate gland.

protection Measures that an individual can take when participating in risky behavior to prevent injury or unwanted risks.

protein A substance that is basically a compound of amino acids; one of the essential nutrients.

protozoa Microscopic animals made up of one cell or a group of similar cells.

psoriasis A chronic skin disorder caused by stress, skin damage, or illness and resulting in scaly, deep-pink, raised patches on the skin.

psychiatric drugs Medications that regulate a persons mental, emotional, and physical functions to facilitate normal functioning.

psychiatric nurse A nurse with special training and experience in mental health care.

psychiatrists Licensed medical doctors with additional training in psychotherapy, psychopharmacology, and treatment of mental disorders.

psychoactive Mood-altering.

psychodynamic Interpreting behaviors in terms of early experiences and unconscious influences.

psychological dependence The emotional or mental attachment to the use of a drug.

psychologists Mental health care professionals who have completed doctoral or graduate pro-

grams in psychology and are trained in a variety of psychotherapeutic techniques, but who are not medically trained and do not prescribe medications.

psychoneuroimmunology A scientific field that explores the relationships between and among the mind, the central nervous system, and the immune system.

psychoprophylaxis See Lamaze method.

psychotherapy Treatment designed to produce a response by psychological rather than physical means, sucn as suggestion, persuasion, reassurance, and support.

psychotropic Mind-affecting.

pyelonephritis Inflammation of the kidney.

quackery Medical fakery; unproven practices claiming to cure diseases or solve health problems.

quadrantectomy The surgical removal of a large portion of the breast and surrounding lymph glands.

quid pro quo A form of harassment in which a person in power or authority makes unwanted sexual advances as a condition for receiving a job, promotion, or favor.

rape Sexual penetration of a female or a male by means of intimidation, force, or fraud.

rapid-eye-movement (REM) sleep Regularly occurring periods of sleep during which the most active dreaming takes place.

receptors Molecules on the surface of neurons on which neurotransmitters bind after their release from other neurons.

recycling The processing or reuse of manufactured materials to reduce consumption of raw materials.

refractory period The period of time following orgasm during which the male cannot experience another orgasm.

rehabilitation medicine The use of surgical procedures, medication, and physical therapy to improve the condition of patients with disabling conditions such as blindness, deafness, and arthritis.

reinforcements Rewards or punishments for a behavior that will increase or decrease one's likelihood of repeating the behaviors.

relapse prevention An alcohol recovery treatment method that focuses on social skills training to develop ways of preventing or minimizing a relapse.

rep (or repetition) In weight training, a single performance of a movement or exercise.

repetitive motion injury (RMI) Inflammation of or damage to a part of the body due to repetition of the same movements.

rescue marriage A marital relationship in which one partner has had a traumatic childhood and views marriage as a way of healing the past.

resting heart rate The number of heartbeats per minute during inactivity.

reuptake Reabsorption by the originating cell of neurotransmitters that have not connected with receptors and have been left in synapses.

rhythm method A birth-control method in which sexual intercourse is avoided during those days of the menstrual cycle in which fertilization is most likely to occur.

romantic marriage A marital relationship in which sexual passion never fades.

rubella An infectious disease that may cause birth defects if contracted by a pregnant woman; also called German measles.

satiety A feeling of fullness after eating.

saturated fat A chemical term indicating that a fat molecule contains as many hydrogen atoms as its carbon skeleton can hold. These fats are normally solid at room temperature.

schizophrenia A general term for a group of mental disorders with characteristic psychotic symptoms, such as delusions, hallucinations, and disordered thought patterns during the active phase of the illness, and a duration of at least six months.

scrotum The external sac or pouch that holds the testes.

seasonal affective disorder (SAD) An annual rhythm of depression that appears to be linked to seasonal variations in light.

secondary sex characteristics Physical changes associated with maleness or femaleness, induced by the sex hormones.

self-actualization A state of wellness and fulfillment that can be achieved once certain human needs are satisfied; living to ones full potential.

self-efficacy Belief in ones ability to accomplish a goal or change a behavior.

self-esteem Confidence and satisfaction in oneself.

self-talk Repetition of positive messages about ones self-worth to learn more optimistic patterns of thought, feeling, and behavior.

semen The viscous whitish fluid that is the complete male ejaculate; a combination of sperm and secretions from the prostate gland, seminal vesicles, and other glands.

seminal vesicles Glands in the male reproductive system that produce the major portion of the fluid of semen.

set A person's expectations or preconceptions about a situation or experience; mind-set.

set-point theory The proposition that every person has an unconscious control system for keeping body fat (and therefore weight) at a predetermined level, or set point.

sets In weight training, the number of repetitions of the same movement or exercise.

sex Maleness or femaleness, resulting from genetic, structural, and functional factors.

sexual addiction A preoccupation with sex so intense and chronic that an individual cannot have a normal sexual relationship with a spouse or lover; sexual compulsion.

sexual coercion Sexual activity forced upon a person by the exertion of psychological pressure by another person.

sexual compulsion See sexual addiction.

sexuality The behaviors, instincts, and attitudes associated with being sexual.

sexually transmitted diseases (STDs) Any of a number of diseases that are acquired through sexual contact.

sexual orientation Sexual attraction to (and behavior with) individuals of ones own sex, the other sex, or both.

sidestream smoke The smoke emitted by a burning cigarette and breathed by everyone in a closed room, including the smoker; contains more tar and nicotine than mainstream smoke.

simple carbohydrates Sugars; like all carbohydrates, they provide the body with glucose.

skin calipers An instrument used to pinch skin folds at the arms, waist, and back to determine the percentage of body fat.

smog A grayish or brownish fog caused by the presence of smoke and/or chemical pollutants in the air.

social isolation A feeling of unconnectedness with others caused by and reinforced by infrequency of social contacts.

social phobia A severe form of social anxiety marked by extreme fears and avoidance of social situations.

sperm The male gamete produced by the testes and transported outside the body through ejaculation.

spermatogenesis The process by which sperm cells are produced.

spinal block An injection of anesthesia directly into the spinal cord to numb the lower body during labor and childbirth.

spiritual health The ability to identify ones basic purpose in life and to achieve ones full potential; the sense of connectedness to a greater power.

sterilization A surgical procedure to end a persons reproductive capability.

stimulant An agent, such as a drug, that temporarily relieves drowsiness, helps in the performance of repetitive tasks, and improves capacity for work.

strength Physical power; the maximum weight one can lift, push, or press in one effort.

stress The nonspecific response of the body to any demands made upon it; may be characterized by muscle tension and acute anxiety, or may be a positive force for action.

stressor Specific or nonspecific agents or situations that cause the stress response in a body.

stroke A cerebrovascular event in which the blood supply to a portion of the brain is blocked.

subcutaneous Under the skin.

suction curettage A procedure in which the contents of the uterus are removed by means of suction and scraping.

sudden infant death syndrome (SIDS) See crib death.

synapse A specialized site at which electrical impulses are transmitted from the axon terminal of one neuron to a dendrite of another.

synergistic Characterized by a combined effect that is greater than the sum of the individual effects.

syphilis A sexually transmitted disease caused by the bacterium *Treponema pallidum*, and characterized by early sores, a latent period, and a final period of life-threatening symptoms including brain damage and heart failure.

systemic disease A pathologic condition that spreads throughout the body.

systole The contraction phase of the cardiac cycle.

tachycardia An abnormally rapid heart rate, over 100 beats per minute.

tar A thick, sticky dark fluid produced by the burning of tobacco, made up of several hundred different chemicals, many of them poisonous, some of them carcinogenic.

target heart rate Sixty to eighty-five percent of the maximum heart rate; the heart rate at which one derives maximum cardiovascular benefit from aerobic exercise.

teratogen Any agent that causes spontaneous abortion or defects or malformations in a fetus.

terminal illness An illness in which death is inevitable.

testes (singular, testis) The male sex organs that produce sperm and testosterone.

testosterone The male sex hormone that stimulates male secondary sex characteristics.

thallium scintigraphy A diagnostic test in which radioactive isotopes are injected into the bloodstream, and images of the rays emitted by the isotopes are captured and then translated into images of the heart as it pumps.

thanatology The discipline of humanitarian care-giving for critically ill patients and their grieving family members and friends.

toxicity Poisonousness; the dosage level at which a drug becomes poisonous to the body, causing either temporary or permanent damage.

toxic shock syndrome (TSS) A disease characterized by fever, vomiting, diarrhea, and often shock, caused by a bacteria that releases toxic waste products into the bloodstream.

traditional marriage A marital relationship in which the roles of the partners are distinct; defined by gender-based cultural norms and expectations.

transcendence The sense of passing into a foreign region or dimension, often experienced by a person near death.

trans fats Fats formed when liquid vegetable oils are processed to make table spreads or cooking fats, and also found in dairy and beef products; considered to be especially dangerous dietary fats.

transgendered Having a gender identity opposite ones biological sex; transsexual.

transient ischemic attack (TIA) A cerebrovascular event in which the blood supply to a portion of the brain is blocked temporarily; repeated attacks are predictors of more severe strokes.

trichomoniasis An infection of the protozoa Trichomonas vaginalis; females experience vaginal burning, itching, and discharge, but male carriers may be asymptomatic.

triglyceride A blood fat that flows through the blood after meals and is linked to increased risk of coronary artery disease.

tubal ligation The suturing or tying shut of the fallopian tubes to prevent pregnancy.

tubal occlusion The blocking of the fallopian tubes to prevent pregnancy.

tuberculosis A highly infectious bacterial disease that primarily affects the lungs and is often fatal.

twelve-step programs Self-help group programs based on the principles of Alcoholics Anonymous.

ulcer A lesion in, or an erosion of, the mucous membrane of an organ.

unsaturated fat A chemical term indicating that a fat molecule contains fewer hydrogen atoms than its carbon skeleton can hold. These fats are normally liquid at room temperature.

urethra The canal through which urine from the bladder leaves the body; in the male, also serves as the channel for seminal fluid.

urethral opening The outer opening of the thin tube that carries urine from the bladder.

urethritis Infection of the urethra.

uterus The female organ that houses the developing fetus until birth.

vagina The canal leading from the exterior opening in the female genital area to the uterus.

vaginal contraceptive film (VCF) A small dissolvable sheet saturated with spermicide that can be inserted into the vagina and placed over the cervix.

vaginal spermicide A substance that kills or neutralizes sperm, inserted into the vagina in the form of a foam, cream, jelly, or suppository.

vaginismus A sexual difficulty in which a woman experiences painful spasms of the vagina during sexual intercourse.

values The criteria by which one makes choices about ones thoughts and actions and goals and ideals.

vas deferens Two tubes that carry sperm from the epididymis into the urethra.

vasectomy A surgical sterilization procedure in which each vas deferens is cut and tied shut to stop the passage of sperm to the urethra for ejaculation.

vector A biological or physical vehicle that carries the agent of infection to the host.

vegans People who eat only plant foods.

ventricle Either of the two lower chambers of the heart, which pump blood out of the heart and into the arteries.

video display terminal (VDT) A screen or monitor that emits electromagnetic fields from all sides; these fields may lead to increased reproductive problems, miscarriages, low birth weights, and cataracts.

virus A submicroscopic infectious agent; the most primitive form of life.

visualization An approach to stress control, self-healing, or motivating life changes by means of guided, or directed, imagery.

vital signs Measurements of physiological functioning; specifically, temperature, blood pressure, pulse rate, and respiration rate.

vitamins Organic substances that are needed in very small amounts by the body and carry out a variety of functions in metabolism and nutrition.

wellness A state of optimal health.

withdrawal Development of symptoms that cause significant psychological and physical distress when an individual reduces or stops drug use.

zero population growth (ZPG) The state at which the number of births equals the number of deaths.

zygote A fertilized egg.

INDEX